REFERENCE VALUES FOR *FREQUENTLY* ASSAYED CLINICAL CHEM... :d)

ANALYTE	SPECIMEN[†]	REFERENCE INTERVAL[‡]		PAGES
		CONVENTIONAL UNITS	RECOMMENDED SI UNITS	
γ-Glutamyltransferase (GGT)	S	Male 6–45 U/L Female 5–30 U/L	$10\text{–}75 \times 10^{-8}$ katal/L $8\text{–}50 \times 10^{-8}$ katal/L	255–256
Glycosylated hemoglobin (GHb)	P	4.5–8.0		277–278
High-density lipoprotein (HDL) cholesterol	S	Male 29–60 mg/dL Female 38–75 mg/dL	0.75–1.6 mmol/L 1.0–1.94 mmol/L	290–292
Immunoglobulins	S	IgG 800–1200 mg/dL IgA 70–312 mg/dL IgM 50–280 mg/dL IgD 0.5–2.8 mg/dL IgE 0.01–0.06 mg/dL	IgG 8–12 g/L IgA 0.7–3.12 g/L IgM 0.5–2.8 g/L IgD 0.005–0.2 g/L IgE 0.1–0.6 mg/L	190
Iron	S	Male 65–170 μg/dL Female 50–170 μg/dL		366–369
Lactate dehydrogenase (LD)	S	(L → P) 100–225 U/L (P → L) 80–280 U/L		248–250
Lactate dehydrogenase isoenzymes (as percentage of total)	S	LD–1 14–26% LD–2 29–39% LD–3 20–26% LD–4 8–16% LD–5 6–16%		248–250
Lipase	S	0–1.0 U/mL		257–258
Magnesium (Mg²⁺)	S U	1.2–2.1 mEq/L 6.0–10.0 mEq/24 hours	0.63–1.0 mmol/L 3.00–5.00 mmol/24 hours	327–330
Osmolality	S U (24-hour)	275–295 mOsm/kg 300–900 mOsm/kg		315–317
Urine/serum ratio		1.0–3.0		
Phosphate	S	2.7–4.5 mg/dL	0.87–1.45 mmol/L	334–336
Potassium (K⁺)	S U (24-hour)	3.4–5.0 mEq/L Neonate 3.7–5.9 mEq/L 25–125 mEq/day	3.4–5.0 mmol/L 3.7–5.9 mmol/L 25–125 mmol/day	322–325
Protein (total)	S CSF	6.5–8.3 g/dL 0.5% of plasma	65–83 g/L	204–205
Sodium (Na⁺)	S U (24-hour) CSF	135–145 mEq/L 40–220 mEq/L 138–150 mEq/L	135–145 mmol/L 40–220 mmol/L 138–150 mmol/L	317–322
Thyroid-stimulating hormone (TSH)	S	0.5–5.0 μU/mL		448–449
Thyroxine (T₄)	S	4.5–13 μg/dL	58–167 nmol/L	448–449
Triglycerides	S	67–157 mg/dL	0.11–2.15 mmol/L	290
Uric acid	S	Male 3.5–7.2 mg/dL Female 2.6–6.0 mg/dL	208–428 μmol/L 155–357 μmol/L	227–230

Reference values listed in this table are not universal. Reference ranges will vary by instrument and laboratory method. Readers should review the procedure manuals of their own laboratories for reference ranges.

*The list represents those analytes most frequently assayed in the clinical chemistry laboratory. For drug therapeutic ranges, refer to Appendix P, Summary Table of Pharmacokinetic Parameters.

†S = serum; P = plasma; U = urine; CSF = cerebrospinal fluid; WB = whole blood.

‡Values may vary according to method and population; values for enzymes are at 37°C unless otherwise noted.

Clinical Chemistry

PRINCIPLES, PROCEDURES, CORRELATIONS

FIFTH EDITION

Clinical Chemistry

PRINCIPLES, PROCEDURES, CORRELATIONS

FIFTH EDITION

Michael L. Bishop, MS, CLS, MT(ASCP)

Application Specialist
Global Customer Service
Knowledge Center 6
bioMérieux
Durham, North Carolina

Edward P. Fody, MD

Chief
Department of Pathology
Erlanger Medical Center
Chattanooga, Tennessee

Larry Schoeff, MS, MT(ASCP)

Director and Associate Professor, Medical Laboratory Science Program
University of Utah School of Medicine
Education Consultant, ARUP Laboratories
Salt Lake City, Utah

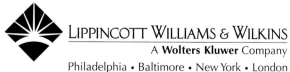

LIPPINCOTT WILLIAMS & WILKINS
A **Wolters Kluwer** Company

Philadelphia • Baltimore • New York • London
Buenos Aires • Hong Kong • Sydney • Tokyo

Acquisitions Editor: Pamela Lappies
Managing Editor: Kevin C. Dietz
Marketing Manager: Mary Martin
Production Editor: Bill Cady
Designer: Doug Smock
Compositor: Graphic World
Printer: Courier (Westford)

Printed in the United States of America

First Edition, 1985   Third Edition, 1996
Second Edition, 1992   Fourth Edition, 2000

Library of Congress Cataloging-in-Publication Data

Clinical chemistry: principles, procedures, correlations / [edited by] Michael L. Bishop,
Edward P. Fody, Larry Schoeff.—5th ed.
p. ; cm.
Includes bibliographical references and index.
ISBN 0-7817-4611-6
1. Clinical chemistry. I. Bishop, Michael L. II. Fody, Edward P. III. Schoeff, Larry E.
[DNLM: 1. Clinical Chemistry Tests. 2. Chemistry, Clinical—methods. QY 90 C6413 2005]
RB40.C576 2005
616.07′56—dc22

2004044148

To purchase additional copies of this book, call our customer service department at **(800) 638-3030** or fax orders to **(301) 824-7390.** International customers should call **(301) 714-2324.**

Visit Lippincott Williams & Wilkins on the Internet: http://www.LWW.com. Lippincott Williams & Wilkins customer service representatives are available from 8:30 am to 6:00 pm, EST.

04 05 06 07 08
1 2 3 4 5 6 7 8 9 10

To Sheila, Chris, and Carson for their support and patience.

MLB

To Nancy, my wife, for her continuing support and dedication.

EPF

To my wife, Anita, for her love and support.

LS

Foreword

It seems only a short time ago that I wrote the Foreword to the fourth edition of this text. Since that time, however, I find that many new diagnostic tests have been introduced and that, under the latest ADA/HSS guidelines, there are new and more demanding roles for some of our old tests, even glucose. Our laboratory has changed most of its analytic systems, installed a new laboratory information system, and reorganized again to meet the ever-increasing needs of a health care system that depends heavily on laboratory testing. Much has changed since the fourth edition, and it is to the credit of the editors and contributors of this book that they are committed to keeping the educational contents current with the changes occurring in laboratory medicine.

Many new tests, methods, and measurement systems continue to be introduced in a health care market that is becoming more and more competitive. Laboratory tests seem easier to perform; however, the testing processes often require complex technology that is more difficult to understand. New tests are evolving as a result of new research findings, together with new measurement processes that, again, often depend on complex technology. The one constant seems to be the increasing knowledge required to understand clinical laboratory science today.

This rapid change and evolution of laboratory testing makes it increasingly difficult to capture the knowledge that defines the current state of practice for clinical laboratory scientists. The task of the laboratory professional becomes more daunting and also more critical with each passing year. Fortunately, the editors and contributors of this text have been willing to tackle this seemingly impossible task to support and advance the profession. I want to both thank and congratulate them!

The fifth edition of *Clinical Chemistry: Principles, Procedures, Correlations* continues its mission of addressing the formal educational needs of our students in clinical laboratory science, as well as the ongoing needs of the professionals in the field. It facilitates the educational process by identifying the learning objectives, focusing on key concepts and ideas, and applying the theory through case studies. It covers the basics of laboratory testing, as well as many special areas of clinical chemistry testing. And, it is still possible to carry this text with you—to class, to the laboratory, to the office, or home to study!

Having personally worked with some of the editors and contributors, I know they have high standards—both in the laboratory and in the classroom. Their interests and backgrounds provide an excellent balance between the academic and the practical, ensuring that both students and practitioners are exposed to a well-developed base of knowledge that has been carefully refined by experience. They provide the sifting and winnowing necessary to separate the wheat from the chaff and to provide the real sustenance for our students and ourselves.

For the many students for whom this book is intended, let me offer some advice from my close friend and mentor, Hagar the Horrible. It seems his young Viking son was embarking on a voyage to the real world of work. Hagar's son asked him, "How do I get to the top?" Hagar's advice was, "You have to start at the bottom and work your way up!" After pondering this for a moment, his son asked, "How do I get to the bottom?" Hagar replied, "You have to know somebody!" As students in clinical laboratory science, you should study and heed the advice offered in this book; however, you should also search for mentors. The authors of this book, as well as your course instructors and your teachers in the laboratory, are keys to getting started in your career. Seek them out and profit from their learning and experience! These professionals know the state of the art and possess current knowledge of the field and, above all, are dedicated to help you.

James O. Westgard, PhD
Professor, Pathology and Laboratory Medicine
University of Wisconsin
Madison, Wisconsin

Preface

Clinical chemistry continues to be one of the most rapidly advancing areas of laboratory medicine. Since the publication of the first edition of this textbook in 1985, many changes have taken place. New technologies and analytic techniques have been introduced, with a dramatic impact on the practice of clinical chemistry. In addition, the health care system is changing. There is increased emphasis on improving quality of patient care, individual patient outcomes, financial responsibility, and total quality management. Point-of-care testing (POCT) is also at the forefront of health care practice and has brought forth both challenges and opportunities to clinical laboratorians. Now, more than ever, clinical laboratorians need to be concerned with disease correlations, interpretations, problem-solving, quality assurance, and cost effectiveness; they need to know not only the *how* of tests but also the *what, why, and when*. The editors of *Clinical Chemistry: Principles, Procedures, Correlations* have designed the fifth edition to be an even more valuable resource to both students and practitioners.

Like the previous four editions, the fifth edition of *Clinical Chemistry: Principles, Procedures, Correlations* is comprehensive, up-to-date, and easy to understand for students at all levels. It is also intended to be a practically organized resource for both instructors and practitioners. The editors have tried to maintain the book's readability and further improve its content. Because clinical laboratorians use their interpretative and analytic skills in the daily practice of clinical chemistry, an effort has been made to maintain an appropriate balance between analytic principles, techniques, and the correlation of results with disease states.

In this fifth edition, the editors have made several significant changes in response to requests from our readers, students, instructors, and practitioners. Chapter outlines, objectives, key terms, and summaries have been updated and expanded. Every chapter now includes current, more frequently encountered case studies and practice questions or exercises. The glossary of key terms has been expanded. To provide a thorough, up-to-date study of clinical chemistry, all chapters have been updated and reviewed by professionals who practice clinical chemistry and laboratory medicine on a daily basis. The basic principles of the analytic procedures discussed in the chapters reflect the most recent or commonly performed techniques in the clinical chemistry laboratory. Detailed procedures have been omitted because of the variety of equipment and commercial kits used in today's clinical laboratories. Instrument manuals and kit package inserts are the most reliable reference for detailed instructions on current analytic procedures. All chapter material has been updated, improved, and rearranged for better continuity and readability. As a new offering, an instructor's CD, with teaching resources, teaching tips, additional references, and teaching aids, is available from the publisher to assist in the use of this textbook.

Michael L. Bishop
Edward P. Fody
Larry Schoeff

Contributors

Dev Abraham, MD
Assistant Professor in Medicine
University of Utah School of Medicine
Salt Lake City, Utah

John J. Ancy, MA, RRT
Director of Respiratory Services
St. Elizabeth's Hospital
Belleville, Illinois

Michael J. Bennett, PhD, FRCPath, FACB, DABCC
Professor of Pathology and Pediatrics
Mary Quincy Parsons and Kelsey Louise Wright Professor of Mitochondrial Disease Research
University of Texas Southwestern Medical Center
Dallas, Texas

Larry H. Bernstein, MD
Chief, Clinical Pathology
New York Methodist Hospital Weill Cornell
Brooklyn, New York

Larry A. Broussard, PhD, DABCC, FACB
Professor
Clinical Laboratory Sciences
LSU Health Sciences Center
New Orleans, Louisiana

Ellen Carreiro-Lewandowski, MS, CLS
Professor
Department of Medical Laboratory Science
University of Massachusetts Dartmouth
North Dartmouth, Massachusetts

George S. Cembrowski, MD, PhD
Associate Professor
Department of Laboratory Medicine and Pathology
University of Alberta
Director, Medical Biochemistry
Regional Laboratory Services
Capital Health Authority
Edmonton, Alberta, Canada

Sharon S. Ehrmeyer, PhD, MT(ASCP)
Professor, Pathology and Laboratory Medicine
Director, MT/CLS
University of Wisconsin
Madison, Wisconsin

Elizabeth L. Frank, PhD
Assistant Professor—Clinical
Department of Pathology
University of Utah Health Sciences Center
Salt Lake City, Utah

Vicki S. Freeman, PhD, MT(ASCP)SC
Chair and Associate Professor
Department of Clinical Laboratory Science
School of Allied Health Science
The University of Texas Medical Branch at Galveston
Galveston, Texas

Lynn R. Ingram, MS
Program Director
Clinical Laboratory Sciences
University of Tennessee, Memphis
Memphis, Tennessee

Robert E. Jones, MD, FACP, FACE
Adjunct Associate Professor of Medicine and Pediatrics
University of Utah School of Medicine
Diabetes Scientific Manager
Aventis Pharmaceuticals
Salt Lake City, Utah

Lauren E. Knecht, BA
Salt Lake City, Utah

Thomas P. Knecht, MD, PhD
Associate Professor of Medicine
Division of Endocrinology
University of Utah School of Medicine
Salt Lake City, Utah

Daniel H. Knodel, MD, FACP, JD
Associate Professor of Medicine—Clinical
Division of Endocrinology and Metabolism
University of Utah School of Medicine
Salt Lake City, Utah

Robin Gaynor Krefetz, MEd, MT(ASCP), CLS(NCA)
CLT Program Director
Community College of Philadelphia
Philadelphia, Pennsylvania

Ronald H. Laessig, PhD
Professor, Population Health
Professor, Pathology and Laboratory Medicine
Director, Wisconsin State Laboratory of Hygiene
University of Wisconsin
Madison, Wisconsin

Louann W. Lawrence, DrPH, CLS(NCA)
Professor and Department Head
Clinical Laboratory Sciences
School of Allied Health Professions
Louisiana State University Health Sciences Center
New Orleans, Louisiana

Barbara J. Lindsey, MS, CLSp(C), C(ASCP), ART(CSLT)
Chair, Department of Clinical Laboratory Sciences
Virginia Commonwealth University
Richmond, Virginia

Roberta A. Martindale, BSc(MLS), MLT, MT(ASCP)
Lecturer/Clinical Instructor
Division of Medical Laboratory Science
Department of Laboratory Medicine and Pathology
University of Alberta
Edmonton, Alberta, Canada

Gwen A. McMillin, PhD
Assistant Professor (Clinical) of Pathology
University of Utah School of Medicine
Medical Director, Clinical Toxicology
ARUP Laboratories, Inc.
Salt Lake City, Utah

Judith R. McNamara, MT
Lipid Metabolism and Cardiovascular Research
  Laboratories
Jean Mayer USDA Human Nutrition Research Center on
  Aging at Tufts University and
Gerald J. and Dorothy R. Friedman School of Nutrition
  Science and Policy
Tufts University
Boston, Massachusetts

A. Wayne Meikle, MD
Professor of Medicine and Pathology
University of Utah School of Medicine
Director, Endocrine Testing Laboratory
ARUP Laboratories
Salt Lake City, Utah

Susan Orton, PhD, MS, MT(ASCP)
Senior Clinical Immunology Fellow
McLendon Clinical Labs
University of North Carolina Healthcare
Chapel Hill, North Carolina

Joan E. Polancic, MSEd, CLS(NCA)
Director of Education & Project Planning
American Society for Clinical Laboratory Science
Bethesda, Maryland

Elizabeth E. Porter, BS, MT(ASCP)
Lab Alliance, Cincinnati, Ohio
Technical Specialist, Point of Care
The Health Alliance, Laboratory Services
Cincinnati, Ohio

Alan T. Remaley, MD, PhD
National Institutes of Health
Senior Staff
Department of Laboratory Medicine
Bethesda, Maryland

William L. Roberts, MD, PhD
Associate Professor
Department of Pathology
University of Utah Health Sciences Center
Salt Lake City, UT

Frank A. Sedor, PhD, DABCC
Director, Clinical Chemistry Services
Duke University Medical Center
Durham, North Carolina

Carol J. Skarzynski, BA, SC(ASCP)
Clinical Instructor
Department of Pathology and Laboratory Medicine
Hartford Hospital School of Allied Health
Hartford, Connecticut

LeAnne Swenson, MD
Division of Endocrinology
Department of Medicine
University of Utah
Salt Lake City, Utah

David P. Thorne, PhD, MT(ASCP)
Medical Technology Program
Michigan State University
East Lansing, Michigan

John G. Toffaletti, PhD
Associate Professor of Pathology
Co-Director of Clinical Chemistry Services
Duke University Medical Center
Durham, North Carolina

Tolmie E. Wachter, SLS(ASCP)
AVP, Director of Corporate Safety
ARUP Laboratories
Salt Lake City, Utah

G. Russell Warnick, MS, MBA
President
Pacific Biometrics Research Foundation
Issaquah, Washington

Alan H. B. Wu, PhD
Director, Clinical Chemistry Laboratory
Hartford Hospital
Hartford, Connecticut

James T. Wu
Professor of Pathology
Department of Pathology
University of Utah Health Sciences Center
Salt Lake City, Utah

Acknowledgments

A project as large as this requires the assistance and support of many individuals. The editors wish to express their appreciation to the contributors of this fifth edition of *Clinical Chemistry: Principles, Procedures, Correlations*—the dedicated laboratory professionals and educators whom the editors have had the privilege of knowing and exchanging ideas with over the years. These individuals were selected because of their expertise in particular areas and their commitment to the education of clinical laboratorians. Many have spent their professional careers in the clinical laboratory, at the bench, teaching students, or consulting with clinicians. In these frontline positions, they have developed a perspective of what is important for the next generation of clinical laboratorians.

We extend appreciation to our students, colleagues, teachers, and mentors in the profession who have helped shape our ideas about clinical chemistry practice and education. Also, we want to thank the many companies and professional organizations that provided product information and photographs or granted permission to reproduce diagrams and tables from their publications. Many National Committee for Clinical Laboratory Standards (NCCLS) documents have been important sources of information also. These documents are directly referenced in the appropriate chapters.

The editors would like to acknowledge the contribution and effort of all individuals to previous editions. Their efforts provided the framework for many of the current chapters. Finally, we gratefully acknowledge the cooperation and assistance of the staff at Lippincott Williams & Wilkins, particularly, Kevin Dietz for his advice and support.

The editors are continually striving to improve future editions of this book. We again request and welcome our readers' comments, criticisms, and ideas for improvement.

Contents

Basic Principles and Practice of Clinical Chemistry

Basic Principles and Practice

Eileen Carreiro-Lewandowski

CHAPTER OUTLINE

- **UNITS OF MEASURE**
- **REAGENTS**
  Chemicals
  Reference Materials
  Water Specifications
  Solution Properties
- **CLINICAL LABORATORY SUPPLIES**
  Thermometers/Temperature
  Glassware and Plasticware
  Desiccators and Desiccants
  Balances
- **BASIC SEPARATION TECHNIQUES**
  Centrifugation
  Filtration
  Dialysis

- **LABORATORY MATHEMATICS AND CALCULATIONS**
  Significant Figures
  Logarithms
  Concentration
  Dilutions
  Water of Hydration
- **SPECIMEN CONSIDERATIONS**
  Types of Samples
  Sample Processing
  Sample Variables
  Chain of Custody
- **SUMMARY**
- **REVIEW QUESTIONS**
- **REFERENCES**

OBJECTIVES

Upon completion of this chapter, the clinical laboratorian should be able to:

- Convert results from one unit format to another using the SI system.
- Describe the specifications for each type of laboratory water.
- Identify the varying chemical grades used in reagent preparation and indicate their correct use.
- Define primary standard, SRM, secondary standard.
- Describe the following terms that are associated with solutions and, when appropriate, provide the respective units: percent, molarity, normality, molality, saturation, colligative properties, redox potential, conductivity, and specific gravity.
- Define a buffer and give the formula for pH and pK calculations.
- Use the Henderson-Hasselbalch equation to determine the missing variable when given either the pK and pH or the pK and concentration of the weak acid and its conjugate base.

- List and describe the types of thermometers used in the clinical laboratory.
- Classify the type of pipet when given an actual pipet or its description.
- Describe two ways to calibrate a pipetting device.
- Define a desiccant and discuss how it is used in the clinical laboratory.
- Perform the laboratory mathematical calculations provided in this chapter correctly.
- Identify and describe the types of samples used in clinical chemistry.
- Outline the general steps for processing blood samples.
- Identify the preanalytic, precollection, collection, and postcollection variables that can adversely affect laboratory results.
- List the proper drawing order for collection tubes.
- Identify the additive or preservative, if present, when given a collection stopper color.

K E Y   T E R M S

Analyte	Dilution	NCCLS	Serial dilution
Anhydrous	Distilled water	Normality	Serum
Arterial blood	EDTA	One-point calibration	Significant figures
Beer's law	Equivalent weight	Osmotic pressure	Solute
Buffer	Evacuated tube	Oxidized	Solution
Buret	Filtrate	Oxidizing agent	Solvent
Centrifugation	Filtration	Paracentesis	Specific gravity
Cerebrospinal fluid (CSF)	Hemolysis	Percent solution	Standard
Character	Henderson-Hasselbalch	pH	Standard reference
Colligative property	Hydrate	Phlebotomy	materials (SRMs)
Conductivity	Hygroscopic	Pipet	Système Internationale
Deionized water	Icterus	pK	d'Unités (SI)
Deliquescent substances	International unit	Primary standard	Thermistor
Delta absorbance	Ionic strength	Ratio	Ultrafiltration
Density	Mantissa	Redox potential	Valence
Desiccant	Molality	Reduced	Venipuncture
Desiccator	Molarity	RO water	Whole blood
Dialysis	Nanofiltration	Secondary standard	

The primary goal of a clinical chemistry laboratory is the correct performance of analytic procedures that yield accurate and precise information, aiding patient diagnosis and treatment. The achievement of reliable results requires that the clinical laboratory scientist be able to correctly use basic supplies and equipment and possess an understanding of fundamental concepts critical to any analytic procedure. The topics in this chapter include units of measure, basic laboratory supplies, introductory laboratory mathematics, plus a brief discussion of specimen collection and processing.

UNITS OF MEASURE[1]

Any meaningful quantitative laboratory result consists of two components. The first component represents the actual value, and the second is a label identifying the units of the expression. The number describes the numeric value, whereas the unit defines the physical quantity or dimension, such as mass, length, time, or volume.

Although several systems of units have traditionally been used by various scientific divisions, the *Système Internationale d'Unités (SI)*, adopted internationally in 1960, is preferred in scientific literature and clinical laboratories and often is the only system used in many countries. This system was devised to give the global scientific community a uniform method when describing physical quantities. The SI system units (referred to as *SI units*) are based on the metric system. Several classifications of units exist in the SI system, one of which is the basic unit. There are seven basic units (Table 1-1), with length (meter), mass (kilogram), and quantity of a substance (mole) being the most frequently encountered. Another set of SI

recognized units are termed *derived units*. A derived unit, as the name implies, is a derivative or a mathematical function of one of the basic units. An example of a SI-derived unit is meter per second (m/s), used to express speed per velocity. However, some non-SI units are so widely used that they have become acceptable for use with SI basic or derived units (Table 1-1). These include certain long-standing units, such as hour, minute, day, gram, liter, and plane angles expressed as degrees. These units, although used and recognized, are not technically categorized as either basic or derived SI units.

Another SI convention is the use of standard prefixes used in combination with a single unit (Table 1-2). Prefixes can be added to indicate decimal fractions or multiples of a given unit. For example, 0.001 liter could be expressed using the prefix *milli*, making it equivalent to one milliliter and written as 1 mL. Note that the SI term for mass is *kilogram;* it is the only basic unit that contains a prefix as part of its naming convention. Generally, the standard prefixes for mass employ the term *gram* rather than kilogram.

Reporting of laboratory results is often expressed in terms of substance concentration (*eg*, moles) or the mass of a substance (*eg*, mg/dL, g/dL, g/L, mEq/L, and IU). These familiar and traditional units can cause confusion during interpretation. It has been recommended that *analytes* be reported using moles of solute per volume of solution (substance concentration) and that the liter be used as the reference volume.[2] Tables listing laboratory reference values provide traditional values as well as SI-recommended values. Appendix D, *Conversion of Traditional Units to SI Units for Common Clinical Chemistry Analytes*, lists both units together with the conversion factor from traditional to SI units for common analytes.

TABLE 1-1. SI UNITS

BASE QUANTITY	NAME	SYMBOL
length	meter	m
mass	kilogram	kg
time	second	s
electric current	ampere	A
thermodynamic temperature	kelvin	K
amount of substance	mole	mol
luminous intensity	candela	cd
Selected Derived		
frequency	hertz	Hz
force	newton	N
Celsius temperature	degree Celsius	°C
catalytic activity	katal	kat
Selected Accepted Non-SI		
minute (time)	(60s)	min
hour	(3600s)	h
day	(86,400s)	d
liter (volume)	($1 \, dm^3 = 10^{-3} \, m^3$)	L
angstrom	($0.1 \, nm = 10^{-10} \, m$)	Å

TABLE 1-2. PREFIXES USED WITH SI UNITS

FACTOR	PREFIX	SYMBOL
10^{-18}	atto	a
10^{-15}	femto	f
10^{-12}	pico	p
10^{-9}	nano	n
10^{-6}	micro	μ
10^{-3}	milli	m
10^{-2}	centi	c
10^{-1}	deci	d
10^{1}	deka	da
10^{2}	hecto	h
10^{3}	kilo	k
10^{4}	mega	M
10^{9}	giga	G
10^{12}	tera	T
10^{15}	peta	P
10^{18}	exa	E

Note: Prefixes are used to indicate a subunit or multiple of a basic SI unit.

REAGENTS

In today's highly automated laboratory, there seems little need for reagent preparation by the clinical laboratory scientist. Most instrument manufacturers also make the reagents, usually in a readily available "kit" form (ie, all necessary reagents and respective storage containers are prepackaged as a unit) or requiring only the addition of water or buffer to the prepackaged reagent components. A heightened awareness of the hazards of certain chemicals and numerous regulatory agency requirements have caused clinical chemistry laboratories to readily eliminate massive stocks of chemicals and opt instead for the ease of using prepared reagents. Periodically, especially in hospital laboratories involved in research and development, specialized analyses, or method validation, the laboratorian may still face preparing various reagents or solutions. As a result of reagent deterioration, supply and demand, or the institution of cost-containment programs, the decision may be made to prepare reagents in-house. Therefore, a thorough knowledge of chemicals, standards, solutions, buffers, and water requirements is necessary.

Chemicals[3]

Analytic chemicals exist in varying grades of purity: analytic reagent grade (AR); ultrapure, chemically pure (CP); United States Pharmacopeia (USP); National For-

mulary (NF); and technical or commercial grade. The American Chemical Society (ACS) has established specifications for analytic reagent grade chemicals, and chemical manufacturers will either meet or exceed these requirements. Labels on these reagents state the actual impurities for each chemical lot or list the maximum allowable impurities. The labels should be clearly printed with the percentage of impurities present and either the initials *AR* or *ACS* or the terms *for laboratory use* or *ACS Standard-Grade Reference Materials*. Chemicals of this category are suitable for use in most analytic laboratory procedures. Ultrapure chemicals have been put through additional purification steps for use in specific procedures such as chromatography, atomic absorption, immunoassays, molecular diagnostics, standardization, or other techniques that require extremely pure chemicals. These reagents may carry designations of HPLC or chromatographic (see below) on their labels.

Because USP and NF grade chemicals are used to manufacture drugs, the limitations established for this group of chemicals are based only on the criterion of not being injurious to individuals. Chemicals in this group may be pure enough for use in most chemical procedures; however, it should be recognized that their purity standards are not based on the needs of the laboratory and, therefore, these may or may not meet all assay requirements.

Reagent designations of CP or pure grade indicate that the impurity limitations are not stated and that preparation of these chemicals is not uniform. Melting point analysis is often used to ascertain the acceptable purity range. It is not recommended that clinical laboratories use these chemicals for reagent preparation unless further purification or a reagent blank is included. Technical- or commercial-grade reagents are used primarily in manufacturing and should never be used in the clinical laboratory.

Organic reagents also have varying grades of purity that differ from those used to classify inorganic reagents. These grades include a practical grade with some impurities; chemically pure, which approaches the purity level of reagent grade chemicals; spectroscopic (spectrally pure) and chromatographic (minimum purity of 99% determined by gas chromatography) grade organic reagents, with purity levels attained by their respective procedures; and reagent grade (ACS), which is certified to contain impurities below certain levels established by the ACS. As in any analytic method, the desired organic reagent purity is dictated by the particular application.

Other than the purity aspects of the chemicals, laws such as the Occupational Safety and Health Act (OSHA)[4] require manufacturers to clearly indicate the lot number, plus any physical or biologic health hazard and precautions needed for the safe use and storage of any chemical. A manufacturer is required to provide technical data sheets for each chemical manufactured on a document called a material safety data sheet (MSDS). A more detailed discussion of this topic may be found in Chapter 2, *Laboratory Safety and Regulations.*

Reference Materials[5–9]

Unlike other areas of chemistry, clinical chemistry is involved in the analysis of biochemical by-products found in *serum,* which makes purifying and providing their exact composition almost impossible. For this reason, traditionally defined standards do not necessarily exist for use in clinical chemistry.

Recall that a *primary standard* is a highly purified chemical that can be measured directly to produce a substance of *exact* known concentration and purity. The ACS purity tolerances for primary standards are $100 \pm 0.02\%$. Because most biologic constituents are unavailable within these limitations, NIST-certified *standard reference materials (SRMs)* are used instead of ACS primary standards.

NIST developed certified reference material (CRMs/SRMs) for use in clinical chemistry laboratories. They are assigned a value after careful analysis, using state-of-the-art methods and equipment. The chemical composition of these substances is then certified; however, they may not possess the purity equivalent of a primary standard. Because each substance has been characterized for certain chemical or physical properties, it can be used in

place of an ACS primary standard in clinical work and is often used to verify calibration or accuracy/bias assessments. Many manufacturers use an NIST SRM when producing calibrator and standard materials and, in this way, these materials are considered "traceable to NIST" and may meet certain accreditation requirements. There are SRMs for a limited number of analytes, including hormones, selected drugs, and blood gases. Human serum SRM 909a and 909b are available, with SRM 909a certified for calcium; chloride; cholesterol; creatinine; glucose; lithium; magnesium; potassium; sodium; urea; uric acid; and the trace metals cadmium, chromium, copper, iron, lead, and vanadium; and SRM 909b adds triglycerides.[10]

A *secondary standard* is a substance of lower purity with concentration determined by comparison with a primary standard. The secondary standard not only depends on its composition, which cannot be directly determined, but also on the analytic reference method. Once again, because physiologic primary standards are generally unavailable, clinical chemists do not by definition have "true" secondary standards. Manufacturers of secondary standards will list the SRM or primary standard used for comparison. This information may be needed during laboratory accreditation processes.

Water Specifications[11]

Water is the most frequently used reagent in the laboratory. Because tap water is unsuitable for laboratory applications, most procedures, including reagent and standard preparation, use water that has been substantially purified. Water solely purified by distillation results in *distilled water;* water purified by ion exchange produces *deionized water.* Reverse osmosis, which pumps water across a semipermeable membrane, produces *RO water.* Water can also be purified by ultrafiltration, ultraviolet light, sterilization, or ozone treatment. Laboratory requirements generally call for *reagent grade water* that, according to the *National Committee for Clinical Laboratory Standards (NCCLS)*, belongs to one of three types (Types I, II, and III). It is recommended that water be referred to as reagent grade, followed by the associated type (I, II, or III) rather than the method of preparation.[12]

Prefiltration can remove particulate matter for municipal water supplies before any additional treatments. Filtration cartridges are composed of glass; cotton; activated charcoal, which removes organic materials and chlorine; and submicron filters (≤0.2 mm), which remove any substances larger than the filter's pores, including bacteria. The use of these filters depends on the quality of the municipal water and the other purification methods used. For example, hard water (containing calcium, iron, and other dissolved elements) may require prefiltration with a glass or cotton filter rather than activated charcoal or submicron filters that quickly become clogged and are expensive to operate. The submicron filter may be better suited after distillation, deionization, or reverse osmosis treatment.

Distilled water has been purified to remove almost all organic materials, using a technique of distillation much like that found in organic chemistry laboratory distillation experiments in which water is boiled and vaporized. The vapor rises and enters into the coil of a condenser, a glass tube that contains a glass coil. Cool water surrounds this condensing coil, lowering the temperature of the water vapor. The water vapor returns to a liquid state, which is then collected. Many impurities do not rise in the water vapor, remaining in the boiling apparatus. The water collected after condensation has less contamination. Because laboratories use thousands of liters of water each day, stills are used instead of small condensing apparatuses; however, the principles are basically the same. Water may be distilled more than once, with each distillation cycle removing additional impurities.

Deionized water has some or all ions removed, although organic material may still be present, so it is neither pure nor sterile. Generally, deionized water is purified from previously treated water, such as prefiltered or distilled water. Deionized water is produced using either an anion or a cation exchange resin, followed by replacement of the removed particles with hydroxyl or hydrogen ions. The ions that are anticipated to be removed from the water will dictate the type of ion exchange resin to be used. One column cannot service all ions present in water. A combination of several resins will produce different grades of deionized water. A two-bed system uses an anion resin followed by a cation resin. The different resins may be in separate columns or in the same column. This process is excellent in removing dissolved ionized solids and dissolved gases.

Reverse osmosis is a process that uses pressure to force water through a semipermeable membrane, producing water that reflects a filtered product of the original water. It does not remove dissolved gases. Reverse osmosis may be used as a pretreatment of water.

Ultrafiltration and nanofiltration, like distillation, are excellent in removing particulate matter, microorganisms, and any pyrogens or endotoxins. Ultraviolet oxidation (removes some trace organic material) or sterilization processes (uses specific wavelengths), together with ozone treatment, can destroy bacteria but may leave behind residual products. These techniques are often used after other purification processes have been used.

Type I grade water production largely depends on the condition of the feed water. Generally, water can be obtained by initially filtering it to remove particulate matter, followed by reverse osmosis, deionization, and a 0.2-mm filter or more restrictive filtration process. Type III water is acceptable for glassware washing but not for analysis or reagent preparation. Type II water is acceptable for most analytic requirements, including reagent, quality control, and standard preparation. Type I water is used for test methods requiring minimum interference, such as trace metal, iron, and enzyme analyses. Use with high-performance liquid chromatography may require less than a 0.2-mm final filtration step. Because Type I water should be used immediately, storage is discouraged because the resistivity changes. Type II water should be stored in a manner that reduces any chemical or bacterial contamination and for short periods.

Testing procedures to determine the quality of reagent grade water include measurements of resistance; pH; colony counts (for assessing bacterial contamination) on selective and nonselective media for the detection of coliforms; chlorine; ammonia; nitrate or nitrite; iron; hardness; phosphate; sodium; silica; carbon dioxide; chemical oxygen demand (COD); and metal detection. Some accreditation agencies[13] recommend that laboratories document culture growth, pH, and specific resistance on water used in reagent preparation. Resistance is measured because pure water, devoid of ions, is a poor conductor of electricity. The relationship of water purity to resistance is linear. Generally, as purity increases, so does resistance. This one measurement does not suffice for determination of true water purity because a nonionic contaminant may be present that has little effect on resistance. Table 1-3 lists reagent water specifications for each type for selected parameters according to the NCCLS guidelines.

Note that reagent water meeting specifications from other organizations, such as the American Society for Testing Materials (ASTM), may not be equivalent to those established for each type by NCCLS and care should be taken to meet the assay procedural requirements for water type requirements. Specialty type water that exceeds Type I specifications may also be required for certain procedures.

Solution Properties

In clinical chemistry, substances found in biologic fluids are measured (*eg*, serum, urine, and spinal fluid). A substance that is dissolved in a liquid is called a *solute*; in

TABLE 1-3. REAGENT WATER

	TYPE I	TYPE II	TYPE III
Maximum colony count (CFU/mL)	≤10	1000	NS
Silicate (mg/L SiO_2)	0.05	0.1	1.0
Resistivity (megaohm·cm)	10 (inline)	1.0	0.1
pH	NS	NS	5.0–8.0

NS = not specified.

laboratory science, these biologic solutes are also known as *analytes*. The liquid in which the solute is dissolved—in this instance, a biologic fluid—is the *solvent*. Together they represent a *solution*. Any chemical or biologic solution is described by its basic properties, including concentration, saturation, colligative properties, redox potential, conductivity, density, pH, and ionic strength.

Concentration

Analyte concentration in solution can be expressed in many ways. Routinely, concentration is expressed as percent solution, molarity, molality, or normality and, because these non-SI expressions are so widely used, they will be discussed here. Note that the SI expression for the amount of a substance is mole.

Percent solutions are equal to parts per hundred or the amount of solute per 100 total units of solution. Three expressions of percent solutions are weight per weight (w/w), volume per volume (v/v), and, most commonly, weight per volume (w/v). For v/v solutions, it is recommended that milliliters per liter (mL/L) be used instead of percent or % (v/v).

Molarity is expressed as the number of moles per 1 L of solution. One mole of a substance equals its gram molecular weight (gmw). The SI representation for the traditional molar concentration is moles of solute per volume of solution, with the volume of the solution given in liters. The SI expression for concentration should be represented as moles per liter (mol/L), millimoles per liter (mmol/L), micromoles per liter (μmol/L), and nanomoles per liter (nmol/L). The familiar concentration term *molarity* has not been adopted by the SI as an expression of concentration.

Molality represents the amount of solute per 1 kg of solvent. Molality is sometimes confused with molarity; however, it can be easily distinguished from molarity because molality is always expressed in terms of weight per weight or moles per kilogram and describes moles per 1000 g (1 kg) of solvent. The preferred expression for molality is moles per kilogram (mol/kg).

Normality is the least likely of the four concentration expressions to be encountered in clinical laboratories, but is often used in chemical titrations and chemical reagent classification. It is defined as the number of gram equivalent weights per 1 L of solution. An *equivalent weight* is equal to the gram molecular weight of a substance divided by its valence. The *valence* is the number of units that can combine with or replace 1 mole of hydrogen ions for acids, hydroxyl ions for bases, and the number of electrons exchanged in oxidation reduction reactions. It is the number of atoms/elements that can combine for a particular compound; therefore, the equivalent weight is the gram combining weight of a material. Normality is always equal to or greater than the molarity of that compound.

Normality was previously used for reporting electrolyte values, *eg*, sodium [Na^+], potassium [K^+], and chloride [Cl^-] expressed as milliequivalents per liter (mEq/L); however, this convention has been replaced with the more familiar units of millimoles per liter (mmol/L).

Solution saturation gives little specific information about the concentration of solutes in a solution. Temperature, as well as the presence of other ions, can influence the solubility constant for a solute in a given solution and thus affect the saturation. Routine terms in the clinical laboratory that describe the extent of saturation are *dilute, concentrated, saturated,* and *supersaturated*. A *dilute solution* is one in which there is relatively little solute. In contrast, a *concentrated solution* has a large quantity of solute in solution. A solution in which there is an excess of undissolved solute particles is a *saturated solution*. As the name implies, a *supersaturated solution* has an even greater concentration of undissolved solute particles than a saturated solution of the same substance. Because of the greater concentration of solute particles, a supersaturated solution is thermodynamically unstable. The addition of a crystal of solute or mechanical agitation disturbs the supersaturated solution, resulting in crystallization of any excess material out of solution. An example is seen when measuring serum osmolality by freezing point depression.

Colligative Properties

The behavior of particles in solution demonstrates four repeatable properties based only on the relative number of each kind of molecule present. The properties of osmotic pressure, vapor pressure, freezing point, and boiling point, are called *colligative properties*. *Vapor pressure* is the pressure at which the liquid solvent is in equilibrium with the water vapor. *Freezing point* is the temperature at which the vapor pressures of the solid and liquid phases are the same. *Boiling point* is the temperature at which the vapor pressure of the solvent reaches one atmosphere.

Osmotic pressure is the pressure that allows solvent to flow through a semipermeable membrane to establish equilibrium between compartments of different osmolality. The osmotic pressure of a dilute solution is proportional to the concentration of the molecules in solution. The expression for concentration is the osmole. One osmole of a substance equals the molarity multiplied by the number of particles at dissociation. When a solute is dissolved in a solvent, these colligative properties change in a predictable manner for each osmole of substance present; the freezing point is lowered by $-1.86°C$, the boiling point is raised by $0.52°C$, the vapor pressure is lowered by 0.3 mm Hg or torr, and the osmotic pressure is increased by a factor of 1.7×10^4 mm Hg or torr. In the clinical setting, freezing point and vapor pressure depression are measured as a function of osmolality.

Redox Potential

Redox potential, or *oxidation-reduction potential,* is a measure of the ability of a solution to accept or donate electrons. Substances that donate electrons are called *reducing agents;* those that accept electrons are considered *oxidizing agents.* The pneumonic—LEO (lose electrons = *oxidized*) the lion says GER (gain electrons = *reduced*)— may prove useful when trying to recall the relationship between reducing/oxidizing agents and redox potential.

Conductivity

Conductivity is a measure of how well electricity passes through a solution. A solution's conductivity quality depends principally on the number of respective charges of the ions present. *Resistivity,* the reciprocal of conductivity, is a measure of a substance's resistance to the passage of electrical current. The primary application of resistivity in the clinical laboratory is for assessing the purity of water. Resistivity or resistance is expressed as ohms and conductivity is expressed as $ohms^{-1}$ or mho.

pH and Buffers

Buffers are weak acids or bases and their related salts that, as a result of their dissociation characteristics, minimize changes in the hydrogen ion concentration. Hydrogen ion concentration is often expressed as pH. A lowercase *p* in front of certain letters or abbreviations operationally means the "negative logarithm of" or "inverse log of" that substance. In keeping with this convention, the term *pH* represents the negative or inverse log of the hydrogen ion concentration. Mathematically, pH is expressed as

$$pH = \log(1/[H^+])$$
$$pH = -\log[H^+] \qquad \text{(Eq. 1–1)}$$

where $[H^+]$ equals the concentration of hydrogen ions in moles per liter.

The pH scale ranges from 0 to 14 and is a convenient way to express hydrogen ion concentration.

A buffer's capacity to minimize changes in pH is related to the dissociation characteristics of the weak acid or base in the presence of its respective salt. Unlike a strong acid or base, which dissociates almost completely, the dissociation constant for a weak acid or base solution tends to be very small, meaning little dissociation occurs.

The ionization of acetic acid (CH_3COOH), a weak acid, can be illustrated as follows:

$$[HA] \leftrightarrow [A^-] + [H^+]$$
$$[CH_3COOH] \leftrightarrow [CH_3COO^-] + [H^+] \qquad \text{(Eq. 1–2)}$$

where HA = weak acid, A^- = conjugate base, and H^+ = hydrogen ions.

Note that the dissociation constant, K_a, for a weak acid may be calculated using the following equation:

$$K_a = \frac{[A^-][H^+]}{[HA]} \qquad \text{(Eq. 1–3)}$$

Rearrangement of this equation reveals

$$[H^+] = K_a \times \frac{[HA]}{[A^+]} \qquad \text{(Eq. 1–4)}$$

Taking the log of each quantity and then multiplying by minus 1 (–1), the equation can be rewritten as

$$-\log[H^+] = -\log K_a \times -\log \frac{[HA]}{[A^+]} \qquad \text{(Eq. 1–5)}$$

By convention, lower case *p* means "negative log of"; therefore, $-\log [H^+]$ may be written as pH, and $-K_a$ may be written as pK_a. The equation now becomes

$$pH = pK_a - \log \frac{[HA]}{[A^+]} \qquad \text{(Eq. 1–6)}$$

Eliminating the minus sign in front of the log of the quantity [HA] / $[A^+]$ results in an equation known as the *Henderson-Hasselbalch* equation, which mathematically describes the dissociation characteristics of weak acids and bases and the effect on pH:

$$pH = pK_a + \log \frac{[A^+]}{[HA]} \qquad \text{(Eq. 1–7)}$$

When the ratio of $[A^+]$ to [HA] is 1, the pH equals the pK and the buffer has its greatest buffering capacity. The dissociation constant K_a, and therefore the pK_a, remains the same for a given substance. Any changes in pH are solely due to the ratio of base/salt $[A^+]$ concentration to weak acid [HA] concentration.

Ionic strength is another important aspect of buffers, particularly in separation techniques. *Ionic strength* is the concentration or activity of ions in a solution or buffer. It is defined[14] as follows:

$$\mu = I = \frac{1}{2} \Sigma C_i Z_i^2 \text{ or}$$

$$\frac{\Sigma\{(C_i) \times (Z_i)^2\}}{2} \qquad \text{(Eq. 1–8)}$$

where C_i is the concentration of the ion, Z_i is the charge of the ion, and Σ is the sum of the quantity $(C_i) \times (Z_i)^2$ for each ion present. In mixtures of substances, the degree of dissociation must be considered. Increasing ionic strength increases the ionic cloud surrounding a compound and decreases the rate of particle migration. It can also promote compound dissociation into ions effectively increasing the solubility of some salts, along with changes in current, which can also effect electrophoretic separation.

CLINICAL LABORATORY SUPPLIES

Many different supplies are required in today's medical laboratory; however, several items are common to most facilities, including thermometers, pipets, flasks, beakers, burets, desiccators, and filtering material. The following is a brief discussion of the composition and general use of these supplies.

Thermometers/Temperature[15,16]

The predominant practice for temperature measurement uses the Celsius (°C) scale; however, Fahrenheit (F) and Kelvin (K) scales are also used. The SI designation for temperature is the Kelvin scale. Appendix C, *Basic Clinical Laboratory Conversions*, lists the various conversion formulas between each scale.

All analytic reactions occur at an optimal temperature. Some laboratory procedures, such as enzyme determinations, require precise temperature control, whereas others work well over a wide range of temperatures. Reactions that are temperature dependent use some type of heating/cooling cell, heating/cooling block, or water/ice bath to provide the correct temperature environment. Laboratory refrigerator temperatures are often critical and need periodic verification. Thermometers are either an integral part of an instrument or need to be placed in the device for temperature maintenance. The three major types of thermometers discussed include liquid-in-glass, electronic thermometer or *thermistor* probe, and digital thermometer; however, several other types of temperature indicating devices are in use. Regardless of being used, all temperature reading devices must be calibrated to ascertain accuracy.

Liquid-in-glass thermometers, using a colored liquid (red or other colored material), are now replacing the more traditional mercury-in-glass devices. The design is essentially the same, with a bulb at one end and a graduated stem. They usually measure temperatures between −20°C to 400°C. Partial immersion thermometers are used for measuring temperatures in units such as heating blocks and water baths and should be immersed to the proper height as indicated by the continuous line etched on the thermometer stem. Total immersion thermometers are used for refrigeration applications, and surface thermometers may be needed to check temperatures on flat surfaces, such as in an incubator or heating oven. Visual inspection of the liquid-in-glass thermometer should reveal a continuous line of liquid, free from separation or gas bubbles. The accuracy range for a thermometer used in clinical laboratories is determined by the specific application but, generally, the accuracy range should equal 50% of the desired temperature range required by the procedure.

Liquid-in-glass thermometers should be calibrated against a NIST-certified, or NIST-traceable thermometer for critical laboratory applications.[17] NIST has a SRM thermometer with various calibration points (0°, 25°, 30°, and 37°C) for use with liquid-in-glass thermometers. Gallium, another SRM, has a known melting point and can also be used for thermometer verification.

As automation advances and miniaturizes, the need for an accurate, fast-reading electronic thermometer (thermistor) has increased and is now routinely incorporated in many devices. The advantages of a thermistor over the more traditional liquid-in-glass thermometers are size and millisecond response time. One disadvantage can be the initial cost, although the use of a thermistor probe attached to an already owned volt–ohm meter (VOM) can be cost effective. Similar to the liquid-in-glass thermometers, the thermistor can be calibrated against a SRM thermometer or the gallium melting point cell.[18,19] When the thermistor is calibrated against the gallium cell, it can be used as a reference for any type thermometer.

Glassware and Plasticware

Until recently, laboratory supplies (*eg*, pipets, flasks, beakers, and burets) consisted of some type of glass and could be correctly termed *glassware*. As plastic material was refined and made available to manufacturers, plastic has been increasingly used to make laboratory utensils. Before discussing general laboratory supplies, a brief summary of the types and uses of glass and plastic commonly seen today in laboratories is given. (See Appendix L, *Characteristics of Types of Glass*; Appendix M, *Characteristics of Types of Plastic*; and Appendix N, *Chemical Resistance of Types of Plastic*.) Regardless of design, most laboratory supplies must satisfy certain tolerances of accuracy. Those that satisfy NIST specifications[20,21] are classified as Class A. Vessels holding or transferring liquid are designed either to contain (TC) or to deliver (TD) a specified volume. As the names imply, the major difference is that TC devices do not deliver that same volume when the liquid is transferred into a container, whereas the TD designation means that the labware will deliver that amount.

Glassware used in the clinical laboratory usually falls into one of the following categories: Kimax/Pyrex (borosilicate), Corex (aluminosilicate), high silica, Vycor (acid- and alkali-resistant), low actinic (amber colored), or flint (soda lime) glass used for disposable material.[22] Whenever possible, routinely used clinical chemistry glassware should consist of high thermal borosilicate or aluminosilicate glass and meet the Class A tolerances recommended by the NIST. Glassware that *does not* meet Type A specifications may have twice the tolerance range despite its appearance being identical to a piece of Type A glassware. The manufacturer is the best source of information about specific uses, limitations, and accuracy specifications for glassware.

Plasticware is beginning to replace glassware in the laboratory setting. The unique high resistance to corrosion and breakage, as well as varying flexibility, has made plasticware most appealing. Relatively inexpensive, it allows most items to be completely disposable after each use. The major types of resins frequently used in the clinical chemistry laboratory are polystyrene, polyethylene, polypropylene, Tygon, Teflon, polycarbonate, and polyvinyl chloride. Again, the individual manufacturer is the best source of information concerning the proper use and limitations of any plastic material.

In most laboratories, glass or plastic that is in direct contact associated with biohazardous material is usually disposable. Should the need arise, however, cleaning of glass or plastic may require special techniques. Immediately rinsing glass or plastic supplies after use, followed by washing with a powder or liquid detergent designed for cleaning laboratory supplies and several distilled water rinses may be sufficient. Presoaking glassware in soapy water is highly recommended whenever immediate cleaning is impractical. Many laboratories use automatic dishwashers and dryers for cleaning. Detergents and temperature levels should be compatible with the material and the manufacturer's recommendations. To ensure that all detergent has been removed from the labware, multiple rinses with Type II water is recommended. Check the pH of the final rinse water and compare it with the initial pH of the prerinse water. Detergent-contaminated water will have a more alkaline pH when compared with the pH of the Type II reagent water. Visual inspection should reveal spotless vessel walls. Any biologically contaminated labware should be disposed according to the precautions followed by that laboratory.

Some determinations, such as those used in assessing heavy metals or assays associated with molecular testing, require scrupulously clean glassware, if not disposable. Some applications may require plastic rather than glass because glass can absorb metal ions. Successful cleaning solutions are acid dichromate and nitric acid. It is suggested that disposable glass and plastic be used whenever possible.

Dirty pipets should be placed immediately in a container of soapy water with the pipet tips up. The container should be long enough to allow the pipet tips to be covered with solution. A specially designed pipet soaking jar and washing/drying apparatus is recommended. For each final water rinse, fresh Type I or II water should be provided. If possible, designate a pipet container for final rinses only. Cleaning brushes are available to fit almost any size glassware and are recommended for any articles that are washed routinely.

Although plastic material is often easier to clean because of its nonwettable surface, it may not be appropriate for some applications involving organic solvents or autoclaving. Brushes or harsh abrasive cleaners should not be used on plasticware. Acid rinses or washes are not required. The initial cleaning procedure described in Appendix O, *Cleaning Labware,* can be adapted for plasticware as well. Ultrasonic cleaners can help remove debris coating the surfaces of glass or plasticware. Properly cleaned glassware should be completely dried before using.

Laboratory Vessels

Flasks, beakers, and graduated cylinders are used to hold solutions. Volumetric and Erlenmeyer flasks are two types of containers in general use in the clinical laboratory.

A Class A *volumetric flask* is calibrated to hold one exact volume of liquid (TC). The flask has a round, lower portion with a flat bottom and a long, thin neck with an etched calibration line. Volumetric flasks are used to bring a given reagent to its final volume with the prescribed diluent and should be Class A quality. When bringing the bottom of the meniscus to the calibration mark, a pipet should be used when adding the final drops of diluent to ensure maximum control is maintained and the calibration line is not missed.

Erlenmeyer flasks and *Griffin beakers* are designed to hold different volumes rather than one exact amount. Because Erlenmeyer flasks and Griffin beakers are often used in reagent preparation, flask size, chemical inertness, and thermal stability should be considered. The Erlenmeyer flask has a wide bottom that gradually evolves into a smaller, short neck. The Griffin beaker has a flat bottom, straight sides, and an opening as wide as the flat base, with a small spout in the lip.

Graduated cylinders are long, cylindrical tubes usually held upright by an octagonal or circular base. The cylinder has calibration marks along its length and is used to measure volumes of liquids. Graduated cylinders do not have the accuracy of volumetric glassware. The sizes routinely used are 10, 25, 50, 100, 500, 1000, and 2000 mL.

All laboratory utensils should be Class A whenever possible to maximize accuracy and precision and thus decrease calibration time. Figure 1-8 illustrates representative laboratory glassware. Table 1-4 lists the Class A tolerances for some commonly used volumes.

Pipets

Pipets are glass or plastic utensils used to transfer liquids; they may be reusable or disposable. Although pipets may transfer any volume, they are usually used for volumes of 20 mL or less; larger volumes are usually transferred or dispensed using automated pipetting devices or jar-style pipetting apparatus. To minimize confusion, Table 1-5 lists the classification scheme further described here. Examples of pipets are found in Figure 1-1.

Similar to many laboratory utensils, pipets are designed to contain (TC) or to deliver (TD) a particular volume of liquid. The major difference is the amount of liquid needed to wet the interior surface of the ware and the amount of any residual liquid left in the pipet tip. Most manufacturers stamp *TC* or *TD* near the top of the pipet to alert the user as to the type of pipet. Like other TC-designated labware, a TC pipet holds or contains a particular volume but does not dispense that exact volume, whereas a TD pipet will dispense the volume indi-

TABLE 1-4. CLASS A TOLERANCES

SIZE (mL)	TOLERANCES (mL)
Burets	
5	± 0.01
10	± 0.02
25	± 0.03
50	± 0.05
100	± 0.10
Pipets (Transfer)	
0.5–2	± 0.006
3–5	± 0.01
10	± 0.02
15–25	± 0.03
50	± 0.05
Volumetric Flasks	
1–10	± 0.02
25	± 0.03
50	± 0.05
100	± 0.08
200	± 0.10
250	± 0.12
500	± 0.20
1000	± 0.30
2000	± 0.50

TABLE 1-5. PIPET CLASSIFICATION

I. Design

   A. To contain (TC)

   B. To deliver (TD)

II. Drainage characteristics

   A. Blowout

   B. Self-draining

III. Type

   A. Measuring or graduated

     1. Serologic

     2. Mohr

     3. Bacteriologic

     4. Ball, Kolmer, or Kahn

     5. Micropipet

   B. Transfer

     1. Volumetric

     2. Ostwald-Folin

     3. Pasteur pipets

     4. Automatic macropipets or micropipets

cated. When using either pipet, the tip must be immersed in the liquid to be transferred to a level that will allow it to remain in solution after the volume of liquid has entered the pipet—without touching the vessel walls. The pipet is held upright, not at an angle (Fig. 1-2). Using a pipet bulb or similar device, a slight suction is applied to the opposite end until the liquid enters the pipet and the meniscus is brought above the desired graduation line (Fig. 1-3A); suction is then stopped. While the meniscus level is held in place, the pipet tip is raised slightly out of the solution and wiped with a laboratory tissue of any adhering liquid. The liquid is allowed to drain until the bottom of the meniscus touches the desired calibration mark (Fig. 1-3B). With the pipet held in a vertical position and the tip against the side of the receiving vessel, the pipet contents are allowed to drain into the vessel (*eg*, test tube, cuvet, flask). A *blowout pipet* has a continuous etched ring or two small, close, continuous rings located near the top of the pipet. This means that the last drop of liquid should be expelled into the receiving vessel. Without these markings, a pipet is *self-draining*, and the user allows the contents of the pipet to drain by gravity. The tip of the pipet should not be in contact with the accu-

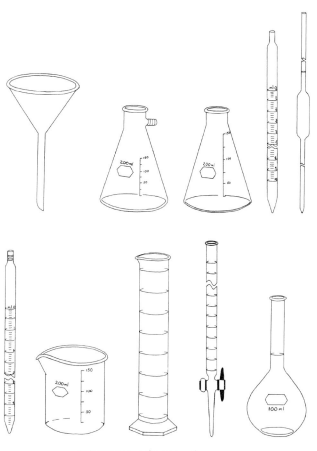

FIGURE 1-1. Laboratory glassware.

Serologic/Mohr

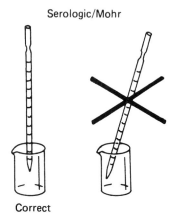

Correct

Volumetric/Ostwald-Folin

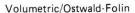

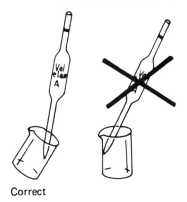

Correct

FIGURE 1-2. Correct and incorrect pipet positions.

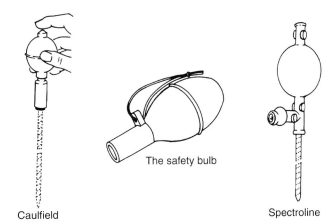

The safety bulb

Caulfield   Spectroline

FIGURE 1-4. Types of pipet bulbs.

can be used to measure 5, 4, 3, 2, or 1 mL of liquid, with further graduations between each milliliter. The pipet is designated as 5 in $^1/_{10}$ increments (Fig. 1-5) and could deliver any volume in tenths of a milliliter, up to 5 mL. Another pipet, such as a 1-mL pipet, may be designed to dispense 1 mL and have subdivisions of hundredths of a milliliter. The markings at the top of a measuring or graduated pipet indicate the volume(s) it is designed to dispense.

The subgroups of measuring or graduated pipets are Mohr, serologic, and micropipets. A *Mohr pipet* does not have graduations to the tip. It is a self-draining pipet, but the tip should not be allowed to touch the vessel while the pipet is draining and its full volume should be used to achieve proper accuracy. A *serologic pipet* has calibration marks to the tip and is generally a blowout pipet. A *micropipet* is a pipet with a total holding volume of less than 1 mL; it may be designed as either a Mohr or serologic pipet.

The next major category is the *transfer pipets*. These pipets are designed to dispense one volume without further subdivisions. *The bulb-like enlargement in the pipet stem easily distinguishes the Ostwald-Folin and volumetric subgroups.* Ostwald-Folin pipets are used with biologic fluids having a viscosity greater than water. They are blowout pipets, indicated by two etched continuous

mulating fluid in the receiving vessel during drainage. With the exception of the Mohr pipet, the tip should remain in contact with the side of the vessel for several seconds after the liquid has drained. The pipet is then removed. Various pipet bulbs are illustrated in Figure 1-4. Mouth pipetting is strictly *forbidden* because of the possibility of aspirating hazardous material.

Measuring or graduated pipets are capable of dispensing several different volumes. Because the graduation lines located on the pipet may vary, they should be indicated on the top of each pipet. For example, a 5-mL pipet

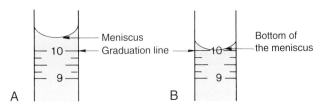

FIGURE 1-3. Pipetting technique. (**A**) Meniscus is brought above the desired graduation line. (**B**) Liquid is allowed to drain until the bottom of the meniscus touches the desired calibration mark.

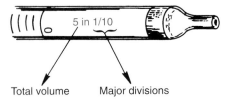

FIGURE 1-5. Volume indication of a pipet.

rings at the top. The volumetric pipet is designed to dispense or transfer aqueous solutions and is always self-draining. This type pipet usually has the greatest degree of accuracy and precision and should be used when diluting standards, calibrators, or quality-control material. *Pasteur pipets* do not have calibration marks and are used to transfer solutions or biologic fluids without consideration of a specific volume. These pipets should not be used in any quantitative analytic techniques.

The *automatic pipet* is the most routinely used pipet in today's clinical chemistry laboratory. Automatic and semiautomatic pipets have many advantages, including safety, stability, ease of use, increased precision, the ability to save time, and less cleaning is required as a result of the contaminated portions of the pipet (*eg*, the tips) often being disposable. Figure 1-6 illustrates many common automatic pipets. A pipet associated with only one volume is termed a *fixed* volume, models able to select different volumes are termed *variable*; however, only one volume may be used at a time. The available range of volumes is 1 μL to 1000 mL. The widest volume range usually seen in a single pipet is 0 to 1 mL. A pipet with a pipetting capability of less than 1 mL is considered a *micropipet*, and a pipet that dispenses greater than 1 mL is called an *automatic macropipet*.

The term *automatic*, as used here, implies that the mechanism that draws up and dispenses the liquid is an integral part of the pipet. It may be fully automated/self-operating, semiautomatic, or a completely manually operated device. There are three general types of automatic pipets: air-displacement, positive-displacement, and dispenser pipets. An *air-displacement pipet* relies on a piston for suction creation to draw the sample into a disposable tip that must be changed after each use. The piston does not come in contact with the liquid. A *positive-displacement pipet* operates by moving the piston in the pipet tip or barrel, much like a hypodermic syringe. It does not require a different tip for each use. Because of carryover concerns, rinsing and blotting between samples may be required. *Dispensers* and *dilutor/dispensers* are automatic pipets that obtain the liquid from a common reservoir and dispense it repeatedly. The dispensing pipets may be bottle-top, motorized, handheld, or attached to a dilutor. The dilutor often combines sampling and dispensing functions. Figure 1-7 provides examples of different types of automatic pipetting devices. These pipets should be used according to the individual manufacturer's directions. Many automated pipets use a wash in between samples to eliminate carryover problems. However, to minimize carryover contamination with manual or semiautomatic pipets, careful wiping of the tip may remove any liquid that adhered to the outside of the tip before dispensing any liquid. Care should be taken to ensure that the orifice of the pipet tip is not blotted, drawing sample from the tip. Another precaution in using manually operated semiautomatic pipets is to move the plunger in a continuous, slow manner.

Disposable, one-use, pipet tips are designed for use with air-displacement pipets. The laboratory scientist should ensure that the pipet tip is seated snugly on the end

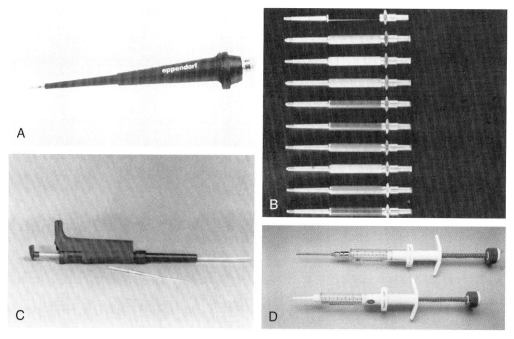

FIGURE 1-6. (**A**) Fixed-volume, ultramicrodigital, air-displacement pipetter with tip ejector. (**B**) Fixed-volume air-displacement pipet. (**C**) Digital electronic positive-displacement pipetter. (**D**) Syringe pipetter.

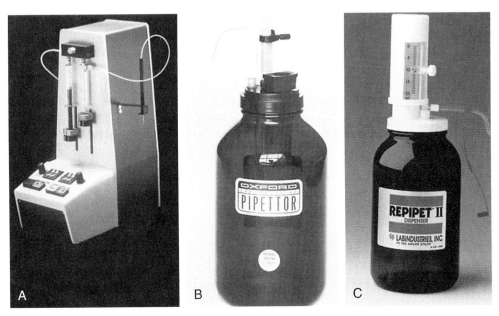

FIGURE 1-7. (**A**) Digital dilutor/dispenser. (**B**) Dispenser. (**C**) Dispenser.

of the pipet and free from any deformity. Plastic tips used on air-displacement pipets are particularly likely to vary. Different brands can be used for one particular pipet but they do not necessarily perform in an identical manner. Plastic burrs may be present that cannot always be detected by the naked eye. A method using a 0.1%-solution of phenol red in distilled water has been used to compare the reproducibility of different brands of pipet tips.[23] When using this method, the pipet and the operator should remain the same so that variation is only a result of changes in the pipet tips. Tips for positive-displacement pipets are made of straight columns of glass or plastic. These tips must fit snugly to avoid carry-over and can be used repeatedly without being changed after each use. As previously mentioned, these devices may need to be rinsed and dried between samples to minimize carryover.

Class A pipets, like all other Class A glassware, do not need to be recalibrated by the laboratory. Automatic pipetting devices, as well as non–Class A materials, do need recalibration. A gravimetric method (see page 15) can accomplish this task by delivering and weighing a solution of known specific gravity, such as water. A currently calibrated analytic balance and at least Class 2 weights should be used. A pipet should only be used if it is within ±1.0% of the expected value.

Although gravimetric validation is the most desirable method, pipet calibration may also be accomplished by using photometric methods, particularly for automatic pipetting devices. When a spectrophotometer is used, the molar extinction coefficient of a compound, such as potassium dichromate, is obtained. After an aliquot of diluent is pipetted, the change in concentration will reflect the volume of the pipet. Another photometric technique used to assess pipet accuracy compares the absorbances of dilutions of potassium dichromate, or another colored liquid with appropriate absorbance spectra, using Class A volumetric glassware versus equivalent dilutions made with the pipetting device.

These calibration techniques are time-consuming and, therefore, impractical for use in daily checks. It is recommended that pipets be checked initially and subsequently three to four times per year, or as dictated by the laboratory's accrediting agency. Many companies offer calibration services; the one chosen should also satisfy any accreditation requirements. A quick, daily check for many larger volume automatic pipetting devices uses volumetric flasks. For example, a bottle-top dispenser that routinely delivers 2.5 mL of reagent may be checked by dispensing four aliquots of the reagent into a 10-mL Class A volumetric flask. The bottom of the meniscus should meet with the calibration line on the volumetric flask.

Burets

A *buret* looks like a wide, long, graduated pipet with a stopcock at one end. A buret's usual total volume ranges from 25 mL to 100 mL of solution and is used to dispense a particular volume of liquid during a titration (Fig. 1-8).

Syringes

Syringes are sometimes used for transfer of small volumes (less than 500 μL) in blood gas analysis or in separation techniques such as chromatography or electrophoresis. The syringes are glass and have fine barrels. The plunger is often made of a fine piece of wire. Tips are

GRAVIMETRIC PIPET CALIBRATION[21,24]

Materials

Pipet.
10–20 pipet tips, if needed.
Balance capable of accuracy and resolution to ±0.1% of dispensed volumetric weight.
Weighing vessel large enough to hold volume of liquid.
Type I water.
Thermometer and barometer.

Procedure

1. Record the weight of the vessel. Record the temperature of the water. It is recommended that all materials be at room temperature. Obtain the barometric pressure.
2. Place a small volume (0.5 mL) of the water into the container. To prevent effects from evaporation, loosely covering each container using a substance such as Parafilm is desirable. Avoid handling of the containers.
3. Weigh each container plus water to the nearest 0.1 mg *or* set the balance to zero.
4. Using the pipet to be tested, draw up the specified amount. Carefully wipe the outside of tip. Care should be taken not to touch the end of the tip. This will cause liquid to be wicked out of the tip, introducing an inaccuracy as a result of technique.
5. Dispense the water into the weighed vessel. Touch the tip to the side.
6. Record the weight of the vessel.
7. Subtract the weight obtained in step 3 from that obtained in step 6. Record the result.
8. If plastic tips are used, change the tip between each dispensing. Repeat steps 1 to 6 for a minimum of nine additional times.
9. Obtain the average or mean of the weight of the water. Multiply the mean weight by the corresponding density of water at the given temperature and pressure. This may be obtained from the *Handbook of Chemistry and Physics*[24a] or in Table 1-3[6] for a quick reference.
10. Determine the accuracy or the ability of the pipet to dispense the expected (selected or stated) volume according to the following formula:

$$\frac{\text{Mean volume}}{\text{Expected volume}} \times 100\% \qquad \text{(Eq. 1–9)}$$

The manufacturer usually gives acceptable limitations for a particular pipet, but they should not be used if the value differs by more than 1.0% from the expected value.

Precision can be indicated as the percent coefficient of variation (%CV) or standard deviation (SD) for a series of repetitive pipetting steps. A discussion of %CV and SD can be found in Chapter 3, *Quality Control and Statistics*. The equations to calculate the SD and %CV are as follows:

$$SD = \sqrt{\frac{\Sigma(x - \bar{x})^2}{n - 1}}$$

$$\%CV = \frac{SD}{\bar{x}} \times 100 \qquad \text{(Eq. 1–10)}$$

Required imprecision is usually ±1 SD. The %CV will vary with the expected volume of the pipet, but the smaller the %CV value, the greater is the precision. When *n* is large, the data are more statistically valid.

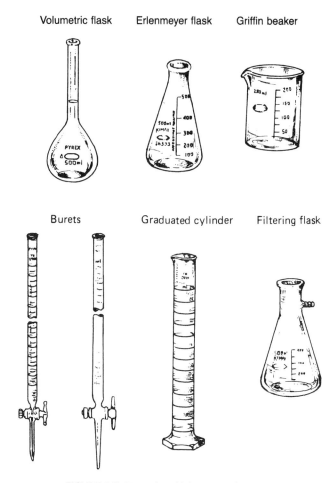

FIGURE 1-8. Examples of laboratory glassware.

not used when syringes are used for injection of sample into a gas chromatographic system. In electrophoresis work, however, disposable Teflon tips may be used. Expected inaccuracies of volumes less than 5 μL is 2%, whereas for greater volumes, the inaccuracy is approximately 1%.

Desiccators and Desiccants

Many compounds combine with water molecules to form loose chemical crystals. The compound and the associated water are called a *hydrate.* When the water of crystallization is removed from the compound, it is said to be *anhydrous.* Substances that take up water on exposure to atmospheric conditions are called *hygroscopic.* Materials that are very hygroscopic can remove moisture from the air as well as from other materials. These materials make excellent drying substances and are sometimes used as *desiccants* (drying agents) to keep other chemicals from becoming hydrated. Commonly used desiccants are listed in Table 1-6, beginning with the most hygroscopic and ending with the least effective drying agent. If these

TABLE 1-6. COMMON DESICCANTS

AGENT	FORMULA
Magnesium perchlorate (Dehydrite)	$Mg(ClO_4)$
Barium oxide	BaO
Alumina	Al_2O_3
Phosphorus pentoxide	P_4O_{10}
Lithium perchlorate	$LiClO_4$
Calcium chloride	$CaCl_2$
Calcium sulfate (Drierite)	$CaSO_4$
Silica gel	SiO_2
Ascarite	NaOH on asbestos

compounds absorb enough water from the atmosphere to cause dissolution, they are called *deliquescent substances*.

Desiccants are most effective when placed in a closed, airtight chamber called a *desiccator* (Fig. 1-9). The desiccant is placed below the perforated platform inside the desiccator. Placing a fine film of lubricant on the rim of the cover seals a glass or plastic desiccator; it is correctly opened or sealed by slowly sliding the lid horizontally. The lubricated seal prevents the desiccator from being opened with a direct upward pull. The desiccator should be opened slowly and with caution because the air pressure inside the desiccator could be below atmospheric pressure. Desiccants containing indicators that signify desiccant exhaustion and that can be regenerated using heat or dried in a microwave oven are particularly helpful. Desiccants that produce dust should also be avoided. In the laboratory, desiccants are primarily used to prevent moisture absorption by chemicals, gases, and instrument components.

Balances

A properly operating balance is essential in producing high-quality reagents and standards. However, because many laboratories discontinued in-house reagent preparation, balances may no longer be as widely used. Balances are classified according to their design, number of pans (single or double), and whether they are mechanical or electronic or classified by operating ranges, as determined by precision balances (readability ~2 µg), analytic balances (readability ~0.001 g), or microbalances (readability ~0.1 µg; Fig. 1-10).

Analytic and electronic balances are currently the most popular in the clinical laboratory. Analytic balances are required for the preparation of any primary standards. The mechanical analytic balance is also known as a *substitution balance*. It has a single pan enclosed by sliding transparent doors, which minimize environmental influences on pan movement. The pan is attached to a series of calibrated weights that are counterbalanced by a single weight at the opposite end of a knife-edge fulcrum. The operator adjusts the balance to the desired mass and places the material, contained within a tared weighing vessel, on the sample pan. An optical scale allows the operator to visualize the mass of the substance. The weight range for certain analytic balances is from 0.01 mg to 160 g.

Electronic balances are single-pan balances that use an electromagnetic force to counterbalance the weighed sample's mass. Their measurements equal the accuracy and precision of any available mechanical balance, with the advantage of a fast response time (less than 10 seconds).

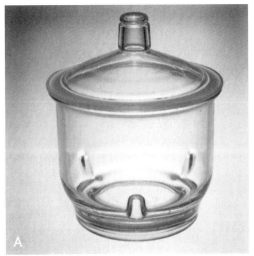 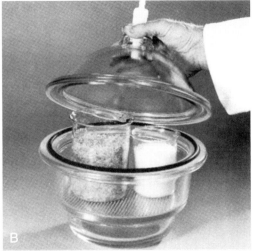

FIGURE 1-9. (**A**) Glass desiccator. (**B**) Glass desiccator with dry seal ring (no grease is necessary to seal cover to body).

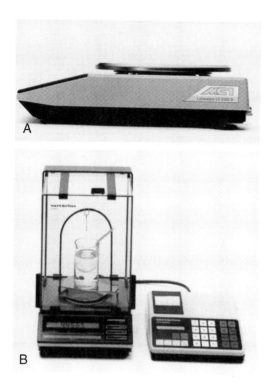

FIGURE 1-10. (**A**) Electronic top-loading balance. (**B**) Electronic analytic balance with printer.

Test weights used for calibrating balances should be selected from the appropriate ANSI/ASTM classes 1 through 4.[25] This system has replaced the former NIST Class S standards used prior to 1993. Class 1 weights provide the greatest precision and should be used for calibrating high-precision analytic balances in the weight range of 0.01 mg to 0.1 mg. Former NBS S standard weights are equivalent to ASTM Class 2 (0.001–0.01 g), and S-1 is equivalent to ASTM Class 3 (0.01–0.1 g). The frequency of calibration is dictated by the accreditation/licensing guidelines for a specific laboratory. Balances should be kept scrupulously clean and be located in an area away from heavy traffic, large pieces of electrical equipment, and open windows. A slab of marble separated from its supporting surface by a flexible material is sometimes placed under a balance to minimize any vibration interference that may occur. The level checkpoint should always be corrected before weighing occurs.

BASIC SEPARATION TECHNIQUES

Contemporary modifications of filtration and dialysis employ matrix-based fibrous material that provides a mechanism of separation in many homogenous immunoassays. These materials may be coated with specific antibody-ligand to foster selection of specific materials or species. Certain labels employ magnetic particles used in conjunction with strong magnets to effect separation. Further discussion of separation mechanisms used in immunoassays may be found in Chapter 6, *Immunoassays and Nucleic Acid Probe Techniques*. Basic universally employed separation mechanisms outside of those incorporated in immunoassay, are centrifugation, filtration, and dialysis.

Centrifugation

Centrifugation is a process in which centrifugal force is used to separate solid matter from a liquid suspension. The *centrifuge* carries out this action. It consists of a head or rotor, carriers, or shields (Fig. 1-11) that are attached to the vertical shaft of a motor and enclosed in a metal covering. The centrifuge always has a lid and an on/off switch; however, many models include a brake or a built-in tachometer, which indicates speed, and some centrifuges are refrigerated. Centrifugal force depends on

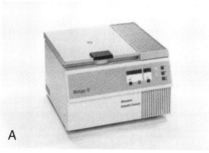

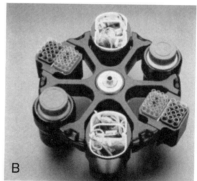

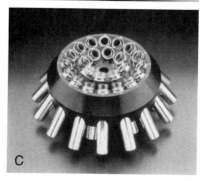

FIGURE 1-11. (**A**) Benchtop centrifuge. (**B**) Swinging-bucket rotor. (**C**) Fixed-head rotor.

three variables: mass, speed, and radius. The speed is expressed in revolutions per minute (rpm), and the centrifugal force generated is expressed in terms of relative centrifugal force (RCF) or gravities (g). The speed of the centrifuge is related to the RCF by the following equation:

$$RCF = 1.118 \times 10^{-5} \times r \times (rpm)^2 \quad \text{(Eq. 1–11)}$$

where 1.118×10^{-5} is a constant, determined from the angular velocity, and r is the radius in centimeters, measured from the center of the centrifuge axis to the bottom of the test-tube shield. The RCF value also may be obtained from a nomogram similar to that found in Appendix H, *Relative Centrifugal Force Nomogram*. Centrifuge classification is based on several criteria, including benchtop or floor model, refrigeration, rotor head (*eg*, fixed, hematocrit, swinging-bucket, or angled; Fig. 1-11), or maximum speed attainable (*ie*, ultracentrifuge). Centrifuges are generally used to separate serum from a blood clot as the blood is being processed; to separate a supernatant from a precipitate during an analytic reaction; to separate two immiscible liquids, such as lipid laden serum; or to expel air.

Centrifuge care includes daily cleaning of any spills or debris, such as blood or glass, and ensuring that the centrifuge is properly balanced (Fig. 1-12) and free from any excessive vibrations. Balancing the centrifuge load is critical. Many newer centrifuges will automatically decrease their speed if the load is not evenly distributed, but more often, the centrifuge will shake and vibrate or make more noise than expected. The centrifuge cover should remain closed until the centrifuge has come to a complete stop to avoid any aerosol contamination. It is recommended that the timer, brushes (if present), and speed be periodically checked. The brushes, which are graphite bars attached to a retainer spring, create an electrical contact in the motor. The specific manufacturer's service manual should be consulted for details on how to change brushes and on lubrication requirements. The speed of a centrifuge is easily checked using a tachometer or strobe light. The hole located in the lid of many centrifuges is designed for speed verification using these devices but may also represent an aerosol biohazard.

Filtration

Filtration can be used instead of centrifugation for the separation of solids from liquids. However, paper filtration is only occasionally used in today's laboratory and, therefore, only the basics are discussed here. Filter material is made of paper, cellulose and its derivatives, polyester fibers, glass, and a variety of resin column materials. Traditionally, filter paper was folded in a manner that allowed it to fit into a funnel. In method A, round filter paper is folded like a fan (Fig. 1-13A); in method B, the paper is folded into fourths (Fig. 1-13B).

Filter paper differs in pore size and should be selected according to separation needs and associated flow rate for given liquids. Filter paper should not be used when using strong acids or bases. When the filter paper is placed inside the funnel, the solution slowly drains through the filter paper within the funnel and into a receiving vessel. The liquid that passes through the filter paper is called the *filtrate*.

Dialysis

Dialysis is another method for separating macromolecules from a solvent or smaller sized substances. It became popular when used in conjunction with the Tech-

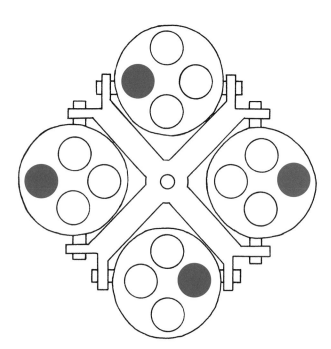

FIGURE 1-12. Properly balanced centrifuge. *Colored circles* represent counterbalanced positions for sample tubes.

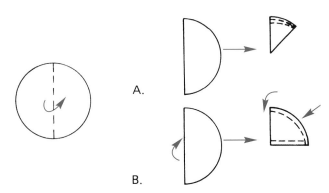

FIGURE 1-13. Methods of folding a filter paper. (**A**) In a fan. (**B**) In fourths.

nicon Autoanalyzer system in the 1970s. Basically, a solution is put into a bag or is contained on one side of a semipermeable membrane. Larger molecules are retained within the sack or on one side of the membrane, while smaller molecules and solvents diffuse out. This process is very slow. Use of columns that contain a gel material have replaced manual dialysis separation in most analytic procedures.

LABORATORY MATHEMATICS AND CALCULATIONS

Significant Figures

Significant figures are the minimum number of digits needed to express a particular value in scientific notation without loss of accuracy. The number 814.2 has four significant figures because in scientific notation it is written as 8.142×10^2. The number 0.000641 has three significant figures, and the scientific notation expression for this value is 6.41×10^{-4}. The zeros are merely holding decimal places and are not needed to express the number in scientific notation.

Logarithms

The base 10 *logarithm* (log) of a positive number N greater than zero is equal to the exponent to which 10 must be raised to produce N. Therefore, it can be stated that N equals 10^x, and the log of N is equal to x. The number N is the antilogarithm (antilog) of x.

The logarithm of a number, which is written in *decimal* format, consists of two parts: the character, or characteristic, and the mantissa. The *character* is the number to the left of the decimal point in the log and is derived from the exponent, and the *mantissa* is that portion of the logarithm to the right of the decimal point and is derived from the number itself. Although several approaches can be taken to determine the log, one approach is to write the number in scientific notation. The number 1424 expressed in scientific notation is 1.424×10^3, making the character a 3. The character can also be determined by adding the number of significant figures and then subtracting 1 from the sum. The mantissa is derived from a log table or calculator having a log function for the remainder of the number. For 1.424, a calculator would give a mantissa of 0.1535, and a log table would reveal what is shown in Table 1-7. Certain calcu-

lators with a log function do not require conversion to scientific notation.

When using a log table, the initial step is to determine N. N is obtained from the first two digits in the number. In this example, N is 14. Locate the number 14 under the N column in the log tables (Table 1-7). The next digit in this example, 1.424, is 2. Continue along the row and read the numbers under 142, which, in this case, are 1523. The last part of the mantissa is obtained from the proportional parts section of the log table and is added to 1523. In this instance (1.424), the remaining digit is 4. The value under 4 in the table is 12. The mantissa becomes $1523 + 12 = 1535$. The logarithm of 1.425×10^3 equals 3.1535. The character is 3, and the mantissa is 1535. Because there are only four significant figures in the original number, only four significant figures should be written in the log. The log now becomes 3.154. For numbers less than 1, the character usually has a bar over the top. The number 2.12×10^{-2} has a log of $\bar{2}.3263$, or $\bar{2}.33$ to satisfy the number of significant figures.

To determine the original number from a log value, the process is done in reverse. This process is termed the *antilogarithm*. Using the previous example, determine the antilogarithm of $\bar{2}.33$. The character $\bar{2}$, which has a bar over the top of it, indicates 10^{-2}. The mantissa, 0.3263, or 0.33, may lead to the number in two ways. The mantissa may be located in a logarithm table, and may determine N. A second approach is to use an antilogarithm table. Table 1-8 illustrates both methods. The rounding of numbers does affect the antilogarithm. Most calculators have logarithm and antilogarithm functions. Consult the specific manufacturer's directions to become acquainted with the proper use of these functions.

Negative or Inverse Logarithms

The character of a log may be positive or negative, but the mantissa is always positive. In certain circumstances, the laboratorian must deal with inverse or negative logs. Such is the case with pH or pK_a. As previously stated, the pH of a solution is defined as minus the log of the hydrogen ion concentration. The following is a convenient formula to determine the negative logarithm when working with pH or pK_a:

$$pH/pK_a = x - \log N \qquad \text{(Eq. 1–12)}$$

where x = negative exponent base ten expressed without the minus sign and N = decimal portion of the scientific notations expression.

TABLE 1-7. PORTION OF A LOGARITHM TABLE

Proportional Parts

N	0	1	2	3	4	5	6	7	8	9	1	2	3	4	5	6	7	8	9
14	1461	1492	1523	1553	1584	1614	1644	1673	1703	1732	3	6	9	12	15	18	21	24	27

TABLE 1-8. ANTILOGARITHM DETERMINATION

A. Log Table

N	0	1	2	3
21	3222	3243	<u>3263</u>	3284

The number, as determined from the mantissa 3263, is 212.

B. Antilog Table

N	0	1	2	3	4	5	6	7	8	9	Proportional Parts 123456789
.32	2089	2094	2099	2104	2109	2113	<u>2118</u>	2123	2128	2133	011223344
.33	<u>2138</u>	2143									

.3263 = 2118 + 1 = 2119 = 2.12.
.33 = 2138 = 2.14.

For example, if the hydrogen ion concentration of a solution is 5.4×10^{-6}, then $x = 6$ and $N = 5.4$. Substitute this information into Eq. 1-12, and it becomes:

$$\text{pH} = 6 - \log 5.4 \qquad \text{(Eq. 1–13)}$$

The logarithm of N (5.4) is equal to 0.7324, or 0.73. The pH becomes

$$\text{pH} = 6 - 0.73 = 5.27 \qquad \text{(Eq. 1–14)}$$

The same formula can be applied to obtain the hydrogen ion concentration of a solution when only the pH is given. Using a pH of 5.27, the equation becomes

$$5.27 = x - \log N \qquad \text{(Eq. 1–15)}$$

In this instance, the x term is always the next largest whole number. For this example, the next largest whole number is 6. Substituting for x, the equation becomes

$$5.27 = 6 - \log N \qquad \text{(Eq. 1–16)}$$

Multiply all the variables by –1:

$$(-1)(5.27) = (-1)(6) - (-1)(\log N).$$
$$-5.27 = -6 + \log N \qquad \text{(Eq. 1–17)}$$

Solve the equation for the unknown quantity by adding a positive 6 to both sides of the equal sign and the equation becomes:

$$6 - 5.27 = \log N \qquad \text{(Eq. 1–18)}$$
$$0.73 = \log N$$

The result is 0.73, which is the antilogarithm value of N, which is 5.37, or 5.4.

$$\text{Antilog } 0.73 = N; N = 5.37 = 5.4 \quad \text{(Eq. 1–19)}$$

The hydrogen ion concentration for a solution with a pH of 5.27 is 5.4×10^{-6}. Many scientific calculators have an inverse function that allows for more direct calculation of inverse or negative logarithms. It is important, however, to fully understand the proper use of the many calculator functions available, keeping in mind that the specific steps vary between manufacturers.

Concentration

A detailed description of each concentration term (eg, molarity, normality) may be found at the beginning of this chapter. The following discussion focuses on the basic mathematical expressions needed to prepare reagents of a stated concentration.

Percent Solution

A percent solution is determined in the same manner regardless of whether weight/weight, volume/volume, or weight/volume units are used. *Percent* implies "parts per 100," which is represented as percent (%) and is independent of the molecular weight of a substance.

Example 1-1: Weight/Weight (w/w)

To make up 100 g of a 5% aqueous solution of hydrochloric acid (using 12 M HCl), multiply the total amount by the percent expressed as a decimal. The calculation becomes

$$5\% = \frac{5}{100} = 0.050 \qquad \text{(Eq. 1–20)}$$

Therefore,

$$0.050 \times 100 = (5 \text{ g of HCl}) \qquad \text{(Eq. 1–21)}$$

Another way of arriving at the answer is to set up a ratio so that

$$\frac{5}{100} = \frac{x}{100}$$
$$x = 5 \qquad \text{(Eq. 1–22)}$$

Example 1-2: Weight/Volume (w/v)

The most frequently used term for a percent solution is weight per volume, which is often expressed as grams per 100 mL of diluent. To make up 1000 mL of a 10% (w/v) solution of NaOH, use the preceding approach. The calculations become

$$\underset{(\% \text{ expressed as a decimal})}{0.10} \quad \times \quad \underset{(\text{total amount})}{1000} \quad = 100 \text{ g}$$

or

$$\frac{10}{100} = \frac{x}{1000}$$

$$x = 100 \qquad \text{(Eq. 1–23)}$$

Therefore, add 100 g of NaOH to a 1000 mL volumetric Class A flask and dilute to the calibration mark with Type II water.

Example 1-3: Volume/Volume (v/v)

Make up 50 mL of a 2% (v/v) concentrated hydrochloric acid solution.

$$0.02 \times 50 = 1 \text{ mL}$$

or

$$\frac{2}{100} = \frac{x}{50}$$

$$x = 1 \qquad \text{(Eq. 1–24)}$$

Therefore, add 40 mL of water to a 50-mL Class A volumetric flask, add 1 mL of HCl, mix, and dilute up to the calibration mark with Type II water. Remember, always add acid to water!

Molarity

Molarity (*M*) is routinely expressed in units of moles per liter (mol/L) or sometimes millimoles per milliliter (mmol/mL). Remember that 1 mol of a substance is equal to the gram molecular weight (gmw) of that substance. When trying to determine the amount of substance needed to yield a particular concentration, initially decide what final concentration *units* are needed. For molarity, the final units will be moles per liter (mol/L) or millimoles per milliliter (mmol/mL). The second step is to consider the existing units and the relationship they have to the final desired units. Essentially, try to put as many units as possible into "like" terms and arrange so that the same units cancel each other out, leaving only those wanted in the final answer. To accomplish this, it is important to remember what units are used to define each concentration term. It is key to understand the relationship between molarity (moles/liter), moles, and gmw.

Example 1-4

How many *grams* are needed to make 1 *L* of a 2 *M* solution of HCl?

Step 1: Which units are needed in the final answer? *Answer:* Grams per liter (g/L).
Step 2: Assess other mass/volume terms used in the problem. In this case, moles are also needed for the calculation: How many grams are equal to 1 mole? The gmw of HCl, which can be determined from the periodic table, will be equal to 1 mole. For HCl, the gmw is 36.5, so the equation may be written as

$$\frac{36.5 \text{ g HCL}}{\text{mol}} \times \frac{2 \text{ mol}}{L} = \frac{73 \text{ g HCl}}{L} \qquad \text{(Eq. 1–25)}$$

Cancel out like units, and the final units should be grams per liter. In this example, 73 g HCl per liter is needed to make up a 2 *M* solution of HCl.

Example 1-5

A solution of NaOH is contained within a Class A 1-L volumetric flask filled to the calibration mark. The content label reads 24 g of NaOH. Determine the molarity.

Step 1: What *units* are ultimately needed? *Answer:* Moles per liter (mol/L).
Step 2: The units that exist are grams and 1 L. NaOH may be expressed as moles and grams. The gmw of NaOH is calculated to equal 40 g/mol. Rearrange the equation so that grams can be canceled and the remaining units reflect those needed in the answer.
Step 3: The equation becomes

$$\frac{24 \text{ g NaOH}}{L} \times \frac{1 \text{ mol}}{40 \text{ g NaOH}} = 0.6 \frac{\text{mol}}{L} \qquad \text{(Eq. 1–26)}$$

By canceling out like units and performing the appropriate calculations, the final answer of 0.6 *M* or 0.6 mol/L is derived.

Example 1-6

Make up 250 mL of a 4.8 *M* solution of HCl.
Step 1: *Units* needed? *Answer:* Grams (g).
Step 2: Determine the gmw of HCl (36.5 g), which is needed to calculate the molarity.
Step 3: Set up the equation, cancel out like units, and perform the appropriate calculations:

$$\frac{36.5 \text{ g HCL}}{\text{mol}} \times \frac{4.8 \text{ mol HCL}}{L} \times \frac{250 \text{ mL} \times 1 \text{ L}}{1000 \text{ mL}} = 43.8 \text{ g HCl}$$

$$\text{(Eq. 1–27)}$$

In a 250-mL volumetric flask, add 200 mL of Type II water. Add 43.8 g of HCl and mix. Dilute up to the calibration mark with Type II water.

Although there are various methods to calculate laboratory mathematical problems, this technique of canceling like units can be used in most clinical chemistry situations, regardless of whether the problem requests molarity, normality, or exchanging one concentration term for another. However, it is necessary to recall the interrelationship between all the units in the expression.

Normality

Normality (*N*) is expressed as the number of equivalent weights per liter (Eq/L) or milliequivalents per milliliter (mEq/mL). Equivalent weight is equal to gmw divided by the valence (*V*). Normality has often been used in acid-base calculations because an equivalent weight of a substance is also equal to its combining weight. Another advantage in using equivalent weight is that an equivalent weight of one substance is equal to the equivalent weight of any other chemical.

Example 1-7

Give the equivalent weight, in grams, for each substance listed below.
1. NaCl (gmw = 58 g, valence = 1)

$$58/1 = 58 \text{ g per equivalent weight} \qquad \text{(Eq. 1–28)}$$

2. HCl (gmw = 36, valence = 1)

$$36/1 = 36 \text{ g per equivalent weight} \qquad \textbf{(Eq. 1–29)}$$

3. H_2SO_4 (gmw = 98, valence = 2)

$$98/2 = 49 \text{ g per equivalent weight} \qquad \textbf{(Eq. 1–30)}$$

A. What is the normality of a 500-mL solution that contains 7 g of H_2SO_4? The approach used to calculate molarity could be used to solve this problem as well.

Step 1: Units needed? *Answer:* Normality expressed as equivalents per liter (Eq/L).

Step 2: Units you have? *Answer:* Milliliters and grams. Now determine how they are related to equivalents per liter. (Hint: There are 49 g per equivalent—see Equation 1-30 above.)

Step 3: Rearrange the equation so that like terms cancel leaving Eq/L. This equation is

$$\frac{7 \text{ g } H_2SO_4}{500 \text{ mL}} \times \frac{1 \text{ Eq}}{49 \text{ g } H_2SO_4} \times \frac{1000 \text{ mL}}{1 \text{ L}}$$

$$= 0.285 \text{ Eq/L} = 0.285 \text{ N} \qquad \textbf{(Eq. 1–31)}$$

Because 500 mL is equal to 0.5 L, the final equation could be written by substituting 0.5 L for 500 mL, eliminating the need to include the 1000 mL/L conversion factor in the equation.

B. What is the normality of a 0.5 M solution of H_2SO_4? Continuing with the previous approach, the final equation is

$$\frac{0.5 \text{ mol } H_2SO_4}{L} \times \frac{98 \text{ g } H_2SO_4}{\text{mol } H_2SO_4} \times \frac{1 \text{ Eq } H_2SO_4}{49 \text{ g } H_2SO_4}$$

$$= 1 \text{ Eq/L} = 1 \text{ N} \qquad \textbf{(Eq. 1–32)}$$

When changing molarity into normality or vice versa, the following conversion formula may be applied:

$$M \times V = N \qquad \textbf{(Eq. 1–33)}$$

where V is the valence of the compound. Using this formula, Example 1-7.3 becomes

$$0.5 \ M \times 2 = 1 \ N \qquad \textbf{(Eq. 1–34)}$$

Example 1-8

What is the molarity of a 2.5 N solution of HCl? This problem may be solved in several ways. One way is to use the stepwise approach in which existing units are exchanged for units needed. The equation is

$$\frac{2.5 \text{ Eq HCl}}{L} \times \frac{36 \text{ g HCl}}{1 \text{ Eq}} \times \frac{1 \text{ mol HCl}}{36 \text{ g HCl}}$$

$$= 2.5 \text{ mol/L HCl} \qquad \textbf{(Eq. 1–35)}$$

The second approach is to use the normality to molarity conversion formula. The equation now becomes

$$M \times V = 2.5 \ N$$
$$V = 1$$
$$M = \frac{2.5 \ N}{1} = 2.5 \ N \qquad \textbf{(Eq. 1–36)}$$

When the valence of a substance is 1, the molarity will equal the normality. As previously mentioned, normality either equals or is greater than the molarity.

Specific Gravity

Density is expressed as mass per unit volume. The specific gravity is the ratio of the density of a material when compared to the density of water at a given temperature. The units for specific gravity are grams per milliliter. Specific gravity is often used with very concentrated materials, such as commercial acids (*eg,* sulfuric and hydrochloric acids).

The density of a concentrated acid can also be expressed in terms of an assay or percent purity. The actual concentration is equal to the *specific gravity* multiplied by the *assay* or *percent purity value* (expressed as a decimal) stated on the label of the container.

Example 1-9

A. What is the actual weight of a supply of concentrated HCl whose label reads specific gravity 1.19 with an assay value of 37%?

$$1.19 \text{ g/mL} \times 0.37 = 0.44 \text{ g/mL of HCl} \qquad \textbf{(Eq. 1–37)}$$

B. What is the molarity of this stock solution? The final units desired are moles per liter (mol/L). The molarity of the solution is

$$\frac{0.44 \text{ g HCl}}{\text{mL}} \times \frac{1 \text{ mol HCl}}{3.5 \text{ g HCl}} \times \frac{1000 \text{ mL}}{L}$$

$$= 12.05 \text{ mol/L or } 12 \ M \qquad \textbf{(Eq. 1–38)}$$

Conversions

To convert one unit into another, the same approach of crossing out like units can be applied. In some instances, a chemistry laboratory may report a given analyte using two different concentration units; for example, calcium. The recommended SI unit for calcium is millimoles per liter. The better known and more traditional units are milligrams per deciliter (mg/dL). Again, it is important to understand the relationship between the units given and those needed in the final answer.

Example 1-10

Convert 8.2 mg/dL calcium to millimoles per liter (mmol/L). The gmw of calcium is 40 g. So, if there are 40 g per mol, then it follows that there are 40 mg per mmol. The units wanted are mmol/L. The equation becomes

$$\frac{8.2 \text{ mg}}{\text{dL}} \times \frac{1 \text{ dL}}{100 \text{ mL}} \times \frac{1000 \text{ mL}}{L} \times \frac{1 \text{ mmol}}{40 \text{ mg}} = \frac{2.05 \text{ mmol}}{L}$$

$$\textbf{(Eq. 1–39)}$$

Once again, the systematic stepwise approach of deleting similar units can be used for this conversion problem.

A frequently encountered conversion problem, or more precisely, a dilution problem occurs when a weaker concentration or different volume is needed than the stock substance available, but the concentration *terms* are the same. The following formula is used:

$$V_1 \times C_1 = V_2 \times C_2 \qquad \textbf{(Eq. 1–40)}$$

This formula is useful only if the concentration and volume units between the substances are the *same* and if three of four variables are known.

Example 1-11

What volume is needed to make 500 mL of a 0.1 *M* solution of tris buffer from a solution of 2 *M* tris buffer?

$$V_1 \times 2\ M = 0.1\ M \times 500\ \text{mL}$$

$$(V_1)(2\ M) = (0.1)(500) = (V_1)(2) = 50 = V_1 = 50/2 = 25$$

(Eq. 1–41)

It requires 25 mL of the 2 *M* solution to make up 500 mL of a 0.1 *M* solution. This problem differs from the other conversions in that it is actually a dilution of a stock solution. A more involved discussion of dilutions follows.

Dilutions

A *dilution* represents the ratio of concentrated or stock material to the total final volume of a solution and consists of the volume or weight of the concentrate plus the volume of the diluent, with the concentration units remaining the same. This ratio of concentrated or stock solution to the total solution volume equals the *dilution factor*. Because a dilution is made by adding a more concentrated substance to a diluent, the dilution is always less concentrated than the original substance. The relationship of the dilution factor to concentration is an inverse one; thus, the dilution factor increases as the concentration decreases. To determine the dilution factor required, simply take the amount needed and divide by the stock concentration, leaving it in a reduced-fraction form.

Example 1-12

What is the dilution factor needed to make a 100 mEq/L sodium solution from a 3000 mEq/L stock solution? The dilution factor becomes

$$\frac{1\cancel{00}}{3\cancel{000}} = \frac{1}{30}$$

(Eq. 1–42)

The dilution factor indicates that the ratio of stock material is 1 part stock made to a *total volume* of 30. To actually make this dilution, 1 mL of stock is added to 29 mL of diluent. Note that the dilution factor indicates the parts per total amount; however, in making the dilution, the sum of the amount of the stock material plus the amount of the diluent must equal the total volume or dilution fraction denominator. The dilution factor may be written as a fraction ($^1/_{30}$) or can be expressed using a colon (1:30). Either format is correct. To avoid confusion, distinction needs to be made between expressions relating to the dilution factor/dilution and those referring to the terms used to make dilutions or the *ratio* of parts versus the *dilution*. A suggested convention[26] when directing the making of a dilution is that a slash (/) used in a fraction refers to a part "in" total volume and represents the dilution. A colon (:) represents the ratio or the parts of the dilution, or the term *to*. For example, a 1:2 or $^1/_2$ dilution of serum has a ratio of one part serum to one part diluent. However, dilute a sample 1:2 would represent one part sample to two parts diluent and a dilution factor of 1:3 or $^1/_3$. It is important in procedures that you fully understand the meaning of these expressions. Sample dilutions should be made using either Type I or II water, saline, or method specific diluent using Class A glassware. The sample and diluent should be thoroughly mixed before use. It is not recommended that sample dilutions be made in smaller volume sample cups or holders. Any total volume can be used as long as the fraction reduces to give the dilution factor.

Example 1-13

If in the preceding example 150 mL of the 100 mEq/L sodium solution was required, the dilution ratio of stock to total volume must be maintained. Set up a ratio between the desired total volume and the dilution factor to determine the amount of stock needed. The equation becomes

$$\frac{1}{30} = \frac{x}{150}$$

$$x = 5$$

(Eq. 1–43)

Note that $^5/_{150}$ reduces to the dilution factor of $^1/_{30}$. To make up this solution, 5 mL of stock is added to 145 mL of the appropriate diluent, making the ratio of *stock volume* to *diluent volume* equal to $^5/_{145}$. Recall that the dilution factor includes the total volume of *both* stock plus diluent.

Simple Dilutions

When making a *simple dilution*, the laboratory scientist must decide on the total volume desired and the amount of stock to be used.

Example 1-14

A 1:10 ($^1/_{10}$) dilution of serum can be achieved by using any of the following approaches. A ratio of 1:9—one part serum and nine parts diluent (saline):

A. 100 μL of serum added to 900 μL of saline.
B. 20 μL of serum added to 180 μL of saline.
C. 1 mL of serum added to 9 mL of saline.
D. 2 mL of serum added to 18 mL of saline.

Note that the ratio of serum to diluent (1:9) needed to make up each dilution satisfies the dilution factor (1:10 or $^1/_{10}$) of stock material to total volume.

The dilution factor is also used to determine the final concentration of a dilution by multiplying the original concentration by the inverse of the dilution factor or the dilution factor denominator when it is expressed as a fraction.

Example 1-15

Determine the concentration of a 200 μmol/mL human chorionic gonadotropin (hCG) standard that was diluted $^1/_{50}$. This value is obtained by multiplying the original concentration, 200 μmol/mL hCG, by the dilution factor, $^1/_{50}$. The result is 4 μmol/mL hCG. Quite often, the concentration of the original material is needed.

Example 1-16

A 1:2 dilution of serum with saline had a creatinine result of 8.6 mg/dL. Calculate the actual serum creatinine concentration.

Dilution factor: $\frac{1}{2}$
Dilution result = 8.6 mg/dL

Because this result represents $\frac{1}{2}$ of the concentration, the actual serum creatinine value is

$$2 \times 8.6 = 17.2 \text{ mg/dL} \qquad \textbf{(Eq. 1–44)}$$

Note: When determining the original stock or undiluted concentration from the dilution, divide by the dilution factor denominator.

Serial Dilutions

A *serial dilution* may be defined as multiple progressive dilutions ranging from more concentrated solutions to less concentrated solutions. Serial dilutions are extremely useful when the volume of concentrate or diluent is in short supply and needs to be minimized or a number of dilutions are required, such as in determining a titer. The volume of patient serum available to the laboratory may be small (*eg*, pediatric samples), and a serial dilution may be needed to ensure that sufficient sample is available. The serial dilution is initially made in the same manner as a simple dilution. Subsequent dilutions will then be made from each preceding dilution. When a serial dilution is made, certain criteria may need to be satisfied. The criteria vary with each situation but usually include such considerations as the total volume desired, the amount of diluent or concentrate available, the dilution factor, the final concentration needed, and the support materials required.

Example 1-17

A serum sample is to be diluted 1:2, 1:4, and, finally, 1:8. It is arbitrarily decided that the total volume for each dilution is to be 1 mL. Note that the least common denominator for these dilution factors is 2. Once the first dilution is made ($\frac{1}{2}$), a 1:2 (least common denominator between 2 and 4), dilution of it will yield

$$\frac{1}{2} \times \frac{1}{2} = \frac{1}{4}$$

(initial dilution factor)(next dilution factor)

$$= \text{(final dilution factor)} \qquad \textbf{(Eq. 1–45)}$$

By making a 1:2 dilution of the first dilution, the second dilution factor of 1:4 is satisfied. Making a 1:2 dilution of the 1:4 dilution will result in the next dilution (1:8). To establish the dilution factor needed for subsequent dilutions, it is helpful to solve the following equation for (x):

Stock/preceding concentration $\times$ (x)

$$= \text{final dilution factor needed} \qquad \textbf{(Eq. 1–46)}$$

To make up these dilutions, three test tubes are labeled 1:2, 1:4, and 1:8, respectively. One mL of diluent is added to each test tube. To make the primary dilution of 1:2, 1 mL of serum is added to test tube number 1. The solution is mixed, and 1 mL of the primary dilution is removed and added to test tube number 2. After mixing, this solution contains a 1:4 dilution. Then 1 mL of the 1:4 dilution from test tube number 2 is added to test tube number 3. Mix and the resultant dilution in this test tube is 1:8, satisfying all of the previously established criteria. Refer to Figure 1-14 for an illustration of this serial dilution.

Example 1-18

Another type of serial dilution combines several dilution factors that are not multiples of one another. In our previous example, 1:2, 1:4, and 1:8 dilutions are all related to one another by a factor of 2. Consider the situation when 1:10, 1:20, 1:100, and 1:200 dilution factors are required. There are several approaches to solving this type of dilution problem. One method is to treat the 1:10 and 1:20 dilutions as one serial dilution problem, the 1:20 and 1:100 dilutions as a second serial dilution, and the 1:100 and 1:200 dilutions as the last serial dilution. Another approach is to consider what dilution factor of the concentrate is needed to yield the final dilution. In this example, the initial dilution is 1:10, with subsequent dilutions of 1:20, 1:100, and 1:200. The first dilution may be accomplished by adding 1 mL of stock to 9 mL of diluent. The total volume of solution is 10 mL. Our initial dilution factor has been satisfied. In making the remaining dilutions, 2 mL of diluent is added to each test tube.

Initial/preceding dilution $\times$ (x) = dilution needed
Solve for (x).

Using the dilution factors listed above and solving for (x), the equations become

1:10 $\times$ (x) = 1:20,
  where (x) = 2 (or 1 part stock to 1 part diluent)

1:20 $\times$ (x) = 1:100,
  where (x) = 5 (or 1 part stock to 4 parts diluent)

1:100 $\times$ (x) = 1:200,
  where (x) = 2 (or 1 part stock to 1 part diluent)

$$\textbf{(Eq. 1–47)}$$

In practice, the 1:10 dilution must be diluted by a factor of 2 to obtain a subsequent 1:20 dilution. Because the second tube already contains 2 mL of diluent, 2 mL of the 1:10 dilution should be added (1 part stock to 1 part diluent). In preparing the 1:100 dilution from this, a 1:5 dilution factor of the 1:20 mixture is required (1 part stock to 4 parts diluent). Because this tube already contains 2 mL, the volume of diluent in the

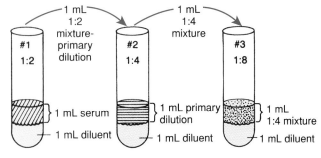

FIGURE 1-14. Serial dilution.

tube is divided by its parts, which is 4; thus, 500 μL, or 0.500 mL, of stock should be added. The 1:200 dilution is prepared in the same manner using a 1:2 dilution factor (1 part stock to 1 part diluent) and adding 2 mL of the 1:100 to the 2 mL of diluent already in the tube.

Water of Hydration

Some compounds are available in a hydrated form. To obtain a correct weight for these chemicals, the attached water molecule(s) must be included.

Example 1-19

How much $CuSO_4 \cdot 5H_2O$ must be weighed to prepare 1 L of 0.5 M $CuSO_4$? When calculating the gmw of this substance, the water weight must be considered so that the gmw is 250 g rather than gmw of $CuSO_4$ alone (160 g). Therefore,

$$\frac{250 \text{ g } CuSO_4 \cdot 5H_2O}{\text{mol}} \times \frac{0.5 \text{ mol}}{1 \text{ L}} = 125 \text{ g/L} \quad \textbf{(Eq. 1–48)}$$

Cancel out like terms to obtain the result of 125 g/L. A reagent protocol often designates the use of an anhydrous form of a chemical; frequently, however, all that is available is a hydrated form.

Example 1-20

A procedure requires 0.9 g of $CuSO_4$. All that is available is $CuSO_4 \cdot 5H_2O$. What weight of $CuSO_4 \cdot 5H_2O$ is needed?

Calculate the percentage of $CuSO_4$ present in $CuSO_4 \cdot 5H_2O$. The percentage is

$$\frac{160}{250} = 0.64, \quad \text{or} \quad 64\% \quad \textbf{(Eq. 1–49)}$$

Therefore, 1 g of $CuSO_4 \cdot 5H_2O$ contains 0.64 g of $CuSO_4$, so the equation becomes:

$$\frac{0.9 \text{ g } CuSO_4 \text{ needed}}{0.64 \text{ } CuSO_4 \text{ in } CuSO_4 \cdot 5H_2O}$$

$$= 1.41 \text{ g } CuSO_4 \cdot 5H_2O \text{ required} \quad \textbf{(Eq. 1–50)}$$

Graphing Beer's Law

The *Beer-Lambert law (Beer's law)* mathematically establishes the relationship between concentration and absorbance in many photometric determinations. Beer's law is expressed as

$$A = abc \quad \textbf{(Eq. 1–51)}$$

where A = absorbance; a = absorptivity constant for a particular compound at a given wavelength under specified conditions of temperature, pH, and so on; b = length of the light path; and c = concentration.

If a method follows Beer's law, then absorbance is proportional to concentration as long as the length of the light path and the absorptivity of the absorbing species remain unaltered during the analysis. In practice, however, there are limits to the predictability of a linear response. Even in automated systems, adherence to Beer's law is often determined by checking the linearity of the

test method over a wide concentration range. The limits of linearity often represent the reportable range of an assay. This term should not be confused with the reference ranges associated with clinical significance of a test. Assays measuring absorbance generally obtain the concentration results by using a Beer's law graph, known as a standard graph or curve. This graph is made by plotting absorbance versus the concentration of known standards (Fig. 1-15). Because most photometric assays set the initial absorbance to zero (0) using a reagent blank, the initial data points are 0,0. Graphs should be labeled properly and the concentration units must be given. The horizontal axis is referred to as the *x*-axis, whereas the vertical line is the *y*-axis. It is not important which variable (absorbance or concentration) is assigned to an individual axis, but it is important that the values assigned to them are uniformly distributed along the axis. By convention, in the clinical laboratory, concentration is usually plotted on the *x*-axis. On a standard graph, only the standard and the associated absorbances are plotted.

Once a standard graph has been established, it is permissible to run just one standard, or calibrator, as long as the system remains the same. *One point calculation* or *calibration* refers to the calculation of the comparison of the known standard/calibrator concentration and its corresponding absorbance to the absorbance of the unknown value according to the following ratio:

$$\frac{\text{Concentration of standard } (Cs)}{\text{Absorbance of standard } (As)}$$

$$= \frac{\text{Concentration of unknown } (Cu)}{\text{Absorbance of unknown } (Au)} \quad \textbf{(Eq. 1–52)}$$

Solving for the concentration of the unknown, the equation becomes:

$$c_u = \frac{(A_u)(C_u)}{A_s} \quad \textbf{(Eq. 1–53)}$$

Example 1-21

The biuret protein assay is very stable and follows Beer's law. Rather than make up a complete new standard graph, one standard (6 g/dL) was assayed. The absorbance of the standard was

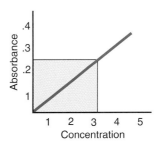

Unknown absorbance = .250
Concentration from graph = 3.2

FIGURE 1-15. Standard curve.

0.400, and the absorbance of the unknown was 0.350. Determine the value of the unknown in g/dL.

$$Cu = \frac{(0.350)(6 \text{ g/dL})}{(0.400)} = 5.25 \text{ g/dL} \quad \textbf{(Eq. 1–54)}$$

This method of calculation is acceptable as long as everything in the system, including the instrument and lot of reagents, remains the same. If anything in the system changes, a new standard graph should be done. Verification of linearity and/or calibration is required whenever a system changes or becomes unstable. Regulatory agencies often prescribe the condition of verification.

Enzyme Calculations

Another application of Beer's law is the calculation of enzyme assay results. When calculating enzyme results, the *rate of absorbance change* is often monitored continuously during the reaction to give the difference in absorbance, known as the *delta absorbance*, or ΔA. Instead of using a standard graph or a one-point calculation, the molar absorptivity of the product is used. If the absorptivity constant and absorbance, in this case ΔA, is given, Beer's law can be used to calculate the enzyme concentration directly without initially needing a standard graph, as follows:

$$A = abc$$
$$C = \frac{A}{ab} \quad \textbf{(Eq. 1–55)}$$

When the absorptivity constant (*a*) is given in units of grams per liter (moles) through a 1-centimeter (cm) light path, the term *molar absorptivity* (ϵ) is used. Substitution of ϵ for *a*, and ΔA for *A* produces the following Beer's law formula:

$$C = \frac{\Delta A}{\epsilon} \quad \textbf{(Eq. 1–56)}$$

Units used to report enzyme activity traditionally have included weight, time, and volume. In the early days of enzymology, method-specific units (*eg*, King-Armstrong, Caraway) were all different and confusing. In 1961, the Enzyme Commission of the International Union of Biochemistry recommended using one unit, the international unit (IU), for reporting enzyme activity. The IU is defined as the amount of enzyme that will catalyze 1 Mmol of substrate/minute/liter. These units were often expressed as units per liter (U/L). The designations IU, U, or IU/L were adopted by many clinical laboratories to represent the IU. Although the reporting unit is the same, unless the analysis conditions are identical, use of the IU does not standardize the actual enzyme activity and, therefore, results between different methods of the same enzyme do not result in equivalent activity of the enzyme. For example, an ALP performed at 37°C will catalyze more substrate than if it is run at lower temperature, such as 25°C, even though the unit of expression, U/L, will be the same. The SI recommended unit is the

katal, which is expressed as mol/L/second. Whichever unit is used, calculation of the activity using Beer's law requires inclusion of the dilution and, depending on the reporting unit, possible conversion to the appropriate term (*eg*, μmol to mol, mL to L, minute to second, and temperature factors). Beer's law for the IU now becomes:

$$C = \frac{(\Delta A)10^{-6}(TV)}{(\epsilon)(b)(SV)} \quad \textbf{(Eq. 1–57)}$$

where TV = total volume of sample plus reagents in mL and SV = sample volume used in mL. The 10-6 converts moles to nmol for the IU. If another unit of activity is used, such as the katal, conversion into liters and seconds would be needed, but the conversion to and from micromoles are excluded.

Example 1-22

The ΔA per minute for an enzyme reaction is 0.250. The product measured has a molar absorptivity of 12.2×10^3 at 425 nm at 30°C. The incubation and reaction temperature are also kept at 30°C. The assay calls for 1 mL of reagent and 0.050 mL of sample. Give the enzyme activity results in international units. Applying Beer's law and the necessary conversion information, the equation becomes:

$$c = \frac{(0.250)(10^{-6})(1.050 \text{ mL})}{(12.2 \times 10^3)(1)(0.050 \text{ mL})} = 430 \text{ U} \quad \textbf{(Eq. 1–58)}$$

Note: *b* is usually given as 1 cm; because it is a constant, it may not be considered in the calculation.

SPECIMEN CONSIDERATIONS

Specimen collection, handling, and processing remains one of the *primary* areas of preanalytic error. Careful attention to each phase is necessary to ensure proper subsequent testing and reporting of meaningful results. All accreditation agencies require laboratories to clearly define and delineate the procedures used for proper collection, transport, and processing of patient samples and the steps used to minimize and detect any errors, along with the documentation of the resolution of any errors. The Clinical Laboratory Improvement Amendments Act of 1988 (CLIA 88)[27] specifies procedures for specimen submission and proper handling, including the disposition of any specimen that does not meet the laboratories' criteria of acceptability, be documented.

Types of Samples

Phlebotomy, or *venipuncture,* is the act of obtaining a blood sample from a vein using a needle attached to a syringe or a stoppered *evacuated tube.* These tubes come in different volume sizes; from pediatric sizes (~150 μL) to larger, 7-mL tubes. The most frequent site for venipuncture is the antecubital of the arm. A tourniquet made of pliable rubber tubing or a strip with Velcro at the end is wrapped around the arm, causing a cessation of blood flow and dilation of the veins, making them easier to detect. The gauge of the needle is inversely related to the size of the needle; the larger the number, the smaller the needle bore and length. An IV infusion set, sometimes referred to as a butterfly because of the appearance of the setup, is used whenever the veins are fragile, small, or hard to reach or find. The butterfly is attached to a piece of tubing, which is then attached to either a hub or tube. Sites adjacent to IV therapy should be avoided; however, if both arms are involved in IV therapy and the IV cannot be discontinued for a short time, a site *below* the IV site should be sought. The initial sample drawn (5 mL) should be discarded because it is most likely contaminated with IV fluid and only subsequent sample tubes used for analytic purposes.

In addition to venipuncture, blood samples can be collected using a skin puncture technique that customarily involves the outer area of the bottom of the foot (a heel stick), the fleshy part of the middle of the last phalanx of the third or fourth (ring) finger (finger stick), or possibly the fleshy portion of the earlobe. A sharp lancet is used to pierce the skin and a capillary tube (*ie*, short, narrow glass tube) is used for sample collection.

Additional information regarding phlebotomy and skin puncture is available,[28,29] plus many accredited training programs in phlebotomy and laboratory science include formal guidelines and procedures for the proper collection of blood samples. Unfortunately, other hospital personnel who may be collecting samples (*eg*, nurses, physicians) may not have the benefit of such training. This lack of training may result in improper collection and an increase in errors.

Analytic testing of blood involves the use of whole blood, serum, or plasma. *Whole blood*, as the name implies, uses both the liquid portion of the blood called *plasma* and the cellular components (red blood cells, white blood cells, and platelets). This requires blood collection into a vessel containing an anticoagulant. Complete mixing of the blood immediately following venipuncture is necessary to ensure the anticoagulant can adequately inhibit the blood's clotting factors. As whole blood sits, the cells fall toward the bottom, leaving a clear yellow supernate on top called *plasma*. If a tube does not contain an anticoagulant, the blood's clotting factors are active to form a clot. The clot is encapsulated by the large protein fibrinogen. The remaining liquid is called *serum* rather than plasma. Most testing in the clinical chemistry laboratory is performed on serum. The major difference between plasma and serum is that serum does not contain fibrinogen (*ie*, there is less protein in serum than plasma) and some potassium is released from platelets (serum potassium is slightly higher in serum than in plasma). It is important that serum samples be allowed to completely clot (about 20 minutes) before being centrifuged.

Centrifuging the sample accelerates the process of separating the plasma and cells. Specimens should be centrifuged for approximately 10 minutes at an RCF of 1000 g to 2000 g but should avoid mechanical destruction of red cells that can result in hemoglobin release, called *hemolysis*.

Arterial blood samples measure blood gases (partial pressures of oxygen and carbon dioxide) and pH. Syringes are used instead of evacuated tubes because of the pressure in an arterial blood vessel. The radial, brachial, and femoral arteries are the primary arterial sites. Arterial punctures are more difficult to perform because of inherent arterial pressure, difficulty in stopping bleeding afterward, and the undesirable development of a hematoma, which cuts off the blood supply to the surrounding tissue. For further information on arterial puncture, see *Procedures for the Handling and Processing of Blood Specimens* (NCCLS, 1999).[29]

Continued metabolism may occur if the serum or plasma remains in contact with the cells for any period. Evacuated tubes may incorporate plastic, gel-like material that serves as a barrier between the cells and the plasma or serum and seals these compartments from one another during centrifugation. Some gels can interfere with certain analytes, notably trace metals, and drugs such as the tricyclic antidepressants.

Any preservatives required for analytic testing can also be incorporated into the collection tubes. Usually, either the collection tube (*ie*, capillary tubes) or the stopper is color coded for easy identification of the presence of an anticoagulant or preservative (Table 1-9). As not all tests have the same sample requirements, the laboratory scientist needs to ascertain the specific collection requirements for each test before sample collection. To prevent contamination, tubes should be drawn starting with blood culture tubes (yellow/black stoppers); followed by tubes without anticoagulants or preservatives (red stoppers); followed by coagulation study tubes containing sodium citrate (light-blue stoppers); followed by tubes containing heparin preservatives (green); and with tubes containing *ethylenediaminetetraacetic acid (EDTA)* (lavender) and sodium fluoride/oxalate (gray) being drawn last, respectively.

Proper patient identification is the first step in sample collection. The importance of using the proper collection tube, avoiding prolonged tourniquet application, drawing tubes in the proper order, and proper labeling of tubes cannot be stressed strongly enough. Prolonged tourniquet application causes a stasis of blood flow and an increase in hemoconcentration and anything bound to proteins or the cells. Having patients open and close their fist during phlebotomy is of no value and may cause an increase in potassium and, therefore, should be avoided. Intravenous contamination should be considered if a large increase occurs in the substances being infused, such as glucose, potassium, sodium, and chloride, with a

TABLE 1-9. COMMONLY USED EVACUATED TUBES

STOPPER COLOR	ADDITIVE	ACTION	USE
Red	None	Allows blood clotting resulting in serum	Most chemistry, blood bank, and immunology assays
Red/gray, red/black	Contains separator material	Allows blood clotting resulting in serum; material serves as a barrier between serum and cells	Most chemistry tests
Lavender	EDTA (Na$_2$ or K$_2$)	Anticoagulant; binds Ca^{++} resulting in whole blood or plasma	CEA, lead, CBC with differential, platelet and reticulocyte counts
Orange	Thrombin	Accelerates clot formation resulting in serum	STAT serum tests (less time needed for clot formation)
Blue	Na Citrate	Anticoagulant; binds Ca^{++} resulting in whole blood or plasma	Coagulation testing; factor assays, fibrinogen, PT, PTT, thrombin time
Gray	a. Na fluoride/K oxalate	Inhibits the glycolytic enzyme enolase and acts as an anticoagulant resulting in whole blood or plasma. Interferes with Na, K, and most BUN (urease) determinations	Glucose (OGTT)/lactate
	b. Iodoacetate	Inhibits the glycolytic enzyme glyceraldehyde-3-phosphate; results in serum; will not interfere with Na, K, or BUN (urease) assays	
Green	Heparin (Na, Li, or NH$_4$); interferes with many ions	Inhibits thrombin activation resulting in whole blood or plasma	Ammonia, carboxy/methemoglobin, lead

decrease of other analytes such as urea and creatinine. In addition, the proper antiseptic must be used. Isopropyl alcohol wipes, for example, are used for cleaning and disinfecting the collection site; however, this is not the proper antiseptic for disinfecting the site when drawing blood alcohol levels.

Blood is not the only sample analyzed in the clinical chemistry laboratory. Urine is the next most common fluid for determination. Most quantitative analyses of urine require a timed sample (usually 24 hours); a complete sample (all urine must be collected in the specified time) can be difficult because many timed samples are collected by the patient in an outpatient situation. Creatinine analysis is often used to assess the completeness of a 24-hour urine sample because creatinine output is relatively free from interference and is stable, with little change in output between individuals. The average adult excretes 1 to 2 g of creatinine per 24 hours. Urine volume differs widely among individuals; however, a 4-L container is adequate (average output is about 2 L). It should be noted that this analysis differs from the creatinine clearance test used to assess glomerular filtration rate, which compares urine creatinine output with that in the serum

in a specified time interval and urine volume (often correcting for the surface area). The generic formula is:

$$UV/P \qquad \text{(Eq 1–59)}$$

where U represents the urine creatinine value in mg/dL, V = urine volume per unit of time expressed in mL/minute, and P represents the plasma or serum creatinine value in mg/dL. Using this formula expresses the creatinine clearance value in mL/min. (See Chapter 24, *Renal Function*.)

Other body fluids analyzed by the clinical chemistry laboratory include *cerebrospinal fluid (CSF)*; *paracentesis* fluids (pleural, pericardial, and peritoneal); and amniotic fluids. The color and characteristics of the fluid *before* centrifugation should be noted for these samples. *Before* centrifugation, a laboratorian should also verify that the sample is designated for clinical chemistry analysis *only* because a single fluid sample may be shared among several departments (ie, hematology or microbiology) and centrifugation could invalidate certain tests in those areas.

CSF is an ultrafiltrate of the plasma and will, ordinarily, reflect the values seen in the plasma. For glucose and protein analysis (total and specific proteins), it is recommended that a blood sample be analyzed concurrently with the analysis of those analytes in the CSF. This will assist in determining the clinical utility of the values obtained on the CSF sample. This is also true for lactate dehydrogenase and protein assays requested on paracentesis fluids. All fluid samples should be handled immediately without delay between sample procurement, transport, and analysis.

Amniotic fluid is used to assess fetal lung maturity (L/S ratio), congenital diseases, hemolytic diseases, genetic defects, and gestational age. The laboratory scientist should verify the specific handling of this fluid with the manufacturer of the testing procedure(s).

Sample Processing

When samples arrive in the laboratory, the samples are then processed. In the clinical chemistry laboratory, this means correctly matching the blood collection tube(s) with the appropriate analyte request and patient identification labels. This is a particularly sensitive area of preanalytic error. Bar code labels on primary sample tubes are a popular means to detect errors and to minimize clerical errors at this point of the processing. In some facilities, samples are numbered or entered into work lists or a second identification system useful during the analytic phase. The laboratory scientist must also ascertain if the sample is acceptable for further processing. The criteria used depend on the test involved, but usually include volume considerations (ie, is there sufficient volume for testing needs); use of proper anticoagulants or preservatives; timing is clearly indicated and appropriate for timed testing; and that the specimen is intact and has been properly transported (eg, cooled or on ice, within a reasonable period, protected from light, properly stoppered). Unless a whole blood analysis is being performed, the sample is then centrifuged as previously described and the serum or plasma should be separated from the cells.

Once processed, the laboratory scientist should note the presence of any serum or plasma characteristics such as *hemolysis* and *icterus* (increased bilirubin pigment) or the presence of turbidity often associated with lipemia (increased lipids). Samples should be analyzed within 4 hours; to minimize the effects of evaporation, samples should be properly capped and kept away from areas of rapid airflow, light, and heat. If testing is to occur after that time, samples should be appropriately stored. For most, this means refrigeration at 4°C for 8 hours. Many analytes are stable at this temperature, with the exception of alkaline phosphatase (increases) and lactate dehydrogenase (decreases as a result of temperature labile fractions four and five). Samples may be frozen at –20°C and stored for longer periods without deleterious effects on the results. Repeated cycles of freezing and thawing, like those that occur in so-called frost-free freezers, should be avoided.

Sample Variables

Sample variables include physiologic considerations; proper patient preparation; and problems in collection, transportation, processing, and storage. Although laboratorians must include mechanisms to minimize the effect of these variables on testing and must document each preanalytic incident, it is often frustrating to try to control the variables that largely depend on individuals outside of the laboratory. The best course of action is to critically assess or predict the weak areas or links, identify potential problems, and put an action plan in place that contains policies, procedures, or checkpoints throughout the sample's journey to the laboratory scientist actually performing the test. Good communication with all personnel involved helps ensure that whatever plans are in place meet the needs of the laboratory and, ultimately, the patient and physician. Most accreditation agencies require that laboratories consider all aspects of preanalytic variation as part of their quality assurance plans, including effective problem solving and documentation.

Physiologic variation refers to changes that occur within the body, such as cyclic changes (diurnal or circadian variation) or those resulting from exercise, diet, stress, gender, age, underlying medical conditions (eg, fever, asthma, obesity), drugs, or posture (Table 1-10). Most samples are drawn on patients who are fasting (usually overnight for at least 8 hours). Because overnight and fasting are relative terms, however, the length of time and what was consumed during that time should be determined before sample procurement for those tests most affected by diet or fasting. Patient preparation for timed samples or those requiring specific diets or other instructions must be well written and verbally explained to patients. Elderly patients often misunderstand or are overwhelmed by the directions given to them by physician office personnel. A laboratory information telephone number listed on these printed directions can often serve as an excellent reference for proper patient preparation.

Drugs can affect various analytes.[30] It is important to ascertain what, if any, medications the patient is taking that may interfere with the test. Unfortunately, many laboratorians do not have either the time or access to this information, and the interest in this type of interference only arises when the physician questions a result. Some frequently encountered influences are smoking, which causes an increase in glucose as a result of the action of nicotine; growth hormone; cortisol; cholesterol; triglycerides; and urea. High amounts or chronic consumption of alcohol causes hypoglycemia, increased triglycerides, and an increase in the enzyme γ-glutamyltransferase and

TABLE 1-10. FACTORS AFFECTING COMMON SERUM CONSTITUENTS

CONSTITUENT	PROLONGED TOURNIQUET APPLICATION	HEMOLYSIS	POSTURE SUPINE TO STANDING	DIURNAL VARIATION	EDTA	MEALS	OTHER
Ammonia	↑	↑				↑	Cigarette smoking; ↑ with exercise
TP/Albumin	↑	↑ (Alb ↓*)	↑				Lipemia
Bilirubin		↓					Light
Iron	↑	↑		✓		↑	Menstruation
Glucose		✓				↑	Caffeine, smoking
Phosphate		↑				↓	
Electrolytes							
Calcium			↑		↓	↑ (ionized)	Marked changes in albumin and pH must be considered in evaluation
Na		↓ (severe)					
K	↓	↑		↑			↑ with opening/closing of hand before collection
Chloride				↓			
Magnesium		↑		↓			Lipemia*
Enzymes							
ALT		↑	↑				↑ with strenuous exercise
AST		↑	↑				↑ with strenuous exercise
Amylase			↑			↓	Serum and only heparinized plasma
CK		↑ (moderate)*					Light and pH sensitive—keep covered to minimize CO_2 loss and in dark
LD		↑					Cold labile fractions
ALP		↑	↑		↓		
ACP		↑		↑			Lipemia; pH stabilized at 5.4 for proper storage
Lipids							
Cholesterol	↑	↑*	↑				
Triglyceride		↑*	↑				
Hormones							
Prolactin				✓		↑(protein)	Stress, ambulation, exercise = ↑
Insulin						↑	
ACTH				✓			Adheres to glass; use polystyrene
Catecholamines		↑		✓		↑	Stress; ↑ with intoxication, tobacco
Cortisol				✓			Caffeine
Gastrin						↑	
GH				✓		↑	↑ with exercise
PTH				✓	✓		Affected by Ca levels; short half-life

TABLE 1-10. FACTORS AFFECTING COMMON SERUM CONSTITUENTS—(CONTINUED)

CONSTITUENT	PROLONGED TOURNIQUET APPLICATION	HEMOLYSIS	POSTURE SUPINE TO STANDING	DIURNAL VARIATION	EDTA	MEALS	OTHER
Renin			✓		✓		Sample should not be chilled; affected by licorice
Aldosterone					✓		Na and K values must be considered
Glucagon						↑	
Thyroid			↑				
TSH				↑			

*Possible interference in assay methods.

other liver function tests. Intramuscular injections increase the enzyme creatine kinase and the skeletal muscle fraction of lactate dehydrogenase. Opiates, such as morphine or meperidine, cause increases in liver and pancreatic enzymes, and oral contraceptives may affect many analytic results. Many drugs affect liver function tests. Diuretics can cause decreased potassium and hyponatremia. Thiazide-type medications can cause hyperglycemia and prerenal azotemia secondary to the decrease in blood volume. Postcollection variations are related to those factors discussed under specimen processing. Clerical errors are the most frequently encountered, followed by inadequate separation of cells from serum, improper storage, and collection.

Chain of Custody

When laboratory tests are likely linked to a crime or accident, they become forensic in nature. In these cases, documented specimen identification is required at each phase of the process. Each facility has its own forms and protocols; however, the patient, and usually a witness, must identify the sample. It should have a tamper-proof seal. Any individual in contact with the sample must document receipt of the sample, the condition of the sample at the time of receipt, and the date and time it was received. In some instances, one witness verifies the entire process and co-signs as the sample moves along. Any analytic test could be used as part of legal testimony; therefore, the laboratory scientist should give each sample—even without the documentation—the same attention given to a forensic sample.

SUMMARY

The primary goal of any clinical chemistry laboratory is to correctly perform analytic procedures that yield accurate and precise information to aid in patient diagnosis. To achieve accurate and reliable results that reflect the patient's physiologic status, the clinical laboratory scientist must be familiar with the use of basic supplies and equipment, with the fundamental understanding of the concepts critical to clinical chemistry testing. This chapter provides the information necessary for the important practice of clinical chemistry, including units of measure; temperature; reagents (chemicals, standards, solutions, water specifications); laboratory supplies (glassware and plasticware, pipets, burets, balances, and desiccants); separation techniques; specimen collection, transport, and processing; and laboratory mathematics and calculations.

REVIEW QUESTIONS

1. Determine each of the following for a solution containing 100 g of NaCl made up to 500 mL with distilled water.
   a. Molarity
   b. Normality
   c. Percent (w/v)
   d. Dilution factor

2. Determine the concentration values for each of the following for a solution containing 10 mg of $CaCl_2$ made with 100 mL of distilled water.
   a. mg/dL
   b. Molarity
   c. Normality

3. You must make 1 L of 0.2 *M* acetic acid (CH$_3$COOH). All you have available is concentrated glacial acetic acid (assay value, 98%; specific gravity, 1.05 g/mL). How many milliliters are needed to make this solution?

4. What is the hydrogen ion concentration of an acetate buffer with a pH of 4.24?

5. Use the Henderson-Hasselbalch equation to solve each of the following buffer problems:
   a. What is the ratio of salt to weak acid for a Veronal buffer with a pH of 8.6 and a pK_a of 7.43?
   b. The pK_a for acetic acid is 4.76. What is the expected pH if the concentration of salt is 5 mmol/L and that of acetic acid is 10 mmol/L?

6. The hydrogen ion concentration of a solution is 0.0000937. What is the pH?

7. You are making up a standard curve for an albumin assay. The standard values needed are:
   1.0 g/dL
   2.0 g/dL
   4.0 g/dL
   6.0 g/dL
   8.0 g/dL
   10.0 g/dL

   You have a 30 g/dL stock solution.
   a. What is the dilution needed to obtain each of the standard values listed?
   b. You need a total volume of 15 mL per standard. List the amount of stock plus the amount of diluent needed to make up each standard.

8. Perform the following conversions.
   8×10^3 mg = _____ μg
   40 μg = _____ mg
   13 dL = _____ mL
   200 μL = _____ mL
   5 μL = _____ mL
   50 mL = _____ L
   4 cm = _____ mm

9. What volume of 14 *N* H$_2$SO$_4$ is needed to make 250 mL of 3.2 *M* H$_2$SO$_4$ solution?

10. A 24-hour urine has a total volume of 1200 mL. A 1:200 dilution of the urine specimen gives a creatinine result of 0.8 mg/dL. The serum value is 1.2 mg/dL.
    a. What is the creatinine concentration for the undiluted urine specimen?
    b. What is the concentration in terms of milligrams per milliliter?
    c. What is the result in terms of grams per 24 hours?
    d. What is the creatinine clearance value? (No correction for surface area)

11. How much CuSO$_4$ · 5H$_2$O is needed to make up 500 mL of 2.5 *M* CuSO$_4$?

12. An enzyme reaction yields a Δ*A* of 0.031 per 30 seconds. The assay calls for 1.5 mL of reagent and 50 μL of sample. The ε of the product is 5.3×10^3. Give the enzyme results in international units.

13. A blood sample is received in the laboratory. The test requests include electrolytes, CK, LD, and AST. After centrifuging, hemolysis is noted. Which tests, if any, are invalid?

14. A blood sample is received in the lab with a label having only a room number written on it. Because it is a private room, only one person is assigned for that room. Is this sample acceptable?

15. A 3-hour glucose tolerance is received from a remote site. This tube uses sodium fluoride as glycolytic inhibitor. The physician's office calls to add a test for urea. Can you satisfy this request?

REFERENCES

1. National Institute of Standards and Technology (NIST). Reference on constants, units, and uncertainty. Adapted from Special Publications (SP) 811 and 330. Washington, D.C.: U.S. Department of Commerce, 1991/1993. Available at http://physics.nist.gov. Accessed April 2003.
2. National Committee for Clinical Laboratory Standards (NCCLS). The reference system for the clinical laboratory: Criteria for development and credentialing of methods and materials for harmonization and results; approved guideline. NCCLS Document NRSCL 13-P. Wayne, PA: NCCLS, 2000.
3. American Chemical Society (ACS). Reagent Chemicals, 9th ed. Washington, D.C.: ACS Press, 2000.
4. Department of Labor and Occupational Safety and Health Administration (OSHA). Occupational exposure to hazardous chemicals in laboratories. Federal Register, 29 CFR, Part 1910.1450. Washington, D.C.: OSHA, 1990.
5. National Institute of Standards and Technology (NIST). Standard reference materials. Publication 260. Washington, D.C.: U.S. Department of Commerce, 1991.
6. International Union of Pure and Allied Chemistry (IUPAC). In: McNaught A, Wilkinson A, eds. Royal Society of Chemistry. Compendium of Chemical Terminology, 2nd ed. Cambridge, UK: Blackwell Scientific, 1997.
7. National Committee for Clinical Laboratory Standards. Development of certified reference materials for the national reference

system for the clinical laboratory. NCCLS Document NRSCL-3A. Villanova, PA: NCCLS, 1991.

8. International Organization for Standardization, European Committee for Standardization (ISO). In vitro diagnostic medical devices—measurement of quantities in samples of biological origin—metrological traceability of values assigned to calibrators and control material. ISO/TC 212/WG2 N65/EN 17511. Geneva, Switzerland: ISO, 2000.

9. Dybaer R. Reference materials and reference measurement systems in laboratory medicine. Harmonization of nomenclature and definitions in reference measurement systems. Eur J Clin Chem Clin Biochem 1995;33:995-998.

10. National Institute of Standards and Technology (NIST). Standard reference materials program. Washington, D.C.: U.S. Department of Commerce. Available at http://ts.nist.gov/srm. Accessed April 2003.

11. Carreiro-Lewandowski E. Basic principles and practice of clinical chemistry. In Bishop M, Duben-Engelkirk J, Fody P, eds. Clinical Chemistry, Principles, Procedures, and Correlations, 4th ed. Baltimore: Lippincott Williams & Wilkins, 2000.

12. National Committee for Clinical Laboratory Standards (NCCLS). Preparation and testing of reagent water in the clinical laboratory. Approved guideline, 3rd ed, C3-A3. Wayne, PA: NCCLS 1997.

13. College of American Pathologists (CAP). General laboratory guidelines; Water Quality. Northfield, IL: College of American Pathologists, July 1999.

14. Skoog D, West D, Holler J, Crouch S, eds. Analytical Chemistry: An Introduction, 7th ed. Stamford, CT: Thompson/Brooks-Cole, 2000.

15. National Committee for Clinical Laboratory Standards (NCCLS). Temperature calibration of water baths, instruments, and temperature sensors. I2-A2, Villanova, PA: NCCLS, 1990.

16. National Institute of Standards and Technology (NIST). Calibration uncertainties of liquid-in-glass thermometers over the range from −20°C to 400°C. Gaithersburg, MD: U.S. Department of Commerce, 2000.

17. National Institute of Standards and Technology (NIST), Wise J. A procedure for the effective recalibration of liquid-in-glass thermometers. (SP)819. Gaithersburg, MD: National Institute of Standards and Technology, August, 1991.

18. Bowers GN, Inman SR. The gallium melting-point standard. Clin Chem 1977;23:733.

19. Bowie L, Esters F, Bolin J, et al. Development of an aqueous temperature-indicated technique and its application to clinical laboratory instruments. Clin Chem 1976;22:449.

20. American Society for Testing and Materials (ASTM). Standards specification for volumetric (transfer) pipets. E969-83. 14.02:500–501. West Conshohocken, PA: ASTM, 1993.

21. American Society for Testing and Materials (ASTM). Calibration of volumetric flasks. E288-94. 14:04. West Conshohocken, PA: ASTM, 2003.

22. Seamonds B. Basic laboratory principles and techniques. In: Kaplan L, Pesce A, Kazmierczak S, eds. Clinical Chemistry. Theory, Analysis, and Correlation, 4th ed. St. Louis: CV Mosby, 2003.

23. Bio-Rad Laboratories. Procedure for comparing precision of pipet tips. Product Information No. 81-0208. Hercules, CO: Bio-Rad Laboratories, 1993.

24. National Committee for Clinical Laboratory Standards (NCCLS). Determining performance of volumetric equipment. NCCLS document 18-P. Villanova, PA: NCCLS, 1984.

24a. Lide DH, ed. Handbook of Chemistry and Physics, 76th ed. Boca Raton, FL: CRC Press, 1995.

25. American Society for Testing and Materials (ASTM). Standard specification for laboratory weights and precision mass standards. E617-97. 14.04. West Conshohocken, PA: ASTM, 2003.

26. Campbell JB, Campbell JM. Laboratory Mathematics: Medical and Biological Applications, 5th ed. St. Louis: CV Mosby, 1997.

27. Clinical Laboratory Improvement Amendments. Centers for Disease Control, Division of Laboratory Systems. CFR Part 493, Laboratory Requirements. Available at http://www.phppo.cdc.gov/clia/regs2/toc.asp. Accessed May 2003.

28. National Committee for Clinical Laboratory Standards (NCCLS). Procedures and devices for the collection of diagnostic blood specimens by skin puncture. Approved standard H4-A4, 4th ed. Wayne, PA: NCCLS, 1999.

29. National Committee for Clinical Laboratory Standards (NCCLS). Procedures for the handling and processing of blood specimens, H11-A3, 3rd ed. Wayne, PA: NCCLS, 1999.

30. Young DS. Effects of Drugs on Clinical Laboratory Tests, 5th ed. Washington, D.C.: AACC Press, 2000.

Laboratory Safety and Regulations

Tolmie E. Wachter

CHAPTER OUTLINE

OBJECTIVES

Upon completion of this chapter, the clinical laboratorian should be able to:
- Discuss safety awareness for clinical laboratory personnel.
- List the responsibilities of employer and employee in providing a safe workplace.
- Identify hazards related to handling chemicals, biologic specimens, and radiologic materials.
- Choose appropriate personal protective equipment when working in the clinical laboratory.

- Identify the classes of fires and the type of fire extinguishers to use for each.
- Describe steps used as precautionary measures when working with electrical equipment, cryogenic materials, and compressed gases and avoiding mechanical hazards associated with laboratory equipment.
- Select the correct means for disposal of waste generated in the clinical laboratory.
- Outline the steps required in documentation of an accident in the workplace.

KEY TERMS

Airborne pathogens
Biohazard
Bloodborne pathogens
Carcinogen
Chemical hygiene plan
Corrosive chemical
Cryogenic material

Fire tetrahedron
Hazard communication
    standard
Hazardous material
High-efficiency
    particulate air (HEPA)
    filter

Laboratory standard
Material safety data
    sheet (MSDS)
Mechanical hazard
Medical waste
National Fire Protection
    Association (NFPA)

Occupational Safety and
    Health Act (OSHA)
Radioactive material
Reactive chemical
Standard precautions
Teratogen

LABORATORY SAFETY AND REGULATIONS

All clinical laboratory personnel, by the nature of the work they perform, are exposed daily to a variety of real or potential hazards: electric shock, toxic vapors, compressed gases, flammable liquids, radioactive material, corrosive substances, mechanical trauma, poisons, and the inherent risks of handling biologic materials, to name a few. Each professional must be "safety conscious" at all times!

Laboratory safety necessitates the effective control of all hazards that exist in the clinical laboratory at any time. Safety begins with the recognition of hazards and is achieved through the application of common sense, a safety-focused attitude, good personal behavior, good housekeeping in all laboratory work and storage areas, and, above all, the continual practice of good laboratory technique. In most cases, accidents can be traced directly to two primary causes: unsafe acts (not always recognized by personnel) and unsafe environmental conditions. This chapter discusses laboratory safety as it applies to the clinical laboratory.

Occupational Safety and Health Act (OSHA)

Public Law 91-596, better known as the *Occupational Safety and Health Act* (OSHA), was enacted by Congress in 1970. The goal of this federal regulation was to provide all employees (clinical laboratory personnel included) with a safe work environment. Under this legislation, the Occupational Safety and Health Administration is authorized to conduct on-site inspections to determine whether an employer is complying with the mandatory standards. Safety is no longer only a moral obligation, but also a federal law.

Other Regulations and Guidelines

There are other federal regulations relating to laboratory safety, such as the Clean Water Act, the Resource Conservation and Recovery Act, and the Toxic Substances Control Act. In addition, clinical laboratories are required to comply with applicable local and state laws, such as fire and building codes. OSHA standards that regulate safety in the laboratory include Bloodborne Pathogen Standard,

Formaldehyde Standard, Laboratory Standard, Hazard Communication Standard, Respiratory Standard, Air Contaminants Standard, and Personal Protective Equipment Standard. Because laws, codes, and ordinances are updated frequently, current reference materials should be reviewed. Assistance can be obtained from local libraries; the Internet; and from federal, state, and local regulatory agencies.

Safety is also an important part of the requirements for accreditation and reaccreditation of health care institutions and laboratories by voluntary accrediting bodies such as the Joint Commission on Accreditation of Health Care Organizations (JCAHO) and the Commission on Laboratory Accreditation of the College of American Pathologists (CAP). JCAHO publishes a yearly accreditation manual for hospitals and *Accreditation Manual for Pathology and Clinical Laboratory Services*, which includes a detailed section on safety requirements. CAP publishes an extensive inspection checklist as part of their *Laboratory Accreditation Program*, which includes a section dedicated to laboratory safety.

SAFETY AWARENESS FOR CLINICAL LABORATORY PERSONNEL

Safety Responsibility

The employer and the employee share safety responsibility. The employer has the ultimate responsibility for safety and delegates authority for safe operations to supervisors. Safety management in the laboratory should start with a written safety policy. Laboratory supervisors, who reflect the attitudes of management toward safety, are essential members of the safety program.

Employer's Responsibilities
- Establish laboratory work methods and safety policies.
- Provide supervision and guidance to employees.
- Provide safety information, training, personal protective equipment, and medical surveillance to employees.
- Provide and maintain equipment and laboratory facilities that are adequate for the tasks required.

The employee also has a responsibility for his or her own safety and the safety of coworkers. Employee conduct in the laboratory is a vital factor in the achievement of a workplace without accidents or injuries.

Employee's Responsibilities

- Know and comply with the established laboratory work safety methods.
- Have a positive attitude toward supervisors, coworkers, facilities, and safety training.
- Give prompt notification of unsafe conditions or practices to the immediate supervisor and ensure that unsafe conditions and practices are corrected.
- Engage in the conduct of safe work practices and use of personal protective equipment.

Signage and Labeling

Appropriate signs to identify hazards are critical, not only to alert laboratory personnel to potential hazards, but also to identify specific hazards that arise because of emergencies such as fire or explosion. The *National Fire Protection Association (NFPA)* developed a standard hazards-identification system (diamond-shaped, color-coded symbol), which has been adopted by many clinical laboratories. At a glance, emergency personnel can assess health hazards (blue quadrant), flammable hazards (red quadrant), reactivity/stability hazards (yellow quadrant), and other special information (white quadrant). In addition, each quadrant shows the magnitude of severity, graded from a low of 0 to a high of 4, of the hazards within the posted area. (Note the NFPA hazard-code symbol in Figure 2-1.)

Manufacturers of laboratory chemicals also provide precautionary labeling information for users. Information indicated on the product label includes statement of the hazard, precautionary measures, specific hazard class, first aid instructions for internal/external contact, the storage code, the safety code, and personal protective gear and equipment needed. This information is in addition to specifications on the actual lot analysis of the chemical constituents and other product notes (Fig. 2-1). All in-house prepared reagents and solutions should be labeled in a standard manner with the chemical identity, concentration, hazard warning, special handling, storage conditions, date prepared, expiration date (if applicable), and preparer's initials.

SAFETY EQUIPMENT

Safety equipment has been developed specifically for use in the clinical laboratory. The employer is required by law to have designated safety equipment available, but it is also the responsibility of the employee to comply with all safety rules and to use safety equipment.

All laboratories are required to have safety showers, eyewash stations, and fire extinguishers and to periodi-

cally test and inspect the equipment for proper operation. It is recommended that safety showers deliver 30–50 gal/min of water at 20–50 psi. Other items that must be available for personnel include fire blankets, spill kits, and first aid supplies.

Mechanical pipetting devices must be used for manipulating all types of liquids in the laboratory, including water. Mouth pipetting is strictly prohibited.

Hoods

Fume Hoods

Fume hoods are required to expel noxious and hazardous fumes from chemical reagents. Fume hoods should be visually inspected for blockages. A piece of tissue paper placed at the hood opening will indicate airflow direction. The hood should never be operated with the sash fully opened. Chemicals stored in hoods should not block airflow. Periodically, ventilation should be evaluated by measuring the face velocity with a calibrated velocity meter. The velocity at the face of the hood (with the sash in normal operating position) must be 100 to 120 ft/min. Smoke testing is also recommended to locate dead or turbulent areas in the working space. Additional monitoring should be in accordance with the chemical hygiene plan of the facility.

Biosafety Hoods

Biohazard hoods remove particles that may be harmful to the employee who is working with infective biologic specimens. The Centers for Disease Control and Prevention (CDC) and the National Institutes of Health have described four levels of biosafety, which consist of combinations of laboratory practices and techniques, safety equipment, and laboratory facilities. The biosafety level of a laboratory is based on the operations performed, the routes of transmission of the infectious agents, and the laboratory function or activity. Accordingly, biohazard hoods are designed to offer various levels of protection, depending on the biosafety level of the specific laboratory (Table 2-1).

Chemical Storage Equipment

Safety equipment is available for the storage and handling of chemicals and compressed gases. Safety carriers should always be used to transport 500-mL bottles of acids, alkalis, or other solvents, and approved safety cans should be used for storing, dispensing, or disposing of flammables in volumes greater than 1 qt. Safety cabinets are required for the storage of flammable liquids, and only specially designed, explosion-proof refrigerators should be used to store flammable materials. Only that amount of chemical needed for the day should be available at the bench. Gas-cylinder supports or clamps must

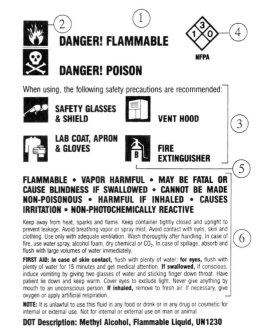

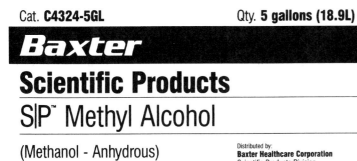

Cat. **C4324-5GL**   Qty. **5 gallons (18.9L)**

Scientific Products

S|P™ Methyl Alcohol

(Methanol - Anhydrous)
CH_3OH FW 32.04
For Laboratory Use
Store at 68-86°F (20-30°C)

Flash Point: 11°C (52°F Closed Cup)
Maximum Limits and Specifications
Methyl Alcohol: 99.8% Minimum by volume
Residue after Evaporation: 0.001% Maximum
Water: 0.10% Maximum
CAS — (67-56-1);

Distributed by:
Baxter Healthcare Corporation
Scientific Products Division
McGaw Park, IL 60085-6787 USA
Rev. 11/04

Made in USA

Lot No. **KEAM**

DANGER! FLAMMABLE

DANGER! POISON

When using, the following safety precautions are recommended:

SAFETY GLASSES & SHIELD   **VENT HOOD**

LAB COAT, APRON & GLOVES   **FIRE EXTINGUISHER**

FLAMMABLE • VAPOR HARMFUL • MAY BE FATAL OR CAUSE BLINDNESS IF SWALLOWED • CANNOT BE MADE NON-POISONOUS • HARMFUL IF INHALED • CAUSES IRRITATION • NON-PHOTOCHEMICALLY REACTIVE

Keep away from heat, sparks and flame. Keep container tightly closed and upright to prevent leakage. Avoid breathing vapor or spray mist. Avoid contact with eyes, skin and clothing. Use only with adequate ventilation. Wash thoroughly after handling. In case of fire, use water spray, alcohol foam, dry chemical or CO_2. In case of spillage, absorb and flush with large volumes of water immediately.

FIRST AID: in case of skin contact, flush with plenty of water; **for eyes,** flush with plenty of water for 15 minutes and get medical attention. **If swallowed,** if conscious, induce vomiting by giving two glasses of water and sticking finger down throat. Have patient lie down and keep warm. Cover eyes to exclude light. Never give anything by mouth to an unconscious person. **If inhaled,** remove to fresh air. If necessary, give oxygen or apply artificial respiration.

NOTE: It is unlawful to use this fluid in any food or drink or in any drug or cosmetic for internal or external use. Not for internal or external use on man or animal.

DOT Description: Methyl Alcohol, Flammable Liquid, UN1230

FIGURE 2-1. Sample chemical label: (**1**) statement of hazard; (**2**) hazard class; (**3**) safety precautions; (**4**) National Fire Protection Agency (NFPA) hazard code; (**5**) fire extinguisher type; (**6**) safety instructions; (**7**) formula weight; and (**8**) lot number.
   Color of the diamond in the NFPA label indicates hazard:
Red = flammable. Store in an area segregated for flammable reagents.
Blue = health hazard. Toxic if inhaled, ingested, or absorbed through the skin. Store in a secure area.
Yellow = reactive and oxidizing reagents. May react violently with air, water, or other substances. Store away from flammable and combustible materials.
White = corrosive. May harm skin, eyes, or mucous membranes. Store away from red-, blue-, and yellow-coded reagents.
Gray = presents no more than moderate hazard in any of categories. For general chemical storage.
Exception = reagent incompatible with other reagents of same color bar. Store separately. *Hazard code* (**4**)—Following the NFPA usage, each diamond shows a red segment (flammability), a blue segment (health; *ie,* toxicity), and yellow (reactivity). Printed over each color-coded segment is a black number showing the degree of hazard involved. The fourth segment, as stipulated by the NFPA, is left blank. It is reserved for special warnings, such as radioactivity. The numeric ratings indicate degree of hazard: 4 = extreme; 3 = severe; 2 = moderate; 1 = slight; and 0 = none according to present data.

be used at all times, and large tanks should be transported using handcarts.

Personal Protective Equipment

The parts of the body most frequently subject to injury in the clinical laboratory are the eyes, skin, and respiratory and digestive tracts. Hence, the use of personal protective equipment is very important. Safety glasses, goggles, visors, or work shields protect the eyes and face from splashes and impact. Contact lenses do not offer eye protection. It is strongly recommended that they not be worn in the clinical chemistry laboratory. If any solution is accidentally splashed into the eye(s), thorough irrigation is required.

Gloves and rubberized sleeves protect the hands and arms when using caustic chemicals. Gloves are required for routine laboratory use; however, polyvinyl or other

nonlatex gloves are an acceptable alternative for people with latex allergies. Certain glove materials offer better protection against particular reagent formulations. Nitrile gloves, for example, offer a wider range of compatibility with organic solvents than latex. Lab coats, preferably with cuffed sleeves, should be full length, buttoned, and made of liquid-resistant material. Proper footwear is required; shoes constructed of porous materials, open-toed shoes, or sandals are considered hazardous.

Respirators are required for various procedures in the clinical laboratory. Whether used for biologic or chemical hazards, the correct type of respirator must be used for the specific hazard. Respirators with *high-efficiency particulate air (HEPA)* filters must be worn when engineering controls are not feasible, for example, when working directly with tuberculosis (TB) patients or performing procedures that may aerosolize specimens of patients with suspected or confirmed cases of TB. Training, mainte-

TABLE 2-1. COMPARISON OF BIOLOGIC SAFETY CABINETS

	CABINETS		APPLICATIONS		
TYPE	FACE VELOCITY (IFPM)	AIRFLOW PATTERN	RADIONUCLIDES/ TOXIC CHEMICALS	BIOSAFETY LEVEL(S)	PRODUCT PROTECTION
Class I,* open front	75	In at front; out rear and top through HEPA filter	No	2,3	No
Class II					
Type A	75	70% recirculated through HEPA; exhaust through HEPA	No	2,3	Yes
Type B1	100	30% recirculated through HEPA; exhaust via HEPA and hard-ducted	Yes (low levels/volatility)	2,3	Yes
Type B2	100	No recirculation; total exhaust via HEPA and hard-ducted	Yes	2,3	Yes
Type B3	100	Same as IIA, but plena under negative pressure to room and exhaust air is ducted	Yes	2,3	Yes
Class III	NA	Supply air inlets and exhaust through 2 HEPA filters	Yes	3,4	

Source: Centers for Disease Control and Prevention and the National Institutes of Health. Biosafety in Microbiological and Biomedical Laboratories, 3rd ed. Washington, D.C.: U.S. Government Printing Office, Table 3, Comparison of Biological Safety Cabinets, 1993.
*Glove panels may be added and will increase face velocity to 150 lfpm; gloves may be added with an inlet air pressure release that will allow work with chemicals/radionuclides.

nance, and written protocol for use of respirators are required according to the respiratory protection standard.

Each employer must provide (at no charge) lab coats, gloves, or other protective equipment to all employees who may be exposed to biologic or chemical hazards. It is the employer's responsibility to clean and maintain all personal protective equipment. All contaminated personal protective equipment must be removed and properly disposed of before leaving the laboratory.

BIOLOGIC SAFETY

General Considerations

All blood samples and other body fluids should be collected, transported, handled, and processed using strict precautions. Gloves, gowns, and face protection must be used if splashing or splattering is likely to occur. Consistent and thorough hand washing is an essential component of infection control.

Centrifugation of biologic specimens produce finely dispersed aerosols that are a high-risk source of infection. Ideally, specimens should remain capped during centrifugation. As an additional precaution, the use of a centrifuge with an internal shield is recommended.

Spills

Any blood, body fluid, or other potentially infectious material spill must be cleaned up and the area or equipment

disinfected immediately. Recommended cleanup includes the following:

- Wear appropriate protective equipment.
- Use mechanical devices to pick up broken glass or other sharp objects.
- Absorb the spill with paper towels, gauze pads, or tissue.
- Clean the spill site using a common aqueous detergent.
- Disinfect the spill site using approved disinfectant or 10% bleach, using appropriate contact time.
- Rinse the spill site with water.
- Dispose of all materials in appropriate biohazard containers.

Bloodborne Pathogen Exposure Control Plan

In December 1991, OSHA issued the final rule for occupational exposure to *bloodborne pathogens*. To minimize employee exposure, each employer must have a written exposure control plan. The plan must be available to all employees whose reasonable anticipated duties may result in occupational exposure to blood or other potentially infectious materials. The exposure control plan must be discussed with all employees and be available to them while they are working. The employee must be provided with adequate training of all techniques described in the exposure control plan at initial work assignment and annually thereafter. All necessary equipment and supplies must be readily available and inspected on a regular basis.

Clinical laboratory personnel are knowingly or unknowingly in frequent contact with potentially biohazardous materials. In recent years, new and serious occupational hazards to personnel have arisen, and this problem has been complicated because of the general lack of understanding of the epidemiology, mechanisms of transmission of the disease, or inactivation of the causative agent. Special precautions must be taken when handling all specimens because of the continual increase of infectious samples received in the laboratory. Therefore, in practice, specimens from patients with confirmed or suspected hepatitis, acquired immunodeficiency syndrome, Creutzfeldt-Jakob disease, or other potentially infectious diseases should be handled no differently than other routine specimens. Adopting a *standard precautions* policy, which considers blood and other body fluids from all patients as potentially infective, is required.

Airborne Pathogens

Because of the recent resurgence of tuberculosis (TB), OSHA issued a statement in 1993 that the agency would enforce the CDC *Guidelines for Preventing the Transmission of Tuberculosis in Health Care Facilities.* The purpose of the guidelines is to encourage early detection, isolation, and treatment of active cases. A TB exposure control program must be established and risks to laboratory workers must be assessed. In 1997, a proposed standard (29 CFR 1910.1035, *Tuberculosis*) was issued by OSHA. The standard mandates the development of a *tuberculosis exposure control plan* by any facility involved in the diagnosis or treatment of cases of confirmed infectious TB. TB isolation areas with specific ventilation controls must be established in health care facilities. Those workers in high-risk areas may be required to wear a respirator for protection. All health care workers considered to be at risk must be screened for TB infection.

Shipping

Clinical laboratories routinely ship regulated material. The U.S. Department of Transportation (DOT) and the International Air Transport Association (IATA) have specific requirements for carrying regulated materials. There are two types of specimen classifications. Known or suspect infectious specimens are labeled *infectious substances* if the pathogen can be readily transmitted to humans or animals and there is no effective treatment available. *Diagnostic specimens* are those tested as routine screening or for initial diagnosis. Each type of specimen has rules and packaging requirements. The DOT guidelines are found in *Code of Federal Regulations 49;* IATA publishes its own manual, *Dangerous Goods Regulations.*

CHEMICAL SAFETY

Hazard Communication

In the August 1987 issue of the *Federal Register,* OSHA published the new *Hazard Communication Standard* (Right to Know Law). The Right to Know Law was developed for employees who may be exposed to hazardous chemicals. Employees must be informed of the health risks associated with those chemicals. The intent of the law is to ensure that health hazards are evaluated for all chemicals that are produced and that this information is relayed to employees.

To comply with the regulation, clinical laboratories must:

- Plan and implement a written hazard communication program.
- Obtain *material safety data sheets* (MSDSs) for each hazardous compound present in the workplace and have the MSDSs readily accessible to employees.
- Educate all employees annually on how to interpret chemical labels, MSDSs, and health hazards of the chemicals and how to work safely with the chemicals.
- Maintain hazard warning labels on containers received or filled on site.

Material Safety Data Sheet (MSDS)

The MSDS is a major source of safety information for employees who may use *hazardous materials* in their occupations. Employers are responsible for obtaining from the chemical manufacturer or developing an MSDS for each hazardous agent used in the workplace. A standardized format is not mandatory, but all requirements listed in the law must be addressed. A summary of the MSDS information requirements includes the following:

- Product name and identification.
- Hazardous ingredients.
- Permissible Exposure Limit (PEL).
- Physical and chemical data.
- Health hazard data and carcinogenic potential.
- Primary routes of entry.
- Fire and explosion hazards.
- Reactivity data.
- Spill and disposal procedures.
- Personal protective equipment recommendations.
- Handling.
- Emergency and first aid procedures.
- Storage and transportation precautions.
- Chemical manufacturer's name, address, and phone number.
- Special information section.

The MSDS must be printed in English and provide the specific compound identity, together with all common names. All information sections must be completed, and the date that the MSDS was printed must be indicated. Copies of the MSDS must be readily accessible to employees during all shifts.

Laboratory Standard

Occupational Exposure to Hazardous Chemicals in Laboratories, also known as the *laboratory standard,* was enacted in May 1990 to provide laboratories specific guidelines for handling hazardous chemicals. This OSHA standard requires each laboratory that uses hazardous chemicals to have a written *chemical hygiene plan.* This plan provides procedures and work practices for regulating and reducing exposure of laboratory personnel to hazardous chemicals. *Hazardous chemicals* are those that pose a physical or health hazard from acute or chronic exposure. Procedures describing how to protect employees against *teratogens* (substances that affect cellular development in a fetus or embryo), carcinogens, and other toxic chemicals must be described in the plan. Training in use of hazardous chemicals to include recognition of signs and symptoms of exposure, location of MSDS, a chemical hygiene plan, and how to protect themselves against hazardous chemicals must be provided to all employees. A chemical hygiene officer must be designated for any laboratory using hazardous chemicals. The protocol must be reviewed annually and updated when regulations are modified or chemical inventory changes. Remember that practicing consistent and thorough hand washing is an essential component of preventative chemical hygiene.

Toxic Effects From Hazardous Substances

Toxic substances have the potential of deleterious effects (local or systemic) by direct chemical action or interference with the function of body systems. They can cause acute or chronic effects related to the duration of exposure (ie, short-term or single contact versus long-term or prolonged, repeated contact). Almost any substance, even the most harmless, can risk damage to a worker's lungs, skin, eyes, or mucous membranes following long- or short-term exposure and can be toxic in excess. Moreover, some chemicals are toxic at very low concentrations. Exposure to toxic agents can be through direct contact (absorption), inhalation, ingestion, or inoculation/injection.

In the clinical chemistry laboratory, personnel should be particularly aware of toxic vapors from chemical solvents, such as acetone, chloroform, methanol, or carbon tetrachloride, that do not give explicit sensory-irritation warnings, as do bromide, ammonia, and formaldehyde. Air sampling or routine monitoring may be necessary to quantify dangerous levels. Mercury is another frequently disregarded source of poisonous vapors. It is highly volatile and toxic and is rapidly absorbed through the skin and respiratory tract. Mercury spill kits should be available in areas where mercury thermometers are used. Most laboratories are phasing out the use of mercury and mercury-containing compounds. Laboratories should have a policy and method for legally disposing of mercury. Laboratory engineering controls, personal protective equipment, and procedural controls must be adequate to protect employees from these substances.

Storage and Handling of Chemicals

To avoid accidents when handling chemicals, it is important to develop respect for all chemicals and to have a complete knowledge of their properties. This is particularly important when transporting, dispensing, or using chemicals that, when in contact with certain other chemicals, could result in the formation of substances that are toxic, flammable, or explosive. For example, acetic acid is incompatible with other acids such as chromic and nitric, carbon tetrachloride is incompatible with sodium, and flammable liquids are incompatible with hydrogen peroxide and nitric acid.

Arrangements for the storage of chemicals will depend on the quantities of chemicals needed and the nature or type of chemicals. Proper storage is essential to prevent and control laboratory fires and accidents. Ideally, the storeroom should be organized so that each class of chemicals is isolated in an area that is not used for routine work. An up-to-date inventory should be kept that indicates location of chemicals, minimum/maximum quantities required, shelf life, and so on. Some chemicals deteriorate over time and become hazardous (eg, ether forms explosive peroxides). Storage should not be based solely on alphabetical order because incompatible chemicals may be stored next to each other and react chemically. They must be separated for storage as shown in Table 2-2.

Flammable/Combustible Chemicals
Flammable and combustible liquids, which are used in numerous routine procedures, are among the most haz-

TABLE 2-2. STORAGE REQUIREMENTS

SUBSTANCE	STORED SEPARATELY
Flammable liquids	Flammable solids
Mineral acids	Organic acids
Caustics	Oxidizers
Perchloric acid	Water-reactive substances
Air-reactive substances	Others
Heat-reactive substances requiring refrigeration	
Unstable substances (shock-sensitive explosives)	

Refer to Appendix F, *Examples of Incompatible Chemicals.*

ardous materials in the clinical chemistry laboratory because of possible fire or explosion. They are classified according to flash point, which is the temperature at which sufficient vapor is given off to form an ignitable mixture with air. A flammable liquid has a flash point below 37.8°C (100°F), and combustible liquids, by definition, have a flash point at or above 37.8°C (100°F). Some commonly used flammable and combustible solvents are acetone, benzene, ethanol, heptane, isopropanol, methanol, toluene, and xylene. It is important to remember that flammable chemicals also include certain gases, such as hydrogen, and solids, such as paraffin.

Corrosive Chemicals

Corrosive chemicals are injurious to the skin or eyes by direct contact or to the tissue of the respiratory and gastrointestinal tracts if inhaled or ingested. Typical examples include acids (acetic, sulfuric, nitric, and hydrochloric) and bases (ammonium hydroxide, potassium hydroxide, and sodium hydroxide).

Reactive Chemicals

Reactive chemicals are substances that, under certain conditions, can spontaneously explode or ignite or that evolve heat or flammable or explosive gases. Some strong acids or bases react with water to generate heat (exothermic reactions). Hydrogen is liberated if alkali metals (sodium or potassium) are mixed with water or acids, and spontaneous combustion also may occur. The mixture of oxidizing agents, such as peroxides, and reducing agents, such as hydrogen, generate heat and may be explosive.

Carcinogenic Chemicals

Carcinogens are substances that have been determined to be cancer-causing agents. OSHA has issued lists of confirmed and suspected carcinogens and detailed standards for the handling of these substances. Benzidine is a common example of a known carcinogen. If possible, a substitute chemical or different procedure should be used to avoid exposure to carcinogenic agents. For regulatory (OSHA) and institutional safety requirements, the laboratory must maintain an accurate inventory of carcinogens.

Chemical Spills

Strict attention to good laboratory technique can help prevent chemical spills. However, emergency procedures should be established to handle any accidents. If a spill occurs, the first step should be to assist/evacuate personnel, then confinement and cleanup of the spill can begin. There are several commercial spill kits available for neutralizing and absorbing spilled chemical solutions (Fig. 2-2). However, no single kit is suitable for all types of spills. Emergency procedures for spills should also include a reporting system.

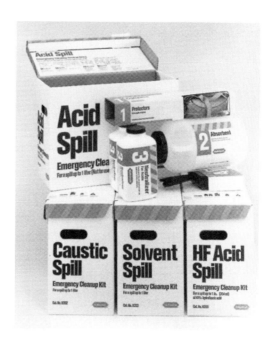

FIGURE 2-2. Spill cleanup kit.

RADIATION SAFETY

Environmental Protection

A radiation safety policy should include environmental and personnel protection. All areas where *radioactive materials* are used or stored must be posted with caution signs, and traffic in these areas should be restricted to essential personnel only. Regular and systematic monitoring must be emphasized, and decontamination of laboratory equipment, glassware, and work areas should be scheduled as part of routine procedures. Records must be maintained as to the quantity of radioactive material on hand as well as the quantity that is disposed. A Nuclear Regulatory Commission (NRC) license is required if the total amount of radioactive material exceeds a certain level. The laboratory safety officer must consult with the institutional safety officer about these requirements.

Personal Protection

It is essential that only properly trained personnel work with radioisotopes and that users are monitored to ensure that the maximal permissible dose of radiation is not exceeded. Radiation monitors must be evaluated regularly to detect degree of exposure for the laboratory employee. Records must be maintained for the length of employment plus 30 years.

Nonionizing Radiation

Nonionizing forms of radiation are also a concern in the clinical laboratory. Equipment often emits a variety of

TABLE 2-3. EXAMPLES OF NONIONIZING RADIATION IN CLINICAL LABORATORIES

TYPE	APPROXIMATE WAVELENGTH	SOURCE EQUIPMENT EXAMPLE	PROTECTIVE MEASURES
Low frequency	1 cm +	RF coil in ICP-mass spectrometer	Engineered shielding and posted pacemaker warning
Microwaves	3 m–3 mm	Energy-beam microwave used to accelerate tissue staining in histology-prep processes	Engineered shielding
Infrared	750 nm–0.3 cm	Heat lamps, lasers	Containment and appropriate warning labels
Visible spectrum	400–750 nm	General illumination and glare	Filters, diffusers, and non-reflective surfaces
Ultraviolet	4–400 nm	Germicidal lamps used in biologic safety cabinets	Eye and skin protection; UV warning labels

wavelengths of electromagnetic radiation that must be protected against through engineered shielding or use of personal protective equipment (Table 2-3). These energies have varying biologic effects, depending on wavelength, power intensity, and duration of exposure. Laboratorians must be knowledgeable regarding the hazards presented by their equipment to protect themselves and ancillary personnel.

FIRE SAFETY

The Chemistry of Fire

Fire is basically a chemical reaction that involves the rapid oxidation of a combustible material or fuel, with the subsequent liberation of heat and light. In the clinical chemistry laboratory, all the elements essential for fire to begin are present—fuel, heat or ignition source, and oxygen (air). However, recent research suggests that a fourth factor is present. This factor has been classified as a reaction chain in which burning continues and even accelerates. It is caused by the breakdown and recombination of the molecules from the material burning with the oxygen in the atmosphere.

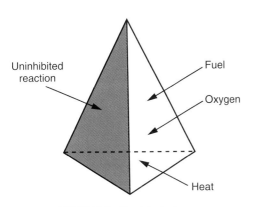

FIGURE 2-3. Fire tetrahedron.

The fire triangle has been modified into a three-dimensional pyramid known as the *fire tetrahedron* (Fig. 2-3). This modification does not eliminate established procedures in dealing with a fire but does provide additional means by which fires may be prevented or extinguished. A fire will extinguish if any of the three basic elements (heat, air, or fuel) are removed.

Classification of Fires

Fires have been divided into four classes based on the nature of the combustible material and requirements for extinguishment:

Class A: ordinary combustible solid materials, such as paper, wood, plastic, and fabric.
Class B: flammable liquids/gases and combustible petroleum products.
Class C: energized electrical equipment.
Class D: combustible/reactive metals, such as magnesium, sodium, and potassium.

Types/Applications of Fire Extinguishers

Just as fires have been divided into classes, fire extinguishers are divided into classes that correspond to the type of fire to be extinguished. Be certain to choose the right type—using the wrong type of extinguisher may be dangerous. For example, do not use water on burning liquids or electrical equipment.

Pressurized-water extinguishers, as well as foam and multipurpose dry-chemical types, are used for Class A fires. Multipurpose dry-chemical and carbon dioxide extinguishers are used for Class B and C fires. Halogenated hydrocarbon extinguishers are particularly recommended for use with computer equipment. Class D fires present special problems, and extinguishment is left to trained firefighters using special dry-chemical extinguishers (Fig. 2-4). Personnel should know the location and type of

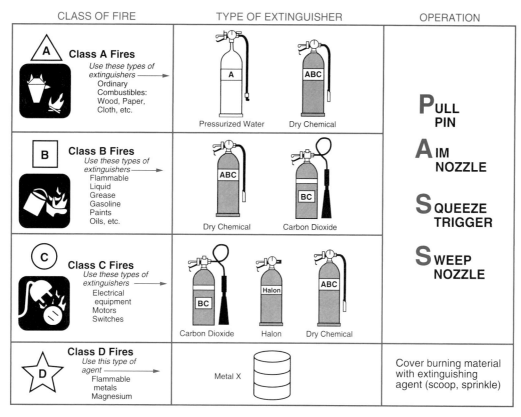

FIGURE 2-4. Proper use of fire extinguishers. (Adapted from the Clinical and Laboratory Safety Department, The University of Texas Health Science Center at Houston.)

portable fire extinguisher near their work area and know how to use an extinguisher before a fire occurs. In the event of a fire, first evacuate all personnel, patients, and visitors who are in immediate danger and then activate the fire alarm, report the fire, and attempt to extinguish the fire, if possible. Personnel should work as a team to carry out emergency procedures. Fire drills must be conducted regularly and with appropriate documentation.

CONTROL OF OTHER HAZARDS

Electrical Hazards

Most individuals are aware of the potential hazards associated with the use of electrical appliances and equipment. Hazards of electrical energy can be direct and result in death, shock, or burns. Indirect hazards can result in fire or explosion. Therefore, there are many precautionary procedures to follow when operating or working around electrical equipment:

- Use only explosion-proof equipment in hazardous atmospheres.
- Be particularly careful when operating high-voltage equipment, such as electrophoresis apparatus.
- Use only properly grounded equipment (three-prong plug).

- Check for frayed electrical cords.
- Promptly report any malfunctions or equipment producing a "tingle" for repair.
- Do not work on "live" electrical equipment.
- Never operate electrical equipment with wet hands.
- Know the exact location of the electrical control panel for the electricity to your work area.
- Use only approved extension cords and do not overload circuits. (Some local regulations prohibit the use of any extension cord.)
- Have ground checks and other periodic preventive maintenance performed on equipment.

Compressed Gases Hazards

Compressed gases, which serve a number of functions in the laboratory, present a unique combination of hazards in the clinical laboratory: danger of fire, explosion, asphyxiation, or mechanical injuries. There are several general requirements for safely handling compressed gases:

- Know the gas that you will use.
- Store tanks in a vertical position.
- Keep cylinders secured at all times.
- Never store flammable liquids and compressed gases in the same area.

- Use the proper regulator for the type of gas in use.
- Do not attempt to control or shut off gas flow with the pressure relief regulator.
- Keep removable protection caps in place until the cylinder is in use.
- Make certain that acetylene tanks are properly piped (the gas is incompatible with copper tubing).
- Do not force a "frozen" or stuck cylinder valve.
- Use a hand truck to transport large tanks.
- Always check tanks on receipt and then periodically for any problems such as leaks.
- Make certain that the cylinder is properly labeled to identify the contents.
- Empty tanks should be marked "empty."

Cryogenic Materials Hazards

Liquid nitrogen is probably one of the most widely used cryogenic fluids (liquefied gases) in the laboratory. There are, however, several hazards associated with the use of any *cryogenic material:* fire or explosion, asphyxiation, pressure buildup, embrittlement of materials, and tissue damage similar to that of thermal burns.

Only containers constructed of materials designed to withstand ultralow temperatures should be used for cryogenic work. In addition to the use of eye/face protection, hand protection to guard against the hazards of touching supercooled surfaces is recommended. The gloves, of impermeable material, should fit loosely so that they can be taken off quickly if liquid spills on or into them. Also, to minimize violent boiling/frothing and splashing, specimens to be frozen should always be inserted into the coolant very slowly. Cryogenic fluids should be stored in well-insulated but loosely stoppered containers that minimize loss of fluid resulting from evaporation by boil-off and that prevent plugging and pressure buildup.

Mechanical Hazards

In addition to physical hazards such as fire and electric shock, laboratory personnel should be aware of the *mechanical hazards* of equipment such as centrifuges, autoclaves, and homogenizers.

Centrifuges, for example, must be balanced to distribute the load equally. The operator should never open the lid until the rotor has come to a complete stop. Safety locks on equipment should never be rendered inoperable.

Laboratory glassware itself is another potential hazard. Agents, such as glass beads, should be added to help eliminate bumping/boilover when liquids are heated. Tongs or gloves should be used to remove hot glassware from ovens, hot plates, or water baths. Glass pipets should be handled with extra care, as should sharp instruments such as cork borers, needles, scalpel blades, and other tools. A glassware inspection program should be in place to detect signs of wear or fatigue that could contribute to breakage or injury. All infectious *sharps* must be disposed in OSHA-approved containers to reduce the risk of injury and infection.

Ergonomic Hazards

Although increased mechanization and automation have made many tedious and repetitive manual tasks obsolete, laboratory processes often require repeated manipulation of instruments, containers, and equipment. These physical actions can, over time, contribute to repetitive strain disorders such as tenosynovitis, bursitis, and ganglion cysts. The primary contributing factors associated with repetitive strain disorders are position/posture, applied force, and frequency of repetition. Remember to consider the design of hand tools (*eg,* ergonomic pipets), adherence to ergonomically correct technique, and equipment positioning when engaging in any repetitive task. Chronic symptoms of pain, numbness, or tingling in extremities may indicate the onset of repetitive strain disorders. Other hazards include acute musculoskeletal injury. Remember to lift heavy objects properly, keeping the load close to the body and using the muscles of the legs rather than the back. Gradually increase force when pushing or pulling, and avoid pounding actions with the extremities.

DISPOSAL OF HAZARDOUS MATERIALS

The safe handling and disposal of chemicals and other materials requires a thorough knowledge of their properties and hazards. Generators of hazardous wastes have a moral and legal responsibility, as defined in applicable local, state, and federal regulations, to protect both the individual and the environment when disposing of waste. There are four basic waste-disposal techniques: flushing down the drain to the sewer system, incineration, landfill burial, and recycling.

Chemical Waste

In some cases, it is permissible to flush water-soluble substances down the drain with copious quantities of water. However, strong acids or bases should be neutralized before disposal. Foul-smelling chemicals should never be disposed of down the drain. Possible reaction of chemicals in the drain and potential toxicity must be considered when deciding if a particular chemical can be dissolved or diluted and then flushed down the drain. For example, sodium azide, which is used as a preservative, forms explosive salts with metals, such as the copper, in pipes. Most institutions restrict the use of sodium azide due to this hazard.

Other liquid wastes, including flammable solvents, must be collected in approved containers and segregated into compatible classes. If practical, solvents such as xylene and acetone may be filtered or redistilled for reuse. If recycling is not feasible, disposal arrangements should be made by specifically trained personnel. Flammable material also can be burned in specially designed incinerators with afterburners and scrubbers to remove toxic products of combustion.

Also, before disposal, hazardous substances that are explosive, such as carcinogens and peroxides, should be transformed to less hazardous forms whenever feasible. Solid chemical wastes that are unsuitable for incineration must be buried in a landfill. This practice, however, has created an environmental problem, and there is now a shortage of safe sites.

Radioactive Waste

The manner of use and disposal of isotopes is strictly regulated by the Nuclear Regulatory Commission (NRC) and depends on the type of waste (soluble or nonsoluble), its level of radioactivity, and the radiotoxicity and half-life of the isotopes involved. The radiation safety officer should always be consulted about policies dealing with radioactive waste disposal. Many clinical laboratories transfer radioactive materials to a licensed receiver for disposal.

Biohazardous Waste

On November 2, 1988, President Reagan signed into law The Medical Waste Tracking Act of 1988. Its purpose was to (1) charge the Environmental Protection Agency with the responsibility to establish a program to track medical waste from generation to disposal, (2) define medical waste, (3) establish acceptable techniques for treatment and disposal, and (4) establish a department with jurisdiction to enforce the new laws. Several states have implemented the federal guidelines and incorporated additional requirements. Some entities covered by the rules are any health care-related facility including, but not limited to, ambulatory surgical centers; blood banks and blood drawing centers; clinics, including medical, dental, and veterinary; clinical, diagnostic, pathologic, or biomedical research laboratories; emergency medical services; hospitals; long-term-care facilities; minor emergency centers; occupational health clinics and clinical laboratories; and professional offices of physicians and dentists.

Medical waste is defined as *special waste from health care facilities* and is further defined as solid waste that, if improperly treated or handled, "may transmit infectious diseases" (For additional information, see the JCAHO Web site: www.jcaho.org). It comprises animal waste, bulk blood and blood products, microbiologic waste, pathologic waste, and sharps. The approved methods for treatment and disposition of medical waste

are incineration, steam sterilization, burial, thermal inactivation, chemical disinfection, or encapsulation in a solid matrix.

Generators of medical waste must implement the following procedures:

- Employers of health care workers must establish and implement an infectious waste program.
- All biomedical waste should be placed into a bag marked with the biohazard symbol and then placed into a leakproof container that is puncture resistant and equipped with a solid, tight-fitting lid. All containers must be clearly marked with the word *biohazard* or its symbol.
- All sharp instruments, such as needles, blades, and glass objects, should be placed into special puncture-resistant containers before placing them inside the bag and container.
- Needles should not be transported, recapped, bent, or broken by hand.
- All biomedical waste must then be disposed of by one of the recommended procedures.
- Potentially biohazardous material, such as blood or blood products and contaminated laboratory waste, cannot be directly discarded. Contaminated combustible waste can be incinerated. Contaminated noncombustible waste, such as glassware, should be autoclaved before being discarded. Special attention should be given to the discarding of syringes, needles, and broken glass that also could inflict accidental cuts or punctures. Appropriate containers should be used for discarding these sharp objects.

ACCIDENT DOCUMENTATION AND INVESTIGATION

Any accidents involving personal injuries, even minor ones, should be reported immediately to a supervisor. Under OSHA regulations, employers are required to maintain records of occupational injuries and illnesses for length of employment plus 30 years. The record-keeping requirements include a first report of injury, an accident investigation report, and an annual summary that is recorded on an OSHA injury log (Form 300).

The first report of injury is used to notify the insurance company and the human resources or employee relations department that a workplace injury has occurred. The employee and the supervisor usually complete the report, which contains information on the employer and injured person, as well as the time and place, cause, and nature of the injury. The report is signed and dated; then it is forwarded to the institution's risk manager or insurance representative.

The investigation report should include information on the injured person; a description of what happened; the cause of the accident (environmental or personal);

other contributing factors; witnesses; the nature of the injury; and actions to be taken to prevent a recurrence. This report should be signed and dated by the person who conducted the investigation.

Annually, a log and summary of occupational injuries and illnesses should be completed and forwarded to the U.S. Department of Labor, Bureau of Labor Statistics (OSHA Injury Log No. 300). The standardized form requests information similar to the first report of injury and the accident investigation report. Information about every occupational death, nonfatal occupational illness, biologic or chemical exposure, and nonfatal occupational injury that involved loss of consciousness, restriction of work or motion, transfer to another job, or medical treatment (other than first aid) must be reported.

Because it is important to determine why and how an accident occurred, an accident investigation should be conducted. Most accidents can be traced to two underlying causes: environmental (unsafe conditions) or personal (unsafe acts). Environmental factors include inadequate safeguards, use of improper or defective equipment, hazards associated with the location, or poor housekeeping. Personal factors include improper laboratory attire, lack of skills or knowledge, specific physical or mental conditions, and attitude. The employee's positive motivation is important in all aspects of safety promotion and accident prevention.

It is particularly important that the appropriate authority be notified immediately if any individual sustains a needle puncture during blood collection or a cut during subsequent specimen processing or handling. For a summary of recommendations for the protection of laboratory workers, refer to *Protection of Laboratory Workers from Instrument Biohazards and Infectious Disease Transmitted by Blood, Body Fluids and Tissue,* Approved Guideline M29-A2 (NCCLS).

SUMMARY

The cardinal safety rules of the clinical laboratory are to develop foresight and accident perception, use common sense, and develop and practice the following:

1. *Good personal behavior/habits.*
   Wear proper attire and protective clothing.
   Tie back long hair.
   Do not eat, drink, or smoke in the work area.
   Never mouth pipet.
   Wash hands frequently.
2. *Good housekeeping.*
   Keep work areas free of chemicals, dirty glassware, and so on.
   Store chemicals properly.
   Label reagents and solutions.
   Post warning signs.
3. *Good laboratory technique.*
   Do not operate new or unfamiliar equipment until you have received instruction and authorization.
   Read all labels and instructions carefully.
   Use the personal safety equipment that is provided.
   For the safe handling, use, and disposal of chemicals, learn their properties and hazards.
   Learn emergency procedures and become familiar with the location of fire exits, fire extinguishers, blankets, and so on.
   Be careful when transferring chemicals from container to container and always add acid to water slowly.

REVIEW QUESTIONS

1. Which of the following standards require that MSDSs are accessible to all employees who come in contact with a hazardous compound?
   a. Bloodborne Pathogen Standard
   b. Hazardous Communication Standard
   c. CDC Regulations
   d. Personal Protection Equipment Standard

2. Chemicals should be stored:
   a. alphabetically, for easy accessibility.
   b. inside a safety cabinet with proper ventilation.
   c. according to their chemical properties and classification.
   d. inside a fume hood, if toxic vapors can be released when opened.

3. Proper personal protective equipment (PPE) in the chemistry laboratory for routine testing includes:
   a. respirators with HEPA filter.
   b. gloves with rubberized sleeves.
   c. safety glasses for individuals not wearing contact lenses.
   d. impermeable lab coat with eye/face protection and appropriate disposable gloves.

4. A fire caused by a flammable liquid should be extinguished by using which type of extinguisher?
   a. Halogen
   b. Class B
   c. Pressurized water
   d. Class C

5. Which of the following is the proper means of disposal for the type of waste?
    a. Xylene into the sewer system
    b. Microbiologic waste by steam sterilization
    c. Mercury by burial
    d. Radioactive waste by incineration

6. What are the major contributing factors to repetitive strain injuries?
    a. Inattention on the part of the laboratorian
    b. Temperature and vibration
    c. Position/posture, applied force, and frequency of repetition
    d. Fatigue, clumsiness, and lack of coordination

7. Which of the following are examples of nonionizing radiation?
    a. Gamma rays and x-rays
    b. Ultraviolet light and microwaves
    c. Alpha and beta radiation
    d. Neutron radiation

SUGGESTED READINGS

Allocca JA, Levenson HE. Electrical and Electronic Safety. Reston, VA: Reston Publishing Company, 1985.

American Chemical Society, Committee on Chemical Safety, Smih GW, ed. Safety in Academic Chemistry Laboratories. Washington, D.C.: American Chemical Society, 1985.

Boyle MP. Hazardous chemical waste disposal management. Clin Lab Sci 1992;5:6.

Brown JW. Tuberculosis alert: An old killer returns. Med Lab Obs 1993;25:5.

Bryan RA. Recommendations for handling specimens from patients with confirmed or suspected Creutzfeldt-Jakob disease. Lab Med 1984;15:50.

Centers for Disease Control and Prevention, National Institutes of Health. Biosafety in Microbiological and Biomedical Laboratories, 3rd ed. Washington, D.C.: U.S. Government Printing Office, 1993.

Chervinski D. Environmental awareness: it's time to close the loop on waste reduction in the health care industry. Adv Admin Lab 1994;3:4.

Committee on Hazardous Substances in the Laboratory, Assembly of Mathematical and Physical Sciences, National Research Council. Prudent practices for handling hazardous chemicals in laboratories. Washington, D.C.: National Academy Press, 1981.

Furr AK. Handbook of Laboratory Safety, 5th ed. Boca Raton, FL: CRC Press, 2000.

Gile TJ. An update on lab safety regulations. Med Lab Obs 1995;27:3.

Gile TJ. Hazard-communication program for clinical laboratories. Clin Lab 1988;1:2.

Hayes DD. Safety considerations in the physician office laboratory. Lab Med 1994;25:3.

Hazard communication. Federal Register 59:27, Feb 4, 1994.

Karcher RE. Is your chemical hygiene plan OSHA proof? Med Lab Obs 1993;25:7.

Le Sueur CL. A three-pronged attack against AIDS infection in the lab. Med Lab Obs 1989;21:37.

Miller SM. Clinical safety: dangers and risk control. Clin Lab Sci 1992;5:6.

National Committee for Clinical Laboratory Standards. Clinical laboratory safety (approved guideline). Villanova, PA: NCCLS, 1996.

National Committee for Clinical Laboratory Standards. Clinical laboratory waste management (approved guideline). Villanova, PA: NCCLS, 1993.

National Committee for Clinical Laboratory Standards. Protection of laboratory workers from instrument biohazards and infectious disease transmitted by blood, body fluids, and tissue (approved guideline, M29-A). Villanova, PA: NCCLS, 1997.

National Institutes of Health, Radiation Safety Branch. Radiation: The National Institutes of Health safety guide. Washington, D.C.: U.S. Government Printing Office, 1979.

National Regulatory Committee, Committee on Hazardous Substances in the Laboratory. Prudent practices for disposal of chemicals from laboratories. Washington, D.C.: National Academy Press, 1983.

National Regulatory Committee, Committee on Hazardous Substances in the Laboratory. Prudent practices for the handling of hazardous chemicals in laboratories. Washington, D.C.: National Academy Press, 1981.

National Regulatory Committee, Committee on the Hazardous Biological Substances in the Laboratory. Biosafety in the laboratory: prudent practices for the handling and disposal of infectious materials. Washington, D.C.: National Academy Press, 1989.

National Safety Council. Fundamentals of Industrial Hygiene, 5th ed. Chicago, IL: National Safety Council, 2002.

Occupational exposure to bloodborne pathogens; final rule. Federal Register Dec 6, 1991;56:235.

OSHA Subpart Z 29CFR 1910.1000–.1450

Otto CH. Safety in health care: prevention of bloodborne diseases. Clin Lab Sci 1992;5:6.

Pipitone DA. Safe Storage of Laboratory Chemicals. New York: Wiley, 1984.

Rose SL. Clinical Laboratory Safety. Philadelphia: JB Lippincott, 1984.

Rudmann SV, Jarus C, Ward KM, Arnold DM. Safety in the student laboratory: a national survey of university-based programs. Lab Med 1993;24:5.

Stern A, Ries H, Flynn D, et al. Fire safety in the laboratory: Part I. Lab Med 1993;24:5.

Stern A, Ries H, Flynn D, et al. Fire safety in the laboratory: Part II. Lab Med 1993;24:6.

Wald PH, Stave GM. Physical and Biological Hazards of the Workplace. New York: Van Nostrand Reinhold, 1994.

Quality Control and Statistics

George S. Cembrowski
Roberta A. Martindale

CHAPTER OUTLINE

OBJECTIVES

Upon completion of this chapter, the clinical laboratorian should be able to:

- Define the following terms: quality assurance, quality control, control, standard, accuracy, precision, descriptive statistics, inferential statistics, reference interval, random error, systematic error, dispersion, delta check, and confidence intervals.
- Calculate the following: sensitivity, specificity, efficiency, predictive value, mean, median, range, variance, and standard deviation.
- Evaluate laboratory data using the multirule system for quality control.
- Graph the data and determine significant constant or proportional errors, given laboratory data.

- Describe the preanalytic and postanalytic phases of quality assurance.
- Determine if there is a trend or a shift, given laboratory data.
- Discuss the role of clinical laboratorians in point-of-care testing.
- Describe the important features/requirements of point-of-care analyzers.
- Discuss the processes involved in method selection and evaluation.
- Discuss proficiency-testing programs in the clinical laboratory.

KEY TERMS

Accuracy	Descriptive statistics	Predictive value theory	Reference method
Analytic variations	Dispersion	Proficiency testing	Shift
CLIA	F-test	Quality assurance	Standard
Control	Histogram	Quality control	Systematic error
Control rule	Inferential statistics	Random error	Trend
Delta check	Precision	Reference interval	t-test

STATISTICAL CONCEPTS

Statistics may be defined as the science of gathering, analyzing, interpreting, and presenting data. The volume of data generated by the clinical chemistry laboratory is enormous and must be summarized to be maximally useful to laboratorian and clinician. The introduction of a new test illustrates the extensive use of statistics in the laboratory. First, the laboratorian should introduce the test only after reviewing the data that document the usefulness of the test for diagnosing or monitoring a disease state. If several methods are available for performing the test, the laboratorian should study the published evaluations and select the most practical, as well as the optimally accurate and precise, method. During in-house evaluation of the method, precision and accuracy must be evaluated. If the method's performance is acceptable, reference-interval (normal range) data must be accumulated to verify the manufacturer's recommended interval or to set up a laboratory-specific reference interval. The clinician can then properly interpret patient data. Once the method is in use, accuracy and precision must be continually assessed to ensure reliable analyses. The following sections review some of the statistical concepts that must be understood by the laboratorian.

Descriptive Statistics

Descriptive statistics are used to summarize the important features of a group of data. Another type of statistics, *inferential statistics,* is used to compare the features of two or more groups of data. The descriptive statistics in this chapter are applied to groups of single observations as well as to groups of paired observations.

Descriptive Statistics of Groups of Single Observations

One of the most useful ways to summarize groups of data is by graphing them. Figure 3-1 shows the results obtained from the repeated analysis of a patient plasma specimen for the analyte antithrombin III (ATT), which is a potent inhibitor of many of the activated clotting factors. The results are plotted as a frequency *histogram*, with the value of the result plotted on the *x*-axis and the frequency (quantity) of each result plotted on the *y*-axis. The frequency histogram of the repeated measurements

should have a bell shape, with most of the results falling close to the center of the distribution. The repeated measurements of the same specimen can be different because of variations in instrument; reagent; operator technique; and even environmental conditions, including temperature. The laboratorian usually classifies these variations as *analytic* variations.

For most assays, the analytic variation is usually much lower than the variation among samples obtained from different individuals (the *interindividual variations*) or among timed samples obtained from the same individual (*the intraindividual variation*). Table 3-1 shows the results of a reference-interval study for ATT. The blood of fasting, healthy, ambulatory subjects was sampled in a standard manner, with the plasma analyzed for ATT. Frequency histograms of the ATT data are shown in Figure 3-2. The scale for the concentration is expressed in intervals of 2 units for Figure 3-2*A* and 5 units for Figure 3-2*B*. With a decreased number of intervals, the shape of the frequency histogram becomes more regular. Both histograms are bell-shaped and almost symmetric. The bell shape of this distribution approximates the shape of a gaussian distribution and allows analysis of the data by standard (parametric) statistical tests. Data that deviate greatly from the gaussian distribution should be analyzed with distribution-free statistics, also known as non-

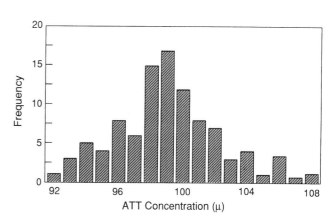

FIGURE 3-1. Frequency histogram of ATT results obtained from the repeated analysis of a single patient specimen ($\bar{x} = 100$; $s = 3$ units).

TABLE 3-1. ANTITHROMBIN III VALUES FROM A REFERENCE INTERVAL*

VALUE	FREQUENCY	CUMULATIVE FREQUENCY	VALUE	FREQUENCY	CUMULATIVE FREQUENCY
88	1	1	111	4	58
92	1	2	112	4	62
93	2	4	113	4	66
95	1	5	114	7	73
96	1	6	115	7	80
97	3	9	116	7	87
98	1	10	117	4	91
99	1	11	118	7	98
100	3	14	120	4	102
101	4	18	121	1	103
102	4	22	122	4	107
103	3	25	124	1	108
104	2	27	125	2	110
105	4	31	126	3	113
106	4	35	127	1	114
107	5	40	129	1	115
108	3	43	133	2	117
109	2	45	138	1	118
110	9	54	140	1	119

*Mean = 111.6; median = 112; mode = 110; s = 9.5 units.

parametric statistics. Small departures from gaussian distributions do not seriously affect the results of parametric statistical tests. The most common type of deviation from the gaussian distribution in clinical laboratory observations is *skewness*, or the presence of increased numbers of observations in one of the tails of the distribution. (An example of a skewed distribution is shown in Figure 3-9.)

Another type of plot is the *cumulative-frequency histogram*. In this plot, the number of observations that are less than or equal to a certain observation are plotted against the value of that observation. Figure 3-3 shows a

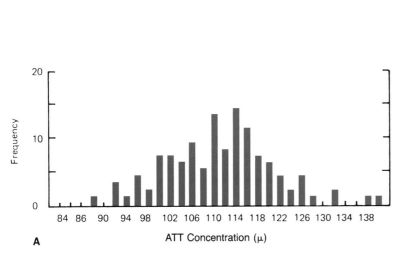

A

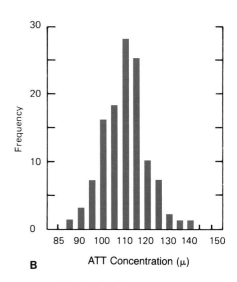

B

FIGURE 3-2. Frequency histograms of antithrombin III concentrations from a reference-interval study. The data in **A** have been grouped in intervals of 2 units. The data in **B** have been grouped by 5 units ($\bar{x}$ = 111.6; *s* = 9.5 units).

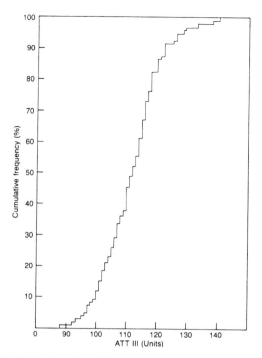

FIGURE 3-3. Cumulative frequency histogram for antithrombin III.

cumulative-frequency histogram for the normal-range ATT data. The cumulative frequencies in Table 3-1 have been divided by the total number of observations (n) and then multiplied by 100 to obtain *relative* cumulative frequencies that range from 0 to 100%.

Groups of gaussian observations can be described by statistics that summarize their location and dispersion. The most common statistical test that summarizes location is the *mean*, which is calculated by summing the observations and dividing by the number of the observations. If the observations are $x_1, x_2, x_3, \ldots, x_n$, then the mean, or $\bar{x}$, is

$$\bar{x} = \frac{x_1 + x_2 + x_3 + \cdots + x_n}{n}$$

$$= \frac{\Sigma x_i}{n} \qquad \text{(Eq. 3-1)}$$

Three other measures of location are commonly used: median, mode, and percentile. The *median* is the value of the observation that divides the observations into two groups, each containing equal numbers of observations. The values in the one group are smaller than the median, and those in the other are larger than the median. If the observations are arranged in increasing order and there are an odd number of observations, the median is the middle observation. If there is an even number of observations, the median is the average of the two innermost observations.

The *mode* is the most frequent observation. For the ATT data, the mean is 111.6, the median is 112, and the mode is 110 units. For data with approximately a gauss-

ian distribution, the mean, mode, and median are approximately equal and, therefore, reporting of the mean is usually sufficient. Data that are significantly non-gaussian should have the mode, median, and mean reported. The *percentile*, the only nonparametric statistic to be described in this chapter, is the value of an observation below which a certain proportion of the observations fall and which may be obtained from the relative cumulative-frequency histogram. Percentiles are often used to define the usual ranges for patient test results. The 5th percentile, or P_5, is the value below which 5% of the observations fall. For ATT, P_5 is 96. The 97.5 percentile, or $P_{97.5}$, is the value below which 97.5% of the observations fall. For ATT, $P_{97.5}$ is 133. The median is, of course, P_{50}. *Dispersion*, or the spread of data around its location, is most simply estimated by the range, which is the difference between the largest and smallest observations. The most commonly used statistic for describing the dispersion of groups of single observations is the *standard deviation*, which is usually represented by the symbol s. The standard deviation of the observations $x_1, x_2, x_3, \ldots, x_n$ is

$$s = \sqrt{\frac{\Sigma(\bar{x} - x_i)^2}{n - 1}} \qquad \text{(Eq. 3-2)}$$

Figure 3-4 shows an idealized frequency histogram of glucose quality control values, which have a mean of 120 and a standard deviation of 5 mg/dL. For these data, as well as for other data with gaussian distributions, approximately 68.2% of the observations will be between the limits of $\bar{x} - s$ and $\bar{x} + s$, 95.5% will be between $\bar{x} - 2s$ and $\bar{x} + 2s$, and 99.7% will be between $\bar{x} - 3s$ and $\bar{x} + 3s$. Additionally, 99% of the observations will be between $\bar{x} - 2.58s$ and $\bar{x} + 2.58s$. Limits can be constructed to include a specific proportion of the population. By convention, the usual limits for patient test results (reference range) include the inner 95% of the population and correspond to $\bar{x} - 1.96s$ and $\bar{x} + 1.96s$. For ATT, the 95% or $\pm 1.96s$ limits would be 92.5–130.6 or 92–131 units (U). The percentile also may be used to express dispersion. The percentile limits that would enclose 95% of the population would be $P_{2.5}$–$P_{97.5}$, or 93–133 U.

In Equation 3-2, calculation of s requires that the mean be calculated first. There is an alternate equation (Eq. 3-3) that does not need prior calculation of the mean:

$$s = \sqrt{\frac{n\Sigma x_i^2 - (\Sigma x_i)^2}{n(n - 1)}} \qquad \text{(Eq. 3-3)}$$

This equation is frequently used in computer programs to minimize computation time. Another way of expressing s is in terms of the coefficient of variation (CV), which is obtained by dividing s by the mean and multiplying by 100 to express it as a percentage:

$$\text{CV (\%)} = \frac{100s}{\bar{x}} \qquad \text{(Eq. 3-4)}$$

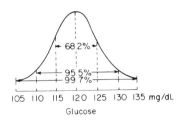

FIGURE 3-4. Idealized gaussian frequency histogram of glucose control values with a mean of 120 and standard deviation of 5 mg/dL. The percentages indicate the area under the curve bounded by the ± 1, ± 2, and ± 3, limits.

The CV, a unitless number, simplifies comparison of standard deviations of test results expressed in different units and concentrations. The CV of the glucose control data of Figure 3-4 is thus 100 times 5 mg/dL divided by 120 mg/dL, or 4.2%. The CV is used extensively to summarize quality control data. The CV of highly precise analyzers can be lower than 1%.

The *mean absolute deviation* (MAD), also known as the *average deviation*, is another measure of dispersion of groups of single observations and is calculated using the following equation:

$$\text{MAD} = \frac{\Sigma|x_i - \bar{x}|}{n} \qquad \text{(Eq. 3–5)}$$

The *standard deviation of the mean*, also called the *standard error of the mean* (SEM), is calculated from the following equation, in which n represents the number of observations averaged to calculate the mean:

$$\text{SEM} = \frac{s}{\sqrt{n}} \qquad \text{(Eq. 3–6)}$$

The SEM is used to calculate the statistical limits for the mean. The SEM can be interpreted as the average error encountered if the sample mean was used to estimate the population mean. The 95% limits for the mean $\bar{x}$ would be $\bar{x} \pm 1.96s/\sqrt{n}$. The SEM decreases as sample size increases, and the mean of a large sample is likely to

$$y = 1.0116x - 0.0071$$
$$R^2 = 0.9948$$

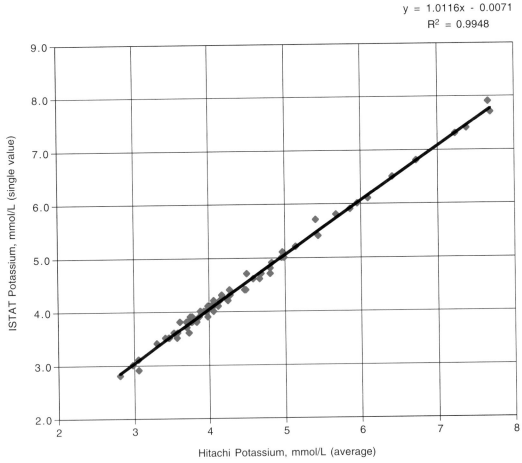

FIGURE 3-5A. Central laboratory ISTAT versus central laboratory Hitachi Graphic presentation of a comparison-of-methods experiment. Potassium measured by the Hitachi 917 (plasma specimen) is compared with potassium measured by the ISTAT (whole blood). Whole blood specimens were obtained from the emergency department, transported to the chemistry laboratory where the whole blood specimens were mixed with pairs of aliquots removed, one for ISTAT testing and the other separated into plasma for Hitachi analysis.

be closer to the true mean than the mean of a small sample.

Descriptive Statistics of Groups of Paired Observations

Perhaps the most informative step in the evaluation of a new analytic method is the comparison-of-methods experiment, in which patient specimens are measured by both the new method and the old, or comparative, method.[1] The data obtained from this comparison consist of two measurements for each patient specimen. Graphing is the simplest way to visualize and summarize the paired-method comparison data. By convention, the values obtained by the old (comparative) method are plotted on the x-axis and the values obtained by the new (test) method are plotted on the y-axis. Figure 3-5A shows a plot of potassium determinations performed using two different instruments: (1) the Hitachi 917, analyzing patient plasma specimens plotted on the x-axis; and (2) a point-of-care analyzer, the ISTAT, analyzing whole blood specimens plotted on the y-axis. There is a linear relationship between the two methods over the entire range of potassium values. There is an alternate approach to visualizing these paired data. Figure 3-5B shows a plot in which the differences between the comparative method and the test method values are plotted against the comparative method value. This plot is also known as an Altman-Bland[3] diagram. This approach per-

mits simple comparison of the differences to previously established maximum limits. In addition, any concentration-dependent differences can easily be seen.

In Figure 3-5A, the agreement between the two methods may be estimated from the straight line that best fits the points. Whereas visual estimation may be used to draw the line, the use of a statistical technique, *linear regression analysis*, will result in an impartial choice of line and will provide the laboratorian with measures of location and dispersion for the line. The straight line through the data will have the equation of

$$y = mx + y_0 \qquad \text{(Eq. 3–7)}$$

The slope of the line will be m; the value of the y intercept (the value of y at $x = 0$) will be y_0. If there is perfect agreement between the two methods, each test method value will be identical to the comparative method value. The equation of this perfect relationship would be $y = x$, with m being 1 and y_0 being 0. Figure 3-6A shows this perfect agreement. Figure 3-6B shows the situation in which values from the test method are consistently higher than those of the comparative method. The best line through the data still has a slope of 1 but a y intercept of 5.0. Figure 3-6C shows the situation in which values from the test method are higher than values from the comparative method for nonzero concentrations; the slope is greater than 1 (1.1), but the y intercept is 0. For increasing concentrations, there are

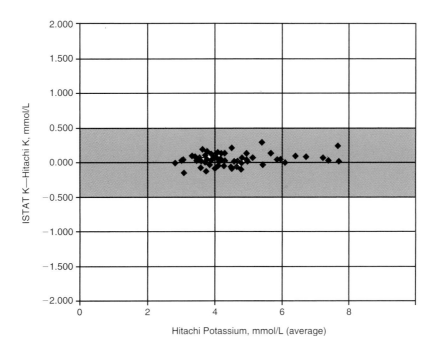

FIGURE 3-5B. Altman-Bland difference plot showing the differences between the ISTAT and the Hitachi 917 potassiums vs. the Hitachi 917 potassium.

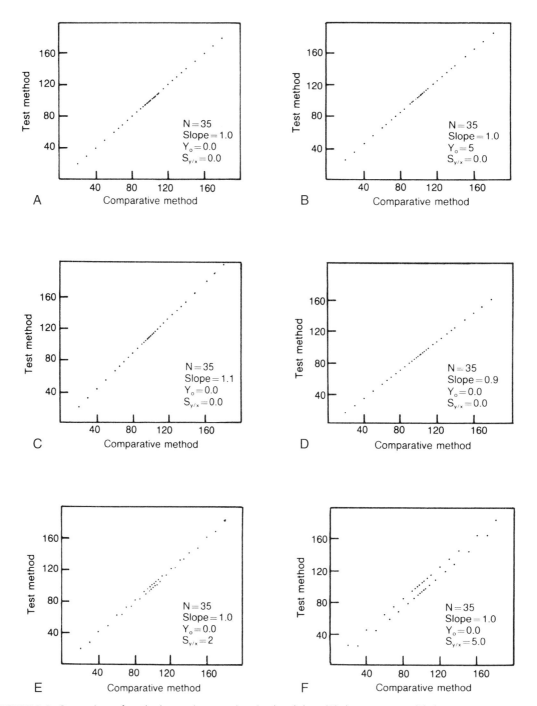

FIGURE 3-6. Comparison-of-methods experiments using simulated data. (**A**) shows no error; (**B**) shows constant error; (**C**) and (**D**) show proportional error; (**E**) and (**F**) show random error.

greater differences between the test and comparative values. In Figure 3-6D, the y intercept is still 0 and the slope is less than 1 (0.9), showing that the test-method values are lower than the comparative-method values for all nonzero values.

Linear regression analysis usually provides unbiased estimates of the slope and y intercept. In linear regression, the line of best fit is one that minimizes the sum of the squares of the vertical distances of the observed points from the line. For the points (x_1, y_1), (x_2, y_2), . . . , (x_i, y_i), . . . , (x_n, y_n), the equation of the slope of the regression line is

$$m = \frac{\Sigma(x_i - \bar{x})(y_i - \bar{y})}{\Sigma(x_i - \bar{x})^2}$$

$$= \frac{n\Sigma x_i y_i - \Sigma x_i \, \Sigma y_i}{n\Sigma x_i^2 - (\Sigma x_i)^2} \qquad \text{(Eq. 3–8)}$$

The y intercept is calculated from m and the means of x_i and y_i:

$$y_0 = \frac{\Sigma y_i}{n} - m\frac{\Sigma x_i}{n}$$

$$= \bar{y} - m\bar{x} \qquad \text{(Eq. 3-9)}$$

Linear regression assumes that there is no measurement error in the comparative method and that the spread (dispersion) of the points around the regression line is due to random errors in the test method. The dispersion of the points about the regression line is referred to as the *standard deviation* of the regression line and is abbreviated as $s_{y/x}$. Another name for this dispersion is the *standard error* of the estimate. It is calculated using the following equation:

$$S_{y/x} = \sqrt{\frac{\Sigma(y_i - Y_i)^2}{n - 2}} \qquad \text{(Eq. 3-10)}$$

The method-comparison plots in Figure 3-6E and F show the influence of increased scatter of points about the regression line. In Figure 3-6E and F, the value of either 2 or 5, respectively, was alternately added to or subtracted from the values of y in Figure 3-6A. The slope and intercept did not change. Only $s_{y/x}$ increased to 2 or 5, respectively.

The *correlation coefficient r* is a measure of the strength of the relationship between the y and x variables. The correlation coefficient can have values from -1 to $+1$, with the sign indicating the direction of relationship between the two variables. A positive r indicates that both variables increase or decrease together, whereas a negative r indicates that as one variable increases, the other decreases. An r value of 0 indicates no relationship. A value of 1.0 indicates a perfect relationship. The usual equation for the calculation of r is

$$r = \sqrt{\frac{n\Sigma x_i y_i - \Sigma x_i \Sigma y_i}{[n\Sigma x_i^2 - (\Sigma x_i)^2] \times [(n\Sigma y_i)^2 - (\Sigma y_i)^2]}} \qquad \text{(Eq. 3-11)}$$

Although many laboratorians equate high positive values of r (0.95 or higher) with excellent agreement between the test and comparative methods, most clinical chemistry comparisons should have correlation coefficients greater than 0.98. The absolute value of the correlation coefficient can be significantly increased by widening the range of samples being compared. The correlation coefficient does have a use, however. When r is less than 0.99, use of the regression formula results in an estimate of the slope that is too small and a y intercept that is too large. Waakers and associates have recommended that if r is less than 0.99, alternate regression statistics should be used to derive more realistic estimates of the regression, slope, and y intercept.[2-4]

Error accounts for the difference between test- and comparative-method results. Two kinds of error are measured in comparison-of-methods experiments: random and systematic. *Random error* is present in all measurements; can be either positive or negative; and is due to instrument, operator, reagent, and environmental variations. The measure of dispersion $s_{y/x}$ provides an estimate of random error. *Systematic error* is an error that influences observations consistently in one direction. Unlike random error, systematic error should not be present in a method. The measures of location, the slope and y intercept, provide measures of the systematic error.

Because $s_{y/x}$ is an estimate of the standard deviation about the regression line, statistical limits can be calculated for any point on the line. The 95% limits of any y value on the regression line are $y \pm 1.96s_{y/x}$. If $mx + y_0$ is substituted for y (Eq. 3-7), then the 95% limits are $mx + y_0 \pm 1.96s_{y/x}$.

There are two types of systematic error: constant error and proportional error. *Constant systematic error* exists when there is a constant difference between the test method and the comparative method values, regardless of the concentration. In Figure 3-6B, there is a constant difference of 5 between the test-method values and the comparative-method values. This constant difference, reflected in the y intercept, is called *constant systematic error*. *Proportional error* exists when the differences between the test method and the comparative method values are proportional to the analyte concentration. In Figures 3-6C and D, the difference between the test method and comparative method is proportional to the measured concentration. This difference, indicated by a slope different from unity, is due to proportional systematic error.

Inferential Statistics

The inferential statistical tests described in this chapter are used to compare the means or standard deviations of two groups of data. The t-*test*, described by Gosset in 1908, is used to determine whether there is a statistically significant difference between the means of two groups of data. The F-*test* is used to determine whether there is a statistically significant difference between the standard deviations of two groups of data. Both tests have limited usefulness in method-evaluation studies.

For both tests, a statistic is calculated and then compared with critical values found in the t and F tables of statistics books. The critical values define the significance level or the probability that the differences are due to chance. By convention, the t- or F-test is said to be *statistically significant* if the probability of the difference occurring due to chance is less than 5%. If the probability of the difference occurring due to chance exceeds 5%, then the difference is usually said to be *not statistically significant*. The lower the probability, the more statistically significant the difference. For example, a difference that occurs 1% of the time due to chance has greater significance than one that occurs 5% due to chance.

TABLE 3-2. CRITICAL *t* VALUES

SIGNIFICANCE LEVEL	TWO-TAILED	ONE-TAILED
5% (0.05)	1.96	1.64
1% (0.01)	2.58	2.33

To apply the *t*-test, the *t* statistic is calculated and compared with a table of critical *t* values for selected significance levels and degrees of freedom. Values of *t* should be obtained from the *t* table if a small number of observations (30 or fewer) are averaged. If more than 30 observations are averaged, the critical values are almost independent of the number of observations and depend primarily on the significance level. The critical values listed in Table 3-2 may be used if more than 30 observations are averaged.

If the calculated *t* statistic exceeds the critical value, then a significant difference is said to exist. The larger the difference, the larger will be the *t* statistic and the lower the probability that the difference is due to chance. The one-tailed critical values are used to test whether one mean of a group of numbers is either significantly greater or less than the other mean. The two-tailed critical values are used to test whether the means are significantly different.

In its simplest application, the *t*-test is used to determine whether the mean of a group of data ($\bar{x}$) is different from the true mean (abbreviated as M). The equation for the calculation of the *t* statistic is

$$t = \frac{|\bar{x} - M|}{s/\sqrt{n}}$$

Degrees of freedom = $n - 1$ **(Eq. 3–12)**

The *t* value is the absolute value of the difference of the true mean and the mean of the data divided by the SEM. For example, if the mean of a group of glucose quality control measurements was statistically evaluated and shown to be different from the usual mean value, the **two-tailed** critical *t* values would be used. If the calculated *t* value were less than 1.96, then the difference between the means would not be considered significant at the 5% level. A *t* value between 1.96 and 2.58 indicates a statistically significant difference; such a difference would occur due to chance, with a probability between 1% and 5%. A difference with a *t* value greater than 2.58 is more statistically significant and has less than a 1% probability of occurring due to chance. Most computer spreadsheet programs provide the *t*-test and the significance level.

The **one-tailed** critical values would be used to determine whether the mean of a group of data is either significantly larger or smaller than the true mean. For example, a laboratory physician may have several cholesterol values from a patient and may wish to determine whether these values are significantly greater than the upper limit of acceptability. After calculating the *t* value, the physician should use the table of one-tailed critical values.

In clinical chemistry, the *t*-test is sometimes applied to method-comparison data obtained by measuring patient specimens by both the test and the comparative methods. The measured values are averaged for each method, with the averages tested for a statistically significant difference. If x_i and y_i are the values obtained by the comparative and test methods, respectively, the *t* value for a group of paired observations $(x_1, y_1), (x_2, y_2), \ldots, (x_i, y_i), \ldots, (x_n, y_n)$ is

$$t = \frac{\dfrac{\Sigma y_i}{n} - \dfrac{\Sigma x_i}{n}}{s_d/\sqrt{n}}$$

$$= \text{bias}/(s_d/\sqrt{n}) \qquad \textbf{(Eq. 3–13)}$$

The numerator of the expression is the difference between the mean of the test method ($\Sigma y_i/n$) and the mean of the comparative method ($\Sigma x_i/n$). This difference between the means is called the *bias*. The symbol s_d stands for the standard deviation of the differences:

$$s_d = \sqrt{\frac{\Sigma[y_i - x_i - \text{bias}]^2}{n - 1}} \qquad \textbf{(Eq. 3–14)}$$

Equation 3-13 shows that the *t* value is the bias, or difference of the means, divided by the standard error of the mean. Westgard et al and Westgard and Hunt have shown that the interpretation of the *t*-test without regard for s_d and n may be misleading.[5,6] A statistically significant bias may exist between the methods, but its size may not be clinically significant. The user is cautioned to verify that the bias is both clinically and statistically significant.[6] Sometimes, the bias and s_d may be clinically large, but the resulting *t* value may be small. When interpreting the results of the *t*-test, all terms, bias, s_d, and *t* value must be critically evaluated.

The second inferential statistical test, the *F*-test, has been used to compare the sizes of the standard deviations of two methods. To calculate the *F* statistic, the square of the larger standard deviation (s_L) is divided by the square of the smaller standard deviation (s_S):

$$F = \frac{(s_L)^2}{(s_S)^2} \qquad \textbf{(Eq. 3–15)}$$

Like the *t*-test, the *F* statistic is then compared with critical *F* values in statistical tables that are tabulated by degrees of freedom and significance level. Because the *F*-test provides information about statistical significance but not clinical significance, Westgard and Hunt recommend that the *F* value should not be used as an indicator of acceptability of a test.[6] Rather, acceptability should depend on the size of random error.

REFERENCE INTERVALS (NORMAL RANGE)

Definition of Reference Interval

Physicians order laboratory tests for various reasons. The most important of these are diagnosis of disease, screening for disease, and monitoring of levels of drugs and endogenous substances such as electrolytes. Other reasons for testing include determining prognosis, confirming a previously abnormal test, physician education, and medicolegal purposes. When a test is used for diagnosis, screening, or prognosis, the test result is usually compared with a reference interval (normal range) that is defined as the usual values for a healthy population. For example, if a patient appears to have signs and symptoms of hypothyroidism, one of the follow-up tests ordered by the attending physician would be the serum thyroid-stimulating hormone (TSH). If the patient's TSH exceeds the upper reference limit, the diagnosis is consistent with primary hypothyroidism. Physicians may require further testing to determine the cause of the hyperthyroidism. When a test is used for monitoring, the test result is usually compared with values that were previously obtained from the same patient. For example, in patients with surgically removed colonic carcinomas, the presence of carcinoembryonic antigen (CEA) is often used to detect recurrence of the carcinoma. In these patients, each new CEA value is compared with previous CEA values. The acceptable range for the CEA values should be derived from the previous test values of each patient.[7]

The International Federation of Clinical Chemistry (IFCC) has recommended use of the term *reference interval* to denote the usual limits of laboratory data.[8] The presence of health is not implied in the definition, therefore, reference intervals may be constructed for ill as well as healthy populations. The IFCC recommends[8] that the following five factors be specified when reference intervals are established: (1) makeup of the reference population with respect to age, sex, and genetic and socioeconomic factors; (2) the criteria used for including or excluding individuals from the reference sample group; (3) the physiologic and environmental conditions by which the reference population was studied and sampled, including time and date of collection, intake of food and drugs, posture, smoking, degree of obesity, and stage of menstrual cycle; (4) the specimen-collection procedure, including preparation of the individual; and (5) the analytic method used, including details of its *precision* and *accuracy*. The IFCC considers the terms *normal values* and *normal range* to be specific reference intervals that correspond to the health-associated (central 95%) reference interval. As this chapter discusses the health-associated reference interval almost exclusively, we will use the terms *normal values, normal range,* and *reference range* and *reference interval* interchangeably. For an

overview of reference intervals, the reader is referred to the author's Web site: www.mylaboratoryquality.com.[9]

In the past, many hospital laboratories have either used the reference interval recommended by the instrument or test manufacturer or the values published in medical or laboratory textbooks. Because of the diversity of instrumentation, methodologies, reagents, and populations, it is important that large hospital laboratories determine their own reference intervals. Smaller laboratories will lack the resources to conduct such work; instead they should analyze far fewer specimens (at least 20) and verify the reference interval specified in the method's package insert, provided by the manufacturer.

The selection of subjects for the reference-interval study is important. Many laboratory data depend on age and sex. For example, plasma testosterone level is low in both prepubertal boys and girls and increases during puberty, attaining higher levels in boys. If a physician obtains a testosterone level to rule out a testosterone-secreting tumor in a pubertal girl, the physician must be able to compare the girl's testosterone value with normal values for girls of her age. Similarly, alkaline phosphatase levels are elevated during growth (Fig. 3-7),[10] as well as in men and women older than 60 years. Ideally, the laboratory should have age- and sex-stratified normal values for all populations tested. Thus, if a laboratory tests many specimens from older adults, proper reference intervals should be provided for this population.

To derive reliable estimates of reference intervals, at least 120 individuals should be tested in each age and sex category. However, it is often necessary to carry out reference range studies using fewer individuals. Sampling of 120 males and females would be adequate for determining the reference interval of an analyte that does not vary substantially with age and sex (eg, sodium). An analyte, such as creatine kinase, in which there are substantial

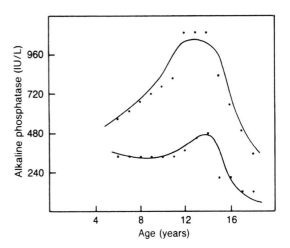

FIGURE 3-7. $P_{2.5} - P_{97.5}$ reference intervals for alkaline phosphatase in healthy boys determined by the Bowers-McComb method.[20]

differences between males and females, would require sampling of at least 120 males and 120 females. If reference intervals were desired for both males and females from birth to age 70 years, and if each age category equaled a 10-year interval, then the minimum number of individuals to be tested would be 100 subjects $\times$ 2 sexes $\times$ 7 age classifications, or 1400 subjects. Systematic testing of such a large number of subjects is almost always prohibitive. Winsten[11] has suggested that four age categories be used: newborns, prepubertal, adult population (postpubertal and premenopausal), and older adult population (males older than age 60 years and postmenopausal females). Although these divisions are not optimal, they reduce the number of tested categories. The dependence of alkaline phosphatase on age (shown in Figure 3-7) indicates that, unless there is further stratification of alkaline phosphatase by age, the prepubertal reference interval may be limited in usefulness.

Reference-interval studies on healthy children are limited because of the psychological and physical pain of phlebotomy. Many such studies are done on pediatric patients for whom serum and plasma samples are already available. Unfortunately, the diseases and treatments of these children can result in systematic shifts in their laboratory data. Use of their laboratory data can result in erroneous reference intervals. Because few centers can undertake systematic reference-interval studies on healthy newborns and children, we recommend that published reference values be used and compared critically with the clinical laboratory's adult reference values. Soldin et al[12] and Meites[13] have compiled reference values for pediatric patients in comprehensive monographs.

Collection of Data for Reference-Interval Studies

If reference-interval data are to be maximally useful, the reference population should consist of individuals in good health. Hospital employees are the most readily available healthy individuals for reference-interval studies but, unfortunately, there is a sampling bias, with the population consisting primarily of young and middle-aged females. Great effort often must be expended to recruit enough male adults. Once the desired reference population is identified, a consent form should be drafted and presented to the hospital's human subject experimentation committee or institutional review board so that volunteers can be recruited for donation of blood or other specimens.

Ideally, all potential donors should be interviewed to gather the following data: age, sex, health status, activity level, height and weight, alcohol consumption, drug usage (including oral contraceptives), smoking history, and stage of menstrual cycle. These interview data can then be used to exclude the donor or to explain an abnormal

value, such as an elevated CK in a training athlete. If a normal-range or health-associated reference interval is desired, pregnant individuals and those with acute or chronic disease should be excluded. The donors should be instructed about preparation before specimen collection. Fasting specimens are usually required, in which case the donor should be instructed not to eat after 10 p.m. and to drink only noncaloric, decaffeinated fluids before blood drawing. All donors should be sampled in a similar fashion, with care taken by the phlebotomist to not apply the tourniquet for longer than 1 minute. It should be noted that many analytes (eg, iron, ACTH [adrenocorticotropic hormone], and cortisol) exhibit significant diurnal variations. The time of sampling for these substances should be controlled.

The obtained samples must be labeled and handled in the same manner as the regular specimens. The instruments used to analyze these specimens should be in good running operation. Ideally, no more than 5–10 subjects should be sampled and analyzed daily. With this longer-term analysis, the normal range will reflect the long-term state of analytic control. Analysis over a short period may introduce *shifts* in the reference range due to transient instrument or reagent differences.

Statistical Analysis of the Reference-Interval Data

Rigorous Definition of the Reference Interval

The analysis of the large amount of data derived from reference-interval studies used to be very laborious. Today this task is simplified by the readily available microcomputer-based spreadsheet or statistical programs. The test data are first entered into the computer along with donor demographic data, such as identifier code, sex, and age. Frequency histograms then are plotted for all the tests. Results for individuals with outlying laboratory data should be forwarded to their physicians. If the reason for the outlying results is known (eg, the elevated CK in the athlete), the outlying results should be eliminated from further analysis.

Until approximately 1990, the standard practice was to plot the reference-interval data as cumulative-frequency histograms on probability paper and then derive reference intervals from the probability plot. Figure 3-2 shows frequency histograms of ATT. Figure 3-3 shows the cumulative-frequency histogram of ATT using a linear scale for the *y*-axis. Figure 3-8 shows a cumulative-frequency histogram for ATT plotted on probability paper. Cumulative frequency probability plots make gaussian distributions linear and enable drawing the best straight line through the points. Most reference-interval data have been used to determine the reference interval, and the effect of outliers is diminished. The outer 2.5% and 97.5% limits of the population are deter-

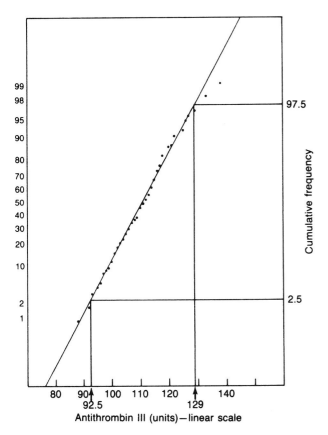

FIGURE 3-8. Probability plot for antithrombin III (linear scale).

mined by selecting values for ATT on the straight line that correspond to cumulative frequencies of 2.5% and 97.5%, respectively. In Figure 3-8, the 2.5–97.5 percentile limits are 92.5–129 U. If the distribution of the population is very smooth and gaussian, then the 95% limits also can be calculated directly from $\bar{x} \pm 1.96s$. In the case of ATT, the limits calculated in this manner are

115.6 $\pm$ 1.96 $\times$ 9.5 U, or 92.5–130.6 U. Alternately, the 95% limits can be determined from the 2.5 and 97.5 percentile limits (Fig. 3-3) or 93–133 U.

If the data are not gaussian, determination of the 95% limits is more difficult. Figure 3-9 shows a frequency histogram for γ-glutamyl transpeptidase (GGTP) in 118 females; Figure 3-10 presents its probability plot. The frequency histogram shows a skewing toward increased GGTP values. The nonlinear probability plot indicates a non-gaussian distribution. As percentiles do not depend on the shape of the distribution, they may be used to determine the 2.5% and 97.5% limits for the population. The 2.5 and 97.5 percentile limits for GGTP are 10 and 35 IU/L.

Since the early 1990s, enthusiasm has waned for deriving reference intervals with probability plots. At least three factors have inspired the laboratorian to use percentiles for setting up reference intervals: (1) the many sets of non-gaussian reference-interval data, (2) the complex nature of the construction and interpretation of probability plots, and (3) the National Committee for Clinical Laboratory Standards (NCCLS) document *Approved Guideline for How to Define and Determine Reference Intervals in the Clinical Laboratory (C28-A)*[14] that promotes the percentile approach.

Reference intervals are occasionally widened to include the lower limit of the analyte. For example, Figure 3-11 shows the frequency histogram and the probability plot for total bilirubin in 228 male and female subjects. The probability plot is nonlinear, so the 2.5 and 97.5 percentile limits are used to define the reference interval: 0.3–1.4 mg/dL. Because the published lower limit of bilirubin is usually 0 and because there are few, if any, pathologic reasons for a bilirubin of 0, the reference interval derived from these data is set as 0–1.4 mg/dL.

Occasionally, the results of a new reference-interval study may be quite different from the old reference inter-

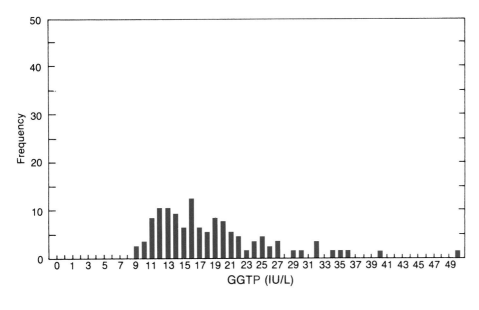

FIGURE 3-9. Frequency histogram of GGTP in 118 females. The corresponding probability plots are shown in Figure 3-10.

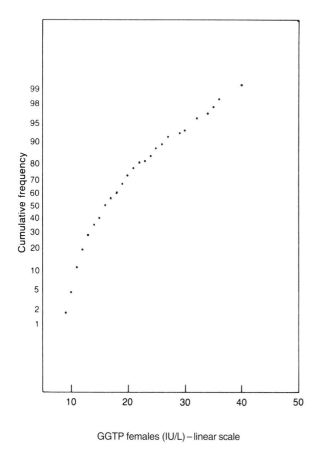

FIGURE 3-10. Probability plot for GGTP: linear scale.

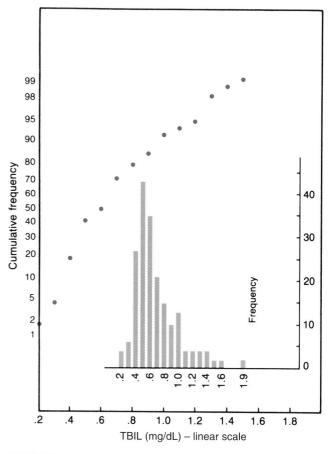

FIGURE 3-11. Frequency histogram of total bilirubin in 228 males and females (*inset*) and the corresponding probability plot (*linear scale*).

vals, even though the same instrument and methodology are used. Before making any adjustments in the reference interval, careful investigation must be undertaken to discover whether the analytic method or reference population has changed.

The distribution of hospitalized patient data has been analyzed by various computational methods in an attempt to derive health-associated reference intervals. Martin and associates have recommended that reference intervals be derived from the numeric analysis of distributions of patient data.[15] Problems exist in this approach to reference-interval determination and account for its lack of acceptance.

A normal range or health-associated reference interval is adequate for most tests. There are a few tests, such as glycosylated hemoglobin (HbA$_{1c}$), for which an alternate reference interval is desirable. HbA$_{1c}$ is a measure of an individual's average blood glucose level over the past 10 weeks; HbA$_{1c}$ is usually measured to determine and improve compliance to diet, exercise, and medication regimes. The frequency histogram in Figure 3-12 compares the HbA$_{1c}$ values of normal subjects with those of patients with diabetes. There is little overlap between nondiabetic and diabetic patients. The upper range of

normal has little significance to diabetic patients; many physicians use a somewhat arbitrary limit of less than 7% to designate excellent diabetic control. For HbA$_{1c}$, the most useful reference interval is probably that based on the patient's previous HbA$_{1c}$ values.

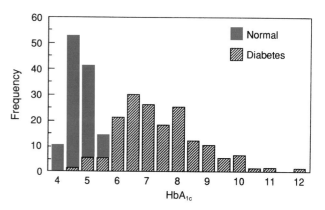

FIGURE 3-12. Comparison of frequency histograms of hemoglobin A$_{1c}$ for subjects with normal fasting glucoses and patients with diabetes.

Validation of the Reference Interval

Many laboratories do not have adequate resources to perform statistically rigorous reference-interval studies. Even without the data entry and analysis steps, the recruitment and sampling of a minimum of 120 subjects is demanding. Most manufacturers of clinical laboratory analyzers provide reference intervals for those analytes measured with their reagents. An individual laboratory does not need to develop its own reference interval for a new analyzer and reagents. Rather, it needs to do a much smaller validation study described in the same NCCLS document *C28-A*.[14] Only 20 reference individuals need to be sampled for analysis on a test instrument if the laboratorian determines that the test instrument and test subject population are similar to those described in the manufacturer's package insert. The manufacturer's reported 95% reference limits may be considered valid if no more than 2 of 20 tested subjects fall outside the original reported limits. If 3 or more test results are outside these limits, another 20 reference specimens should be obtained; if no more than 2 of these new results are outside the manufacturer's limits, then the manufacturer's limits can be used. If the second attempt at validation fails, the laboratorian should reexamine the analytic procedure and identify any differences between the laboratory's population and the population used by the manufacturer for the package insert information. If no differences are identified, the laboratory may need to do the full 120 individual reference-interval study.

DIAGNOSTIC EFFICACY

The material in this section allows the reader to analyze patient test data and to calculate a test's diagnostic sensitivity and specificity and predictive value. The reader also will be able to compare the diagnostic efficacies of various laboratory tests and to determine the most useful test.

Predictive Value Theory

Whereas the terms *diagnostic sensitivity, specificity,* and *predictive value* were used by radiologists beginning in the early 1950s, it was not until the 1970s that laboratorians became familiar with their meanings. Diagnostic sensitivity should not be confused with analytic sensitivity. For a test that is used to diagnose a certain disease, the *diagnostic sensitivity* is the proportion of individuals with that disease who test positively with the test. Sensitivity is usually expressed as a percentage:

$$\text{Sensitivity (\%)} = \frac{100 \times \text{the number of diseased individuals with a positive test}}{\text{total number of diseased individuals tested}}$$

(Eq. 3–16)

The specificity of a test is defined as the proportion of individuals without the disease who test negatively for the disease. The specificity (%) is defined as follows:

$$\text{Specificity (\%)} = \frac{100 \times \text{the number of individuals without the disease with a negative test}}{\text{total number of individuals tested without the disease}}$$

(Eq. 3–17)

Ideally, sensitivity and specificity should each be 100%. The sensitivity and specificity of a test depend on the distribution of test results for the diseased and nondiseased individuals and also the test values that define the abnormal levels. Figure 3-13 shows frequency histograms of prostate-specific antigen (PSA) of two patient populations. These two populations are subsets of a group of 4962 male volunteers, aged 50 years or older who were evaluated for the presence of prostate cancer by digital rectal examination of the prostate and a PSA measurement.[16] Of these volunteers, 770 had abnormal findings. The upper frequency histogram represents the subset of 578 patients with abnormal PSA values or abnormal digital rectal examinations who were biopsied for possible prostate cancer and found to be cancer-free. The lower frequency histogram represents the subset of 192 patients with abnormal PSA values or abnormal digital rectal examinations who were biopsied and found to have prostate cancer. It can be seen that, although patients with prostate carcinoma tend to have higher values of PSA, there is a great deal of overlap between the two populations.

The sensitivity and specificity can be calculated for any value of PSA. If high values of PSA are used to indicate the presence of disease (*ie,* if values exceeding 35 ng/mL are used to indicate prostate cancer), then the specificity of the test will be 100% (all the patients without prostate cancer are classified as negative using the test). The sensitivity, however, is low (2.6%), with only 5 of the 192 patients with carcinoma having PSA values greater than 35 ng/mL. The sensitivity can be increased by decreasing the test value. Therefore, if values of PSA in excess of 4.0 ng/mL (the accepted upper reference limit) are used to diagnose carcinoma, the sensitivity increases to 79%. The specificity, however, decreases to 46%. There are few laboratory tests with sensitivities and specificities close to 100%. The sensitivity and specificity of the MB fraction of creatine kinase for the diagnosis of myocardial infarction are approximately 95% each. Troponin, although having roughly the same sensitivity for diagnosing myocardial infarction, has an improved specificity, roughly 98%. Urine and serum human chorionic gonadotropin (hCG) pregnancy tests used in the clinical laboratory have sensitivities and specificities approaching 100%. Many tests have sensitivities and specificities that are close to 50%. Galen

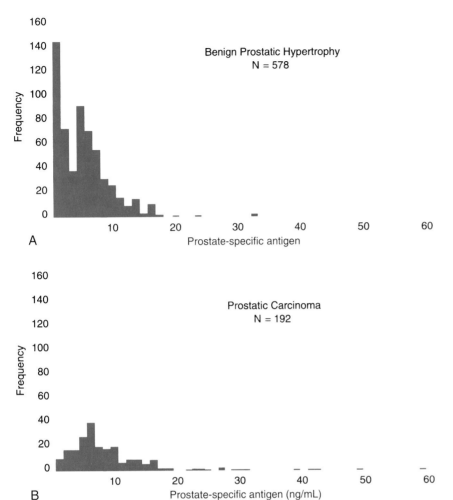

FIGURE 3-13. Frequency histograms of PSA results (Hybritech Tandem assay) of patients evaluated for possible prostate cancer. (**A**) The top plot shows the PSA of patients being biopsied without prostate cancer; (**B**) the bottom shows the PSA of patients with biopsy-positive prostate cancer. (Adapted from Catalona WJ, Richie JP, deKernion JB, et al. Comparison of prostate specific antigen concentration versus prostate specific antigen density in the early detection of prostate cancer: Receiver operating characteristic curves. J Urol 1994;152:2031.)

and Gambino have stated that if the sum of the sensitivity and specificity of a test is approximately 100%, the test is no better than a coin toss.[17]

The sensitivity and specificity may be calculated from simple ratios. Patients with disease who are correctly classified by a test to have the disease are called *true positives* (TP). Patients without the disease who are classified by the test not to have the disease are called *true negatives* (TN). Patients with the disease who are classified by the test as disease-free are called *false negatives* (FN). Patients without the disease who are incorrectly classified as having the disease are called *false positives* (FP). The sensitivity may be calculated from the formula 100 TP/(TP + FN). Specificity may be calculated from 100 TN/(TN + FP).

Three other ratios are important in evaluating diagnostic tests: predictive value of a positive test (PV+), predictive value of a negative test (PV−), and the efficiency. PV+ is that fraction of positive tests that are true positives: PV+ (%) = 100 TP/(TP + FP). PV− is that fraction of negative tests that are true negatives: PV−a (%) = 100 TN/(TN + FN). The efficiency of a test is the fraction of

all test results that are either true positives or true negatives: efficiency (%) = 100(TP + TN)/(TP + TN + FP + FN). The calculations for sensitivity, specificity, and predictive values for PSA exceeding 4.0 ng/mL are shown in Table 3-3. If a patient has a negative test result, he has an 87% probability of not having cancer. The probability that a patient has cancer if he has a positive test is rather low—approximately 33%.

The predictive value of a test can be expressed as a function of sensitivity, specificity, and disease prevalence, or the proportion of individuals in the population who have the disease:

$$PV^+ = \frac{\text{prevalence} \times \text{sensitivity}}{(\text{prevalence})(\text{sensitivity}) + (1 - \text{prevalence})(1 - \text{specificity})} \quad \textbf{(Eq. 3–18)}$$

The PV+ for PSA for various prevalences and a cutoff of 4.0 ng/mL (sensitivity =, specificity =) are shown in Table 3-4. It can be seen that, even in the situation in which disease has a high prevalence (0.2, or one fifth of

TABLE 3-3. SAMPLE CALCULATION OF SENSITIVITY, SPECIFICITY, PV⁺, PV⁻, AND EFFICIENCY CALCULATED FOR VALUES OF PSA OF >4.0 NG/ML

	NUMBER OF PATIENTS WITH POSITIVE PSA (>4.0 ng/mL)	NUMBER OF PATIENTS WITH NEGATIVE PSA (4.0 ng/mL)
Number of patients with prostate cancer	TP (151)	FN (41)
Number of patients without prostate cancer	FP (313)	TN (265)

Sensitivity = 100 × TP/(TP + FN) = 100 × 151/192 = 79%.
Specificity = 100 × TN/(TN + FP) = 100 × 265/578 = 46%.
PV⁺ = 100 × TP/(TP + FP) = 100 × 154/464 = 33%.
PV⁻ = 100 × TN/(TN + FN) = 100 × 265/306 = 87%.

the population), the probability that a positive test truly indicates carcinoma is only 27%.

Because the selection of a cutoff level to define disease has too often been arbitrary, it is preferable to calculate and plot sensitivity and specificity for all values of a test. This allows comparison of sensitivities of two or more tests at defined specificities or comparison of specificities for certain sensitivities. Receiver operating characteristic (ROC) curves, which are plots of sensitivity (true-positive rate) versus 1– specificity (false-positive rate), have been used to compare different laboratory tests.[18] Figure 3-14 illustrates two different ROC curves. Curve A is an ROC curve for a test in which there is wide separation between the test values of the diseased and nondiseased patients. Curve B illustrates the ROC curve obtained from a test for which there is little separation between diseased and nondiseased patients. The lower left part of the curve, where the false-positive rate is close to 0 (100% specificity) and the true-positive rate is close to 0 (0% sensitivity), corresponds to extreme test values in the diseased population. The upper right part of the curve, in which both the true-positive rate and the false-positive rate are high, corresponds to typical test values in the nondiseased population. For intermediate test values, a good test should have a high sensitivity (high true-positive rate) and a high specificity (low false-positive rate) and will form a ROC curve with points close to the

upper left-hand corner of the plot. Curve A corresponds to such a test. The test represented by curve B, in which the false-positive rate is equal to the true-positive rate, conveys no useful diagnostic information. Increasingly, clinical evaluations of diagnostic tests are being presented in the form of ROC curves. The NCCLS has published guidelines for clinically evaluating laboratory tests, including a comprehensive guide to ROC curves.[19]

Figure 3-15 shows the ROC curve of the PSA data of Figure 3-13. Also shown are the PSA concentrations at which the sensitivity and specificity were calculated. It can be seen that no PSA value offers both a high sensitivity and high specificity. Urologists are now recommending a more specific variant of the PSA test: the percentage of free PSA.[20]

TABLE 3-4. DEPENDENCE OF PREDICTIVE VALUE ON DISEASE PREVALENCE*

PREVALENCE OF DISEASE	PV⁺
0.001	0.1%
0.01	1.5%
0.10	14.0%
0.2	26.8%
0.5	59.4%

*Sensitivity = 79%; specificity = 46%.

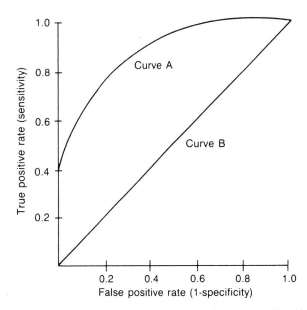

FIGURE 3-14. ROC curves. *Curve A* corresponds to a test with wide separation between the diseased and nondiseased patients. *Curve B* corresponds to a test that provides no additional information.

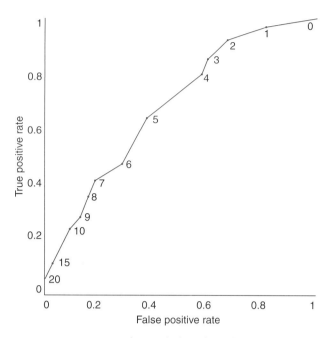

FIGURE 3-15. ROC curve for PSA (Hybritech Tandem assay) for the diagnosis of prostate cancer. (Adapted from Catalona WJ, Richie JP, deKernion JB, et al. Comparison of prostate specific antigen concentration versus prostate specific antigen density in the early detection of prostate cancer: receiver operating characteristic curves. J Urol 1994;152:2031.)

METHOD SELECTION AND EVALUATION

Method Selection

Before a new test or methodology is introduced into the laboratory, both managerial and technical information must be compiled and carefully considered. The information should be collected from many different sources, including manufacturer and sales representatives, colleagues, scientific presentations, and the scientific literature. The managerial information should include instrument cost, throughput, sample volume, personnel requirements, cost per test, specimen types, instrument size, and power and environmental requirements. The technical information must include analytic sensitivity, analytic specificity, detection limit, linear range, interfering substances, and estimates of imprecision and inaccuracy.

The *analytic sensitivity* or *detection limit* refers to the smallest concentration that can be measured accurately. One professional group has defined the *detection limit* as equal to three times the standard deviation of the blank, or as located three standard deviations above the measured blank.[21] *Specificity* refers to a method's ability to measure only the analyte of interest. The *linear range* (sometimes called the *analytic* or *dynamic range*) is the concentration range over which the measured concentration is equal to the actual concentration without modification of the method. The wider the linear range, the less

frequent will be specimen dilutions. Estimates of the inaccuracy of instruments may be obtained by studying the summaries of proficiency-testing programs that use fresh plasma or serum (misleading comparisons can be made from proficiency programs that analyze reconstituted lyophilized product). Estimates of intrainstrument imprecision are available from the group summary reports provided by vendors of quality control products.

Method Evaluation

When a method or instrument is brought in-house, the laboratorian must become proficient in its use. In advance of the complete evaluation, a short, initial evaluation should be carried out. This preliminary evaluation should include the analysis of a series of *standards* to verify the linear range and the replicate analysis (at least 8 measurements) of two controls to obtain estimates of short-term imprecision. If any results fall short of the specifications published in the method's product information sheet (package insert), the method's manufacturer should be consulted. Without improvement in the method, more extensive evaluations are pointless.[22] Figure 3-16 shows a simple data input form that can be used to simplify collection of method evaluation data.

When the method evaluation data are collected, the imprecision and inaccuracy of a method are estimated and compared with the maximum allowable error, which usually is based on medical criteria. If the imprecision or inaccuracy exceeds this maximum allowable error, the method is judged as unacceptable and must be modified and reevaluated or rejected. *Imprecision,* the dispersion of repeated measurements about the mean, is due to the presence of random analytic error. Imprecision is estimated from studies in which aliquots of a specimen with a constant concentration of analyte are analyzed repetitively. *Inaccuracy,* the difference between a measured value and its true value, is due to the presence of systematic analytic error, which can be either constant or proportional. Inaccuracy can be estimated from three studies: recovery, interference, and a comparison-of-methods study.

Measurement of Imprecision

The first step in method evaluation is the *precision* study. This study estimates the random error associated with the test method and points out any problems affecting reproducibility. It is recommended that this study be done over a 10- to 20-day period, incorporating one or two analytic runs per day.[23,24] An *analytic run* is defined as a group of patient specimens and control materials that are analyzed, evaluated, and reported together. Imprecision should be measured at more than one concentration, with control materials spanning the clinically meaningful range of concentrations. For example, glucose should be

PATIENT COMPARISONS:

COMPARATIVE METHOD: _____

TEST METHOD: _____

MID RANGE

	DATE	COMP	TEST
1			
2			
3			
4			
5			
6			
7			
8			
9			
10			
11			
12			
13			
14			
15			
16			
17			
18			
19			
20			
21			
22			
23			
24			
25			
26			
27			
28			
29			
30			

LO RANGE

	DATE	COMP	TEST
31			
32			
33			
34			
35			
36			
37			
38			
39			
40			
41			
42			
43			
44			
45			
46			
47			
48			
49			
50			
51			
52			
53			
54			
55			
56			
57			
58			
59			
60			

HI RANGE

	DATE	COMP	TEST
61			
62			
63			
64			
65			
66			
67			
68			
69			
70			
71			
72			
73			
74			
75			
76			
77			
78			
79			
80			
81			
82			
83			
84			
85			
86			
87			
88			
89			
90			

LINEARITY:

	A	B	C	D	E
TARGET					
1					
2					
3					
MEASURED					

PRECISION:

WITHIN RUN

	LO	MID	HI
1			
2			
3			
4			
5			
6			
7			
8			
9			
10			
$\overline{X}$			
SD			
CV			

CONTROL PRODUCT:_____
I: _____
II: _____
III: _____

BETWEEN RUN

	DATE	I	II	III
1				
2				
3				
4				
5				
6				
7				
8				
9				
10				
11				
12				
13				
14				
15				
16				
17				
18				
19				
20				
$\overline{X}$				
SD				
CV				

FIGURE 3-16. Data input form for method evaluation experiment. (Courtesy of Kristen Lambrecht.)

studied in the hypoglycemic (~50 mg/dL), and hyperglycemic (~150 mg/dL ranges).

Once the precision data are collected, the mean, standard deviation, and coefficient of variation are calculated. The random error or imprecision associated with the test procedure is indicated by the standard deviation and the coefficient of variation. The within-run imprecision is indicated by the standard deviation of the controls analyzed within one run. The total imprecision may be obtained from the standard deviation of control data with one or two data points accumulated per day. A statistical technique, analysis of variance, may be used to analyze all the available precision data to provide estimates of the within-run, between-run, and total imprecision.[25]

Measurement of Inaccuracy

When the short-term imprecision of the method is estimated and deemed adequate, the accuracy experiments[24] can begin. *Accuracy* can be estimated in three ways: recovery, interference, and patient-sample comparison studies. Recovery and interference studies should be performed and documented by the manufacturer. Because these two types of studies can be prohibitive in terms of effort and materials, they are usually performed in larger clinical laboratories. Recovery experiments will show whether a method measures all or only part of the analyte. In a recovery experiment, a test sample is prepared by adding a small aliquot of concentrated analyte in diluent to the patient sample. Another sample of the patient specimen is diluted by adding the same volume of diluent alone. Both diluted specimens are then analyzed by the test method. The amount recovered is the difference between the two measured values. Care should be taken to ensure that the original patient samples are diluted by no more than 10%; in this way, the solution matrix of the samples is minimally affected. The comparative method can also be used to measure the diluted specimens,[24] and, therefore, assure appropriate specimen preparation. Table 3-5 shows a sample calculation of recovery; the results are expressed as percentage recovered.

The interference experiment is used to measure systematic errors caused by substances other than the analyte. An interfering material can cause systematic errors several ways. The interferent may react with the analytic reagent or it may alter the reaction between the analyte and the analytic reagents. Hemolysis and turbidity can obscure the absorbance of the measured analyte. In the interference experiment,[26] the potential interferent is added to the patient sample. A sample calculation of interference is shown in Table 3-6. The concentration of the potentially interfering material should be in the maximally elevated range. If an effect is observed, its concentration should be lowered to discover the concentration at which test results are first invalidated. Materials to be tested should be selected from literature reviews and recent method-specific references.

Young[27] and Siest and Galteau[28] have published extensive listings of the effects of drugs on laboratory tests. Common interferences (eg, hemoglobin, lipids, bilirubin, anticoagulants, and preservatives) also should be tested by the manufacturer. Glick and Ryder[29,30] have presented "interferographs" for various chemistry instruments—these graphs relate analyte concentration measured versus interferent concentration. They have demonstrated that tens of thousands of dollars of rework can be saved by the acquisition of instruments that minimize hemoglobin, triglyceride, and bilirubin interference.[31]

Comparison-of-Methods Experiment

In a comparison-of-methods study, patient samples are analyzed by the method being evaluated (test method) and a comparative method. The quality of the comparative method will affect the interpretation of the experimental results. The best comparative method is the *reference method*; a method with negligible inaccuracy in comparison with its imprecision. Reference methods may be laborious and time-consuming (eg, the reference method for cholesterol). Because most laboratories are not staffed and equipped to perform reference methods, the results of the test method are usually compared with those of the method routinely in use. The routine method will have certain inaccuracies, both known and unknown, depending on how well the laboratory has studied them or how well the method is documented in the literature. If the test method will be replacing the comparative method, the differences between the two methods should be well characterized.

TABLE 3-5. EXAMPLE OF A RECOVERY STUDY

Sample Preparation

Sample 1: 2.0 mL serum + 0.1 mL H₂O

Sample 2: 2.0 mL serum + 0.1 mL 20 mg/dL calcium standard

Sample 3: 2.0 mL serum + 0.1 mL 50 mg/dL calcium standard

Concentration

	CALCIUM MEASURED	CALCIUM ADDED	CALCIUM RECOVERED	% RECOVERY
Sample 1	7.50 mg/dL			
Sample 2	8.35 mg/dL	0.95 mg/dL	0.85 mg/dL	89
Sample 3	9.79 mg/dL	2.38 mg/dL	2.29 mg/dL	96

Calculation of Recovery

$$\text{Concentration added} = \text{standard concentration} \times \frac{mL\ standard}{mL\ standard + mL\ serum}$$

$$\text{Concentration recovered} = \text{concentration (diluted test)} - \text{concentration (baseline)}$$

$$Recovery = \frac{\text{concentration recovered}}{\text{concentration added}} \times 100\%$$

TABLE 3-6. EXAMPLE OF AN INTERFERENCE STUDY

Sample Preparation

Sample 1: 1.0 mL serum + 0.1 mL H$_2$O

Sample 2: 1.0 mL serum + 0.1 mL of 10 mg/dL magnesium standard

Sample 3: 1.0 mL serum + 0.1 mL of 20 mg/dL magnesium standard

	CALCIUM MEASURED	MAGNESIUM ADDED	INTERFERENCE
Sample 1	9.80 mg/dL		
Sample 2	10.53 mg/dL	0.91 mg/dL	0.73 mg/dL
Sample 3	11.48 mg/dL	1.81 mg/dL	1.68 mg/dL

Calculation of Interference

$$\textit{Concentration added} = \textit{standard concentration} \times \frac{\textit{mL standard}}{\textit{mL standard} + \textit{mL serum}}$$

Inference = concentration (diluted test) − concentration (baseline)

Westgard et al[24] and the NCCLS[32] recommend that between 40 and 100 samples be run by both methods, spanning the clinical range and representing many different pathologic conditions. Duplicate analyses of each sample by each method are recommended, with the duplicate samples analyzed in different runs and in a different order of analysis on the two runs. Analysis by both methods should be performed on the same day, preferably within 4 hours.

If duplicates are not analyzed, the validity of the experimental results must be checked by comparing the test and comparative-method results immediately after analysis, identifying those samples with large differences, and, if necessary, repeating the analyses. If 40 specimens are compared, two to five patient specimens should be analyzed daily for a minimum of 8 days. If 100 specimens are compared, the comparison study should be carried out during the 20-day replication study.

A graph of the test-method data (plotted on the y-axis) versus the comparative-method data (plotted on the x-axis) helps to visualize the method comparison data (Fig. 3-5). Data should be plotted on a daily basis and inspected for linearity and outliers. In this way, original samples can be available for reanalysis. Visual confirmation of linearity is usually adequate; in some cases, however, it may be necessary to evaluate linearity more quantitatively.[33] Many analysts have used the F-test, the paired t-test, and the correlation coefficient for the interpretation of the experimental data. The F-test is used to compare the magnitude of the imprecision of the test method with that of the imprecision of the comparative method. The paired t-test is used to compare the magnitude of the bias (the difference between the means of the test and that of the comparative method) with that of the random error. Both the F-test and t-test indicate only whether a statistically significant difference exists between the two standard deviations or means, respectively.

They provide no information about the magnitude of the existing error relative to the clinically allowable limits of error.[6]

Despite regular admonishments about the misuse of the correlation coefficient r, laboratorians continue to use it as an indicator of the acceptability of the test method. The value of r can be increased by increasing the range of the patient specimens. The main application of the correlation coefficient in method-evaluation studies should be in determining the type of regression analysis to be used. If the correlation coefficient is 0.99 or greater, the range of patient samples is adequate for the standard linear regression analysis described in the statistics section. If r is less than 0.99, then alternate regression analysis should be used.[1,34,35] Linear regression analysis is far more useful than the t-test and F-test for evaluating method-comparison data.[6] The constant systematic error can be estimated from the y intercept, proportional systematic error from the slope, and random error from the standard error of the estimate ($s_{y/x}$). If there is a nonlinear relationship between the test and comparative values, then linear regression can only be used over the linear range. Because outlying points are weighted more heavily in linear regression, it is important to ensure that these outliers are genuine and not the result of laboratory error.

When all of the imprecision and inaccuracy estimates are calculated, they are compared with predefined limits of medically allowable analytic error.[36] If the random and systematic error is smaller than the allowable error, the performance is considered acceptable. If the error is larger than the allowable error, the errors must be reduced or the method rejected.

The allowable analytic error represents total error and includes components of both random and systematic error. Many approaches have been used to estimate medically allowable error, including using multiples of the ref-

TABLE 3-7. PERFORMANCE STANDARDS FOR COMMON CLINICAL CHEMISTRY ANALYTES AS DEFINED BY THE CLIA[41]

Calcium, total	Target ± 1.0 mg/dL
Chloride	Target ± 5%
Cholesterol, total	Target ± 10%
Cholesterol, HDL	Target ± 30%
Glucose	Greater of target ± 6 mg/dL or ± 10%
Potassium	Target ± 0.5 mmol/L
Sodium	Target ± 4 mmol/L
Total protein	Target ± 10%
Triglycerides	Target ± 25%
Urea nitrogen	Greater of target ± 2 mg/dL or ± 9%
Uric acid	Target ± 17%

erence interval,[37] using pathologist opinions,[38] and physiologic variation.[39,40] Under federal law, the Clinical Laboratory Improvement Amendments of 1988 (*CLIA* 88), the Health Care Financing Administration (HCFA) has published allowable errors for a wide array of clinical laboratory tests.[41] Although the CLIA-allowable error limits are used to specify the maximum error allowable in federally mandated *proficiency testing*, these limits are now being used as guidelines to determine the acceptability of clinical chemistry analyzers.[42,43] Table 3-7 shows the CLIA limits for common clinical chemistry tests. Westgard et al[36] have recommended two different sets of criteria for the evaluation of error: *confidence-interval* criteria and single-value criteria. Because of the complexity of confidence-interval criteria, the reader is referred to the original description.[44] The single-value criteria are found in Table 3-8. In using the single-value criteria, estimates of the random error and systematic error are calculated and

TABLE 3-8. SINGLE-VALUE CRITERIA OF WESTGARD ET AL[58]

ANALYTIC ERROR	CRITERION
Random error (RE)	$2.58\,s < E_A$
Proportional error (PE)	$|\,(\text{Recovery} - 100) \times X_0/100)\,| < E_A$
Constant error (CE)	$|\,\text{Bias}\,| < E_A$
Systematic error (SE)	$|\,(y_0 + mX_c) - X_0\,| < E_A$
Total error	$2.58\,s + |\,(y_0 + mX_c) - X_c\,| < E_A$
(TE = RE + SE)	

E_A = medically allowable error.
X_c = critical concentration.

then compared to the allowable error. The error estimates depend on the concentration of analyte measured and are usually calculated at critical concentrations of the analyte. In applying these performance criteria, the random and systematic error must be less than the allowable error for a method to be judged acceptable. Otherwise, the analytic method must be rejected or modified to reduce the error. As an ultimate criterion, Westgard et al[36] suggested a total-error criterion, which combines random and systematic components of error, to estimate the magnitude of error that can be expected when a patient specimen is measured. The use of the single-value criteria is illustrated in Table 3-9, in which whole blood potassium measured by a point-of-care method is compared with central laboratory plasma potassium. The method-evaluation experiment for this comparison is plotted in Figure 3-5. The CLIA error limit for potassium is 0.5 mmol/L.

Currently, there is disagreement regarding the selection of the multiplier of the standard deviation in the random error calculation. Westgard et al originally suggested 1.96, which permits 5% of observations to be outside of the allowable error limits. Choice of just a slightly larger multiplier would allow considerable fewer outliers; for example, if the multiplier was 2.58, no more than 1% of the observations could be outside the allowable error limits. The CLIA regulations forced laboratorians to reevaluate the proportion of acceptable outliers that they would accept, which fell outside of the CLIA limits. Clinical laboratories are at high risk of failing proficiency testing if they use analyzers that produce 5% of results that deviate by more than the CLIA limits. In our laboratory, we are now using 2.58 and are recommending all laboratories use a multiplier of at least 2.58 to calculate random error. Although some authors have proposed multipliers as high as 4.0, most of today's instruments cannot achieve such performance. Before a method can be put into routine use, the manufacturer's reference range must be validated or even reestablished, the procedure must be written or updated, and personnel should be trained to use the method. A statistical quality control program should be implemented for the procedure, using the accumulated control data to establish quality-control limits. It may be necessary to adjust the control limits once the procedure is in routine service.

Because of constraints of personnel, time, and budget, a laboratory may be unable to perform comprehensive comparison-of-methods experiments on every new method introduced. An understanding of the principles of method evaluation and a familiarity with statistical tests will allow the laboratory supervisor to choose a method that would probably fit the laboratory's performance criteria.[45] A series of abbreviated experiments could then be undertaken to estimate imprecision and inaccuracy.[3]

The NCCLS recently published guidelines for just such an abbreviated application. This protocol, the User

TABLE 3-9. EXAMPLE OF THE APPLICATION OF THE SINGLE-VALUE CRITERIA OF WESTGARD ET AL[36] TO POTASSIUM EVALUATION DATA*

1. Random error (RE) = 2.58 s.
   Random error is estimated from analyzing a control product once daily for 20 days.

   $$X = 5.5 \text{ mmol/L, } s = 0.07 \text{ mmol/L}$$
   $$RE = 2.58 \times s$$
   $$= 2.58 \times 0.07 \text{ mmol/L}$$
   $$= 0.18$$

   Because RE $<E_A$, RE is acceptable.

2. Proportional error (PE) = | (Recovery − 100) × $(X_c/100)$ |.
   Proportional error is estimated from a series of recovery experiments, after which the average recovery is calculated.

   $$\text{Average recovery for potassium} = 99\%$$
   $$PE = | (99 - 100) \times (5.5/100) |$$
   $$= 0.05 \text{ mmol/L}$$

3. Constant Error (CE) = bias.
   Constant error is estimated from the bias | $Y − X$ |, derived from the comparison-of-methods experiment.

   $$CE = | Y - X |$$
   $$= | 5.31 - 5.28 |$$
   $$= 0.03 \text{ mmol/L}$$

   Because CE E_A, CE is acceptable.

4. Systematic Error (SE) = | $(Y_o + mX_c) − X_c$ |.

   Systematic error is estimated from the above equation in which Y_o and m are derived from a comparison-of-methods experiments (Fig. 3-5).

   $$Y_0 = -0.057, \, m = 1.02$$
   $$SE = | (-0.057 + 1.02 \times 5.5) - 5.5 |$$
   $$= | 5.55 - 5.5 |$$
   $$= 0.05$$

   Because SE E_A, SE is acceptable.

5. Total error (TE) = RE + SE.
   Total error is estimated from the sum of RE and SE as calculated above.

   $$TE = 0.18 + 0.05$$
   $$= 0.23 \text{ mmol/L}$$

   Because TE $<E_A$, the method is acceptable.

*Allowable error (E_A) for potassium, as defined in the CLIA Regulations, is 0.5 mmol/L.

Demonstration of Precision and Accuracy, can be used to demonstrate that a laboratory can obtain precision and accuracy performance consistent with the manufacturer's claims. Because these precision and accuracy studies can be completed in 5 working days, it is likely many laboratories will use the guidelines for setting up new methods.

QUALITY ASSURANCE AND QUALITY CONTROL

The *quality control system* is the laboratory's system for recognizing and minimizing analytic errors.[46,47] Quality control is one component of the *quality assurance system,* which has been defined as all systematic actions necessary to provide adequate confidence that laboratory services will satisfy given medical needs for patient care.[48] The quality assurance system encompasses preanalytic, analytic, and postanalytic factors. The monographs *Laboratory Quality Management* (Cembrowski and Carey),[49] *Cost-Effective Quality Control* (Westgard and Barry),[50] and *Basic QC Practices* (Westgard)[1] provide detailed information about quality control and quality assurance practices in the clinical chemistry laboratory.

There are many preanalytic factors that can influence analytic results, including patient preparation, sample collection, sample handling, and storage. Young provides the most comprehensive reviews of preanalytic factors on chemistry tests.[27,51] Preanalytic factors are difficult to monitor and control because most occur outside the laboratory. Health care professionals, especially physicians and nurses, should become more aware of the importance of patient preparation and how it can affect laboratory tests. Patient preparation for a test is critical. For example, nutritional status, a recent meal, alcohol, drugs,[27] smoking, exercise, stress, sleep, and posture all affect various laboratory tests. The laboratory must provide instructions, usually in the form of a procedure manual,[52] for proper patient preparation and specimen acquisition. This procedure manual should be found in all nursing units and, therefore, be available to all medical personnel. Additionally, easy-to-understand patient handouts must be available for outpatients.

Specimen-collection procedures should follow specific guidelines such as those established by the NCCLS.[53–56] Blood-collection teams should be periodically inserviced about the guidelines for duration of application of tourniquets and the types of specimen-collection tubes and anticoagulants to be used. Methods of specimen transport, separation, aliquoting, and storage are critical.[57,58] The length of time elapsed between drawing and separation of the serum or plasma from the cells can be a factor in analytic testing. For example, leukocytes and erythrocytes metabolize glucose and cause a steady decrease in glucose concentration in clotted, uncentrifuged blood. The centrifuging and aliquoting of samples to secondary containers may be critical.[55,58] Contamination of the specimen may occur at this point, rendering a suboptimal specimen for analytic testing. For example, secondary containers for specimens submitted for lead analysis must be scrupulously clean because of the ubiquitous presence of lead and the low levels of lead that must be accurately measured.

Specimen storage also may lead to errors in the reported results. Guidelines on storage requirements for specimens should be established for each analyte. Specimens may be affected by evaporation (eg, electrolytes), exposure to light (eg, bilirubin), refrigeration (eg, lactate dehydrogenase [LD]), and freezing. Clerical errors may occur at any step in the processing of specimens. Although the use of computers has simplified clerical tasks, one specimen may still be mistaken for another. Obviously, such mistakes should be minimized.

The laboratorian can at least control the analytic factors, which primarily depend on instrumentation and reagents. A schedule of daily and monthly preventive maintenance is essential for each piece of equipment. Routinely performed instrument function checks should be detailed in the procedure manual and their performance should be documented. The NCCLS has developed standards for monitoring variables such as water quality,[59] calibration of analytic balances, calibration of volumetric glassware and pipets, stability of electrical power,[60] and the temperature of thermostatically controlled instruments.[61] Reagents and kits should be dated when received and also when opened. New lots of reagents should be run in parallel with old reagent lots before being used for analysis.

If the reagents are to be used as standards or calibrators, the most highly purified chemicals, reagent grade or American Chemical Society (ACS) grade, should be used. Different types of standards are available. A *primary standard* is a stable, nonhygroscopic (does not absorb water), highly purified substance that can be dried, preferably at 104°C to 110°C without a change in composition. Primary standards can thus be dried and then weighed to prepare solutions of selected concentrations. When purchased, primary standards are supplied with a record of analysis for contaminating elements, which should not exceed 0.05% by weight. Some standards have been certified to be pure by various official bodies such as the National Institute for Standardization and Technology (NIST) and the College of American Pathologists (CAP).

A *primary standard* is the most highly purified substance currently available that can be accurately weighed analytically. A *secondary standard* is one whose concentration is usually determined by analysis by an acceptable reference method that is calibrated with a primary standard. Its concentration cannot be determined directly from the weight of solute and volume of solution. Calibrators are used in calibration processes to establish concentrations of patient specimens. Calibration materials should meet the identity, labeling, and performance requirements of NCCLS guideline *Tentative Guideline for Calibration Materials in Clinical Chemistry* (C22).[62] Whenever possible, calibrators should have their concentrations assigned through the use of either reference methods or other very specific methods. The compara-

tive analytic response of the calibrator and the specimens provides the basis for calculating values for patient specimens. The same material should not serve as calibrator and control.

Laboratory error can be minimized if attention is paid to proper laboratory procedures and techniques. The quality control system for individual test methodologies can focus on controlling the test-specific variables. The postanalytic factors consist of the recording and reporting of the patient data to the physician within the appropriate time interval. With automation and computer-generated patient reports, the incidence of errors in the postanalytic phase has decreased greatly.

Quality Control

The purpose of the quality control system is to monitor analytic processes, detect analytic errors during analysis, and prevent the reporting of incorrect patient values. Analytic methods are usually monitored by measuring stable control materials and then comparing the measured values with their expected value. The laboratory's budget must reflect the importance of quality control. The monetary commitment is important to ensure an adequate system for monitoring and improving the laboratory's performance. The statistical system used to interpret the measured concentrations of the controls is called the *statistical quality control system*. The principles of statistical quality control were established by Shewhart[63] early in the last century. In 1950, Levey and Jennings[64] used these same basic principles when they introduced statistical quality control to the clinical laboratory. Since 1950, statistical quality control systems in the laboratory have undergone many modifications.

Analytic error may be separated into random-error and systematic-error components (Fig. 3-17). *Random error* affects precision and is the basis for varying differences between repeated measurements. Increases in random error may be caused by variations in technique. *Systematic error* arises from factors that contribute a constant difference, either positive or negative. Systematic error can be caused by several factors, including poorly made standards or reagents, failing instrumentation, and poorly written procedures.

Quality control materials should behave like real specimens, be available in sufficient quantity to last a minimum of 1 year, be stable during that period, be available in convenient vial volumes, and vary minimally in concentration and composition from vial to vial.[65] The *control* material should closely resemble the specimen it is simulating both physically and chemically. The control material should be tested in the same manner as patient specimens. Control materials should span the clinically important range of the analyte's concentrations. Levels of the control should be at appropriate decision levels; for

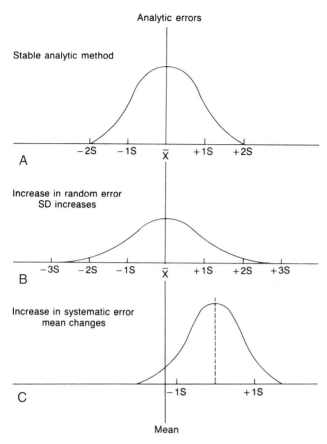

Analytic errors

Stable analytic method

A   −2S   −1S   X̄   +1S   +2S

Increase in random error
SD increases

B   −3S   −2S   −1S   X̄   +1S   +2S   +3S

Increase in systematic error
mean changes

C   −1S   +1S

Mean

FIGURE 3-17. Schematic representation of distributions of control data. (**A**) represents the situation with no analytic error; (**B**) represents increased random error; (**C**) represents systematic shift.

example, for sodium, they might be at 130 and 150 mmol/L, levels that define hyponatremia and hypernatremia. For general chemistry quality control, two levels of control are typically used; for immunochemistry, three levels are often used. The control manufacturer may assay its controls with various instruments and methodologies and then make available target ranges for its control products. While these "assayed" controls are more expensive, they can be used as external checks for accuracy.

Most commercially prepared control materials are lyophilized and require reconstitution before use. In reconstitution, the diluent should be carefully added and mixed. Incomplete mixing yields a partition of supernatant liquid and underlying sediment and will result in incorrect control values. Frequently, the reconstituted material will be more turbid (cloudy) than the actual patient specimen. Stabilized frozen controls do not require reconstitution but may behave differently from patient specimens in some analytic systems. It is important to carefully evaluate these stabilized controls with any new instrument system.

At one time, chemistry laboratories prepared all their control materials.[66] Compared with commercial controls,

these "homemade" control materials are more susceptible to deterioration and contamination. It is difficult to minimize the infectious disease risk of such materials. On occasion, it is necessary to prepare control pools for selected analytes, such as uncommonly assayed drugs. Proper procedures should be followed,[66] but the task is more manageable because far smaller quantities are required than for a laboratory-wide pool.

Most control materials are produced from human serum. With greater emphasis placed on cost containment, more laboratories are using bovine-based control materials, which are lower in price than the human-based materials. The stability of bovine-based control materials is similar to that of human-based materials. For most analytes, bovine material meets the necessary requirements for monitoring imprecision.[67] Because bovine proteins differ greatly from human proteins, bovine material is inappropriate for immunochemistry assays of specific proteins. Similarly, bovine material is inappropriate for some dye-binding procedures for albumin and certain bilirubin methods. Bovine-based material can be used as a control in electrophoresis, but its electrophoretic pattern differs from that of human control serum and resembles a polyclonal gammopathy.

General Operation of a Statistical Quality Control System

The statistical quality control system in the clinical laboratory is used to monitor and control the analytic variations that occur during testing. In certain instances, these variations may be systematic and are caused by procedural errors due to technique, instrumentation, or failures of reagents or other materials. In other instances, however, increased random variations may appear despite tightly controlled, well-calibrated analytic methods.

The statistical quality control program can be thought of as a three-stage process:

1. Establishing allowable statistical limits of variation for each analytic method.
2. Using these limits as criteria for evaluating the quality control data generated for each test.
3. Taking remedial action when indicated (*eg*, finding causes of errors, rectifying them, and reanalyzing control and patient data).

To establish statistical quality control on a new instrument or on new lots of control material, the different levels of control material must be analyzed between 5 and 20 days. For assays that are highly precise (CV ≤1%) like blood gases, 5 days are adequate; for less precise assays, 10–20 days are needed. The means (x̄) and standard deviations (s) of these control data are then calculated. Because of the small number of observations and possible outliers in the new control data, these initial estimates may not be totally reliable and should be revised as more data become available. When changing to a new lot of similar material, many laboratorians use the newly obtained mean as the target mean but retain the previous standard deviation used. As more data are obtained, all of the data should be averaged to derive the best estimates of the mean and standard deviation.[68]

Control values may be compared numerically or visually with statistical limits on a control chart. This chart is simply an extension of a gaussian distribution curve (Fig. 3-18), with time expressed on the x-axis. The y-axis usually is scaled to provide concentrations made from $\bar{x} - 3s$ to $\bar{x} + 3s$. Horizontal lines corresponding to multiples of s are drawn around the x-axis. The 2s lines correspond to the 95.5% limits for the control. If the analytic process is in control, approximately 95% of the points will be within these limits and approximately 5% of the points will be outside these limits. The 3s limits correspond to approximately the 99.7% limits. If the process is in control, no more than 0.3% of the points will be outside the 3s limits. An analytic method is considered to be in control when there is symmetrical distribution of control values about the mean and there are few control values outside the 2s control limits. Some laboratories define an analytic method to be out of control if a control value fell outside its 2s limits. Other laboratories have used the 2s limits as warning limits and 3s limits as error limits. For these laboratories, a control value between 2s and 3s would alert the technologist to a potential problem. A point outside the 3s limits would require corrective action.

Different criteria have been used to judge whether control results indicate out-of-control situations. Westgard and Grothhave studied the error-detection capabilities of most of these criteria.[69] They used the term *control rule* to indicate the criterion for judging whether the analytic process is out of control. To simplify comparison of the various control rules, Westgard and associates used abbreviations for the different control rules. Table 3-10 frequently used control rules and their abbreviations. The abbreviations have the form A_L, where A is a symbol for a statistic or is the number of control observations per analytic run and L is the control limit.[70] For example, a 1_{2s} rule violation indicates the situation in which one control observation is outside the $\bar{x} \pm 2s$ limits. An *analytic run* is defined as a set of control and patient specimens assayed, evaluated, and reported together.

Ideally, if a method is in control, none of the control rules should be violated and there should be no rejection of the analytic run. Unfortunately, some analytic runs will be rejected as out of control even when there is no additional analytic error. For example, when the 1_{2s} control rule is used with only one control being analyzed per analytic run, then 5% of the runs will be outside the 2s limits when only the usual analytic variation is present. When more than one control is analyzed in an analytic run and no additional error is present, the probability becomes higher that at least one control is outside the 2s limits. When two controls are used, there is approximately a 10% chance that at least one control will be outside the 2s limits; when four controls are used, there is a 17% chance. For this reason, many analysts usually do not investigate the analytic method if a single control exceeds the 2s limits when two or more controls are used. They merely re-assay the controls or the entire analytic run.

Unfortunately, this intuitive approach to quality control achieves an unknown level of quality. What is needed is a control system that will reliably signal the presence of significant analytic error but will not respond to small errors. Defining such a control system requires an understanding of the response of control rules to analytic error.

Response of Control Rules to Error

Westgard and associates[69] have studied the response of control rules, either singly or in groups, to the presence of error, either systematic or random. Different control procedures (groups of control rules) have distinct re-

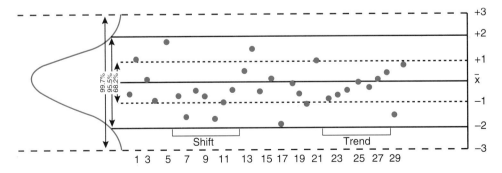

FIGURE 3-18. Control chart showing the relationship of control limits to the gaussian distribution. Daily control values are graphed, and they show examples of a shift, an abrupt change in the analytic process, and a *trend,* a gradual change in the analytic process.

TABLE 3-10. POPULAR CONTROL RULES

1_{2s}	Use as a rejection or warning when one control observation exceeds the $\bar{x} \pm 2s$ control limits; usually used as a warning.	Overused. Should only be used with manual assays with low number of analytes/control materials
1_{3s}	Reject a run when one control observation exceeds the $\bar{x} \pm 3s$ control limits.	Detects random error and large systematic error
2_{2s}	Reject a run when two consecutive control observations are on the same side of the mean and exceed the $\bar{x} + 2s$ or $\bar{x} - 2s$ control limits.	Detects systematic error
4_{1s}	Reject a run when four consecutive control observations are on the same side of the mean and exceed either the $\bar{x} + 1s$ or $\bar{x} - 1s$ control limits.	Detects small systematic error; very few applications
$10_{\bar{x}}$	Reject a run when ten consecutive control observations are on the same side of the mean.	Detects very small errors; do not use
R_{4s}	Reject a run if the range or difference between the maximum and minimum control observation out of the last 4–6 control observations exceeds $4s$.	Detects random errors; use within run
$\bar{x}_{0.01}$	Reject a run if the mean of the last N control observations exceeds the control limits that give a 1% frequency of false rejection ($P_{fr} = 0.01$).	Underutilized
R0.01	Reject a run if the range of the last N control observations exceeds the control limits that give a 1% frequency of false rejection ($P_{fr} = 0.01$).	Underutilized

s, standard deviation; $\bar{x}$, mean.

sponses, depending on the control rules and number of control observations (n) used. Westgard and Groth[71] simulated the analysis of control materials by instruments with varying levels of error. A large number of simulations were done at each error level, with the proportion of out-of-control situations tabulated and then plotted against the size of the error. The resulting graphs, depicting probability of rejection versus size of analytic error, are called *power functions*. Ideally, a control rule should have a 0% probability of detecting small errors and a 100% probability of detecting significant error. Figure 3-19A shows a graph of a family of power functions for the detection of systematic error by the 1_{2s} control rule. The probability of rejection is plotted against the size of the systematic error. The size of the systematic error ranges from 0 to 5s, where s is the standard deviation. The different lines correspond to different numbers of controls analyzed. When one control is used and there is no error, the probability of rejection in the absence of error is approximately 5%. The probability of rejection when no error is present is called the probability of false rejection (P_{fr}). The probability of error detection (P_{ed}) is the probability of rejecting an analytic run as out of control when an error exists. The P_{ed} can be determined for any size error by locating the size of the error on the *x*-axis and erecting a vertical line that intersects the power-function curve for the desired n. From this intersection,

a horizontal line is drawn to the *y*-axis. The value of the probability on the *y*-axis is the P_{ed}. In Figure 3-19A, P_{ed} for the 1_{2s} control rule and a systematic error of 2s is 0.5 if one control is analyzed. The power-function graphs may be used to determine the effectiveness of various control procedures in detecting analytic errors. Two sets of power functions are necessary, one for systematic error (shift of the mean) and one for the random error (increase in imprecision). Figure 3-19B shows a family of power functions for the detection of random error by the 1_{2s} control rule. Because analytic processes always contain random error, the *x*-axis originates at 1s. In Figure 3-19B, P_{ed} for the 1_{2s} control rule and a doubling of the random error is 0.3 if one control is analyzed. The best control procedure is the one with the lowest P_{fr} and the highest P_{ed} for detecting analytic errors of a size that can compromise the quality of analytic results. Figure 3-19 shows the power function for ideal procedure. Although the 1_{2s} control rule results in a high detection of moderate-sized systematic errors, its P_{fr} is unacceptably high. Figures 3-20A and B show power functions for the 1_{3s} control rule for systematic and random error, respectively. The 1_{3s} control rule is less responsive to moderate increases in systematic error but has a low P_{fr}.

Westgard and associates have suggested a manual implementation of a combination of control rules with at least two control observations per analytic run.[68] In addi-

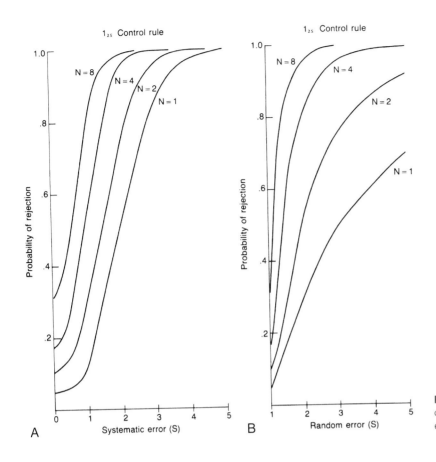

FIGURE 3-19. Power function curves for the 1_{2s} control rule for systematic error (**A**) and random error (**B**). (Provided by P. Douville)

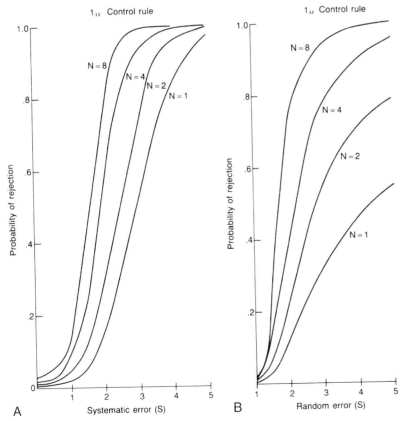

FIGURE 3-20. Power function curves for the 1_{3s} control rule for systematic error (**A**) and random error (**B**). (Provided by P. Douville)

tion to using the 1_{2s} rule as a warning rule and the 1_{3s} rule for rejection, this system also included the 2_{2s}, R_{4s}, 4_{1s}, and $10_{\bar{x}}$ rules. The counting rules (the 2_{2s}, 4_{1s}, and $10_{\bar{x}}$ rules) are effective in detecting systematic error. *As the 4_{1S} and 10_x rules detect small, usually clinically unimportant shifts that are exhibited by most analyzers, we do not recommend their use.* The R_{4s} and 1_{3s} rules are effective in detecting random error. The 1_{3s} rule also can detect systematic error. Examples of the violations of all of the above rules are shown in Figure 3-21.

To apply the classic Westgard multirule control procedure manually, all new control results are evaluated to ensure that they are within their $\pm2s$ limits. If they are,

there is no further inspection. Otherwise, the other rules are applied in this order: 2_{2s}, 4_{1s}, $10_{\bar{x}}$, and R_{4s}. The 2_{2s} rule is invoked whenever two consecutive control observations on the same side of the mean exceed either the $\bar{x} + 2s$ or $\bar{x} - 2s$ control limits. This rule responds most often to systematic errors. The 2_{2s} rule is initially applied to the control observations within the most recent analytic run (across materials and within run). The rule can then be applied to the last two observations on the same control material but from consecutive runs (within materials and across runs) or it can be applied on the last two consecutive observations of the different control materials (across materials and across runs).

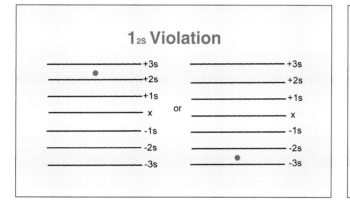

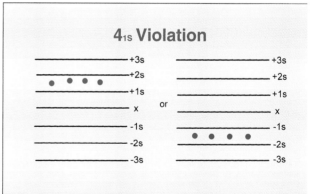

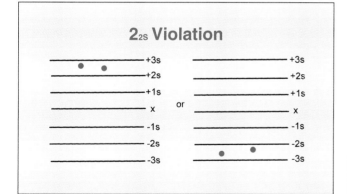

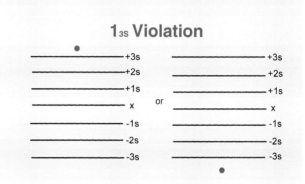

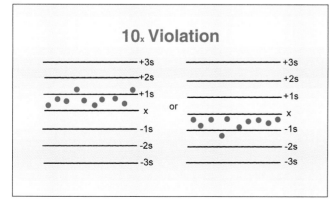

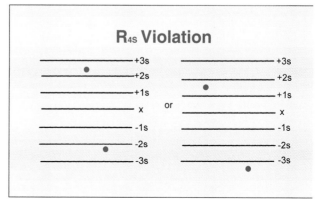

FIGURE 3-21. Examples of violations of the 6 rules comprising the Westgard multirule control procedure.

The 4_{1s} rule is violated when four consecutive control observations on the same side of the mean exceed the $\bar{x} + 1s$ or $\bar{x} - 1s$ control limits. It is most responsive to systematic errors. This rule is applied within and across materials and runs. The $10_{\bar{x}}$ rule is sensitive to systematic error and is violated when 10 consecutive control observations fall on one side of the mean. This rule is applied within materials and across runs, as well as across materials and across runs.

The R_{4s} rule is violated when the range or difference between the highest and lowest control observations within the run exceeds 4_s. This rule is most responsive to random error or increased imprecision. The rule is invoked when one control observation material exceeds a $+2s$ limit and the other observation exceeds a $-2s$ limit. The two observations are outside 2s limits but in opposite directions, resulting in a range that exceeds 4s. The range rule is intended for use within a single run with a maximum of four to six control observations, not across runs.

The combination of the 1_{2s}, 1_{3s}, 2_{2s}, 4_{1s}, $10_{\bar{x}}$, and R_{4s} control rules used in conjunction with a control chart has been called the *multirule Shewhart procedure*. The power functions for this multirule procedure are shown in Figure 3-22. This multirule procedure yields increased error detection over the use of the 1_{3s} rule alone. The inclusion of the 1_{3s} and R_{4s} rules improves the detection of random error, and the 2_{2s}, 4_{1s}, and $10_{\bar{x}}$ rules increase the detection of systematic error. When used with imprecise

systems, this multirule procedure has provided the laboratory with improved error detection and less false rejection of analytic runs. It was easily adapted to existing control procedures and has become extremely popular since its initial description in 1981.

Implementation of the multirule procedure involves the following:

1. Calculation of the means and standard deviations of the different concentrations of control materials.
2. Construction of control charts, with lines indicating the 0, ± 1, 2, and 3 standard deviation limits.
3. Analysis of the different levels of control material in each analytic run, with plotting of the control data on the appropriate chart.
4. Accepting the analytic run if each observation falls within 2s limits.
5. Checking the 1_{3s}, 2_{2s}, R_{4s}, 4_{1s}, and $10_{\bar{x}}$ rules for violations if one of the control materials is outside its 2s limits. If none of the rules is violated, the run is accepted. If a violation has occurred, the run is rejected, with the most likely type of error determined (random versus systematic). Once the error condition is identified and corrected, the patient and control specimens are reanalyzed.

Figure 3-23 shows a two-level control chart that simplifies implementation of the multirule procedure. Application of the multirule procedure to a two-level control

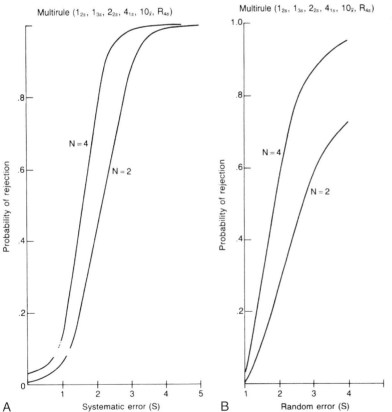

FIGURE 3-22. Power functions for the multirule control procedure for systematic error (**A**) and random error (**B**). (Provided by P. Douville)

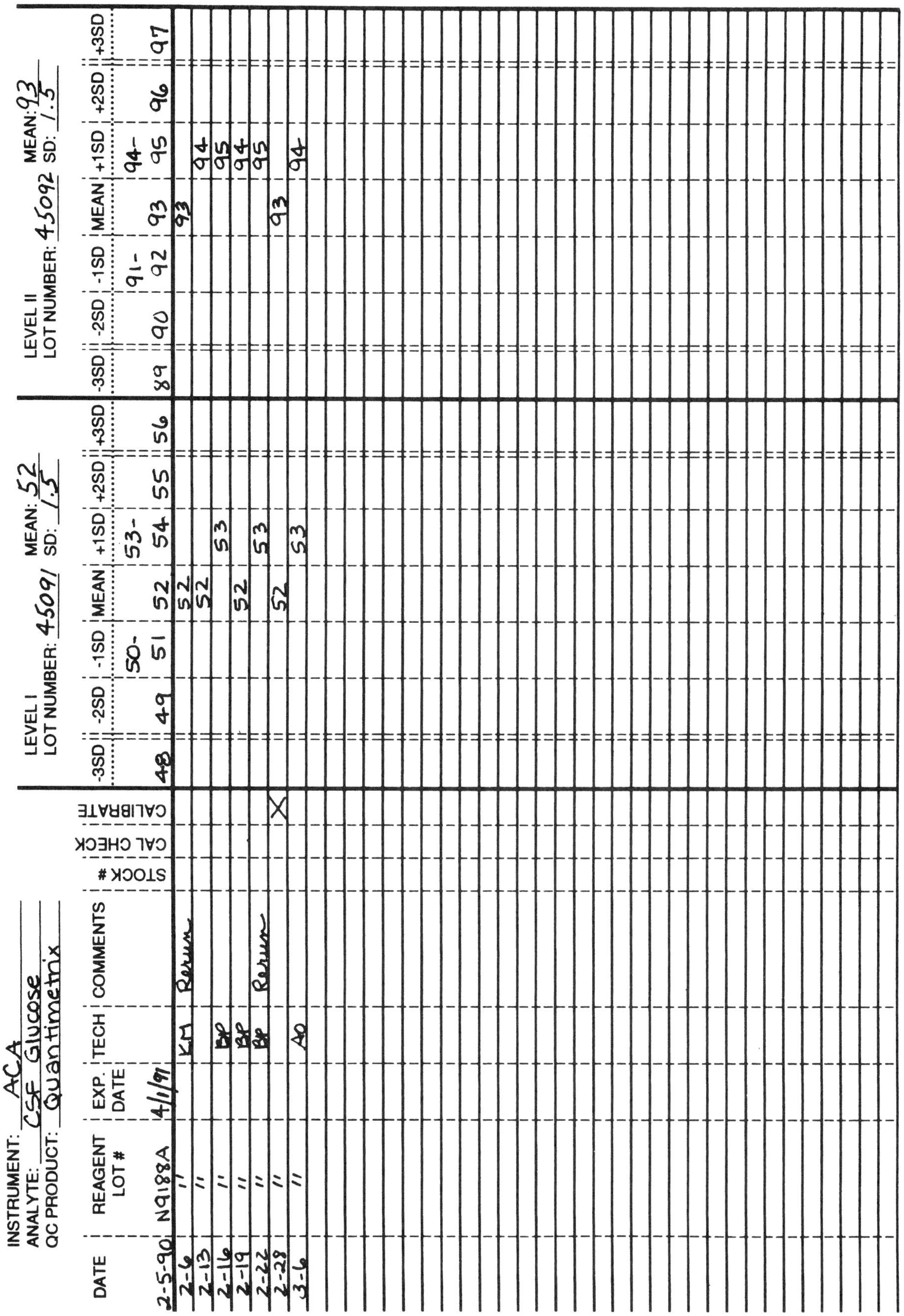

FIGURE 3-23. Two-level control chart for implementing multirule procedures.

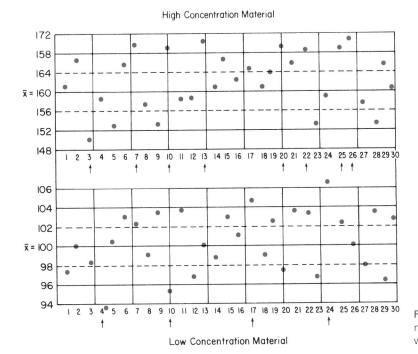

FIGURE 3-24. Control data to illustrate use of the multirule procedure. The *arrows* correspond to days in which there are violations of at least one rule.

system is illustrated in Figure 3-24. Interpretation of the control data is summarized in Table 3-11. Note that the R_{4s} rule is not applied across runs. The astute reader will note that the multirule procedure will detect $10_{\bar{x}}$ or 4_{1s} rule violations only if there is a 1_{2s} rule violation. On occasion, the $10_{\bar{x}}$ and 4_{1s} rules may be violated without the activation of the 1_{2s} warning rule. Such occurrences will be infrequent and would be indicative of small, systematic errors that would eventually be detected by the multirule procedure.

Automated implementations of the multirule procedure should not use the 1_{2s} screening rule. Westgard orig-

inally recommended the 1_{2s} screening rule to reduce the number of control observations that the medical technologist had to evaluate with the other control rules. The 1_{2s} screening rule thus decreased the technologist's labor. Today, the analysis of a single control product on a large, multianalyte chemistry analyzer will result in 20–30 different control results, one for each analyte. Even in the absence of increased analytic error, there is a greater than 50% chance that at least one of those analytes will be outside its +2s limits. As today's instruments are more precise than those used when the multirule control procedure was first described, the 1_{2s} rule violation should be

TABLE 3-11. INTERPRETATION OF THE MULTIRULE SHEWHART CONTROL CHARTS (FIG. 3-22) FOR HIGH- AND LOW-CONCENTRATION MATERIALS

CONTROL MATERIAL	DAY	RULE VIOLATION
High	Day 3	1_{2s} rule violation—warning—accept run
Low	Day 4	1_{3s} rule violation—reject run
High + low	Day 7	4_{1s} rule violation—reject run—across runs and materials
High + low	Day 10	R_{4s} rule violation—reject run—within run, across materials
High	Day 13	1_{2s} rule violation—warning—accept run
Low	Day 17	1_{2s} rule violation—warning—accept run
Low	Day 20	1_{2s} rule violation—warning—accept run
High	Day 22	$10_{\bar{x}}$ rule violation—reject run—within materials, across runs
Low	Day 24	1_{3s} rule violation—reject run
High	Day 25	1_{2s} rule violation—warning—accept run
High	Day 26	2_{2s} rule violation—reject run—within materials, across runs

ignored, unless it is associated with a 2_{2s} or 1_{3s} rule violation. Too often the detection of the 1_{2s} outlier is often followed by rerunning the out-of-control analyte, an expensive, delaying and non–value-added procedure. It is our recommendation that 1_{2s} rule not be used whenever quality control data are interpreted by a computer program.

The power functions in Figure 3-22 show that when the multirule procedure is used with four control observations, it will detect moderate-sized errors (*eg*, a 2s shift or a doubling of the random error) with a probability of approximately 50%. Smaller errors cannot be reliably detected. More sensitive control procedures are required for assays in which a 2s shift or a doubling of the standard deviation will cause misclassifications of clinical status. For example, the standard deviation of many calcium assays is 0.15 mg/dL for a normal range calcium. A positive shift of 0.30 mg/dL can easily place many normocalcemic patients into the hypercalcemic category. The sensitivity of the multirule procedure can be increased to detect smaller systematic errors by increasing the number of observations considered. Other control procedures can be used. The mean and range control procedure[72] has significantly greater power for the detection of error if each control material is analyzed in duplicate in each analytic run. Practically, this procedure requires computer implementation because calculations of the mean and range are required with each analytic run.

The *cumulative summation (cusum) technique* has been described for routine laboratory use[73]; it also requires computer implementation. The cusum procedure is responsive to systematic error and can be used with the 1_{3s} rule. Cusum is sensitive to small, persistent shifts that commonly occur in the modern, low-calibration-frequency analyzer. There are other control procedures that use exponentially smoothed averages and standard deviations.[71,74] These procedures have been implemented on several commercially available laboratory information quality control systems.

Many of today's analyzers are capable of very high accuracy and precision. The magnitude of the analytic standard deviation may be small when compared with that of the medically allowable error (*eg*, the standard deviation of glucose on certain analyzers approaches 1–2 mg/dL, which is much smaller than the medically allowable error of 10 mg/dL). Only very large errors need be detected when these analyzers measure analytes such as glucose. The sensitivity of the control procedure must be reduced rather than increased. One way to do this is by incorporating fewer observations; for example, using the 1_{3s} control rule or even expanding the control limits (for example, using ±3.5s control limits [ie, the $1_{3.5s}$ control rule]).[75] Koch et al showed that the application of optimized analyte-specific quality control practices reduced the frequency of falsely rejected runs, reduced quality control expenses, and increased the efficiency of their Hi-

tachi high-volume chemistry analyzer.[76] Their current analyte specific quality control program comprises the $1_{3.5s}$ rule for sodium, potassium, glucose, and blood urea nitrogen; the $1_{2.5s}$ rule for albumin, chloride, and carbon dioxide; and the $1_{2.5s}$ rule for calcium tests, which are run in duplicate and averaged.

A variety of approaches can be used to derive these analyte-specific control rules (Fig. 3-25). A commercially available computer program[77] allows the laboratorian to specify an analyte, its imprecision, and the medically allowable error (usually the proficiency test limits as specified by CLIA 88). The program then proposes optimal quality control procedures for that analyte. Today, most laboratories just use the same subset of the multirule control procedure for all of their analytes: the 1_{3s} rule for detecting random error and the 2_{2s} rule for detecting systematic error. This two-rule combination is probably the most common control procedure used in North American clinical laboratories.

Use of Patient Data for Quality Control

Various algorithms have been proposed for manipulating patient data to determine whether processing or preanalytic errors have occurred. This section focuses on two different control procedures that use patient data: the average of patient data and delta checks. Other quality control procedures that use patient data include the review of individual outlying results to identify gross clerical errors (sometimes called *limit checks*) and the routine analysis of duplicate specimens, as is frequently done in endocrinology assays. Some laboratories use duplicate analyses of another type: patient-sample comparisons. These comparisons require the regular analysis of split samples on instruments that measure the same analyte. Differences between instruments that exceed predetermined limits are investigated and corrected.

The use of patient data averages was described by Hoffman and Waid in 1965.[78] In their "average of normals" method, an error condition was signaled when the average of consecutive centrally distributed patient data was beyond the control limits established for the average of the patient data. The assumption underlying the average of normals is that the patient population is stable. Any shift would thus be secondary to a systematic analytic error. Cembrowski, Chandler, and Westgard studied the use of average of patients with computer simulations and found that its error-detection capabilities depended on several factors.[79] The most important were the number of patient results averaged and the ratio of the standard deviation of the patient population (s_p) to the standard deviation of the analytic method (s_a). Other important factors included the limits for evaluating the mean (control limits), the limits for determining which patient data are averaged (truncation limits), and the

Westgard Multirule QC Selection Grid		Process Stability (Frequency of Errors, *f*)		
		>10%	2% – 10%	<2%
Process Capability (Magnitude of errors, SEc)	<2.0s	1_{3S} / 2_{2S} / R_{4S} / 4_{1S} / $12\bar{x}$ N = 6	1_{3S} / 2_{2S} / R_{4S} / 4_{1S} / $8\bar{x}$ N = 4	1_{3S} / 2_{2S} / R_{4S} / 4_{1S} N = 2
	2.0s to 3.0s	1_{3S} / 2_{2S} / R_{4S} / 4_{1S} / $8\bar{x}$ N = 4	1_{3S} / 2_{2S} / R_{4S} / 4_{1S} N = 2	1_{3S}/2_{2S}/R_{4S}/(4_{1S} W) N = 2
	>3.0s	1_{3S} / 2_{2S} / R_{4S} / 4_{1S} N = 2	1_{3S}/2_{2S}/R_{4S}/(4_{1S} W) N = 2	1_{3S}/(4_{1S} W) N = 2

FIGURE 3-25. QC selection grid for Westgard multirule algorithm. (Reproduced with permission from J.O. Westgard.)

magnitude of the population lying outside the truncation limits. Cembrowski et al recommended that computer implementations of the technique could be used to supplement reference-sample quality control and recommended computer implementation. Douville, Cembrowski, and Strauss evaluated the averages of patient endocrine data and demonstrated high error-detection capabilities for thyroid testing.[80]

Cembrowski et al investigated the use of the anion gap for quality control and found that the practice of reanalyzing single specimens with abnormally high or low anion gaps usually resulted in the needless repetition of analyzing patient specimens.[81] More often, these single specimens had genuinely abnormal anion gaps. An improved control procedure consists of averaging eight consecutive patient anion gaps and comparing the average with the control limits for the anion-gap average.[82]

One other quality control approach uses patient data, the *delta check*, in which the most recent result of a patient is compared to the previous value. The difference between consecutive laboratory data (deltas) is calculated and compared to previously established limits.[83,84] A difference that exceeds these limits is investigated; this difference is either the result of specimen mix-up or real changes in the patients' test results. The difference is usually calculated in two ways: as a numerical difference (current value minus last value) and as a percentage difference (numerical difference times 100 divided by the current value). Wheeler and Sheiner evaluated the performance of several delta check methods and classified each delta check investigated as either a true or false positive.[85] They found that the percentage of true positives ranged from 5 to 29% and concluded that the delta check methods could detect errors otherwise overlooked but at the cost of investigating many false positives. In their tertiary-care hospital population, there were many false positives caused by large excursions in laboratory values secondary to disease or therapy.

External Quality Control

Proficiency-testing programs periodically provide samples of unknown concentrations of analytes to participating laboratories. Participation in these programs is mandated by the U.S. government under CLIA 88. CAP and the American Association of Bioanalysts are the two largest providers of proficiency testing programs in the United States. They provide samples for all major qualitative and quantitative chemistry areas, including general chemistry, protein chemistry, urinalysis, toxicology, and endocrinology. Samples for quantitative analysis contain multiple analytes and are usually provided as lyophilized materials. Once a laboratory receives its samples, it must analyze and return its results within a specified time to a computer center for compilation and comparison with the results of other participating laboratories. The computer center establishes target values and ranges of acceptable results based on either the average of the participants' values or reference laboratories' values.

For the CAP proficiency program, the means and standard deviations of all results from peer laboratories (similar instrument and methodology) are computed. Then values beyond three standard deviations from the mean are discarded, and the mean and standard deviation are recomputed. A participant result is classified as acceptable if the difference between the result and the target answer (usually the peer mean) is less than the allowable error. CLIA 88 has defined allowable errors for a large number of regulated analytes[41]; some are shown in Table 3-7. These allowable errors are sometimes referred to as "fixed limits" and are expressed either in measurement units of the analyte (eg, ±0.5 mmol/L from the mean for potassium) or as percentages (eg, ±10% for total cholesterol).

For a far smaller number of analytes (eg, thyroid-stimulating hormone), CLIA 88 has statistically defined limits of acceptability. For these analytes, the participant result is acceptable if it falls within ± 3 standard deviation indices (SDI) of the group mean. The comparison with statistical limits requires calculation of the deviation of the survey results from the mean, which is expressed in numbers of SDI above or below the mean. The SDI is the numeric difference between an individual laboratory's results and the mean, divided by the standard deviation. A deviation outside ± 3 SDIs usually is considered unacceptable because such deviations will occur only 0.3% of the time as a result of chance.

Compared with statistical limits, the violations of fixed-limits criteria will more often demonstrate the need for replacement of outmoded or unreliable instrumentation. Ehrmeyer and Laessig have used computer simulations to evaluate the ability of many different proficiency-testing schemes to detect poorly performing laboratories. The performance of all of these schemes is imperfect, with some good laboratories being judged as poor and some poor laboratories escaping detection.[86,87]

Cembrowski et al and Cembrowski, Hackney, and Carey have proposed a multirule system to evaluate the HCFA-mandated proficiency test result.[88–90] The multirule is illustrated in Figure 3-26. When significant deviations are detected in a set of five survey results (one or more observations exceeding ± 3 SDIs, the range of the observations exceeding 4 SDIs, or the mean of the 5 results exceeding ± 1.5 SDIs), the laboratory records, including the internal quality control results, should be reviewed. Mix-ups of proficiency specimens or of profi-

ciency and clinical specimens should be ruled out. Whenever possible, aliquots of the survey specimens should be frozen and saved. If the survey results differ significantly from peer instruments, these aliquots should be re-assayed. Results that still deviate significantly after retesting indicate a long-term bias. If the deviations are variable in magnitude and direction, there may be a problem with imprecision (random error). In the event that repeat analysis yields satisfactory results, the error probably represented a random error or transient bias encountered during the testing period. Figure 3-27 shows a survey form that can be used by the Chemistry Technologist to review proficiency surveys.

External proficiency testing is also used to determine estimates of the state-of-the-art of interlaboratory performance. The CAP regularly publishes summaries of its interlaboratory comparisons in the *Archives of Pathology and Laboratory Medicine.*

Point-of-Care Testing: The Newest Challenge

Point-of-care testing (POCT) is defined as analytic testing performed outside the confines of the central laboratory, usually by nonlaboratorian personnel (eg, nurses, respiratory therapists). Synonyms for POCT include near-patient testing, decentralized testing, bedside testing, and alternate site testing. The most common POCT involves the use of portable whole blood glucose meters for the management of patients with diabetes.[91] Many different analytes can now be measured accurately and quickly near the patient, whether the patient is in a hospital, an ambulance, or even in an airplane. Part of the of success of POCT arises from the inability of the centralized clinical laboratory to respond to clinician demands for faster turnaround times (TATs).[92,93] The rapid provision of test results can increase the throughput of patients through bottleneck areas, such as emergency departments, and might even decrease a patient's length of stay and reduce the total cost of patient care.[94]

A successful POCT program requires careful planning, implementation, and ongoing evaluation of equipment, education, and quality control. The first step to implementing a POCT program is forming a POCT steering committee. Committee membership should include the director of laboratory medicine (chair holder); the POCT coordinator (usually a laboratory technologist); and clinician, nursing, and respiratory care representatives. If possible, information systems and finance personnel should also attend. Meeting attendance will depend on agenda items. This collaboration sets the stage for communication and the resolution of POCT problems. Before the POCT steering committee can recommend any POCT device, they must evaluate all available systems and then choose the one that best meets the needs of the requesting area. The quality requirements of POCT ana-

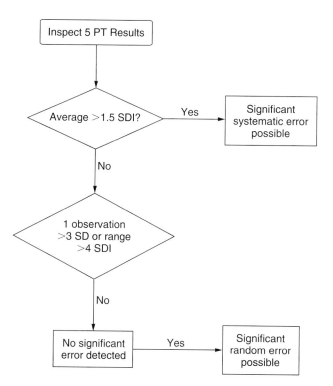

FIGURE 3-26. Screening PT results. Flow chart to investigate groups of 5 proficiency results for significant systematic and random error.

PROFICIENCY RESULTS REVIEW

Lab: ☐ Core ☐ Spec Inv ☐ HDIP ☐ Tox
Proficiency Sample Name: _____
Cycle _____ Sample _____

Date of Analysis: _____
Sample ID No: _____
Lab Accn No: _____

Analyte	1-2 Specimens/Analyte Rule Violated	3-5 Specimens/Analyte Rule Violated	Mean (SDIs)	Investigation Sources of test errors	Comments and Corrective Action	Senior Staff Comments
	☐ 1 >2.5 SDI ☐ X >1.5 SDI ☐ 2 consecutive >2 SDI	☐ Screening rule: 2/5 > ±1.0 SD Systematic error: ☐ Mean >1.5 SDI Random error: ☐ 1-3SDI ☐ R-4SDI		☐ Calibration drift ☐ Method bias ☐ Reporting range error ☐ Instability ☐ Random event ☐ Other		
	☐ 1 >2.5 SDI ☐ X >1.5 SDI ☐ 2 consecutive >2 SDI	☐ Screening rule: 2/5 > ±1.0 SD Systematic error: ☐ Mean >1.5 SDI Random error: ☐ 1-3SDI ☐ R-4SDI		☐ Calibration drift ☐ Method bias ☐ Reporting range error ☐ Instability ☐ Random event ☐ Other		
	☐ 1 >2.5 SDI ☐ X >1.5 SDI ☐ 2 consecutive >2 SDI	☐ Screening rule: 2/5 > ±1.0 SD Systematic error: ☐ Mean >1.5 SDI Random error: ☐ 1-3SDI ☐ R-4SDI		☐ Calibration drift ☐ Method bias ☐ Reporting range error ☐ Instability ☐ Random event ☐ Other		
	☐ 1 >2.5 SDI ☐ X >1.5 SDI ☐ 2 consecutive >2 SDI	☐ Screening rule: 2/5 > ±1.0 SD Systematic error: ☐ Mean >1.5 SDI Random error: ☐ 1-3SDI ☐ R-4SDI		☐ Calibration drift ☐ Method bias ☐ Reporting range error ☐ Instability ☐ Random event Other		
	☐ 1 >2.5 SDI ☐ X >1.5 SDI ☐ 2 consecutive >2 SDI	☐ Screening rule: 2/5 > ±1.0 SD Systematic error: ☐ Mean >1.5 SDI Random error: ☐ 1-3SDI ☐ R-4SDI		☐ Calibration drift ☐ Method bias ☐ Reporting range error ☐ Instability ☐ Random event ☐ Other		

Calibration drift: significant systematic error, recalibration resolves the error
Method bias: significant systematic error, inherent method bias identified
Reporting range error: significant analytical bias near limits of reportable range for method, non-linear
Instability: random error, a component (ie, sample probe, cells, reagents) was not performing optimally, acceptable upon repeat
Random event: unable to replicate error or identify possible sources

Reviewed by:

	Sign	Date
Core:		
Tox:		
HDIP:		
Spec Inv:		

Reviewed by Laboratory Director: Dr. G. C _____ Date _____

	Sign	Date
Dr. C.P		
Dr. D.L		
Dr. F.B		

Revised: May 2, 2001 by T h

FIGURE 3-27. Survey form for reviewing proficiency survey results.

TABLE 3-12. QUALITY REQUIREMENTS OF POINT-OF-CARE ANALYZERS

Speed (test[s] should be completed within minutes of sample introduction)

Accuracy and precision approaching that of the central laboratory analyzer

Small and portable equipment

Ability to analyze an "unprepared specimen" (eg, whole blood)

Low sample size

Flexible test menu

Broad dynamic range to minimize repeats, dilutions, and confirmatory tests

Ease of use by nonlaboratory personnel

Lock-out ability

   To prevent testing by unauthorized users

   When patient identification is not entered

   When quality control is not entered

Cost per test approaching that provided by the main laboratory

Low capital equipment outlay

Quantitative readout (no subjectivity on the part of the observer)

Automatic calibration

Automated quality control interpretation

Seamless interface with laboratory or hospital information system (communication by wireless system: infrared or radio frequency)

Low maintenance

Minimal troubleshooting requirements

High reliability with minimum downtime

Backup capability

Bar code reading capabilities

Use of either no reagent or ready-for-use reagents

Minimal waste production

Minimal and recyclable disposables.

Source: Cembrowski GS, Kiechle FL. Point-of-care testing: Critical analysis and practical application. Adv Pathol Lab Med 1994;7:3–26.

lyzers are summarized in Table 3-12. Many criteria must be considered before a POCT program can be approved, including the perceived need for POCT; potential for improvements in patient outcome; as well as testing frequency, method reliability, and training and staffing requirements. It is important to choose an analyzer that is relatively simple to operate and control. It is almost impossible to fit extensive POCT training programs into clinicians' already hectic schedules. Data management ca-

pabilities must also be considered. The interfacing of POCT analyzers to the laboratory information system can provide institution-wide access to the patient data.

The overall POCT cost depends on the volume of samples tested and the personnel performing the testing (nurse vs. technician).[95] When calculating cost per test at the point-of-care or the central laboratory, it is important to include labor costs, instrumentation costs, supplies, training, and depreciation and indirect costs (ie, reporting costs or hospital overhead). In most cases, central laboratory testing will be less expensive on a cost-per-test basis than alternate site testing. Although it may appear less expensive to perform analysis in the central laboratory, one must consider the impact of TAT on patient throughput efficiency and length of stay. Selective use of POCT in critical care areas can result in long-term cost savings to the health care facility.

Toward Quality Patient Care

Much of this chapter has focused on the delivery of *accurate* laboratory test results. Accuracy in laboratory testing is only one quality characteristic that is required of the clinical chemistry laboratory.[49] Other equally important quality characteristics include effective test request forms; clear instructions for patient preparation and specimen handling; appropriate turnaround times for specimen processing, testing, and result reporting; appropriate reference ranges; and intelligible result reports. Most clinical laboratories provide accurate laboratory testing. We are just beginning to appreciate that most laboratory failures or mistakes occur in the preanalytic or postanalytic realm.

For example, Ross and Boone reviewed 363 incidents that occurred in a large tertiary-care hospital in 1987.[96] Of the 336 medical records investigated, they found that preanalytic and postanalytic mistakes accounted for 46% and 47% of the total incidents, respectively. Preanalytic mistakes included missed or incorrectly interpreted laboratory orders, improper patient preparation, incorrect patient identification, wrong specimen container, and mislabeled or mishandled specimen. Postanalytic mistakes included delayed, unavailable, or incomplete results. Nonlaboratory personnel were responsible for 29% of the mistakes.

Most of these errors were interdepartmental; prevention of such errors requires a coordinated, interdepartmental group approach. Committed representation of all relevant players is a prerequisite for success, whether they be physician, nurse, ward clerk, phlebotomist, or analyst. These individuals can form a *quality team* or *improvement team* which would meet regularly to define the problem and, eventually, to make recommendations for its solution. The group should use various statistical and group techniques. For these *group processes* to succeed, there must be total commitment from management. Management must be trained in this "quality-improvement process"[97,98] and must support its growth throughout the institution. Such approaches have been successfully transferred to American businesses and even the hospital and clinic environment.[99,100] It is only through such quality-improvement efforts that we can significantly improve total patient care.

PRACTICE PROBLEMS

Problem 3-1: Calculation of Sensitivity and Specificity

Alpha-fetoprotein (AFP) levels are used by obstetricians to help diagnose neural tube defects (NTD) in early pregnancy. For the following data, calculate the sensitivity, specificity, and efficiency of AFP for detecting NTD, as well as the predictive value of a positive AFP.

NUMBER OF PREGNANCIES INTERPRETATION OF AFP FINDINGS

OUTCOME OF PREGNANCY	POSITIVE (NTD)	NEGATIVE (NO NTD)	TOTAL
NTD	5	3	8
No NTD	4	843	847
Total	9	846	855

Problem 3-2: A Management Decision in Quality Control

You are in charge of the clinical laboratory when a technologist presents you with the technologist's glucose worksheet. A 2_{2s} rule violation has occurred across runs and within materials on the high-concentration material. You ask to see the patient data and the previous control data. They follow:

GLUCOSE WORKSHEET JANUARY 8

SAMPLES	RESULTS	JANUARY GLUCOSE CONTROL VALUES		
		DATE	LOW	HIGH
Control—High	224	1/1	86	215
Patient	117	1/2	82	212
Patient	85	1/3	83	218
Patient	98	1/4	87	214
Patient	74	1/5	85	220
Patient	110	1/6	81	217
Control—Low	83	1/7	88	223
Patient	112	1/8	83	224
Patient	120			
Patient	97			
Patient	105			

1. Plot these control data.
2. What do you observe about these control data?
3. What might be a potential problem?
4. Should you report the patient data for today? Why or why not?

See Figure 3-28.

Problem 3-3: Interdepartmental Communication

You are having a problem with the medical intensive care unit (MICU) and the arterial blood gas specimens they submit to the laboratory. In the past 3 weeks, you have refused to perform blood gas analyses on six different MICU specimens because of small clots found in the specimens. The MICU staff is furious with the rejection policy, yet you believe the analyses will be incorrect if these specimens are used.

1. Outline where the problem lies.
2. What can be done to remedy this problem?
3. Why would your present quality-control system not detect this sort of error?

The following problems represent the steps in a method-evaluation study. An abbreviated data set is used to encourage hand calculations by the student. Perform the calculations for the following experimental data, which were obtained from a glucose study. The test method is a coupled glucose oxidase procedure. The

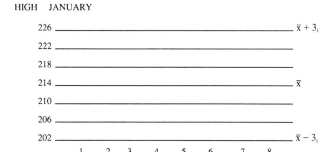

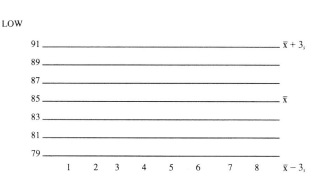

FIGURE 3-28. Blank control chart for Practice Problem 3-2.

comparative method is the hexokinase method currently in use.

Problem 3-4: Precision (Replication)

For the following precision data, calculate the mean, standard deviation, and coefficient of variation for each of the two control solutions A and B. These control solutions were chosen because their concentrations were close to medical decision levels (X_c) for glucose: 120 mg/dL for control solution A and 300 mg/dL for control solution B. Control solution A was analyzed daily, and the following values were obtained:

118, 120, 121, 119, 125, 118, 122, 116, 124, 123, 117, 117, 121, 120, 120, 119, 121, 123, 120, and 122 mg/dL

Control solution B was analyzed daily and gave the following results:

295, 308, 296, 298, 304, 294, 308, 310, 296, 300, 295, 303, 305, 300, 308, 297, 297, 305, 292, and 300 mg/dL

Problem 3-5: Recovery

For the recovery data below, calculate the percent recovery for each of the individual experiments and the average of all the recovery experiments. The experiments were performed by adding two levels of standard to each of five patient samples (A through E) with the following results:

SAMPLE	0.9 mL SERUM + 0.1 mL WATER	0.9 mL SERUM + 0.1 mL 500 mg/dL STD	0.9 mL SERUM + 0.1 mL 1000 mg/dL STD
A	59	110	156
B	63	112	160
C	76	126	175
D	90	138	186
E	225	270	320

What do the results of this study indicate?

Problem 3-6: Interference

For the interference data that follow, calculate the concentration of ascorbic acid added, the interference for each individual sample, and the average interference for the group of patient samples. The experiments were performed by adding 0.1 mL of a 150-mg/dL ascorbic acid standard to 0.9 mL of five different patient samples (A through E). A similar dilution was prepared for each patient sample using water as the diluent. The results follow:

SAMPLE	0.9 mL SERUM + 0.1 mL WATER	0.9 mL SERUM + 0.1 mL 150 mg/dL STD
A	54	46
B	99	91
C	122	112
D	162	152
E	297	286

What do the results of this study indicate?

Problem 3-7: Linear Regression

The following method-comparison data were obtained (mg/dL):

SAMPLE	BY HEXOKINASE (mg/dL)	BY COUPLED GLUCOSE OXIDASE (mg/dL)
1	191	192
2	97	96
3	83	85
4	71	72
5	295	299
6	63	61
7	127	131
8	110	114
9	320	316
10	146	141

1. Graph these results. From inspection of the graph, determine whether there is significant constant or proportional error.
2. Calculate the linear regression statistics as follows:
   a. Set up a table with the following column headings: $x_1, y_1, x^2i, y^2i, x_iy_i, Y_i$
   b. Enter the x_i and y_i data into the table (remember that x is the comparative method and y the test method) and calculate Σx_i, Σy_i, Σx^2i, Σy^2i, and Σx_iy_i. Enter these data into the table.
   c. From the summations in (b), calculate $\bar{x}$ and $\bar{y}$. Use Equations 3–8 and 3–9 to calculate the slope m and the y intercept (y_0), respectively.
   d. Using the regression equation $Y = mx + y_0$, calculate y_i for each x_i, enter the Y_i values in the Y_i column, and then calculate: $(y_i - Y_i)$, $(y_i - Y_i)^2$, and $\Sigma (y_i - Y_i)^2$

Enter these data into the table.

   e. From the summation in (d) and Equation 3–10, calculate $s_{y/x}$.
   f. From the summations in (b) and Equation 3–11, calculate r.
3. Report the following statistics for the comparison of methods experiment: m, y_0, $s_{y/x}$, and r.

Problem 3-8: Interpretation

Use the statistics calculated in Problem 3-7 to answer the following questions. Explain your answers by referring to the statistical value you used to arrive at your answer. Where appropriate, calculate errors at the two medical decision levels $X_{c1} = 120$ mg/dL and $X_{c2} = 300$ mg/dL.

1. What is the random error (RE) of the test method? What is the magnitude of the statistic that quantitates RE *between* the methods?
2. What is the constant error (CE) and the proportional error (PE)?
3. Calculate the systematic error (SE) at both X_c. What is the predominant nature of the SE (refer to item 2)?

4. What is the total error (TE = RE + SE) of the method? *Note:* Linear regression statistics should be used for error estimates only within the concentration range studied; we should have collected data up to 300 mg/dL in the comparison-of-methods experiment.

5. a. What is the statistic that quantitates random error between methods? b. What value did you calculate for this statistic?

6. Judge the acceptability of the performance of the test method. To reach your judgment, apply the following criteria:
   a. For the method to be accepted, all errors must be less than the allowable error (E_a) for a given X_c.
   b. The following are the E_a for glucose:
      $X_{c1} = 120$ mg/dL $E_{a1} = 10$ mg/dL
      $X_{c2} = 300$ mg/dL $E_{a2} = 25$ mg/dL

Problem 3-9: Point-of-Care Testing

1. You are appointed as a clinical laboratorian to a point-of-care (POC) work team. Who else might serve on this team?

2. What needs to be in place before implementing a POC testing protocol to ensure accurate and precise patient results?

3. Once you decide to provide physicians and patients with POC testing, what are important features or requirements of POC analyzers?

Problem 3-10: Sample Labeling

You receive a urine specimen in the lab with a request for a complete urinalysis. The cup is labeled and you begin your testing. You finish the testing and report the results to the ward. Several minutes later, you receive a phone call from the ward informing you that the urine was reported on the wrong patient. You are told that the cup was labeled incorrectly before it was brought to the lab.

1. What is the problem in this case and where did it occur?

2. Would your lab's QC system be able to detect or prevent this type of problem?

Problem 3-11: QC Program for POCT Testing

Your lab is in charge of overseeing the QC program for the glucometers (POCT) in use at your hospital. You notice that the ward staff is not following proper procedure for running QC. For example, in this case, the glucometer QC was rerun three times in a row in an effort to have the results in control. The first two runs were both 1_{3s}. The last run did return to less than 2 SD. Explain the correct follow up procedure for dealing with the out of control results.

Problem 3-12: QC Rule Interpretation

Explain the R_{4s} rule, including what type of error it detects?

REVIEW QUESTIONS

1. A gaussian distribution is usually
   a. rectangular.
   b. bell-shaped.
   c. uniform.
   d. skewed.

2. The following chloride (mmol/L) results were obtained using a point-of-care analyzer in the emergency department:

l06	111	l04	106	112	110
115	127	85	110	108	109
83	119	105	106	108	114
120	100	107	110	109	102

   What is the mean?
   a. 105
   b. 108
   c. 109
   d. 107

   What is the median?
   e. 105
   f. 108
   g. 109
   h. 107

3. The correlation coefficient should be used
   a. for determining method acceptability.
   b. for determining regression type used to derive slope and y intercept.
   c. always expressed as R_2.
   d. to express method imprecision.

4. On doing a correlation study, the test method and reference method generate equal data points. When plotted, the slope equals ____ and the y intercept equals ____.
   a. 0.0, 1.0
   b. 1.0, 1.0
   c. 1.0, 0.0
   d. 0.0, 0.0

5. Using the following ROC curve, which is the best test?
    a. Test A
    b. Test B
    c. Test C
    d. Test D

6. Interference studies typically use _____ as an interferent.
    a. Hemolyzed red blood cells
    b. Intralipid
    c. Highly icteric specimens
    d. All of the above

7. Which Westgard rule detects random error?
    a. 1_{3s}
    b. 4_{1s}
    c. 2_{2s}
    d. 10_0

8. Which of the following rule(s) probably detect small systematic error and should hardly be used?
    a. R_{4s}
    b. 10_x
    c. 2_{2s}, 4_{1s}
    d. 1_{3s}

9. Which rules can be used to evaluate sets of five proficiency testing results?
    a. Mean >1.0 SDI
    b. 1 result > 2 SDI
    c. 5/5 results > ±1.0 SDI and mean > 1.5 SDI
    d. 1 result > 3 SDI

10. The primary reason for implementing POCT is
    a. reduced testing cost.
    b. enhanced outcomes of patient care.
    c. lower central laboratory workload.
    d. use of nonlaboratorians as analysts.

11. True or False (If the answer is false, explain why.)
    a. A trend occurs when QC results fall on one side of the mean or the other over a period of 6-7 consecutive days.
    b. Diagnostic sensitivity refers to the probability that only people who do not have the disease will test negative for the disease.
    c. Random error relates to method precision and systematic error relates to method accuracy.

REFERENCES

1. Westgard JO. Precision and accuracy: concepts and assessment by method evaluation testing. Crit Rev Clin Lab Sci 1981;13:28c.
2. Westgard, JO. Basic QC Practices, 2nd ed. Madison, WI: Westgard Quality Corporation, 2002.
3. Bland JM, Altman DG. Statistical methods for assessing agreement between two methods of clinical measurement. Lancet 1986;1(8476):307-310.
4. Waakers PJM, Hellendoorn HBA, Op De Weegh GH, et al. Applications of statistics in clinical chemistry: a critical evaluation of regression lines. Clin Chem Acta 1975;64:173.
5. Westgard JO, deVos DJ, Hunt MR, et al. Concepts and practices in the evaluation of clinical chemistry methods: III. Statistics. Am J Med Tech 1978;44:552.
6. Westgard JO, Hunt MR. Use and interpretation of common statistical tests in method-comparison studies. Clin Chem 1973;19:49.
7. Harris EK, Cooil BK, Shakarji G, et al. On the use of statistical models of within person variation in long-term studies of healthy individuals. Clin Chem 1980;26:383.
8. Grasbeck R, Siest G, Wilding P, et al. Provisional recommendation on the theory of reference values: I. The concept of reference values. Clin Chem 1979;25:1506.
9. Author's Web site available at: www.mylaboratoryquality.com
10. Fleisher GA, Eickelberg ES, Elveback LR. Alkaline phosphatase activity in the plasma of children and adolescents. Clin Chem 1977;23:469.
11. Winsten S. The ecology of normal values in clinical chemistry. Crit Rev Clin Lab Sci 1976;6:319.
12. Soldin WJ, Hicks JM, Gunter KC, et al. Pediatric Reference Ranges, 2nd ed. Washington, D.C.: American Association for Clinical Chemistry, 1997.
13. Meites S, ed. Pediatric Clinical Chemistry: Reference (Normal) Values. Washington, D.C.: American Association of Clinical Chemistry, 1989.
14. National Committee for Clinical Laboratory Standards. Approved guideline for how to define and determine reference intervals in the clinical laboratory. Document C28-A2. Villanova, PA: NCCLS, 2000
15. Martin HF, Gudzinowicz BJ, Driscoll JL. An algorithm for the selection of proper group intervals for histograms representing clinical laboratory data. Am J Clin Pathol 1975;64:327.
16. Catalona WJ, et al. Comparison of prostate specific antigen concentration versus prostate specific antigen density in the early detection of prostate cancer: receiver operating characteristic curves. J Urol 1994;152:203.
17. Galen RS, Gambino SR. Beyond Normality: The Predictive Value and Efficacy of Medical Diagnoses. New York: Wiley, 1975.
18. Robertson EA, Zweig MH, Van Steirteghem AC. Evaluating the clinical efficacy of laboratory tests. Am J Clin Pathol 1983; 79:78.
19. National Committee for Clinical Laboratory Standards. Approved guideline for assessment of clinical sensitivity and specificity of laboratory tests using receiver operating characteristic (ROC) plots. Document GP10-A. Villanova, PA: NCCLS, 1995.
20. Catalona WJ, et al. Use of the percentage of free prostate-specific antigen to enhance differentiation of prostate cancer from benign prostatic disease. JAMA 1998;279:1542–1547.
21. American Chemical Society, Committee on Environmental Improvement, Subcommittee on Environmental Analytic Chemistry. Guidelines for data acquisition and data quality evaluation in environmental chemistry. Anal Chem 1980;52:2242.

22. Westgard JO, deVos DJ, Hunt MR, et al. Concepts and practices in the evaluation of clinical chemistry methods: I. Background and approach. Am J Med Tech 1978;44:290.

23. National Committee for Clinical Laboratory Standards. Approved guideline for precision performance of clinical chemistry devices. Document EP05-A. Villanova, PA: NCCLS, 1999.

24. Westgard JO, deVos DJ, Hunt MR, et al. Concepts and practices in the evaluation of clinical chemistry methods: II. Experimental procedures. Am J Med Tech 1978;44:420.

25. Krouwer JS, Rabinowitz R. How to improve estimates of imprecision. Clin Chem 1984;30:290.

26. National Committee for Clinical Laboratory Standards. Proposed guideline for interference testing in clinical chemistry. Document EP07-A. Villanova, PA: NCCLS, 1986 (www.nccls.org).

27. Young DS. Effects of Drugs on Clinical Laboratory Tests, 4th ed. Washington, D.C.: American Association for Clinical Chemistry, 1995.

28. Siest G, Galteau MM. Drug Effects on Laboratory Test Results. Littleton, MA: PSG Publishing, 1988.

29. Glick MR, Ryder KW, Jackson SA. Graphical comparisons of interferences in clinical chemistry instrumentation. Clin Chem 1986;32:470.

30. Glick MR, Ryder KW. Analytical systems ranked by freedom from interferences. Clin Chem 1987;33:1453.

31. Ryder KW, Glick MR. Erroneous laboratory results from hemolyzed, icteric, and lipemic specimens. Clin Chem 1993;39:175–176.

32. National Committee for Clinical Laboratory Standards. Approved guideline for method comparison and bias estimation using patient samples. Document EP09-A2. Villanova, PA: NCCLS, 2002.

33. National Committee for Clinical Laboratory Standards. Proposed guideline for evaluation of linearity of quantitative analytical methods. Document EP6-P2. Villanova, PA: NCCLS, 2001.

34. Cornbleet PJ, Gochman N. Incorrect least-squares regression coefficients in method-comparison analysis. Clin Chem 1979;25:432.

35. Feldman U, Schmeider B, Klinkers H. A multivariate approach for the biometric comparison of analytical methods in clinical chemistry. Clin Biochem 1981;19:121.

36. Westgard JO, deVos DJ, Hunt MR, et al. Concepts and practices in the evaluation of clinical chemistry methods: IV. Decisions of acceptability. Am J Med Tech 1978;44:727.

37. Tonks D. A study of the accuracy and precision of clinical chemistry determinations in 170 Canadian laboratories. Clin Chem 1963;9:217.

38. Barnett RN. Medical significance of laboratory results. Am J Clin Pathol 1968;50:671.

39. Fraser CG: Data on biological variation: essential prerequisites for introducing new procedures. Clin Chem 1994;40:1671–1673.

40. Fraser CG: Biological Variation: From Principles to Practice. Washington, D.C.: AACC Press, 2001.

41. U.S. Department of Health and Human Services. Medicare, Medicaid, and CLIA programs. Regulations implementing the clinical laboratory improvement amendments of 1988 (CLIA) final rule. Federal Register 1992;57:7002.

42. Ehrmeyer SS, et al. Medicare/CLIA final rules for proficiency testing: minimum intra-laboratory performance characteristics (CV and bias) need to pass. Clin Chem 1990;36:1736.

43. Westgard JO, Seehafer JJ, Barry PL. European specifications for imprecision and inaccuracy compared with operating specifications that assure the quality required by U.S. CLIA proficiency-testing criteria. Clin Chem 1994;40:1228.

44. Westgard JO, Carey RN, Wold S. Criteria for judging precision and accuracy in method development and evaluation. Clin Chem 1974;20:825.

45. Westgard JO, deVos DJ, Hunt MR, et al. Concepts and practices in the evaluation of clinical chemistry methods: V. Applications. Am J Med Tech 1978;44:803.

46. National Committee for Clinical Laboratory Standards. User demonstration of performance for precision and accuracy: proposed guideline. Document EP15-A. Wayne, PA: NCCLS, 2001.

47. Buttner J, Borth R, Boutwell JH, et al. Provisional recommendation on quality control in clinical chemistry. Clin Chem 1976;22:532.

48. Elin RJ. Elements of cost management for quality assurance. Pathologist 1980;34:182.

49. Cembrowski GS, Carey RN. Laboratory Quality Management. Chicago: ASCP Press, 1989.

50. Westgard JO, Barry PD. Cost-Effective Quality Control: Managing the Quality and Productivity of Analytical Processes. Washington, D.C.: AACC Press, 1986.

51. Young DS. Effects of Pre-Analytical Variables on Clinical Laboratory Tests, 2nd ed. Washington, D.C.: American Association for Clinical Chemistry, 1997.

52. National Committee for Clinical Laboratory Standards. Approved guideline for clinical laboratory procedure manuals, 4th ed. Document GP02-A4. Wayne, PA: NCCLS, 2002.

53. National Committee for Clinical Laboratory Standards. Approved standard for procedures for the collection of diagnostic blood specimens by venipuncture, 4th ed. Document H03-A4. Wayne, PA: NCCLS, 1998.

54. National Committee for Clinical Laboratory Standards. Approved standard for procedures for the collection of diagnostic blood specimens by skin puncture, 4th ed. Document H04-A4. Wayne, PA: NCCLS, 1999.

55. National Committee for Clinical Laboratory Standards. Approved standard for the percutaneous collection of arterial blood for laboratory analysis, 2nd ed. Document H11-A2. Villanova, PA: NCCLS, 1992.

56. National Committee for Clinical Laboratory Standards. Approved guideline for devices for collection of skin puncture specimens, 2nd ed. NCCLS Document H14-A2. Villanova, PA: NCCLS, 1990.

57. National Committee for Clinical Laboratory Standards. Approved standard for procedures for the handling and transport of domestic diagnostic specimens and etiologic agents, 3rd ed. Document H5-A3. Villanova, PA: NCCLS, 1985.

58. National Committee for Clinical Laboratory Standards. Approved guideline for procedures for the handling and processing of blood specimens. Document H18-A2. Wayne, PA: NCCLS, 1999.

59. National Committee for Clinical Laboratory Standards. Approved guideline for preparation and testing of reagent water in the clinical laboratory, 3rd ed. Document C3-A3. Villanova, PA: NCCLS, 1997.

60. National Committee for Clinical Laboratory Standards. Approved standard for power requirements for clinical laboratory instruments and for laboratory power sources. Document I5-A. Villanova, PA: NCCLS, 1980.

61. National Committee for Clinical Laboratory Standards. Approved standard for temperature calibration of water baths, instruments, and temperature sensors, 2nd ed. Document I2-A2. Villanova, PA: NCCLS, 1990.

62. National Committee for Clinical Laboratory Standards. Tentative guideline for calibration materials in clinical chemistry. Document C22-T. Villanova, PA: NCCLS, 1982.

63. Shewhart WA. Economic Control of Quality of the Manufactured Product. New York: Van Nostrand, 1931.

64. Levey S, Jennings ER. The use of control charts in the clinical laboratories. Am J Clin Pathol 1950;20:1059.

65. National Committee for Clinical Laboratory Standards. Tentative guideline for control materials in clinical chemistry. Document C23-T. Villanova, PA: NCCLS, 1982.

66. Bowers GN, Burnett RW, McComb RB. Preparation and use of human serum control materials for monitoring precision in clinical chemistry. In: Selected Methods for Clinical Chemistry, Vol. 8. Washington, D.C.: American Association of Clinical Chemists, 1977;21.

67. Caputo MJ, et al. Bovine-based serum as quality control material: a comparative analytical study of bovine vs. human controls. Fullerton, CA: Hyland Diagnostics, 1981.

68. Westgard JO, Barry PL, Hunt MR, et al. A multirule Shewhart chart for quality control in clinical chemistry. Clin Chem 1981;27:493.

69. Westgard JO, Groth T. Power functions for statistical control rules. Clin Chem 1979;25:863.

70. Westgard JO, Groth T, Aronsson T, et al. Performance characteristics of rules for internal quality control: probabilities for false rejection and error detection. Clin Chem 1977;23:1857.

71. Westgard JO, Groth T. Design and evaluation of statistical control procedures: applications of a computer "quality control simulator" program. Clin Chem 1981;27:1536.

72. Hainline A Jr. Quality assurance: theoretical and practical aspects. In: Selected Methods for the Small Clinical Chemistry Laboratory. Washington, D.C.: American Association of Clinical Chemistry, 1982;17.

73. Westgard JO, Groth T, Aronsson T, et al. Combined Shewhart-cusum control chart for improved quality control in clinical chemistry. Clin Chem 1977;23:1881.

74. Cembrowski GS, Westgard JO, Eggert AA, et al. Trend detection in control data: optimization and interpretation of Trigg's technique for trend analysis. Clin Chem 1975;21:139.

75. Cembrowski GS, Carey RN. Considerations for the implementation of clinically derived quality control procedures. Lab Med 1989;20:400.

76. Koch DD, Oryall JJ, Quam EF, et al. Selection of medically useful quality control procedures for individual tests on a multi-test analytical system. Clin Chem 1990;36:230–233.

77. Westgard JO: Charts of operational process specifications ("OP-Specs charts") for assessing the precision, accuracy, and quality control needed to satisfy proficiency testing performance criteria. Clin Chem 1992;38:1226–1233.

78. Hoffman RG, Waid ME. The "average of normals" method of quality control. Am J Clin Pathol 1965;43:134.

79. Cembrowski GS, Chandler EP, Westgard J. Assessment of "average of normals" quality control procedures and guidelines for implementation. Am J Clin Pathol 1984;81:492.

80. Douville P, Cembrowski GS, Strauss J. Evaluation of the average of patients, application to endocrine assays. Clin Chim Acta 1987;167:173.

81. Cembrowski GS, Westgard JO, Kurtycz DFI. Use of anion gap for the quality control of electrolyte analyzers. Am J Clin Pathol 1983;79:688.

82. Bockelman HW, et al. Quality control of electrolyte analyzers: evaluation of the anion gap average. Am J Clin Pathol 1984;81:219.

83. Ladenson JH. Patients as their own controls: use of the computer to identify "laboratory error." Clin Chem 1975;21:1648.

84. Sheiner LB, Wheeler LA, Moore JK. The performance of delta check methods. Clin Chem 1979;25:2034.

85. Wheeler LA, Sheiner LB. A clinical evaluation of various delta check methods. Clin Chem 1981;27:5.

86. Ehrmeyer SS, Laessig RH, Schell K. Use of alternate rules (other than the 1_{2s}) for evaluating interlaboratory performance data. Clin Chem 1988;34:250.

87. Ehrmeyer SS, Laessig RH. External proficiency testing. In: Cembrowski GS, Carey RN, eds. Laboratory Quality Management. Chicago, IL: ASCP Press, 1989;227.

88. Cembrowski GS, Anderson PG, Crampton CA, et al. Pump up your PT IQ. Med Lab Observer 1996;28(1):46–51.

89. Cembrowski GS, Crampton C, Byrd J, et al. Detection and classification of proficiency testing errors in HCFA regulated analytes. Application to ligand assays. J Clin Immunoassay 1995;17:210.

90. Cembrowski GS, Hackney JR, Carey N. The detection of problem analytes in a single proficiency test challenge in the absence of the Health Care Financing Administration rule violations. Arch Pathol Lab Med 1993;117:437.

91. Emergency Care Research Institute. Portable blood glucose monitors. Health Devices 1992;21:43–79.

92. Cembrowski GS, Kiechle FL. Point of care testing: critical analysis and practical application. Adv Pathol Lab Med 1994;7:3.

93. Goldsmith BM. New POCT guide establishes testing uniformity. MLO Aug 1995;50–52.

94. Tsai WW, Nash DB, Seamonds B, et al. Point-of-care versus central laboratory testing: an economic analysis in an academic medical center. Clin Therap 1994;16:898–910.

95. Bailey TM, Topham TM, Wantz S, et al. Laboratory process improvement through point-of-care testing. J Quality Improvement 1997;23:363–380.

96. Ross JW, Boone DJ. Assessing the effect of mistakes in the total testing process on the quality of patient care. [Abstract] Presented at the 1989 Institute on Critical Issues in Health Laboratory Practice, sponsored by the Centers for Disease Control and the University of Minnesota. Minneapolis, MN: April 9–12, 1989.

97. Harrington HJ. The Improvement Process. New York: McGraw-Hill, 1987.

98. Westgard JO, Barry PL. Total quality control: evolution of quality management systems. Lab Med 1989;20:377.

99. Berwick DM. Continuous improvement as an ideal in health care. N Engl J Med 1989;320:53.

100. Laffel G, Blumenthal D. The case for using industrial quality management science in health care organizations. JAMA 1989;262:2869.

Analytic Techniques and Instrumentation

Alan H. B. Wu

OBJECTIVES

Upon completion of this chapter, the clinical laboratorian should be able to:
- Explain the general principles of each analytic method.
- Discuss the limitations of each analytic technique.
- Compare and contrast the various analytic techniques.
- Discuss existing clinical applications for each analytic technique.
- Describe the operation and component parts of the following instruments: spectrophotometer, atomic absorption spectrometer, fluorometer, gas chromatograph, osmometer, ion-selective electrode, and pH electrode.
- Outline the quality assurance and preventive maintenance procedures involved with the following instruments: spectrophotometer, atomic absorption spectrometer, fluorometer, gas chromatograph, osmometer, ion-selective electrode, and pH electrode.

KEY TERMS

Atomic absorption	Electrophoresis	Ion-selective electrodes	Point-of-care testing
Chemiluminescence	Fluorometry	Liquid chromatography	(POCT)
Electrochemistry	Gas chromatography		Spectrophotometry

Analytic techniques and instrumentation provide the foundation for all measurements made in a modern clinical chemistry laboratory. The majority of techniques fall into one of four basic disciplines within the field of analytic chemistry: spectrometry (including spectrophotometry, atomic absorption, and mass spectrophotometry); luminescence (including fluorescence, chemiluminescence, and nephelometry); electroanalytic methods (including electrophoresis, potentiometry, and amperometry); and chromatography (including gas, liquid, and thin-layer). With the improvements in optics, electronics, and computerization, instrumentation has become miniaturized. This miniaturization has enabled the development of point-of-care testing (POCT) devices that produce results as accurate as large laboratory-based instrumentation.

SPECTROPHOTOMETRY AND PHOTOMETRY

The instruments that measure electromagnetic radiation have several concepts and components in common. Shared instrumental components are discussed in some detail in a later section. Photometric instruments measure light intensity without consideration of wavelength. Most instruments today use filters (photometers), prisms, or gratings (spectrometers) to select (isolate) a narrow range of the incident wavelength. Radiant energy that passes through an object will be partially reflected, absorbed, and transmitted.

Electromagnetic radiation is described as photons of energy traveling in waves. The relationship between wavelength and energy E is described by Planck's formula:

$$E = h\nu \qquad \text{(Eq. 4–1)}$$

where h = a constant (6.62×10^{-27} erg sec), known as Planck's constant
ν = frequency

Because the frequency of a wave is inversely proportional to the wavelength, it follows that the energy of electromagnetic radiation is inversely proportional to wavelength. Figure 4-1A shows this relationship. Electromagnetic radiation includes a spectrum of energy from short-wavelength, highly energetic gamma and x-rays on the left in Figure 4-1B to long-wavelength radio frequencies on the right. Visible light falls in between, with the color violet at 400 nm and red at 700 nm wavelength being the approximate limits of the visible spectrum.

The instruments discussed in this section measure either absorption or emission of radiant energy to determine concentration of atoms or molecules. The two phenomena, absorption and emission, are closely related. For a ray of electromagnetic radiation to be absorbed, it must have the same frequency as a rotational or vibrational frequency in the atom or molecule that it strikes. Levels of energy that are absorbed move in discrete steps, and any particular type of molecule or atom will absorb only certain energies and not others. When energy is absorbed, valence electrons move to an orbital with a higher energy level. Following energy absorption, the excited electron will fall back to the ground state by emitting a discrete amount of energy in the form of a characteristic wavelength of radiant energy.

Absorption or emission of energy by atoms results in a line spectrum. Because of the relative complexity of molecules, they absorb or emit a bank of energy over a large region. Light emitted by incandescent solids (tungsten or deuterium) is in a continuum. The three types of spectra are shown in Figure 4-2.[1–3]

Beer's Law

The relationship between absorption of light by a solution and the concentration of that solution has been described by Beer and others. Beer's Law states that the concentration of a substance is directly proportional to the amount of light absorbed or inversely proportional to the

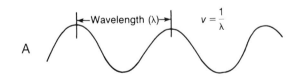

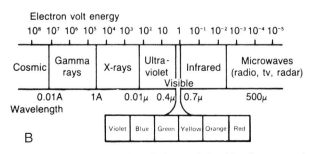

FIGURE 4-1. Electromagnetic radiation—relationship of energy and wavelength.

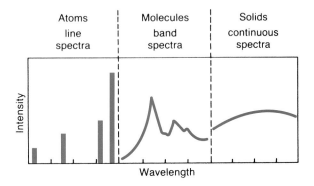

FIGURE 4-2. Characteristic absorption or emission spectra. (From Coiner D. Basic Concepts in Laboratory Instrumentation. Bethesda, MD: ASMT Education and Research Fund, 1975–1979.)

logarithm of the transmitted light. Percent transmittance (% T) and absorbance (A) are related photometric terms that are explained in this section.

Figure 4-3A shows a beam of monochromatic light entering a solution. Some of the light is absorbed. The remainder passes through, strikes a light detector, and is converted to an electric signal. *Percent transmittance* is the ratio of the radiant energy transmitted (T) divided by the radiant energy incident on the sample (I). All light absorbed or blocked results in 0% T. A level of 100% T is obtained if no light is absorbed. In practice, the solvent without the constituent of interest is placed in the light path, as in Figure 4-3B. Most of the light is transmitted, but a small amount is absorbed by the solvent and cuvet or is reflected away from the detector. The electrical readout of the instrument is set arbitrarily at 100% T, while the light is passing through a "blank" or reference. The sample containing absorbing molecules to be measured is placed in the light path. The dif-

ference in amount of light transmitted by the blank and that transmitted by the sample is due only to the presence of the compound being measured. The % T measured by commercial spectrophotometers is the ratio of the sample transmitted beam divided by the blank transmitted beam.

Equal thicknesses of an absorbing material will absorb a constant fraction of the energy incident upon the layers. For example, in a tube containing layers of solution (Fig. 4-4A), the first layer transmits 70% of the light incident upon it. The second layer will, in turn, transmit 70% of the light incident upon it. Thus, 70% of 70% (49%) is transmitted by the second layer. The third layer transmits 70% of 49%, or 34% of the original light. Continuing on, successive layers transmit 24% and 17%, respectively. The % T values, when plotted on linear graph paper, yield the curve shown in Figure 4-4B. Considering each equal layer as many monomolecular layers, we can translate layers of material to concentration. If semilog graph paper is used to plot the same figures, a straight line is obtained (Fig. 4-4C), indicating that, as concentration increases, % T decreases in a logarithmic manner.

Absorbance A is the amount of light absorbed. It cannot be measured directly by a spectrophotometer, but rather is mathematically derived from % T as follows:

$$\% \ T = \frac{I}{I_0} \times 100 \qquad \text{(Eq. 4–2)}$$

where I_0 = incident light
I = transmitted light

Absorbance is defined as

$$A = -\log(I/I_0) = \log (100\%) - \log \% \ T = 2 - \log \% \ T$$

(Eq. 4–3)

According to Beer's Law, absorbance is directly proportional to concentration (Fig. 4-4D):

$$A = \epsilon \times b \times c \qquad \text{(Eq. 4–4)}$$

where ϵ = molar absorptivity, the fraction of a specific wavelength of light absorbed by a given type of molecule
b = length of light path through the solution
c = concentration of absorbing molecules

Absorptivity depends on molecular structure and the way in which the absorbing molecules react with different energies. For any particular molecular type, absorptivity changes as wavelength of radiation changes. The amount of light absorbed at a particular wavelength depends on molecular and ion types present and may vary with concentration, pH, or temperature.

Because the path length and molar absorptivity are constant for a given wavelength,

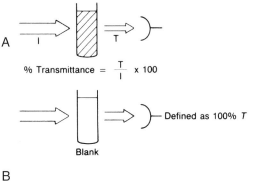

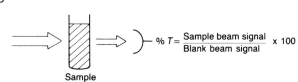

FIGURE 4-3. Percent transmittance (% T) defined.

$$A \propto C \qquad \text{(Eq. 4–5)}$$

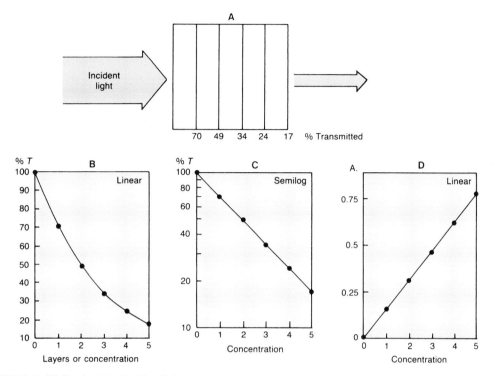

FIGURE 4-4. (**A**) % of original incident light transmitted by equal layers of light-absorbing solution; (**B**) % *T* versus concentration on linear graph paper; (**C**) % *T* versus concentration on semilog graph paper; (**D**) *A* versus concentration on linear graph paper.

Unknown concentrations are determined from a calibration curve that plots absorbance at a specific wavelength versus concentration for standards of known concentration. For calibration curves that are linear and have a zero *y* intercept, unknown concentrations can be determined from a single calibrator. Not all calibration curves result in straight lines. Deviations from linearity are typically observed at high absorbances. The stray light within an instrument will ultimately limit the maximum absorbance that a spectrophotometer can achieve; typically 2.0 absorbance units.

Spectrophotometric Instruments

A spectrophotometer is used to measure the light transmitted by a solution to determine the concentration of the light-absorbing substance in the solution. Figure 4-5 illustrates the basic components of a single-beam spectrophotometer, which are described in subsequent sections.

Components of a Spectrophotometer

Light Source

The most common source of light for work in the visible and near-infrared region is the incandescent tungsten or tungsten-iodide lamp. Only about 15% of radiant energy emitted falls in the visible region, with most emitted as near-infrared.[1–3] Often, a heat-absorbing filter is inserted between the lamp and sample to absorb the infrared radiation.

The lamps most commonly used for ultraviolet work are the deuterium-discharge lamp or the mercury-arc lamp. Deuterium provides continuous emission down to 165 nm. Low-pressure mercury lamps emit a sharp-line spectrum, with both ultraviolet and visible lines. Medium and high-pressure mercury lamps emit a continuum from ultraviolet to the midvisible region. The most important factors for a light source are range, spectral distribution within the range, the source of ra-

FIGURE 4-5. Single-beam spectrophotometer.

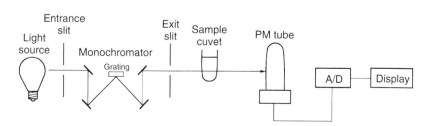

diant production, stability of the radiant energy, and temperature.

Monochromators

Isolation of individual wavelengths of light is an important and necessary function of a monochromator. The degree of wavelength isolation is a function of the type of device used and the width of entrance and exit slits. The bandpass of a monochromator defines the range of wavelengths transmitted and is calculated as width at more than half the maximum transmittance (Fig. 4-6).

Numerous devices are used for obtaining monochromatic light. The least expensive are colored-glass filters. These filters usually pass a relatively wide band of radiant energy and have a low transmittance of the selected wavelength. Although not precise, they are simple, inexpensive, and useful.

Interference filters produce monochromatic light based on the principle of constructive interference of waves. Two pieces of glass, each mirrored on one side, are separated by a transparent spacer that is precisely one-half the desired wavelength. Light waves enter one side of the filter and are reflected at the second surface. Wavelengths that are twice the space between the two glass surfaces will reflect back and forth, reinforcing others of the same wavelengths, and finally passing on through. Other wavelengths will cancel out because of phase differences (destructive interference). Because interference filters also transmit multiples of the desired wavelengths, they require accessory filters to eliminate these harmonic wavelengths. Interference filters can be constructed to pass a very narrow range of wavelengths with good efficiency.

The prism is another type of monochromator. A narrow beam of light focused on a prism is refracted as it enters the more dense glass. Short wavelengths are refracted more than long wavelengths, resulting in dispersion of white light into a continuous spectrum. The prism can be rotated, allowing only the desired wavelength to pass through an exit slit.

Diffraction gratings are most commonly used as monochromators. A diffraction grating consists of many parallel grooves (15,000 or 30,000 per inch) etched onto a polished surface. Diffraction, the separation of light into component wavelengths, is based on the principle that wavelengths bend as they pass a sharp corner. The degree of bending depends on the wavelength. As the wavelengths move past the corners, wave fronts are formed. Those that are in phase reinforce one another, whereas those not in phase cancel out and disappear. This results in complete spectra. Gratings with very fine line rulings produce a widely dispersed spectrum. They produce linear spectra, called *orders*, in both directions from the entrance slit. Because the multiple spectra have a tendency to cause stray light problems, accessory filters are used.

Sample Cell

The next component of the basic spectrophotometer is the sample cell or cuvet, which may be round or square. The light path must be kept constant to have absorbance proportional to concentration. This is easily checked by preparing a colored solution to read midscale when using the wavelength of maximum absorption. Fill each cuvet to be tested, take readings, and save those that match within an acceptable tolerance (*eg,* ±0.25% T). Because it is difficult to manufacture round tubes with uniform diameters, they should be etched to indicate the position for use. Cuvets are sold in matched sets. Square cuvets have plane-parallel optical surfaces and a constant light path. They have an advantage over round cuvets in that there is less error from the lens effect, orientation in the spectrophotometer, and refraction. Cuvets with scratched optical surfaces scatter light and should be discarded. Inexpensive glass cuvets can be used for applications in the visible range, but they absorb light in the ultraviolet region. Quartz cuvets must, therefore, be used for applications requiring ultraviolet radiation.

Photodetectors

The purpose of the detector is to convert the transmitted radiant energy into an equivalent amount of electrical energy. The least expensive of the devices is known as a *barrier-layer cell,* or *photocell.* The photocell is composed of a film of light-sensitive material, frequently selenium, on a plate of iron. Over the light-sensitive material is a thin, transparent layer of silver. When exposed to light, electrons in the light-sensitive material are excited and released to flow to the highly conductive silver. In comparison with the silver, a moderate resistance opposes the electron flow toward the iron, forming a hypothetical barrier to flow in that direction. Consequently, this cell

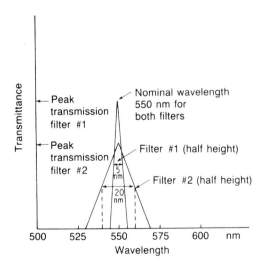

FIGURE 4-6. Spectral transmittance of two monochromators with band pass at half height of 5 nm and 20 nm.

generates its own electromotive force, which can be measured. The produced current is proportional to incident radiation. Photocells require no external voltage source but rely on internal electron transfer to produce a current in an external circuit. Because of their low internal resistance, the output of electrical energy is not easily amplified. Consequently, this type of detector is used mainly in filter photometers with a wide bandpass, producing a fairly high level of illumination so that there is no need to amplify the signal. The photocell is inexpensive and durable; however, it is temperature-sensitive and nonlinear at very low and very high levels of illumination.

A *phototube* (Fig. 4-7) is similar to a barrier-layer cell in that it has photosensitive material that gives off electrons when light energy strikes it. It differs in that an outside voltage is required for operation. Phototubes contain a negatively charged cathode and a positively charged anode enclosed in a glass case. The cathode is composed of a material (*eg*, rubidium or lithium) that acts as a resistor in the dark but emits electrons when exposed to light. The emitted electrons jump over to the positively charged anode, where they are collected and return through an external, measurable circuit. The cathode usually has a large surface area. Varying the cathode material changes the wavelength at which the phototube gives its highest response. The photocurrent is linear, with the intensity of the light striking the cathode as long as voltage between the cathode and anode remains constant. A vacuum within the tubes avoids scattering of the photoelectrons by collision with gas molecules.

The third major type of light detector is the *photomultiplier* (PM) *tube*, which detects and amplifies radiant energy. As shown in Figure 4-8, incident light strikes the coated cathode, emitting electrons. The electrons are attracted to a series of anodes, known as *dynodes,* each having a successively higher positive voltage. These dynodes

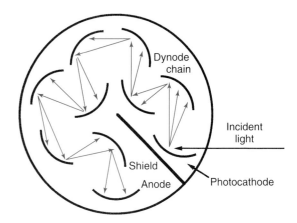

FIGURE 4-8. Dynode chain in a photomultiplier.

are of a material that gives off many secondary electrons when hit by single electrons. Initial electron emission at the cathode triggers a multiple cascade of electrons within the PM tube itself. Because of this amplification, the PM tube is 200 times more sensitive than the phototube. PM tubes are used in instruments designed to be extremely sensitive to very low light levels and light flashes of very short duration. The accumulation of electrons striking the anode produces a current signal, measured in amperes, that is proportional to the initial intensity of the light. The analog signal is converted first to a voltage and then to a digital signal through the use of an analog-to-digital (A/D) converter. Digital signals are processed electronically to produce absorbance readings.

In a *photodiode,* absorption of radiant energy by a reversed-biased *pn*-junction diode (*pn*, positive-negative) produces a photocurrent that is proportional to the incident radiant power. Although photodiodes are not as sensitive as PM tubes because of the lack of internal amplification, their excellent linearity (6–7 decades of radiant power), speed, and small size make them useful in applications where light levels are adequate.[4] *Photodiode array* (PDA) detectors are available in integrated circuits containing 256–2048 photodiodes in a linear arrangement. A linear array is shown in Figure 4-9. Each photodiode responds to a specific wavelength, and as a result, a complete UV/visible spectrum can be obtained in less than 1 second. Resolution is 1–2 nm and depends on the number of discrete elements. In spectrophotometers using PDA detectors, the grating is positioned *after* the sample cuvet and disperses the *transmitted* radiation onto the PDA detector (Fig. 4-9).

For single-beam spectrophotometers, the absorbance reading from the sample must be blanked using an appropriate reference solution that does not contain the compound of interest. Double-beam spectrophotometers permit automatic correction of sample and reference absorbance, as shown in Figure 4-10. Because the intensities of light sources vary as a function of wavelength, double-beam

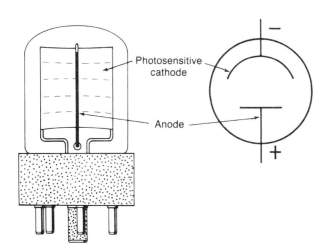

FIGURE 4-7. Phototube drawing and schematic.

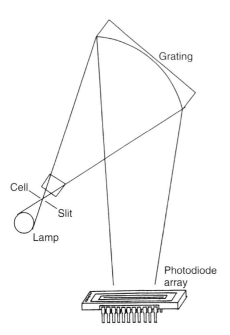

FIGURE 4-9. Photodiode array spectrophotometer illustrating the placement of the sample cuvet before the monochromator.

spectrophotometers are necessary when the absorption spectrum for a sample is to be obtained. Computerized, continuous zeroing, single-beam spectrophotometers have replaced most double-beam spectrophotometers.

Spectrophotometer Quality Assurance

Performing at least the following checks should validate instrument function: wavelength accuracy, stray light, and linearity. *Wavelength accuracy* means that the wavelength indicated on the control dial is the actual wavelength of light passed by the monochromator. It is most commonly checked using standard absorbing solutions or filters with absorbance maxima of known wavelength. Didymium or holmium oxide in glass is stable and frequently used as filters. The filter is placed in the light path and the wavelength control is set at the wavelength at which maximal absorbance is expected. The wavelength control is then rotated in either direction to locate

the actual wavelength that has maximal absorbance. If these two wavelengths do not match, the optics must be adjusted to calibrate the monochromator correctly.

Some instruments with narrow bandpass use a mercury-vapor lamp to verify wavelength accuracy. The mercury lamp is substituted for the usual light source, and the spectrum is scanned to locate mercury emission lines. The wavelength indicated on the control is compared with known mercury emission peaks to determine the accuracy of the wavelength indicator control.

Stray light refers to any wavelengths outside the band transmitted by the monochromator. The most common causes of stray light are reflection of light from scratches on optical surfaces or from dust particles anywhere in the light path and higher-order spectra produced by diffraction gratings. The major effect is absorbance error, especially in the high-absorbance range. Stray light is detected by using cutoff filters, which eliminate all radiation at wavelengths beyond the one of interest. To check for stray light in the near-ultraviolet region, for example, insert a filter that does not transmit in the region of 200 nm to 400 nm. If the instrument reading is greater than 0% *T*, stray light is present. Certain liquids, such as $NiSO_4$, $NaNO_2$, and acetone, absorb strongly at short wavelengths and can be used in the same way to detect stray light in the UV range.

Linearity is demonstrated when a change in concentration results in a straight-line calibration curve, as discussed under Beer's law. Colored solutions may be carefully diluted and used to check linearity, using the wavelength of maximal absorbance for that color. Sealed sets of different colors and concentrations are available commercially. They should be labeled with expected absorbance for a given bandpass instrument. Less than expected absorbance is an indication of stray light or of a bandpass that is wider than specified. Sets of neutral-density filters to check linearity over a range of wavelengths are also commercially available.

A routine system should be devised for each instrument to check and record each parameter. The probable cause of a problem and the maintenance required to eliminate it are generally described in the instrument's manual.

FIGURE 4-10. Double-beam spectrophotometer.

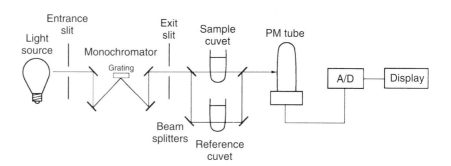

Atomic Absorption Spectrophotometer

The *atomic absorption* spectrophotometer is used to measure concentration by detecting absorption of electromagnetic radiation by atoms rather than by molecules. The basic components are shown in Figure 4-11. The usual light source, known as a *hollow-cathode lamp,* consists of an evacuated gas-tight chamber containing an anode; a cylindrical cathode; and an inert gas, such as helium or argon. When voltage is applied, the filler gas is ionized. Ions attracted to the cathode collide with the metal, knock atoms off, and cause the metal atoms to be excited. When they return to the ground state, light energy is emitted that is characteristic of the metal in the cathode. Generally, a separate lamp is required for each metal (*eg,* a copper hollow-cathode lamp is used to measure Cu).

Electrodeless discharge lamps are a relatively new light source for atomic absorption spectrophotometers. A bulb is filled with argon and the element to be tested. A radiofrequency generator around the bulb supplies the energy to excite the element, causing a characteristic emission spectrum of the element.

The analyzed sample must contain the reduced metal in the atomic vaporized state. Commonly, this is done by using the heat of a flame to break the chemical bonds and form free, unexcited atoms. The flame is the sample cell in this instrument, rather than a cuvet. There are various designs; however, the most common burner is the *premix long-path burner.* The sample, in solution, is aspirated as a spray into a chamber, where it is mixed with air and fuel. This mixture passes through baffles, where large drops fall and are drained off. Only fine droplets reach the flame. The burner is a long, narrow slit, to permit a longer path length for absorption of incident radiation.

Light from the hollow-cathode lamp passes through the sample of ground-state atoms in the flame. The amount of light absorbed is proportional to the concentration. When a ground-state atom absorbs light energy, an excited atom is produced. The excited atom then returns to the ground state, emitting light of the same energy as it absorbed. The flame sample thus contains a dynamic population of ground-state and excited atoms, both absorbing and emitting radiant energy. The emitted energy from the flame will go in all directions, and it will be a steady emission. Because the purpose of the instrument is to measure the amount of light absorbed, the light detector must be able to distinguish between the light beam emitted by the hollow-cathode lamp and that emitted by excited atoms in the flame. To do this, the hollow-cathode light beam is modulated by inserting a mechanical rotating chopper between the light and the flame or by pulsing the electric supply to the lamp. Because the light beam being absorbed enters the sample in pulses, the transmitted light also will be in pulses. There will be less light in the transmitted pulses because part of it will be absorbed. There are, therefore, two light signals from the flame—an alternating signal from the hollow-cathode lamp and a direct signal from the flame emission. The measuring circuit is tuned to the modulated frequency. Interference from the constant flame emission is electronically eliminated by accepting only the pulsed signal from the hollow cathode.

The monochromator is used to isolate the desired emission line from other lamp emission lines. In addition, it serves to protect the photodetector from excessive light emanating from flame emissions. A PM tube is the usual light detector.

Flameless atomic absorption requires an instrument modification that uses an electric furnace to break chem-

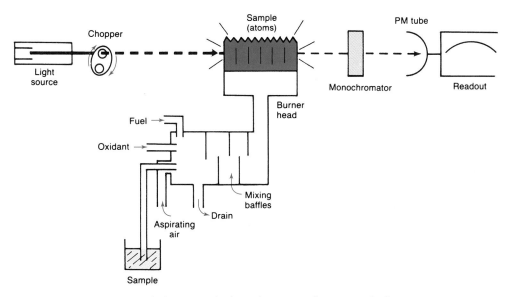

FIGURE 4-11. Single-beam atomic absorption spectrophotometer—basic components.

ical bonds (electrothermal atomization). A tiny graphite cylinder holds the sample, either liquid or solid. An electric current passes through the cylinder walls, evaporates the solvent, ashes the sample and, finally, heats the unit to incandescence to atomize the sample. This instrument, like the spectrophotometer, is used to determine the amount of light absorbed. Again, Beer's law is used for calculating concentration. A major problem is that background correction is considerably more necessary and critical for electrothermal techniques than for flame-based atomic absorption methods. Currently, the most common approach uses a deuterium lamp as a secondary source and measures the difference between the two absorbance signals. However, there has also been extensive development of background correction techniques based on the Zeeman effect.[1] The presence of an intense magnetic field will cause the wavelength of the emitted radiation to shift slightly; this shift in wavelength is the Zeeman effect.

Atomic absorption spectrophotometry is sensitive and precise. It is routinely used to measure concentration of trace metals that are not easily excited. It is generally more sensitive than flame emission because the vast majority of atoms produced in the usual propane or air-acetylene flame remain in the ground state available for light absorption. It is accurate, precise, and specific. One disadvantage, however, is the inability of the flame to dissociate samples into free atoms. For example, phosphate may interfere with calcium analysis by formation of calcium phosphate. This may be overcome by adding cations that compete with calcium for phosphate. Routinely, lanthanum or strontium is added to samples to form stable complexes with phosphate. Another possible problem is the ionization of atoms following dissociation by the flame, which can be decreased by reducing the flame temperature. Matrix interference, due to the enhancement of light absorption by atoms in organic solvents or formation of solid droplets as the solvent evaporates in the flame, can be another source of error. This interference may be overcome by pretreatment of the sample by extraction.[5]

Recently, inductively coupled plasma (ICP) has been used to increase sensitivity for atomic emission. The torch, an argon plasma maintained by the interaction of a radiofrequency field and an ionized argon gas, is reported to have used temperatures between 5500°K and 8000°K. Complete atomization of elements is thought to occur at these temperatures. Use of inductively coupled plasma as a source is recommended for determinations involving refractory elements such as uranium, zirconium, and boron. ICP with mass spectrometer detection is the most sensitive and specific assay technique for all elements on the periodic hart. Atomic absorption spectrophotometry is used less frequently because of this newer technology.

Flame Photometry

The flame-emission photometer, which measures light emitted by excited atoms, was widely used to determine concentration of Na^+, K^+, or Li^+. With the development of ion selective electrodes for these analytes, flame photometers are no longer routinely used in clinical chemistry laboratories. Discussion of this technique, therefore, is no longer included in this edition; the reader should refer to previous editions of this book.

Fluorometry

As seen with the spectrophotometer, light entering a solution may pass mainly on through or may be absorbed partly or entirely, depending on the concentration and the wavelength entering that particular solution. Whenever absorption occurs, there is a transfer of energy to the medium. Each molecular type possesses a series of electronic energy levels and can pass from a lower energy level to a higher level only by absorbing an integral unit (quantum) of light that is equal in energy to the difference between the two energy states. There are additional energy levels owing to rotation or vibration of molecular parts. The excited state lasts about 10^{-5} seconds before the electron loses energy and returns to the ground state. Energy is lost by collision, heat loss, transfer to other molecules, and emission of radiant energy. Because the molecules are excited by absorption of radiant energy and lose energy by multiple interactions, the radiant energy emitted is less than the absorbed energy. The difference between the maximum wavelengths, excitation, and emitted fluorescence is called *Stokes shift*. Both excitation (absorption) and fluorescence (emission) energies are characteristic for a given molecular type; for example, Figure 4-12 shows the absorption and fluorescence spectra of quinine in 0.1 N sulfuric acid. The dashed line on the left shows the short-wavelength excitation energy that is maximally absorbed, whereas the solid line on the

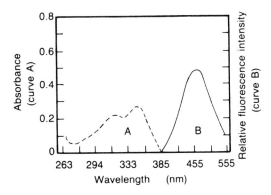

FIGURE 4-12. Absorption and fluorescence spectra of quinine in 0.1 N sulfuric acid. (From Coiner D. Basic Concepts in Laboratory Instrumentation. Bethesda, MD: ASMT Education and Research Fund, 1975–1979.)

right is the longer-wavelength (less energy) fluorescent spectrum.

Basic Instrumentation

Filter fluorometers measure the concentrations of solutions that contain fluorescing molecules. A basic instrument is shown in Figure 4-13. The source emits short-wavelength high-energy excitation light. A mechanical attenuator controls light intensity. The primary filter, placed between the radiation source and the sample, selects the wavelength that is best absorbed by the solution to be measured. The fluorescing sample in the cuvet emits radiant energy in all directions. The detector (placed at right angles to the sample cell) and a secondary filter that passes the longer wavelengths of fluorescent light prevent incident light from striking the photodetector. The electrical output of the photodetector is proportional to the intensity of fluorescent energy. In spectrofluorometers, the filters are replaced by prisms or grating monochromators.

Gas-discharge lamps (mercury and xenon-arc) are the most frequently used sources of excitation radiant energy. Incandescent tungsten lamps are seldom used because they release little energy in the ultraviolet region. Mercury-vapor lamps are commonly used in filter fluorometers. Mercury emits a characteristic line spectrum. Resonance lines at 365 nm to 366 nm are commonly used. Energy at wavelengths other than the resonance lines is provided by coating the inner surface of the lamp with a material that absorbs the 254-nm mercury radiation and emits a broad band of longer wavelengths. Most spectrofluorometers use a high-pressure xenon lamp. Xenon has a good continuum, which is necessary for determining excitation spectra.

Monochromator fluorometers use grating, prisms, or filters for isolation of incident radiation. Light detectors are almost exclusively PM tubes because of their higher sensitivity to low light intensities. Double-beam instruments are used to compensate for instability due to electric-power fluctuation.

Fluorescence concentration measurements are related to molar absorptivity of the compound, intensity of the incident radiation, quantum efficiency of the energy emitted per quantum absorbed, and length of the light path. In dilute solutions with instrument parameters held constant, fluorescence is directly proportional to concentration. Generally, a linear response will be obtained until the concentration of the fluorescent species is so high that the sample begins to absorb significant amounts of excitation light. A curve demonstrating nonlinearity as concentration increases is shown in Figure 4-14. The solution must absorb less than 5% of the exciting radiation for a linear response to occur.[6] As with all quantitative measurements, a standard curve must be prepared to demonstrate that the concentration used falls in a linear range.

In fluorescence polarization, radiant energy is polarized in a single plane. When the sample (fluorophor) is excited, it emits polarized light along the same plane as the incident light if the fluorophor is attached to a large molecule. In contrast, a small molecule emits depolarized light because it will rotate out of the plane of polarization during its excitation lifetime. This technique is widely used for the detection of therapeutic and abused drugs. In the procedure, the sample analyte is allowed to compete with a fluorophor-labeled analyte for a limited antibody to the analyte. The lower the concentration of the sample analyte, the higher the macromolecular anti-

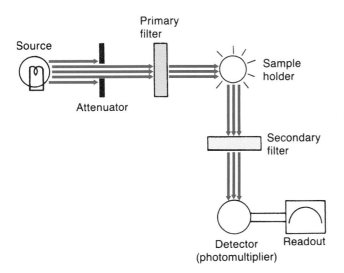

FIGURE 4-13. Basic filter fluorometer. (From Coiner D. Basic Concepts in Laboratory Instrumentation. Bethesda, MD: ASMT Education and Research Fund, 1975–1979.)

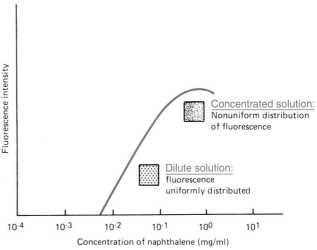

FIGURE 4-14. Dependence of fluorescence on the concentration of fluorophor. (From Guilbault GG. Practical Fluorescence, Theory, Methods and Techniques. New York: Marcel Dekker, 1973.)

body-analyte-fluorophor formed and the lower the depolarization of the radiant light.

Advantages and Disadvantages of Fluorometry

Fluorometry has two advantages over conventional spectrophotometry: specificity and sensitivity. Fluorometry increases specificity by selecting the optimal wavelength for *both* absorption and fluorescence, rather than just the absorption wavelength seen with spectrophotometry.

Fluorometry is approximately one thousand times more sensitive than most spectrophotometric methods.[6] One reason is because emitted radiation is measured directly; it can be increased simply by increasing the intensity of the exciting radiant energy. In addition, fluorescence measures the amount of light intensity present over a zero background. In absorbance, however, the quantity of absorbed light is measured indirectly as the difference between the transmitted beams. At low concentrations, the small difference between 100% *T* and the transmitted beam is difficult to measure accurately and precisely, limiting the sensitivity.

The biggest disadvantage is that fluorescence is very sensitive to environmental changes. Changes in pH affect availability of electrons, and temperature changes the probability of loss of energy by collision rather than fluorescence. Contaminating chemicals or a change of solvents may change the structure. Ultraviolet light used for excitation can cause photochemical changes. Any decrease in fluorescence resulting from any of these possibilities is known as *quenching*. Because so many factors may change the intensity or spectra of fluorescence, extreme care is mandatory in analytic technique and instrument maintenance.

Chemiluminescence

In *chemiluminescence* reactions, part of the chemical energy generated produces excited intermediates that decay to a ground state with the emission of photons.[7] The emitted radiation is measured with a PM tube, and the signal is related to analyte concentration. Chemiluminescence is different than fluorescence in that no excitation radiation is required and no monochromators are needed because the chemiluminescence arises from one species. Most importantly, chemiluminescence reactions are oxidation reactions of luminol, acridinium esters, and dioxetanes characterized by a rapid increase in intensity of emitted light followed by a gradual decay. Usually, the signal is taken as the integral of the entire peak. Enhanced chemiluminescence techniques increase the chemiluminescence efficiency by including an enhancer system in the reaction of a chemiluminescent agent with an enzyme. The time course for the light intensity is much longer (60 minutes) than for conventional chemiluminescent reactions, which last for about 30 seconds (Fig. 4-15).

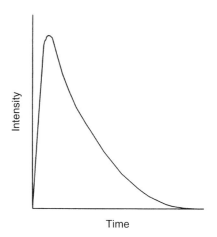

FIGURE 4-15. Representative intensity versus time curve for a transient chemiluminescence signal.

Advantages of chemiluminescence assays include subpicomolar detection limits, speed (with flash-type reactions, light is only measured for 10 seconds), ease of use (most assays are one-step procedures), and simple instrumentation.[7] The main disadvantage is that impurities can cause background signal that degrades sensitivity and specificity.

Turbidity and Nephelometry

Turbidimetric measurements are made with a spectrophotometer to determine concentration of particulate matter in a sample. The amount of light blocked by a suspension of particles depends not only on concentration, but also on size. Because particles tend to aggregate and settle out of suspension, sample handling becomes critical. Instrument operation is the same as for any spectrophotometer.

Nephelometry is similar, except that light scattered by the small particles is measured at an angle to the beam incident on the cuvet. Figure 4-16 demonstrates two possible optical arrangements for a nephelometer. Light scattering depends on wavelength and particle size. For macromolecules with a size close to or larger than the wavelength of incident light, sensitivity is increased by measuring forward light scatter.[8] Instruments are available with detectors placed at various forward angles, as well as at 90° to the incident light. Monochromatic light obtains uniform scatter and minimizes sample heating. Certain instruments use lasers as a source of monochromatic light; however, any monochromator may be used.

Measuring light scatter at an angle other than at 180° in turbidimetry minimizes error from colored solutions and increases sensitivity. Because both methods depend on particle size, some instruments quantitate initial change in light scatter rather than total scatter. Reagents must be free of any particles, and cuvets must be free of any scratches.

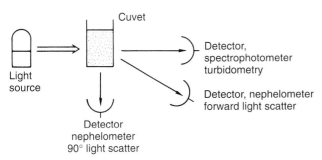

FIGURE 4-16. Nephelometer versus spectrophotometer—optical arrangements.

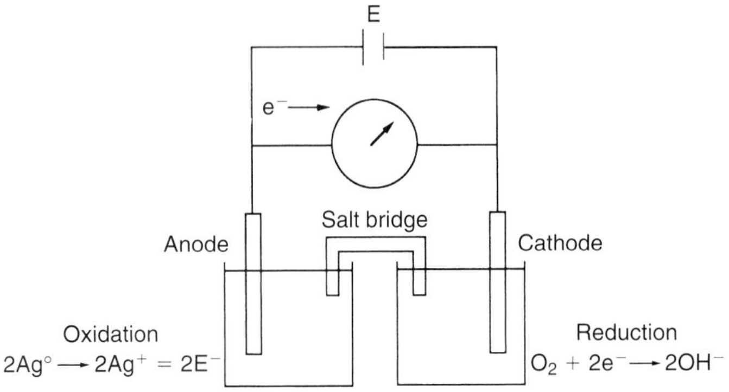

FIGURE 4-17. Electrochemical cell.

Laser Applications

Light amplification by stimulated emission of radiation (LASER) is based on the interaction of radiant energy and suitably excited atoms or molecules. The interaction leads to stimulated emission of radiation. The wavelength, direction of propagation, phase, and plane of polarization of the emitted light are the same as those of the incident radiation. Laser light is polarized and coherent and has narrow spectral width and small cross-sectional area with low divergence. The radiant emission can be very powerful and either continuous or pulsating.

Laser light can serve as the source of incident energy in a spectrometer or nephelometer. Some lasers produce bandwidths of a few kilohertz in both the visible and infrared regions, making these applications about three to six orders more sensitive than conventional spectrometers.[9]

Laser spectrometry also can be used for the determination of structure and identification of samples, as well as for diagnosis. Quantitation of samples depends on the spectrometer used. An example of the clinical application of the laser is the Coulter counter, which is used for differential analysis of white blood cells.[10]

ELECTROCHEMISTRY

Many types of electrochemical analyses are used in the clinical laboratory, including potentiometry, amperometry, coulometry, and polarography. The two basic electrochemical cells involved in these analyses are galvanic and electrolytic cells.

Galvanic and Electrolytic Cells

An electrochemical cell can be set up as shown in Figure 4-17. It consists of two half-cells and a salt bridge, which can be a piece of filter paper saturated with electrolytes. Instead of two as shown, the electrodes can be immersed in a single, large beaker containing a salt solution. In such a setup, the solution serves as the salt bridge.

In a galvanic cell, as the electrodes are connected, there is spontaneous flow of electrons from the elec-

trode with the lower electron affinity (oxidation; *eg*, silver). These electrons pass through the external meter to the cathode (reduction), where OH^- ions are liberated. This reaction continues until one of the chemical components is depleted; at which point, the cell is "dead" and cannot produce electrical energy to the external meter.

Current may be forced to flow through the dead cell only by applying an external electromotive force E. This is called an *electrolytic cell*. In short, a galvanic cell can be built from an electrolytic cell. When the external E is turned off, accumulated products at the electrodes will spontaneously produce current in the opposite direction of the electrolytic cell.

Half-Cells

It is impossible to measure the electrochemical activity of one half-cell; two reactions must be coupled and one reaction compared with the other. To rate half-cell reactions, a specific electrode reaction is arbitrarily assigned 0.00 V. Every other reaction coupled with this arbitrary zero reaction is either positive or negative, depending on the relative affinity for electrons. The electrode defined as 0.00 V is the standard hydrogen electrode: H_2 gas at 1 atmosphere (atm). The hydrogen gas in contact with H^+ in solution develops a potential. The hydrogen electrode coupled with a zinc half-cell is cathodic, with the reaction $2H^+ + 2e^- \rightarrow H_2$, because H_2 has a greater affinity than Zn for electrons. Cu, however, has a greater affinity than H_2 for electrons, and thus the anodic reaction $H_2 \rightarrow 2H^+ + 2e^-$ occurs when coupled to the Cu-electrode half-cell.

The potential generated by the hydrogen-gas electrode is used to rate the electrode potential of metals in 1 mol/L solution. Reduction potentials for certain metals are shown in Table 4-1.[11] A hydrogen electrode is used to determine the accuracy of reference and indicator electrodes, the stability of standard solutions, and the potentials of liquid junctions.

TABLE 4-1. STANDARD REDUCTION POTENTIALS

	POTENTIAL, V
$Zn^{2+} + 2e \leftrightarrow Z$	−0.7628
$Cr^{2+} + 2e \leftrightarrow Cr$	−0.913
$Ni^{2+} + 2e \leftrightarrow Ni$	−0.257
$2H^+ + 2e \leftrightarrow H_2$	0.000
$Cu^{2+} + 2e \leftrightarrow Cu$	0.3419
$Ag^+ + e \leftrightarrow Ag$	0.7996

Data presented are examples from Lide DR. CRC Handbook of Chemistry and Physics, 83rd ed. Boca Raton, FL: CRC Press, 2003–2004.

Ion-Selective Electrodes (ISE)

Potentiometric methods of analysis involve the direct measurement of electrical potential due to the activity of free ions. ISEs are designed to be sensitive toward individual ions.

pH Electrodes

An ISE universally used in the clinical laboratory is the pH electrode. The basic components of a pH meter are presented in Figure 4-18.

Indicator Electrode
The pH electrode consists of a silver wire coated with AgCl, immersed into an internal solution of 0.1 mmol/L HCl and placed into a tube containing a special glass membrane tip. This membrane is only sensitive to hydrogen ions. Glass membranes that are selectively sensitive to H^+ consist of specific quantities of lithium, cesium, lanthanum, barium, or aluminum oxides in silicate. When the pH electrode is placed into the test solution, movement of H^+ ions near the tip of the electrode produces a potential difference between the internal solution and the test solution, which is measured as pH and read by a voltmeter. The combination pH electrode also contains a built-in reference electrode, either Ag/AgCl or calomel (Hg/Hg_2Cl_2) immersed in a solution of saturated KCl.

The specially formulated glass continually dissolves from the surface. The present concept of the selective mechanism that causes formation of electromotive force at the glass surface is that an ion-exchange process is involved. Cationic exchange occurs only in the gel layer—there is no penetration of H^+ through the glass. Although the glass is constantly dissolving, the process is slow, and the glass tip generally lasts for several years. pH electrodes are highly selective for hydrogen ions; however, other cations in high concentration interfere, the most common of which is sodium. Electrode manufacturers should list the concentration of interfering cations that may cause error in pH determinations.

Reference Electrode
The reference electrode commonly used is the calomel electrode. Calomel, a paste of predominantly mercurous chloride, is in direct contact with metallic mercury in an electrolyte solution of potassium chloride. As long as the electrolyte concentration and the temperature remain constant, a stable voltage is generated at the interface of the mercury and its salt. A cable connected to the mercury leads to the voltmeter. The filling hole is needed for adding potassium chloride solution. A tiny opening at the bottom is required for completion of electric contact between the reference and indicator electrodes. The liquid junction consists of a fiber or ceramic plug that allows a small flow of electrolyte filling solution.

Construction varies, but all reference electrodes must generate a stable electrical potential. Reference electrodes generally consist of a metal and its salt in contact with a solution containing the same anion. Mercury/mercurous chloride, as in this example, is a frequently used reference electrode; the disadvantage is that it is slow to reach a new stable voltage following temperature change and it is unstable above 80°C.[1,2] Ag/AgCl is another common reference electrode. It can be used at high temperatures, up to 275°C, and the AgCl-coated Ag wire makes a more compact electrode than that of mercury. In measurements in which chloride contamination must be avoided, a mercury sulfate and potassium sulfate reference electrode may be used.

Liquid Junctions
Electrical connection between the indicator and reference electrodes is achieved by allowing a slow flow of electrolyte from the tip of the reference electrode. A junction potential is always set up at the boundary between

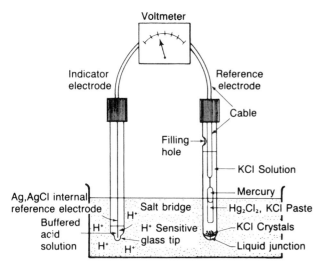

FIGURE 4-18. Necessary components of a pH meter.

two dissimilar solutions because of positive and negative ions diffusing across the boundary at unequal rates. The resultant junction potential may increase or decrease the potential of the reference electrode. Therefore, it is important that the junction potential be kept to a minimum reproducible value when the reference electrode is in solution.

KCl is a commonly used filling solution because K⁺ and Cl⁻ ions have nearly the same mobilities. When KCl is used as the filling solution for Ag/AgCl electrodes, the addition of AgCl is required to prevent dissolution of the AgCl salt. One way of producing a lower junction potential is to mix K^+, Na^+, NO_3^-, and Cl^- in appropriate ratios.

Readout Meter

Electromotive force produced by the reference and indicator electrodes is in the millivolt range. Zero potential for the cell indicates that each electrode half-cell is generating the same voltage, assuming there is no liquid junction potential. The isopotential is that potential at which a temperature change has no effect on the response of the electrical cell. Manufacturers generally achieve this by making midscale (pH, 7.0) correspond to 0 V at all temperatures. They use an internal buffer whose pH changes due to temperature compensate for the changes in the internal and external reference electrodes.

Nernst Equation

The electromotive force generated because of H⁺ at the glass tip is described by the Nernst equation, which is shown in a simplified form:

$$\epsilon = \Delta pH \times \frac{RT \ln 10}{F} = \Delta pH \times 0.059 \text{ V}$$

(Eq. 4–6)

where ϵ = the electromotive force of the cell
F = Faraday's constant (96,500 C/mol)
R = the molar gas constant
T = temperature, in degrees Kelvin

As the temperature increases, hydrogen ion activity increases and the potential generated increases. Most pH meters have a temperature-compensation knob that amplifies the millivolt response when the meter is on pH function. pH units on the meter scale are usually printed for use at room temperature. On the voltmeter, 59.16 is read as 1 pH unit change. The temperature compensation changes millivolt response to compensate for changes due to temperature from 54.2 at 0°C to 66.10 at 60°C. However, most pH meters are manufactured for greatest accuracy in the 10°C to 60°C range.

Calibration

The steps necessary to standardize a pH meter are fairly straightforward. First, balance the system with the electrodes in a buffer with a 7.0 pH. The balance or intercept

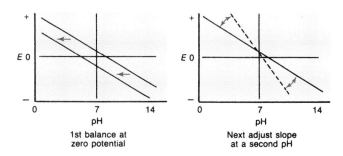

FIGURE 4-19. pH meter calibration. (From Willard HH, Merritt LL, Dean JA, Settle FA. Instrumental Methods of Analysis. Belmont, CA: Wadsworth, 1981.)

control shifts the entire slope, as shown in Figure 4-19. Next, replace the buffer with one of a different pH. If the meter does not register the correct pH, amplification of the response changes the slope to match that predicted by the Nernst equation. If the instrument does not have a slope control, the temperature compensator performs the same function.

pH Combination Electrode

The most commonly used pH electrode has both the indicator and reference electrodes combined in one small probe, which is convenient when small samples are tested. It consists of an Ag/AgCl internal reference electrode sealed in a narrow glass cylinder with a pH-sensitive glass tip. The reference electrode is an Ag/AgCl wire wrapped around the indicator electrode. The outer glass envelope is filled with KCl and has a tiny pore near the tip of the liquid junction. The solution to be measured must completely cover the glass tip. Examples of other ISEs are shown in Figure 4-20. The reference electrode, electrometer, and calibration system described for pH measurements are applicable to all ISEs.

There are three major ISE types: inert-metal electrodes in contact with a redox couple, metal electrodes that par-

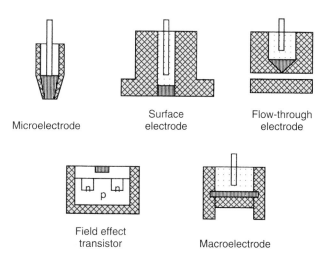

FIGURE 4-20. Other examples of ion-selective electrodes.

ticipate in a redox reaction, and membrane electrodes. The membrane can be solid material (*eg*, glass), liquid (*eg*, ion-exchange electrodes), or special membrane (*eg*, compound electrodes), such as gas-sensing and enzyme electrodes.

The standard hydrogen electrode is an example of an inert-metal electrode. The Ag/AgCl electrode is an example of the second type. The electrode process AgCl + $e^- \to Ag^+ + Cl^-$ produces an electrical potential proportional to Cl^- ion activity. When the chloride ion is held constant, the electrode is used as a reference electrode. The electrode in contact with varying Cl^- concentrations is used as an indicator electrode to measure chloride concentration.

The H^+ sensitive gel layer of the glass pH electrode is considered a membrane. A change in the glass formulation makes the membrane more sensitive to sodium ions than to hydrogen ions, creating a sodium ISE. Other solid-state membranes consist of either a single crystal or fine crystals immobilized in an inert matrix such as silicone rubber. Conduction depends on a vacancy defect mechanism, and the crystals are formulated to be selective for a particular size, shape, and change; for example, F^- selective electrodes of LaF, Cl^- sensitive electrodes with AgCl crystals, and AgBr electrodes for the detection of Br^-.

The calcium ISE is a liquid-membrane electrode. An ion-selective carrier, such as dioctyphenyl phosphate dissolved in an inert water-insoluble solvent, diffuses through a porous membrane. Because the solvent is insoluble in water, the test sample cannot cross the membrane, but Ca^{2+} ions are exchanged. The Ag/AgCl internal reference in a filling solution of $CaCl_2$ is in contact with the carrier by means of the membrane.

Potassium-selective liquid membranes use the antibiotic valinomycin as the ion-selective carrier. Valinomycin membranes show great selectivity for K^+. Liquid-membrane electrodes are recharged every few months to replace the liquid ion exchanger and the porous membrane.

Gas-Sensing Electrodes

Gas electrodes are similar to pH glass electrodes but are designed to detect specific gases (*eg*, CO_2 and NH_3) in solutions and are usually separated from the solution by a thin, gas-permeable hydrophobic membrane. Figure 4-21 shows a schematic illustration of the PCO_2 electrode. The membrane in contact with the solution is permeable only to CO_2, which diffuses into a thin film of sodium bicarbonate solution. The pH of the bicarbonate solution is changed as follows:

$$CO_2 + H_2O \leftrightarrow H_2CO_3 \leftrightarrow H^+ + HCO_3^- \qquad \text{(Eq. 4–7)}$$

The change in pH of the HCO_3^- is detected by a pH electrode. The PCO_2 electrode is widely used in clinical

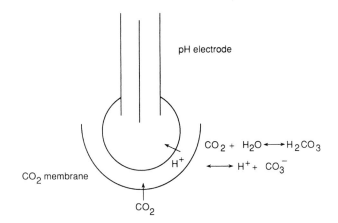

FIGURE 4-21. The PCO_2 electrode.

laboratories as a component of instruments for measuring serum electrolytes and blood gases.

In the NH_3 gas electrode, the bicarbonate solution is replaced by ammonium chloride solution, and the membrane is permeable only to NH_3 gas. As in the PCO_2 electrode, NH_3 changes the pH of NH_4Cl as follows:

$$NH_3 + H_2O \leftrightarrow NH_4^+ + OH^- \qquad \text{(Eq. 4–8)}$$

The amount of OH^- ions produced varies linearly with the log of the partial pressure of NH_3 in the sample.

Other gas-sensing electrodes function on the basis of an amperometric principle; that is, measurement of the current flowing through an electrochemical cell at a constant applied electrical potential to the electrodes. Examples are the determination of PO_2, glucose, and peroxidase.

The chemical reactions of the PO_2 electrode (Clark electrode), an electrochemical cell with a platinum cathode and an Ag/AgCl anode, are illustrated in Figure 4-17. The electrical potential at the cathode is set to -0.65 V and will not conduct current without oxygen in the sample. The membrane is permeable to oxygen, which diffuses through to the platinum cathode. Current passes through the cell and is proportional to the PO_2 in the test sample.

Glucose determination is based on the reduction in PO_2 during glucose oxidase reaction with glucose and oxygen. Unlike the PCO_2 electrode, the peroxidase electrode has a polarized platinum anode and its potential is set to $+ 0.6$ V. Current flows through the system when peroxide is oxidized at the anode as follows:

$$H_2O_2 \to 2H^+ + 2e^- + O_2 \qquad \text{(Eq. 4–9)}$$

Enzyme Electrodes

The various ISEs may be covered by immobilized enzymes that can catalyze a specific chemical reaction. Selection of the ISE is determined by the reaction product of the immobilized enzyme. Examples include urease, which is used for the detection of urea, and glucose oxidase, which is used for glucose detection. A urea electrode must have an ISE that is selective for NH_4^+ or NH_3, whereas glucose oxidase is used in combination with a pH electrode.

Coulometric Chloridometers and Anodic Stripping Voltametry

Chloride ISEs have largely replaced coulometric titrations for determination of chloride in body fluids. Anodic stripping voltametry was widely used for analysis of lead and is best measured by electrothermal (graphite furnace) atomic absorption spectroscopy or, preferably, ICP-MS.

ELECTROPHORESIS

Electrophoresis is the migration of charged solutes or particles in an electrical field. *Iontophoresis* refers to the migration of small ions, whereas *zone electrophoresis* is the migration of charged macromolecules in a porous support medium such as paper, cellulose acetate, or agarose-gel film. An electrophoretogram is the result of zone electrophoresis and consists of sharply separated zones of a macromolecule. In a clinical laboratory, the macromolecules of interest are proteins in serum, urine, cerebrospinal fluid, and other biologic body fluids and erythrocytes and tissue.

Electrophoresis consists of five components: the driving force (electrical power), the support medium, the buffer, the sample, and the detecting system. A typical electrophoretic apparatus is illustrated in Figure 4-22.

Charged particles migrate toward the opposite charged electrode. The velocity of migration is controlled by the net charge of the particle, the size and shape of the particle, the strength of the electric field, chemical and physical properties of the supporting medium, and the electrophoretic temperature. The rate of mobility[12] of the molecule (μ) is given by

$$\mu = \frac{Q}{k} \times r \times n \qquad \text{(Eq. 4–10)}$$

where Q = net charge of particle
k = constant
r = ionic radius of the particle
n = viscosity of the buffer

From the equation, the rate of migration is directly proportional to the net charge of the particle and inversely proportional to its size and the viscosity of the buffer.

Procedure

The sample is soaked in hydrated support for approximately 5 minutes. The support is put into the electrophoresis chamber, which was previously filled with the buffer. Enough buffer must be added to the chamber to maintain contact with the support. Electrophoresis is carried out by applying a constant voltage or constant current for a specific time. The support is then removed and placed in a fixative or rapidly dried to prevent diffusion of the sample. This is followed by staining the zones with appropriate dye. The uptake of dye by the sample is proportional to sample concentration. After excess dye is washed away, the supporting medium may need to be placed in a clearing agent. Otherwise, it is completely dried.

Power Supply

Power supplies operating at either constant current or constant voltage are available commercially. In electrophoresis, heat is produced when current flows through a medium that has resistance, resulting in an increase in thermal agitation of the dissolved solute (ions) and leading to a decrease in resistance and an increase in current. The increase leads to increases in heat and evaporation of water from the buffer, increasing the ionic concentration of the buffer and subsequent further increases in the current. The migration rate can be kept constant by using a power supply with constant current. This is true because, as electrophoresis progresses, a decrease in resistance as a result of heat produced also decreases the voltage.

Buffers

Two buffer properties that affect the charge of ampholytes are pH and ionic strength. The ions carry the applied electric current and allow the buffer to maintain constant pH during electrophoresis. An ampholyte is a molecule, such as protein, whose net charge can be either positive or negative. If the buffer is more acidic than the isoelectric point (pI) of the ampholyte, it binds H^+ ions, becomes positively charged, and migrates toward the

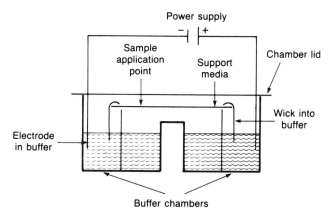

FIGURE 4-22. Electrophoresis apparatus—basic components.

cathode. If the buffer is more basic than the pI, the ampholyte loses H^+ ions, becomes negatively charged, and migrates toward the anode. A particle without a net charge will not migrate, remaining at the point of application. During electrophoresis, ions cluster around a migrating particle. The higher the ionic concentration, the higher the size of the ionic cloud and the lower the mobility of the particle. Greater ionic strength produces sharper protein-band separation but leads to increased heat production. This may cause denaturation of heat-labile proteins. Consequently, the optimal buffer concentration should be determined for any electrophoretic system. Generally, the most widely used buffers are made of monovalent ions because their ionic strength and molality are equal.

Support Materials

Cellulose Acetate

Paper electrophoresis use has been replaced by cellulose acetate or agarose gel in clinical laboratories. Cellulose is acetylated to form cellulose acetate by treating it with acetic anhydride. Cellulose acetate, a dry, brittle film composed of about 80% air space, is produced commercially. When the film is soaked in buffer, the air spaces fill with electrolyte and the film becomes pliable. After electrophoresis and staining, cellulose acetate can be made transparent for densitometer quantitation. The dried transparent film can be stored for long periods. Cellulose acetate prepared to reduce electroendosmosis is available commercially. Cellulose acetate is also used in isoelectric focusing.

Agarose Gel

Agarose gel is another widely used supporting medium. Used as a purified fraction of agar, it is neutral and, therefore, does not produce electroendosmosis. After electrophoresis and staining, it is detained (cleared), dried, and scanned with a densitometer. The dried gel can be stored indefinitely. Agarose-gel electrophoresis requires small amounts of sample (approximately 2 μL); it does not bind protein and, therefore, migration is not affected.

Polyacrylamide Gel

Polyacrylamide-gel electrophoresis involves separation of protein on the basis of charge and molecular size. Layers of gel with different pore sizes are used. The gel is prepared before electrophoresis in a tubular-shaped electrophoresis cell. The small-pore separation gel is at the bottom, followed by a large-pore spacer gel and, finally, another large-pore gel containing the sample. Each layer of gel is allowed to form a gelatin before the next gel is poured over it. At the start of electrophoresis, the protein molecules move freely through the spacer gel to its boundary with the separation gel, which slows their movement. This allows for concentration of the sample before separation by the small-pore gel. Polyacrylamide-gel electrophoresis separates serum proteins into 20 or more fractions rather than the usual 5 fractions separated by cellulose acetate or agarose. It is widely used to study individual proteins (*eg*, isoenzymes).

Starch Gel

Starch-gel electrophoresis separates proteins on the basis of surface charge and molecular size, as does polyacrylamide gel. The procedure is not widely used because of technical difficulty in preparing the gel.

Treatment and Application of Sample

Serum contains a high concentration of protein, especially albumin and, therefore, serum specimens are routinely diluted with buffer before electrophoresis. In contrast, urine and cerebrospinal fluid (CSF) are usually concentrated. Hemoglobin hemolysate is used without further concentration. Generally, preparation of a sample is done according to the suggestion of the manufacturer of the electrophoretic supplies.

Cellulose acetate and agarose-gel electrophoresis require approximately 2 to 5 μL of sample. These are the most common routine electrophoreses performed in clinical laboratories. Because most commercially manufactured plates come with a thin plastic template that has small slots through which samples are applied, overloading of agarose gel with sample is not a frequent problem. After serum is allowed to diffuse into the gel for approximately 5 minutes, the template is blotted to remove excess serum before being removed from the gel surface. Sample is applied to cellulose acetate with a twin-wire applicator designed to transfer a small amount.

Detection and Quantitation

Separated protein fractions are stained to reveal their locations. Different stains come with different plates from different manufacturers. The simplest way to accomplish detection is visualization under UV light, whereas densitometry is the most common and reliable way for quantitation. Most densitometers will automatically integrate the area under a peak, and the result is printed as percentage of the total. A schematic illustration of a densitometer is shown in Figure 4-23.

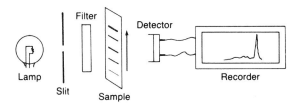

FIGURE 4-23. Densitometer—basic components.

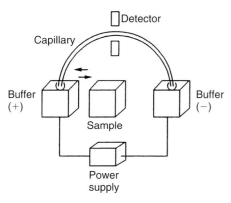

FIGURE 4-24. Schematic of capillary electrophoresis instrumentation. Sample is loaded on the capillary by replacing the anode buffer reservoir with the sample reservoir. (From Heiger DN. High-Performance Capillary Electrophoresis. Waldbronn, Germany: Hewlett-Packard, 1992.)

Electroendosmosis

The movement of buffer ions and solvent relative to the fixed support is called *endosmosis* or *electroendosmosis*. Support media, such as paper, cellulose acetate, and agar gel, take on a negative charge from adsorption of hydroxyl ions. When current is applied to the electrophoresis system, the hydroxyl ions remain fixed while the free positive ions move toward the cathode. The ions are highly hydrated, resulting in net cathodic movement of solvent. Molecules that are nearly neutral are swept toward the cathode with the solvent. Support media such as agarose and acrylamide gel are essentially neutral, eliminating electroendosmosis. The position of proteins in any electrophoresis separation depends not only on the nature of the protein, but also on all other technical variables.

Isoelectric Focusing

Isoelectric focusing is a modification of electrophoresis. An apparatus is used similar to that shown in Figure 4-24. Charged proteins migrate through a support medium that has a continuous pH gradient. Individual proteins move in the electric field until they reach a pH equal to their isoelectric point, at which point they have no charge and cease to move.

Capillary Electrophoresis

In capillary electrophoresis (CE), separation is performed in narrow-bore fused silica capillaries (inner diameter, 2575 mm). Usually, the capillaries are only filled with buffer, although gel media can also be used. A CE instrumentation schematic is shown in Figure 4-24. Initially, the capillary is filled with buffer and then the sample is loaded; applying an electric field performs the separation. Detection can be made near the other end of the capillary directly through the capillary wall.[13]

A fundamental CE concept is the *electro-osmotic flow* (EOF). EOF is the bulk flow of liquid toward the cathode upon application of electric field and it is superimposed on electrophoretic migration. EOF controls the amount of time solutes remain in the capillary. Cations migrate fastest because both EOF and electrophoretic attraction are toward the cathode; neutral molecules are all carried by the EOF but are not separated from each other; and anions move slowest because, although they are carried to the cathode by the EOF, they are attracted to the anode and repelled by the cathode (Fig. 4-25). Widely used for monitoring separated analytes, UV-visible detection is performed directly on the capillary; however, sensitivity is poor because of the small dimensions of the capillary, resulting in a short path-length. Fluorescence, laser-induced fluorescence, and chemiluminescence detection can be used for higher sensitivity.

CE has been used for the separation, quantitation, and determination of molecular weights of proteins and peptides; for the analysis of polymerase chain reaction (PCR) products; and for the analysis of inorganic ions, organic acids, pharmaceuticals, optical isomers, and drugs of abuse in serum and urine.[14]

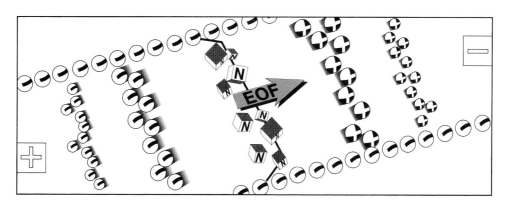

FIGURE 4-25. Differential solute migration superimposed on electro-osmotic flow in capillary zone electrophoresis. (From Heiger DN. High-Performance Capillary Electrophoresis. France: Hewlett-Packard, 1992.)

CHROMATOGRAPHY

Chromatography refers to the group of techniques used to separate complex mixtures on the basis of different physical interactions between the individual compounds and the stationary phase of the system. The basic components in any chromatographic technique are the mobile phase (gas or liquid), which carries the complex mixture (sample); the stationary phase (solid or liquid), through which the mobile phase flows; the column holding the stationary phase; and the separated components (eluate).

Modes of Separation

Adsorption

Adsorption chromatography, also known as *liquid-solid chromatography*, is based on the competition between the sample and the mobile phase for adsorptive sites on the solid stationary phase. There is an equilibrium of solute molecules being adsorbed to the solid surface and desorbed and dissolved in the mobile phase. The molecules that are most the soluble in the mobile phase, move fastest; the least soluble, move slowest. Thus, a mixture is typically separated into classes according to polar functional groups. The stationary phase can be either acidic polar (*eg*, silica gel), basic polar (*eg*, alumina), or nonpolar (*eg*, charcoal). The mobile phase can be a single solvent or a mixture of two or more solvents, depending on the analytes to be desorbed. Liquid-solid chromatography is not widely used in clinical laboratories because of technical problems with the preparation of a stationary phase that has homogeneous distribution of absorption sites.

Partition

Partition chromatography is also referred to as *liquid-liquid chromatography*. Separation of solute is based on relative solubility in an organic (nonpolar) solvent and an aqueous (polar) solvent. In its simplest form, partition (extraction) is performed in a separatory funnel. Molecules containing polar and nonpolar groups in an aqueous solution are added to an immiscible organic solvent. After vigorous shaking, the two phases are allowed to separate. Polar molecules remain in the aqueous solvent; nonpolar molecules are extracted in the organic solvent. This results in the partitioning of the solute molecules into two separate phases.

The ratio of the concentration of the solute in the two liquids is known as the *partition coefficient:*

$$K = \frac{\text{solute in stationary phase}}{\text{solute in mobile phase}} \quad \textbf{(Eq. 4–11)}$$

Modern partition chromatography uses pseudoliquid stationary phases that are chemically bonded to the support or high-molecular-weight polymers that are insoluble in the mobile phase.[15] Partition systems are considered *normal phase* when the mobile solvent is less polar than the stationary solvent and *reverse phase* when the mobile solvent is more polar.

Partition chromatography is applicable to any substance that may be distributed between two liquid phases. Because ionic compounds are generally soluble only in water, partition chromatography works best with nonionic compounds.

Steric Exclusion

Steric exclusion, a variation of liquid-solid chromatography, is used to separate solute molecules on the basis of size and shape. The chromatographic column is packed with porous material, as shown in Figure 4-26. A sample containing different-sized molecules moves down the column dissolved in the mobile solvent. Small molecules enter the pores in the packing and are momentarily trapped. Large molecules are excluded from the small pores and so move quickly between the particles. Intermediate-sized molecules are partially restricted from entering the pores and, therefore, move through the column at an intermediate rate that is between those of the large and small molecules.

Early methods used hydrophilic beads of cross-linked dextran, polyacrylamide, or agarose, which formed a gel when soaked in water. This method was termed *gel filtration*. A similar separation process using hydrophobic gel beads of polystyrene with a nonaqueous mobile phase was called *gel permeation chromatography*. Current porous packing uses rigid inorganic materials such as silica or glass. The term *steric exclusion* includes all these variations. Pore size is controlled by the manufacturer, and packing materials can be purchased with different pore sizes, depending on the size of the molecules being separated.

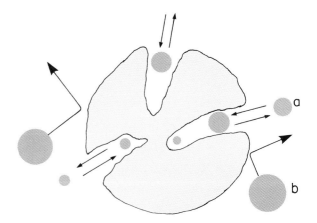

FIGURE 4-26. Pictorial concept of steric exclusion chromatography. Separation of sample components by their ability to permeate pore structure of column-packing material. Smaller molecules (**a**) permeating the interstitial pores; large excluded molecules (**b**). (From Parris NA. Instrumental Liquid Chromatography: A Practical Manual on High Performance Liquid Chromatographic Methods. New York: Elsevier, 1976.)

Ion-Exchange Chromatography

In ion-exchange chromatography, solute mixtures are separated by virtue of the magnitude and charge of ionic species. The stationary phase is a resin, consisting of large polymers of substituted benzene, silicates, or cellulose derivatives, with charge functional groups. The resin is insoluble in water, and the functional groups are immobilized as side chains on resin beads that are used to fill the chromatographic column. Figure 4-27A shows resin with sulfonate functional groups. H^+ ions are loosely held and free to react. This is an example of a cation-exchange resin. When a cation such as Na^+ comes in contact with these functional groups, an equilibrium is formed, following the law of mass action. Because there are many sulfonate groups, Na^+ ions are effectively and completely removed from solution. The Na^+ ions that are concentrated on the resin column can be eluted from the resin by pouring acid through the column, driving the equilibrium to the left.

Anion-exchange resins are made with exchangeable hydroxyl ions such as the diethylamine functional group illustrated in Figure 4-27B. They are used like cation-exchange resins, except that hydroxyl ions are exchanged for anions. The example shows Cl^- ions in sample solution exchanged for OH^- ions from the resin functional group. Anion and cation resins mixed together (mixed-bed resin) are used to deionize water. The displaced protons and hydroxyl ions combine to form water. Ionic functional groups other than the illustrated examples are used for specific analytic applications. Ion-exchange chromatography is used to remove interfering substances from a solution, to concentrate dilute ion solutions, and to separate mixtures of charged molecules, such as amino acids. Changing pH and ionic concentration of the mobile phase allows separation of mixtures of organic and inorganic ions.

Chromatographic Procedures

Thin-Layer Chromatography (TLC)

TLC is a variant of column chromatography. A thin layer of *sorbent*, such as alumina, silica gel, cellulose, or cross-linked dextran, is uniformly coated on a glass or plastic plate. Each sample to be analyzed is applied as a spot near one edge of the plate, as shown in Figure 4-28. The mobile phase (solvent) is usually placed in a closed container until the atmosphere is saturated with solvent vapor. One edge of the plate is placed in the solvent, as shown. The solvent migrates up the thin layer by capillary action, dissolving and carrying sample molecules. Separation can be achieved by any of the four processes previously described, depending on the sorbent (thin layer) and solvent chosen. After the solvent reaches a predetermined height, the plate is removed and dried. Sample components are identified by comparison with standards on the same plate. The distance a component migrates, compared with the distance the solvent front moves, is called the *retention factor R_f*:

$$R_f = \frac{\text{distance leading edge of component moves}}{\text{total distance solvent front moves}}$$

(Eq. 4–12)

Each sample-component R_f is compared with the R_f of standards. Using Figure 4-28 as an example, standard A has an R_f value of 0.4, standard B has an R_f value of 0.6, and standard C is 0.8. The first unknown contains A and C, because the R_f values are the same. This ratio is valid only for separations run under identical conditions. Because R_f values may overlap for some components, further identifying information is obtained by spraying different stains on the dried plate and comparing colors of the standards.

TLC is most commonly used as a semiquantitative screening test. Technique refinement has resulted in the development of semiautomated equipment and the ability to quantitate separated compounds. For example, sample applicators apply precise amounts of sample extracts in concise areas. Plates prepared with uniform sorbent thickness, finer particles, and new solvent systems have resulted in the technique of high-performance thin-layer

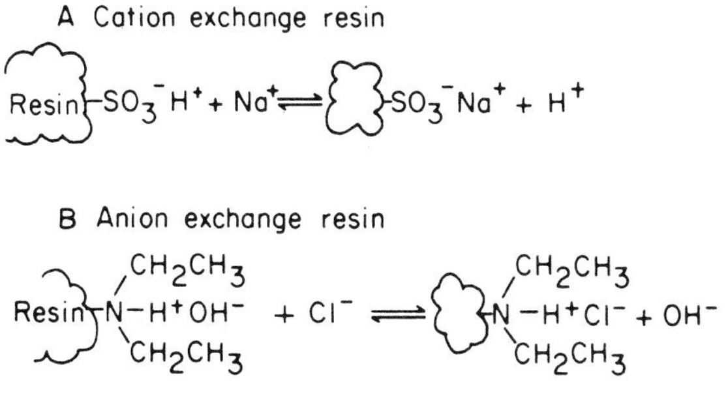

FIGURE 4-27. Chemical equilibrium of ion-exchange resins. (**A**) Cation exchange resin. (**B**) Anion exchange resin.

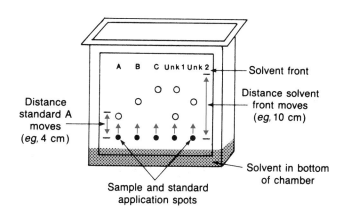

FIGURE 4-28. TLC plate in chromatographic chamber.

chromatography (HPTLC).[16] Absorbance of each developed spot is measured using a densitometer, and the concentration is calculated by comparison with a reference standard chromatographed under identical conditions.

High-Performance Liquid Chromatography (HPLC)

Modern liquid chromatography uses pressure for fast separations, controlled temperature, in-line detectors, and gradient elution techniques.[17,18] Figure 4-29 illustrates the basic components.

Pumps

A pump forces the mobile phase through the column at a much greater velocity than that accomplished by gravity-flow columns and include pneumatic, syringe, reciprocating, or hydraulic amplifier pumps. The most widely used pump today is the mechanical reciprocating pump, which is now used as a multihead pump with two or more reciprocating pistons. During pumping, the pistons operate out of phase (180° for two heads, 120° for three heads) to provide constant flow. Pneumatic pumps are used for preoperative purposes; hydraulic amplifier pumps are no longer commonly used.

Columns

The stationary phase is packed into long stainless steel columns. HPLC is usually run at ambient temperatures, although columns can be put in an oven and heated to enhance the rate of partition. Fine, uniform column packing results in much less band broadening but requires pressure to force the mobile phase through. The packing also can be either pellicular (an inert core with a porous layer), inert and small particles, or macroporous particles. The most common material used for column packing is silica gel. It is very stable and can be used in different ways. It can be used as solid packing in liquid-solid chromatography or coated with a solvent, which serves as the stationary phase (liquid-liquid). As a result of the short lifetime of coated particles, molecules of the mobile-phase liquid are now bonded to the surface of silica particles.

Reversed-phase HPLC is now popular; the stationary phase is nonpolar molecules (eg, octadecyl C-18 hydrocarbon) bonded to silica-gel particles. For this type of column packing, the mobile phase commonly used is acetonitrile, methanol, water, or any combination of solvents. A reversed-phase column can be used to separate ionic, nonionic, and ionizable samples. A buffer is used to produce the desired ionic characteristics and pH for separation of the analyte. Column packings vary in size (3 mm to 20 mm), using smaller particles mostly for analytic separations and larger ones for preparative separations.

Sample Injectors

A small syringe can be used to introduce the sample into the path of the mobile phase that carries it into the col-

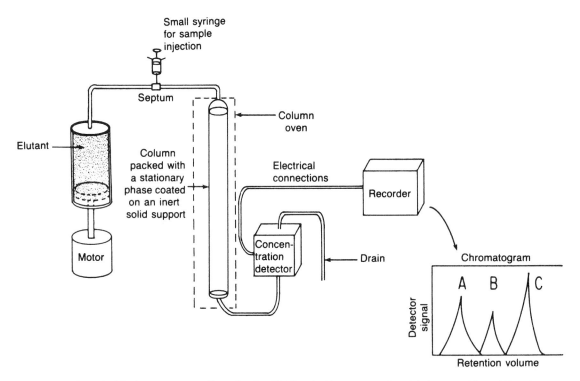

FIGURE 4-29. HPLC basic components. (From Bender GT. Chemical Instrumentation: A Laboratory Manual Based on Clinical Chemistry. Philadelphia: WB Saunders, 1972.)

umn (Fig. 4-29). The best and most widely used method, however, is the loop injector. The sample is introduced into a fixed-volume loop. When the loop is switched, the sample is placed in the path of the flowing mobile phase and flushed onto the column.

Loop injectors have high reproducibility and are used at high pressures. Many HPLC instruments have loop injectors that can be programmed for automatic injection of samples. When the sample size is less than the volume of the loop, the syringe containing the sample is often filled with the mobile phase to the volume of the loop before filling the loop. This prevents the possibility of air being forced through the column because such a practice may reduce the lifetime of the column packing material.

Detectors

Modern HPLC detectors monitor the eluate as it leaves the column and, ideally, produce an electronic signal proportional to the concentration of each separated component. Spectrophotometers that detect absorbances of visible or ultraviolet light are most commonly used. PDA and other rapid scanning detectors are also used for spectral comparisons and compound identification and purity. These detectors have been used for drug analyses in urine. Obtaining an ultraviolet scan of a compound as it elutes from a column can provide important information as to its identity. Unknowns can be compared against library spectra in a similar manner as mass spectrometry. Unlike gas chromatography/mass spectrometry, which requires volatilization of targeted compounds, liquid chromatography/photodiode array (LC/PDA) enables direct injection of aqueous urine samples.

Because many biologic substances fluoresce strongly, fluorescence detectors are also used, involving the same principles discussed in the section on spectrophotometric measurements. Another common HPLC detector is the amperometric or electrochemical detector, which measures current produced when the analyte of interest is either oxidized or reduced at some fixed potential set between a pair of electrodes.

A mass spectrometer (MS) can also be used as a detector, not only for the identification and quantitation of compounds but also for structural information and molecular weight determination.[19] The sample in an MS is first volatilized and then ionized to form charged molecular ions and fragments that are separated according to their mass-to-charge (m/z) ratio; the sample is then measured by a detector, which gives the intensity of the ion current for each species. Molecule identification is based on the formation of characteristic fragments. Coupling a liquid chromatograph to a mass spectrometer is difficult because of the large amount of solvent in the eluate. The electrospray (ES) technique allows ions to be transferred from solution to the gas phase.[20] The sample is passed through a metal capillary tip and converted, under the influence of a high electric field (10^6 V/m), to a fine mist of positively charged droplets, from which the solvent rapidly evaporates. The solute ions that remain are then transferred to a mass spectrometer to be analyzed.

Recorders

The recorder is used to record detector signal versus the time the mobile phase passed through the instrument, starting from the time of sample injection. The graph is called a *chromatogram* (Fig. 4-30). The retention time is used to identify compounds when compared with standard retention times run under identical conditions. Peak area is proportional to concentration of the compounds that produced the peaks.

When the elution strength of the mobile phase is constant throughout the separation, it is called *isocratic elution*. For samples containing compounds of widely differing relative compositions, the choice of solvent is a compromise. Early eluting compounds may have retention times close to zero, producing a poor separation (resolution), as shown in Figure 4-30A. Basic compounds often have low retention times because C-18 columns cannot tolerate high pH mobile phases. The addition of cation-pairing reagents to the mobile phase (*eg*, octane sulfonic acid) can result in better retention of negatively charged compounds onto the column.

The late-eluting compounds may have long retention times, producing broad bands resulting in decreased sensitivity. In some cases, certain components of a sample may have such a great affinity for the stationary phase that they do not elute at all. Gradient elution is an HPLC technique that can be used to overcome this problem. The composition of the mobile phase is varied to provide a continual increase in the solvent strength of the mobile phase entering the column (Fig. 4-30B). The same gradient elution can be performed with a faster change in concentration of the mobile phase (Fig. 4-30C).

Gas Chromatography

Gas chromatography is used to separate mixtures of compounds that are volatile or can be made volatile.[21] Gas chromatography may be gas-solid chromatography (GSC), with a solid stationary phase, or gas-liquid chromatography (GLC), with a nonvolatile liquid stationary phase. GLC is commonly used in clinical laboratories. Figure 4-31 illustrates the basic components of a gas chromatographic system. The setup is similar to HPLC, except that the mobile phase is a gas and samples are partitioned between a gaseous mobile phase and a liquid stationary phase. The carrier gas can be nitrogen, helium, or argon. The selection of a carrier gas is determined by the detector used in the instrument. The instrument can be operated at a constant temperature or programmed to run at different temperatures if a sample has components

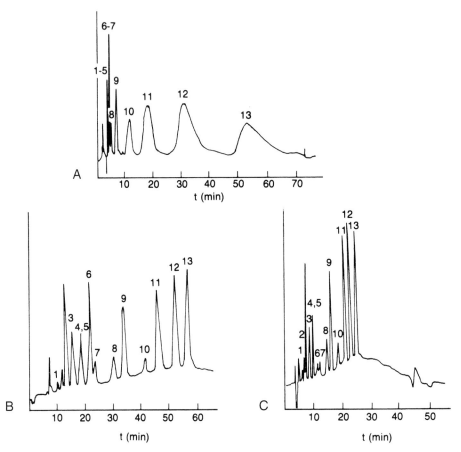

FIGURE 4-30. Chromatograms: (**A**) Isocratic ion-exchange separation-mobile phase contains 0.055 M NaNO₃. (**B**) Gradient elution-mobile phase gradient from 0.01 to 0.1 M NaNO₃ at 2%/minute. (**C**) Gradient elution—5%/minute. (From Horváth C. High Performance Liquid Chromatography, Advances and Perspectives. New York: Academic Press, 1980.)

with different volatilities. This is analogous to gradient elution described for HPLC.

The sample, which is injected through a septum, must be injected as a gas or the temperature of the injection port must be above the boiling point of the components

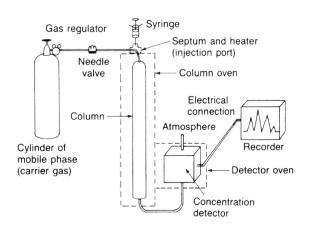

FIGURE 4-31. GLC basic components. (From Bender GT. Chemical Instrumentation: A Laboratory Manual Based on Clinical Chemistry. Philadelphia: WB Saunders, 1972.)

so that they vaporize upon injection. Sample vapor is swept through the column partially as a gas and partially dissolved in the liquid phase. Volatile compounds that are present mainly in the gas phase will have a low partition coefficient and will move quickly through the column. Compounds with higher boiling points will move slowly through the column. The effluent passes through a detector that produces an electric signal proportional to the concentration of the volatile components. As in HPLC, the chromatogram is used both to identify the compounds by the retention time and to determine their concentration by the area under the peak.

Columns

GLC columns are generally made of glass or stainless steel and are available in a variety of coil configurations and sizes. Packed columns are filled with inert particles such as diatomaceous earth or porous polymer or glass beads coated with a nonvolatile liquid (stationary) phase. These columns are usually ⅛ to ¼ inch wide and 3 to 12 feet long. Capillary-wall coated open tubular columns have inside diameters in the range of 0.25 mm to 0.50 mm and are up to 60 m long. The liquid layer is coated on the walls of the column. A solid support coated with a liquid stationary phase may in turn be coated on column walls.

The liquid stationary phase must be nonvolatile at the temperatures used, must be thermally stable, and must not react chemically with the solutes to be separated. The stationary phase is termed *nonselective* when separation is primarily based on relative volatility of the compounds. Selective liquid phases are used to separate polar compounds based on relative polarity (as in liquid-liquid chromatography).

Detectors

Although there are many types of detectors, only thermal conductivity (TC) and flame ionization detectors are discussed because they are the most stable (Fig. 4-32). TC detectors contain wires (filaments) that change electrical resistance with change in temperature. The filaments form opposite arms of a Wheatstone bridge and are heated electrically to raise their temperature. Helium, which has a high thermal conductivity, is usually the carrier gas. Carrier gas from the reference column flows steadily across one filament, cooling it slightly. Carrier

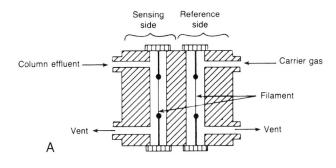

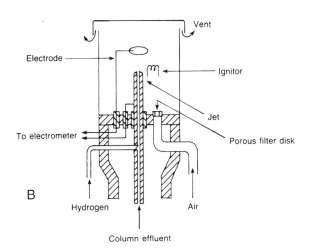

FIGURE 4-32. (**A**) Schematic diagram of a thermal conductivity detector. (**B**) Schematic diagram of a flame ionization detector. (From Tietz NW, ed. Fundamentals of Clinical Chemistry. Philadelphia: WB Saunders, 1987.)

gas and separated compounds from the sample column flow across the other filament. The sample components usually have a lower thermal conductivity, increasing the temperature and resistance of the sample filament. The change in resistance results in an unbalanced bridge circuit. The electrical change is amplified and fed to the recorder. The electrical change is proportional to the concentration of the analyte.

Flame ionization detectors are widely used in the clinical laboratory. They are more sensitive than TC detectors. The column effluent is fed into a small hydrogen flame burning in excess air or atmospheric oxygen. The flame jet and a collector electrode around the flame have opposite potentials. As the sample burns, ions form and move to the charged collector. Thus, a current proportional to the concentration of the ions is formed and fed to the recorder.

Mass Spectrometry

Definitive identification of samples eluting from gas chromatographic columns are possible when a mass spectrometer is used as a detector.[20] A block diagram of quadrupole and ion trap mass spectrometers are shown in Figures 4-33A and B. Substances separated from a gas chromatogram enter the source where samples are bombarded by electrons to form charged molecular ions and fragments. Molecules break down into characteristic fragments according to their molecular structure (Fig. 4-34). These particles are focused to enter the mass filtering sector where they are sorted according to their mass-to-charge (*m/z*) ratio and counted by an electron multiplier. Both quadrupole and ion trap detectors contain rods or plates that are charged with varying AC and DC voltages to form electric fields. In the quadrupole, ions selectively form stable sinusoidal orbits and traverse the filtering sector where they reach the detector and are measured. The ion trap, ions also form stable orbits, but are selectively destabilized in order to reach the detector. The characteristic fragmentation patterns produced by these ions are used for identification. Computerized libraries and matching algorithms are available within the instrument to compare mass spectral results of an unknown substance obtained from a sample to the reference library. GC/MS systems are widely used for measuring drugs of abuse in urine toxicology confirmations. Figure 4-35 illustrates the mass spectrum of Δ^9 9-carboxytetrahydrocannabinol, a metabolite of marijuana. Drugs and metabolites must be extracted from body fluids and typically reacted with derivatizing reagents to form compounds that are more volatile for the gas chromatography process.

Tandem mass spectrometers (GC/MS/MS), obtained by the addition of a second mass spectrometer to a GC/MS system, can be used for greater selectivity and lower detection limits. The first mass spectrometer al-

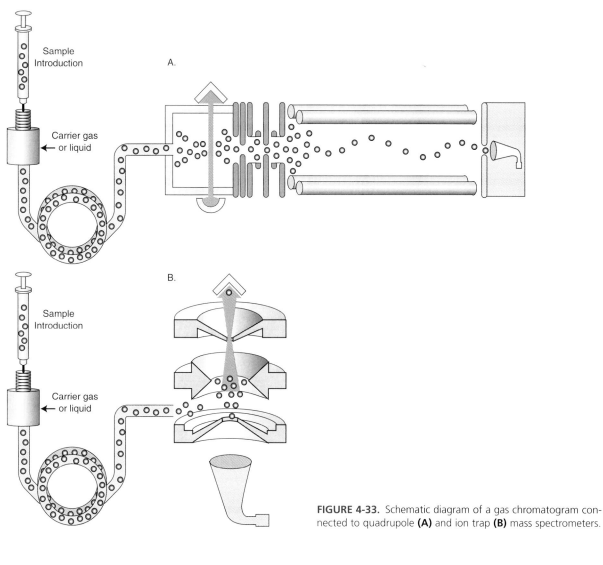

FIGURE 4-33. Schematic diagram of a gas chromatogram connected to quadrupole **(A)** and ion trap **(B)** mass spectrometers.

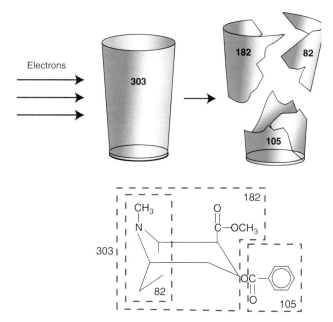

FIGURE 4-34. Electron bombardment breaks cocaine into fragments, with number and size quantified. Unlike the illustrative glass tumbler, the result of mass fragmentation of cocaine or other chemical compounds is both predictable and reproducible.

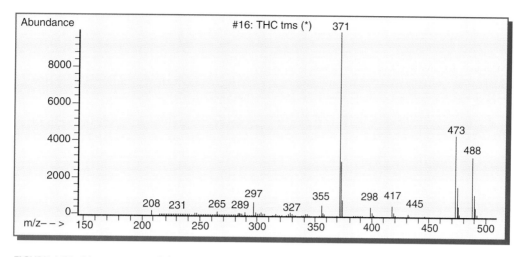

FIGURE 4-35. Mass spectrum of the trimethylsilane derivative of Δ^9 9-carboxytetrahydrocannabinol (marijuana metabolite).

lows only ions of a specific *m/z* ratio to pass to the second mass spectrometer, where they are further fragmented and analyzed (Fig. 4-36).

INSTRUMENTATION FOR PROTEOMICS

The next generation of biomarkers for human diseases will be discovered using techniques found within the research fields of genomics and proteomics. Genomics use the known sequences of the entire human genome for determining the role of genetics in certain human diseases. Proteomics is the investigation of the protein products encoded by these genes. Protein expression is equal to and, in many cases, more important for disease detection than genomics because these products determine

what is *currently* occurring within a cell, rather than the genes, which indicate what a cell *might* be capable of performing. Moreover, many (posttranslational) changes can occur to the protein, as influenced by other proteins and enzymes, that cannot be easily predicted by knowledge at the genomic level.

A "shotgun" approach is often used in the discovery of new biochemical markers. The proteins from samples (eg, serum, urine, tissue extract) from normal individuals are compared with those derived from patients with the disease being studied. Techniques such as two-dimensional electrophoresis can be used to separate proteins into individual spots or bands. Proteins that only appear in either the normal or diseased specimens are further studied. Computer programs are available that

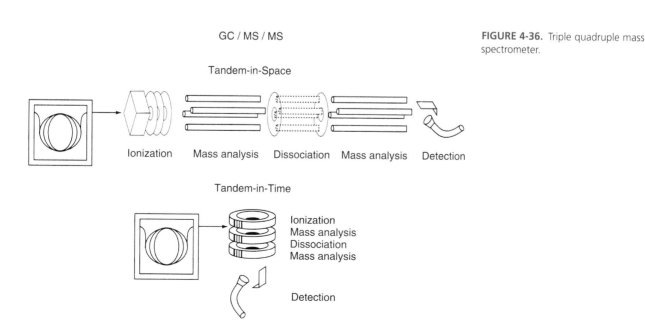

FIGURE 4-36. Triple quadruple mass spectrometer.

digitally compare gels to determine spots or areas that are different. When candidate proteins have been found, the spots can be isolated and subjected to sophisticated mass spectrometric analysis to identify the protein and possibly any posttranslational modifications that may have occurred. Using this approach, the researcher does not have any preconceptions or biases as to what directions or particular proteins to look for.

Two-Dimensional Electrophoresis

This electrophoresis assay combines two different electrophoresis dimensions to separate proteins from complex matrices such as serum or tissue. In the first dimension, proteins are resolved according to their isoelectric points (pIs), using immobilized pH gradients. Commercial gradients are available in a variety of pH ranges. In the second dimension, proteins are separated according to their relative size (molecular weight), using sodium dodecyl sulfate-polyacrylamide gel electrophoresis (SDS-PAGE). A schematic of this procedure is shown in Figure 4-37. Gels can be run under denaturing or nondenaturing conditions (*eg*, for the maintenance of enzyme activity) and visualized by a variety of techniques, including the use of colorimetric dyes (*eg*, Coomassie blue or silver stain), radiographic, fluorometric, or chemiluminescence of appropriately labeled polypeptides. These latter techniques are considerably more sensitive than the colorimetric dyes.

MALDI-TOF and SELDI-TOF Mass Spectrometry

Matrix-assisted laser desorption ionization time-of-flight mass spectrometry (MALDI-TOF) is used for the analysis of biomolecules, such peptides and proteins. Protein samples, such as those isolated from a two-dimensional electrophoretogram, are mixed with an appropriate matrix solvent and spotted onto a stainless steel plate. The solvent is dried and the plate is introduced into the vacuum system of the MALDI-TOF analyzer. As shown in Figure 4-38, a laser pulse irradiates the sample causing desorption and ionization of both the matrix and sample. Because the monitored mass spectral range is high (>500 daltons), the ionization of the low molecular weight matrix can be readily distinguished from high molecular weight peptides and proteins and do not interfere with the assay of the protein. Ions from the sample are focused into the mass spectrum. The time required for a mass to reach the detector is a nonlinear function of the mass, with larger ions requiring more time than smaller ions. The molecular weight of the proteins acquired by mass spectrum is used to determine the identity of the sample and is helpful in determining posttranslational modifica-

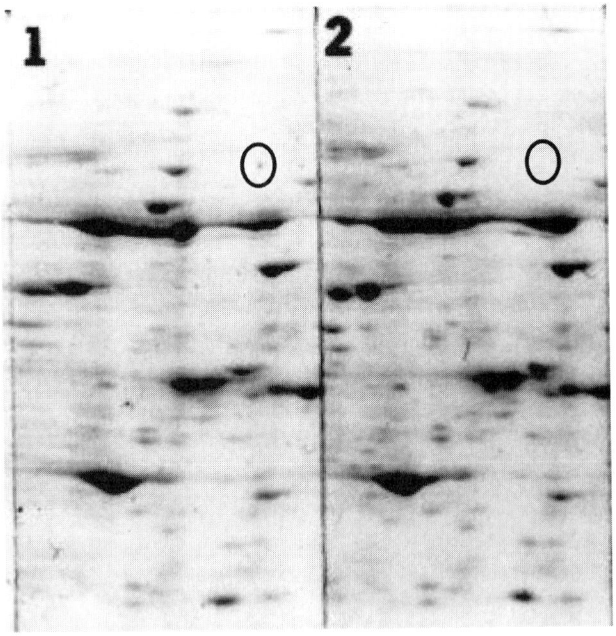

FIGURE 4-37. Hypothetical example of a two-dimensional electrophoretogram from a patient with a disease (panel 1) compared with a normal subject (panel 2). The patient exhibits a protein (oval) that is not expressed in the normal subject. This protein might be a potential marker for this disease. (Gels courtesy of Kendrick Laboratories, Madison, WI.)

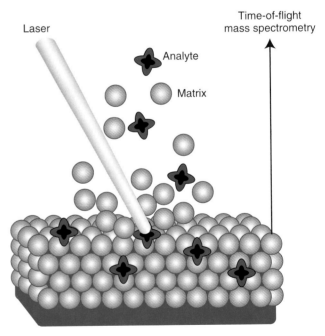

FIGURE 4-38. Sample desorption process prior to MALDI-TOF analysis. (Diagram courtesy of Stanford Research Systems, Sunnyvale, CA.)

tions that may have occurred. For very large proteins, samples can be pretreated with trypsin, which cleaves peptide bonds between lysine and arginine, to produce lower molecular weight fragments that can then be measured. The detection limit of this assay is about 10^{-15} to 10^{-18} moles. A modification of MALDI-TOF mass spectrometry is surface-enhanced laser desorption ionization time-of-flight (SELDI-TOF) mass spectrometry, in which proteins are directly captured on a chromatographic biochip without the need of sample preparation. Figure 4-39 illustrates the SELDI-TOF process.

OSMOMETRY

An osmometer is used to measure the concentration of solute particles in a solution. The mathematic definition is

$$\text{Osmolality} = \varphi \times n \times C \qquad \textbf{(Eq. 4–13)}$$

where φ = osmotic coefficient

n = number of dissociable particles (ions) per molecule in the solution

C = concentration in moles per kilogram of solvent

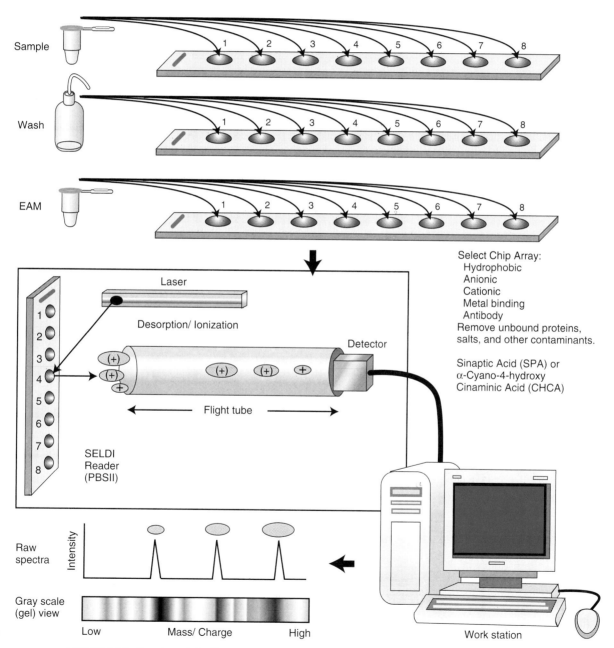

FIGURE 4-39. Overview of the SELDI-TOF process. (Diagram courtesy of Ciphergen Biosystems, Fremont, CA.)

1. Apply supernatant from CD8⁺ cells

Supernatant from stimulated and unstimulated CD8⁺ cell cultures from Normal, LTPN, and Progressors is added to a Protein Chip Array. Proteins bind to chemical or biological "docking" sites on the array surface through an affinity interaction.

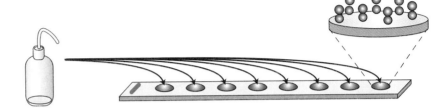

2. Wash Protein Chip Array

Proteins that bind non-specifically and buffer contaminants are washed away, eliminating sample noise.

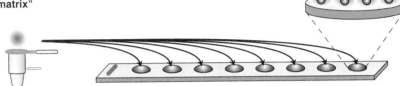

3. Add energy absorbing molecules or "matrix"

After sample processing, the array is dried and EAM is applied to each spot to facilitate desorption and ionization.

4. Analyze in a Protein Chip Reader

The proteins that are retained on the array are detected on the Protein Chip Reader.

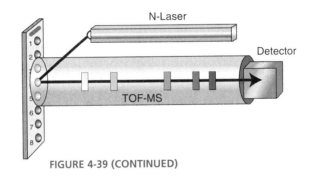

B

FIGURE 4-39 (CONTINUED)

The osmotic coefficient is an experimentally derived factor to correct for the fact that some of the molecules, even in a highly dissociated compound, exist as molecules rather than ions.

The four physical properties of a solution that change with variations in the number of dissolved particles in the solvent are osmotic pressure, vapor pressure, boiling point, and freezing point. Osmometers measure osmolality indirectly by measuring one of these colligative properties, which change proportionally with osmotic pressure. Osmometers in clinical use measure either freezing-point depression or vapor-pressure depression; results are expressed in milliosmolal per kilogram (mOsm/kg) units.

Freezing-Point Osmometer

Figure 4-40 illustrates the basic components of a freezing-point osmometer. The sample in a small tube is lowered into a chamber with cold refrigerant circulating from a cooling unit. A thermistor is immersed in the sample. To measure temperature, a wire is used to gently stir the sample until it is cooled to several degrees below its freezing point. It is possible to cool water to as low as –40°C and still have liquid water, provided no crystals or particulate matter are present. This is referred to as a *supercooled solution*. Vigorous agitation when the sample is supercooled results in rapid freezing. Freezing also can be started by "seeding" a supercooled solution with crys-

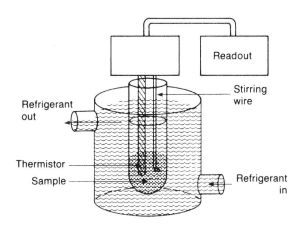

FIGURE 4-40. Freezing-point osmometer. (From Coiner D. Basic Concepts in Laboratory Instrumentation. Bethesda, MD: ASMT Education and Research Fund, 1975–1979.)

tals. When the supercooled solution starts to freeze as a result of the rapid stirring, a slush is formed and the solution actually warms to its freezing-point temperature. The slush, an equilibrium of liquid and ice crystals, will stay at the freezing-point temperature until the sample freezes solid and drops below its freezing point.

Impurities in a solvent will lower the temperature at which freezing or melting occurs by reducing the bonding forces between solvent molecules so that the molecules break away from each other and exist as a fluid at a lower temperature. The decrease in the freezing-point temperature is proportional to the number of dissolved particles present.

The thermistor is a material that has less resistance when the temperature increases. The readout uses a Wheatstone bridge circuit that detects temperature change as proportional to change in thermistor resistance. Freezing-point depression is proportional to the number of solute particles. Standards of known concentration are used to calibrate the instruments in mOsm/kg.

ANALYTIC TECHNIQUES FOR POCT

Point-of-care testing devices are widely used for a variety of clinical applications, including physician offices, emergency departments, intensive care units, and even for self-testing. Because analyses can be done at patient-side by primary caregivers, the major attraction of POCT is the reduced turnaround time needed to deliver results. In some cases, total costs can be reduced if the devices eliminate the need for laboratory-based instrumentation or if increased turnaround times lead to shorter hospital stays. POCT relies on the same analytic techniques as laboratory-based instrumentation: spectrometry, electroanalytic techniques, and chromatography. As such, the same steps needed to perform an analysis from the central laboratory are needed for POCT, including instrument validation, periodic assay calibration, quality control testing, operator training, and proficiency testing. Chapter 7, *Point-of-Care Testing,* provides an in-depth discussion of this technology. The analytic techniques used in these devices are given in this section.

The most commonly used POCT devices used at bedside, in physician offices, and at home are the fingerstick blood glucose monitors. The first generation devices use a photometric approach, whereby glucose produces hydrogen peroxide with glucose oxidase immobilized onto test strips. The H_2O_2 is coupled to peroxidase to produce a color whose intensity is measured as a function of concentration and measured using reflectance photometry. A schematic of this technique is shown in Figure 4-41. These strips are measured for glucose concentration without the need to wipe the blood off the strips.

The strip technology in a POCT platform can also be used to measure proteins and enzymes, such as cardiac markers. The separation of analytes from the matrix is accomplished by paper chromatography, in which specific antibodies immobilized onto the chromatographic surface capture the target analyte as it passes through. For qualitative analysis, detection is made by visual means. Reflectance meters similar to those used for glucose are also available for quantitative measurements.

The next generation of POCT devices use biosensors.[22] A biosensor couples a specific biodetector, such as an enzyme, antibody, or nucleic acid probe, to a transducer for the direct measurement of a target analyte without the need to separate it from the matrix (Fig. 4-42).

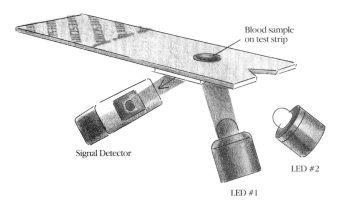

FIGURE 4-41. Dual-wavelength reflectance photometry used in a point-of-care glucose monitors. A microporous hydrophilic membrane is used as a reservoir of the sample to filter out solid cellular material from the reservoir and provide a smooth, optical surface for reflectance measurements. (Figure courtesy of Lifescan Inc. One touch system technology. Challenges in Diabetes Management: Clinical Protocols for Professional Practice. New York: Health Education Technologies, 1988.)

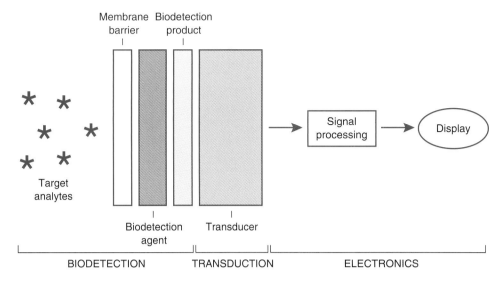

FIGURE 4-42. Schematic diagram of a biosensor. (From Rosen A. Biosensors: where do we go from here? MLO Med Lab Obs 1995;27(3):24.)

The field has exploded in recent years with the development of microsilicon chip fabrication because biosensors can be miniaturized and made available at low costs. An array of biosensors can be produced onto a single silicon wafer to produce a multipanel of results, such as an electrolyte profile. Commercial POCT devices use electrochemical (such as *microion-selective electrodes*) and optical biosensors for the measurement of glucose, electrolytes, and arterial blood gases. With the immobilization of antibodies and specific DNA sequences, biosensor probes will soon be available for detection of hormones, drugs and drugs of abuse, and hard-to-culture bacteria and viruses such as *Chlamydia,* tuberculosis, or human immunodeficiency virus.[22]

SUMMARY

The techniques and general principles used in a clinical chemistry laboratory are identical to those used in other analytic testing laboratories. Clinical laboratories do have special needs that require analyzers to have high throughput and sample turnaround times. The current generation of chemistry analyzers operates under the "random access" mode; that is, any combination of tests can be performed on a sample from an onboard menu of analytes. For general chemistry analytes, such as glucose or phosphorus, spectrophotometry is the most widely used technique. For electrolytes, such as sodium and potassium, ion-specific electrodes are extensively used and have largely replaced flame photometers. Atomic absorption spectrophotometry is still used for metals such as zinc

and copper and remains the reference method for calcium and magnesium. However, colorimetric assays and ISEs are now used routinely for these latter two metals.

Electrophoresis is still an important technique in clinical laboratories, although the development of new assays has challenged its role. For example, lipoprotein electrophoresis has been largely replaced by direct measurement of high-density lipoprotein (HDL) cholesterol and calculation of low-density lipoprotein (LDL) cholesterol. The development of a specific assay for LDL cholesterol will further diminish the role of electrophoresis. With the development of specific immunoassays for isoenzyme creatine kinase form MB (CK-MB) and inhibition assays for lactate dehydrogenase form 1 (LD1), electrophoresis is not as commonly used as before; however, an automated electrophoresis assay has recently been released for CK-MB isoforms. Electrophoresis will play a critical role in the area of molecular pathology for the identification of gene products and mutations. Two-dimensional electrophoresis enables the separation of complex mixtures and is an important tool for the discovery of new biomarkers for disease (proteomics). The identity of specific proteins can be performed by laser-assisted desorption mass spectrometer instruments. Capillary electrophoresis is an emerging technology that promises to have many clinical applications. With the development of immunoassays, the role of liquid chromatography has shifted away from therapeutic drug monitoring toward toxicology. HPLCs with rapid scanning UV detectors are being used for comprehensive drug screens. GC/MS is the mainstay for confirmation.

REVIEW QUESTIONS

1. Which of the following is NOT necessary for obtaining the spectrum of a compound from 190–500 nm?
   a. Deuterium light source
   b. Double-beam spectrophotometer
   c. Quartz cuvets
   d. Tungsten light source
   e. Photomultiplier

2. Stray light in a spectrophotometer places limits on:
   a. sensitivity.
   b. upper range of linearity.
   c. photometric accuracy below 0.1 absorbance units.
   d. ability to measure in the UV range.
   e. use of a grating monochromator.

3. Which of the following light sources is used in atomic absorption spectrophotometry?
   a. Hollow cathode lamp
   b. Xenon arc lamp
   c. Tungsten light
   d. Deuterium lamp
   e. Laser

4. Which of the following is true concerning fluorometry?
   a. Emission wavelengths are always set at lower wavelengths than excitation.
   b. The detector is always placed at right angles to the excitation beam.
   c. All compounds undergo fluorescence.
   d. Fluorescence is an inherently more sensitive technique than absorption.
   e. Fluorometers require special detectors.

5. Which of the following techniques has the highest potential sensitivity?
   a. Chemiluminescence
   b. Fluorescence
   c. Turbidimetry
   d. Nephelometry
   e. Phosphorescence

6. Which electrochemical assay measures current at fixed potential?
   a. Anodic stripping voltametry
   b. Amperometry
   c. Coulometry
   d. Analysis with ion selective electrodes
   e. Electrophoresis

7. Which of the following refers to the movement of buffer ions and solvent relative to the fixed support?
   a. Isoelectric focusing
   b. Iontophoresis
   c. Zone electrophoresis
   d. Electroendosmosis
   e. Plasmapheresis

8. Reverse-phase liquid chromatography refers to:
   a. a polar mobile phase and nonpolar stationary phase.
   b. a nonpolar mobile phase and polar stationary phase.
   c. distribution between two liquid phases.
   d. size used to separate solutes instead of charge.
   e. charge used to separate solutes instead of size.

9. Which of the following is NOT an advantage of capillary electrophoresis?
   a. Very small sample size
   b. Rapid analysis
   c. Use of traditional detectors
   d. Multiple samples can be assayed simultaneously on one injection
   e. Cations, neutrals, and anions move in the same direction at different rates

10. Tandem mass spectrometers:
    a. are two mass spectrometers placed in series with each other.
    b. are two mass spectrometers placed in parallel with each other.
    c. require use of a gas chromatograph.
    d. require use of an electrospray interface.
    e. do not require an ionization source.

11. Which of the following is FALSE concerning the principles of point-of-care testing devices?
    a. They use principles that are identical to laboratory-based instrumentation.
    b. Biosensors have enabled miniaturization particularly amendable for POC testing.
    c. Devices do not require quality control testing.
    d. Onboard microcomputers control instrument functions and data reduction.
    e. Whole blood analysis is the preferred specimen.

12. Which is the most sensitive detector for spectrophotometry?
    a. Phototube
    b. Photomultiplier
    c. Electron multiplier
    d. Photodiode array
    e. All are equally sensitive

13. Which of the following is Beer's law?
    a. $\% T = I/I_o \times 100$
    b. $E = h\nu$
    c. $\epsilon = \Delta pH \times 0.59V$
    d. $A = \epsilon \times b \times c$
    e. $Osmolality = \phi \times n \times C$

14. Which of the following correctly ranks electromagnetic radiation from low energy to high energy?
    a. Cosmic, gamma, x-rays, UV, visible, infrared, microwaves
    b. UV, visible, infrared, microwaves, x-rays, cosmic, gamma
    c. UV, visible, infrared, cosmic, gamma, microwaves, x-rays
    d. Microwaves, infrared, visible, UV, x-rays, gamma, cosmic
    e. Visible, UV, infrared, cosmic, gamma, microwaves, x-rays

15. What is the purpose of the chopper in an atomic absorption spectrophotometer?
    a. Correct for the amount of light emitted by the flame
    b. Correct for the fluctuating intensity of the light source
    c. Correct for the fluctuating sensitivity of the detector
    d. Correct for differences in the aspiration rate of the sample
    e. Correct for the presence of stray light

16. Which of the following best describes the process of fluorescence?
    a. Atoms emit a photon when the electrons are excited.
    b. Molecules emit a photon when the electrons are excited.
    c. Molecules emit a photon at the same energy when excited electrons return to the ground state.
    d. Molecules emit a photon at higher energy when excited electrons return to the ground state.
    e. Molecules emit a photon at lower energy when excited electrons return to the ground state.

17. Which is most accurate concerning ion selective electrodes?
    a. The pH electrode uses a solid-state membrane.
    b. The calcium electrode does not require a reference electrode.
    c. Gas-specific membranes are necessary for oxygen and carbon dioxide electrodes.
    d. The sodium electrode uses an ion-selective carrier (valinomycin).
    e. The ISE for urea uses immobilized urease.

18. Which of the following regarding mass spectrometry is FALSE?
    a. Ions are formed by the bombardment of electrons.
    b. Quadrupole and ion trap sectors separate ions according to their mass to charge ratio.
    c. Each chemical compound has a unique mass spectrum.
    d. Mass spectrometry detects for gas and liquid chromatography.
    e. Mass spectrometers can be used to sequence DNA.

19. Which of the following is not an objective of proteomics research?
    a. Identifying novel proteins as potential new biomarkers for disease
    b. Identifying posttranslational modifications of proteins
    c. Understanding the mechanism of diseases
    d. Identifying specific gene mutations
    e. Determining which genes are expressed and which genes are dormant

20. Which of the following procedures is not currently or routinely used for point-of-care testing devices?
    a. Immunochromatography
    b. Biosensors
    c. Colorimetric detection
    d. Electrochemical detection
    e. Polymerase chain reaction

REFERENCES

1. Christian GD, et al. Instrumental Analysis, 2nd ed. Boston: Allyn and Bacon, 1986.
2. Willard HH, et al. Instrumental Methods of Analysis. Belmont, CA: Wadsworth, 1981.
3. Coiner D. Basic Concepts in Laboratory Instrumentation. Bethesda, MD: ASMT Education and Research Fund, 1975–1979.
4. Ingle JD, Crouch SR. Spectrochemical Analysis. Upper Saddle River, NJ: Prentice-Hall, 1988.
5. Holland JF, et al. Mass spectrometry on the chromatographic time scale: realistic expectations. Anal Chem 1983;55:997A.
6. Guilbault GG. Practical Fluorescence, Theory, Methods and Techniques. New York: Marcel Dekker, 1973.
7. Kricka LJ. Chemiluminescent and bioluminescent techniques. Clin Chem 1991;37:1472.
8. Wild D. The Immunoassay Handbook. London: Macmillan Press, 1994.
9. Svelto O, et al. Principles of Lasers, 2nd ed. New York: Plenum Press, 1982.

10. Coulter Hematology Analyzer: Multidimensional Leukocyte Differential Analysis, Vol. 11 (1). Miami: Beckman Coulter, 1989.

11. Weast RC. CRC Handbook of Chemistry and Physics, 61st ed. Cleveland: CRC Press, 1981.

12. Burtis CA. Tietz Textbook of Clinical Chemistry, 2nd ed. Philadelphia: WB Saunders, 1993.

13. Heiger DN. High-Performance Capillary Electrophoresis: An Introduction, 2nd ed. Waldbronn, Germany: Hewlett-Packard, 1992.

14. Monnig CA, Kennedy RT. Capillary electrophoresis. Anal Chem 1994;66:280R.

15. Parris NA. Instrumental Liquid Chromatography: A Practical Manual on High Performance Liquid Chromatographic Methods. New York: Elsevier, 1976.

16. Jurk H. Thin-Layer Chromatography. Reagents and Detection Methods, Vol. 1a. Weinheim, Germany: Verlagsgesellschaft, 1990.

17. Bender GT. Chemical Instrumentation: A Laboratory Manual Based on Clinical Chemistry. Philadelphia: WB Saunders, 1972.

18. Horváth C. High Performance Liquid Chromatography, Advances and Perspectives. New York: Academic Press, 1980.

19. Constantin E, et al. Mass Spectrometry. New York: Ellis Horwood, 1990.

20. Kebarle E, Liang T. From ions in solution to ions in the gas phase. Anal Chem 1993;65:972A.

21. Karasek FW, Clement RE. Basic Gas Chromatography: Mass Spectrometry. New York: Elsevier, 1988.

22. Rosen A. Biosensors: where do we go from here? MLO Med Lab Obs 1995;27(3):24.

CHAPTER 5

Principles of Clinical Chemistry Automation

William L. Roberts

OBJECTIVES

Upon completion of this chapter, the clinical laboratorian should be able to:

- Define the following terms: automation, channel, continuous flow, discrete analysis, dwell time, flag, random access, and throughput.
- Discuss the history of the development of automated analyzers in the clinical chemistry laboratory.
- List four driving forces behind the development of new automated analyzers.
- Name three basic approaches to sample analysis used by automated analyzers.
- Explain the major steps in automated analysis.
- Provide examples of commercially available discrete chemistry analyzers and modular systems.

- Compare the different approaches to automated analysis used by instrument manufacturers.
- Discriminate between an open versus a closed reagent system.
- Relate three considerations in the selection of an automated analyzer.
- Explain the concept of total laboratory automation.
- Differentiate the three phases of the laboratory testing process.
- Discuss future trends in automated analyzer development.

KEY TERMS

Automation
Bar code
Channel
Closed tube sampling

Continuous flow
Discrete analysis
Dry chemistry slide
Flag

Modular
Probe
Random access
Robotics

Rotor
Total laboratory
  automation

The modern clinical chemistry laboratory uses a high degree of automation. Many steps in the analytic process that were previously performed manually can now be performed automatically, permitting the operator to focus on tasks that cannot be readily automated and increasing both efficiency and capacity. The analytic process can be divided into three major phases—preanalytic, analytic, and postanalytic, corresponding to sample processing, chemical analysis, and data management, respectively. Substantial improvements have occurred in all three areas during the past decade. Seven major diagnostics vendors sell automated analyzers and reagents. These vendors are continually refining their products to make them more functional and user friendly. The analytic phase is the most automated and more research and development efforts are now focusing on increasing automation of the preanalytic and postanalytic processes.

HISTORY OF AUTOMATED ANALYZERS

Following the introduction of the first automated analyzer by Technicon in 1957, automated instruments proliferated from many manufacturers.[1] This first "AutoAnalyzer" (AA) was a continuous-flow, single-*channel*, sequential batch analyzer capable of providing a single test result on approximately 40 samples per hour. The next generation of Technicon instruments to be developed was the Simultaneous Multiple Analyzer (SMA) series. SMA-6 and SMA-12 were analyzers with multiple channels (for different tests), working synchronously to produce 6 or 12 test results simultaneously at the rate of 360 or 720 tests per hour. It was not until the mid-1960s that these continuous-flow analyzers had any significant competition in the marketplace.

In 1970, the first commercial centrifugal analyzer was introduced as a spin-off technology from NASA outer space research. Dr. Norman Anderson developed a prototype in 1967 at the Oak Ridge National Laboratory as an alternative to continuous-flow technology, which had significant carryover problems and costly reagent waste. He wanted to perform analyses in parallel and also take advantage of advances in computer technology. The second generation of these instruments (1975) was more successful, as a result of miniaturization of computers and advances in the polymer industry for high-grade, optical plastic cuvets.

The next major development that revolutionized clinical chemistry instrumentation occurred in 1970 with the introduction of the Automatic Clinical Analyzer (ACA) (DuPont [now, Dade Behring]). It was the first noncontinuous flow, discrete analyzer, as well as the first instrument to have *random access* capabilities, whereby *STAT* specimens could be analyzed out of sequence from the batch as needed. Plastic test packs, positive patient iden-

tification, and infrequent calibration were among the unique features of the ACA. Other major milestones were the introduction of thin film analysis technology in 1976 and the production of the Kodak Ektachem (now, Vitros) Analyzer (now, Ortho-Clinical Diagnostics) in 1978. This instrument was the first to use microsample volumes and reagents on slides for dry chemistry analysis and to incorporate computer technology extensively into its design and use.

Since 1980, several primarily discrete analyzers have been developed that incorporate such characteristics as ion selective electrodes (ISE), fiber optics, polychromatic analysis, continually more sophisticated computer hardware and software for data handling, and larger test menus. The popular and more successful analyzers using these and other technologies since 1980 are Astra (now, Synchron) analyzers (Beckman Coulter) that extensively used ISEs; Paramax (Dade) that uses reagent tablet dispensing and primary tube sampling; the Hitachi analyzers (Boehringer Mannheim; now, Roche Diagnostics) with reusable reaction disks and fixed diode arrays for spectral mapping; and the Chem 1 by Technicon (now, Bayer), which used encapsulated oil segments of sample and reagents in a single continuous-flow tube. Automated systems that are commonly used in clinical chemistry laboratories today are Aeroset and ARCHITECT analyzers (Abbott Laboratories), Advia analyzers (Bayer), Synchron analyzers (Beckman Coulter), Dimension analyzers (Dade Behring), AU analyzers (Olympus), Vitros analyzers (Ortho-Clinical Diagnostics), and several Roche analyzer lines.

Many manufacturers of these instrument systems have adopted the more successful features and technologies of other instruments, where possible, to make each generation of their product more competitive in the marketplace. The differences among the manufacturers' instruments, operating principles, and technologies are less distinct now than in the beginning years of laboratory automation.

DRIVING FORCES TOWARD MORE AUTOMATION

Since 1995, the pace of changes with current routine chemistry analyzers and the introduction of new ones have slowed down considerably, compared with the first half of the 1990s. Certainly, analyzers are faster and easier to use as a result of continual reengineering and electronic refinements. Methods are more precise, sensitive, and specific, although some of the same principles are found in today's instruments as in earlier models. Manufacturers have worked successfully toward automation with "walk away" capabilities and minimal operator intervention.[2] Manufacturers have also responded to the physicians' desire to bring laboratory testing to the patient. The introduction of small, portable, easy-to-operate benchtop analyzers in physician office laboratories (POL), as well as in surgical and critical care units that demand immediate lab results, has resulted in a hugely successful domain of point-of-care (POC) analyzers.[3] Another specialty area with a rapidly developing arsenal of analyzers is immunochemistry. Immunologic techniques for assaying drugs, specific proteins, tumor markers, and hormones have evolved to an increased level of automation. Instruments that use techniques such as fluorescence-polarization immunoassay (FPIA), nephelometry, and competitive and noncompetitive immunoassay with chemiluminescent detection have become popular in laboratories.

The most recent milestone in chemistry analyzer development has been the combination of chemistry and immunoassay into a single *modular* analyzer. The Dimension RxL analyzer with a heterogeneous immunoassay module was introduced in 1997. This design permits further workstation consolidation with consequent improvements in operational efficiency and further reductions in turnaround time. Modular analyzers combining chemistry and immunoassay capabilities are now available from several vendors (Fig. 5-1).

Other forces are also driving the market toward more focused automation. Higher volume of testing and faster turnaround time have resulted in fewer and more centralized core labs performing more comprehensive testing.[4] The use of laboratory panels or profiles has declined, with more diagnostically directed individual tests as dictated by recent policy changes from Medicare and Medicaid. Researchers have known for many years that chemistry

panels only occasionally lead to new diagnoses in patients who appear healthy.[5] The expectation of quality results with higher accuracy and precision is ever present with the regulatory standards set by the Clinical Laboratory Improvement Amendments (CLIA), Joint Commission on Accreditation of Healthcare Organizations (JCAHO), College of American Pathologists (CAP), and others. Intense competition among instrument manufacturers has driven automation into more sophisticated analyzers with creative technologies and unique features. Furthermore, escalating costs have spurred health care reform and, more specifically, managed care and capitation environments within which laboratories are forced to operate.

BASIC APPROACHES TO AUTOMATION

There are many advantages to automating procedures. One purpose is to increase the number of tests performed by one laboratorian in a given period. Labor is an expensive commodity in clinical laboratories. Through mechanization, the labor component devoted to any single test is minimized and this effectively lowers the cost per test. A second purpose is to minimize the variation in results from one laboratorian to another. By reproducing the components in a procedure as identically as possible, the coefficient of variation is lowered and reproducibility is increased. Accuracy is then not dependent on the skill or workload of a particular operator on a particular day. This allows better comparison of results from day to day and week to week. Automation, however, cannot correct for deficiencies inherent in methodology. A third advantage is gained because automation eliminates the potential errors of manual analyses such as volumetric pipetting steps, calculation of results, and transcription of results. A fourth advantage accrues because instruments can use very small amounts of samples and reagents. This allows less blood to be drawn from each patient. In addition, the use of small amounts of reagents decreases the cost of consumables.

There are three basic approaches with instruments: continuous flow, centrifugal analysis, and discrete analysis. All three can use batch analysis (*ie*, large number of specimens in one run), but only discrete analyzers offer random access, or *STAT* capabilities.

In *continuous flow*, liquids (reagents, diluents, and samples) are pumped through a system of continuous tubing. Samples are introduced in a sequential manner, following each other through the same network. A series of air bubbles at regular intervals serve as separating and cleaning media. Continuous flow, therefore, resolves the major consideration of uniformity in performance of tests because each sample follows the same reaction path. Continuous flow also assists the laboratory that needs to run many samples requiring the same procedure. The more sophisticated continuous-flow analyzers

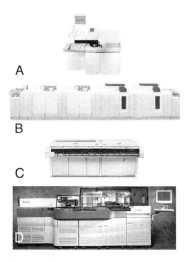

FIGURE 5-1. Modular chemistry/immunoassay analyzers. (**A**) Dade Behring Dimension RxL (photograph courtesy of Dade Behring); (**B**) Roche MODULAR *ANALYTICS* (photograph courtesy of Roche Diagnostics); (**C**) Abbott ARCHITECT ci8200 (photograph courtesy of Abbott Diagnostics); and (**D**) Beckman Coulter Synchron LXi 725 (photograph courtesy of Beckman Coulter).

used parallel single channels to run multiple tests on each sample; for example, SMA, and SMAC. The major drawbacks that contributed to the eventual demise of traditional continuous-flow analyzers (*ie,* AA, SMA, and SMAC) in the marketplace were significant carryover problems and wasteful use of continuously flowing reagents. Technicon's answer to these problems was a noncontinuous-flow discrete analyzer (the RA1000), using random-access fluid (a hydrofluorocarbon liquid to reduce surface tension between samples/reagents and their tubing) and, thereby, reducing carryover. Later, the Chem 1 was developed by Technicon to use Teflon tubing and Teflon oil, virtually eliminating carryover problems. The Chem 1 is a continuous-flow analyzer but only remotely comparable to the original continuous-flow principle.

Centrifugal analysis uses the force generated by centrifugation to transfer and then contain liquids in separate cuvets for measurement at the perimeter of a spinning *rotor.* Centrifugal analyzers are most capable of running multiple samples, one test at a time, in a batch. Batch analysis is their major advantage because reactions in all cuvets are read virtually simultaneously, taking no longer to run a full rotor of about 30 samples than it would take to run a few. Laboratories with a high workload of individual tests for routine batch analysis may use these instruments. Again, each cuvet must be uniformly matched to each other to maintain quality handling of each sample. The Cobas-Bio (Roche Diagnostics), with a xenon flash lamp and longitudinal cuvets,[6] and the IL Monarch, with a fully integrated walkaway design, are two of the more successful centrifugal analyzers.

Discrete analysis is the separation of each sample and accompanying reagents in a separate container. Discrete analyzers have the capability of running multiple tests one sample at a time or multiple samples one test at a time. They are the most popular and versatile analyzers and have almost completely replaced continuous-flow and centrifugal analyzers. However, because each sample is in a separate reaction container, uniformity of quality must be maintained in each cuvet so that a particular sample's quality is not affected by the particular space that it occupies. The analyzers listed in Table 5-1 are all examples of current discrete analyzers with random access capabilities.

STEPS IN AUTOMATED ANALYSIS

In clinical chemistry, *automation* is the mechanization of the steps in a procedure. Manufacturers design their instruments to mimic manual techniques. The major steps in a procedure may be listed as follows:

- Specimen preparation and identification
- Specimen measurement and delivery

- Reagent systems and delivery
- Chemical reaction phase
- Measurement phase
- Signal processing and data handling.

Each step of automated analysis is explained in this section, and several different applications are discussed. Several instruments have been chosen because they have components that represent either common features used in chemistry instrumentation or a unique method of automating a step in a procedure. None of the representative instruments is completely described, but rather the important components are described in the text as examples.

Specimen Preparation and Identification

Preparation of the sample for analysis has been and remains a manual process in most laboratories. The clotting time (if using serum), centrifugation, and the transferring of the sample to an analyzer cup (unless using primary tube sampling) cause delay and expense in the testing process. One alternative to manual preparation is to automate this process by using *robotics*, or front-end automation, to "handle" the specimen through these steps and load the specimen onto the analyzer. Another option is to bypass the specimen preparation altogether by using whole blood for analysis; for example, Abbott-Vision. Robotics for specimen preparation has already become a reality in some clinical laboratories in the United States and other countries. Another approach is to use a plasma separator tube and perform primary tube sampling with heparin plasma. This eliminates the need both to wait for the sample to clot and to aliquot the sample. More discussion about preanalytic specimen processing, or front-end automation, appears later in this chapter.

The sample must be properly identified and its location in the analyzer must be monitored throughout the test. The simplest means of identifying a sample is by placing a manually labeled sample cup in a numbered analysis position on the analyzer, in accordance with a manually prepared worksheet or a computer-generated load list. The most sophisticated approach that is commonly used today employs a *bar code* label affixed to the primary collection tube. This label contains patient demographics and also may include test requests.

The bar code-labeled tubes are then transferred to the loading zone of the analyzer, where the bar code is scanned and the information is stored in the computer's memory. The analyzer is then capable of monitoring all functions of identification, test orders and parameters, and sample position. Certain analyzers may take test requests downloaded from the laboratory information system and run them when the appropriate sample is identified and ready to be pipetted.

TABLE 5-1. SUMMARY OF FEATURES FOR SELECTED CLINICAL CHEMISTRY ANALYZERS

VENDOR	ABBOTT DIAGNOSTICS AEROSET	BAYER ADVIA 1650	BECKMAN COULTER SYNCHRON LX20 PRO	DADE BEHRING DIMENSION RXL	OLYMPUS AMERICA AU640	ORTHO-CLINICAL DIAGNOSTICS VITROS 950	ROCHE COBAS INTEGRA 800	ROCHE DIAGNOSTICS MODULAR ANALYTICS P MODULE
First sold in U.S.	1998	1999	2001	1997	2002	1995	2001	1998
Throughput (tests/hr, depends on test mix)	1600	600–1200	360–540	288–500	800	600–700	472–708	600–1200
Assays onboard simultaneously	59	49	41/71	48/95	51	75	72	47
Open channels	100	62	41/71	10	95	Closed system	Utility channels available	5
Ion selective electrode channels	3	3	5	4	3	3	4	3
Minimum sample volume aspirated	2 µL	2 µL	3 µL	2 µL	1 µL	6 µL	2 µL	2 µL
Pediatric sample cup dead volume	50 µL	50 µL	40 µL	20 µL	Not available	30 µL	50 µL	50 µL
Primary tube cap piercing	No	No	Yes	No	No	No	No	No
Minimum final reaction volume	160 µL	80 µL	210 µL	350 µL	150 µL	Not applicable	200 µL	180 µL
Short sample detection	Yes	Yes	Yes	Yes	Yes	Yes	Yes	Yes
Clot detection	No	Yes	Yes	Yes	Yes	Yes	Yes	No
Index measurements	Yes	Yes	Yes	No	Yes	No	No	Yes
Automatic patient sample dilution and retest	Yes	Yes	Yes	Yes	Yes	No	Yes	Yes
Onboard test automatic inventory	Yes	Yes	Yes	Yes	Yes	Yes	Yes	Yes
Remote troubleshooting by modem	No	Yes	Yes	Yes	Yes	No	Yes	Yes

Information obtained from Aller RD. Chemistry analyzers branching out. CAP Today 2002;July:84–106(34) and directly from vendors.

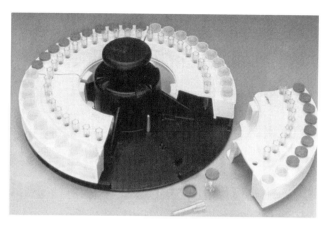

FIGURE 5-2. Vitros. The four quadrant trays, each holding ten samples, fit on a tray carrier. (Photograph courtesy of Ortho-Clinical Diagnostics.)

Specimen Measurement and Delivery

Most instruments use either circular carousels or rectangular racks as specimen containers for holding disposable sample cups or primary sample tubes in the loading or pipetting zone of the analyzer. These cups or tubes hold standards, controls, and patient specimens to be pipetted into the reaction chambers of the analyzers. The slots in the trays or racks are usually numbered to aid in sample identification. The trays or racks move automatically in 1-position steps at preselected speeds. The speed determines the number of specimens to be analyzed per hour. As a convenience, the instrument can determine the slot number containing the last sample and terminate the analysis after that sample. The instrument's microprocessor holds the number of samples in memory and aspirates only in positions containing samples.

On the Vitros analyzer, sample cup trays are quadrants that hold 10 samples each in cups with conical bottoms. The four quadrants fit on a tray carrier (Fig. 5-2). Al-

though the tray carrier accommodates only 40 samples, more trays of samples can be programmed and then loaded in place of completed trays while tests on other trays are in progress. A disposable sample tip is hand-loaded adjacent to each sample cup on the tray. Roche/Hitachi analyzers can use 5 position racks to hold samples (Fig. 5-3). A modular analyzer can accommodate as many as 60 of these racks at one time.

In centrifugal analyzers, the loading of the samples and reagents is accomplished by pipetting the appropriate liquid into a rotor with 20 or more positions. Each position contains a sample compartment, a reagent compartment, and a cuvet located at the periphery of the rotor (Fig. 5-4).

The Paramax allows sampling from primary collection tubes, or for limited samples, there are microsample tubes. The tubes are placed in a circular tray that holds 96 specimens at one time. Bar code labels for each sample, which include the patient name and identification number, can be printed on demand by the operator (Fig. 5-5). This allows samples to be loaded in any order. The loading carousel dispenses the tubes to a transfer carousel, from which the sampling occurs, and then the samples are transferred to an unloading carousel (Fig. 5-6). Both the Paramax and Dimension analyzers make use of a continuous belt of flexible, disposable plastic cuvets carried through the analyzer's water bath on a main drive track. The cuvets are loaded onto the analyzer from a continuous spool. These cuvets index through the instrument at the rate of one every 5 seconds and are cut into sections or groups as required. A schematic of the

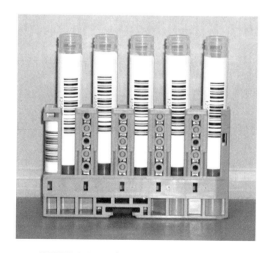

FIGURE 5-3. Roche/Hitachi 5-position rack.

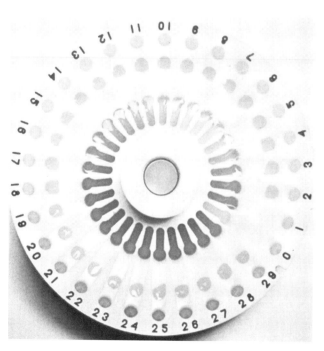

FIGURE 5-4. Centrifugal analyzer rotor.

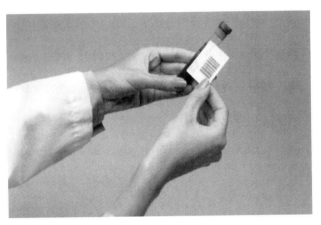

FIGURE 5-5. Paramax. Sample collection tubes are identified with barcode labels. (Photograph courtesy of Dade International.)

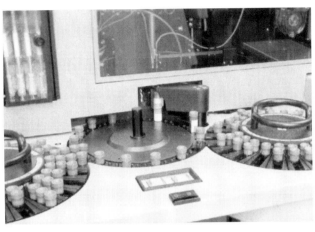

FIGURE 5-6. Paramax. The loading carousel dispenses tubes to a transfer carousel, from which the sampling occurs, and then the samples are transferred to an unloading carousel. (Photograph courtesy of Dade International.)

Dimension RxL cuvet production and reading system are shown in Figure 5-7. Exposure of the sample to air can lead to sample evaporation and produce errors in analysis. Evaporation of the sample may be significant and may cause the concentration of the constituents being analyzed to rise 50% in 4 hours.[7] With instruments measuring electrolytes, the carbon dioxide present in the samples will be lost to the atmosphere, resulting in low carbon dioxide values. Manufacturers have devised a variety of mechanisms to minimize this effect; for example, lid covers for trays and individual caps that can be pierced, which includes *closed tube sampling* from primary collection tubes.[8]

The actual measurement of each aliquot for each test must be very accurate. This is generally done through aspiration of the sample into a *probe*. When the discrete instrument is in operation, the probe automatically dips into each sample cup and aspirates a portion of the liquid. After a preset, computer-controlled time interval, the probe quickly rises from the cup. Sampling probes on instruments using specific sampling cups are programmed or adjusted to reach a prescribed depth in those cups to maximize use of available sample. Those analyzers capable of aspirating sample from primary collection tubes usually have a parallel liquid level-sensing probe that will control entry of the sampling probe to a minimal depth below the surface of the serum, allowing full aliquot aspiration while avoiding clogging of the probe with serum separator gel or clot (Fig. 5-8).

In continuous-flow analyzers, when the sample probe rises from the cup, air is aspirated for a specified time to produce a bubble in between sample and reagent plugs of liquid. Then the probe descends into a container where wash solution is drawn into the probe and through the system. The wash solution is usually deionized water, possibly with a surfactant added. Remembering that all samples follow the same reaction path, the necessity for the wash solution between samples becomes obvious. Immersion of the probe into the wash reservoir cleanses the outside, whereas aspiration of an aliquot of solution cleanses the lumen. The reservoir is continually replenished with an excess of fresh solution. The wash aliquot, plus the previously mentioned air bubble, maintains sample integrity and minimizes sample carryover.

Certain pipetters use a disposable tip and an air-displacement syringe to measure and deliver reagent. When this is used, the pipetter may be reprogrammed to measure sample and reagent for batches of different tests comparatively easily. Besides eliminating the effort of priming the reagent delivery system with the new solution, no reagent is wasted or contaminated because nothing but the pipet tip contacts it.

The cleaning of the probe and tubing after each dispensing to minimize the carryover of one sample into the next is a concern for many instruments. In some systems, the reagent or diluent is also dispersed into the cuvet through the same tubing and probe. Deionized water may be dispensed into the cuvet after the sample to produce a specified dilution of the sample and also to rinse the dispensing system. In the Technicon (now, Bayer) RA1000, a random-access fluid is the separation medium. The fluorocarbon fluid is a viscous, inert, immiscible, nonwetting substance that coats the delivery system. The coating on the sides of the delivery system prevents carryover due to the wetting of the surfaces and, forming a plug of the solution between samples, prevents carryover by diffusion. A small amount (10 μL) of this fluid is dispensed into the cuvet with the sample. Surface tension leaves a coating of the fluid in the dispensing system.

If a separate probe or tip is used for each sample and discarded after use, as in the Vitros, the issue of carryover is a moot point. Vitros has a unique sample-dispensing

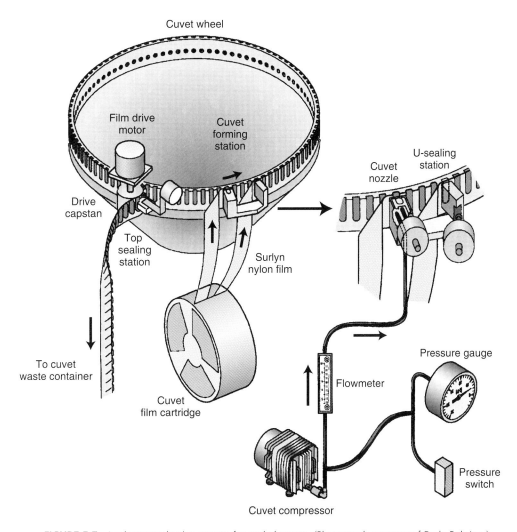

FIGURE 5-7. Analyzer production system for sealed cuvets. (Photograph courtesy of Dade Behring.)

FIGURE 5-8. Dual sample probes of the Hitachi 736 analyzer. Note the liquid level sensor to the left of probes. (Photograph courtesy of Boehringer Mannheim.)

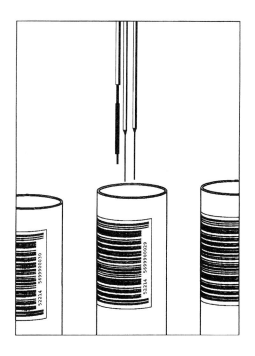

system. A proboscis presses into a tip on the sample tray, picks it up, and moves over the specimen to aspirate the volume required for the tests programmed for that sample. The tip is then moved over to the slide-metering block. When a slide is in position to receive an aliquot, the proboscis is lowered so that a dispensed 10-µL drop touches the slide, where it is absorbed from the nonwetting tip. A stepper motor-driven piston controls aspiration and drop formation. The precision of dispensing is specified at ±5%.

In several discrete systems, the probe is attached by means of nonwettable tubing to precision syringes. The syringes draw a specified amount of sample into the probe and tubing. Then the probe is positioned over a cuvet, into which the sample is dispensed. The Hitachi 736 uses two sample probes to simultaneously aspirate a double volume of sample in each probe immersed in one specimen container and, thereby, deliver sample into four individual test channels, all in one operational step (Fig. 5-9). The loaded probes pass through a fine mist shower bath before delivery to wash off any sample residue adhering to the outer surface of the probes. After delivery, the probes move to a rinse bath station for cleaning the inside and outside surfaces of the probes.

The ACA Star (Dade) filling station puts the appropriate amounts of sample and diluent into each analytic test pack. A filled sample cup is followed in the loading tray by the test packs for the tests required on the specimen. When the system is activated, a shuttle pushes the first sample cup left to the sampling position. While the specimen is moving left, a spring-loaded pack pusher pushes the first test pack onto the filling station rail below a decoder plate. The decoder senses the binary code on the top of the test pack. This code, when translated, provides the instrument with instructions, including the sample volume, type of diluent, and special handling characteristics. The pump flushes with the diluent to be used for the particular method to purge the lines and needle before diluent intake. The sample needle is positioned over the sample cup, dips down into the cup, and aspirates the proper volume of specimen. The needle rises out of the sample cup and moves right to a position over the test pack. The sample and diluent are injected into the test pack through a special pack-fill opening. After the pack is filled, the needle, tubing, and pump are flushed. The test pack is moved onto the transport system. The instrument also transfers the patient sample-identification number on the sample pack to the results-reporting system.

The Paramax uses computer-controlled stepping motors to drive both the sampling and washout syringes. Every 5 seconds, the sampling probe enters a specimen container, withdraws the required volume, moves to the cuvet, and dispenses the aliquot with a volume of water to wash the probe. The washout volume is adjusted to yield the final reaction volume. If a procedure's range of linearity is exceeded, the system will retrieve the original sample tube, repeat the test using one-fourth the original sample volume for the repeat test, and calculate a new result, taking the dilution into consideration.

Economy of sample size is a major consideration in developing automated procedures, but methodologies have limitations to maintain proper levels of sensitivity and specificity. The factors governing sample and reagent measurement are interdependent. Generally, if sample size is reduced, then either the size of the reaction cuvet and final reaction volume must be decreased or the reagent concentration must be increased to ensure sufficient color development for accurate photometric readings.

Reagent Systems and Delivery

Reagents may be classified as liquid or dry systems for use with automated analyzers. Liquid reagents may be purchased in bulk volume containers or in unit dose packaging as a convenience for *STAT* testing on some analyzers. Dry reagents are packaged in various forms. They may be bottled as lyophilized powder, which requires reconstitution with water or a buffer. Unless the manufacturer provides the diluent, the water quality available in the laboratory is important. Other dry reagents may be in tablet form, such as those used by the ACA Star and Paramax. The ACA Star crushes and dis-

FIGURE 5-9. Sampling operation of the Hitachi 736 analyzer. (Courtesy of Boehringer Mannheim.)

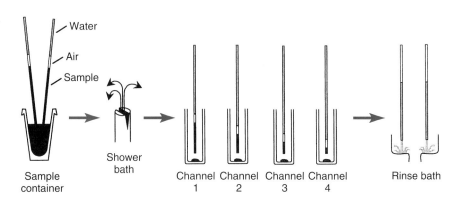

solves reagent tablets in the plastic test pouch on board the instrument. Paramax uses an ultrasonic horn to break up and dissolve the tablet in a plastic cuvet filled with water. A third and unique type of dry reagent is the multilayered *dry chemistry slide* for the Vitros analyzer. These slides have microscopically thin layers of dry reagents mounted on a plastic support. The slides are approximately the size of a postage stamp and not much thicker.

Reagent handling varies according to instrument capabilities and methodologies. Many test procedures use sensitive, short-lived working reagents; so contemporary analyzers use a variety of techniques to preserve them. One technique is to keep all reagents refrigerated until the moment of need and then quickly preincubate them to reaction temperature or store them in a refrigerated compartment on the analyzer that feeds directly to the dispensing area. Another means of preservation is to provide reagents in a dried, tablet form and reconstitute them when the test is to be run. A third is to manufacture the reagent in two stable components that will be combined at the moment of reaction. If this approach is used, the first component also may be used as a diluent for the sample. The various manufacturers often use combinations of these reagent-handling techniques.

Reagents also must be dispensed and measured accurately. Many instruments use bulk reagents to decrease the preparation and changing of reagents. Instruments that do not use bulk reagents have unique reagent packaging. In continuous-flow analyzers, reagents and diluents are supplied from bulk containers into which tubing is suspended. The inside diameter, or bore, of the tubing governs the amount of fluid that will be dispensed. A proportioning pump, along with a manifold, continuously and precisely introduces, proportions, and pumps liquids and air bubbles throughout the continuous-flow system.

To deliver reagents, many discrete analyzers use techniques similar to those used to measure and deliver the samples. Syringes, driven by a stepping motor, pipet the reagents into reaction containers. Piston-driven pumps, connected by tubing, may also dispense reagents. Another technique for delivering reagents to reaction containers uses pressurized reagent bottles connected by tubing to dispensing valves. The computer controls the opening and closing of the valves. The fill volume of reagent into the reaction container is determined by the precise amount of time the valve remains open.

The Vitros analyzers use slides to contain their entire reagent chemistry system. Multiple layers on the slide are backed by a clear polyester support. The coating itself is sandwiched in a plastic mount. There are three or more layers: (1) a spreading layer, which accepts the sample; (2) one or more central layers, which can alter the aliquot; and (3) an indicator layer, where the analyte of

interest may be quantified (Fig. 5-10). The number of layers varies depending on the assay to be performed. The color developed in the indicator layer varies with the concentration of the analyte in the sample. Physical or chemical reactions can occur in one layer, with the product of these reactions proceeding to another layer, where subsequent reactions can occur. Each layer may offer a unique environment and the possibility to carry out a reaction comparable to that offered in a chemistry assay or it may promote an entirely different activity that does not occur in the liquid phase. The ability to create multiple reaction sites allows the possibility of manipulating and detecting compounds in ways not possible in solution chemistries. Interfering materials can be left behind or altered in upper layers.

All reagents for the ACA analyzers are contained in special test packs, which are compartmentalized plastic envelopes. A separate pack is used for each test performed on a specimen (Fig. 5-11). Compartments along the top of the envelope contain liquid or tablet reagents. The code name and a binary code depicting the test are printed on a plastic bar at the top of each test pack. All of the test packs require refrigerated storage.

Chemical Reaction Phase

This phase consists of mixing, separation, incubation, and reaction time. In most discrete analyzers, the chemical reactants are held in individual moving containers

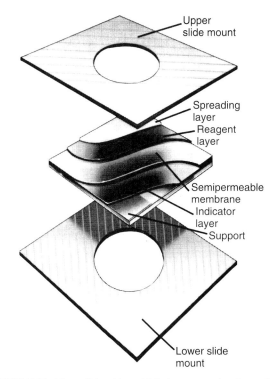

FIGURE 5-10. Vitros slide with multiple layers contains the entire reagent chemistry system. (Courtesy of Ortho-Clinical Diagnostics.)

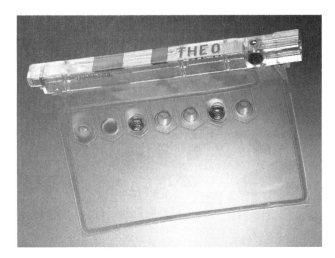

FIGURE 5-11. ACA. A test pack with binary code on a bar at the top. (Photograph courtesy of Dade Behring.)

that are either disposable or reusable. These reaction containers also function as the cuvets for optical analysis. If the cuvets are reusable, then wash stations are set up immediately after the read stations to clean and dry these containers (Fig. 5-12). This arrangement allows the analyzer to operate continuously without replacing cuvets. Examples of this approach include Advia (Bayer Health), Aeroset (Abbott Laboratories), Hitachi (Roche Diagnostics), AU (Olympus), and Synchron (Beckman Coulter) analyzers. Alternatively, the reactants may be placed in a stationary reaction chamber (*eg*, Astra) in which a flow-through process of the reaction mixture occurs before and after the optical reading. In continuous-flow systems, flow-through cuvets are used and optical readings

are taken during the flow of reactant fluids. The Chem 1 uses this approach with its single analytic pathway Teflon tube (Fig. 5-13).

Mixing

A vital component of each procedure is the adequate mixing of the reagents and sample. Instrument manufacturers go to great lengths to ensure complete mixing. Nonuniform mixtures can result in noise in continuous-flow analysis and in poor precision in discrete analysis.

Mixing is accomplished in continuous-flow analyzers (*eg*, the Chem 1) through the use of coiled tubing. When the reagent and sample stream goes through coiled loops, the liquid rotates and tumbles in each loop. The differential rate of liquids falling through one another produces mixing in the coil.

RA1000 uses a rapid start–stop action of the reaction tray. This causes a sloshing action against the walls of the cuvets, which mixes the components. Centrifugal analyzers may use a start–stop sequence of rotation or bubbling of air through the sample and reagent to mix them while these solutions are moving from transfer disk to rotor. This process of transferring and mixing occurs in just a few seconds. The centrifugal force is responsible for the mixing as it pushes sample from its compartment, over a partition into a reagent-filled compartment and, finally, into the cuvet space at the perimeter of the rotor.

In the Vitros slide technology, the spreading layer provides a structure that permits a rapid and uniform spreading of the sample over the reagent layer(s) for even color development.

The ACA analyzers have components specially designed for mixing: the breaker-mixers. Platens press selectively against and collapse the reagent compartments along the top of the test pack, releasing the reagents into the interior environment of the pack. Meanwhile, a lower platen presses against the bottom portion of the test-pack envelope to force the fluids up into the ruptured reagent

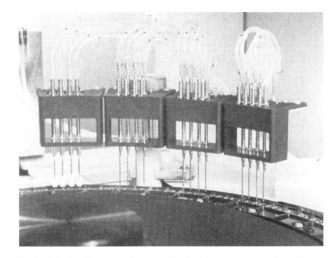

FIGURE 5-12. Wash stations on Hitachi 736 analyzer perform the following: (1) aspirate reaction waste and dispense water; (2) aspirate and dispense rinse water; (3) aspirate rinse water and dispense water for measurement of cell blank; (4) aspirate cell blank water to dryness. (Photograph courtesy of Boehringer Mannheim.)

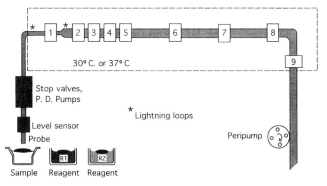

FIGURE 5-13. Technicon system overview. Chem 1 analytic pathway of single Teflon tube. (Courtesy of Bayer.)

compartments. Then, with a patting motion, the breaker-mixer thoroughly mixes the reagents with the fluids.

Paramax uses ultrasonic sound waves for 45 seconds to dissolve the reagent tablets in the deionized water in each cuvet. Ultrasound is also used to mix the sample with the previously prepared reagents and to mix, if necessary, the contents of the cuvets after a second reagent addition.

The Hitachi analyzers use stirring paddles that dip into the reaction container for a few seconds to stir sample and reagents, after which they return to a wash reservoir (Fig. 5-14). Other instruments, such as Astra, use magnetic stir bars lying in the bottom of the reaction container that, when activated, produce a whirling motion to mix. Still others use forceful dispensing to accomplish mixing.

Separation

In chemical reactions, undesirable constituents that will interfere with an analysis may need to be separated from the sample before the other reagents are introduced into the system. Protein causes major interference in many analyses. One approach without separating protein is to use a very high reagent-to-sample ratio (the sample is highly diluted) so that any turbidity caused by precipitated protein is not sensed by the spectrophotometer. Another approach is to shorten reaction time to eliminate slower reacting interferents.

In the older continuous-flow systems, a dialyzer was the separation or filtering module. It performed the equivalent of the manual procedures of precipitation, centrifugation, and filtration, using a fine-pore cellophane membrane. In the Vitros slide technology, the spreading layer of the slide traps cells, crystals, and other small particulate matter but also retains large molecules,

such as protein. In essence, what passes through the spreading layer is a protein-free filtrate.

Many discrete analyzers have no automated methodology by which to separate interfering substances from the reaction mixture. Therefore, methods have been chosen that have few interferences or that have known interferences that can be compensated for by the instrument (*eg*, using correction formulas).

The use of automated column chromatography in some methods gives the ACA the ability to remove from the sample substances that might adversely influence the reaction. Three types of columns can be used: gel filtration, ion exchange, and protein-removal. The column is located at the top of the test pack, immediately under the plastic pack header. If the test pack contains a chromatographic column, the sample and a prescribed quantity of diluent are injected into the column fill site opposite the usual sample and diluent fill site. The sample is moved through the column by the pressure of the diluent and into the test pack for analysis.

Incubation

A heating bath in discrete or continuous-flow systems maintains the required temperature of the reaction mixture and provides the delay necessary to allow complete color development. The principal components of the heating bath are the heat-transfer medium (*ie*, water or air), the heating element, and the thermoregulator. A thermometer is located in the heating compartment of an analyzer and is monitored by the system's computer. On many discrete analyzer systems, the multicuvets incubate in a water bath maintained at a constant temperature of usually 37°C.

Slide technology incubates colorimetric slides at 37°C. There is a precondition station to bring the temperature of each slide close to 37°C before it enters the incubator. The incubator moves the slides at 12-second intervals in such a manner that each slide is at the incubator exit four times during the 5-minute incubation time. This feature is used for two point-rate methods and enables the first point reading to be taken part way through the incubation time. Potentiometric slides are held at 25°C. The slides are kept at this temperature for 3 minutes to ensure stability before reading.

Reaction Time

Before the optical reading by the spectrophotometer, the reaction time may depend on the rate of transport through the system to the "read" station, timed reagent additions with moving or stationary reaction chambers, or a combination of both processes. An environment conducive to the completion of the reaction must be maintained for a sufficient length of time before spectrophotometric analysis of the product is made. Time is a definite limitation. To sustain the advantage of speedy multiple analyses, the instrument must produce results as quickly as possible.

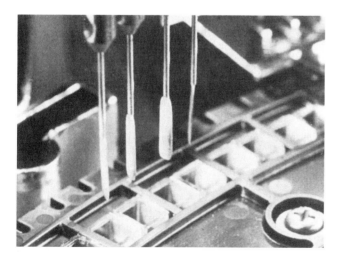

FIGURE 5-14. Stirring paddles on Hitachi 736 analyzer. (Photograph courtesy of Boehringer Mannheim.)

It is possible to monitor not only completion of a reaction but also the rate at which the reaction is proceeding. The instrument may delay the measurement for a predetermined time or may present the reaction mixtures for measurement at constant intervals of time. Use of rate reactions may have two advantages: the total analysis time is shortened and interfering chromogens that react slowly may be negated. Reaction rate is controlled by temperature; therefore, the reagent, timing, and spectrophotometric functions must be coordinated to work in harmony with the chosen temperature.

The ACA has five delay stations located in the pack-processing area. At these points, the instrument performs no operations on the test packs. This interval allows enough reaction time for endpoint or blank reactions to go to completion. The entire pack-processing area is maintained at 37°C in a closed environment with circulating fans.

The Paramax has eight photometric stations located along the cuvet track. The addition of the sample initiates each reaction, which is monitored from 40 seconds to 10 minutes by the photometric stations for rate or endpoint reactions. The environment of the cuvets is maintained at a constant temperature by a water bath in which the cuvets move.

Measurement Phase

After the reaction is completed, the formed products must be quantified. Almost all available systems for measurement have been used, such as ultraviolet, fluorescent, and flame photometry; ion-specific electrodes; gamma counters; and luminometers. Still, the most common is visible and ultraviolet light spectrophotometry, although adaptations of traditional fluorescence measurement, such as fluorescence polarization, chemiluminescence, and bioluminescence, have become popular. The Abbott AxSYM, for example, is a popular instrument for drug analysis that uses fluorescence polarization to measure immunoassay reactions.

Analyzers that measure light require a monochromator to achieve the desired component wavelength. Traditionally, analyzers have used filters or filter wheels to separate light. The old AutoAnalyzers used filters that were manually placed in position in the light path. Many instruments still use rotating filter wheels that are microprocessor controlled so that the appropriate filter is positioned in the light path. However, newer and more sophisticated systems offer the higher resolution afforded by diffraction gratings to achieve light separation into its component colors. Many instruments now use such monochromators with either a mechanically rotating grating or a fixed grating that spreads its component wavelengths onto a fixed array of photo diodes; for ex-

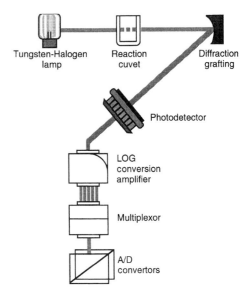

FIGURE 5-15. Photometer for Hitachi 736 analyzer. Fixed diffraction grating separates light into specific wavelengths and reflects them onto a fixed array of 11 specific photodetectors. Photometer has no moving parts. (Courtesy of Boehringer Mannheim.)

ample, Hitachi analyzers (Fig. 5-15). This latter grating arrangement, as well as rotating filter wheels, easily accommodates polychromatic light analysis, which offers improved sensitivity and specificity over monochromatic measurement. By recording optical readings at different wavelengths, the instrument's computer can then use these data to correct for reaction mixture interferences that may occur at adjacent, as well as desired, wavelengths.

Many newer instruments use fiber optics as a medium to transport light signals from remote read stations back to a central monochromator detector box for analysis of these signals. The Paramax has fiber optic cables, or "light pipes" as they are sometimes called, attached from multiple remote stations where the reaction mixtures reside, to a centralized filter wheel/detector unit that, in conjunction with the computer, sequences and analyzes a large volume of light signals from multiple reactions (Fig. 5-16).

The containers holding the reaction mixture also play a vital role in the measurement phase. The reagent volume and, therefore, sample size, speed of analysis, and sensitivity of measurement are some aspects influenced by the method of analysis. A flow-through cuvet is used in continuous-flow analysis. The reagent stream under analysis flows continuously through the flow-cell tubing. The Chem 1 "captures" absorbance signals in between air bubbles of the flowing stream (Fig. 5-17). This means that no debubbling is required as in the older continuous-flow analyzers. As the stream flows through the flow-cell, a steady beam of light is focused through the stream.

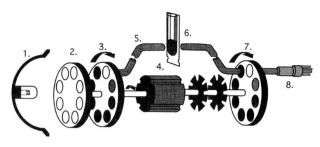

FIGURE 5-16. Paramax instrument photo optical system: (**1**) Source with reflector, (**2**) fixed focusing lens, (**3**) filter wheel, (**4**) double shafted motor, (**5**) fiber optic bundle, (**6**) cuvet, (**7**) filter wheel, (**8**) photomultiplier tube. (Courtesy of Dade International.)

The amount of light that exits from the flow-cell is dictated primarily by the absorbance of light by the stream. The exiting light strikes a photodetector, which converts the light into electrical energy. Filters and light-focusing components permit the desired light wavelength to reach the photodetector. The photometer continuously senses the sample photodetector output voltage and, as is the process in most analyzers, compares it with a reference output voltage. The electrical impulses are sent to a read-out device, such as a printer or computer, for storage and retrieval.

In discrete analyzers, such as Hitachi, Synchron, or ACA systems, the cuvet used for analysis is also the reaction vessel in which the entire procedure has occurred.

The ACA Star photometer consists of a cuvet-forming device and a photometric system for making absorbance measurements. When compressed by the photometer jaws, the test pack forms a cuvet between quartz windows. A wetting solution is introduced between the quartz windows and the test-pack walls to achieve a good optical interface.

Centrifugal analysis measurement occurs while the rotor is rotating at a constant speed of approximately 1000 rpm. Consecutive readings are taken of the sample, the dark current (readings between cuvets), and the reference cuvet. Each cuvet passes through the light source every few milliseconds. After all the data points have been determined, centrifugation stops and the results are printed. The rotor is removed from the analyzer and discarded. For endpoint analyses, an initial absorbance is measured before the constituents have had time to react, usually a few seconds, and is considered a blank measurement. After enough time has elapsed for the reaction to be completed, another absorbance reading is taken. For rate analyses, the initial absorbance is measured, and then a lag time is allowed (preset into the instrument for each analysis). For each assay, several data points are determined at a programmed time interval. The instrument monitors the absorbance measurements at each data point and calculates a result.

Slide technology depends on reflectance spectrophotometry, as opposed to traditional transmittance photometry, to provide a quantitative result. The amount of chromogen in the indicator layer is read after light passes through the indicator layer, is reflected from the bottom of a pigment-containing layer (usually the spreading layer), and is returned through the indicator layer to a light detector. For colorimetric determinations, the light source is a tungsten-halogen lamp. The beam focuses on a filter wheel holding up to eight interference filters, which are separated by a dark space. The beam is focused at a 45° angle to the bottom surface of the slide, and a silicon photodiode detects the portion of the beam that reflects down. Three readings are taken for the computer to derive reflectance density. The three recorded signals taken are (1) the filter wheel blocking the beam, (2) reflectance of a reference white surface with the programmed filter in the beam, and (3) reflectance of the slide with the selected filter in the beam (Fig. 5-18).

After a slide is read, it is shuttled back in the direction from which it came, where a trap door allows it to drop into a waste bin. If the reading was the first for a two-point rate test, the trap door remains closed, and the slide reenters the incubator.

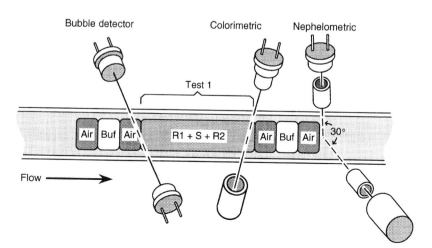

FIGURE 5-17. In-line reaction detector. Flow-through cuvet for Chem 1 Analyzer. (Courtesy of Bayer.)

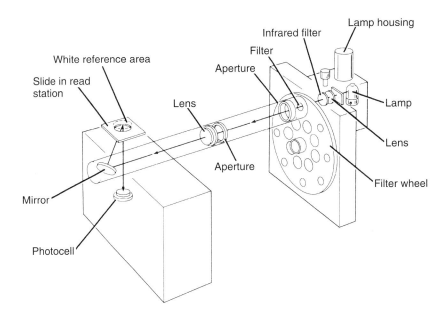

FIGURE 5-18. Components of the system for making colorimetric determinations with slide technology. (Courtesy of Ortho-Clinical Diagnostics.)

The Advia Centaur (Bayer), a fully automated, random access immunoassay system (Fig. 5-19), uses chemiluminescence technology for reaction analysis. In chemiluminescence assays, quantification of an analyte is based on emission of light resulting from a chemical reaction.[9] The principles of chemiluminescent immunoassays are similar to those of radioimmunoassay (RIA), except that an acridinium ester is used as the tracer and paramagnetic particles are used as the solid phase. Sample, tracer, and paramagnetic particle reagent are added and incubated in disposable plastic cuvets, depending on the assay protocol. After incubation, magnetic separation and washing of the particles is performed automatically. The cuvets are then transported into a light-sealed luminometer chamber, where appropriate reagents are added to initiate the chemiluminescent reaction. On injection of the reagents into the sample cuvet, the system luminometer detects the chemiluminescent signal. Luminometers are similar to gamma counters in that they use a photomultiplier tube detector; however, unlike gamma counters, luminometers do not require a crystal to convert gamma rays to light photons. Light photons from the sample are detected directly, converted to electrical pulses, and then counted.

Signal Processing and Data Handling

Because most automated instruments print the results in reportable form, accurate calibration is essential to obtaining accurate information. There are many variables that may enter into the use of calibration standards. The matrices of the standards and unknowns may be different. Depending on the methodology, this may or may not present problems. If secondary standards are used to calibrate an instrument, the methods used to derive the standard's constituent values should be known. Standards containing more than one analyte per vial may cause interference problems. Because there are no primary standards available for enzymes, either secondary standards or calibration factors based on the molar extinction coefficients of the products of the reactions may be used.

Many times, a laboratory will have more than one instrument capable of measuring a constituent. Unless there are different normal ranges published for each method, the instruments should be calibrated so that the results are comparable. The advantage of calibrating an automated instrument is the long-term stability of the standard curve, which requires only monitoring with controls on a daily basis. Some analyzers use low- and high-concentration standards at the beginning of each run and then use the absorbances of the reactions produced by the standards to produce a standard curve elec-

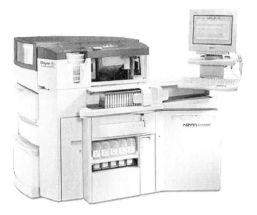

FIGURE 5-19. Advia Centaur Automated Chemiluminescence System. (Photo courtesy of Bayer Diagnostics.)

tronically for each run. Other instruments are self-calibrating after analyzing standard solutions.

The original continuous-flow analyzers used six standards assayed at the beginning of each run to produce a calibration curve for that particular batch. Now, continuous-flow analyzers use a single-level calibrator to calibrate each run with water used to establish the baseline.

The centrifugal analyzer uses standards pipetted into designated cuvets in each run for endpoint analyses. After the delta absorbance for each sample has been obtained, the computer calculates the results by determining a constant for each standard. The constants are derived by dividing the concentration of the standard (preentered into the computer) by the delta absorbance and averaging the constants for each of the standards to obtain a factor. The concentration of each control and unknown is determined by multiplying the delta absorbance of the unknown by the factor. If the concentration of an unknown exceeds the range of the standards, the result is printed with a *flag*. Enzyme activity is derived by a linear regression fit of the delta absorbance versus time. The slope of the produced line is multiplied by the enzyme factor (preentered) to calculate the activity.

Slide technology requires more sophisticated calculations to produce results. The calibration materials require a protein-based matrix because of the necessity for the calibrators to behave as serum when reacting with the various layers of the slides. Calibrator fluids are bovine serum based, and the concentration of each analyte is determined by reference methods. Endpoint tests require three calibrator fluids, blank-requiring tests need four calibrator fluids, and enzyme methods require three calibrators. Colorimetric tests use spline fits to produce the standardization. In enzyme analysis, a curve-fitting algorithm estimates the change in reflection density per unit time. This is converted to either absorbance or transmission-density change per unit time. Then, a quadratic equation converts the change in transmission density to volume activity (U/L) for each assay.

The ACA Star retains the calibrations for each lot of a particular method until the laboratorian programs the instrument for recalibration. Instrument calibration is initiated or verified by assaying a minimum of three levels of primary standards or, in the case of enzymes, reference samples. The values obtained are compared with the known concentrations by using linear regression, with the x-axis representing the expected values and the y-axis representing the mean of the values obtained. The slope (scale factor) and y intercept (offset) are the adjustable parameters on the ACA. On earlier models of this instrument, the parameters were determined and entered manually into the instrument computer by the operator; however, on later, more automated models, the instrument performs calibration automatically on operator request. After calibration has been performed and the

chemical or electrical analysis of the specimen is either in progress or completed, the instrument's computer goes into data acquisition and calculation mode. The process may involve signal averaging, which may entail hundreds of data pulses per second, as with a centrifugal analyzer, and blanking and correction formulas for interferents that are programmed into the computer for calculation of results.

All advanced automated instruments have some method of reporting printed results with a link to sample identification. In sophisticated systems, the demographic-sample information is entered in the instrument's computer together with the tests required. Then the sample identification is printed with the test results. The Paramax prints bar code labels for sample identification after the operator enters the patient information and tests requested into the computer terminal. When the label is applied to the sample, the sample can be loaded on the analyzer. Microprocessors control the tests, reagents, and timing, while verifying the bar code for each sample. This is the link between the results reported and the specimen identification. Even the simplest of systems sequentially number the test results to provide a connection with the samples.

Because most instruments now have either a built-in or attached video monitor, the sophisticated software programs that come with the instrument can be displayed for determining the status of different aspects of the testing process. Computerized monitoring is available for such parameters as reaction and instrument linearity, quality control data with various options for statistical display and interpretation, short sample sensing with flags on the printout, abnormal patient results flagged, clot detection, reaction vessel or test chamber temperature, and reagent inventories. The printer can also display patients' results as well as various warnings previously mentioned. Most instrument manufacturers offer computer software for preventive maintenance schedules and algorithms for diagnostic troubleshooting. Some manufacturers also install phone modems on the analyzer for a direct communication link between the instrument and their service center for instant troubleshooting and diagnosis of problems.

SELECTION OF AUTOMATED ANALYZERS

Each manufacturer's approach to automation is unique. The instruments being evaluated should be rated according to previously identified needs. One laboratory may need a *STAT* analyzer, whereas another's need may be a batch analyzer for high-test volumes. When considering cost, the price of the instrument and, even more important, the total cost of consumables, are significant. The high capital cost of an instrument may actually be small when divided by the large number of samples to be processed. It is also important to calculate the total cost per test for each instrument that is considered. Moreover, a break-even analysis to study the relationship of fixed costs, variable costs, and profits can be helpful in analyzing the financial justification and economic impact on a laboratory. Of course, the mode of acquisition, that is, purchase, lease, rental, and so on, must also be factored into this analysis. The variable cost of consumables will increase as more tests are performed or samples are analyzed. The ability to use reagents produced by more than one supplier (open vs. closed reagent systems) can provide a laboratory with the ability to customize testing and, possibly, save money. The labor component also should be evaluated. Older instruments may have the CAP's workload recording units assigned; this provides an excellent basis for comparison, using time-motion studies. Unfortunately, the newest instruments on the market may not have been timed for labor and, therefore, this judgment may be more subjective than desired. With the large number of instruments available on the market, the goal is to find the right instrument for each situation.[10]

Another major concern toward the selection of an instrument is its analytic capabilities. What is the instrument's performance characteristics for accuracy, precision, linearity, specificity, and sensitivity (which may be method dependent), calibration stability, and stability of reagents (both shelf life and onboard or reconstituted)? The best way to verify these performance characteristics of an analyzer before making a decision on an instrument is to see it in operation. Ideally, if a manufacturer will place an instrument in the prospective buyer's laboratory on a trial basis, then its analytic performance can be evaluated to the customer's satisfaction with studies to verify accuracy, precision, and linearity. At the same time, laboratory personnel can observe such design features as its test menus, true walkaway capability, user friendliness, and the space that the instrument and its consumables occupy in their lab.

Clinical chemistry instrumentation provides speed and precision for assays that would otherwise be performed manually. The chosen methodologies and adherence to the requirements of the assay provide accuracy. No one may assume that the result produced is the correct value. Automated methods must be evaluated completely before being accepted as routine. It is important to understand how each instrument actually works.

TOTAL LABORATORY AUTOMATION[11]

The pressures of health care reform and managed care have caused increasing interest in improving productivity of the preanalytic and postanalytic phases of laboratory testing. As for the analytic process itself, routine analyzers in clinical chemistry today have nearly all the

mechanization they need. The next generation of automation will replicate the Japanese practice of "black box" labs, in which the sample goes in at one end and the printed result comes out the other end.[12] Much effort has been expended during the past decade on the development of automated "front-end" feeding of the sample into the analytic "box" and computerized/automated management of the data that come out the back end of the box. There have been many developments in the three phases of the laboratory testing process; that is, preanalytic (sample processing), analytic (chemical analyses), and postanalytic (data management) as they merge closer into an integrated *total laboratory automation* (TLA) system. Automation equipment vendors are developing open architecture components that provide more flexibility in automation implementation.[13]

Preanalytic Phase (Sample Processing)

The sample handling protocol currently available on all major chemistry analyzers is to use the original specimen collection tube (primary tube sampling) of any size (after plasma or serum separation) as the sample cup on the analyzer and to use bar code readers, also on the analyzer, to identify the specimen. An automated process is gradually replacing manual handling and presentation of the sample to the analyzer. Increasing efficiency while decreasing costs has been a major impetus for laboratories to start integrating some aspect of total laboratory automation into their operations. Conceptually, TLA refers to automated devices and robots integrated with existing analyzers to perform all phases of laboratory testing. Most attention to date has been devoted to development of the front-end systems that can identify and label specimens, centrifuge the specimen and prepare aliquots, and sort and deliver samples to the analyzer or to storage.[14] Back-end systems may include removal of specimens from the analyzer and transport to storage, retrieval from storage for retesting, realiquoting, or disposal, as well as comprehensive management of the data from the analyzer and interfacing with the laboratory's information system (LIS).

Dr. Sasaki and colleagues installed the first fully automated clinical laboratory in the world at Koshi Medical School in Japan[15]; since then, the concept has gradually, but steadily, become a reality in the United States. The University of Nebraska and the University of Virginia have been pioneers for TLA system development. In 1992, a prototype of a laboratory automation platform was developed at the University of Nebraska, the key components being a conveyance system, bar coded specimens, and a computer software package to control specimen movement and tracking, and coordination of robots with the instruments as work cells.[16] Some of the first automated laboratories in the United States have reported their experiences with front-end automation with a wealth of information for others interested in the technology.[17,18] The first hospital laboratory to install an automated system was The University of Virginia Hospital in Charlottesville in 1995. Their Medical Automation Research Center cooperated with Johnson & Johnson and Coulter Corporation to use a Vitros 950 attached to a Coulter/IDS "U" lane for direct sampling from a specimen conveyor without using intervening robotics.[19] The first commercially available turnkey system was the Hitachi Clinical Laboratory Automation System (CLAS) (Boehringer-Mannheim Diagnostics; now, Roche Diagnostics). It couples the Hitachi line of analyzers to a conveyor belt system to provide a completely operational system with all interfaces.[20]

Robotics and front-end automation are changing the face of the clinical laboratory.[21] Much of the benefit derivable from TLA can be realized merely by automating the front end. The planning, implementation, and performance evaluation of an automated transport and sorting system by a large reference laboratory have been described in detail.[22,23] Several instrument manufacturers are currently working on or are already marketing interfacing front-end devices together with software for their own chemistry analyzers. Johnson & Johnson introduced the Vitros 950 AT (Automation Technology) system in 1995 with an open architecture design to allow laboratories to select from many front-end automation systems rather than being locked into a proprietary interface. A Lab-Track interface is now available on the Dimension RxL from Dade Behring Chemistry Systems that is compatible with major laboratory automation vendors and allows for direct sampling from a track system. Also, the technology now exists for microcentrifugal separators to be integrated into clinical chemistry analyzers.[24] Several other systems are now on the market, including the Advia LabCell system (Bayer), which uses a modular approach to automation. The Power Processor Core System (Beckman Coulter) performs sorting, centrifugation, and cap removal. The enGen Series Automation System (Ortho-Clinical Diagnostics) provides sorting, centrifugation, decapping, and sample archiving functions and interface directly with a Vitros 950 AT analyzer. Three automation systems are available from Olympus that can perform sorting, centrifugation, decapping, aliquoting, and direct instrument interface capabilities. The Genesis FE500 (Tecan) is an example of a stand-alone front-end system that sorts, centrifuges, decaps, and aliquots. Some laboratories have taken a modular phased-end approach with devices for only certain automated functions. Ciba-Corning Clinical Laboratories installed Coulter/IDS robotic systems in several regional laboratories.[19] The bottom line is that robotics and front-end automation are here to stay. As more and more clinical laboratories reengineer for total laboratory automation, they are building core labs containing all of their automated analyzers as the necessary first step to more easily link the different instruments into one TLA system.[25]

Analytic Phase (Chemical Analyses)

There have been changes and improvements that are now common to many general chemistry analyzers. They include ever smaller microsampling and reagent dispensing with multiple additions possible from randomly replaced reagents; expanded onboard and total test menus, especially drugs and hormones; accelerated reaction times with chemistries for faster throughput and lower dwell time; higher resolution optics with grating monochromators and diode arrays for polychromatic analysis; improved flow-through electrodes; enhanced user-friendly interactive software for quality control, maintenance, and diagnostics; integrated modems for on-line troubleshooting; LIS interfacing data management systems; reduced frequencies of calibration and controls; automated modes for calibration, dilution, rerun, and maintenance; as well as ergonomic and physical design improvements for operator ease, serviceability, and maintenance reduction. According to recent CAP survey data, the eight most popular general chemistry analyzers are Aeroset (Abbott Diagnostics); Advia (Bayer Health); AU systems (Olympus); Dimension (Dade Behring); Hitachi systems (Roche Diagnostics); Integra systems (Roche Diagnostics); Synchron systems (Beckman Instruments); and Vitros (Ortho-Clinical Diagnostics).[26] Features and specifications of these eight systems are summarized in Table 5-1. One main advantage of modular chemistry analyzers is scalability. As workload increases, additional modules can be added to increase throughput. A schematic of the MODULAR *ANALYTICS* system (Roche) is shown in Figure 5-20. This system can accommodate from one to four D, P, or E modules. This provides flexibility to adapt to changing workloads. Chemistry and immunoassay testing can be combined, obviating the need to split samples. Repeat testing can be accomplished automatically using the rerun buffer, which holds the samples until all testing is completed.

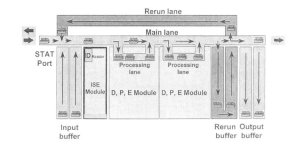

FIGURE 5-20. Schematic drawing of Roche MODULAR *ANALYTICS* system. (Photo courtesy of Roche Diagnostics.)

Postanalytic Phase (Data Management)

Although most of the attention in recent years in total laboratory automation concept has been devoted to front-end systems for sample handling, several manufacturers have been developing and enhancing back-end handling of data. Bidirectional communication between the analyzer(s) and the host computer or LIS has become an absolutely essential link to request tests and enter patient demographics, automatically transfer this customized information to the analyzer(s), as well as post the results in the patient's record. Evaluation and management of data from the time of analysis until posting has become more sophisticated and automated with the integration of work station managers into the entire communication system.[27] Most data management devices are personal computer–based modules with manufacturers' proprietary software that interfaces with one or more of their analyzers and the host LIS. They offer automated management of quality control data with storage and evaluation of quality control results against the lab's predefined quality control perimeters with multiple plotting, displaying, and reporting capabilities. Review and editing of patient results before verification and transmission to the host is enhanced by user-defined perimeters for reportable range limits, panic value limits, delta checks, and quality control comparisons for clinical change, repeat testing, and algorithm analysis. Reagent inventory and quality control, along with monitoring of instrument functions, are also managed by the workstation's software. Most LIS vendors have interfacing software available for all the major chemistry analyzers.

Some data handling needs associated with automation cannot be adequately handled by most current LIS's. For example, most current analyzers are capable of assessing the degree of sample hemolysis, icterus, and lipemia (Table 5-1). However, making this information available and useful to either the clinician or laboratorian in an automated fashion requires additional manipulation of the data. Ideally, the tests ordered on the sample, the threshold for interference of each test by each of the three agents, and whether the interference is positive or negative needs to be determined. In the case of lipemia, the results for affected tests need to be held until the sample can be clarified and the tests rerun. It is difficult or impossible for current LIS systems to perform this latter task. There is a need for a "gap-filler" between the instrument and the LIS. One company, Data Innovations, has developed a system called Instrument Manager, which links the analyzer to the LIS and provides the ability for the user to define rules for release of information to the LIS. In addition, flags can be displayed to the instrument operator to perform additional operations, such as sample clarification and reanalysis. The ability to fully automate data review using rules based analysis is a key factor in moving toward TLA.

FUTURE TRENDS IN AUTOMATION

Clinical chemistry automation will continue to evolve at a rapid pace from 2004 to 2010 as it has in the 1990s. With most of the same forces driving the automation market through 2005, as those discussed in this chapter, analyzers will continue to perform more cost effectively and efficiently. More integration and miniaturization of components and systems will persist to accommodate more sophisticated portable analyzers for the successful point-of-care testing market. Effective communication among all automation stakeholders for a given project is key to successful implementation.[28]

More new tests for expanded menus will be developed, with a mixture of measurement techniques used on the analyzers to include more immunoassays and PCR-based assays. Spectral-mapping, or multiple wavelength monitoring, with high-resolution photometers in analyzers will be routine for all specimens and tests as more instruments are designed with the monochromator device in the light path after the cuvet, not before. Spectral mapping capabilities will allow simultaneous analysis of multiple chemistry analytes in the same reaction vessel. This will have a tremendous impact on throughput and turn-around time of test results. Mass spectrometry and capillary electrophoresis will be used more extensively in clinical laboratories for identification and quantification of elements and compounds in extremely small concentrations. In the coming years, more system and workflow integration will occur with robotics and data management for more inclusive total laboratory automation.[29] To accomplish this, more companies will form alliances to place their instrumentation products in the laboratories. The incorporation of artificial intelligence into analytic systems will evolve, using both experts systems and neural networks.[30,31] This will greatly advance the technologies of robotics, digital processing of data, computer-assisted diagnosis, and data integration with electronic patient records.

Finally, technologic advances in chip technology and biosensors will accelerate the development of noninvasive, in vivo testing.[32–34] Transcutaneous monitoring is already available with some blood gases. "True" or dynamic values from in vivo monitoring of constituents in blood and other body fluids will revolutionize laboratory medicine as we know it today. It sounds futuristic, but so did the first AutoAnalyzer 50 years ago.

SUMMARY

Since the introduction of the first automated analyzer by Technicon, automated instruments have proliferated in the clinical chemistry laboratory. The driving forces behind the development and improvement of automated analyzers included the increased volume of testing, faster turnaround time, and escalating costs. Automated analyzers can use one of three basic approaches to sample analysis: continuous flow, centrifugal analysis, and discrete analysis, with most now using discrete analysis. Manufacturers have designed their instruments to mimic the steps in a manual procedure to include specimen preparation and identification, specimen measurement and delivery, reagent systems and delivery, chemical reaction phase, measurement phase, and signal processing and data handling. Each manufacturer's approach to automation is unique.

When selecting an automated analyzer for the clinical chemistry laboratory, several factors need to be considered: laboratory needs, cost, method of acquisition, consumables, analytic capabilities, space, and user friendliness. Clinical chemistry automation will continue to evolve. TLA now provides integration of all three phases of laboratory testing, linking the front-end sample processing and back-end data management with the analytic phase. Future trends will undoubtedly include more computer power, more portability, increased use of robotics, spectral mapping, continuous improvement in computer software, and the development of artificially intelligent computer systems. New technologies, such as polymerase chain reactions and noninvasive in vivo testing, will also have a large impact.

REVIEW QUESTIONS

1. Which of the following is NOT a driving force for more automation?
   a. High-volume testing
   b. Fast turnaround time
   c. Expectation of high-quality, accurate results
   d. Increased use of chemistry panels

2. Which of the following approaches to analyzer automation can use mixing paddles to stir?
   a. Centrifugal analysis
   b. Continuous flow
   c. Discrete analysis
   d. Dry chemistry slide analysis

3. Which of the following types of analyzers offers random access capabilities?
   a. Continuous-flow analyzers
   b. Centrifugal analyzers
   c. Discrete analyzers
   d. None of the above

4. All of the following are primary considerations in the selection of an automated chemistry analyzer EXCEPT:
   a. the cost of consumables.
   b. total instrument cost.
   c. the labor component.
   d. how reagents are added or mixed.

5. An example of an automated immunoassay analyzer would be the:
   a. Advia Centaur.
   b. Paramax.
   c. Synchron.
   d. Vitros.

6. *Dwell time* refers to the:
   a. number of tests an instrument can handle in a specified time.
   b. ability of an instrument to perform a defined workload in a specified time.
   c. time between initiation of a test and the completion of the analysis.
   d. None of the above.

7. The first commercial centrifugal analyzer was introduced in what year?
   a. 1957
   b. 1967
   c. 1970
   d. 1976

8. All of the following are advantages to automation EXCEPT:
   a. increased number of tests performed.
   b. minimized labor component.
   c. correction for deficiencies inherent in methodologies.
   d. use of small amounts of samples and reagents in comparison to manual procedures.

9. Which of the following steps in automation generally remains a manual process in most laboratories?
   a. Preparation of the sample
   b. Specimen measurement and delivery
   c. Reagent delivery
   d. Chemical reaction phase

10. Which of the following chemistry analyzers uses slides to contain the entire reagent system?
    a. Vitros analyzers
    b. ACA analyzers
    c. Paramax analyzers
    d. None of the above

REFERENCES

1. Hodnett J. Automated analyzers have surpassed the test of time. Adv Med Lab 1994;8.
2. Schoeff L, et al. Principles of Laboratory Instruments. St. Louis: Mosby-Year Book, 1993.
3. Jacobs E, Simson E. Point of care testing and laboratory automation: the total picture of diagnostic testing at the beginning of the next century. Clin Lab News 1999;December:12-4.
4. Boyce N. Why hospitals are moving to core labs. Clin Lab News 1996;22(11):1–2.
5. Boyce N. Why labs should discourage routine testing. Clin Lab News 1996;22(12):1, 9.
6. Eisenwiener H, Keller M. Absorbance measurement in cuvets lying longitudinal to the light beam. Clin Chem 1979;25(1):117–121.
7. Burtis CA. Factors influencing evaporation from sample cups, and assessment of their effect on analytic error. Clin Chem 1975;21:1907–1917.
8. Burtis CA, Watson JS. Design and evaluation of an anti-evaporative cover for use with liquid containers. Clin Chem 1992;38:768–775.
9. Dudley RF. Chemiluminescence immunoassay: an alternative to RIA. Lab Med 1990;21(4):216.
10. Haboush L. Lab equipment management strategies: balancing costs and quality. Clin Lab News 1997;23(6):20–21.
11. Schoeff L. Clinical instrumentation (general chemistry analyzers). Anal Chem 1997;69(12):200R–203R.
12. Ringel M. National survey results: automation is everywhere. MLO Med Lab Obs 1996;28:38–43.
13. Douglas L. Redefining automation: perspectives on today's clinical laboratory. Clin Lab News 1997;23(7):48–49.
14. Felder R. Front-end automation. In: Kost G, ed. Handbook of Clinical Laboratory Automation and Robotics. New York: Wiley, 1995.
15. Sasaki M. A fully automated clinical laboratory. Lab Inform Mgmt 1993;21:159–168.
16. Markin R, Sasaki M. A laboratory automation platform: the next robotic step. MLO Med Lab Obs 1992;24:24–29.
17. Bauer S, Teplitz C. Total laboratory automation: a view of the 21st century. MLO Med Lab Obs 1995;27:22–25.
18. Bauer S, Teplitz C. Laboratory automation, Part 2. Total lab automation: system design. MLO Med Lab Obs 1995;27:44–50.
19. Felder R. Cost justifying laboratory automation. Clin Lab News 1996;22(4):10–11, 17.
20. Felder R. Laboratory automation: strategies and possibilities. Clin Lab News 1996;22(3):10–11.
21. Boyd J, Felder R, Savory J. Robotics and the changing face of the clinical laboratory. Clin Chem 1996;42(12):1901–1910.
22. Hawker CD, Garr SB, Hamilton LT, Penrose JR, Ashwood ER, Weiss RL. Automated transport and sorting system in a large reference laboratory: Part 1. Evaluation of needs and alternatives and development of a plan. Clin Chem 2002;48(10):1751–1760.
23. Hawker CD, Roberts WL, Garr SB, Hamilton LT, Penrose JR, Ashwood ER, Weiss RL. Automated transport and sorting system in a large reference laboratory: Part 2. Implementation of the system and performance measures over three years. Clin Chem 2002;48(10):1761–1767.
24. Richardson P, Molloy J, Ravenhall R, et al. High speed centrifugal separator for rapid online sample clarification in biotechnology. J Biotechnol 1996;49(1–3):111–118.
25. Zenie F. Re-engineering the laboratory. Autom Chem 1996;18(4):135–141.
26. CAP Surveys, Proficiency Testing Program. Northfield, IL: College of American Pathologists, 2002.
27. Saboe T. Managing laboratory automation. J Autom Chem 1995;17(3):83–88.
28. Fisher JA. Laboratory automation: communicating with all stakeholders is the key to success. Clin Lab News 2000;July:38–40.
29. Brzezicki L. Workflow integration: does it make sense for your lab? Adv Lab 1996;23:57–62.
30. Place J, Truchaud A, Ozawa K, et al. Use of artificial intelligence in analytical systems for the clinical laboratory. J Autom Chem 1995;17(1):1–15.
31. Boyce N. Neural networks in the lab: new hope or just hype? Clin Lab News 1997;23(1):2–3.
32. Boyce N. Tiny "lab chips" with huge potential? Clin Lab News 1996;22(12):21.
33. Rosen S. Biosensors: where do we go from here? MLO Med Lab Obs 1995;27:24–29.
34. Aller RD. Chemistry analyzers branching out. CAP Today 2002;July:84–106.

Immunoassays and Nucleic Acid Probe Techniques

Susan Orton

OBJECTIVES

Upon completion of this chapter, the clinical laboratorian should be able to:
- State the principle of each of the following methods:
  - Double diffusion
  - Radial immunodiffusion
  - Immunoelectrophoresis
  - Immunofixation electrophoresis
  - Nephelometry
  - Turbidimetry
  - Competitive immunoassay
  - Noncompetitive immunoassay
  - Immunoblot
  - Direct immunocytochemistry
  - Indirect immunocytochemistry
  - Immunophenotyping by flow cytometry
  - Polymerase chain reaction
  - Southern blot
  - In situ hybridization
  - Restriction fragment length polymorphism
- Compare and contrast the general types of labels used in immunoassays.

- Classify an immunoassay, given its format, as homogeneous or heterogeneous, competitive or noncompetitive, and by its label.
- Explain how the concentration of the analyte in the test sample is related to the amount of bound-labeled reagent for competitive and noncompetitive immunoassays.
- Describe the three methods used to separate unbound-labeled reagent from bound-labeled reagent.
- Describe the data reduction in the classic competitive radioimmunoassay.
- Compare and contrast EMIT, DELFIA, MEIA, RIA, FPIA, ELISA, CEDIA, ICON, and OIA methodologies.
- Explain the principles of hybridization.
- State the role of reverse transcriptase, polymerase, and restriction endonuclease in nucleic acid probe assays.
- Describe the principle of fluorescence resonance energy transfer as it is used in a real time polymerase chain reaction assay.

KEY TERMS

Affinity
Amplicon
Anneal
Antibody
Antigen
Avidity
Competitive
    immunoassay
Counterimmunoelectro-
    phoresis
Cross-reactivity
Direct
    immunofluorescence
    (DIF)
DNA index (DI)
Duplex
Epitope

Flow cytometry
Fluorescence resonance
    energy transfer (FRET)
Hapten (Hp)
Heterogeneous
    immunoassay
Homogeneous
    immunoassay
Hybridization
Immunoblot
Immunocytochemistry
Immunoelectrophoresis
    (IEP)
Immunofixation
    electrophoresis (IFE)
Immunohistochemistry
Immunophenotyping

Indirect
    immunofluorescence
    (IIF)
In situ hybridization
Ligase chain reaction
    (LCR)
Monoclonal
Nephelometry
Noncompetitive
    immunoassay
Northern blot
Nucleic acid probe
Polyclonal
Polymerase chain
    reaction (PCR)
Postzone
Prozone

Radial immunodiffusion
    (RID)
Restriction fragment
    length polymorphism
Reverse transcriptase-
    polymerase chain
    reaction (RT-PCR)
Rocket technique
Self-sustained sequence
    replication (3SR)
Solid phase
Southern blot
Tracer
Turbidimetry
Western blot

This chapter introduces two generic analytic methods used in the clinical laboratory: one involves the binding of antibody to antigen and the other relies on the binding of a nucleic acid sequence to its complimentary target nucleic acid sequence. Common to both methods are the complementary nature of the reactants, which determines the specificity, and the detector system, which indicates the extent of the binding reaction and is related to the analytic sensitivity. In immunoassays, an antigen binds to an antibody. The antigen–antibody interactions may involve unlabeled reactants in less analytically sensitive techniques or a labeled reactant in more sensitive techniques. The design, label, and detection system combine to create many different assays, which enable the measurement of a wide range of molecules.

In nucleic acid binding, typically, a probe will bind to a complementary nucleic acid sequence. The target nucleic acid may or may not be amplified prior to detection and/or quantitation. Thus, nucleic acid–based methods are designed to detect changes at the DNA or RNA level rather than to detect a synthesized gene product, such as a protein detected in immunoassays. Again, many assay designs use probes. To give a clearer explanation, immunoassays will be considered separately from nucleic acid probe assays. This chapter reviews the concepts of binding, describes the nature of the reagents used, and discusses basic assay design of selected techniques used in the clinical laboratory; as such, it is intended to be an overview rather than an exhaustive review.

IMMUNOASSAYS

General Considerations

In an immunoassay, an *antibody* molecule recognizes and binds to an *antigen*. The molecule of interest may be either an antigen or antibody. This binding is related to the concentration of each reactant, the specificity of the antibody for the antigen, the affinity and avidity for the pair, and the environmental conditions. Although this chapter focuses on immunoassays that use an antibody molecule as the binding reagent, other assays, such as receptor assays and competitive binding protein assays, use receptor proteins or transport proteins as the binding reagent, respectively. The same principles apply to these assays. An antibody molecule is an immunoglobulin with a functional domain known as F(ab); this area of the immunoglobulin protein binds to a site on the antigen. An antigen is relatively large and complex and usually has multiple sites that can bind to antibodies with different specificities; each site on the antigen is referred to as an antigenic determinant or *epitope*. Some confusion exists in the terminology used: some immunologists refer to an *immunogen* as the molecule that induces the biologic response and synthesis of antibody, and some use *antigen* to refer to that which binds to antibody. However, all agree that the antigenic site to which an F(ab) can bind is the epitope.

The degree of binding is an important consideration in an immunoassay. The binding of an antibody to an antigen is directly related to the affinity and avidity of the antibody for the epitope, as well as the concentration of the antibody and epitope. Under standard conditions, the *affinity* of an antibody is measured using a *hapten (Hp)* because the hapten is a low molecular weight antigen considered to have only one epitope. The affinity for the hapten is related to the likelihood to bind or to the degree of complementary nature of each. The reversible reaction is summarized in Equation 6-1:

$$\text{Hapten} + \text{antibody} \rightleftharpoons \text{hapten–antibody complex}$$

(Eq. 6–1)

The binding between a hapten and the antibody obeys the law of mass action and is expressed mathematically in Equation 6-2:

$$K_a = \frac{k_1}{k_2} = \frac{[\text{Hp} - \text{Ab}]}{[\text{Hp}][\text{Ab}]} \qquad \textbf{(Eq. 6–2)}$$

K_a is the affinity or equilibrium constant and represents the reciprocal of the concentration of free hapten when 50% of the binding sites are occupied. The greater the affinity of the hapten for the antibody, the smaller the concentration of hapten needed to saturate 50% of the binding sites of the antibody. For example, if the affinity constant of a monoclonal antibody is 3×10^{11} L/mole, it means that a hapten concentration of 3×10^{-11} moles/L is needed to occupy half of the binding sites. Typically, the affinity constant of antibodies used in immunoassay procedures ranges from 10^9 to 10^{11} L/mole, whereas the affinity constant for transport proteins ranges from 10^7 to 10^8 L/mole and the affinity for receptors ranges from 10^8 to 10^{11} L/mole.

As with all chemical (molecular) reactions, the initial concentrations of the reactants and the products affect the extent of complex binding. In immunoassays, the reaction moves forward (to the right) (Equation 6-1) when the concentration of reactants (Ag and Ab) exceeds the concentration of the product (Ag–Ab complex) and when there is a favorable affinity constant.

The forces that bring an antigenic determinant and an antibody together are noncovalent, reversible bonds that result from the cumulative effects of hydrophobic, hydrophilic, and hydrogen bonding and van der Waals forces. The most important factor that affects the cumulative strength of bonding is the goodness (or closeness) of fit between the antibody and the antigen. The strength of most of these interactive forces is inversely related to the distance between the interactive sites. The closer the antibody and antigen can physically approach one another, the greater the attractive forces.

After the antigen–antibody complex is formed, the likelihood of separation (which is inversely related to the tightness of bonding) is referred to as *avidity*. The avidity represents a value-added phenomenon in which the strength of binding of all antibody–epitope pairs exceeds the sum of single antibody–epitope binding. In general, the stronger the affinity and avidity, the greater the possibility of cross-reactivity.

The specificity of an antibody is most often described by the antigen that induced the antibody production, the homologous antigen. Ideally, this antibody would react only with that antigen. However, an antibody can react with an antigen that is structurally similar to the homologous antigen; this is referred to as *cross-reactivity*. Considering that an antigenic determinant can be five or six amino acids or one immunodominant sugar, it is not surprising that antigen similarity is common. The greater the similarity between the cross-reacting antigen and the homologous antigen, the stronger the bond with the antibody.[1] Reagent antibody production is achieved by polyclonal or monoclonal techniques. In *polyclonal* antibody production, the stimulating antigen is injected in an animal responsive to the antigen; the animal detects this foreign antigen and mounts an immune response to eliminate the antigen. If part of this immune response includes strong antibody production, then blood is collected and antibody is harvested, characterized, and purified to yield the commercial antiserum reagent. This polyclonal antibody reagent is a mixture of antibody specificities. Some antibodies react with the stimulating epitopes and some are endogenous to the host. Multiple antibodies directed against the multiple epitopes on the antigen are present and can cross-link the multivalent antigen. Polyclonal antibodies are often used as "capture" antibodies in sandwich or indirect immunoassays.

In contrast, an immortal cell line produces *monoclonal* antibodies; each line produces one specific antibody. This method developed as an extension of the hybridoma work published by Kohler and Milstein in 1975.[2] The process begins by selecting cells with the qualities that will allow the synthesis of a homogeneous antibody. First, a host (commonly, a mouse) is immunized with an antigen (the one to which an antibody is desired); later, the sensitized lymphocytes of the spleen are harvested. Second, an immortal cell line (usually a nonsecretory mouse myeloma cell line that is hypoxanthine guanine phosphoribosyltransferase deficient) is required to ensure that continuous propagation in vitro is viable. These cells are then mixed in the presence of a fusion agent, such as polyethylene glycol, that promotes the fusion of two cells to form a hybridoma. In a selective growth medium, only the hybrid cells will survive. B cells have a limited natural life span in vitro and cannot survive, and the unfused myeloma cells cannot survive due to their enzyme deficiency. If the viable fused cells synthesize antibody, then the specificity and isotype of the antibody are evaluated. Monoclonal antibody reagent is commercially produced by growing the hybridoma in tissue culture or in compatible animals. An important feature about monoclonal antibody reagent is that the antibody is homogeneous (a single antibody, not a mixture of antibodies). Therefore, it recognizes only one epitope on a multivalent antigen and cannot cross-link a multivalent antigen.

Unlabeled Immunoassays

Immune Precipitation in Gel

In one of the simplest unlabeled immunoassays introduced into the clinical laboratory, unlabeled antibody was layered on top of unlabeled antigen (both in the fluid phase); during the incubation period, the antibody and antigen diffused and the presence of precipitation was recorded. The precipitation occurred because each antibody recognized an epitope and that multivalent antigens were cross-linked by multiple antibodies. When the antigen–antibody complex is of sufficient size, the interaction with water is limited so that the complex becomes insoluble and precipitates.

It has been observed that if the concentration of antigen is increased while the concentration of antibody remains constant, the amount of precipitate formed is related to the ratio of antibody to antigen. As shown in Figure 6-1, there is an optimal ratio of the concentration of antibody to the concentration of antigen that results in the maximal precipitation; this is the zone of equivalence. Outside the zone of equivalence, the amount of precipitate is diminished or absent because the ratio of antibody to antigen is out of proportion and the cross-linking of antigen is decreased. When antibody concentration is in excess and cross-linking is decreased, the assay is in *prozone*. Conversely, when antigen concentration is in excess and cross-linking is decreased, the assay is in *postzone*. Although originally described with precipitation reactions, this concept applies to other assays in which the ratio of antibody to antigen is critical.

Precipitation reactions in gel are commonly performed in the clinical laboratory today. Gel is dilute agarose (typically less than 1%) dissolved in an aqueous buffer. This provides a semisolid medium through which soluble antigen and antibody can easily pass. Precipitated immune complexes are easier to discern in gel versus a liquid suspension. Immune precipitation methods in gel can be classified as passive methods or those using electrophoresis and are summarized in Table 6-1. The simplest and least sensitive method is double diffusion (the

TABLE 6-1. IMMUNE PRECIPITATION METHODS

Gel
Passive
Double diffusion (Ouchterlony technique)
Single diffusion (radial immunodiffusion)
Electrophoresis
Counterimmunoelectrophoresis
Immunoelectrophoresis
Immunofixation electrophoresis
Rocket electrophoresis
Soluble Phase
Turbidimetry
Nephelometry

Ouchterlony technique).[3] Agarose is placed on a solid surface and allowed to solidify. Wells are cut into the agarose. A common template is six antibody wells, surrounding a single antigen well in the center. Soluble antigen and soluble antibody are added to separate wells and diffusion occurs. The intensity and pattern of the precipitation band are interpreted. As shown in Figure 6-2, the precipitin band of an unknown sample is compared with the precipitin band of a sample known to contain the antibody. A pattern of identity confirms the presence of the antibody in the unknown sample. Patterns of partial identity and nonidentity are ambiguous. This technique is used to detect antibodies associated with autoimmune

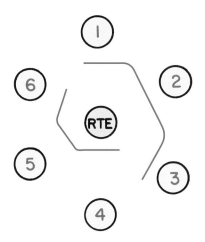

FIGURE 6-2. A schematic demonstrating the pattern of identity. The center well contains the antigen, rabbit thymus extract. Well 1 is filled with a serum known to contain Sm antibody. Test sera are in Wells 2 and 3; the pattern of identity, the smooth continuous line between the 3 wells, confirms the presence of Sm antibody in the test sera. Well 4 is filled with a serum known to contain U1-RNP antibody. Test sera in Wells 5 and 6 also contain U1-RNP antibody confirmed by the pattern of identity between the known serum and the test sera.

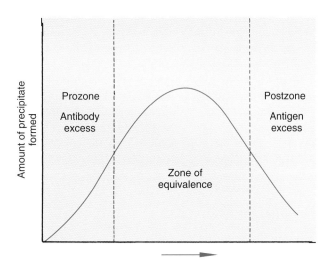

FIGURE 6-1. Precipitin curve showing the amount of precipitate versus antigen concentration. The concentration of antibody is constant.

diseases, such as Sm and RNP detected in systemic lupus erythematosus, SSA and SSB in Sjögren's syndrome, and Scl-70 in progressive systemic sclerosis.

The single-diffusion technique, *radial immunodiffusion (RID)*, is an immune precipitation method used to quantitate protein (the antigen). In this method, monospecific antiserum is added to the liquefied agarose; then the agarose is poured into a plate and cooled. Wells are cut into the solidified agarose. Multiple standards, one or more quality control samples, and patient samples are added to the wells. The antigen diffuses from the well in all directions, binds to the soluble antibody in the agarose, and forms a complex seen as a concentric precipitin ring (Fig. 6-3). The diameter of the ring is related to the concentration of the antigen that diffused from the well. A standard curve is constructed to determine the concentration in the quality control and patient samples. The usable analytic range is between the lowest and highest standards. If the ring is greater than the highest standard, the sample should be diluted and retested. If the ring is less than the lowest standard, the sample should be run on a low-level plate. Two variations exist: the end point (Mancini) method[4] and the kinetic (Fahey-McKelvey) method.[5] The end point method requires that all antigen diffuse from the well and the concentration of the antigen is related to the square of the diameter of the precipitin ring; the standard curve is plotted on linear graph paper and is the line of best fit. To ensure that all antigen has diffused, the incubation time is 48 to 72 hours, depending on the molecular weight of the antigen; for example, IgG quantitation requires 48 hours, IgM requires 72 hours. In contrast, the kinetic method requires that all rings be measured at a fixed time of 18 hours; a sample with a greater concentration will diffuse at a faster rate and will be larger at a fixed time. Using semilogarithmic graph paper, the concentration of the antigen is plotted against the diameter of the precipitin ring; the line is drawn point to point. For those performing RID, the end point method is favored because of its stability and indifference to temperature variations; however, turnaround time is longer compared with the kinetic method.

Counterimmunoelectrophoresis is an immune precipitation method that uses an electrical field to cause the antigen and antibody to migrate toward each other. Two parallel lines of wells are cut into agarose; antibody is placed in one line and antigen is placed in the other. Antibody will migrate to the cathode and the antigen to the anode; a precipitin line forms where they meet. This qualitative test is useful to detect bacterial antigens in cerebrospinal fluid and other fluids when a rapid laboratory response is needed.

Immunoelectrophoresis (IEP) and *immunofixation electrophoresis (IFE)* are two methods used in the clinical laboratory to characterize monoclonal proteins in serum and urine. In 1964, Grabar and Burtin published methods for examining serum proteins using electrophoresis coupled with immunochemical reactions in agarose.[6] Serum proteins are electrophoretically separated and then reagent antibody is placed in a trough running parallel to the separated proteins. The antibody reagent and separated serum proteins diffuse; when the reagent antibody recognizes the serum protein and the reaction is in the zone of equivalence, a precipitin arc is seen (Fig. 6-4). The agarose plate is stained (typically, with a protein stain such as Amido black 10), destained, and dried to enhance the readability of precipitin arcs, especially

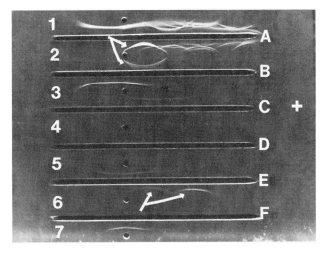

FIGURE 6-4. Immunoelectrophoresis. *Wells 1, 3, 5,* and *7* contain normal human serum, and *wells 2, 4,* and *6* contain the test serum. Antiserum reagent is in the troughs: **A** contains antihuman whole serum; **B** contains antihuman IgG; **C** contains antihuman IgA; **D** contains antihuman IgM; **E** contains antihuman κ; **F** contains antihuman λ. The *arrows* at the *top* point to an abnormal γ chain that reacts with the anti-IgG reagent. A similar band is shown at the bottom with the anti-κ reagent. There is also a pattern of identity with the anti-κ reagent that shows free κ chains in the test serum.

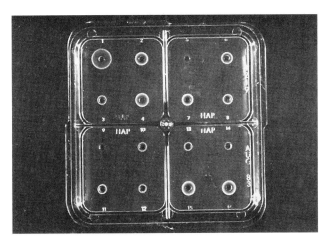

FIGURE 6-3. A radial immunodiffusion plate to detect haptoglobin. The diameter of the precipitin circle is related to the concentration of haptoglobin in the serum.

weak arcs. The size, shape, density, and location of the arcs aid in the interpretation of the protein. All interpretation is made by comparing the arcs of the patient sample with the arcs of the quality control sample, a normal human serum. Because IEP is used to evaluate a monoclonal protein, the heavy chain class and light chain type must be determined. To evaluate the most common monoclonal proteins, the following antisera are used: antihuman whole serum (which contains a mixture of antibodies against the major serum proteins), antihuman IgG (γ chain specific), antihuman IgM (μ chain specific), antihuman IgA (α chain specific), antihuman λ (λ chain specific), and antihuman κ (κ chain specific). The test turnaround time and the subtlety in interpretation have discouraged IEP as the primary method to evaluate monoclonal antibodies.

IFE[7] has replaced IEP in many laboratories. A serum, urine, or cerebrospinal fluid sample is placed in all six lanes of an agarose gel and electrophoresed to separate the proteins. Cellulose acetate (or some other porous material) is saturated with antibody reagent and then applied to one lane of the separated protein. If the antibody reagent recognizes the protein, an insoluble complex is formed. After staining and drying the agarose film, interpretation is based on the migration and appearance of bands. As shown in Figure 6-5, the monoclonal protein will appear as a discrete band (with both a heavy and a light chain monospecific antiserum occurring at the same position). Polyclonal proteins will appear as a diffuse band. The concentration of patient sample may need

adjustment to assure the reaction is in the zone of equivalence.

The last immune precipitation method in gel discussed is the *rocket technique* (Laurell technique, or electroimmunoassay).[8,9] In this quantitative technique, reagent antibody is mixed with agarose; antigen is placed in the well and electrophoresed. As the antigen moves through the agarose, it reacts with the reagent antibody and forms a "rocket," with stronger precipitation along the edges. The height of the rocket is proportional to the concentration of antigen present; the concentration is determined based on a calibration curve. The narrow range of linearity may require dilution or concentration of the unknown sample.

Detection of Fluid-Phase Antigen–Antibody Complexes

A different strategy to quantitate antigen–antibody complexes is to use an instrument to detect the soluble antigen–antibody complexes as they interact with light. When antigen and antibody combine, complexes are formed that act as particles in suspension and thus can scatter light. The size of the particles determines the type of scatter that will dominate when the solution interacts with nearly monochromatic light.[10] When the particle, such as albumin or IgG, is relatively small compared with the wavelength of incident light, the particle will scatter light symmetrically, both forward and backward. A minimum of scattered light is detectable at 90° from the incident light. Larger molecules and antigen–antibody complexes have diameters that approach the wavelength of incident light and scatter light with a greater intensity in the forward direction. The wavelength of light is selected based on its ability to be scattered in a forward direction and the ability of the antigen–antibody complexes to absorb the wavelength of light.

Turbidimetry measures the light transmitted and *nephelometry* measures the light scattered. Turbidimeters (spectrophotometers or colorimeters) are designed to measure the light passing through a solution so the photodetector is placed at an angle of 180° from the incident light. If light absorbance is insignificant, turbidity can be expressed as the absorbance, which is directly related to the concentration of suspended particles and path length. Nephelometers measure light at an angle other than 180° from the incident light; most measure forward light scattered at less than 90° because the sensitivity is increased (see Chapter 4, *Analytic Techniques and Instrumentation*). The relative concentration of the antibody reagent and antigen is critical to ensure that the size of the complex generated is best detected by the nephelometer or turbidimeter and that the immune reaction is not in postzone or prozone. Therefore, it may be important to test more than one concentration of patient sample, to monitor the presence of excess antibody, or to add

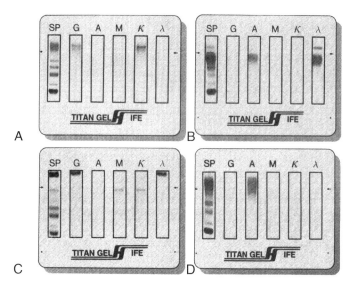

FIGURE 6-5. Immunofixation electrophoresis. **A.** IgG κ monoclonal immunoglobulin. **B.** IgA κ monoclonal immunoglobulin with free κ light chains. **C.** IgG λ and IgM κ biclonal immunoglobulins. **D.** Diffuse IgA heavy chain band without a corresponding light chain.

additional antiserum and monitor the peak rate. Excess antibody would indicate that there is little antigen and that the reaction is underestimated.

For both turbidimetry and nephelometry, all reagents and sera must be free of particles that could scatter the light. Pretreatment of serum with polyethylene glycol, a nonionic, hydrophilic polymer, enhances the antigen–antibody interaction. Because the polymer is more hydrophilic than the antigen or antibody, water is attracted from the antigen and antibody to the polyethylene glycol. This results in a faster rate and greater quantity of antigen–antibody complex formation.

Both methods can be performed in an end point or kinetic mode. In the end point mode, a measurement is taken at the beginning of the reaction (the background signal) and one is taken at a set time later in the reaction (plateau or end point signal); the concentration is determined using a calibration curve. In the kinetic mode, the rate of complex formation is continuously monitored and the peak rate is determined. The peak rate is directly related to the concentration of the antigen, although this is not necessarily linear. Thus, a calibration curve is required to determine concentration in unknown samples.

Labeled Immunoassays

General Considerations

In all labeled immunoassays, a reagent (antigen or antibody) is usually labeled by attaching a particle or molecule that will better detect lower concentrations of antigen–antibody complexes. Therefore, the label improves analytic sensitivity. All assays have a binding reagent, which can bind to the antigen or ligand. If the binding reagent is an antibody, the assay is an immunoassay. If the binding agent is a receptor (*eg*, estrogen or progesterone receptor), the assay is a receptor assay. If the binding reagent is a transport protein (*eg*, thyroxine-binding globulin or transcortin), the assay may be called competitive protein-binding assay. Immunoassays are used today almost exclusively, with two notable exceptions: estrogen and progesterone receptor assays and the thyroid hormone-binding ratio, which uses thyroxine-binding globulin.

Immunoassays may be described based on the label; which reactant is labeled, the relative concentration and source of the antibody, the method used to separate free-from bound-labeled reagents, the signal that is measured, and the method used to assign the concentration of analyte in the sample. Immunoassay design, therefore, has many variables to consider, leading to diverse assays.

Labels

The simplest way to identify an assay is by the label used. Table 6-2 lists the commonly used labels and the methods used to detect the label.

Radioactive Labels. Atoms with unstable nuclei that spontaneously emit radiation are radioactive and referred to as radionuclides. The emission is known as radioactive decay and is independent of chemical or physical parameters, such as temperature, pressure, or concentration. Of the three forms of radiation, only beta and gamma are used in the clinical laboratory. In beta emission, the nucleus can emit negatively charged electrons or positively charged particles called positrons. The emitted electrons are also known as beta particles. Tritium (^{3}H) is the ra-

TABLE 6-2. LABELS AND DETECTION METHODS

IMMUNOASSAY	COMMON LABEL	DETECTION METHOD
RIA	^{3}H	Liquid scintillation counter
	^{125}I	Gamma counter
EIA	Horseradish peroxidase	Photometer, fluorometer, luminometer
	Alkaline phosphatase	Photometer, fluorometer, luminometer
	β-D-Galactosidase	Fluorometer, luminometer
	Glucose-6-phosphate dehydrogenase	Photometer, luminometer
CLA	Isoluminol derivative	Luminometer
	Acridinium esters	Luminometer
FIA	Fluorescein	Fluorometer
	Europium	Fluorometer
	Phycobiliproteins	Fluorometer
	Rhodamine B	Fluorometer
	Umbelliferone	Fluorometer

RIA, radioimmunoassay; EIA, enzyme immunoassay; CLA, chemiluminescent assay; FIA, fluorescent immunoassay.

dionuclide commonly used in cellular immunology assays for diagnosis and research.

Gamma emission is electromagnetic radiation with very short wavelengths originating from unstable nuclei. As a radionuclide releases energy and becomes more stable, it disintegrates or decays, releasing energy. A specific spectrum of energy levels is associated with each radionuclide. The standardized unit of radioactivity is the becquerel (Bq), which is equal to one disintegration per second. The traditional unit is the curie (Ci), which equals 3.7×10^{10} Bq; 1μCi = 37 kBq. The half-life of the radionuclide is the time needed for 50% of the radionuclide to decay and become more stable. The longer the half-life, the more slowly it decays, increasing the length of time it can be measured. For radioactive substances used in diagnostic tests, it is preferable that the emission have an appropriate energy level and that the long half-life be relatively long; ^{125}I satisfies these requirements and is the most commonly used gamma-emitting radionuclide in the clinical laboratory.

Gamma-emitting nuclides are detected using a crystal scintillation detector (also known as a gamma counter). The energy released during decay excites a fluor, such as thallium-activated sodium iodide. The excited fluor releases a photon of visible light, which is amplified and detected by a photomultiplier tube; the amplified light energy is then translated into electrical energy. Detectable decay of the radionuclide is expressed as counts per minute (CPM).

In immunoassays, one reactant is radiolabeled. In competitive assays, the antigen is labeled and called the *tracer*. The radiolabel must allow the tracer to be fully functional and to compete equally with the unlabeled antigen for the binding sites. When the detector antibody is radiolabeled, the antigen-combining site must remain biologically active and unhindered.

Enzyme Labels. Enzymes are commonly used to label the antigen/hapten or antibody.[11,12] Horseradish peroxidase (HRP), alkaline phosphatase (ALP), and glucose-6-phosphate dehydrogenase are used most often. Enzymes are biologic catalysts that increase the rate of conversion of substrate to product and are not consumed by the reaction. As such, an enzyme can catalyze many substrate molecules, amplifying the amount of product generated. The enzyme activity may be monitored directly by measuring the product formed or by measuring the effect of the product on a coupled reaction. Depending on the substrate used, the product can be photometric, fluorometric, or chemiluminescent. For example, a typical photometric reaction using HRP-labeled antibody (Ab-HRP) and the substrate (a peroxide) generate the product (oxygen). The oxygen can then oxidize a reduced chromogen (reduced orthophenylenediamine [OPD]) to produce a colored compound (oxidized OPD), which is measured using a photometer.

$$Ab - HRP + peroxide \rightarrow Ab = HRP + O_2$$

$$O_2 + reduced\ OPD \rightarrow oxidized\ OPD + H_2O \quad \textbf{(Eq. 6–3)}$$

Fluorescent Labels. Fluorescent labels (fluorochromes or fluorophores) are compounds that absorb radiant energy of one wavelength and emit radiant energy of a longer wavelength in less than 10^{-4} seconds. Generally, the emitted light is detected at an angle of 90° from the path of excitation light using a fluorometer or a modified spectrophotometer. The difference between the excitation wavelength and emission wavelength (Stokes shift) usually ranges between 20 nm and 80 nm for most fluorochromes. Some fluorescence immunoassays simply substitute a fluorescent label (such as fluorescein) for an enzyme label and quantitate the fluorescence.[13] Another approach, time-resolved fluorescence immunoassay, uses a highly efficient fluorescent label, such as a europium chelate,[14] which fluoresces approximately 1000 times slower than the natural background fluorescence and has a wide Stokes shift. The delay allows the fluorescent label to be detected with minimal interference from background fluorescence. The long Stokes shift facilitates measurement of emission radiation while excluding the excitation radiation. The resulting assay is highly sensitive and time-resolved, with minimized background fluorescence.

Luminescent Labels. Luminescent labels emit a photon of light as the result of an electrical, biochemical, or chemical reaction.[15,16] Some organic compounds become excited when oxidized and emit light as they revert to the ground state. Oxidants include hydrogen peroxide, hypochlorite, or oxygen. Sometimes a catalyst is needed, such as peroxidase, alkaline phosphatase, or metal ions.

Luminol, the first chemiluminescent label used in immunoassays, is a cyclic diacylhydrazide that emits light energy under alkaline conditions in the presence of peroxide and peroxidase. Because peroxidase can serve as the catalyst, assays may use this enzyme as the label; the chemiluminogenic substrate, luminol, will produce light that is directly proportional to the amount of peroxidase present (Equation 6-4):

$$Luminol + 2H_2O_2 + OH^- \xrightarrow{Peroxidase}$$

$$3\text{-aminophthalate} + light\ (425\ nm) \quad \textbf{(Eq. 6–4)}$$

A popular chemiluminescent label, acridinium esters, is a triple-ringed organic molecule linked by an ester bond to an organic chain. In the presence of hydrogen peroxide and under alkaline conditions, the ester bond is broken and an unstable molecule (N-methylacridon) remains. Light is emitted as the unstable molecule reverts to its more stable ground state.

$$Acridinium\ ester + 2H_2O_2 + OH^- \rightarrow$$

$$N\text{-methylacridon} + CO_2 + H_2O + light\ (430\ nm)$$

$$\textbf{(Eq. 6–5)}$$

Alkaline phosphatase commonly conjugated to an antibody has been used in automated immunoassay analyzers to produce some of the most sensitive chemiluminescent assays. ALP catalyzes adamantyl 1,2-dioxetane aryl phosphate substrates (AMPPD) to release light at 477 nm. The detection limit approaches 1 zmol, or approximately 602 enzyme molecules.[17,18]

Assay Design

Competitive Immunoassays. The earliest immunoassay was a *competitive immunoassay* in which the radiolabeled antigen (Ag*; also called the tracer) competed with unlabeled antigen (Ag) for a limited number of binding sites (Ab) (Fig. 6-6). The proportion of Ag and Ag* binding with the Ab is related to the Ag and Ag* concentration and requires limited antibody in the reaction. In the competitive assay, the Ag* concentration is constant and limited. As the concentration of Ag increases, more binds to the antibody, resulting in less binding of Ag*. These limited reagent assays were very sensitive because low concentrations of unlabeled antigen yielded a large measurable signal from the bound-labeled antigen. If the competitive assay is designed to reach equilibrium, the incubation times are often long.

The antigen–antibody reaction can be accomplished in one step when labeled antigen (Ag*), unlabeled antigen (Ag), and reagent antibody (Ab) are simultaneously incubated together to yield bound-labeled antigen (Ag*Ab), bound-unlabeled antigen (AgAb), and free-label (Ag*) as shown in Figure 6-6 and Equation 6-6:

$$\text{Ag* (fixed reagent)} + \text{Ag} + \text{Ab (limited reagent)} \rightarrow$$

$$\text{Ag*Ab} + \text{AgAb} + \text{Ag*} \qquad \textbf{(Eq. 6–6)}$$

A generic, heterogeneous, competitive simultaneous assay begins by pipetting the test sample (quality control, calibrator, or patient) into test tubes. Next, labeled antigen and antibody reagents are added. After incubation

and separation of free-labeled (unbound) antigen, the bound-labeled antigen is measured.

Alternatively, the competitive assay may be accomplished in sequential steps. First, labeled antigen is incubated with the reagent antibody and then labeled antigen is added. After a longer incubation time and a separation step, the bound-labeled antigen is measured. This approach increases the analytic sensitivity of the assay.

Consider the example in Table 6-3. A relatively small, yet constant, number of Ab combining sites is available to combine with a relatively large, constant amount of Ag* (tracer) and calibrators with known antigen concentrations. Because the amount of tracer and antibody are constant, the only variable in the test system is the amount of unlabeled antigen. As the concentration of unlabeled antigen increases, the concentration (or percentage) of free tracer increases.

By using multiple calibrators, a dose response curve is established. As the concentration of unlabeled Ag increases, the concentration of tracer that binds to the Ab decreases. In the example presented in Table 6-3, if the amount of unlabeled antigen is zero, maximum tracer will combine with the antibody. When no unlabeled antigen is present, maximum binding by the tracer is possible; this is referred to as B_0, B_{max}, maximum binding, or the zero standard. When the amount of unlabeled antigen is the same as the tracer, each will bind equally to the antibody. As the concentration of antigen increases in a competitive assay, the amount of tracer that complexes with the binding reagent decreases. If the tracer is of low molecular weight, free tracer is often measured. If the tracer is of high molecular weight, the bound tracer is measured. The data may be plotted in one of three ways: bound/free versus the arithmetic dose of unlabeled antigen; percentage bound versus the log dose of unlabeled antigen; and logit Bound/B_0 versus the log dose of the unlabeled antigen (Fig. 6-7).

The bound fraction can be expressed in several different formats. Bound/free (B/F) is CPM of the bound fraction compared with the CPM of the free fraction. Percent bound (% B) is the CPM of the bound fraction compared with the CPM of maximum binding of the tracer (B_0) times 100. Logit B/B_0 transformation is the natural log of $(B/B_0)/(1 - B/B_0)$.

When using logit-log graph paper on which B/B_0 is plotted on the ordinate and the log dose of the unlabeled antigen is plotted on the abscissa, a straight line with a negative slope is produced. More often, microcomputers calculate the best straight line using linear regression; patient values may then be calculated by the computer using this relationship.

It is important to remember that the best type of curve-fitting technique is determined by experiment and that there is no assurance that a logit-log plot of the data will always generate a straight line. To determine the best method, several different methods of data plotting

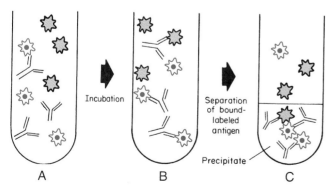

FIGURE 6-6. Competitive labeled immunoassay. During simultaneous incubation, labeled antigen (⊛) and unlabeled antigen (⊛) compete for the antibody-binding sites (⊰). The bound label in the precipitate is frequently measured.

TABLE 6-3. COMPETITIVE BINDING ASSAY EXAMPLE

Ag	+	Ag*	+	Ab	→	AgAb	+	Ag*Ab	+	Ag*
CONCENTRATION OF REACTANTS						**CONCENTRATION OF PRODUCTS**				
Ag		*Ag**		*Ab*		*AgAb*		*Ag*Ab*		*Ag**
0		200		100		0		100		100
50		200		100		20		80		120
100		200		100		34		66		134
200		200		100		50		50		150
400		200		100		66		34		166

SAMPLE CALCULATIONS

DOSE OF [Ag]	% B	B/F
0	$\dfrac{100}{200} = 50$	$\dfrac{100}{100} = 1$
50	$\dfrac{80}{200} = 40$	$\dfrac{80}{120} = .67$
100	$\dfrac{66}{200} = 33$	$\dfrac{66}{134} = .49$
200	$\dfrac{50}{200} = 25$	$\dfrac{50}{150} = .33$
400	$\dfrac{34}{200} = 17$	$\dfrac{34}{166} = .20$

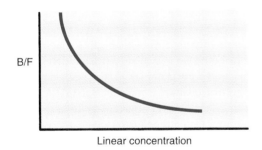

Linear concentration

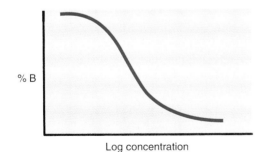

Log concentration

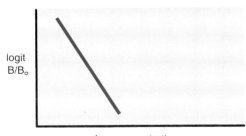

Log concentration

should be tried when a new assay is introduced. Every time the assay is performed, a dose response curve should be prepared to check the performance of the assay. Remember that the relative error for all radioimmunoassay (RIA) dose response curves is minimal when B/B_0 is 0.5 and increases at both high and low concentrations of the plot. As shown in the plot of B/B_0 versus log of the antigen concentration (Fig. 6-7), a relatively large change in the concentration at either end of the curve produces little change in the B/B_0 value. Patient values derived from a B/B_0 value greater than 0.9 or less than 0.1 should be interpreted with caution. When the same data are displayed using the logit-log plot, it is easy to overlook the error at either end of the straight line.

Noncompetitive Immunoassays. Sometimes known as immunometric assays, *noncompetitive immunoassays* use a labeled reagent antibody to detect the antigen. Excess labeled antibody is required to assure that the labeled antibody reagent does not limit the reaction. The concentration of the antigen is directly proportional to the bound-labeled antibody as shown in Figure 6-8. The relationship is linear up to a limit and then is subject to the high-dose hook effect.

FIGURE 6-7. Dose response curves in a competitive assay. B = bound-labeled antigen. F = free-labeled antigen. B_0 = maximum binding. % B = $B/B_0 \times 100$.

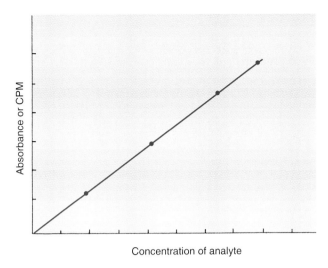

FIGURE 6-8. Dose response curve in a noncompetitive immunoassay.

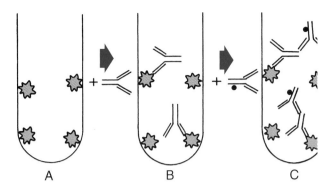

FIGURE 6-10. Two-site noncompetitive sandwich assay to detect antibody. Immobilized antigen (✱) captures the antibody (⊰). Then labeled antibody (⊰•) is added, binds to the captured antibody, and is detected.

In the sandwich assay to detect antigen (also known as an antigen capture assay), immobilized unlabeled antibody captures the antigen. After washing to remove unreacted molecules, the labeled detector antibody is added. After another washing to remove free-labeled detector antibody, the signal from the bound-labeled antibody is proportional to the antigen captured. This format relies on the ability of the antibody reagent to react with a single epitope on the antigen. The specificity and quantity of monoclonal antibodies has allowed the rapid expansion of diverse assays. A schematic is shown in Figure 6-9.

The sandwich assay is another noncompetitive assay used to detect antibody, in which the immobilized antigen captures specific antibody. After washing, the labeled detector antibody is added and binds to the captured antibody. The amount of bound-labeled antibody is directly proportional to the amount of specific antibody present (Fig. 6-10). This assay can be modified to determine the immunoglobulin class of the specific antibody present in serum. For example, if the detector antibody were labeled and monospecific (*eg*, rabbit antihuman IgM [μ-chain specific]), it would detect and quantitate only human IgM captured by the immobilized antigen.

Separation Techniques

All immunoassays require that free-labeled reactant be distinguished from bound-labeled reactant. In *heterogeneous assays*, physical separation is necessary and is achieved by adsorption, precipitation, or interaction with a solid phase as listed in Table 6-4. The better the separation of bound from free reactant, the more reliable the assay will be. This is in contrast to *homogeneous assays* in which the activity or expression of the label depends on whether the labeled reactant is free or bound. No physical separation step is needed in homogeneous assays.

Adsorption. Adsorption techniques use particles to trap small antigens, labeled or unlabeled. A mixture of charcoal and cross-linked dextran is most commonly used. Charcoal is porous and readily combines with small molecules to remove them from solution; dextran prevents nonspecific protein binding to the charcoal. The size of the dextran influences the size of the molecule that can be adsorbed; the lower the molecular weight of dextran used, the smaller the molecular weight of free antigen that can be adsorbed. Other adsorbents include silica, ion exchange resin, and Sephadex. After adsorption and centrifugation, the free-labeled antigen is found in the precipitate.

Precipitation. Nonimmune precipitation occurs when the environment is altered affecting the solubility of protein. Compounds such as ammonium sulfate, sodium sulfate, polyethylene glycol, and ethanol precipitate protein nonspecifically; both free-antibody and antigen–antibody complexes will precipitate. Ammonium sulfate and sodium sulfate "salt out" free globulins and antigen–antibody complexes. Ethanol denatures protein

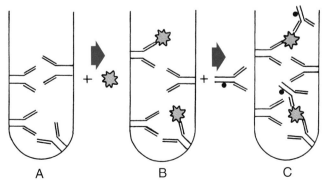

FIGURE 6-9. Two-site noncompetitive sandwich assay to detect antigen. Immobilized antibody (⊰) captures the antigen (✱). Then labeled antibody (⊰•) is added, binds to the captured antigen, and is detected.

TABLE 6-4. CHARACTERISTICS OF SEPARATION TECHNIQUES

SEPARATION TECHNIQUE	EXAMPLE	ACTION
Adsorption	Charcoal and dextran	Traps free-labeled antigen
	Silica	Separation by centrifugation
	Ion exchange resin	
	Sephadex	
Precipitation		
Nonimmune	Ethanol	Denatures bound-labeled antigen
	Ammonium sulfate	Separation by centrifugation
	Sodium sulfate	
	Polyethylene glycol	
Immune	Second antibody	Primary antibody is recognized and forms an insoluble complex
	Staph protein A	
Solid phase	Polystyrene	Separation by centrifugation
	Membranes	One reactant is adsorbed or covalently attached to the inert surface
	Magnetized particles	Separation by washing

and antigen–antibody complexes, causing precipitation. Polyethylene glycol precipitates larger protein molecules with or without the antigen attached. Ideally, after centrifugation, all bound-labeled antigen will be in the precipitate, leaving free-labeled antigen in the supernatant.

Soluble antigen–antibody complexes can be precipitated by a second antibody that recognizes the primary antibody in the soluble complex. The result is a larger complex that becomes insoluble and precipitates. Centrifugation is again used to aid in the separation. This immune precipitation method is also known as the double-antibody or second-antibody method. For example, in a growth hormone assay, the primary or antigen-specific antibody produced in a rabbit recognizes growth hormone. The second antibody, produced in a sheep or goat, would recognize rabbit antibody. Labeled antigen–antibody complexes, unlabeled antigen–antibody complexes, and free primary antibodies are precipitated by the second antibody. This separation method is more specific than nonimmune precipitation because only the primary antibody is precipitated. A similar separation occurs when staphylococcal protein A (SPA) replaces the second antibody. SPA binds to human IgG causing precipitation.

Solid Phase. The use of a *solid phase* to immobilize reagent antibody or antigen provides a method to separate free from bound-labeled reactant after washing. The solid-phase support is an inert surface to which reagent antigen or antibody is attached. The solid-phase support may be, but is not limited to, polystyrene surfaces, membranes, and magnetic beads. The immobilized antigen or antibody may be adsorbed or covalently bound to the solid-phase support; covalent linkage prevents spontaneous release of the immobilized antigen or antibody.

Immunoassays using solid-phase separation are easier to perform and to automate and require less manipulation and time to perform than other immunoassays. However, a relatively large amount of reagent antibody or antigen is required to coat the solid-phase surface and consistent coverage of the solid phase is difficult to achieve. Solid-phase assays are more expensive to produce and require greater technical skill to perform to minimize intra-assay and interassay variability. Insufficient washing is a common source of error.

Examples of Labeled Immunoassays
Particle-enhanced turbidimetric inhibition immunoassay (PETINIA) is a homogeneous competitive immunoassay in which low-molecular-weight haptens bound to particles compete with unlabeled analyte for the specific antibody. The extent of particle agglutination is inversely proportional to the concentration of unlabeled analyte and is assessed by measuring the change in transmitted light in an Automatic Clinical Analyzer (ACA) (DuPont; now, Dade).[19]

Enzyme-linked immunosorbent assays (ELISA), a popular group of heterogeneous immunoassays, have an enzyme label and use a solid phase as the separation technique. Four formats are available: a competitive assay using labeled antigen, a competitive assay using labeled antibody, a noncompetitive assay to detect antigen, and a noncompetitive assay to detect antibody.

One of the earliest homogeneous assays was enzyme multiplied immunoassay technique (EMIT), an enzyme immunoassay currently produced by Syva Corporation.[20] As shown in Figure 6-11, the reactants in most test systems include an enzyme-labeled antigen (commonly, a

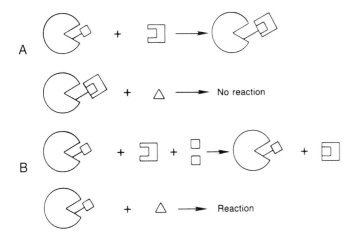

FIGURE 6-11. Enzyme multiplied immunoassay technique. (**A**) When enzyme labeled antigen is bound to the antibody, the enzyme activity is inhibited. (**B**) Free patient antigen binds to the antibody and prevents antibody binding to the labeled antigen. The substrate indicates the amount of free-labeled antigen.

low-molecular-weight analyte, such as a drug), an antibody directed against the antigen, the substrate, and test antigen. The enzyme is catalytically active when the labeled antigen is free (not bound to the antibody). It is thought that when the antibody combines with the labeled antigen, the antibody sterically hinders the enzyme. The conformational changes that occur during antigen–antibody interaction inhibit the enzyme activity. In this homogeneous assay, the unlabeled antigen in the sample competes with the labeled antigen for the antibody-binding sites; as the concentration of unlabeled antigen increases, less enzyme-labeled antigen can bind to the antibody. Therefore, more labeled antigen is free, and the enzymatic activity is greater.

Cloned enzyme donor immunoassays (CEDIA) are competitive, homogeneous assays in which the genetically engineered label is β-galactosidase.[21] The enzyme is in two inactive pieces: the enzyme acceptor and the enzyme donor. When these two pieces bind together, enzyme activity is restored. In the assay, the antigen labeled with the enzyme donor and the unlabeled antigen in the sample compete for specific antibody-binding sites. When the antibody binds to the labeled antigen, the enzyme acceptor cannot bind to the enzyme donor; therefore, the enzyme is not restored and the enzyme is inactive. More unlabeled antigen in the sample results in more enzyme activity.

Microparticle capture enzyme immunoassay (MEIA) is an automated assay available on the IMx (Abbott Laboratories). The microparticles serve as the solid phase, and a glass fiber matrix separates the bound-labeled reagent. Both competitive and noncompetitive assays are available. Although the label is an enzyme (alkaline phosphatase), the substrate (4-methyllumbelliferyl phosphate) is fluorogenic.

Solid-phase fluorescence immunoassays (SPFIA) are analogous to the ELISA methods except that the label fluoresces. Of particular note is FIAX (BioWhittaker, Walkersville, MD). In this assay, fluid-phase unlabeled antigen is captured by antibody on the solid phase; after washing, the detector antibody (with a fluorescent label attached) reacts with the solid-phase captured antigen.

Particle concentration fluorescence immunoassay (PCFIA) is a heterogeneous, competitive immunoassay in which particles are used to localize the reaction and concentrate the fluorescence. Labeled antigen and unlabeled antigen in the sample compete for antibody bound to polystyrene particles. The particles are trapped and the fluorescence is measured. The assay can also be designed so that labeled antibody and unlabeled antibody compete for antigen fixed onto particles.

Fluorescence excitation transfer immunoassay (FETI) is a competitive, homogeneous immunoassay using two fluorophores (such as fluorescein and rhodamine).[22] When the two labels are in close proximity, the emitted light from fluorescein will be absorbed by rhodamine. Thus, the emission from fluorescein is quenched. Fluorescein-labeled antigen and unlabeled antigen compete for rhodamine-labeled antibody. More unlabeled antigen lessens the amount of fluorescein-labeled antigen that binds; therefore, more fluorescence is present (less quenching).

Substrate-level fluorescence immunoassay (SLFIA) is another competitive, homogeneous assay. This time, the hapten is labeled with a substrate; when catalyzed by an appropriate enzyme, fluorescent product is generated. Substrate-labeled hapten and unlabeled hapten in the sample compete with antibody; the bound-labeled hapten cannot be catalyzed by the enzyme.

Fluorescence polarization immunoassay (FPIA) is another assay that uses a fluorescent label.[23,24] This homogeneous immunoassay uses polarized light to excite the fluorescent label. Polarized light is created when light passes through special filters and consists of parallel light waves oriented in one plane. When polarized light is used to excite a fluorescent label, the emitted light could be polarized or depolarized. Small molecules, such as free fluorescent-labeled hapten, rotate rapidly and randomly, interrupting the polarized light. Larger molecules, such as those created when the fluorescent-labeled hapten binds to an antibody, rotate more slowly and emit polarized light parallel to the excitation polarized light. The polarized light is measured at a 90° angle compared with the path of the excitation light. In a competitive FPIA, fluorescent-labeled hapten and unlabeled hapten in the sample compete for limited antibody sites. When no unlabeled hapten is present, the labeled hapten binds maximally to the antibody, creating large complexes that rotate slowly and emit a high-level of polarized light. When hapten is present, it competes with the labeled hapten for the antibody sites; as the hapten concentration increases, more labeled hapten is displaced and is free. The free-labeled hapten rotates rapidly and emits less polarized light. The degree of labeled hapten displacement is inversely related to the amount of unlabeled hapten present.

Dissociation-enhanced lanthanide fluoroimmunoassay (DELFIA) is an automated system (Pharmacia) that measures time-delayed fluorescence from the label europium. The assay can be designed as a competitive, heterogeneous assay or a noncompetitive (sandwich), heterogeneous assay.[25]

The classic RIA is a heterogeneous, competitive assay with a tracer.[26] When bound tracer is measured, the signal from the label (counts per minute) is inversely related to the concentration of the unlabeled antigen in the sample.

Rapid Immunoassay

The sensitivity and specificity of automated labeled assays and the trend for decentralized laboratory testing have led to the development of assays that are easy to use, simple (many classified as waived or moderately complex related to the Clinical Laboratory Improvement Amendments of 1988), fast, and site-neutral and requiring no instrumentation. Those discussed here are representative of currently available commercial kits; however, this discussion is not intended to be exhaustive. Three categories of rapid immunoassays emerge: (1) latex particles for visualization of the reaction, (2) fluid flow and labeled reactant, and (3) changes in a physical or chemical property following antigen–antibody binding.

The earliest rapid tests were those in which a latex particle suspension was added to the sample; if the immunoreactive component attached to the particle recognized its counterpart in the sample, macroscopic agglutination occurred. Colored latex particles are now available to facilitate reading the reaction.

Self-contained devices that use the liquid-nature of the specimen have evolved. In flow-through systems, a capture reagent is immobilized onto a membrane, the solid phase. The porous nature of membranes increases the surface area to which the capture reagent can bind. The more capture reagent that binds to the membrane, the greater the potential assay sensitivity. After the capture reagent binds to the membrane, other binding sites are saturated with a nonreactive blocking chemical to reduce nonspecific binding by substances in the patient sample. In the assay, the sample containing the analyte is allowed to pass through the membrane and the analyte is bound to the capture reagent. Commonly, the liquid is attracted through the membrane by an absorbent material. The analyte is detected by a labeled reactant, as well as the signal from the labeled reactant.

The next step in the development of self-contained, single-use devices was to incorporate internal controls.

One scheme to detect human chorionic gonadotropin, the ImmunoConcentration Assay (ICON; Hybritech),[27,28] creates three zones in which specifically treated particles are deposited. In the assay zone, particles are coated with reagent antibody specific for the assay; in the negative control zone, particles are coated with nonimmune antibody; and, in the positive control zone, particles are coated with an immune complex specific for the assay. The patient sample (serum or urine) passes through the membrane, and the analyte is captured by the specific reagent antibody in the assay zone. Next, a labeled antibody passes through the membrane, which fixes to the specific immune complex formed in the assay zone or the positive control zone. Following color development, a positive reaction is noted when the assay and positive zones are colored.

A second homogeneous immunoassay involves the tangential flow of fluid across a membrane. The fluid dissolves and binds to the dried capture reagent; the complex flows to the detection area, where it is concentrated and viewed.

A third homogeneous immunoassay, enzyme immunochromatography, involves vertical flow of fluid along a membrane.[29] This is quantitative and does not require any instrumentation. A dry paper strip with immobilized antibody is immersed in a solution of unlabeled analyte and an enzyme-labeled analyte; the liquid migrates up the strip by capillary action. As the labeled and unlabeled analyte migrate, they compete and bind to the immobilized antibody. A finite amount of labeled and unlabeled analyte mixture is absorbed. The migration distance of the labeled analyte is visualized when the strip reacts with a substrate reagent and develops a colored reaction product. Comparing the migration distance of the sample with the calibrator allows the concentration of the unlabeled ligand to be assigned.

The next generation of rapid immunoassays involves change in physical or chemical properties after an antigen–antibody interaction occurs. One example is the Optical Immunoassay (OIA).[30] A silicon wafer is used to support a thin film of optical coating; this is then topped with the capture antibody. Sample is applied directly to the device. If an antigen–antibody complex forms, the thickness of the optical surface increases and changes optical path of light. The color changes from gold to purple. Some studies suggest that this method has better analytic sensitivity compared with immunoassays, which rely on the fluid flow.

Immunoblots

Most assays described this far are designed to measure a single analyte. In some circumstances, it is beneficial to separate multiple antigens by electrophoresis so as to be able to simultaneously detect multiple serum antibodies. The *Western blot* is a transfer technique used to detect specific antibodies. As shown in Figure 6-12, multiple protein antigens (such as those associated with the human immunodeficiency virus [HIV]) are isolated, denatured, and separated by sodium dodecyl sulfate-polyacrylamide gel electrophoresis (SDS-PAGE). SDS denatures the protein and adds an overall negative charge proportional to the molecular weight of the protein. The PAGE of SDS-treated proteins allows the separation of protein based on molecular weight. The separated proteins are then transferred to a new medium (eg, nylon, nitrocellulose, or polyvinylidene difluoride membrane). The separated proteins will be fixed on the new medium and may be stained to assure separation. Each lane on the membrane is then incubated with patient or control sample. The antibody recognizes and binds to the antigen forming an insoluble complex. After washing, a labeled antibody reagent detects the complex. Depending on the label, it may yield a photometric, fluorescent, or chemiluminescent product that appears as a band. The bands from the patient sample are compared with those from the control containing antibody that will react with known antigens. Molecular weight markers are also separated and stained to provide a guide for interpretation of molecular weight.

Immunocytochemistry and Immunohistochemistry

When antibody reagents are used to detect antigens in cells or tissue, the methods are known as *immunocytochemistry* and *immunohistochemistry,* respectively. When the antigen is an integral part of the cell or tissue, this is direct testing. A second strategy, indirect testing, uses cells or tissue as a substrate (the source of antigen) to capture serum antibody; this complex is then detected using a labeled antibody reagent.

Fluorescent labels are most commonly used in immunocytochemistry and immunohistochemistry. When used to microscopically identify bacteria or constituents in tissue (such as immune complexes deposited in vivo), the method is called *direct immunofluorescence (DIF)* or direct fluorescence assay (DFA). A specially configured fluorescence microscope is necessary. Appropriate wavelengths of light are selected by a filter monochromator to excite the fluorescent label; the fluorescent label emits light of a second wavelength that is selected for viewing by a second filter monochromator. Examples of DFA include detection of *Treponema pallidum* in lesional fluid or detection of immune complexes in glomerulonephritis associated with Goodpasture's syndrome and lupus nephritis.

When a fluorescent label is used in indirect testing, this is *indirect immunofluorescence (IIF)* or an indirect immunofluorescence assay (IFA). The substrate is placed on a microscopic slide, serum is overlaid and allowed to react with the antigen, and the bound antibody is detected by the labeled antihuman globulin reagent. The slide is viewed using a fluorescence microscope. The most common IFA performed in the clinical laboratory detects antibodies to nuclear antigens (ANA). Both the titer and pattern of fluorescence provide useful information to diagnose connective tissue disease. Other autoantibodies and antibodies to infectious disease can be detected by IFA.

Immunophenotyping

An important and more recent advance in immunocytochemistry is the use of a flow cytometer to detect intracellular and cell surface antigens. This technique, *immunophenotyping,* is used to classify cell lineage and identify the stage of cell maturation. In particular, immunophenotyping aids in the diagnosis of leukemias and

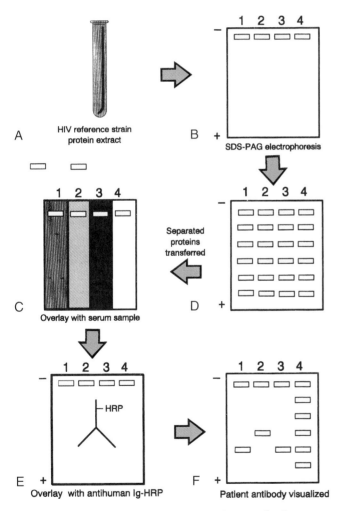

FIGURE 6-12. Immunoblot (Western blot) to detect antibodies to HIV antigens. (**A**) The HIV is disrupted and extracted to generate its antigens. (**B**) The HIV antigens are separated by sodium dodecyl sulfate polyacrylamide gel electrophoresis. (**C**) The separated antigens are visualized and then transferred to a membrane. (**D**) Each lane of the membrane is overlaid with a patient or control serum. (**E**) After incubation and washing, a labeled antibody reagent is overlaid onto all lanes. (**F**) The bound-labeled antibody is detected.

lymphomas. Differentiating between acute myelogenous leukemia and acute lymphoblastic leukemia is difficult morphologically and requires additional information to identify the phenotypically expressed molecules. In lymphoid leukemias and lymphomas, identification of tumor cells as either T or B lymphocytes can be an important predictor of clinical outcome. Another application is to determine the CD4/CD8 ratio (the ratio of the number of helper T lymphocytes to cytotoxic T lymphocytes) and, more recently, the absolute number of CD4 positive cells. This is the standard method to diagnose infection and to initiate and monitor treatment although viral load quantitation is considered by many to be a better marker.

Immunophenotyping begins with a living cell suspension. The cells may come from peripheral blood, bone marrow, or solid tissue. Leukocytes or mononuclear cells can be isolated using density gradient separation (centrifugation through Ficoll-Hypaque) or by red blood cell lysis. Tissue, such as lymph node and bone marrow, requires mechanical removal of cells from the tissue to collect a cell suspension. Based on patient history and type of specimen, a panel of fluorochrome-labeled monoclonal antibodies (MAbs) is used. Fluorochromes commonly used in immunophenotyping include fluorescein isothiocyanate, phycoerythrin, peridinin chlorophyll, CY-5, allophycocyanin, and tetramethyl rhodamine isothiocyanate. An aliquot of the cell suspension is incubated with one or more MAb, depending on the design of the flow cytometer. If the cell expresses the antigen, then the labeled MAb binds and the fluorescent label can be detected. *Flow cytometry* is based on cells transported under fluidic pressure passing one by one through a laser beam. The forward light scatter, side light scatter, and light emitted from fluorescent labels are detected by photomultiplier tubes. Forward light scatter is related to the size of the cell, and side light scatter is related to the granularity of the cell. When these two parameters are used together in a scattergram (2-parameter histogram), the desired cell population can be electronically selected. This cell population is also evaluated for emission from the labeled MAb. For a single parameter, the frequency of cells versus the intensity of fluorescence (the channel number) is recorded and displayed as a single-parameter histogram. Alternatively, if two parameters are evaluated on the same cell, then a scattergram is generated that diagrams the expression of two antigens simultaneously. By using a panel of MAbs, the cell can be identified and the relative or absolute number of the cell can be determined.

DNA Analysis by Flow Cytometry

In flow cytometry, another use of the flow cytometer is to measure the nuclear deoxyribonucleic acid (DNA) content and proliferative capacity of malignant cells. This helps to distinguish between benign and malignant disease, to monitor disease progression, and to predict response to treatment. Resting normal cells are in G_0 and G_1 phase of the cell cycle, and the nuclear DNA content is 2 sets of 23 chromosomes, known as *diploid*. As a cell prepares to replicate, the DNA is synthesized (S phase) and the DNA content is aneuploid. Mitosis (M phase) and cell division follow. The ploidy status reflected in the *DNA index (DI)* compares the amount of measured DNA in tumor cells with that in normal cells (Equation 6-7):

$$DI = \frac{\text{peak channel number of aneuploid } G_0/G_1 \text{ peak}}{\text{peak channel number of diploid } G_0/G_1 \text{ peak}}$$

(Eq. 6–7)

If normal diploid cells were measured, then the DI is one. If the DI is not one, then the cells are aneuploid. If the DI is less than one, the cells are hypodiploid; conversely a DI greater than one is hyperploid. The percentage of cells in S phase is also determined and normally is less than 5%.

Fresh, alcohol-fixed cells or rehydrated cells removed from a paraffin block may be used. The cells are treated with a detergent to enable the stain to enter the nucleus. Stains, such as propidium iodide or ethidium bromide, intercalate the DNA and the fluorescence is measured using the flow cytometer. The DNA content is related to the fluorescence intensity (channel number). Measuring the DI and % S phase cells are prognostic indicators in breast, ovarian, bladder, and colorectal cancer.

NUCLEIC ACID PROBES

Molecular testing is a rapidly expanding area in the clinical laboratory. Research labs have used these techniques for many years; however, development of FDA-approved assays for the detection and quantitation of DNA and RNA in clinical samples has only developed recently. Key quality issues to be addressed in any clinical DNA-based assays include sample quality and preparation, sensitivity of reagents to inactivating contaminants, amplification bias and variability, selection of appropriate controls, restriction enzyme efficiency, and reproducibility and cross-contamination of amplification reactions.[31] Nucleic acids store all genetic information and direct the synthesis of specific proteins. By evaluating nucleic acids, insight into cellular changes may be realized before specific protein products are detectable. Genetically based diseases, presence of infectious organisms, differences between individuals for forensic and transplantation purposes, and altered cell growth regulation are areas that have been investigated using nucleic acid hybridization. The most recent development is the use of molecular arrays (up to 10^5 to 10^6 probes per single array) for high-speed analysis of multiple ligands and the analysis of gene expression.

Nucleic Acid Chemistry

DNA stores human genetic information and dictates the amino acid sequence of peptides and proteins. DNA is composed of two strands of nucleotides; each strand is a polymer of deoxyribose molecules linked by strong 3' 5' phosphodiester bonds that join the 3' hydroxyl group of one sugar to the 5' phosphate group of a second sugar. A purine or pyrimidine base is also attached to each sugar. The two strands are arranged in a double helix with the bases pointing toward the center. The strands are antiparallel, so that the 3' 5' end of one strand bonds with a strand in the 5' 3' direction. Because the phosphate esters are strong acids and dissociated at neutral pH, the strand has a negative charge that is proportional to its length. The purine bases (adenine [A] and thymine [T]) and the pyrimidine bases (cytosine [C] and guanine [G]) maintain the double helix by forming hydrogen bonds between base pairs as shown in Figure 6-13. Adenine pairs with thymine with two hydrogen bonds and cytosine pairs with guanine with three hydrogen bonds. The strands are complementary due to the fixed manner by which the base pairs bond.

Under physiologic conditions, the helical structure of double-stranded DNA (dsDNA) is stable due to the numerous, although weak, hydrogen bonds between base pairs and the hydrophobic interaction between the bases in the center of the helix. However, the weak bonds can be broken in vitro by changing environmental conditions; the strands are denatured and separate from each other. Once denatured, the negative charge of each strand causes the strands to repel each other. The two complementary strands can be reassociated or reannealed if the conditions change and favor this. The renaturation will follow the rules of base pairing so the original DNA molecule is recovered.

Ribonucleic acid (RNA) is also present in human cells and is chemically similar to DNA. RNA differs from DNA in three ways: (1) ribose replaces deoxyribose as the sugar; (2) uracil replaces thymine as a purine base; and (3) RNA is single-stranded. DNA and RNA work together to synthesize proteins. Genomic dsDNA is enzymatically split into its two strands, one of which serves as the template for synthesis of complementary messenger RNA (mRNA). As mRNA is released from the template DNA, the DNA strands reanneal. The mRNA specifies the amino acid to be added to the peptide chain by transfer RNA, which transports the amino acid to the ribosome, where peptide chain elongates.

This discussion of protein synthesis highlights that physiologically DNA routinely is denatured, binds to RNA, and reanneals to reestablish the original DNA, always following base pair rules. These processes form the foundation of nucleic acid *hybridization* assays in which complementary strands of nucleic acid from unrelated sources bind together to form a hybrid or *duplex*. Molecular testing in the clinical laboratory consists of two major areas: (1) the use of DNA probes to directly detect or characterize a specific target, and (2) the use of nucleic acid amplification technologies to detect or characterize a specific target DNA or RNA. Procedures that use probes include solid-phase assays (capture hybridization, Southern and Northern blotting), solution-based assays (protection assays, hybrid capture assays), and in situ hybridization assays. Amplification procedures include nucleic acid amplification (polymerase chain reaction, nucleic acid-based sequence amplification, transcription-mediated amplification, strand displacement amplification), probe amplification (ligase chain reaction), and signal amplification (branched-chain DNA assay).

Hybridization Techniques

A *nucleic acid probe* is a short strand of DNA or RNA of a known sequence that is well characterized and complementary for the base sequence on the test target. Probes may be fragments of genomic nucleic acids, cloned DNA (or RNA), or synthetic DNA. The genomic nucleic acids are isolated from purified organisms. Some probes are molecularly cloned in a bacterial host. First, the sequence of DNA to be used as the probe must be isolated using bacterial restriction endonucleases to cut the DNA at a specific base sequence. The desired base sequence (the probe) is inserted into a plasmid vector, circular ds-

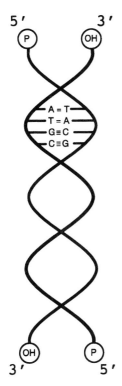

FIGURE 6-13. Representation of a DNA molecule.

DNA. The vector with the insert is incorporated into a host cell, such as *Escherichia coli,* where the vector replicates. The replicated desired base sequence is then isolated and purified. For short DNA segments, an oligonucleotide probe can be synthesized using an automated process; if the amino acid sequence of the protein is known, it is possible to determine the base sequence based on amino acid sequence.

In a hybridization reaction, the probe must be detected. The probe can be labeled directly with a radionuclide (such as ^{32}P), enzyme, or biotin. ^{32}P is detected by autoradiography when the radioactive label exposes x-ray film wherever the probe is located. If the probe is directly labeled with an enzyme, an appropriate substrate must be added to generate a colorimetric, fluorescent, or chemiluminescent product. Biotin labeled probes can bind to avidin, which is complexed to an enzyme (*eg,* ALP or HRP); the enzyme activity can then be detected. Alternatively, the biotinylated probe can be detected by a labeled avidin antibody reagent.

The probe techniques to be discussed are listed in Table 6-5. A classic method for DNA analysis, attributed to EM Southern,[31] is the *Southern blot.* In this method, DNA is extracted from a sample using a phenolic reagent and then enzymatically digested using restriction endonucleases to produce DNA fragments. These fragments are then separated by agarose gel electrophoresis. The separated DNA fragments are denatured and transferred to a solid support medium; most commonly, nitrocellulose or a charged nylon membrane. The transfer oc-

curs by the capillary action of a salt solution, transferring DNA to the membrane or using an electric current to transfer the DNA. When the DNA is on the membrane, a labeled probe is added that binds to the complementary base sequence and appears as a band. In a similar method, the *Northern blot,* RNA is extracted, digested, electrophoresed, blotted, and finally probed.

The *polymerase chain reaction (PCR)* developed by KB Mullis of Cetus Company[32,33] is an amplified hybridization technique that enzymatically synthesizes millions of identical copies of the target DNA to increase the analytic sensitivity. The test reaction mixture includes the test DNA sample (lysed cells or tissue enzymatically digested with RNAse and proteinase and then extracted), oligonucleotide primers, thermostable DNA polymerase (*eg, Taq* polymerase, from *Thermus aquaticus*), and nucleotide triphosphates (ATP, GTP, CTP, and TTP) in a buffer. The process, shown in Figure 6-14, begins by heating the tar-

TABLE 6-5. PROBE TECHNIQUES

Unamplified

Southern blot

Northern blot

In situ hybridization

Restriction fragment length polymorphism (RFLP)

Target Amplification

Polymerase chain reaction (PCR)

Reverse transcriptase-polymerase chain reaction (RT-PCR)

Self-sustained sequence replication (3SR)

Probe Amplification

Q-beta replicase

Ligase chain reaction (LCR)

Signal Amplification

Multiple labels per probe

Multiple probes per target

Two-tiered probe system

Branched DNA assay (bDNA)

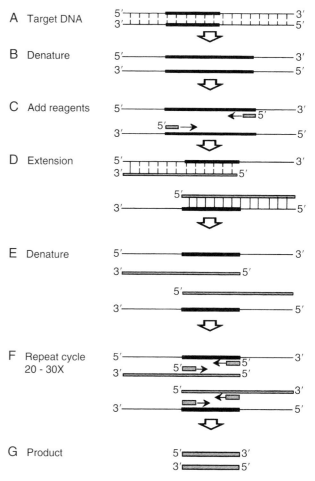

FIGURE 6-14. Polymerase chain reaction. (**A**) The target DNA sequence is indicated by the bold line; (**B**) the double stranded DNA is denatured (separated) by heating; (**C**) reagents are added, and the primer binds to the target DNA sequence; (**D**) polymerase extends the primers; and (**E–G**) heating, annealing of the primer, and extension are repeated.

get DNA to denature it, separating the strands. Two oligonucleotide primers (probes) that recognize the edges of the target DNA are added and anneal to the target DNA. Thermostable DNA polymerase and nucleotide triphosphates extend the primer. The process of heat denaturation, cooling to allow the primers to anneal and heating again to extend the primers, is repeated many fold (15 to 30 times or more). PCR is an exponential amplification reaction in which after n cycles there is $(1 + x)^n$ times as much target as was present initially, where x is the mean efficiency of the reaction for each cycle. Theoretically, as few as 20 cycles would yield approximately 1 million times the amount of target DNA initially present. However, in reality, the theoretical maxima are never reached and more cycles are necessary to achieve such levels of amplification.

The amplified target DNA sequences, known as *amplicons*, can be analyzed by gel electrophoresis, Southern blot, or using directly labeled probes. When the target is microbial RNA or mRNA, the RNA must be enzymatically converted to DNA by reverse transcriptase; the product, complementary DNA (cDNA), can then be analyzed by PCR. This method is referred to a *reverse transcriptase-polymerase chain reaction (RT-PCR)*. Initially, PCR was a qualitative assay, but assays have been developed that allowed for quantitation of amplicons. Quantitative RT-PCR is used to measure viral loads in HIV- and hepatitis C-infected patients. These numbers allow physicians to determine disease status and evaluate efficacy of antiviral treatments. The latest PCR innovation is the development of "real-time" RT-PCR, which allows for direct measurement of amplicon accumulation during the exponential phase of the reaction. Two important findings led to the discovery of real-time PCR. First, finding that the *Taq* polymerase possesses $5' \rightarrow 3'$-exonuclease activity[34,35]; second, the construction of dual-labeled oligonucleotide probes that emit a fluorescence signal only on cleavage, based on the principle of *fluorescence resonance energy transfer (FRET)*.[36] FRET involves the nonradioactive transfer of energy from a donor molecule to an acceptor molecule. Probe-based systems, such as Taq-Man probes,[37] molecular beacons,[38] and Scorpion primers,[39] rely on the close proximity of donor fluorophores and nonfluorophore acceptor molecules (quenchers) in the unhybridized probe, so that little or no signal is generated as the fluorescence of the donor is quenched by the acceptor. Upon hybridization to the target, the fluorphore and quencher become separated through either conformational changes (Molecular Beacons and Scorpion primers) or enzymatic cleavage of the fluorphore from the quencher as a result of the 5' to 3' nuclease activity of *Taq* polymerase. Real-time detection occurs when the fluorescence emission of the reporter probe (driven by the accumulation of amplicons) is monitored cycle by cycle. The results are available immediately and, more impor-

tantly, there is no manipulation of the postamplification sample, reducing the chance of contaminating other samples with amplified products.

PCR is limited by expense, the need for special thermocyclers, potential aerosol contamination from one sample to another, nonspecific annealing, and degree of stringency. Stringency is related to the stability of the bonding between target DNA or RNA and the probe and is based on the degree of match and the length of the probe. Stability of the duplex is strongly influenced by temperature, pH, and ionic strength of the hybridization solution. Under low stringency conditions (low temperature or increased ionic strength), imperfect binding occurs.

Other techniques have evolved to overcome some of these shortcomings, to standardize methods for use in clinical laboratories, or to provide new proprietary approaches. Amplification of the target, probe, and signal have been described. The classic target amplification method, PCR, increases the number of target nucleic acids so that simple signal detection systems can be used. Another target amplification method is *self-sustained sequence replication (3SR)*, which detects target RNA and involves continuous isothermic cycles of reverse transcription.[40,41] One primer (T7RNA polymerase) attaches to the RNA and reverse transcriptase extends the annealed primer. Ribonuclease H then degrades the RNA and allows the second primer to bind, followed by synthesis of the cDNA and RNA sequences. The cDNA serves as a template for the production of multiple copies of antisense RNA, which are converted to cDNA. Thus, the cycle is self-perpetuating.

The *ligase chain reaction (LCR)* is a probe amplification technique that uses two pairs of labeled probes that are complementary for two, short-target DNA sequences in close proximity.[42] After hybridization, the DNA ligase interprets the break between the ends as a nick and links the probe pairs.

Q-beta replicase system uses Q-beta replicase to synthesize additional copies of the MDV-1 sequence of the single-stranded Q-beta RNA.[43] After target DNA or RNA is heated to denature it, a probe with the target-specific sequence and the MDV-1 sequence is added and hybridizes. Unbound probe is removed, the Q-beta replicase and excess ribonucleotide bases are added, and amplification follows.

Signal amplification methods are designed to increase the signal strength by increasing the concentration of the label. A probe may have multiple labels attached or several short probes complementary for the target each could be labeled. A two-tiered probe system has been developed in which part of the primary probe attaches to the target DNA and part of the primary probe extends away from the target DNA. Labeled secondary probes are added that hybridize the portion of the primary probe, which is not bound to the target DNA. A powerful signal amplification system uses multiple probes. Multiple primary probes are used to bind to the target DNA. One arm of a secondary probe can recognize one end of the primary probe; the other secondary probe arms are recognized by an enzyme-labeled tertiary probe. The branched DNA (bDNA) assay is an example of the last method.[44]

In situ hybridization is performed on cells, tissue, or chromosomes that are fixed on a microscope slide.[45] After the DNA is heat denatured, a labeled probe is added and will hybridize the target sequence after the slide is cooled. Colorimetric or fluorescent products are generally used. A strength of this method is the morphologic context in which the localization of target DNA is viewed.

Restriction fragment length polymorphism (RFLP) is a technique that evaluates differences in genomic DNA sequences.[46] This technique can help establish identity or nonidentity in forensic or paternity testing or to identify a gene associated with a disease. Genomic DNA is extracted from a sample (*eg,* peripheral blood leukocytes) and is purified and quantitated. A restriction endonuclease, which cleaves DNA sequences at a specific site, is added. If there is a mutation or change in the DNA sequence, this may cause the length of the DNA fragment to be different than usual. Southern blotting can be used to identify the different lengths of the DNA fragments. A labeled specific probe could be used to identify a specific aberration. PCR can be used to amplify the target DNA sequence before RFLP analysis.

Nucleic Acid Probe Applications

Nucleic acid probes are used to detect infectious organisms; to detect gene rearrangements, chromosomal translocations, or chromosomal breakage; to detect changes in oncogenes and tumor suppressor factors; to aid in prenatal diagnosis of an inherited disease or carrier status; to identify polymorphic markers used to establish identity or nonidentity; and to aid in donor selection. Nucleic acid probes are useful in identifying microorganisms in a patient specimen or confirming an organism isolated in culture. Probes are currently available to confirm *Mycobacterium* species, *Legionella* species, *Salmonella,* diarrheogenic *Escherichia coli* strains, *Shigella,* and *Campylobacter* species. Probes also are available to identify fungi such as *Blastomyces dermatitidis, Coccidioides immitis, Cryptococcus neoformans,* and *Histoplasma capsulatum.* Direct identification of microorganisms in patient specimens includes *Chlamydia trachomatis, Neisseria gonorrhea,* cytomegalovirus, Epstein-Barr virus, and herpes simplex virus. In addition, viral load testing for HIV and the hepatitis C virus are detected using probe technology.

Gene rearrangement studies by Southern blot are helpful to distinguish between T and B lymphocyte lineage.[47] Also, the chromosome translocation associated with most follicular, non-Hodgkin's lymphomas and certain diffuse, large cell lymphomas have been detected and monitored. The Philadelphia chromosome in chronic myelogenous leukemia is associated with the translocation that results in the detection of the bcr/abl fusion gene.[48]

Prenatal diagnosis of genetic diseases such as sickle cell anemia, cystic fibrosis,[49] Huntington's chorea,[50] Duchenne-type muscular dystrophy,[51] and von Willebrand's disease[52] have been made possible using probe technology. In addition, the carrier status in Duchenne-type muscular dystrophy and von Willebrand's disease can be determined.

PCR has been used to detect major histocompatibility complex class I and class II polymorphism.[53] The increased accuracy of detecting differences in the genes, rather than the gene product, has been used to improve transplant compatibility.

Molecular arrays are ordered sets of unique DNA probe molecules attached to a solid support.[54] Arrays consist of hundreds-to-thousands of DNA probes at precisely determined locations on the fixed substrate. Molecular arrays evolved from Southern's work in the 1970s, which demonstrated that labeled DNA probes could be used to interrogate DNA molecules attached to a solid support.[31] Microarrays are used for two major applications, (1) determination of DNA sequences and mutation detection, and (2) determination of gene expression. Currently, Affymetrix, Inc., has developed Gene-Chips, proprietary, high-density microarrays that contain 10,000 to 400,000 different short DNA probes on a 1.2-by 1.2-cm glass wafer. GeneChips are available for HIV-1 genotyping,[55] human p53 tumor suppressor gene mutation analysis, and human cytochrome p450 gene mutation analysis, with other GeneChips currently under development.

SUMMARY

This chapter introduced the foundations of immunoassays and nucleic acid probe techniques. All immunoassays use antibodies to detect target analytes. Unlabeled immunoassays in gel include methods to characterize monoclonal proteins and to identify specific antibodies to nuclear components. Unlabeled immunoassays in the soluble phase are typified by nephelometry and turbidimetry. Labeled immunoassays have increased analytic sensitivity. The variety of assay designs, improved and reliable specificity of monoclonal antibodies, and automation have made immunoassays increasingly popular in the clinical laboratory. Immunoassays are described in terms of the label used, the method to detect the label, the need for separation (homogeneous or heterogeneous), competitive or noncompetitive binding, and qualitative or quantitative measurement. Specialized techniques using antibodies include *immunoblots,* immunocytochemistry, immunohisto-chemistry, and flow cytometry.

Nucleic acid probes, used to detect DNA or RNA sequences in human, bacterial, or viral genomes, are a diverse group of methods that are highly specific under stringent conditions. Unamplified techniques are generally used to identify qualitative changes. Amplified techniques that increase the amount of target nucleic acid, probe, or signal are used to increase analytic sensitivity.

The future of immunoassays and nucleic acid probe technology will be to do more tests simultaneously on a single sample in a single reaction vessel or on a single chip surface. The ability to detect different labels and to recognize capture molecules will allow the simultaneous detection of an exponential number of analytes or sequences. Multiplex testing will replace the test panel, which now consists of separately performed individual tests.

REVIEW QUESTIONS

1. The strength of binding between an antigen and antibody is related to the:
   a. concentration of antigen and antibody.
   b. source of antibody production because monoclonal antibodies bind better.
   c. goodness of fit between the epitope and the F(ab).
   d. specificity of the antibody.

2. In monoclonal antibody production, the specificity of the antibody is determined by the:
   a. myeloma cell line.
   b. sensitized B lymphocytes.
   c. sensitized T lymphocytes.
   d. selective growth medium.

3. Which unlabeled immune precipitation method in gel is used to quantitate a serum protein?
   a. Double diffusion
   b. Radial immunodiffusion
   c. Counterimmunoelectrophoresis
   d. Immunofixation electrophoresis

4. In immunofixation electrophoresis, discrete bands appear at the same electrophoretic location; one reacted with antihuman IgA (α chain specific) reagent and the other reacted with antihuman λ reagent. This is best described as:
   a. an IgA λ monoclonal protein.
   b. an IgA λ polyclonal protein.
   c. IgA biclonal proteins.
   d. cross-reactivity.

5. In nephelometry, the antigen–antibody complex formation is enhanced in the presence of:
   a. high ionic strength saline solution.
   b. normal saline.
   c. polyethylene glycol.
   d. complement.

6. In a classic competitive, heterogeneous RIA to measure T_4, which statements are true and which are false?
   _____ a. The assay requires a separation step.
   _____ b. The tracer is T_4 with a radiolabel.
   _____ c. The detector molecule is radiolabeled anti-T_4.
   _____ d. As the concentration of analyte in the test sample increases, the concentration of bound-labeled molecule decreases.

7. Which homogeneous immunoassay relies on inhibiting the activity of the enzyme label when bound to antibody reagent to eliminate separating free- from bound-labeled reagent?
   a. EMIT
   b. CEDIA
   c. MEIA
   d. ELISA

8. Number the steps in a Western blot in the order performed. Step 1 is the first step in the assay.
   _____ a. Protein antigens are isolated and denatured.
   _____ b. Test serum is incubated with the proteins.
   _____ c. Proteins are transferred to a nitrocellulose membrane.
   _____ d. Proteins are separated by SDS-PAGE.
   _____ e. Labeled antiserum reagent that reacted is evaluated.

9. In flow cytometry, the side scatter is related to the:
   a. DNA content of the cell.
   b. granularity of the cell.
   c. size of the cell.
   d. number of cells in G_0 and G_1.

10. Reagents that are required for a PCR reaction are:
   a. thermostable DNA polymerase.
   b. individual deoxyribonucleotides.
   c. oligonucleotide primers.
   d. *Taq* polymerase.
   e. All of the above.

11. The nucleic acid technique in which RNA is converted to cDNA, which is then amplified, is known as:
    a. PCR.
    b. RT-PCR.
    c. RFLP.
    d. in situ hybridization.

12–14. Match the method with the appropriate description.

    _____ 12. Southern blot

    _____ 13. Northern blot

    _____ 14. Western blot
    a. Single-stranded DNA is the target
    b. Messenger RNA is the target
    c. Proteins are the target.

REFERENCES

1. Sheehan C. An overview of antigen–antibody interaction and its detection. In: Sheehan C, ed. Clinical Immunology: Principles and Laboratory Diagnosis, 2nd ed. Philadelphia: Lippincott-Raven Publishers, 1997:109.
2. Kohler G, Milstein C. Continuous cultures of fused cells secreting antibody of predefined specificity. Nature 1975;256:495.
3. Ouchterlony O. Antigen–antibody reactions in gel. Acta Pathol Microbiol Scand 1949;26:507.
4. Mancini G, Carbonara AO, Heremans JF. Immunochemical quantitation of antigens by single radial immunodiffusion. Immunochemistry 1965;2:235.
5. Fahey JL, McKelvey EM. Quantitative determination of serum immunoglobulins in antibody-agar plates. J Immunol 1965;98:84.
6. Grabar P, Burtin P. Immunoelectrophoresis. Amsterdam, The Netherlands: Elsevier, 1964.
7. Alper CC, Johnson AM. Immunofixation electrophoresis: a technique for the study of protein polymorphism. Vox Sang 1969; 17:445.
8. Laurell CB. Quantitative estimation of proteins by electrophoresis in agarose gel containing antibodies. Anal Biochem 1966;15:45.
9. Laurell CB. Electroimmunoassay. Scand J Clin Lab Invest 1972;29(suppl 124):21.
10. Kusnetz J, Mansberg HP: Optical considerations: nephelometry. In: Ritchie RF, ed. Automated Immunoanalysis. Part 1. New York: Marcel Dekker, 1978.
11. Engvall E, Perlmann P. Immunochemistry 1971;8:871.
12. Van Weemen BK, Schuurs AHWM. Immunoassay using antigen-enzyme conjugates. FEBS Lett 1971;15:232.
13. Nakamura RM, Bylund DJ. Fluorescence immunoassays. In: Rose NR, deMarcario EC, Folds JD, Lane HC, Nakamura RM, eds. Manual of Clinical Laboratory Immunology, 5th ed. Washington, D.C.: ASM Press 1997;39.
14. Diamandis EP, Evangelista A, Pollack A, et al. Time-resolved fluoroimmunoassays with europium chelates as labels. Am Clin Lab 1989;8(8):26.
15. Kricka LJ. Chemiluminescent and bioluminescent techniques. Clin Chem 1991;37:1472.
16. Kricka LJ. Selected strategies for improving sensitivity and reliability of immunoassays. Clin Chem 1994;40:347.
17. Bronstein I, Juo RR, Voyta JC. Novel chemiluminescent adamantyl 1,2-dioxetane enzyme substrates. In: Stanley PE, Kricka LJ, eds. Bioluminescence and Chemiluminescence: Current Status. Chichester, England: Wiley, 1991;73.
18. Edwards B, Sparks A, Voyta JC, et al. In: Campbell AK, Kricka LJ, Stanley PE, eds. Bioluminescence and Chemiluminescence: Fundamentals and Applied Aspects. Chichester, England: Wiley, 1994.
19. Litchfield WJ. Shell-core particles for the turbidimetric immunoassays. In: Ngo TT, ed. Nonisotopic Immunoassay. New York: Plenum Press, 1988.

20. Rubenstein KE, Schneider RS, Ullman EF. "Homogeneous" enzyme immunoassay. A new immunochemical technique. Biochem Biophys Res Commun 1972;47:846.
21. Henderson DR, Freidman SB, Harris JD, et al. CEDIA, a new homogeneous immunoassay system. Clin Chem 1986;32:1637.
22. Ullman EF, Schwartzberg M, Rubinstein KD. Fluorescent excitation transfer assay: a general method for determination of antigen. J Biol Chem 1976;251:4172.
23. Dandliker WB, Dandiker BJ, Levison SA, et al. Fluorescence methods for measuring reaction equilibria and kinetics. Methods Enzymol 1978;48:380.
24. Dandliker WB, Kelly RJ, Dandiker BJ, et al. Fluorescence polarization immunoassay: theory and experimental methods. Immunochemistry 1973;10:219.
25. Diamandis EP. Immunoassays with time-resolved fluorescence spectroscopy: principles and applications. Clin Biochem 1988;21:139.
26. Yalow RS, Berson SA. Immunoassay of endogenous plasma insulin in man. J Clin Invest 1960;39:1157.
27. Valkirs GE, Barton R. ImmunoConcentration: a new format for solid-phase immunoassays. Clin Chem 1985;31:1427.
28. Rubenstein AS, Hostler RD, White CC, et al. Particle entrapment: application to ICON immunoassay. Clin Chem 1986;32:1072.
29. Zuk RF, Ginsberg VK, Houts T, et al. Enzyme immunochromatography: a quantitative immunoassay requiring no instrumentation. Clin Chem 1985;31:1144.
30. Harbeck RJ, Teague J, Crossen GR, et al. Novel, rapid optical immunoassay technique for detection of group A streptococci from pharyngeal specimens: comparison with standard culture methods. J Clin Microbiol 1993;31:839.
31. Southern EM. Detection of specific sequences among DNA fragments separated by gel electrophoresis. J Mol Biol 1975;98:503.
32. Mullis KB, Faloona FA. Specific synthesis of DNA in vitro via a polymerase-catalyzed chain reaction. Methods Enzymol 1987; 155:335.
33. Mullis KB. The unusual origin of the polymerase chain reaction. Sci Am 1990;262:56.
34. Foy CA, Parkes HC. Emerging homogenous DNA-based technologies in the clinical laboratory. Clin Chem 2001;47(6):990.
35. Holland PA, Abramson RD, Watson R, Gelfand DH. Detection of specific polymerase chain reaction by utilizing the 5' to 3' exonuclease activity of Thermus aquaticus DNA polymerase. Proc Natl Acad Sci USA 1991;88:7276.
36. Szollosi J, Damjanovich S, Matyus L. Application of fluorescence resonance energy transfer in the clinical laboratory: routine and research. Cytometry 1998;15:159.
37. Livak K, Flood S, Marmaro J, Giusti W, Deetz K. Oligonucleotides with fluorescent dyes at opposite ends provide a quenched probe system useful for detecting PCR product and nucleic acid hybridization. PCR Meth Appl 1995;4:357.

38. Tyagi S, and Kramer F. Molecular Beacons: probes that fluoresce upon hybridization. Nat Biotechnol 1996;14:303.

39. Whicombe D, Theaker J, Guy S, Brown T, Little S. Detection of PCR products using self-probing amplicons and fluorescence. Nat Biotechnol 1999;17:804.

40. Guatelli JC, Whitfield KM, Kwoh DY, et al. Isothermal in vitro amplification of nucleic acids by a multienzyme reaction modeled after retroviral replication. Proc Natl Acad Sci USA 1990;87:1874.

41. Fahy E, Kwoh DY, Gingeras TR. Self-sustained sequence replication (3SR): an isothermal transcription-based amplification system alternative to PCR. PCR Meth Appl 1991;1:25.

42. Barany F. Genetic disease detection and DNA amplification using cloned thermostable ligase. Proc Natl Acad Sci USA 1991;88:189.

43. Klinger JD, Pritchard CG. Amplified probe-based assay: possibilities and challenges in clinical microbiology. Clin Microbiol Newsletter 1990;12:133.

44. Wiedbrauk DL. Molecular methods for virus detection. Lab Med 1992;23:737.

45. Hankin RC. In situ hybridization: principles and applications. Lab Med 1992;23:764.

46. Bishop JE, Waldholz M. Genome. New York: Simon & Schuster, 1990.

47. Farkas DH. The Southern blot: application to the B- and T-cell gene rearrangement test. Lab Med 1992;23:723.

48. Ni H, Blajchman MA. Understanding the polymerase chain reaction. Transfusion Med Rev 1994;8:242.

49. Gasparini P, Novelli G, Savoia A, et al. First-trimester prenatal diagnosis of cystic fibrosis using the polymerase chain reaction: report of eight cases. Prenat Diag 1989;9:349.

50. Thies U, Zuhlke C, Bockel B, et al. Prenatal diagnosis of Huntington's disease (HD): experience with six cases and PCR. Prenat Diag 1992;12:1055.

51. Clemens PR, Fenwick RG, Chamberlain JS, et al. Carrier detection and prenatal diagnosis in Duchenne and Becker muscular dystrophy families, using dinucleotide repeat polymorphism. Am J Hum Genet 1991;49:951.

52. Peake IR, Bowen D, Bignell P. Family studies ad prenatal diagnosis in severe von Willebrand disease by polymerase chain reaction amplification of variable number tandem repeat region of the von Willebrand factor gene. Blood 1990;76:555.

53. Erlich H, Tugawan T, Begovich AB, et al. HLA-DR, DQ, and DP typing using PCR amplification and immobilized probes. Eur J Immunogenet 1991;18:33.

54. Southern E, Mir K, and Shchepinov M. Molecular interactions on microarrays. Natl Genet 1999;21(Suppl):5.

55. Vahey M, Nau ME, Barrick S, et al. Performance of the Affymetrix GeneChip HIV PRT 440 platform for antiretroviral drug resistance genotyping of human immunodeficiency virus type 1 clades and viral isolates with length polymorphisms. J Clin Microbiol 1999;37:2533.

Point-of-Care Testing

Elizabeth E. Porter

OBJECTIVES

Upon completion of this chapter, the clinical laboratorian should be able to:
• Define point-of-care testing (POCT).
• Explain what basic structure is required to manage a POCT program.
• Explain the nuts and bolts process of implementing a POC test.

• State the basic principles behind these common POC applications:
  ▪ POC glucose
  ▪ POC chemistries and blood gases
  ▪ POC hematology
  ▪ POC coagulation
  ▪ POC connectivity

KEY TERMS

Clinical Laboratory
  Improvement
  Amendments of 1988
  (CLIA 88)

Connectivity
Highly complex testing
Moderately complex
  testing

Performance
  improvement
Point-of-care testing
  (POCT)

Standardization
Waived testing

Point-of-care testing (POCT) has been defined by the College of American Pathologists (CAP) as "those analytical patient-testing activities provided within the institution, but performed outside the physical facilities of the clinical laboratories."[1]

Nursing, perfusion, or respiratory therapy staff or resident or attending physicians may perform POCT. These health care staff members are not usually specifically trained in clinical laboratory science. Clinical laboratory and professional laboratory scientists are uniquely qualified to support, assist, and provide oversight for such testing. In so doing, the quality of POCT results and the quality of patient care are improved and enhanced. Today's laboratories, laboratorians, and health care institutions can accomplish this by:

1. Building an **administration and structure** to support and facilitate quality POCT.
2. Maintaining the **knowledge and skill base** to appropriately implement POCT.
3. Bringing preexisting POCT into regulatory compliance and production of high-quality patient results.

ADMINISTRATION AND STRUCTURE

The components essential for establishing a POCT program are included in Box 7-1.

CLIA License and Regulation

There is a common misconception that POCT may at times be exempt from the body of regulation that applies to testing performed in the clinical laboratory. All testing, regardless of location, falls within the scope of the *Clinical Laboratory Improvement Amendments of 1988 (CLIA 88)*. CLIA 88 is a body of United States' federal regulation. Historically, CLIA 88 was implemented, in part, as a response to the perceived Papanicolaou (pap) test "scandal" of the 1980s. Certain clinical laboratories and physician office laboratories had problematic testing operations, including lack of documentation and poor quality test results that resulted in a lack of clinician confidence.

BOX 7.1 POCT PROGRAM COMPONENTS

Appropriate CLIA license(s)
Chosen inspecting/certifying agency
Support staff
Standardization
A structure defining authority, responsibility, and accountability
Interdisciplinary communication and relationships (Network!)

CLIA 88 oversight and enforcement occurs via the Food and Drug Administration (FDA) and Centers for Medicare and Medicaid Services (CMS), formerly HCFA. CLIA 88 includes quality control regulations and personnel standards and divides testing into basic complexity categories.

Waived testing consists of "simple" tests. The original waived test list only contained methodologies for nine analytes; now, many additional analytes are included. Table 7-1 lists currently waived tests. *Moderately complex testing* includes about 75% of approximately 12,000 test methods. These tests are not modified from the manufacturer's instructions, reagents are readily available, and few operator decision-making steps are required. The remaining 25% are highly complex test methods. *Highly complex testing* may be either modified from the manufacturer's instructions or developed within the individual laboratory or may require significant operator skill and decision-making.

The CLIA license must fit the testing that is actually being performed (*ie*, appropriate complexity). The institution also must make several choices regarding CLIA licensure. The institution may choose to perform POCT under the Clinical Laboratory's license. Alternatively, a separate CLIA license may be obtained for POCT.

The institution must decide which inspecting and certifying agencies apply to their POCT program. Some agencies have "deemed" status, which means that accreditation awarded by these agencies is acceptable under CLIA 88. These include Joint Commission on Accreditation of Healthcare Organizations (JCAHO), College of American Pathologists (CAP), and Commission of Office Laboratory Accreditation (COLA). All institutions, and particularly institutions not accredited by a deemed agency, are subject to CMS or state inspection of testing (Table 7-2).

Provider-Performed Microscopy (PPM) Testing Requirements

PPM is a subcategory of moderate complexity testing. These tests require use of a microscope. Quality control materials usually do not exist for these tests. Generally, the specimens are labile and cannot survive transport to clinical laboratory. The site must have PPM certification (at the minimum). Competency may be assumed for physicians or dentists within the scope of their specialty. Midlevel personnel (*ie*, personnel who are not physicians or dentists) must have a minimum of a high school diploma, together with specific training and orientation to perform the test.

Support Staff

The following positions are useful in establishing and maintaining a quality POCT program.

- **Director.** A PhD, MD, or DO laboratory scientist or pathologist usually fills this position. Responsibilities

TABLE 7-1. CURRENTLY WAIVED ANALYTES

ANALYTE NAME	ANALYTE NAME
Alanine aminotransferase (ALT) (SGPT)	Influenza B
Albumin, urinary	Ketone, blood
Alcohol, saliva	Ketone, urine
Amine	Lactic acid (lactate)
Amphetamine	Luteinizing hormone (LH)
Bladder tumor associated antigen	Lyme disease antibodies (*Borrelia burgdorferi* ABS)
Cannabinoid (THC)	Methamphetamine/amphetamine
Catalase, urine	Methamphetamines
Cholesterol	Microalbumin
Cocaine metabolite	Morphine
Collagen type I cross-link, N-telopeptides (NTX)	Nicotine and/or metabolites
Creatinine	Opiates
Erythrocyte sedimentation rate, nonautomated waived	Ovulation test (LH) by visual color comparison
Estrone-3 glucuronide	pH
Ethanol (alcohol)	Phencyclidine (PCP)
Fecal occult blood	Prothrombin time (PT)
Fern test, saliva	Semen
Follicle-stimulating hormone (FSH)	Spun microhematocrit
Fructosamine	Streptococcus, Group A
Gastric occult blood	Triglyceride
Gastric pH	Urine dipstick or tablet analytes, nonautomated
Glucose	Urine HCG by visual color comparison tests
Glucose monitoring device (FDA cleared/home use)	Urine qualitative dipstick, ascorbic acid
Glucose, fluid (FDA approved for prescription home use)	Urine qualitative dipstick, bilirubin
Glycosylated hemoglobin (HbA$_{1c}$)	Urine qualitative dipstick, blood
hCG, urine	Urine qualitative dipstick, chemistries
HDL cholesterol	Urine qualitative dipstick, creatinine
Helicobacter pylori	Urine qualitative dipstick, glucose
Helicobacter pylori antibodies	Urine qualitative dipstick, ketone
Hematocrit	Urine qualitative dipstick, leukocytes
Hemoglobin by copper sulfate, nonautomated	Urine qualitative dipstick, nitrite
HGB, single analyte inst. w/self-cont.	Urine qualitative dipstick, pH
HIV-1 antibody	Urine qualitative dipstick, protein
Infectious mononucleosis antibodies (MONO)	Urine qualitative dipstick, specific gravity
Influenza A	Urine qualitative dipstick, urobilinogen
Influenza A/B	Vaginal pH

Source: www.fda.gov/cdrh/clia. Database updated 8/03.

include policy, administrative, financial, and technical decisions. The director provides liaison with high-level administration for the health care institution. A good director will be skilled at problem resolution, involving both technical issues and personnel interactions.

- **Point-of-Care Coordinator (POCC).** The point-of-care coordinator is responsible for implementing and coordinating point-of-care patient testing and facilitating compliance with procedures and policies and regulatory requirements. The POCC performs on-site

TABLE 7-2. CMS OR STATE INSPECTION OF TESTING

WAIVED	MODERATE	HIGH
CLIA waiver certificate required.	Certificate of accreditation required.	Certificate of accreditation required.
Personnel have specific training and orientation to perform the test.	Personnel have specific training and orientation to perform the test. Continuing competency must be documented. Personnel must have minimum of high school diploma. Must have a lab director/technical consultant/clinical consultant.	Personnel have specific training and orientation to perform the test. Continuing competency must be documented. Personnel must have minimum of Associate Degree or equivalent. Must have a lab director/technical consultant/clinical consultant.
Must follow the manufacturer's instructions when performing the test.	Must follow the manufacturer's instructions when performing the test. At least 2 levels of control material daily. Calibration verification every 6 months. Proficiency testing. Defined standards: procedure manual, corrective action, record-keeping.	If manufacturer's instructions are not followed, many requirements must be met to validate the test. At least 2 levels of control material daily. Calibration verification every 6 months. Proficiency testing. Defined standards: procedure manual, corrective action, record-keeping. Many additional stringent standards, which are difficult to meet outside of the clinical laboratory. Seldom performed as POCT.

review of patient testing, quality control, and maintenance logs and reports problems and regulatory noncompliance to appropriate management personnel. The POCC facilitates and ensures documentation of competency training and oversees completion of proficiency testing programs. The POCC coordinates problem resolution for POCT and provides on-site technical resource assistance to point-of-care personnel for problem solving related to quality control and instrument performance. The POCC facilitates communication between the POCT testing personnel and the clinical laboratory staff. The POCC facilitates adequate point-of-care inventory control. The POCC should exhibit excellent customer service skills, including superior communication skills and good analytic and problem-solving skills. Time management, planning, and organizational skills are also important. Any individual seeking the position of POCC should be self-motivated and not require continual oversight by management to ensure job performance. The POCC must exhibit high-level technical skills and have excellent interpersonal skills.

- **Designated contacts or trainers in nonlaboratory departments.** For each unit/floor/clinic that performs POCT, it is important to have a designated contact person or trainer. This person greatly facilitates the ef-

ficient POCT program and is a communication link between the POCC and the testing staff. They also help ease training and competency activities when a "train-the-trainer" process is used. (In the train-the-trainer process, the POC coordinator may train the designated contact/trainer, who then trains other POC staff in the department.) This is especially helpful for issues involving off-shifts and weekends.

Standardization

Standardization is the consistent use of the same instrument/reagent/test method for any particular analyte throughout the designated health care system. Standardization produces the following benefits:

- Comparability of results across locations produces improved patient care. This reduces clinician confusion about interpretation of varying test results for the same analyte, regardless of where the test is performed.
- Saves cost. Nearly all vendors negotiate pricing based on expected test volumes. When standardization is present, the test volumes will be higher for the chosen vendor than if multiple vendors were used. Major cost savings may be achieved.
- Saves work and time. With standardization, there is only one test method, rather than multiple test methods, for

which procedures, training and recertification checklists, paper logs, and comparabilities must be maintained.

- Facilitates regulatory compliance. Multiple methods present in a single institution cause difficulty maintaining the above-mentioned factors and also make consistent regulatory compliance nearly impossible with regard to test result comparability.

Oversight Structure

It is important to establish a structure for POCT that defines authority, responsibility, and accountability. The purposes of such a structure are:

- To facilitate timely and accurate performance of patient testing when such testing is being performed outside the laboratory.
- To facilitate compliance with regulatory agencies (eg, JCAHO, CAP, CLIA 88).
- To facilitate a process of standardization across the multiple facilities and sites performing POCT, resulting in improved quality of testing, efficiency, and cost containment.
- To coordinate and facilitate communication between the laboratory; nursing; and vendors of point-of-care instruments, supplies, reagents, or quality control materials.
- To facilitate the education of POCT personnel by providing materials for training and/or recertification.

The components of such a structure usually include methods and/or steering committees. Such committees may oversee compliance, utilization, method/instrument selection, standardization, procedural issues, and decisions on expansion or limitation of testing. These committees function best when they are multidisciplinary and multihospital where applicable (ie, hospital systems). Their structure and function should be documented by written policy.

COMMUNICATION

The structure described above comprises the formal portion of the program. Networking is the informal portion of the program. Networking is equally important to a fully functional POCT program and should cross disciplines (eg, lab, nursing, perfusion, respiratory therapy). Networking is facilitated when staff is skilled in communication and diplomacy, as well as technical issues. The effective POCT program places a high priority on building and maintaining relationships.

Handling a Request for New or Additional POCT

Document the request, preferably via a standardized request form. Box 7-2 indicates some needed information. Evaluate the request, using the program structure previously described. There may be a variety of clinical justification(s) for implementing POCT. Prior to establishing any POC test, it is important to consider whether comparable testing is available in the central clinical laboratory. Some questions to consider include:

- What is the average turnaround time and average cost for testing performed by the clinical laboratory versus POCT?
- If POCT can reduce turnaround time, will the shorter turnaround time result in decreased length of stay or increased patient satisfaction?
- Will a shorter turnaround time result in improved operational efficiency for the department?
- What other option(s) exist for achieving the desired objectives, in addition to performance of the test as POC?

Institutions should also consider other options, such as transporting specimens to the central laboratory by pneumatic tube systems, using "runners" to transport specimens, or reengineering the workflow. It is important to determine whether POCT can achieve a favorable cost-to-benefit ratio. For example, if the expected test volume is small, it may not be cost effective to train personnel, maintain and document competency, purchase quality control reagents, as well as oversee the testing.

Preliminary Selection of Devices/Methods

Make a preliminary selection of method and instrumentation to perform the requested testing. Review the multiple options that are on the market and limit your selection to several methods or instruments. Criteria for selection may include ease of use, cost, test menu, comparability to clinical laboratory instrumentation, buying group contracts, and software features. Data management and connectivity (see POC Connectivity in this chapter) are important criteria for consideration, with an emphasis on the ability to interface the data produced by the POC device.

BOX 7.2 INFORMATION REQUIREMENTS FOR NEW OCT REQUEST

Test(s) requested.
Objective(s).
Who will perform the test?
Estimated test volume.
How will test results be documented and/or charged?
Is this test presently being performed by another method? If so, what are the problems with the current method?

Perform a literature search for existing data on the performance of the method/instrument. Vendor literature may be helpful, but should always be verified with additional data. Also, contact other users for references and possible sharing of validation data. Perform a preliminary, limited validation, including a minicorrelation to your clinical laboratory instrumentation. You can review proficiency test provider literature for expected coefficient of variation (CV). Precision and linearity studies may also be useful on a limited basis. At this point, a test method/instrument selection should be made, preferably using the POC program structure previously described.

Validation

The importance of method validation cannot be overemphasized. Besides the regulatory requirements that must be met, method validation is necessary to insure the reliable test results that are necessary for quality patient care. Method validation includes the following (as applicable):

- Accuracy (clinically correct result).
- Precision (clinically same result repeatedly).
- Sensitivity and specificity, including interfering substances (the likelihood that a positive test is truly positive and a negative test is truly negative).
- Reportable range/linearity (upper and lower limits of the test).
- Reference range (expected results for a normal individual).
- Split-sample correlation versus reference method.

Methods and instruments should also be validated. Perform split-sample correlations to determine agreement between POCT and the methods used in the lab. Be aware of variability between products from different vendors. Agreement between POCT and clinical laboratory testing is more likely if both venues are using products from the same vendor. However, even when the same vendor is used, there may be variation between different instruments. When performing validations, it is important to include both positive and negative samples or high and low values for all analytes that will be reported. Moreover, to obtain the most reliable results, any delay between the analysis on the laboratory instrument and the POC instrument should be minimized.

Contract Negotiation

Only after the test method has been fully validated should a contract be negotiated with the vendor. Most institutions have purchasing departments to assist with this process. Many institutions are also part of buying or purchasing groups; these contracts must be considered throughout the process.

Implementation

Collect Materials

The following materials should be collected before beginning the implementation process:

- Instrument manual(s).
- Package insert(s) for reagents.
- Package insert(s) for quality controls.
- Materials safety data sheet (MSDS).
- Sample procedure from vendor.
- Sample training materials from vendor.
- Other institution's procedure for test.
- Applicable regulatory or certifying standards (ie, NCCLS [National Committee for Clinical Laboratory Standards] standards, JCAHO laboratory standards, CAP checklist).

Procedure/Policy

The first step in the implementation process is the writing of the procedure/policy for the test or method. Start with your institution's format template. (Note: POCT procedures frequently must comply with the format requirements of nonlaboratory departments in addition to meeting the basic requirements with which laboratorians are familiar.) Do not make assumptions about the testing process, but detail the required steps. The level of writing should be understood by a nonlaboratorian. NCCLS format should also be followed.

- **Principle.** Briefly state the type of reaction(s) that is occurring. It is also helpful to include the clinical reason for performing the test.
- **Testing personnel.** Describe who is qualified to perform the test (job category, competency requirements, color discrimination). CLIA 88 regulations and the institution's inspecting agency regulations must be followed. For waived testing, personnel must have specific training and orientation to perform the test. For moderately complex testing, personnel must have a high school diploma and the administration must designate lab director/technical consultant/clinical consultant positions. As always, all of this must be documented. Each institution must determine whether all staff—including nurses and nursing assistants—will receive training or if training will be limited to certain areas of responsibility and qualifications. The smaller the staff and the more frequently a staff member performs testing, the higher the quality of testing is likely to be. However, staffing and scheduling needs must also be considered. It may be useful to have the nursing department designate trainers (eg, train-the-trainer approach).
- **Specimen.** Include requirements for patient preparation, type of specimen required, stability and storage requirements (or the requirement to run the specimen immediately), criteria for specimen acceptability, and handling considerations.

- **Reagents, supplies, and equipment.** List all required reagents, supplies, and equipment. Include storage and stability requirements, including dating and labeling requirements and any applicable safety warnings.
- **Maintenance.** Provide instructions for maintaining the instrument, including required frequency.
- **Power.** Describe the power source(s) for the instrument (AC vs. battery, or both). If batteries are used, identify them. If rechargeable batteries are applicable, explain how to recharge.
- **Calibration/calibration verification.** Identify required materials and required frequency.
- **Quality control (QC).** Identify QC materials, frequency, the process for performing QC, how to determine QC success or failure, and the process for troubleshooting QC failure. (Be sure to include both liquid QC and electronic QC instructions when appropriate.)
- **Patient testing procedure.** Write detailed instructions in a stepwise manner. Do not omit simple steps on the basis of assumption.
- **Reference and therapeutic ranges, technical limits, critical values.** These values (preferably in table format) must be included.
- **Reporting results.** Describe in specific detail how your institution will record and report patient results.
- **Data transfer, electronic documentation, configurations.** It is helpful to document these items (specific to your institution) in the procedure. This will serve as a useful reference tool and will also facilitate standardization, especially in multihospital systems.
- **Limitations, notes.** Include interfering substances and test limitations. Special precautions may be listed. Information regarding possible sources of error, clinical situations influencing results, and clinical applications may be included.
- **Proficiency testing.** Document the proficiency testing requirements and process.
- Reagent and control lot receipt: Identify the process to be followed for receipt of reagents and controls.
- **Quality improvement (QI).** Describe your institutions QI process for the test/method.
- Troubleshooting: Explain how to troubleshoot unexpected results, errors, and instrument problems.
- **Alternative method.** State the process to be followed if the instrument or test is not available. For POCT, this usually involves borrowing a spare or replacement instrument or sending the specimen to the clinical laboratory for testing.
- **References.** Include the manufacturer's product literature, textbook references used, standards publications, and any applicable scientific literature references.

Training Checklist

Start with your checklist template. The training checklist must be clear and sufficiently detailed that nonlaboratory trainer will be reminded to explain clearly all training items. The training checklist should document all operator training. It is most efficient to use a 2-copy system: One copy for the employee's continuing-education file and the second copy for the POC office.

The following items should be included in the training checklist:

- Read procedure.
- Maintenance.
- Reagents.
- Quality control.
- Specimen requirements.
- Direct observation (perform a "mock" patient test).
- Reporting results: software and/or paper documentation, reference and critical ranges.
- Safety.
- Operator information (name, operator ID#, floor).
- Trainer signature.
- May supplement with quiz.

Recertification Checklist

CLIA and other certifying agencies also require documentation of continuing competency for personnel performing testing, or recertification. The recertification checklist may be shorter than the training checklist. It should be tailored or modified to the problems and issues observed as testing is performed. Wait until testing has been in progress for a while so these issues can be observed.

Create Paper Forms/Logs

Unless the test/instrument has full electronic documentation/connectivity, paper forms will be necessary for compliance and monitoring. Some, or all, of the following forms may be needed:

- Quality control log.
- Patient testing log.
- Problem/corrective action log.
- Quality improvement form.

Most, if not all, of these forms may be eliminated with good connectivity.

PROFICIENCY TESTING

Proficiency testing is a part of good laboratory practice that verifies the ability to produce reliable patient test results. It also is required by many regulatory and certifying agencies. To meet these objectives, the following steps facilitate organization and documentation:

- Be sure to have a structure.
- Order the appropriate testing.
- Document receipt of PT shipments.
- Schedule distribution.
- Distribute to POC department.

- Report results to PT supplier.
- Maintain documentation.

Communication

Before implementing the new test or method, it is important to notify all affected parties and users of the implementation, including physicians, nursing departments, administrators, and clinical laboratorians. The notification should include a short description of the test or method and the expected uses.

Keeping Up

Certain clerical or administrative processes should be monitored to ensure regulatory compliance and good basic laboratory practices, including:

- Adding serial numbers to your instrument list.
- Adding to your schedule for comparabilities and calibration verifications.
- Adding required reagents/supplies to your ordering information list.
- Adding the test to your test volume tally log.
- Adding the test to proficiency testing schedule.

Performance Improvement

As with all laboratory testing, a *performance improvement* (PI) process should be in place to ensure quality. Items that should be monitored include quality control (QC). Was QC performed? Was it within acceptable range? Mean and standard deviation should be monitored regularly. The QC items are important because QC evaluates the instrument, reagents, operator (person performing the test), and testing process. The same personnel who are testing patient samples should perform QC. It should be noted that QC for POCT is equally important as clinical laboratory testing. Basic QC theory states that when a test is working properly and specimens of known concentration are run over time, there is a Gaussian distribution of values.[2] It is not the function of this chapter to detail the QC process (for additional information, refer to Chapter 3, *Quality Assurance and Statistics*).

Performance should also be observed for non-QC monitors. Competency of persons performing POCT (*ie,* valid operators) should be monitored. Use of correct patient identification in performing POCT should be documented. Track to ensure that instrument maintenance is performed appropriately.

The performance improvement process should include communication with the POC unit/manager, a corrective action process, and clear follow-up. This process will facilitate operator confidence in the test results produced and clinician confidence in patient test results.

Reporting Results

Patient test and quality control results must be documented. Manual testing generally implies documentation on paper logs, although some electronic systems for

recording manual testing are in development. Manual recording in patient charts introduces the possibility of transcription errors. Results must be recorded in a manner that complies with applicable regulations, including date and time of testing, person performing the test, units of measure, and reference ranges. This all requires training and cooperation from those performing the tests. Today, much instrumented testing has the capability of electronic transfer to a data manager and, possibly, an interface to the laboratory information system (LIS). A detailed discussion follows in the POC connectivity section of this chapter.

POC APPLICATIONS

POC Glucose

POC glucose is the highest volume POC test in most health care institutions. It is frequently used to monitor the glucose level for patients with diabetes, but may be used for other purposes. Most of today's institutional POC glucose meters include the ability to document testing electronically. Many home-use glucose meters are also available; glucose is the most frequently used home POC test.

A small drop of blood, most frequently obtained by capillary puncture, is applied to a test strip. A reaction occurs between the blood and reagents in the test strip. The meter measures the reaction and converts the reaction to a quantitative result. The actual reaction varies among manufacturers.

POC Chemistries and Blood Gases

Several different manufacturers offer instrumentation designed to measure POC chemistries (most frequently electrolytes) and/or blood gases. Most operate on the principle of measuring potentiometric, amperometric, or conductometric changes via sensors (electrodes). This has been accomplished by both nondisposable and disposable sensors. Instruments with disposable sensors may be configured for multispecimen analysis before disposal of the multisample reagent pack, which includes the sensors as well as all required reagents. Alternatively, some POC instruments use a single-sample disposable cartridge that contains all of the system's components (reagents, sensors, and waste container). In these devices, the instrument itself receives the outputs from the sensors as an electrical output and converts the electrical output to a result.

POC Coagulation

The most common POC coagulation test is activated clotting time (ACT). ACT, first described by Hattersley in 1966,[3] is used for monitoring heparin therapy. Although heparin therapy is essential in maintaining hemostasis during many medical procedures, patients can vary greatly in their response to heparin. Overdosing heparin can result in bleeding and underdosing heparin can cause a blood clot to form. This may be avoided by monitoring heparin therapy with an ACT.

In vivo coagulation occurs as the result of a complex interaction of vascular, cellular, and noncellular (coagulation cascade) components. ACT provides an in vitro, nonspecific measurement of the cellular and noncellular components of the coagulation process.

The first POC clotting times were performed by drawing fresh whole blood, then periodically manually mixing or inverting the tube and visually observing for clot formation. More recently, the large variability in this process has been reduced by: (1) the addition of an activator (Celite, silica, kaolin, or glass particles), (2) maintenance of a stable temperature (37°C) during the clotting/measuring process, and (3) a mechanical agitation and/or clot detection system. The newest POC coagulation instruments with microsampling techniques further reduce variability by further automation of the process, requiring less operator technique to perform the test. Newer POC coagulation instruments may also have the capability to perform additional tests, such as PT-INR and aPTT.

POC Hematology

At the present time, only minimal hematology POCT has been available. In past years, the spun hematocrit was the most common POC hematology test. More recently, many institutions are eliminating the spun hematocrit due to safety concerns and because the variability in operator technique can result in significant variation in test results. Many institutions now use a system consisting of disposable cuvets and an analyzer. The cuvet cavity contains reagents deposited on its inner walls that hemolyze the red cells when the blood sample is drawn into the cavity by capillary action. The released hemoglobin is converted to azide methemoglobin. The cuvet is then placed in the analyzer, where absorbance is measured and the hemoglobin level is calculated.[4]

POC Connectivity

Connectivity has been the most significant recent development in POCT. Traditionally, POCT results have been written manually in the patient's medical record or, occasionally, recorded via an instrument printout that has been placed in the medical record. *Connectivity* is the ability to electronically document testing. Generally, the instrument itself has the ability to store a certain amount of data. This is the *device* segment of connectivity. Multiple instruments can then upload data via computer network to a centrally located workstation. This workstation is the *data management* portion of connectivity. The next step in the connectivity process is transmittal of test results from the data manager to the laboratory information system (LIS) and/or hospital information system (HIS). This is the *interface* portion of connectivity. Standards exist for POCT connectivity, known as POCT1-A standards.[5] POCT 1-A standards apply to instrumentation (devices) as well as to data management workstations and interfaces.[6,7]

Many connectivity systems are vendor- or instrument-specific. However, the newer, more sophisticated systems manage results from multiple vendors via a single integrated system. Such a system allows the point-of-care coordinator to oversee testing, QC, instruments, and operators for multiple types of equipment from a single workstation. Some advantages of such a system are:

- Electronic documentation of patient results reduces errors in transcription and ensures that all patient test results are correctly documented in the medical record.
- Electronic documentation allows a practical system for billing for POCT.
- Standardized instrument configurations can be maintained throughout the system.
- Regulatory compliance is improved.
- Paper recording is eliminated or greatly reduced.
- Practically and time-effectively monitoring all testing results in improved quality.
- All test results can run through a single interface.
- Operators for many different devices from many different locations, together with their appropriate competency documentation, can be managed in an integrated manner.

SUMMARY

Point-of-care testing is analytic patient-testing activities provided within the institution, but performed outside the physical facilities of the clinical laboratories. Quality patient service, as well as regulatory compliance, is facilitated by the existence of a structured POCT program within the institution. Laboratorians may provide assistance and support to testing personnel. When POCT is implemented, several preparatory steps must be completed. The end result of careful attention to these details will be a quality POCT program that, in turn, produces quality patient testing results.

POCT is a rapidly growing area of laboratory medicine. As outlined in this chapter, POCT provides numerous opportunities for laboratorians and other health professionals to work collaboratively to provide high quality, consistent, and reliable results wherever testing is performed.

REVIEW QUESTIONS

1. Which of the following does not apply to waived testing?
   a. Uses simple instruments.
   b. Reagents must be mixed or prepared by the operator.
   c. Follows manufacturer's package insert.
   d. Personnel must have specific training to perform the test.

2. Which of the following positions is not part of a well-organized POCT program?
   a. POC trainer
   b. Point-of-care coordinator
   c. Manufacturer representative
   d. Director

3. Information needed to determine whether POCT should be used include all of the following EXCEPT:
   a. Who will perform the test?
   b. Does the point-of-care coordinator get along with the unit manager?
   c. How many tests will be performed per month?
   d. How will the test results be documented?

4. Standardization produces all of the following results except:
   a. decreased work.
   b. comparability of test results between separate locations in the hospital.
   c. increased cost.
   d. improved regulatory compliance.

5. Validation includes:
   a. split-sample correlation versus reference method.
   b. precision evaluation.
   c. reportable range verification.
   d. All of the above.

6. Which of the following statements is correct?
   a. When performing validations, it is important to include both positive and negative samples for all the analytes that will be reported.
   b. The results from approved POCT instruments always correlate well with clinical laboratory methods.
   c. Validation is not needed for POCT because the test methods are simple.
   d. Regulations do not require validation of POCT methods.

7. The federal regulation with which institutions must comply when implementing a POCT system is the:
   a. National Accrediting Agency for Clinical Laboratory Science.
   b. Clinical Laboratory Improvement Amendments.
   c. National Committee for Clinical Laboratory Standards.
   d. American Society for Clinical Laboratory Science.

8. Fill in the following blanks:
   ACT stands for _____ .
   ACT results are used to monitor _____ therapy.
   ACT measures cellular and noncellular components of the _____ process.
   The automation found in newer POC coagulation instruments reduces operator _____ when performing ACT testing.

REFERENCES

1. CAP Commission on Laboratory Accreditation, Laboratory Accreditation Program, Point-of-care Testing Checklist. 2002.
2. Basic QC Practices. Madison, WI: Westgard QC, 2002. Available at: www.westgard.com.
3. Hattersley P. Activated coagulation time of whole blood. JAMA 1966:136–436.
4. Hemoglobin data management analyzer operating manual. Mission Viejo, CA: HemoCue, 2003.
5. Point-of-care connectivity; approved standard. NCCLS document POCT1-A, Vol. 21, No. 24 (ISBN 1-56238-450-3). Wayne, PA: NCCLS, December 2001.
6. 2002-2003 Standards for Pathology and Clinical Laboratory Services. Oakbrook Terrace, IL: Joint Commission on Accreditation of Healthcare Organizations, 2002.
7. Price CP, Hicks JM, eds. Point-of-Care Testing. Washington, D.C.: AACC Press, 1999.

Clinical Correlations and Analytic Procedures

Amino Acids and Proteins

Barbara J. Lindsey

OBJECTIVES

Upon completion of this chapter, the clinical laboratorian should be able to:

- Describe the structures and general properties of amino acids and proteins, including both conjugated and simple proteins.
- Outline protein synthesis and catabolism.
- Discuss the general characteristics of the aminoacidopathies, including the metabolic defect in each and the procedure used for detection.
- Briefly discuss the function and clinical significance of the following proteins:
  - prealbumin
  - albumin
  - α_1-antitrypsin
  - α_1-fetoprotein
  - haptoglobin
  - ceruloplasmin
  - transferrin
  - fibrinogen
  - C-reactive protein
  - immunoglobulin
  - troponin

- Discuss at least five general causes of abnormal serum protein concentrations.
- List the reference intervals for total protein and albumin and discuss any nonpathologic factors that influence the levels.
- Describe and compare methodologies used in the analysis of total protein, albumin, and protein fractionation. Include the structural characteristics or chemical properties that are relevant to each measurement and the clinical usage of each.
- Recognize and name the fractions, interpret any abnormality in the pattern, and associate these patterns with common disease states given a densitometric scan of a serum protein electrophoresis using the routine method (five zones).
- Differentiate the types of proteinuria on the basis of etiology and type of protein found in the urine and describe the principle of the methods used for both qualitative and quantitative determination and identification of urine proteins.
- Describe the diseases associated with alterations in cerebrospinal fluid proteins.

KEY TERMS

Albumin	Denaturation	Monoclonal	Phenylketonuria (PKU)
Amino acid	Globulins	immunoglobulin	Principal fetal protein
Aminoacidopathies	Hyperproteinemia	Nitrogen balance	Proteinuria
Amphoteric	Hypoproteinemia	Opsonization	Quaternary structure
Conjugated protein	Isoelectric point (pI)	Peptide bond	Simple protein

In 1839, the Dutch chemist G.J. Mulder was investigating the properties of a substance found in milk and egg whites that coagulated when heated. The Swedish scientist J.J. Berzelius suggested to Mulder that these substances should be called *proteins* (from the Greek word *proteis*, meaning first rank of importance) because he suspected that they might be the most important of all biologic substances. Mulder thought that all protein substances were the same because they contained carbon, nitrogen, and sulfur. This was found to be untrue when C. Dumas discovered slightly varying nitrogen content in protein obtained from different sources.[1]

Today we know that proteins are macromolecules composed of polymers of covalently linked amino acids and that they are involved in every cellular process. This chapter discusses the general properties of amino acids and proteins, abnormalities related to each, and methods of analysis.

AMINO ACIDS

Basic Structure

α-*Amino acids* are small biomolecules containing at least one amino group (–NH₂) and one carboxyl group (–COOH) bonded to the α-carbon. They differ from one another by the chemical composition of their R groups (side chains). The general structure of an α-amino acid is depicted in Figure 8-1. Twenty different amino acids are used as building blocks for protein. The R groups found on these α-amino acids are shown in Table 8-1.

Metabolism

About half of the 20 amino acids needed by humans cannot be synthesized at a rapid enough rate to support growth. These nine nutritionally essential amino acids must be supplied by the diet in the form of proteins. Under normal circumstances, proteolytic enzymes, such as pepsin and trypsin, completely digest dietary proteins into their constituent amino acids. Amino acids are then rapidly absorbed from the intestine into the portal blood and subsequently become part of the body pool of amino acids. Other contributors to the amino acid pool are newly synthesized amino acids and those released by the normal breakdown of body proteins.

The amino acid pool is drawn on primarily for the synthesis of body proteins, including plasma, intracellular, and structural proteins. Amino acids are also used for the synthesis of nonprotein nitrogen-containing compounds such as purines, pyrimidines, porphyrins, creatine, histamine, thyroxine, epinephrine, and the coenzyme NAD. In addition, protein provides 12–20% of the total daily body energy requirement. The amino group is removed from amino acids by either deamination or transamination. The resultant ketoacid can enter into a common metabolic pathway with carbohydrates and fats. Those amino acids that generate precursors of glucose, for example, pyruvate or a citric acid cycle intermediate, are referred to as *glucogenic*. Examples include alanine, which can be deaminated to pyruvate; arginine, which is converted to α-ketoglutarate; and aspartate, which is converted to oxaloacetate. Amino acids that are degraded to acetyl-CoA or acetoacetyl-CoA, such as leucine or lysine, are termed *ketogenic* because they give rise to ketone bodies. Some amino acids can be both ketogenic and glucogenic because some of their carbon atoms emerge in ketone precursors and others appear in potential precursors of glucose. Figure 8-2 shows the points of entry of the carbon atoms of amino acids into the metabolic pathways of carbohydrates and fats. The ammonium ion that is produced during deamination of the amino acids is converted into urea by the urea cycle in the liver.

Aminoacidopathies

Aminoacidopathies are rare, inherited disorders of amino acid metabolism. The abnormalities exist in either the activity of a specific enzyme in the metabolic pathway or in the membrane transport system for amino acids. More than 100 diseases have been identified that result from inborn errors of amino acid metabolism.

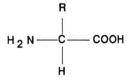

FIGURE 8-1. General structure of an α-amino acid.

TABLE 8-1. AMINO ACIDS REQUIRED IN THE SYNTHESIS OF PROTEINS

AMINO ACID	R	AMINO ACID	R
Glycine (Gly)	—H	Glutamine (Gln)	—CH₂—CH₂—C(=O)—NH₂
Alanine (Ala)	—CH₃	Serine (Ser)	—CH₂—OH
Valine (Val)*	—CH(—CH₃)—CH₃	Threonine (Thr)*	—CH(OH)—CH₃
Leucine (Leu)*	—CH₂—CH(CH₃)—CH₃	Tyrosine (Tyr)	—CH₂—⬡—OH
Isoleucine (Ile)*	—CH(CH₃)—CH₂—CH₃	Lysine (Lys)*	—CH₂—CH₂—CH₂—CH₂—NH₂
Cysteine (Cys)	—CH₂—SH	Arginine (Arg)	—CH₂—CH₂—CH₂—NH—C(=NH₂)—NH₂
Methionine (Met)*	—CH₂—CH₂—S—CH₃	Histidine (His)*	imidazole
Tryptophan (Trp)*	indole	Aspartate (Asp)	—CH₂—COOH
Phenylalanine (Phe)*	—CH₂—phenyl	Glutamate (Glu)	—CH₂—CH₂—COOH
Asparagine (Asn)	—CH₂—C(=O)—NH₂	Proline (Pro)†	pyrrolidine—COOH

The R group is the group attached to the α carbon.
* Nutritionally essential.
† Exception to α attachment of R group is proline.

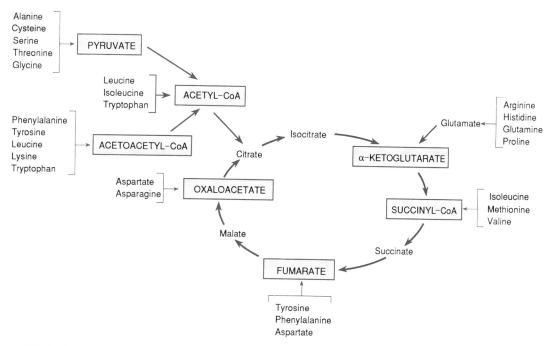

FIGURE 8-2. Conversion of the carbon skeletons of amino acids into pyruvate, acetyl-CoA, or TCA cycle derivatives for further catabolism.

Phenylketonuria

Phenylketonuria (PKU) is inherited as an autosomal recessive trait and occurs in approximately 1 of 15,000 births. The biochemical defect in the classic form of PKU is an almost total absence of activity of the enzyme phenylalanine hydroxylase (PAH) (also called phenylalanine-4-mono-oxygenase), which catalyzes the conversion of phenylalanine to tyrosine (Fig. 8-3). In the absence of the enzyme, phenylalanine accumulates to levels exceeding 1200 µmol/L and is metabolized by an alternate degradative pathway. The catabolites include phenylpyruvic acid, which is the product of deamination of phenylalanine; phenyllactic acid, which is the reduction product of phenylpyruvic acid; phenylacetic acid, which is produced by decarboxylation and oxidation of phenylpyruvic acid; and phenylacetylglutamine, which is the glutamine conjugate of phenylacetic acid. Although phenylpyruvic acid is the primary metabolite, all these compounds are seen in both the blood and the urine of a phenylketonuric patient, giving the urine a characteristic musty odor. Variants of the disease result from partial deficiencies of PAH activity and are typically classified as mild PKU if phenylalanine levels are between 600 and 1200 µmol/L or non-PKU mild hyperphenylalaninemia, which presents with phenylalanine levels in the range of 180–600 µmol/L and no accompanying accumulation of phenylketones.

In infants and children with this inherited defect, retarded mental development occurs as a result of the toxic effects on the brain of phenylpyruvate or one of its metabolic by-products. The deterioration of brain function begins in the second or third week of life. Brain damage can be avoided if the disease is detected at birth and the infant is maintained on a diet containing very low levels of phenylalanine. In the past, the diet was terminated when the child reached age 5 or 6 years. This was based on the belief that, at that age, the brain was no longer vulnerable to damage from hyperphenylalaninemia. However, it has been reported that there is a slight reduction in IQ after discontinuation of the diet. Also, offspring of women with PKU that were untreated during pregnancy were almost always microcephalic and mentally retarded. The fetal effects of maternal PKU are preventable if the mother is maintained on a phenylalanine-restricted diet from before conception through term. For these reasons, it is now recommended that the PKU patient continue dietary treatment indefinitely.[2]

There are cases of hyperphenylalaninemia, however, that are not responsive to dietary treatment. The defect in these cases is a deficiency in the enzymes needed for the regeneration and synthesis of tetrahydrobiopterin (BH$_4$). BH$_4$ is a cofactor required for the enzymatic hydroxylation of the aromatic amino acids phenylalanine, tyrosine, and tryptophan. A deficiency of BH$_4$ results in elevated blood levels of phenylalanine and deficient production of neurotransmitters from tyrosine and tryptophan. Examination of urinary proteins is helpful in diagnosis. Although cofactor defects account for only 1–5% of all cases of elevated phenylalanine levels, they must be identified so that appropriate treatment can be initiated. Patients must be given the active cofactor along with the neurotransmitter precursors L-DOPA and 5-OH tryptophan.[3]

Today, all states have enacted legislation to enforce screening programs so that early therapeutic measures can be taken to prevent the resulting disability and mortality associated with hyperphenylalaninemia. A common screening procedure is the Guthrie bacterial inhibition assay. In this test, spores of the organism *Bacillus subtilis* are incorporated into an agar plate that contains β$_2$-thienylalanine, a metabolic antagonist to *B. subtilis* growth. A filter paper disk impregnated with blood from the infant is placed on the agar. If the blood level of phenylalanine exceeds a range of 2–4 mg/dL, the phenylalanine counteracts the antagonist and bacterial growth occurs. To avoid false-negative results, the infant must be at least 24 hours old to ensure adequate time for enzyme and amino acid levels to develop. Furthermore, the sample should be taken before administration of antibiotics or transfusion of blood or blood products. Premature infants can show false-positive results due to the immaturity of the liver's enzyme systems.

Another approach to the screening for PKU involves a microfluorometric assay for the direct measurement of phenylalanine in dried blood filter disks. This method yields quantitative rather than the semiquantitative results of the Guthrie test, is more adaptable to automation, and is not affected by the presence of antibiotics. The procedure is based on the fluorescence of a complex formed of phenylalanine-ninhydrin-copper in the presence of a dipeptide (*ie*, L-leucyl-L-alanine). The test requires pretreatment of the filter paper specimen with trichloroacetic acid (TCA). The extract is then reacted in a microtiter plate with a mixture of ninhydrin, succinate, and leucylalanine in the presence of copper tartrate. The fluorescence of the complex is measured using excitation/emission wavelengths of 360 nm and 530 nm, respectively.[4]

Any positive results on these screening tests must be verified. The reference method for quantitative serum phenylalanine is HPLC; however, both fluorometric and enzymatic methods are available. The normal limits for serum phenylalanine levels for full-term, normal weight newborns range from 1.2 to 3.4 mg/dL (70–200 µmol/L).

Recently, tandem mass spectrometry (MS/MS) has been used in screening for inherited disorders in newborns. The MS/MS system comprises two quadrupole mass spectrometers separated by a collision chamber that induces molecules to fragment. Blood from a filter paper disk is eluted, then the eluate is esterified with butanol.

The derivatized specimen is injected into the system where it is ionized using a low energy or "soft" ionization technique such as electrospray. The first mass spectrometer separates and determines the masses of the different molecules in the specimen and transmits them to the collision chamber. Here collision of the molecules with an inert gas under pressure causes fragmentation. The fragments pass to a second mass spectrometer that separates them according to mass and charge. Computer scanning of the two mass spectrometers links the fragment ions with their original intact molecular ions and allows for the simultaneous identification and quantitation of amino acids as well as other molecules such as acylcarnitines (which identify disorders of organic and fatty acids).[5] Therefore, both the increase in phenylalanine and the decrease in tyrosine levels seen in PKU can be identified and the ratio of phenylalanine to tyrosine (Phe/Try) calculated. Using the ratio between metabolites rather than an individual level has increased the specificity of the measurement and lowered the false-positive rate for PKU to less than 0.01%. Additionally, the sensitivity of the method detects lower levels of phenylalanine, allowing for diagnosis of PKU as early as the first day of life. Since MS/MS has the ability to detect more than 25 different genetic disorders with a single specimen, this method potentially could replace the multiple procedures currently used in newborn screening programs.

Urine testing for phenylpyruvic acid, although not considered an initial screening procedure, can be used for diagnosis in questionable cases and for monitoring of dietary therapy. The test, which may be performed by tube or reagent strip test (Phenistix, Miles Diagnostics, Elkhart, IN), involves the reaction of ferric chloride with phenylpyruvic acid in urine to produce a green color.

Prenatal diagnosis and detection of carrier status in families with PKU is now available using deoxyribonucleic acid (DNA) analysis. Molecularly, PKU results from multiple independent mutations (more than 400 identified) at the phenylalanine hydroxylase (PAH) locus. Analysis, using cloned human PAH cDNA as a probe, has revealed the presence of numerous restriction fragment length polymorphisms in the PAH gene. Because the restriction fragment patterns and the disease state have been proven to be tightly linked in PKU families, these polymorphisms can be used for prenatal diagnosis.[6] However, although the majority of PAH mutations result in predictable phenotypes, there have been inconsistencies reported in which similar PAH genotypes produced significant variations in the level of activity of PAH.[7]

Tyrosinemia and Related Disorders

A range of familial metabolic disorders of tyrosine catabolism is characterized by excretion of tyrosine and tyrosine catabolites in urine. Normally, the major path of tyrosine metabolism involves the removal of an amine group by tyrosine aminotransferase forming *p*-hydroxyphenylpyruvic acid (PHPPA), which is oxidized to homogentisic acid (HGA). HGA is further metabolized in a series of reactions to fumarate and acetoacetate, as shown in Figure 8-3. The defect in inherited tyrosine abnormalities is either a deficiency in tyrosine aminotransferase, resulting in *tyrosinemia II*; a deficiency of 4-hydroxyphenylpyruvic acid oxidase, leading to *tyrosinemia type III*; or, more commonly, a deficiency in fumarylacetoacetate FAA hydrolase, resulting in *tyrosinemia I*. FAA hydrolase cleaves fumarylacetoacetic acid to fumaric and acetoacetic acids. The absence of these enzymes results in abnormally high levels of tyrosine and, in some cases, increases in PHPPA and methionine. The elevated tyrosine leads to liver damage, which may be fatal in infancy, or to cirrhosis and liver cancer later in life. The incidence of tyrosinemia I is approximately 1 of 100,000 births. Diagnostic criteria include an elevated tyrosine level using

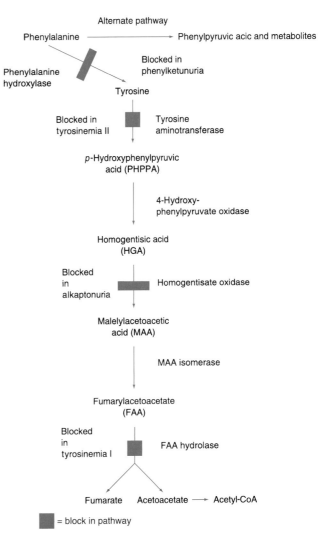

FIGURE 8-3. Metabolism of phenylalanine and tyrosine.

MS/MS coupled with a confirmatory test for an elevated level of the abnormal metabolite succinylacetone.[5]

Alkaptonuria

This disorder is of considerable historical interest in that it was one of the original "inborn errors of metabolism" described. At the turn of the 20th century, Archibald Garrod, a pediatrician, recognized that the syndrome, which had been called alkaptonuria, showed a pattern of familial inheritance. He proposed that alkaptonuria and certain other disorders were due to genetic defects, each of which resulted in the lack of activity of a particular metabolic enzyme.[8] Forty-five years later, it was confirmed that the biochemical defect in alkaptonuria is a lack of homogentisate oxidase in the tyrosine catabolic pathway (Fig. 8-3). This disorder occurs in about 1 of 250,000 births. A predominant clinical manifestation of alkaptonuria is the darkening of urine upon standing exposed to the atmosphere. The phenomenon is due to an accumulation in the urine of HGA, which oxidizes to produce a dark polymer. Alkaptonuric patients have no immediate problems; however, late in the disease, the high level of HGA gradually accumulates in connective tissue, causing generalized pigmentation of these tissues (ochronosis) and an arthritis-like degeneration.

Maple Syrup Urine Disease

As the name implies, the most striking feature of this hereditary disease is the characteristic maple syrup or burnt sugar odor of the urine, breath, and skin. *Maple syrup urine disease (MSUD)* results from an absence or greatly reduced (<2%) activity of the enzyme, branched-chain α-ketoacid decarboxylase, blocking the normal metabolism of the three essential branched-chain amino acids leucine, isoleucine, and valine. Specifically, this enzyme is responsible for catalyzing the oxidative decarboxylation of all three branched-chain α-ketoacids to CO_2 and their corresponding acyl-CoA thioesters (Fig. 8-4). The result of this enzyme defect is an accumulation of the branched-chain amino acids and their corresponding ketoacids in the blood, urine, and cerebrospinal fluid (CSF).

Typically, infants with this inherited abnormality appear normal at birth but, by age 4–7 days, develop lethargy, vomiting, and signs of failure to thrive. Central nervous system (CNS) symptoms follow, including muscle rigidity, stupor, and respiratory irregularities. If left untreated, the disease causes severe mental retardation, convulsions, acidosis, and hypoglycemia. In the classic form of the disease, death usually occurs during the 1st year; however, intermediate forms have been reported. In these less severe variants, the activity of the decarboxylase is approximately 25% of normal. Although this still results in a persistent elevation of the branched-chain amino acids, the levels frequently can be controlled by limiting dietary protein intake.

Although the incidence of MSUD is low—occurring in only 1 of 216,000 births—early diagnosis is important to begin dietary treatment. Therefore, testing for MSUD is included in many of the metabolic screens required by law in certain states. A modified Guthrie test is commonly used for this neonatal screening. The metabolic inhibitor to *B. subtilis*, included in the growth media, is 4-azaleucine. In a positive test for MSUD, an elevated level of leucine from a filter paper disk impregnated with the infant's blood will overcome the inhibitor and bacterial growth occurs. Alternately, a microfluorometric assay for branched-chain amino acids, using leucine dehydrogenase (EC 1.4.1.9), can be used for mass screening. In

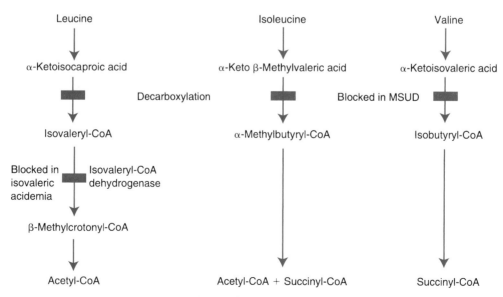

FIGURE 8-4. Metabolism of the branched-chain amino acids.

this procedure, the filter paper specimen is treated with a solvent mixture of methanol and acetone to denature the hemoglobin. Leucine dehydrogenase is added to an aliquot of this sample extract. The fluorescence of the NADH produced in the subsequent reaction is measured at 450 nm, using an excitation wavelength of 360 nm.[4] A confirmed diagnosis is based on finding increased plasma and urinary levels of the three branched-chain amino acids and their ketoacids, with leucine being in highest concentration. A leucine level above 4 mg/dL is indicative of MSUD. The presence of alloisoleucine, an unusual metabolite of isoleucine, is characteristic. Measurement of leucine and its metabolites is also possible using tandem mass spectrometry. MSUD can be diagnosed prenatally by measuring the decarboxylase enzyme concentration in cells cultured from amniotic fluid.

Isovaleric Acidemia

Isovaleric acidemia results from a deficiency of the enzyme isovaleryl-CoA dehydrogenase in the degradative pathway of leucine (Fig. 8-4). The resultant elevation of the glycine conjugate of isovaleric acid, isovalerylglycine, produces a characteristic "sweaty feet" odor. The abnormal organic acid levels can be identified by chromatography or MS/MS.

Homocystinuria

Homocysteine is an intermediate amino acid in the synthesis of cysteine from methionine. The synthesis of cysteine from methionine is illustrated in Figure 8-5. The usual cause of the hereditary disease, homocystinuria, is an impaired activity of the enzyme cystathionine β-synthase, which results in elevated plasma and urine levels of the precursors homocysteine and methionine. Newborns show no abnormalities, but physical defects develop gradually with age. Associated clinical findings in late childhood include thrombosis resulting from the toxicity of homocysteine to the vascular endothelium; osteoporosis; dislocated lenses in the eye resulting from the lack of cysteine synthesis essential for collagen formation; and, frequently, mental retardation.

The enzyme cystathionine β-synthase requires vitamin B_6 (pyridoxine) as its cofactor. Slightly different genetic defects lead to two forms of the disease: a vitamin B_6-responsive form, in which treatment consists of therapeutic doses of vitamin B_6; and a vitamin B_6-unresponsive form, in which the treatment is a diet low in methionine and high in cystine.

The incidence of homocystinuria is approximately 1 of 200,000 births. Neonatal screening can be accomplished with a Guthrie test using L-methionine sulfoximine as the metabolic inhibitor. Increased plasma methionine levels from affected infants will result in bacterial growth. A level of methionine greater than 2 mg/dL using an HPLC procedure confirms positive results on the screening test. Alternately, screening pro-

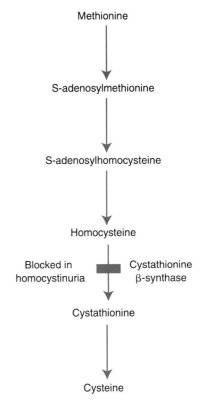

FIGURE 8-5. Cysteine synthesis.

grams can use MS/MS to test for methionine levels. Elevations in urinary homocystine can be detected by the cyanide-nitroprusside spot test. Cystine and homocystine are reduced by sodium cyanide to their free-thiol forms, cysteine and homocysteine, which can then react with sodium nitroprusside to produce a red-purple color. Because cystine also produces a positive result, the presence of homocystine must be confirmed with a silver-nitroprusside test. Silver nitrate reduces homocystine but not cystine, allowing only homocystine to react with the nitroprusside and produce a reddish color. Cystine remains in the oxidized form, which does not react with sodium nitroprusside.

Elevations of homocysteine are also of interest in the investigation of cardiovascular risk. It was found that approximately 50% of individuals with untreated homocystinuria with significantly elevated levels of plasma homocysteine (200–300 μmol/L) had experienced a thromboembolic event before the age of 30. Furthermore, mild homocysteine elevation (>15 μmol/L) occurs in 20–30% of patients with atherosclerotic disease. In addition to cystathionine β-synthase deficiency described above, hyperhomocystinemia can be caused by low folate concentrations; vitamin B_{12} deficiency; decline in renal function; and a genetic alteration in the enzyme, methylenetetrahydrofolate reductase (MTHFR), which converts homocysteine back to methionine. Although there is evidence of endothelial dysfunction in patients with elevated homocysteine levels, there is disagreement on whether mild hyperhomocystinemia is a causative factor in the development of atherosclerotic disease or a consequence of the disease process.[8,9] A more detailed discussion of cardiac risk factors is found in Chapter 23, *Cardiac Function.*

Argininosuccinic Aciduria and Citrullinemia

These amino acid disorders result from inherited enzyme deficiencies in the urea cycle. Argininosuccinic aciduria results from a deficiency in argininosuccinic acid (ASA) lyase, and a decrease in activity of ASA synthetase causes citrullinemia. There are also several related disorders caused by deficiencies in the other enzymes required for urea synthesis. Symptoms include vomiting and high ammonia levels, and mental retardation is associated with some of the conditions. Typically these disorders were not included in the newborn screening programs; however, MS/MS technology has allowed measurement of the affected metabolites. Citrulline is the diagnostic marker for both citrullinemia and argininosuccinic aciduria. Citrulline is dramatically elevated in citrullinemia; in argininosuccinic aciduria, the increase in citrulline is milder and increases in ornithine and arginine are seen in older infants.[5]

Cystinuria

This inherited aminoacidopathy is caused by a defect in the amino acid transport system rather than a metabolic enzyme deficiency. Normally, amino acids are freely filtered by the glomerulus and then actively reabsorbed in the proximal renal tubules. In cystinuria, there is a 20- to 30-fold increase in the urinary excretion of cystine as a result of a genetic defect in the renal resorptive mechanism. The transport mechanism is not specific for cystine. Excretion of the other diamino acids, lysine, arginine, and ornithine, is also significantly elevated as a result of deficient resorption.

Of the four, cystine is the amino acid that causes complications of the disease. Because cystine is relatively insoluble, when it reaches these high levels in the urine, it tends to precipitate in the kidney tubules and form urinary calculi. The formation of cystine calculi can be minimized by a high fluid intake and alkalinizing the urine, which makes cystine relatively more soluble. If this does not succeed, treatment with regular doses of penicillamine can be initiated.[10]

Cystinuria can be diagnosed by testing the urine for cystine using cyanide-nitroprusside, which produces a red-purple color on reaction with sulfhydryl groups. False-positive results as a result of homocystine must be ruled out.

Amino Acid Analysis

Blood samples for amino acid analysis should be drawn after at least a 6- to 8-hour fast to avoid the effect of ab-

sorbed amino acids originating from dietary proteins. The sample is collected in heparin, and the plasma is promptly removed from the cells, taking care not to aspirate the layer of platelets and leukocytes. If this step is not performed with caution, the plasma becomes contaminated with platelet or leukocyte amino acids, in which the contents of aspartic acid and glutamic acid, for example, are about 100-fold higher than those in plasma. Hemolysis should be avoided for the same reason. Deproteinization should be performed within 30 minutes of sample collection, and analysis should be performed immediately or the sample should be stored at −20°C to −40°C.

Urinary amino acid analysis can be performed on a random specimen for screening purposes; however, for quantitation, a 24-hour urine preserved with thymol or organic solvents is required. Amniotic fluid also may be analyzed.

For preliminary screening, the method of choice is thin-layer chromatography. The application of either one- or two-dimensional separations depends on the purpose of the analysis. If one is searching for a particular category of amino acids, such as branched-chain amino acids, or even a single amino acid, usually one-dimensional separations are sufficient. Separation conditions can be selected in such a way as to offer good resolution of the amino acid in question.

For more general screening, two-dimensional maps are essential. In two-dimensional chromatography, the amino acids are allowed to migrate along one solvent front, and then the chromatogram is rotated 90° and a second solvent migration occurs. A variety of solvents have been used, including butanol–acetic acid–water and ethanol–ammonia–water mixtures. The chromatogram is visualized by staining with ninhydrin, which gives most amino acids a blue color.

When the possibility of an amino acid disorder has been indicated in the preliminary steps, amino acids can be separated and quantitated by cation-exchange chromatography using a gradient buffer elution, a HPLC reversed-phase system equipped with fluorescence detection,[11] or capillary electrophoresis. Another technique that provides a highly specific and sensitive method for the measurement of amino acids is tandem mass spectrometry.

PROTEINS

General Characteristics

Proteins are an essential class of compounds comprising 50–70% of the cell's dry weight. Proteins are found in all cells of the body, as well as in all fluids, secretions, and excretions.

Molecular Size

Biologically active proteins are macromolecules that range in molecular weight from approximately 6000 for insulin to several million for some structural proteins.

CASE STUDY 8-1

A 13-month-old boy was admitted to a small, rural hospital.[1] He had been in a normal state of health until 10 days prior, at which time he developed an upper respiratory tract infection. He experienced increasing problems with his balance and became lethargic. These symptoms prompted his mother to seek medical attention at the hospital where pertinent laboratory results at admission showed a serum glucose level of 23 mg/dL and moderate ketones in the urine and serum. An intravenous solution of 5% dextrose was initiated to correct the low glucose level. Because the clinical picture resembled Reye's syndrome, the child was transferred to a medical center hospital for a definitive diagnosis. Laboratory results on admission to the medical center hospital appear in Case Study Table 8-1.1.

1. Campbell P. Case studies. J Med Tech 1985;2:9.

Questions

1. Which laboratory result can be useful in ruling out the diagnosis of Reye's syndrome?

2. What correlations can be made using the blood pH, PCO_2 serum glucose, and serum and urine ketone findings?

3. What other laboratory tests should be performed to verify a defect in protein metabolism?

CASE STUDY TABLE 8-1.1. ADMISSION LABORATORY RESULTS

HEMATOLOGY		URINALYSIS	
Hct	37%	Specific gravity	1.022
WBC	128 × 10⁹/L	Protein	Trace
Bands	28%	Acetone	3+
Segmented	46%	Blood	1+
Lymphocytes	21%		
Monocytes	5%		
CHEMISTRY (REFERENCE RANGE)			
Glucose	133 mg/dL (65–105)	Alk phos	129 U/L (20–70)
BUN	21 mg/dL (7–18)	AST	154 U/L (10–30)
Na	136 mmol/L (136–145)	ALT	133 U/L (8–20)
K	4.3 mmol/L (3.6–5.1)	CK	36 U/L (25–90)
TCO₂	10 mmol/L (23–29)	LD	119 U/L (45–90)
Cl	112 mmol/L (98–106)	Ketone	Moderate
NH₃	48 μmol/L (40–80)		
ARTERIAL BLOOD GASES			
	pH	7.17	
	PCO₂	23 mm Hg	
	PO₂	90 mm Hg	

Structure

All proteins comprise covalently linked polymers of amino acids. The amino acids are linked in a head-to-tail fashion; in other words, the carboxyl group of one amino acid combines with the amino group of another amino acid (Fig. 8-6). During this reaction, a water molecule is removed and the bond that is created is called a *peptide bond*. The amino acid that has the amino group free is the *N-terminal end*, and the amino acid that has the carboxyl group free is the *C-terminal end*. When two amino acids are joined, the molecule is called a *dipeptide*; three amino acids are called a *tripeptide*; and four together is a *tetrapeptide*. As the chain increases further, it is called a *polypeptide*. In human serum, proteins average about 100–150 amino acids in the polypeptide chains.

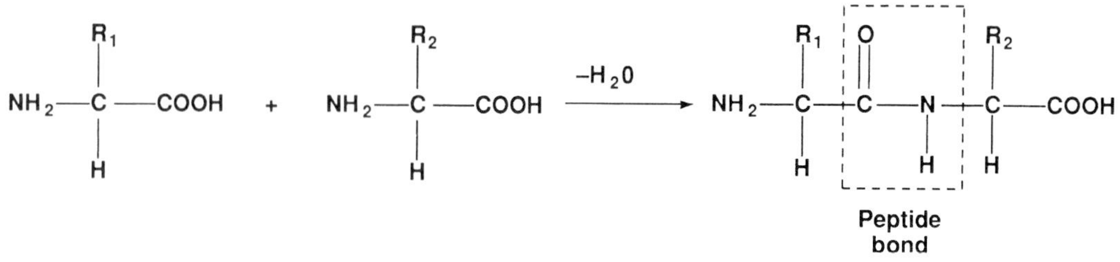

FIGURE 8-6. Formation of a dipeptide.

The conformation (shape) of a protein is determined by interaction between a polypeptide and its aqueous environment in which the polypeptide attains a stable three-dimensional structure. There are four aspects of the structure of a protein that relate to its conformation. The number and kinds of amino acids, as well as their sequence in the polypeptide chain, constitute the primary structure of a protein. The covalent peptide linkage is the only type of bonding involved at this level. The primary structure is crucial for the function and molecular characteristics of the protein. Any change in the amino acid composition can significantly alter the protein. For example, when the amino acid valine is substituted for glutamic acid in the β chain of hemoglobin A, hemoglobin S is formed, which results in sickle cell anemia.

The secondary structure is the winding of the polypeptide chain. The usual pattern that is formed by the globular proteins (most serum proteins) is a helix requiring 3.6 amino acids to make one turn in the coil. A β-pleated sheet or a stable but irregular pattern also can be seen. The secondary structure is maintained by hydrogen bonds between the NH and CO groups of the peptide bonds either within the same chain or between different chains within the same molecule. Figure 8-7 schematically pictures the secondary structure.

The next level of structure, the tertiary structure, refers to the way in which the twisted chain folds back on itself to form the three-dimensional structure. The spe-

cific convolutions a polypeptide undergoes are determined by the interaction of the R groups in the molecule. The reactions of the R groups include disulfide linkages, electrostatic attractions, hydrogen bonds, hydrophobic interactions, and van der Waals forces. The tertiary structure is responsible for many of the physical and chemical properties of the protein.

In addition to these first three levels that can exist in molecules comprising a single polypeptide chain, some proteins display a fourth level of organization called the *quaternary structure*. Quaternary structure is the arrangement of two or more polypeptide chains to form a functional protein molecule. Albumin, which is composed of a single polypeptide chain, would thus have no quaternary structure. However, hemoglobin comprises four globin chains, lactate dehydrogenase consists of five peptide chains, and creatine kinase has two chains joined. The polypeptide chains are united by noncovalent attractions such as hydrogen bonds and electrostatic interactions.

When the secondary, tertiary, or quaternary structure of a protein is disturbed, the protein may lose its functional and molecular characteristics. This loss of its native or original character is called *denaturation*. Denaturation can be caused by heat, hydrolysis by strong acid or alkali, enzymatic action, exposure to urea or other substances, or exposure to ultraviolet light.

Nitrogen Content

Proteins comprise the elements carbon, oxygen, hydrogen, nitrogen, and sulfur. It is the nitrogen content that sets proteins apart from pure carbohydrates and lipids, which contain no nitrogen atoms. The nitrogen content of serum protein varies somewhat; the average is approximately 16%. This characteristic is used in one method of total protein measurement.

Charge and Isoelectric Point

Because of their amino acid composition, proteins can bear positive and negative charges (ie, they are *amphoteric*). The reactive acid or basic groups that are not involved in the peptide linkage can exist in different charged forms, depending on the pH of the surrounding environment. Aspartic acid and lysine are examples of amino acids that have free carboxyl or amino groups, respectively (Table 8-1). Figure 8-8 shows these two amino

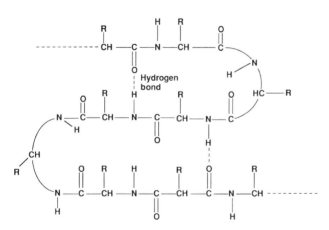

FIGURE 8-7. Secondary structure of proteins.

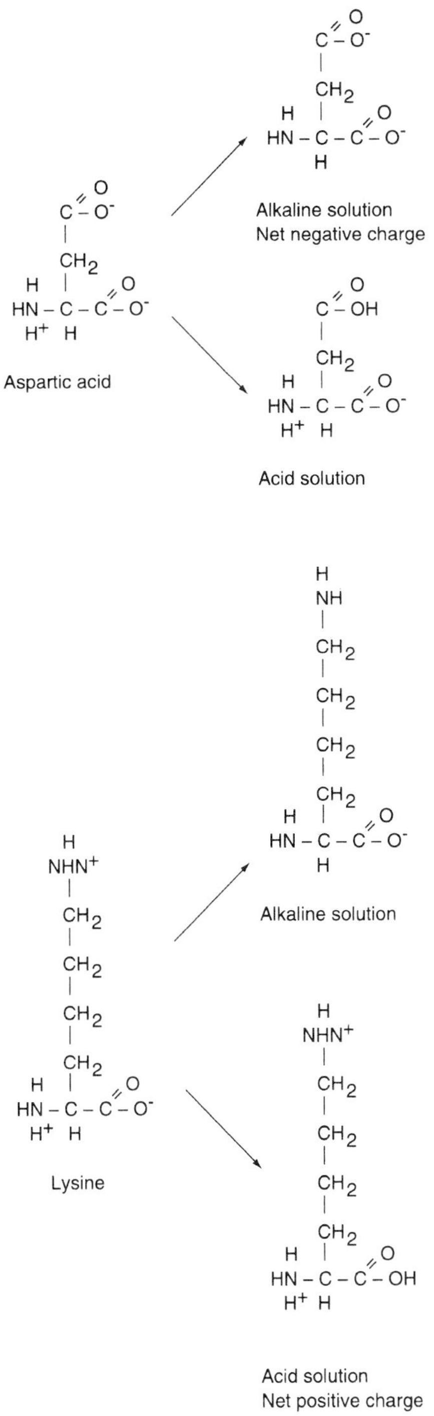

FIGURE 8-8. Charged states of amino acids.

acids and the charges they would have in solutions that are alkaline or acid.

At a pH of 2.98, L-aspartic acid has no net charge (equal or no ionization of the amino and carboxyl groups); whereas, in an alkaline pH (pH, 9.47), aspartic acid has a net negative charge. L-Lysine has no net charge at a pH of 9.47 but, in an acid environment, the gain in

protons results in a net positive charge. The pH at which an amino acid or protein has no net charge is known as its *isoelectric point (pI)*. In other words, for a protein comprising several amino acids, the pI is the point at which the number of positively charged groups equals the number of negatively charged groups. If a protein is placed in a solution that has a pH greater than the pI, the protein will be negatively charged; at a pH less than the pI, the protein will be positively charged. Proteins differ in the number and type of constituent amino acids; they also differ in their pI values. For example, albumin has a pI of 4.9. The pIs of some serum proteins are given in Table 8-2. Because of the different pI values, proteins will carry different net charges at any given pH. This difference in magnitude of the charge is the basis for several procedures for separating and quantitating proteins, such as electrophoresis. The procedure is discussed later in this chapter.

Solubility
Proteins in aqueous solution swell and enclose water. Natelson and Natelson[1] have advised that, for this reason, it is necessary when reconstituting lyophilized serum to mix the reconstituted vial gently for at least 30 minutes to complete the swelling process. Protein solutions are *colloidal emulsoids* or *micelles* because they are charged and because each molecule of protein has an envelope of water around it.

The solubility of proteins is promoted by a high dielectric character of the solvent and a high concentration of free water. Thus, low concentrations of salt (0.1 M) have been used for *salting in* globulins into solution. When the dielectric nature or the amount of free water is decreased, the charges on the protein promote aggregation. In a high salt concentration (~2 M), ionic salts compete with protein for water and thus decrease the amount of water available for hydration of the protein. The resultant precipitation of the globulins is called *salting out*. By using a range of salt concentrations, a wide array of specific proteins can be separated from a mixture. Albumin remains in solution even in high salt concentrations because it has a higher dipole and holds water tighter and, because of its smaller size in relation to the globulins, does not require as much water to keep hydrated.

Water-miscible, neutral organic solvents also can be used to separate proteins based on their solubility. These solvents have a dielectric constant less than water, which suppresses the ionization of the R groups on the protein surface and, thereby, decreases the solubility.

Immunogenicity
Because of their molecular mass, their content of tyrosine, and their specificity by species, proteins can be effective antigens. When injected into another species (eg, rabbit, goat, or chicken), human serum proteins elicit the

TABLE 8-2. CHARACTERISTICS OF SELECTED PLASMA PROTEINS

	REFERENCE VALUE (ADULT, g/L)	MOLECULAR MASS (D)	ISOELECTRIC POINT, pI	ELECTROPHORETIC MOBILITY, pH 8.6, I = 0.1	COMMENTS
Prealbumin	0.1–0.4	55,000	4.7	7.6	Indicator of nutrition; binds thyroid hormones and retinol-binding protein
Albumin	35–55	66,300	4.9	5.9	Binds bilirubin, steroids, fatty acids; major contributor to oncotic pressure
α_1-Globulins					
α_1-Antitrypsin	2–4	53,000	4.0	5.4	Acute-phase reactant; protease inhibitor
α_1-Fetoprotein	1×10^5	76,000	2.7	6.1	Principal fetal protein
α_1-Acid glycoprotein (orosomucoid)	0.55–1.4	44,000		5.2	Acute-phase reactant
α_1-Lipoprotein (HDL)	2.5–3.9	200,000		4.4–5.4	Transports lipids
α_1-Antichymo-trypsin	0.3–0.6	68,000		Inter α	Inhibits serine proteinases (ie, chymotrypsin)
Inter-α-trypsin inhibitor	0.2–0.7	160,000		Inter α	Inhibits proteinases (ie, trypsin)
Gc-globulin	0.2–0.55	59,000		Inter α	Binds vitamin D and actin
α_2-Globulins Haptoglobins					
Type 1-1	1.0–2.2	100,000		4.5	Acute-phase reactant; binds hemoglobin
Type 2-1	1.6–3.0	200,000	4.1	3.5–4.0	Binds hemoglobin
Type 2-2	1.2–1.6	400,000		3.5–4.0	Binds hemoglobin
Ceruloplasmin	0.15–0.60	134,000	4.4	4.6	Peroxidase activity; contains copper
α_2-Macro-globulin	1.5–4.2	725,000	5.4	4.2	Inhibits thrombin, trypsin, pepsin
β-Globulins					
Pre-β-lipoprotein (VLDL)	1.5–2.3	250,000		3.4–4.3	Transports lipids (primarily triglyceride)
Transferrin	2.04–3.60	76,000	5.9	3.1	Transports iron
Hemopexin	0.5–1.0	57,000–80,000		3.1	Binds heme
β-Liproprotein (LDL)	2.5–4.4	3,000,000		3.1	Transports lipids (primarily cholesterol)
β_2-Microglobulin (B2M)	0.001–0.002	11,800		β_2	Component of human leukocyte antigen (HLA) molecules class 1
C_4 complement	0.20–0.65	206,000		0.8–1.4	Immune response
C_3 complement	0.55–1.80	180,000		0.8–1.4	Immune response
C_1 q complement	0.15	400,000			Immune response
Fibrinogen	2.0–4.5	341,000	5.8	2.1	Precursor of fibrin clot
C-reactive protein (CRP)	0.01	118,000	6.2		Acute-phase reactant; motivates phagocytosis in inflammatory disease
γ-Globulins					
Immunoglobulin G	8.0–12.0	150,000	5.8–7.3	0.5–2.6	Antibodies
Immunoglobulin A	0.7–3.12	180,000		2.1	Antibodies (in secretions)
Immunoglobulin M	0.5–2.80	900,000		2.1	Antibodies (early response)
Immunoglobulin D	0.005–0.2	170,000		1.9	Antibodies
Immunoglobulin E	6×10^4	190,000		2.3	Antibodies (reagins, allergy)

formation of antibodies specific for each of the proteins present in the serum. When it became possible to obtain these antibodies for each of the serum proteins, methods using antigen–antibody reactions that are very specific were introduced into the clinical laboratory. Some of the methods commonly used are described in Chapter 6, *Immunoassays and Nucleic Acid Probe Techniques.*

Synthesis

Most plasma proteins are synthesized in the liver and secreted by the hepatocyte into the circulation. The immunoglobulins are exceptions because they are synthesized in plasma cells.

The amino acids of a polypeptide chain are placed in a sequence determined by a corresponding sequence of bases (guanine, cytosine, adenine, and thymine) in the DNA that constitutes the appropriate gene. The double-stranded DNA unfolds in the nucleus, and one strand is used as a template for the formation of a complementary strand of messenger RNA (mRNA). The mRNA, now carrying the genetic code from the DNA, moves to the cytoplasm, where it attaches to ribosomes. A sequence of three bases (*codon*) on the mRNA is required to specify the amino acid to be transcribed. The code on the mRNA also contains initiation and termination codons for the peptide chain.

The next step in protein synthesis is getting the amino acid to the ribosomes. First, the amino acid is activated in a reaction that requires energy and a specific enzyme for each amino acid. This activated amino acid complex is then attached to another kind of RNA, transfer RNA (tRNA), with the subsequent release of the activating enzyme and adenosine monophosphate (AMP). The tRNA is a short chain of RNA that occurs free in the cytoplasm. Each amino acid has a specific tRNA that contains three bases that correspond to the three bases in the mRNA. The tRNA carries its particular amino acid to the ribosome and attaches to the mRNA in accordance with the matching codon. In this manner, the amino acids are aligned in sequence. As each new tRNA brings in the next amino acid, the preceding amino acid is transferred onto the amino group of the new amino acid and enzymes located in the ribosomes form a peptide bond. The tRNA is released into the cytoplasm, where it can pick up another amino acid, and the cycle repeats. When the terminal codon is reached, the peptide chain is detached and the ribosome and mRNA dissociate. Figure 8-9 illustrates protein synthesis. Intracellular proteins are generally synthesized on free ribosomes, whereas proteins made by the liver for secretion are made on ribosomes attached to the rough endoplasmic reticulum. Protein synthesis occurs at the rate of approximately 2–6 peptide bonds per second. Synthesis

FIGURE 8-9. Schematic summary of protein synthesis.

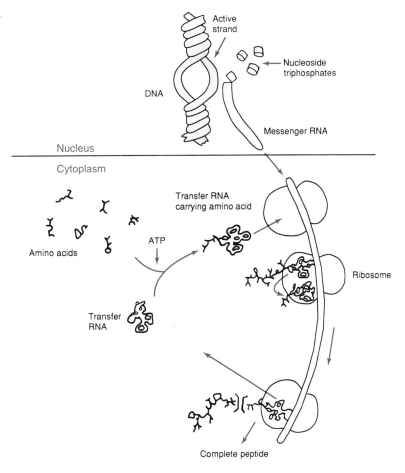

is controlled at two steps: selection of genes for transcription to mRNA and selection of mRNA for translation into proteins. Certain hormones are involved in controlling protein synthesis. Thyroxine, growth hormone, insulin, and testosterone promote synthesis, whereas glucagon and cortisol have a catabolic effect.

Proteins that are excreted after synthesis are thought to have a short sequence of amino acids, a secretory piece that attracts the protein to the Golgi apparatus for consequent secretion by exocytosis. The secretory piece is removed during the secretion process. Secreted proteins, therefore, usually exist as precursor proteins within the cells from which they arise.

Catabolism and Nitrogen Balance

Most proteins in the body are constantly being repetitively synthesized and then degraded. It has been demonstrated that over a wide range of rates of synthesis, protein catabolism and synthesis are equal. Normally, this turnover totals about 125–220 g of protein each day. The rate of protein turnover, however, varies widely for individual proteins. For example, the plasma proteins and most intracellular proteins are rapidly degraded, having half-lives of hours or days; some of the structural proteins, such as collagen, are metabolically stable and have half-lives of years. The disintegration of protein occurs in the digestive tract, kidneys, and, particularly, the liver. During catabolism, proteins are hydrolyzed to their constituent amino acids. The amino acids are deaminated, producing ammonia and ketoacids. The ammonia is converted to urea by the hepatocytes and excreted in the urine. The ketoacids are oxidized by means of the citric acid cycle and converted to glucose or fat.

Ordinarily, a balance exists between protein anabolism (synthesis) and catabolism. In nutritional terms, this is called the *nitrogen balance*. When protein catabolism exceeds protein anabolism, the nitrogen excreted exceeds that ingested. This is "negative" nitrogen balance, and it occurs in conditions in which there is excessive tissue destruction, such as burns, wasting diseases, continual high fevers, or starvation. The converse, "positive" nitrogen balance, is seen when anabolism is greater than catabolism. A positive balance is found during growth, pregnancy, and repair processes.

Classification

Proteins are generally classified into two major groups based on composition: simple and conjugated.

Simple Proteins
Simple proteins contain peptide chains that on hydrolysis yield only amino acids. Simple proteins may be globular or fibrous in shape. Globular proteins are relatively symmetrical, with compactly folded and coiled polypeptide chains. Albumin is an example of a globular protein. Fibrous proteins are more elongated and asymmetrical and have a higher viscosity. Collagen and troponin are examples of fibrous proteins.

Conjugated Proteins
Conjugated proteins comprise a protein (apoprotein) and a nonprotein moiety (prosthetic group). The prosthetic group may be lipid, carbohydrate, porphyrins, metals, and so on. These groups impart certain characteristics to the proteins. Most of the names given to these conjugated proteins are self-descriptive. The *metalloproteins* have a metal ion attached to the protein, either directly, as in ferritin (which contains iron) and ceruloplasmin (which contains copper), or as complex metals (metal plus another prosthetic group), such as hemoglobin and flavoproteins. The metal (iron) in hemoglobin is first attached to protoporphyrin, which is then attached to the globin chains; in flavoprotein, the metal is first attached to FMN or FAD.

When lipids such as cholesterol and triglyceride are linked to proteins, the molecules are called *lipoproteins*. When carbohydrates are joined to proteins, several terms may be used to describe the results. Generally, those molecules with 10–40% carbohydrate are called *glycoproteins*.[1] Examples of glycoproteins are haptoglobin and α_1-antitrypsin. When the percentage of carbohydrate linked to protein is higher, the proteins are often called *mucoproteins* or *proteoglycans* when heparan, keratan, or chondroitin sulfate are also present. An example of a mucoprotein is mucin, a compound that lubricates organ linings. *Nucleoproteins* are those proteins that are combined with nucleic acids (DNA or RNA) (eg, chromatin).

General Function of Proteins

The broad array of molecules that make up proteins may function in general ways or, as individual molecules, may have some unique function. Plasma proteins and tissue proteins share the same amino acid pool, therefore, alterations in one group eventually affect the other. This is why the plasma proteins are important in tissue nutrition. The plasma proteins can be hydrolyzed to amino acids, which can be used for the production of energy by means of the citric acid cycle.

Another general function of plasma proteins is the distribution of water among the compartments of the body. Starling's law attributes a colloid osmotic force to plasma proteins, which, because of their size, cannot cross the capillary membranes. This osmotic force results in the absorption of water from the tissue into the venous end of the capillaries. When the concentration of plasma proteins is significantly decreased, the concomitant decrease in the plasma colloidal osmotic (oncotic) pressure results in increased levels of interstitial fluid and edema. This is often seen in renal disease when proteinuria results in a decreased plasma protein concentration and swelling of the face, hands, and feet occur.

The amphoteric nature of proteins provides the mechanism for their participation as buffers within the plasma and interstitial tissue. The ionizable R groups can either bind or release excess hydrogen ions as needed.

Many plasma proteins function as specific transporters of metabolic substances. Examples include thyroxine-binding globulin, which carries thyroxine; haptoglobin, which binds free hemoglobin; and albumin, which transports free fatty acids, unconjugated bilirubin, calcium, sulfa drugs, and many other endogenous and exogenous compounds. In addition to transporting the molecules to the location where they can be used, proteins, through the binding process, serve to maintain the bound substance in a soluble state, provide a storage site for excess substance (transcobalamin II), and prevent the loss of small molecular mass compounds through the kidney (ie, transferrin in conserving iron).

Several proteins are glycoproteins. One major function of glycoproteins is to distinguish which cells are native and which are foreign to the body. These are notably evident as histocompatibility antigens and erythrocyte blood groups. Antigens can stimulate the synthesis of antibodies, which are also proteins. Antibodies and components of the complement system help protect the body against infection.

Many cellular proteins act as receptors for hormones. The receptor binds to its specific hormone and allows the hormonal message to be transmitted to the cell. In addition, certain hormones (eg, growth hormone and adrenocorticotropic hormone [ACTH]) are themselves proteins.

Proteins also serve a structural role. Collagen is the most abundant protein in mammals, constituting a quarter of their total weight. Collagen is the major fibrous element of skin, bone, tendon, cartilage, blood vessels, and teeth. Elastin and proteoglycans are two other connective-tissue proteins.

Another important biologic property of some proteins (enzymes) is their ability to catalyze biochemical reactions. Other proteins (clotting factors) aid in the maintenance of hemostasis. The vast array of functions attributed to various proteins is summarized in Table 8-3.

Plasma Proteins

Although the proteins in all fluid compartments play a major physiologic function, the plasma proteins are the most frequently analyzed. More than 500 plasma proteins have been identified. The properties of a few selected plasma proteins are discussed in the following section.

Prealbumin (Transthyretin)

Prealbumin is so named because it migrates ahead of albumin in the customary electrophoresis of serum or

TABLE 8-3. FUNCTIONS OF PROTEINS

Tissue nutrition

Maintenance of water distribution between cells and tissue, interstitial compartments, and the vascular system of the body

Participation as buffers to maintain pH

Transportation of metabolic substances

Part of defense system (antibodies)

Hormones and receptors

Connective-tissue structure

Biocatalysts (enzymes)

Participation in the hemostasis and coagulation of blood

plasma proteins. The molecular characteristics of prealbumin can be seen in Table 8-2. It is rarely observed as a distinct band on routine cellulose acetate electrophoretic patterns of serum, although it can be exhibited by high-resolution electrophoresis (HRE) or immunoelectrophoresis. It is rich in tryptophan and contains 0.5% carbohydrate. Prealbumin combines with thyroxine and triiodothyronine to serve as the transport mechanism for these thyroid hormones. Prealbumin also binds with retinol-binding protein to form a complex that transports retinol (vitamin A). Prealbumin is decreased in hepatic damage, acute phase inflammatory response, and tissue necrosis. A low prealbumin level is also a sensitive marker of poor protein nutritional status. When dietary intake of protein-calories is deficient, hepatic synthesis of proteins is reduced and catabolism increases. This results in a decrease in the level of the proteins originating in the liver, including prealbumin, albumin, and β-globulins such as transferrin and complement C3. Prealbumin, because of its short half-life of approximately 2 days, will decrease more rapidly than the other proteins. Prealbumin is increased in patients receiving steroids, in alcoholism, and in chronic renal failure.

Albumin

Albumin is the protein present in highest concentration in the serum (Table 8-2). It is synthesized in the liver. The earliest method for its determination involved the salting out of the globulins with sodium sulfate, leaving the albumin in solution. The albumin was then determined by the Kjeldahl method and, later, by the biuret color development. The method commonly used today involves dye binding and the shift in color when a dye is bound by albumin. When more information about proteins is needed, an electrophoretic pattern is obtained, and the albumin is calculated as a percentage of the total protein (usually, approximately 60%). At birth, the reference value for serum albumin averages 39 g/L. The concentration falls to 28.4 g/L at about 9 months and then begins to increase slowly until adult values of 35–55 g/L are reached.[12] The serum albumin level after age 60 years averages 38.3 g/L.[13]

Albumin has two well-known functions. One is the contribution albumin makes to the colloid osmotic pressure of the intravascular fluid. Because of its high concentration, albumin is responsible for nearly 80% of this pressure, which maintains the appropriate fluid in the tissue. The other prime function is its propensity to bind various substances in the blood. For example, albumin binds bilirubin, salicylic acid, fatty acids, calcium and magnesium ions, cortisol, and some drugs. This characteristic is also exhibited with certain dyes, providing a method for the quantitation of albumin.

Decreased concentrations of serum albumin may be caused by the following:

- An inadequate source of amino acids, which is seen in malnutrition and muscle-wasting diseases.
- Liver disease, resulting in the inability of hepatocytes to synthesize albumin. The increase in globulins that occurs in early cirrhosis, however, will balance the loss in albumin to give a total protein concentration within acceptable limits. The decline in serum albumin is insignificant in viral hepatitis.
- Gastrointestinal loss as interstitial fluid leaks out in inflammation and disease of the intestinal mucosa.

- Loss in the urine in renal disease. Albumin is normally excreted in very small amounts. This excretion is increased when the glomerulus no longer functions to restrict the passage of proteins from the blood.

Abnormalities in serum albumin are also exhibited by the absence of albumin (*analbuminemia*) or the presence of albumin that has unusual molecular characteristics—this abnormality is called *bisalbuminemia* and is demonstrated by the presence of two albumin bands instead of the single band usually seen by electrophoresis. Analbuminemia is an abnormality of genetic origin resulting from an autosomal recessive trait. These conditions are rare.

Increased serum albumin levels are seen in dehydration. This increase is a relative increase, because the albumin is contained in a reduced volume of serum. Administering fluids to treat the dehydration will decrease serum albumin levels back to normal.

Globulins

The *globulin* group of proteins consists of α_1, α_2, β, and γ fractions. Each fraction consists of a number of different proteins with different functions. The following subsections describe selected examples of the globulins.

α_1-**Antitrypsin.** α_1-Antitrypsin is an acute-phase reactant. Its main function is to neutralize trypsin-like enzymes (*ic*, elastase) that can cause hydrolytic damage to

---

CASE STUDY 8.2

Immediately following the birth of a baby girl, the attending physician requested a protein electrophoretic examination of the mother's serum. This was done on a sample that was obtained on the mother's admission to the hospital the previous day. An electrophoretic examination was also performed on the cord-blood specimen. Laboratory reports are shown in Case Study Table 8-2.1.

The appearance of the mother's electrophoretic pattern was within that expected for a healthy person. The electrophoretic pattern of the cord-blood serum resembled the one shown in Figure 8-13C.

Questions

1. What protein fraction(s) is/are abnormal in the mother's serum and the cord-blood serum?

2. An abnormality in this/these fraction(s) is/are most often associated with what disease?

3. What other test(s) may be done to confirm this abnormality?

CASE STUDY TABLE 8-2.1 ELECTROPHORESIS (VALUES g/dL)

	ADULT REFERENCE VALUES	MOTHER'S SERUM	CORD BLOOD
Albumin	3.5–5.0	4.2	3.3
α_1-Globulins	0.1–0.4	0.3	0.0
α_2-Globulins	0.3–0.8	1.2	0.4
β-Globulins	0.6–1.1	1.3	0.7
γ-Globulins	0.5–1.7	1.3	1.0

structural protein. α_1-Antitrypsin is a major component (approximately 90%) of the fraction of serum proteins that migrates electrophoretically immediately following albumin. Molecular characteristics are seen in Table 8-2.

A deficiency of α_1-antitrypsin is associated with severe, degenerative, emphysematous pulmonary disease. The lung disease is attributed to the unchecked proteolytic activity of proteases from leukocytes in the lung during periods of inflammation. Juvenile hepatic cirrhosis is also a correlative disease in α_1-antitrypsin deficiency. The protein is synthesized but not released from the hepatocyte.

Several phenotypes of α_1-antitrypsin deficiency have been identified. The most common phenotype is *MM* (allele *Pi*^{M}) and is associated with normal antitrypsin activity. Other alleles are *Pi*^{S}, *Pi*^{Z}, *Pi*^{F}, and *Pi*$^-$ (null). The homozygous phenotype *ZZ* individual is in serious jeopardy of liver and lung disease from a deficiency of α_1-antitrypsin while those with the SZ phenotype exhibit only about 35% of normal activity of α_1-antitrypsin. Individuals with the *MZ* or *MS* phenotype are usually not affected but should be counseled about having offspring who may be *ZZ* or *Z*$^-$ and in danger. The *Pi*^{Z} allele occurs in 1 of 1500 Caucasians. Factors other than α_1-antitrypsin are also involved in disease because some people who have abnormal phenotypes and low concentrations of proteins do not develop overt disease. Increased levels of α_1-antitrypsin are seen in inflammatory reactions, pregnancy, and contraceptive use.

The discovery of abnormal α_1-antitrypsin levels is most often made by the lack of an α_1-globulin band on protein electrophoresis. This discovery is followed with one of the quantitative methods. A widely used method is radial immunodiffusion. Immunonephelometric assays by automated instrumentation are also available. Phenotyping can be accomplished by immunofixation.

α_1-Fetoprotein. α_1-Fetoprotein (AFP) is synthesized initially by the fetal yolk sac and then by the parenchymal cells of the liver. In 1956, it was first discovered in fetal serum to have an electrophoretic mobility between that of albumin and α_1-globulin. It peaks in the fetus at about 13 weeks' gestation (3 mg/mL) and recedes at 34 weeks' gestation.[14] At birth, it recedes rapidly to adult concentrations, which are normally very low (Table 8-2). The methods commonly used for AFP determinations are radioimmunoassay and enzyme-labeled immunoassay.

The physiologic function of AFP is not well established. It has been proposed that the protein protects the fetus from immunolytic attack by its mother, modulates cell growth, transports compounds such as steroids, and is required for the functional development of the female reproductive system.[15] AFP is detectable in the maternal blood up to month 7 or 8 of pregnancy because it is transmitted across the placenta. Therefore, measurement of the level of AFP in maternal serum is a screening test for any fetal conditions in which there is increased passage of fetal proteins into the amniotic fluid. Conditions associated with an elevated AFP level include spina bifida and neural tube defects, atresia of the gastrointestinal tract, and fetal distress in general. Its use in determining neural tube defects before term is an important reason for its assay. It is also increased in ataxia-telangiectasia, tyrosinosis, and hemolytic disease of the newborn. It is interesting that maternal serum AFP is also increased in the presence of twins. Low levels of maternal AFP indicate an increased risk for Down's syndrome and trisomy 18.

The normal time for screening is between 15 and 20 weeks' gestational age. The maternal AFP increases gradually during this period; therefore, interpretation requires accurate dating of the pregnancy. Maternal AFP levels are also affected by maternal weight, which reflects blood volume (inverse relationship), race (10% higher in African Americans), and diabetes (lowered value); therefore, test results need to be adjusted for these variables. It has been found that reporting AFP in multiples of the median (MoM) leads to good correlation with infant risk. MoM is calculated by dividing the patient's AFP value by the median reference value for that gestational age. Most screening programs use 2.0 MoM as the upper limit and 0.5 MoM as the lower limit for maternal serum AFP.

Serum levels of AFP can also be used as a tumor marker. High concentrations of AFP are found in many cases of hepatocellular carcinoma (approximately 80%) and certain gonadal tumors in adults (see Chapter 30, *Circulating Tumor Markers*).

α_1-Acid Glycoprotein (Orosomucoid). α_1-Acid glycoprotein comprises five carbohydrate units attached to a polypeptide chain. Owing to its low pI (2.7), it is negatively charged even in acid solutions, a fact that led to its name. Other molecular characteristics are seen in Table 8-2. Sequences of haptoglobin, immunoglobulins, and α_1-acid glycoprotein show considerable homology, leading to speculation that these proteins share a precursor in the evolutionary past. α_1-Acid glycoprotein is implicated in the formation of certain membranes and fibers in association with collagen and may inactivate basic hormones such as progesterone.

The analytic methods used most commonly for the determination of orosomucoid are radial immunodiffusion and nephelometry. Immunofixation has been used to study inherited variants.

Increased concentration of this protein is the major cause of an increased glycoprotein level in the serum during inflammation. It is also increased in cancer, pneumonia, rheumatoid arthritis, and other conditions associated with cell proliferation.

α_1-Antichymotrypsin. α_1-Antichymotrypsin (α_1-ACT) is a serine proteinase with cathepsin G, pancreatic elastase, mast cell chymase, and chymotrypsin as target enzymes.[16] α_1-ACT carries four oligosaccharide side chains. It migrates between the α_1 and α_2 zones on high-resolution serum protein electrophoresis. Elevations are seen in inflammation, and it appears that the complex formed between plasma α_1-ACT and its target enzymes plays a major role in signaling acute phase protein synthesis in response to injury. Hereditary deficiency of α_1-ACT is associated with asthma and liver disease.

Inter-α-trypsin Inhibitor. Inter-α-trypsin (ITI) inhibitor comprises at least three distinct polypeptide subunits: two heavy chains designated H_1 and H_2 and a light chain designated L or *bikunin*. The light chain is responsible for the inhibition of the proteases trypsin, plasmin, and chymotrypsin.[17] On high-resolution serum electrophoresis, ITI migrates in the zone between the α_1 and α_2 fractions. Elevations are seen in inflammatory disorders.

Gc-globulin (Group-Specific Component; Vitamin D–Binding Protein). Gc-globulin is another protein that migrates in the α_1–α_2 interzone. This protein exhibits a high binding affinity for Vitamin D compounds and actin, the major constituent of the thin filaments of muscle. Due to genetic polymorphism, several phenotypes of Gc-globulin exist. Elevations of Gc-globulin are seen in the third trimester of pregnancy and in patients taking estrogen oral contraceptives. Severe liver disease and protein-losing syndromes are associated with low levels.

Haptoglobin. Haptoglobin, an α_2 glycoprotein, is synthesized in the hepatocytes and, to a small extent, in cells of the reticuloendothelial system. Haptoglobin comprises two kinds of polypeptide chains: two α chains and one β chain. There are three possible α chains and only one form of β chain. On starch-gel electrophoresis, haptoglobin exhibits three types of patterns, which illustrates the polymorphism in the α chains. Homozygous haptoglobin 1-1 gives 1 band. The peptide chains form polymers with each other and with haptoglobin 1 chains to provide the other two electrophoretic patterns, which have been designated as Hp 2-1 and Hp 2-2 phenotypes. Other characteristics are seen in Table 8-2.

Haptoglobin increases from a mean concentration of 0.02 g/L at birth to adult levels within the first year of life. As old age is approached, haptoglobin levels increase, with a more marked increase being seen in males. Radial immunodiffusion and immunonephelometric methods have been used for the quantitative determination of haptoglobin.

The function of haptoglobin is to bind free hemoglobin by its α chain. Abnormal hemoglobin, such as Bart's and hemoglobin H, has no α chains and cannot be bound. The reticuloendothelial cells remove the haptoglobin–hemoglobin complex from circulation within minutes of its formation. Thus, haptoglobin prevents the loss of hemoglobin and its constituent iron into the urine.

Serum haptoglobin concentration is increased in inflammatory conditions. It is one of the proteins used to evaluate the rheumatic diseases. Increases are also seen in conditions such as burns and nephrotic syndrome when large amounts of fluid and lower-molecular-weight proteins have been lost. Determination of a decreased free haptoglobin level (or haptoglobin-binding capacity) has been used to evaluate the degree of intravascular hemolysis that has occurred in transfusion reactions or hemolytic disease of the newborn. Mechanical breakdown of red cells during athletic trauma may result in a temporary lowering of haptoglobin levels.

Haptoglobin phenotype has also been reported as an independent risk factor for cardiovascular disease (CVD) in individuals with type 2 diabetes mellitus. Haptoglobin 2-2 phenotype is associated with a 5.0 times greater risk as compared with phenotype 1-1. Haptoglobin phenotype 2-1 is reported to carry an intermediate risk of developing CVD in the patient with diabetes.[18]

Ceruloplasmin. Ceruloplasmin is a copper-containing, α_2-glycoprotein that has enzymatic activities (*ie*, copper oxidase, histaminase, and ferrous oxidase). It is synthesized in the liver, where six to eight atoms of copper, half as cuprous (Cu^+) and half as cupric (Cu^{2+}) ions, are attached to an apo-ceruloplasmin. Ninety percent or more of total serum copper is found in ceruloplasmin. Molecular characteristics are given in Table 8-2.

The early analytic method of ceruloplasmin determination was based on its copper oxidase activity. Most assays today use immunochemical methods, including radial immunodiffusion and nephelometry.

Low concentrations of ceruloplasmin at birth gradually increase to adult levels and slowly continue to rise with age. Adult females have higher concentrations than males and pregnancy, inflammatory processes, malignancies, oral estrogen, and contraceptives cause an increased serum concentration.

Certain diseases or disorders are associated with low serum concentrations. In Wilson's disease (hepatolenticular degeneration), an autosomal recessive inherited disease, the levels are typically low (0.1 g/L). Total serum copper is decreased, but the direct reacting fraction is elevated and the urinary excretion of copper is increased. The copper is deposited in the skin, liver, and brain, resulting in hepatic cirrhosis and neurologic damage. Copper also deposits in the cornea, producing the characteristic Kayser-Fleischer rings. Low ceruloplasmin is also seen in malnutrition; malabsorption; severe liver disease; nephrotic syndrome; and Menkes syndrome (kinky hair disease), in which a decreased absorption of copper results in a decrease in ceruloplasmin.

α_2-Macroglobulin. α_2-Macroglobulin, a dimeric, large protein (Table 8-2), is synthesized by hepatocytes. Because its movement is restricted due to size, it is found principally in the intravascular spaces. However, much lower concentrations of α_2-macroglobulin can be found in other body fluids, such as CSF. On binding with and inhibiting proteases, it is removed by the reticuloendothelial tissues. The analytic methods that have been used for the satisfactory assay of this protein are radial immunodiffusion and immunonephelometry.

This protein reaches a maximum serum concentration at the age of 2–4 years and then decreases to about one-third of that concentration at about age 45 years. Later in life, a moderate increase is seen. This change with age is more pronounced in males than in females.[19] There is a distinct difference in the reference values for males and females, adult females having higher values than males.

α_2-Macroglobulin inhibits proteases such as trypsin, pepsin, and plasmin. It also contributes more than one-fourth of the thrombin inhibition normally present in the blood. Little is known of its correlation with disease or disorders, except in the case of renal disease.

In nephrosis, the levels of serum α_2-macroglobulin may increase as much as 10 times because its large size aids in its retention. The protein is also increased in diabetes and liver disease. Use of contraceptive medications and pregnancy increase the serum levels by 20%.

Transferrin (Siderophilin). Transferrin, a glycoprotein, is synthesized primarily by the liver. Two molecules of ferric iron can bind to each molecule of transferrin. Normally, only about 33% of the iron-binding sites on transferrin are occupied. Transferrin is the major component of the β-globulin fraction and appears as a distinct band on high-resolution serum protein electrophoresis. Genetic variation of transferrin has been demonstrated by electrophoresis on polyacrylamide gel. Other characteristics of transferrin are given in Table 8-2.

The analytic methods used for the quantitation of transferrin are immunodiffusion and immunonephelometry. Both are considered to give precise and accurate results.

The major functions of transferrin are the transport of iron and the prevention of loss of iron through the kidney. Its binding of iron prevents iron deposition in the tissue during temporary increases in absorbed iron or free iron. Transferrin transports iron to its storage sites, where it is incorporated into apoferritin, another protein, to form ferritin. Transferrin also carries iron to cells, such as bone marrow, that synthesize hemoglobin and other iron-containing compounds.

The most common form of anemia is iron deficiency anemia, a hypochromic, microcytic anemia. In this type of anemia, transferrin in serum is normal or increased. A decreased transferrin level generally reflects an overall decrease in synthesis of protein, such as seen in liver disease or malnutrition, or it may be seen in protein-losing disorders such as nephrotic syndrome. Transferrin, a negative acute phase protein, is also decreased in inflammation. A deficiency of plasma transferrin may result in the accumulation of iron in apoferritin or in histiocytes or it may precipitate in tissue as hemosiderin. Patients with hereditary transferrin deficiencies have been shown to have significant hypochromic anemia. An increase of iron bound to transferrin is found in a hereditary disorder of iron metabolism, hemochromatosis, in which excess iron is deposited in the tissue, especially the liver and the pancreas. This disorder is associated with bronze skin, cirrhosis, diabetes mellitus, and low plasma transferrin levels.

Hemopexin. The parenchymal cells of the liver synthesize hemopexin, which migrates electrophoretically in the β-globulin region. Other characteristics are seen in Table 8-2. Hemopexin can be determined by radial immunodiffusion. The function of hemopexin is to remove circulating heme. When free heme (ferroprotoporphyrin IX) is formed during the breakdown of hemoglobin, myoglobin, or catalase, it binds to hemopexin in a 1:1 ratio. The heme–hemopexin complex is carried to the liver, where the complex is destroyed. Hemopexin also removes ferriheme and porphyrins.

The level of hemopexin is very low at birth but reaches adult values within the first year of life. Pregnant mothers have increased plasma hemopexin levels. Increased concentrations are also found in diabetes mellitus, Duchenne-type muscular dystrophy, and some malignancies, especially melanomas. In hemolytic disorders, serum hemopexin concentrations decrease. Administration of diphenylhydantoin also results in decreased concentrations.

Lipoproteins. Lipoproteins are complexes of proteins and lipids whose function is to transport cholesterol, triglycerides, and phospholipids in the blood. Lipoproteins are subclassified according to the apoprotein and specific lipid content. On high-resolution serum protein electrophoresis, high-density lipoproteins (HDL) migrate between the albumin and α_1-globulin zone; very-low-density lipoproteins (VLDL) migrate at the beginning of the β-globulin fraction (pre-β); and the low-density lipoproteins (LDL) appear as a separate band in the β-globulin region. For a more detailed discussion of structure and methods of analysis, refer to Chapter 12, *Lipids and Lipoproteins.*

β_2-Microglobulin. β_2-Microglobulin (B2M) is the light chain component of the major histocompatibility complex (HLA). This protein is found on the surface of most nucleated cells and is present in high concentrations on lymphocytes. Because of its small size (MW, 11,800), B2M is filtered by the renal glomerulus but most (>99%) is reabsorbed and catabolized in the proximal tubules. Elevated serum levels are the result of impaired clearance by the kidney or overproduction of the protein that occurs in a number of inflammatory diseases, such as rheumatoid arthritis and systemic lupus erythematosus. In patients with human immunodeficiency virus, a high B2M level in the absence of renal failure indicates a large lymphocyte turnover rate, which suggests the virus is killing lymphocytes. B2M may sometimes be seen on HRE but, because of its low concentration, it is usually measured by immunoassay.

Complement. *Complement* is a collective term for several proteins that participate in the immune reaction and serve as a link to the inflammatory response. Molecular characteristics of selected complement components are listed in Table 8-2. These proteins circulate in the blood as nonfunctional precursors. In the classic pathway, activation of these proteins begins when the first complement factor, C1q, binds to an antigen–antibody complex. The binding occurs at the Fc, or constant, part of the IgG or IgM molecule. Each complement protein (C2–C9) is then activated sequentially and can bind to the membrane of the cell to which the antigen–antibody complex is bound. The final result is lysis of the cell. In addition, complement is able to enlist the participation of other humoral and cellular effector systems in the process of inflammation. An alternate pathway (properdin pathway) for complement activation exists in which the early components are bypassed and the process begins with C3. This pathway is triggered by different substances (does not require the presence of an antibody), however, the lytic attack on membranes is the same (sequence C5–C9). Analytic methods have included a measurement of the titer of complement using complement activity in a hemolytic system and by immunochemical methods such as radial immunodiffusion and nephelometry.

Complement is increased in inflammatory states and decreased in malnutrition, lupus erythematosus, and disseminated intravascular coagulopathies. Inherited deficiencies of individual complement proteins also have been described. In most cases, the deficiencies are associated with recurrent infections.

Fibrinogen. Fibrinogen is one of the largest proteins in blood plasma. It is synthesized in the liver, and it is classified as a glycoprotein because it has considerable carbohydrate content. Other molecular characteristics are given in Table 8-2. On plasma electrophoresis, fibrinogen is seen as a distinct band between the β- and γ-globulins. The function of fibrinogen is to form a fibrin clot when activated by thrombin; therefore, fibrinogen is virtually all removed in the clotting process and is not seen in serum.

Fibrinogen customarily has been determined as clottable protein. Fibrinogen concentration is proportional to the time required to form a clot after the addition of thrombin to citrated plasma. Fibrin split products (degradation products of fibrinogen and fibrin) are determined by immunoassay methods such as radial immunodiffusion, nephelometry, and radioimmunoassay.

Fibrinogen is one of the *acute-phase reactants,* a term that refers to proteins that are significantly increased in plasma during the acute phase of the inflammatory process. Fibrinogen levels also rise with pregnancy and

the use of birth control pills. Decreased values generally reflect extensive coagulation, during which the fibrinogen is consumed.

C-Reactive Protein. C-Reactive protein (CRP) is synthesized in the liver and appears in the blood of patients with diverse inflammatory diseases. Other characteristics are found in Table 8-2. CRP was so named because it precipitates with the C substance, a polysaccharide of pneumococci. However, it was found that CRP rises sharply whenever there is tissue necrosis, whether the damage originates from a pneumococcal infection or some other source. This led to the discovery that CRP recognizes and binds to molecular groups found on a wide variety of bacteria and fungi. CRP bound to bacteria promotes the binding of complement, which facilitates their uptake by phagocytes. This process of protein coating to enhance phagocytosis is known as *opsonization.*

CRP is generally measured by immunologic methods, including nephelometry and enzyme immunoassay (EIA). The traditional methods have a sensitivity of approximately 3–5 mg/L. The more recently developed monoclonal antibody-based CRP methods can detect CRP levels below 1.0 mg/L and have been termed "high-sensitivity CRP" (hsCRP).

CRP is one of the first acute phase proteins to rise in response to inflammatory disease. It is significantly elevated in acute rheumatic fever, bacterial infections, myocardial infarcts, rheumatoid arthritis, carcinomatosis, gout, and viral infections. CRP has also been recognized as an independent risk factor in cardiovascular disease based on the findings that atherothrombosis, in addition to being a disease of lipid accumulation, also represents a chronic inflammatory process. Using the hsCRP assay, levels of <1, 1–3, and >3 mg/L correspond to low-, moderate- and high-risk groups for future cardiovascular events.[20] Elevated levels of CRP stimulate the production of tissue factor that initiates coagulation, activates complement, and binds to LDL in the atherosclerotic plaque; evidence that points to a causal relationship between CRP levels and cardiovascular disease.[21] Furthermore, interventions such as weight loss, diet, exercise, and smoking cessation and administration of pharmacologic agents such as statins all lead to both reduced CRP levels and reduced vascular risk.[20,21] A more detailed discussion of cardiac risk factors is found in Chapter 23, *Cardiac Function.*

Immunoglobulins (Igs). There are five major groups of immunoglobulins in the serum: IgA, IgG, IgM, IgD, and IgE. They are synthesized in plasma cells. Their synthesis is stimulated by an immune response to foreign particles and microorganisms. The immunoglobulins are not synthesized to any extent by the neonate. IgG crosses the placenta; the IgG present in the newborn's serum is that synthesized by the mother. IgM does not cross the placenta but rather is the only immunoglobulin synthesized by the neonate. The concentration of IgM initially is 0.21 g/L, but this increases rapidly to adult levels by about age 6 months. IgA is virtually lacking at birth (0.003 g/L), increases slowly to reach adult values at puberty, and continues to increase during the lifetime. IgD and IgE levels are undetectable at birth by customary methods and increase slowly until adulthood. IgA is generally higher in males than in females; IgM and IgG levels are somewhat higher in females. IgE levels vary with the allergic condition of the individual.

The immunoglobulins comprise two long polypeptide chains (heavy, or H, chains) and two short polypeptides (light, or L, chains), joined by disulfide bonds. An individual is capable of producing 1 million different immunoglobulin molecules. The differences among these molecules are found in a region of the molecule called the *variable region*. This variable region is located on the end of the molecule that contains both the light and heavy chains and is the site at which the immunoglobulin (antibody) combines with the antigen. In this way, there are many different antibodies that are relatively specific for corresponding antigens.

The differences in the heavy chains (H) are called *idiotypes* and are designated IgG, IgA, IgM, IgD, and IgE. The heavy chains are called γ, α, μ, δ, and ε, respectively. The light chains (L) for all the immunoglobulin classes are of two kinds, either κ or λ. Each immunoglobulin or antibody molecule has two identical H chains and two identical L chains. For example, IgG has two λ type H chains and two identical L chains (either κ or λ).

When a foreign substance (antigen) is injected into an animal (*eg*, rabbit or goat), an antibody that will react with that antigen is synthesized. This reaction is relatively specific; that is, the antibodies will react specifically and selectively with the antigen used to raise them. Proteins and polysaccharides are strong antigens. Antibodies can be raised in rabbits and other animals to the human immunoglobulins as well as the other serum proteins. These rabbit antihuman immunoglobulin antibodies are used to detect and to quantitatively assay IgG, IgA, IgM, IgD, and IgE. The immunoglobulins have been determined using radial immunodiffusion and radioimmunoassay. Fluorescent immunoassay techniques and immunonephelometric assays also have been used. The automated immunonephelometric method is available for IgG, IgA, and IgM.

A molecule of immunoglobulin derived from the proliferation of one plasma cell (clone) is called a *monoclonal immunoglobulin* or *paraprotein*. A marked increase in such a monoclonal Ig is found in the serum of patients who have plasma cell malignancy (myeloma). Monoclonal increases are seen on electrophoretic patterns as spikes. Although these immunoglobulins are typically in the β or λ fractions, on occasion, one may appear in the α₂ area. The monoclonal immunoglobulin is typed by the immunofixation method to determine it as IgG, IgA, or IgM, and identify κ or λ light chains. Increases in IgD or IgE, or heavy chain disease should be considered if there is no reaction with the typical immunofixation electrophoresis antisera.

IgG is increased in liver disease, infections, and collagen disease. A decrease in IgG is associated with an increased susceptibility to infections and monoclonal gammopathy of one of the other idiotypes.

IgA is the idiotypic immunoglobulin present in the respiratory and gastrointestinal mucosa. IgA in fluids other than serum has an additional secretory peptide, called a *J piece*. This piece enables the IgA to appear in secretions. Polyclonal increases in the serum IgA (without the J piece) are found in liver disease, infections, and autoimmune diseases. Decreased serum concentrations are found in depressed protein synthesis, ataxia-telangiectasia, and hereditary immunodeficiency disorders.

IgM is the first antibody that appears in response to antigenic stimulation. IgM also is the type of antibody that acts as anti-A and anti-B antibody to red cell antigens, rheumatoid factors, and heterophile antibodies. Increased IgM concentration is found in toxoplasmosis, cytomegalovirus, rubella, herpes, syphilis, and various bacterial and fungal diseases. A monoclonal increase is seen in Waldenström's macroglobulinemia. This increase is seen as a spike in the vicinity of the late β zone of a protein electrophoretic pattern. Decreases are seen in protein-losing conditions and immunodeficiency disorders.

IgD is the immunoglobulin with the fourth highest concentration in normal serum. Its concentration is increased in infections, liver disease, and connective-tissue disorders. IgD multiple myeloma also has been reported with a monoclonal spike in the late β zone of the electrophoretic pattern.

IgE is the idiotypic immunoglobulin associated with allergic and anaphylactic reactions. Polyclonal increases are seen in allergies, including asthma and hay fever. Monoclonal increases are seen in IgE myeloma, a rare disease.

Miscellaneous Proteins

Myoglobin

Myoglobin is a heme protein found in striated skeletal and cardiac muscles. It accounts for approximately 2% of total muscle protein. A minor portion of the myoglobin found in cells is structurally bound but most of it is dissolved in the cytoplasm. It comprises one polypeptide chain containing 153 amino acids, coupled to a heme group. In size, myoglobin, with a molecular weight of 17,800 daltons, is slightly larger than one-fourth of a hemoglobin molecule. It can reversibly bind oxygen in a manner similar to the hemoglobin molecule, but myo-

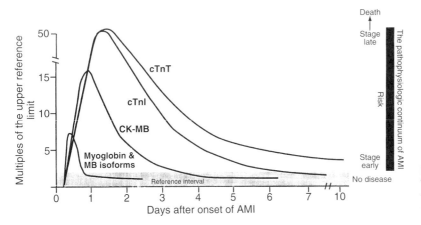

FIGURE 8-10. Current cardiac markers: relative level versus time of onset after AMI. (Source: Alan Wu, PhD, and Robert Jesse, MD, PhD; developed for a wall chart sponsored by Behring Diagnostics, San Jose, CA.)

globin requires a very low oxygen tension to release the bound oxygen. The serum baseline level varies with physical activity and muscle mass and is in the range of 30–90 ng/mL (μg/L) for adult males. Females typically show myoglobin concentrations of less than 50 ng/mL.

When striated muscle is damaged, myoglobin is released, elevating the blood levels. In an acute myocardial infarction (AMI), this increase is seen within 1–3 hours of onset and reaches peak concentration in 5–12 hours. For the diagnosis of AMI, serum myoglobin should be measured serially. If a repeated myoglobin level doubles within 1–2 hours after the initial value, it is highly diagnostic of an AMI.[22] The degree of elevation indicates the size of the infarct. Because myoglobin is a small molecule, the kidney freely filters it, and blood levels return to normal in 18–30 hours after the AMI. Therefore, an increase in myoglobin in the circulation is an early indicator of myocardial infarction and is useful in determining patients who would benefit from thrombolytic therapy. Because of the speed of appearance and clearance of myoglobin, it also is a useful marker for monitoring the success or failure of reperfusion. Figure 8-10 shows the relative level versus time of onset after an AMI for certain current cardiac markers. Although the diagnostic sensitivity of myoglobin elevations following an AMI has been reported to be between 75% and 100%, myoglobin is not cardiac specific. Elevations are also seen in conditions such as progressive muscular dystrophy and crushing injury in which skeletal muscle is damaged. As myoglobin is eliminated from the circulation through the kidneys, renal failure can also elevate the level of serum myoglobin. Table 8-4 lists some of the causes of a myoglobin elevation.

Latex agglutination, enzyme-linked immunosorbent assay (ELISA), immunonephelometry, and fluoroimmunoassays for myoglobin have been developed. A qualitative spot test using immunochromatography is also available.

Troponin

Troponin is a complex of three proteins that bind to the thin filaments of striated muscle (cardiac and skeletal) but are not present in smooth muscle. The complex consists of troponin T (TnT), troponin I (TnI), and troponin C (TnC). Together, they function to regulate muscle contraction. The muscle contraction cycle begins with a release of calcium in response to nerve impulses. Troponin C (MW, 18,000) binds the calcium, causing a conformational change in the troponin–tropomyosin complex. Tropomyosin is a rod-shaped protein that stretches the entire length of the actin backbone (actin is the major constituent of thin filaments). This movement allows the head of the myosin molecule, which forms the thick filaments of muscle, to interact with actin. The binding of myosin and actin accelerates the myosin ATPase activity, and the result is muscle contraction. With the hydrolysis

TABLE 8-4. CAUSES OF MYOGLOBIN ELEVATIONS

Acute myocardial infarction
Angina without infarction
Rhabdomyolysis
Multiple fractures; muscle trauma
Renal failure
Myopathies
Vigorous exercise
Intramuscular injections
Open heart surgery
Tonic–clonic seizures
Electric shock
Arterial thrombosis
Certain toxins

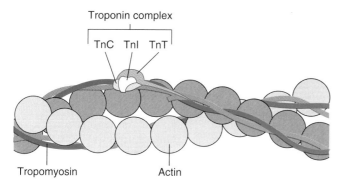

FIGURE 8-11. Schematic of a muscle thin filament.

of ATP, the myosin head returns to its original position and the cycle can begin again. Troponin I (MW, 24,000) regulates this striated muscle contraction by preventing the binding of the myosin head to actin and inhibiting myosin ATPase activity. TnI also serves to bind the actin filament to TnC. The function of troponin T (MW, 37,000) is to bind to tropomyosin and position the troponin complex along the actin filament. The structure of the muscle thin filament is shown in Figure 8-11.

Three genes code for TnT: one each in cardiac muscle and fast- and slow-skeletal muscle. TnI, also encoded by three genes, has similar isoforms, whereas TnC, encoded by two genes, has only a cardiac and slow-skeletal muscle form. The isoforms have different amino acid structures and are biochemically distinct and, therefore, can be differentiated from one another. Of particular interest are the cardiac isoforms of troponin T (cTnT) and troponin I (cTnI). Cardiac troponin T levels in serum begin to rise within 3–4 hours following the onset of myocardial damage, peak in 10–24 hours, and remain elevated for 10–14 days following AMI (Fig. 8-10). Because cardiac TnT is specific for heart muscle, and even small amounts of cardiac necrosis cause release of discernible amounts of cTnT into the serum, measurement of this protein is a valuable aid in the diagnosis of AMI. Cardiac TnT is also useful in monitoring the effectiveness of thrombolytic therapy in myocardial infarction patients. The ratio of peak cardiac TnT concentration on day 1 to cardiac TnT concentration at day 4 discriminates between patients with successful (ratio >1) and failed (ratio ≤1) reperfusion.[23] Another use of cTnT is in the risk assessment of patients with acute myocardial ischemia.[24,25] The prognosis of these patients is variable. The duration, frequency, and timing of ischemic symptoms can be used to determine the severity of unstable angina but are not predictive of events such as infarction, cardiogenic shock, heart failure, ventricular arrhythmia, or even death. However, elevated cTnT values have been shown to be associated with an increased incidence of adverse outcomes, and the higher the cTnT value, the greater the risk. The prognostic value of cTnT is inde-

pendent of age, hypertension, number of antianginal drugs, and electrocardiographic changes. The identification of patients at risk of developing severe complications allows for institution of long-term antithrombotic protection. One disadvantage of cTnT that has been reported is the potential for false-positive elevations in renal failure patients.[26]

Cardiac troponin I is also highly specific for myocardial tissue.[27] Because cTnI, like cTnT, does not normally circulate in the blood and it is 13 times more abundant in the myocardium than CK-MB on a weight basis, cTnI is a very sensitive indicator of even a minor amount of cardiac necrosis. Following an AMI, cTnI levels begin to rise in 3–6 hours, reach peak concentration in 14–20 hours, and return to normal in 5–10 days (Fig. 8-10). The relative increase in cTnI is greater than CK-MB or myoglobin following thrombolytic therapy reperfusion studies. Elevated cardiac troponin I is also associated with increased risk of mortality and morbidity in patients with ischemic heart disease. In evaluating cTnT and cTnI, both offered comparable information.

Although single measurements are useful for risk stratification, serial measurements are needed for accurate diagnosis of AMI. Sequential cardiac troponin determinations on samples drawn at 3- to 8-hour intervals over a period of 48 hours following an AMI will demonstrate the classic rise and fall seen with other cardiac markers. Cardiac troponins can be measured on serum or heparinized plasma by ELISA or immunoenzymometric assays using two monoclonal antibodies directed against different epitopes on the protein. The reference interval for cTnT is <0.1 ng/mL (mg/L). The cutoff concentration for cTnI immunoassays varies 0.1–3.1 ng/mL (mg/L). This difference can be explained, at least partly, by different specificities of the monoclonal antibodies used in the assays. Data have indicated that the largest portion of troponin I released into the bloodstream following myocardial tissue damage is in the form of a complex with cTnC, whereas only a small part is the free form.[28] The ratio of total to free cTnI varies during the period the troponin circulates in the bloodstream and is different in samples from different patients. Cardiac TnC, when complexed with cTnI, causes structural and chemical changes in cTnI that can mask certain epitopes and diminish the interaction of cTnI with certain monoclonal antibodies. In other assays, the pairs of antibodies used recognize epitopes that are not perturbed or sterically shielded by other troponin complexes. These antibodies will react equally with free and complexed cTnI, resulting in higher cutoff values.

There are also rapid immunochromatographic drystrip assays available. Immobilized antibodies bind troponin and produce a purplish band in the test window. The intensity and speed at which the color forms are related to the concentration of the specific troponin.

Fibronectin

Fibronectin is a glycoprotein composed of two nearly identical subunits. Although fibronectin is the product of a single gene, the resulting protein can exist in multiple forms due to splicing of a single pre-mRNA.[29] The variants demonstrate a wide variety of cellular interactions, including roles in cell adhesion, tissue differentiation, growth, and wound healing. These proteins are found in plasma and on cell surfaces and can be synthesized by the liver hepatocytes, endothelial cells, peritoneal macrophages and fibroblasts. Plasma fibronectin has been used as a nutritional marker.

Recently, interest has focused on a unique fibronectin, fetal fibronectin (fFN), as a predictor for preterm delivery. Fetal fibronectin is normally present in amniotic fluid and placental tissue. It exists in the extracellular matrix where the implanted ovum and placental membranes come in contact with the uterine wall and functions to maintain the adherence of the placenta to the uterus. When labor begins, the membranes rupture and there is an increase in the fetal fibronectin level in cervical and vaginal secretions. Therefore, impending preterm delivery due to conditions that cause disruption of the membranes, such as stress, infection, or hemorrhage, can be identified by detection of fFN in cervicovaginal secretions. After collection of these secretions using a swab, fetal fibronectin concentrations are determined by immunoassay. In a normal pregnancy, after the gestational sac attaches to the endometrium at 20–22 weeks gestation, fFN levels in cervicovaginal secretions are <50 ng/mL and undetectable by routine assays. Therefore, the presence of fFN in detectable concentrations, a positive test, indicates a high risk for premature delivery.[30] A quantitative assay is also available.

Amyloid

Amyloid is a protein–polysaccharide complex produced and deposited in tissue during some chronic infections, malignancies, and rheumatologic disorders. It is a homogenous substance staining readily with Congo red. Amyloid fibrils may infiltrate many organs, including the heart and blood vessels, brain and peripheral nerves, kidneys, liver, spleen, and intestines, causing localized or widespread organ failure. Therefore, clinical manifestations of the resultant disorder, amyloidosis, are enormously varied.

Total Protein Abnormalities

Measurement of total plasma protein content provides general information reflecting disease states in many organ systems.

Hypoproteinemia

A total protein level less than the reference interval—*hypoproteinemia*—occurs in any condition where a negative nitrogen balance exists. One cause of a low level of plasma proteins is excessive loss. Plasma proteins can be lost by excretion in the urine in renal disease (ie, nephrotic syndrome); leakage into the gastrointestinal tract in inflammation of the digestive system; and the loss of blood in open wounds, internal bleeding, or extensive burns. Another circumstance producing hypoproteinemia is decreased intake either because of deficiency of protein in the diet (malnutrition) or through intestinal malabsorption due to structural damage (ie, sprue). Without adequate dietary intake of proteins, there is a deficiency of certain essential amino acids and protein synthesis is impaired. A decrease in serum proteins as a result of decreased synthesis is also seen in liver disease (site of all nonimmune protein synthesis) or in inherited immunodeficiency disorders, in which antibody production is diminished. Additionally, hypoproteinemia may result from accelerated catabolism of proteins, such as occurs in burns, trauma, or other injuries.

Hyperproteinemia

An increase in total plasma proteins—*hyperproteinemia*—is not seen as commonly as hypoproteinemia. One condition in which an elevation of all protein fractions is observed is dehydration. When excess water is lost from the vascular system, the proteins, because of their size, remain within the blood vessels. Although the absolute quantity of proteins remains unchanged, the concentration is elevated due to a decreased volume of solvent water. Dehydration results from a variety of conditions, including vomiting, diarrhea, excessive sweating, diabetic acidosis, and hypoaldosteronism. In addition to dehydration, hyperproteinemia may be a result of excessive production, primarily of the γ-globulins.

Some disorders are characterized by the appearance of a monoclonal protein or paraprotein in the serum and often in the urine as well. This protein is an intact immunoglobulin molecule, or occasionally, κ or λ light chains only. The most common disorder is multiple myeloma, in which the neoplastic plasma cells proliferate in the bone marrow. The paraprotein in this case is usually IgG, IgA, or κ or λ light chains. IgD and IgE paraproteins rarely occur. Paraproteins in multiple myeloma may reach a serum concentration of several grams per deciliter.

Not all paraproteins are associated with multiple myeloma. IgM paraprotein is often found in patients with Waldenström's macroglobulinemia, a more benign condition. Many disorders, including chronic inflammatory states, collagen vascular disorders, and other neoplasms, may be asscciated with paraproteins. Polyclonal increases in immunoglobulins, which would be represented by increases in both κ or λ chains, are seen in the serum and urine in many chronic diseases.

Table 8-5 summarizes the disease states affecting total protein levels with the relative changes in the albumin and globulin fractions.

CASE STUDY 8-3

A 76-year-old woman was admitted to the hospital with gangrene of her right toe. She was disoriented and had difficulty finding the right words to express herself. On evaluation, it was revealed she lived alone and was responsible for her own cooking. A daughter who lived in the area said her mother was a poor eater, even with much encouragement. An ECG, performed on admission, showed possible ectopic rhythm with occasional premature supraventricular contractions. The cardiologist suspected a possible inferior myocardial infarction of undetermined age. Lab results are shown in Case Study Table 8-3.1.

Questions

1. In this patient, what is the clinical value of the troponin I measurements?

2. What is a possible explanation for the elevated myoglobin?

3. What condition is indicated by the low prealbumin value?

CASE STUDY TABLE 8-3.1 LABORATORY RESULTS

Day 1		
CK-total	187 U/L	(40–325)
CK-MB Mass	6 µg/L	(<8)
Troponin I	16.3 µg/L	(0–2)
Prealbumin	15 mg/dL	(17–42)
Albumin	2.7 g/dL	(3.7–4.9)
Repeat (5 Hours Later)		
CK-total	180 U/L	
CK-MB mass	5.4 µg/L	
Troponin I	17.5 µg/L	
Day 2		
CK-total	177 U/L	
CK-MB mass	4.5 µg/L	
Troponin I	13.7 µg/L	
Myoglobin	<500 µg/L	(<76)

Methods of Analysis

Total Nitrogen

A total nitrogen determination measures all chemically bound nitrogen in the sample. The method can be applied to various biologic samples, including plasma and urine. In plasma, both the total protein and nonprotein nitrogenous compounds, such as urea and creatinine, are measured. The analysis of total nitrogen level is useful in assessing nitrogen balance. Monitoring the nitrogen nutritional status is particularly important in patients receiving total parenteral nutrition, such as individuals

TABLE 8-5. PROTEIN LEVELS IN SELECTED DISEASE STATES

TOTAL PROTEIN	ALBUMIN	GLOBULIN	DISEASE
N, ↓	↓	↑	Hepatic Damage • Cirrhosis β-γ bridging • Hepatitis ↑ γ-globulins • Obstructive jaundice ↑ α_2-, β-globulins Burns, Trauma Infections • Acute ↑ α_1-, α_2-globulins • Chronic ↑ α_1-, α_2-, γ-globulins
↓	↓	N	Malabsorption Inadequate Diet Nephrotic Syndrome ↑ α_2-, β-globulins; ↓ γ-globulins
↓	N	↓	Immunodeficiency Syndromes
↓	↓	↓	Salt Retention Syndrome
↑	↑	↑	Dehydration
↑	N	↑	Multiple Myeloma Monoclonal and Polyclonal Gammopathies

↑ = increased; ↓ = decreased; N = normal levels.

with neurologic injuries who are sustained on intravenous fluids for an extended period.

The method for total nitrogen analysis uses chemiluminescence. The sample, in the presence of oxygen, is heated to a high temperature ($1100 \pm 20°C$). Any chemically bound nitrogen is oxidized to nitric oxide. The nitric oxide is then mixed with ozone (O_3) to form an excited nitrogen dioxide molecule (NO_2^*). When this molecule decays to the ground state, it emits a photon of light. The amount of light emitted is proportional to the concentration of nitrogen in the sample. This chemiluminescence signal is compared with that of a standard for quantitation.

Total Proteins

The specimen most often used to determine the total protein is serum rather than plasma. The specimen need not be collected when the patient is fasting, although interferences in some of the methods occur with the presence of lipemia. Hemolysis will falsely elevate the total protein result because of the release of RBC proteins into the serum. Clear serum samples, tightly stoppered, are stable for a week or longer at room temperature, for a month at $2°–4°C$, and for at least 2 months at $–20°C$.[31]

The reference interval for serum total protein is 6.5–8.3 g/dL (65–83 g/L) for ambulatory adults. In the recumbent position, the serum total protein concentration is 6.0–7.8 g/dL (60–78 g/L). This lower normal range is a result of shifts in water distribution in the extracellular compartments. The total protein concentration is lower at birth, reaching adult levels by age 3 years. There is a slight decrease with age. Lower total protein levels are also seen in pregnancy. Methods for the determination of total protein are described below and summarized in Table 8-6.

Kjeldahl. The classic method for quantitation of total protein is the Kjeldahl method. Because it is precise and accurate, it is used as a standard by which other methods are compared. In this method, nitrogen is determined; an average of 16% nitrogen mass in protein is assumed to calculate the protein concentration.

The serum proteins are precipitated with an organic acid such as TCA or tungstic acid. The nonprotein nitrogen is removed with the supernatant. The protein pellet is digested in H_2SO_4 with heat ($340°–360°C$) and a catalyst, such as cupric sulfate, to speed the reaction. Potassium sulfate is also introduced to increase the boiling point to improve the efficiency of digestion. The H_2SO_4 oxidizes the C, H, and S in protein to CO_2, CO, H_2O, and SO_2. The nitrogen in the protein is converted to ammonium bisulfite (NH_4HSO_4), which is then measured by adding alkali and distilling the ammonia into a standard boric acid solution. The ammonium borate ($NH_4H_2BO_3$) formed is then titrated with a standard solution of HCL to determine the amount of nitrogen in the original protein solution.

This method is not used in the clinical laboratory because it is time consuming and too tedious for routine use. The nitrogen content of each individual protein may differ from the 16% assumed in the Kjeldahl calculation described. The actual nitrogen content of serum proteins varies 15.1–16.8%. Thus, if one uses a protein standard (calibrated with the Kjeldahl) that differs in composition from the serum specimen to be analyzed, an error is introduced because the percentage of nitrogen will not be the same. It is also necessary to assume that no proteins of significant concentration in the unknown specimen are lost in the precipitation step. Despite these assumptions, the Kjeldahl method is still considered by some to be the reference method for proteins.

Refractometry. Refractometry is useful when a rapid method that requires a small volume of serum is needed. The velocity of light is changed as it passes the boundary between two transparent layers (ie, air and water), causing the light to be bent (refracted). When a solute is added to the water, the refractive index at $20°C$ of 1.330 for pure water is increased by an amount proportional to the concentration of the solute in solution. This proportionality holds fairly well over a 2- to 3-fold increase in concentration (ie, from 520 g/dL). Because the majority of the solids dissolved in serum are protein, the refractive index reflects the concentration of protein. However, in

TABLE 8-6. TOTAL PROTEIN METHODS

METHOD	PRINCIPLE	COMMENT
Kjeldahl	Digestion of protein; measurement of nitrogen content	Reference method; assume average nitrogen content of 16%
Refractometry	Measurement of refractive index due to solutes in serum	Rapid and simple; assume nonprotein solids are present in same concentration as in the calibrating serum
Biuret	Formation of violet-colored chelate between Cu^{2+} ions and peptide bonds	Routine method; requires at least two peptide bonds and an alkaline medium
Dye-binding	Protein binds to dye and causes a spectral shift in the absorbance maximum of the dye	Research use

addition to protein, serum contains several nonprotein solids, such as electrolytes, urea, and glucose, that contribute to the refractive index of serum. Therefore the built-in scale in the refractometer must be calibrated with a serum of a known protein concentration that also has the nonprotein constituents present. An assumption is made that the test samples contain these other solutes in nearly the same concentration as in the calibrating serum. Error is introduced when these substances are increased or when the serum is pigmented (from bilirubin), lipemic, or hemolyzed. The refractive index is also temperature dependent, and some refractometers incorporate a built-in temperature correction.

The total protein is commonly measured with a hand-held refractometer. A drop of serum is placed by capillary action between a coverglass and the prism. The refractometer is held so that light is refracted through the serum layer. The refracted rays cause part of the field of view to be light, producing a point at which there is a sharp line between light and dark. The number of grams per liter at this line on the internal scale is read. The temperature is corrected in the TS meter (American Optical Corp, Scientific Instruments Division; Buffalo, NY) by a liquid crystal system.

The measurement of total protein by refractometry is easy and fast. The accuracy is acceptable,[32] with a reported agreement of $\pm 3\%$ with the biuret method, but it is subject to false-positive interferences.

Biuret. The biuret procedure is the most widely used method and the one recommended by the International Federation of Clinical Chemistry expert panel for the determination of total protein. In this reaction, cupric ions (Cu^{2+}) complex with the groups involved in the peptide bond. In an alkaline medium and in the presence of at least two peptide bonds, a violet-colored chelate is formed. The reagent also contains sodium potassium tartrate to complex cupric ions to prevent their precipitation in the alkaline solution, and potassium iodide, which acts as an antioxidant. The absorbance of the colored chelate formed is measured at 540 nm. When small peptides react, the color of the chelate produced has a different shade than that seen with larger peptides. The color varies from a pink to a reddish violet. However, there is no discernible difference in the reaction given by the proteins normally seen in plasma. Over a wide range of concentrations, therefore, the color that is formed is proportional to the number of peptide bonds present and reflects the total protein level. However, in the presence of abnormally small proteins, such as those seen in multiple myeloma, the concentration of the protein would be underestimated due to the lighter shade of color produced. If lipemic sera must be analyzed, a method for overcoming this problem is available.[33]

In addition to the NHCO group that occurs in the peptide bond, cupric ions will react with any compound that has two or more of the following groups: $NHCH_2$ and NHCS. The method was named because a substance called biuret ($NH_2CONHCONH_2$) reacted with cupric ions in the same manner. There must be a minimum of two of the reactive groups; therefore, amino acids and dipeptides will not react.

Dye Binding. The dye-binding methods are based on the ability of most proteins in serum to bind dyes, although the affinity with which they bind may vary. Bromphenol blue, Ponceau S, amido black 10B, lissamine green, and Coomassie brilliant blue have been used to stain protein bands after electrophoresis. Additionally a dye-binding method for the determination of total protein using Coomassie brilliant blue 250 has been described. The binding of Coomassie brilliant blue 250 to protein causes a shift in the absorbance maximum of the dye from 465 to 595 nm. The increase in absorbance at 595 is used to determine the protein concentration. Although the method is simple and fast, the unequal dye-binding responses of individual proteins has prompted a recommendation for caution when applying this test to the complex mixture of protein found in serum.

Ultraviolet Absorption. Serum proteins also have been estimated by the use of ultraviolet spectrophotometry. Proteins absorb light at 280 nm and at 210 nm. The absorptivity (absorbance of a 1% solution in a 1-cm light path) at 280 nm is related to the absorbance of tyrosine, tryptophan, and phenylalanine amino acids in the protein. Human albumin has only one tryptophan residue in the molecule and has an absorptivity of 5.31 compared with fibrinogen, which has 55 tryptophan residues and an absorptivity of 15.1.

The absorbance of proteins at 210 nm is a result of the absorbance of the peptide bond at that wavelength. The wavelength at which maximal absorbance occurs depends to a small degree on the conformation of the protein. These methods have rarely been used in clinical laboratories but are used routinely in research laboratories to monitor eluates of protein separations from columns. To use these methods, the assumptions must remain that the composition of the unknown serum specimen is near that of the calibrating solution.

Fractionation, Identification, and Quantitation of Specific Proteins

In the assay of total serum proteins, useful diagnostic information can be obtained by determining the albumin fraction and the globulins. A reversal or significant change in the ratio of albumin and total globulin was first noticed in diseases of the kidney and liver. To determine the albumin/globulin (A/G) ratio, it is common to determine total protein and albumin. Globulins are calculated by subtracting the albumin from the total protein (total protein/albumin = globulins).

TABLE 8-7. ALBUMIN METHODS

METHOD	PRINCIPLE	COMMENT
Salt precipitation	Globulins are precipitated in high salt concentrations; albumin in supernatant is quantitated by biuret reaction	Labor intensive
Dye binding		
Methyl orange	Albumin binds to dye; causes shift in absorption maximum	Nonspecific for albumin
HABA [2(4'-hydroxyazobenzene)-benzoic acid]	Albumin binds to dye; causes shift in absorption maximum	Many interferences (salicylates, bilirubin)
BCG (bromcresol green)	Albumin binds to dye; causes shift in absorption maximum	Sensitive; overestimates low albumin levels; most commonly used dye
BCP (bromcresol purple)	Albumin binds to dye; causes shift in absorption maximum	Specific, sensitive, precise
Electrophoresis	Proteins separated based on electric charge	Accurate; gives overview of relative changes in different protein fractions

When an abnormality is found in the total protein or albumin, an electrophoretic analysis is usually performed. Serum proteins are separable into five or more fractions by the customary electrophoretic methods. If an abnormality is seen on the electrophoretic pattern, an analysis of the individual proteins within the area of abnormality is made.

The methods for measuring protein fractions are described in the following text. Table 8-7 lists the types of analyses used in quantitating albumin levels.

Salt Fractionation. Fractionation of proteins has been accomplished by various procedures using precipitation. Globulins can be separated from albumin by salting out using sodium salts. Salts, by decreasing the water available for hydration of hydrophilic groups, will cause precipitation of the globulins. Several different concentrations (26–28% w/v) of different salts (eg, Na_2SO_4, Na_2SO_3) have been used. The albumin that remains in solution in the supernatant can then be measured by any of the routine total protein methods. Salting out is not used to separate the albumin fraction in most laboratories today because direct methods are available that react specifically with albumin in a mixture of proteins.

Dye Binding. The most widely used methods for determining albumin are dye-binding procedures. The pH of the solution is adjusted so that albumin is positively charged. Then, by electrostatic forces, the albumin is attracted to and binds to an anionic dye. When bound to albumin, the dye has a different absorption maximum than the free dye. The amount of albumin can be quantitated by measurement of the absorbance of the albumin–dye complex. A variety of dyes have been used, including

methyl orange, 2-4'-hydroxy-azobenzene)-benzoic acid (HABA), bromocresol green (BCG), and bromcresol purple (BCP). Methyl orange is nonspecific for albumin; β-lipoproteins and some α_1- and α_2-globulins also will bind to this dye. HABA, although more specific for albumin, has a low sensitivity. In addition, several compounds, such as salicylates, penicillin, conjugated bilirubin, and sulfonamides, interfere with the binding of albumin to the dye. BCG is not affected by interfering substances such as bilirubin and salicylates; however, hemoglobin can bind to the dye. For every 100 mg/dL of hemoglobin, the albumin is increased by 0.1 g/dL.[34] Measurement of albumin by BCG has also been reported to overestimate low albumin values. This was particularly observed in patients when the low albumin level was accompanied by an elevated α-globulin fraction, such as occurs in nephrotic syndrome or end-stage renal disease.[35] It was found that the α-globulins, such as ceruloplasmin and α_1-acid glycoprotein, would react with BCG, giving a color whose intensity is approximately one-third of the reaction seen with albumin. This reaction of the α-globulins contributed significantly to the absorbance of the test only after incubation times exceeded 5 minutes. Therefore, the specificity of the reaction for albumin can be improved by taking absorbance readings within a standardized short interval after mixing.[36] The times used have varied 0.5 second to 30 seconds after mixing.

Bromcresol purple (BCP) is an alternate dye that may be used for albumin determinations. Binding specifically to albumin, BCP is not subject to most interferences and is precise and exhibits excellent correlation with immunodiffusion reference methods. Analysis of albumin by the BCP method, however, is not without its disadvantages. In patients with renal insufficiency, the BCP method underestimates the serum albumin.[37] The serum of these patients appears to contain either a substance tightly bound to albumin or a structurally altered albumin that affects the binding of BCP. Similarly, BCP binding to albumin is impaired in the presence of covalently bound bilirubin. BCG binding is unaffected in these situations. Today, both the BCG and BCP methods are commonly used to quantitate albumin.

Determination of Total Globulins. Another approach to fractionation of proteins is the measurement of total globulins. Albumin can then be calculated by subtraction of the globulin from total protein. The total globulin level in serum is determined by a direct colorimetric method using glyoxylic acid. Glyoxylic acid, in the presence of Cu^{2+} and in an acid medium (acetic acid and H_2SO_4), condenses with tryptophan found in globulins to produce a purple color. Albumin has approximately 0.2% tryptophan, compared with 2–3% for the serum globulins. When calibrated using a serum of known albumin and globulin concentrations, the total globulins can be determined. The measurement of globulins based on their tryptophan content has never come into common use because of the ease and simplicity of the dye-binding methods for albumin.

Electrophoresis. Electrophoresis separates proteins on the basis of their electric charge densities. The charge characteristics of protein were discussed earlier in this chapter. Protein, when placed in an electric current, will move according to their charge density, which is determined by the pH of a surrounding buffer. At a pH greater than the pI, the protein is negatively charged, and vice versa. The direction of movement depends on whether the charge is positive or negative; cations (positive net charge) migrate to the cathode (negative terminal), whereas anions (negative net charge) migrate to the anode (positive terminal). The speed of the migration largely depends on the degree of ionization of the protein at the pH of the buffer. This can be estimated from the difference between the pI of the protein and the pH of the buffer. The more the pH of the buffer differs from the pI, the greater the magnitude of the net charge of that protein and the faster it will move in the electric field. In addition to the charge density, the velocity of the movement also depends on the electric field strength, size, and shape of the molecule; temperature; and the characteristics of the buffer (ie, pH, qualitative composition, and ionic strength). The specific electrophoretic mobility μ of a protein can be calculated by:

$$\mu = \frac{(s/t)}{F} \qquad \text{(Eq. 8–1)}$$

where

s = distance traveled in cm
t = time of migration in seconds
F = field strength in V cm^{-1}

Tiselius developed electrophoresis using an aqueous medium. This is known as *moving-boundary* or *free electrophoresis*. Later, in the clinical laboratory, paper was used. The term given to the use of a solid medium is *zone electrophoresis*. Paper has been largely replaced by cellulose acetate or agarose gel as the support media used today.

Serum Protein Electrophoresis

In the standard method for serum protein electrophoresis (SPE), serum samples are applied close to the cathode end of a support medium strip that is saturated with an alkaline buffer (pH, 8.6). The support strip is connected to two electrodes and a current is passed through the

---

CASE STUDY 8-4

A 32-year-old woman developed progressive fatigue and, later, edema in her ankles and in other dependent regions of her body when she lay down for prolonged periods. Although she produced near normal volumes of urine, dipstick urinalysis revealed 4-plus protein. Her serum albumin was below the reference range and her serum cholesterol was significantly elevated. Urine protein loss was in the range of 10–15 g/24 hours. Renal biopsy showed extensive glomerular involvement.

Serum protein electrophoresis showed reduced amounts of albumin (2.27 g/dL), α_1-globulins, and γ-globulins. The α_2 fraction was significantly elevated (34.4% of the total) as was the band of β-lipoprotein.

The total serum protein was 4.7 g/dL. The patient became a candidate for renal transplantation. (*Case 8-4 courtesy of Dr. R. McPherson, Chairman, Clinical Pathology, Medical College of Virginia Hospitals, Virginia Commonwealth University Health System.*)

Questions

1. What disease state is the most likely explanation for the patient's symptoms and laboratory results?

2. In this condition, why are the α_2- and β-globulin fractions elevated?

3. Why is the patient edematous?

strip to separate the proteins. All major serum proteins carry a net negative charge at pH 8.6 and will migrate toward the anode. Using the standard methods, the serum proteins arrange themselves into five bands: albumin travels farthest to the anode followed by α_1-globulins, α_2-globulins, β-globulins, and γ-globulins, in that order. The width of the band of proteins in a fraction depends on the number of proteins with slightly different molecular characteristics that are present in that fraction. Homogenous protein gives a narrow band.

After separation, the protein fractions are fixed by immersing the support strip in an acid solution (eg, acetic acid) to denature the proteins and immobilize them on the support medium. The proteins are then stained. A variety of dyes have been used, including Ponceau S, Amido black, or Coomassie blue. The protein appears as bands on the support medium. Typical cellulose acetate electrophoretic patterns are shown in Figure 8-12B, whereas Figure 8-12A shows the patterns obtained using agarose gel as the support medium.

Visual inspection of the membrane is made or the cleared transparent strip is placed in a scanning densitometer. Reflectance measurements also may be made on the uncleared membranes; however, scanning densitometry is more commonly used. The pattern on the membrane is made to move past a slit through which light is transmitted to a phototube to record the absorbance of the dye that is bound to each fraction. Usually this absorbance is recorded on a strip-chart recorder to obtain a pattern of the fractions (Fig. 8-13).

Many scanning densitometers compute the area under the absorbance curve for each band and the percentage of total dye that appears in each fraction. The concentration is then calculated as a percentage of the total protein that was determined by one of the protein methods, such as the biuret procedure.

The computation also may be made by cutting out the small bands from the membrane and eluting the dye from each band in 0.1 M NaOH. The absorbances are added to obtain the total absorbance, and the percentage of the total absorbance found in each fraction is then calculated.

A reference serum control should be run with each electrophoretic run (Fig. 8-13A), and the results should be monitored to maintain 95% confidence limits for the fractions. Reference values for each fraction are as follows: albumin, 53–65% of the total protein (3.5–5.0 g/dL); α_1-globulin, 2.5–5% (0.1–0.3 g/dL); α_2-globulin, 7–13% (0.6–1.0 g/dL); β-globulin, 8–14% (0.7–1.1 g/dL); and γ-globulin, 12–22% (0.8–1.6 g/dL).

Inadvertent use of plasma will result in a narrow band in the β_2-globulin region because of the presence of fibrinogen. The presence of free hemoglobin will cause a blip in the pattern in the late α_2 or early β zone, and the presence of hemoglobin–haptoglobin complexes will cause a small blip in the α_2 zone.

Often the information obtained by quantitation of each fraction is approximately equal to that obtained by visual inspection. The great advantage of electrophoresis compared with the quantitation of specific proteins is the overview it provides. The electrophoretic pattern can give information about the relative increases and decreases within the protein population, as well as information about the homogeneity of a fraction.

Probably the most significant finding from an electrophoretic pattern is monoclonal immunoglobulin disease. The densitometric scan will show a sharp peak if the increase in immunoglobulins is a result of a monoclonal increase (Fig. 8-13B). A spike in the γ, β, or, sometimes, α_2 region signals the need for examination of the immunoglobulins and observation for clinical signs of myelomatosis. Likewise, a deficiency of the predominant immunoglobulin, IgG, is seen as a much paler stain in the γ area. Another significant finding is a decrease in α_1-antitrypsin (Fig. 8-13C).

In nephrotic syndrome, the patient loses serum albumin and low-molecular-weight proteins in the urine. Some IgG is also lost. At the same time, an increase occurs in α_2-macroglobulin, β-lipoprotein, complement components, and haptoglobin. These two events lead to a dramatic decrease in the relative amount of albumin and a significant increase in the relative amounts of α_2-globulin and β-globulin fractions (Fig. 8-13D).

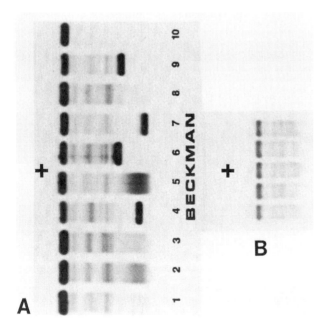

FIGURE 8-12. Serum protein electrophoretic patterns on agarose and cellulose acetate. (**A**) Agarose gel—note the monoclonal γ-globulin; (**B**) cellulose acetate. (Courtesy of Department of Laboratory Medicine, The University of Texas M.D. Anderson Hospital, Drs. Liu, Fritsche, and Trujillo, and Ms. McClure, Supervisor.)

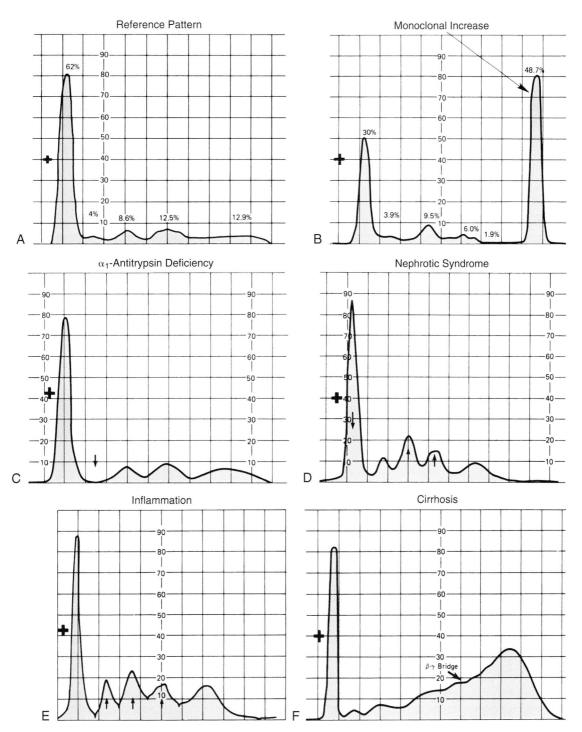

FIGURE 8-13. Selected densitometric patterns of protein electrophoresis. Albumin is at the anodal (+) end followed by α_1-, α_2-, β-, and γ-globulin fractions. *Arrows* indicate decrease or increase in fractions. (**A**) Reference pattern (agarose). (**B**) Monoclonal increase in γ area (agarose). (**C**) α_1-Antitrypsin deficiency (cellulose acetate). (**D**) Nephrotic syndrome (cellulose acetate). (**E**) Inflammation (cellulose acetate). (**F**) Cirrhosis (cellulose acetate). (*A* and *B* are courtesy of Drs. Liu and Fritsche and Jose Trujillo, Director, and Ms. McClure of the Department of Laboratory Medicine, The University of Texas M.D. Anderson Hospital. Others are courtesy of Dr. Wu of the Hermann Hospital Laboratory/The University of Texas Medical School.)

An inflammatory pattern indicating an inflammatory condition is seen when there is a decrease in albumin and an increase in the α_1-globulins (α_1-acid glycoprotein, α_1-antitrypsin), α_2-globulins (ceruloplasmin and haptoglobin), and β-globulin band (C-reactive protein; see Fig. 8-13E). This type of pattern, also called an *acute-phase reactant pattern,* is seen in trauma, burns, infarction, malignancy, and liver disease. Acute-phase reactants are so named because they are increased in the serum within days following trauma or exposure to inflammatory agents. Fibrinogen, haptoglobin, ceruloplasmin, and serum amyloid A increase severalfold, whereas CRP and α_2-macrofetoprotein are increased several hundredfold. Interleukin-1, a protein factor from leukocytes, is recognized as an important mediator of the synthesis of acute-phase proteins by hepatocytes. These acute-phase reactants are thought to play some role in immunoregulatory mechanisms. Chronic infections also produce a decrease in the albumin, but the globulin increase is found in the γ fraction as well as the α_1, α_2, and β fractions.

The electrophoretic pattern of serum proteins in liver disease shows the decrease in serum albumin concentration and the increase in γ-globulin. The pattern in cirrhosis of the liver is rather characteristic, with the abnormalities cited previously; however, in addition, there are some fast moving γ-globulins that prevent resolution of the β- and γ-globulin bands. This is known as the β–γ bridge of cirrhosis (Fig. 8-13F).

In infectious hepatitis, the γ-globulin fraction rises with increasing hepatocellular damage. In obstructive jaundice, there is an increase in the α_2- and β-globulins. Also noted in obstructive jaundice is an increased concentration of lipoproteins, which is an indicator of its biliary origin. This is especially the case when there is little or no decrease of the serum albumin.

High-Resolution Protein Electrophoresis

Standard SPE separates the protein into five distinct zones, which comprise many individual proteins. By modifying the electrophoretic parameters, these fractions may be further resolved into as many as 12 zones. This modification, known as *high-resolution electrophoresis (HRE)*, is accomplished by use of a higher voltage coupled with a cooling system in the electrophoretic apparatus and a more concentrated buffer. The support medium most commonly used is agarose gel. To obtain the HRE patterns, samples are applied on the agarose gel, electrophoresed in a chamber cooled by a gel block, stained, and then visually inspected. Each zone is compared with the same zone on a reference pattern for color density, appearance, migration rates, and appearance of abnormal bands or regions of density. A normal serum HRE pattern is shown in Figure 8-14. In addition, the patterns may be scanned with a densitometer to obtain semiquantitative estimates of the protein found in each zone. HRE is par-

ticularly useful in detecting small monoclonal bands and differentiating unusual bands or prominent increases of normal bands that can masquerade as a monoclonal gammopathy. For example, in patients with nephrotic syndrome, an increased α_2-macroglobulin band in the α_2 region may be confused with a migrating monoclonal protein such as an IgA monoclonal protein gammopathy.[38]

Capillary Electrophoresis

Capillary electrophoresis (CE) is a collection of techniques in which the separation of molecules takes place in small-bore fused silica capillaries. The capillaries are typically 30–50 centimeters long, with an internal diameter between 25 and 100 µm. In capillary zone electrophoresis, the capillaries are filled with a conducting solution, usually an aqueous buffer. One end of the capillary is grounded (detection end) and the other—the sample injection end—is connected to a high voltage

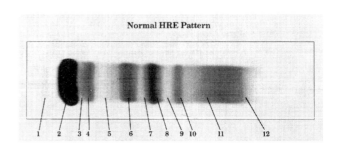

Normal HRE Pattern

Zones	Serum proteins found in zones
1. PREALBUMIN ZONE	-Prealbumin
2. ALBUMIN ZONE	-Albumin
3. ALBUMIN-α_1 INTERZONE	-α-Lipoprotein (α-Fetoprotein)
4. α_1 ZONE	-α_1-Antitrypsin, α_1-Acid glycoprotein
5. α_1-α_2 INTERZONE	-Gc-globulin, inter-α-trypsin inhibitor, α_1-antichymotrypsin
6. α_2 ZONE	-α_2-Macroglobulin, Haptoglobin
7. α_2-β_1 INTERZONE	-Cold insoluble globulin, (Hemoglobin)
8. β_1 ZONE	-Transferrin
9. β_1-β_2 INTERZONE	-β-Lipoprotein
10. β_2 ZONE	-C3
11. γ_1 ZONE	-IgA (Fibrinogen), IgM (Monoclonal Igs, light chains)
12. γ_2 ZONE	-IgC (C-reactive protein) (Monoclonal Igs, light chains)

Proteins listed in ( ) are normally found in too low a concentration to be visible in a normal pattern.

FIGURE 8-14. High-resolution electrophoretic pattern of serum. (Courtesy of Helena Laboratories, Beaumont, TX.)

CASE STUDY 8-5

A 45-year-old man was undergoing continuing evaluation of possible recurrence of a plasmacytoma that had originally presented with a compression fracture of a vertebra. He had been treated with local radiation and chemotherapy. His serum protein electrophoresis showed normal amounts of albumin, α_1, α_2, and β fractions. The γ fraction demonstrated a slight monoclonal band in the fast γ region (close to β). Protein electrophoresis of concentrated urine showed a single monoclonal band that migrated slightly less than the serum band. (*Case 8-5 courtesy of Dr. R. McPherson, Chairman, Clinical Pathology,*

Medical College of Virginia Hospitals, Virginia Commonwealth University Health System)

Questions

1. Does the presence of the monoclonal band in the serum indicate the recurrence of the patient's tumor?

2. What further information is obtained from a urine protein electrophoresis?

3. What other test is needed to confirm the type of urinary protein?

---

power supply. When a positive voltage is applied, the positively charged buffer molecules flow to the detection end, which is grounded and therefore negative relative to the injection end. The net flow of buffer is called electroosmotic flow (EOF). When sample is injected, all molecules will have a tendency to move toward the detector (negative) end of the capillary due to EOF; however, the negatively charged molecules in the specimen will also have a tendency to migrate back toward the injector (positive) end. This is referred to as electrophoretic mobility. EOF is usually stronger than electrophoretic mobility and all ions (positively charged, neutral, and negatively charged) will migrate to the detector end but with different net mobilities based on size and charge differences. The separated molecules are detected by their absorbance as they pass through a small window near the detection end of the capillary. Use of the small-bore capillaries allows heat to be effectively dissipated, which means that higher operating voltages can be used and, therefore, analysis times are faster. Additionally, the sample size required is small (nanoliters).

Isoelectric Focusing

Isoelectric focusing (IEF) is zone electrophoresis that separates proteins on the basis of pI. IEF uses constant power and polyacrylamide or agarose gel, which contains a pH gradient. The pH gradient is established by the incorporation of small polyanions and polycations (ampholytes) in the gel. The varying pIs of the polyions cause them, in the presence of an electric field, to seek their place in the gradient and to remain there. The pH gradient may range from 3.5 to 10.

When a protein is electrophoresed in the gel, it will migrate to a place on the gel where the pH is that of its pI. The protein becomes focused there because, if it should diffuse in either direction, it leaves its pI and gains a net charge. When this occurs, the electric current

once again carries it back to its point of no charge, or its pI.

The clinical applications of IEF have included phenotyping of α_1-antitrypsin deficiencies, determination of genetic variants of enzymes and hemoglobins, detection of paraproteins in serum and oligoclonal bands in CSF, and isoenzyme determinations.

Immunochemical Methods

Specific proteins may be identified by immunochemical assays in which the reaction of the protein (antigen) and its antibody is measured. Methods using various modifications of this principle include RID, immunoelectrophoresis (IEP), immunofixation electrophoresis, electroimmunodiffusion, immunoturbidimetry, and immunonephelometry. These techniques are discussed in Chapter 6, *Immunoassays and Nucleic Acid Probe Techniques*.

Proteins in Other Body Fluids

The kinds of body fluids being studied for their protein content have increased. This is partly a result of the increased sensitivity of the test methods now available. This section includes a discussion of the two fluids whose protein contents are studied most often: urine and CSF.

Urinary Protein

The majority of proteins found in the urine arise from the blood; however, urinary proteins can also originate from the kidney and urinary tract and from extraneous sources such as the vagina and prostate. The proteins in the blood appear in the urine because they have passed through the renal glomerulus and have not been reabsorbed by the renal tubules. The qualitative tests for proteinuria are most commonly performed using a reagent test strip. These methods are based on the change in the response of an indicator dye in the presence of protein, known as protein error of indicators. In an acid pH, the indicator that is yellow in the absence of protein, progresses through various shades of green and finally to blue as the concentration of protein increases. A protein concentration of 6 mg/dL or greater produces a color change.

Most quantitative assays are performed on urine specimens of 12 hours or 24 hours. The 24-hour timing allows for circadian rhythmic changes in excretion at certain times of day. The patient should void, completely emptying the bladder, and discard this urine. Urine is collected from that time for the next 24 hours. At the end of the 24-hour period, the bladder is completely emptied and that urine included in the sample. The volume of the timed specimen is measured accurately and recorded. The results are reported generally in terms of weight of protein per 24 hours by calculating the amount of protein present in the total volume of urine collected during that time.

Several methods have been proposed for the determination of total protein in urine and other body fluids, including the measurement of turbidity when urinary proteins are mixed with an anionic organic acid such as sulfosalicylic acid, TCA, or benzethonium chloride. These methods are sensitive, but the reagent does not react equally with each protein fraction. This is particularly true of sulfosalicylic acid, which produces 4 times more turbidity with albumin than with α-globulin.

A method considered to give more accurate results consists of precipitation of the urine proteins, dissolution of the protein precipitate, and color formation with biuret reagent. Another chemical procedure for urinary protein uses the Folin-Ciocalteau reagent, which is a phosphotungstomolybdic acid solution, frequently called phenol reagent because it oxidizes phenolic compounds. The reagent changes color from yellow to blue during re-

action with tyrosine, tryptophan, and histidine residues in protein. This method is about 10 times more sensitive than the biuret method. Lowry and associates increased the sensitivity of the Folin-Ciocalteau reaction by incorporating a biuret reaction as the initial step. After the binding of the Cu^{2+} to the peptide bonds, the Folin-Ciocalteau reagent is added. As the Cu^{2+} protein complex is oxidized, the reagent is reduced, forming the chromogens tungsten blue and molybdenum blue. This increased the sensitivity to 100 times greater than that of the biuret method alone. Another modification uses a pyrogallol red–molybdate complex that reacts with protein to produce a blue-purple complex. This procedure is easily automated.

Dye-binding methods also have been used to determine the total protein content of body fluids. Methods are available using dyes such as Coomassie blue and Ponceau S. Table 8-8 summarizes the various methods for measurement of urinary total protein.[39]

The reference values or intervals for urinary proteins are highly method dependent, ranging from 100 to 250 mg/24 hours. Because of ease of use, speed, and sensitivity, the techniques used most frequently today are turbidimetric procedures.

Physiologic Significance of Proteinuria. *Proteinuria* in renal disease may be classified as resulting from either glomerular or tubular dysfunction. Glomerular proteinuria is a consequence of loss of glomerular membrane integrity, which normally keeps proteins from passing through to the urine because of their large molecular weight. In early selective glomerular proteinuria, the proteins responsible for the increase are typically albumin (>80%) and transferrin. As the glomerular lesion becomes more severe, the membrane

TABLE 8-8. URINE PROTEIN METHODS

METHOD	PRINCIPLE	COMMENT
Turbidimetric methods (sulfosalicylic acid, trichloroacetic acid, or benzethonium chloride)	Proteins are precipitated as fine particles, turbidity is measured spectrophotometrically	Rapid, easy to use; unequal sensitivity for individual proteins
Biuret	Proteins are concentrated by precipitation, redissolved in alkali, then reacted with Cu^{2+}; Cu^{2+} form colored complex with peptide bonds	Accurate
Folin-Lowry	Initial biuret reaction; oxidation of tyrosine, tryptophan, and histidine residues by Folin phenol reagent (mixture of phosphotungstic and phosphomolybdic acids): measurement of resultant blue color	Very sensitive
Dye-binding (Coomassie blue, Ponceau S)	Protein binds to dye, causes shift in absorption maximum	Limited linearity; unequal sensitivity for individual proteins

CASE STUDY 8-6

A 55-year-old man, with no history of illness, suffered a blow on the head. He was unconscious when admitted to the hospital and remained in that state until his death 15 days later. A nasogastric tube was inserted to administer the required nutrients (protein, carbohydrates, fat, minerals, and vitamins). The total water intake was 1500 mL/day. Starting on day 5, his blood pressure gradually fell. The 24-hour urine volumes recorded from an indwelling catheter were as follows:

DAY AFTER ADMISSION	URINE VOLUME (mL/24 HOURS)
6	1500
8	1300
10	1200
12	1100
14	900

The patient's hemoglobin and hematocrit were elevated.

Blood chemistry analysis on day 13 revealed the following:

Total protein	9.4 g/dL
Albumin	6.0 g/dL
BUN	80 mg/dL
Na	175 mmol/L
K	4.0 mmol/L
Cl	134 mmol/L

Questions

1. What is the probable cause of the elevated proteins?

2. What other results support this conclusion?

3. Why is the BUN elevated?

becomes nonselective, and proteins of all sizes, including immunoglobulins, pass into the urine. Damage to the glomerular membrane occurs in diseases such as diabetes, amyloidosis, and dysglobulinemia and collagen disorders. The presence in the blood of toxic agents, such as mercury or heroin, may also result in loss of glomerular integrity. An early indicator of glomerular dysfunction is the presence of microalbuminuria. The term *microalbuminuria* is used to describe albumin concentrations in the urine that are greater than normal but not detectable with common urine dipstick assays (albumin levels less than lower limit of detection). Studies of patients with diabetes mellitus show that microalbuminuria precedes the nephropathy associated with diabetes, particularly in type 1 (insulin-dependent diabetes mellitus) diabetes.[40] Progression from microalbuminuria to clinical nephropathy can be delayed with intensive therapy to normalize blood glucose and blood pressure. It is recommended, therefore, that all diabetics be tested annually for microalbuminuria. The normal albumin excretion rate is <20 μg/minute or <30 mg/day. Microalbuminuria can be measured by radioimmunoassay, radial immunodiffusion, immunonephelometry, and enzyme immunoassay.

Tubular proteinuria is a result of the renal tubules being unable to perform their usual function of reabsorption because of dysfunction or because the amount of protein appearing in the tubular fluid exceeds the absorptive capability of a normal functioning tubule. In tubular proteinuria, small protein molecules that normally pass through the glomerulus and are reabsorbed, such as β_2-microglobulin (MW, 11,800), retinol-binding protein (MW, 21,000), and α_1-microglobulin (MW, 30,000), appear in the urine.

Overflow proteinuria is an overabundance of proteins from the serum that appear in such high concentrations in the glomerular filtrate that the tubules are overwhelmed in their capacity to absorb them. This type of proteinuria is typified by the increased concentration of immunoglobulin light chains in multiple myeloma (Bence Jones protein). The determination of specific proteins yields much more information than total urinary protein, particularly in the study of tubular proteinuria.

To determine the type of proteins being excreted, most methods require initial concentration of the urine. This is accomplished by precipitation, ultrafiltration, dialysis, or gel filtration techniques. The urine can then be electrophoresed by a method similar to that described for serum. Quantitative measurement of specific urine proteins can be made by use of immunochemical methods, such as radioimmunoassay, radial immunodiffusion, electroimmunoassay, and immunonephelometry.

A protein normally found in urine but not in serum is Tamm-Horsfall protein, a mucoprotein produced in the

An 84-year-old woman resident of a nursing home was admitted to the hospital for treatment of lower back pain resulting from a fall. Radiologic examination revealed a vertebral compression fracture. Because she demonstrated signs of general deterioration, further medical evaluation was performed. A neurologic examination and CT scan were normal. Serologic examinations for collagen vascular disease were also negative, although the erythrocyte sedimentation rate showed a modest increase. Serum protein electrophoresis was done to rule out multiple myeloma. The serum protein fractions were as follows: albumin, 3.2 g/dL; α_1-globulins, 0.31 g/dL; α_2-globulins, 1.59 g/dL (elevated in a tight band); β-globulins, 0.72 g/dL; and γ-globulins, 0.96 g/dL.

Questions

1. What would the next step be in the evaluation of this patient?

2. Given the following additional result, what condition would explain her abnormal protein electrophoresis pattern?

   • Haptoglobin: 416 mg/dL

3. What other proteins would you expect to be abnormal?

renal tubules. It is the major protein constituent of urinary casts. Its concentration in urine is 40.0 mg/day. An IgA (secretory) is also produced in the kidney, and 1.1 mg/day is excreted.

Cerebrospinal Fluid Proteins

CSF is formed in the choroid plexus of the ventricles of the brain by ultrafiltration of the blood plasma. Protein measurement is one test that is usually requested on CSF, in addition to glucose level and differential cell count, culture, and sensitivity. The accepted reference interval for patients between 10 and 40 years of age is 15–45 mg/dL of CSF protein.

The total CSF protein may be determined by several of the more sensitive chemical or optical methods referred to earlier in the discussion on urinary proteins. The most frequently used procedures are turbidimetric using TCA, sulfosalicylic acid with sodium sulfate, or benzethonium chloride. Also available are dye-binding methods (ie, Coomassie brilliant blue), a kinetic biuret reaction, and the Lowry method using a Folin phenol reagent.

Physiologic Significance of CSF Protein Analysis. Abnormally increased total CSF proteins may be found in conditions in which there is an increased permeability of the capillary endothelial barrier through which ultrafiltration occurs. Examples of such conditions include bacterial, viral, and fungal meningitis; traumatic tap; multiple sclerosis; obstruction; neoplasm; disk herniation; and cerebral infarction. The degree of permeability can be evaluated by measuring the CSF albumin and comparing it with the serum albumin. Albumin is usually used as the reference protein for permeability because it is not synthesized to any degree in the CNS. The reference value for the CSF albumin/serum albumin ratio is less than 2.7–7.3. A value greater than this indicates that the increase in the CSF albumin came from serum due to a damaged blood-brain barrier. Low CSF protein values are found in hyperthyroidism and when fluid is leaking from the CNS.

Although total protein levels in the CSF are informative, diagnosis of specific disorders often requires measurement of individual protein fractions. The pattern of types of proteins present can be seen by electrophoresis of CSF that has been concentrated about 100-fold. This may be performed on cellulose acetate or agarose gel. The pattern obtained normally from adult lumbar CSF shows prealbumin, a prominent albumin band, α_1-globulin composed predominantly of α_1-antitrypsin, an α_2 band consisting primarily of haptoglobin and ceruloplasmin, a β_1 band composed principally of transferrin, and a CSF-specific transferrin that is deficient in carbohydrate, referred to as τ protein, in the β_2 zone. The globulin present in the γ band is typically IgG with a small amount of IgA.

Electrophoretic patterns of CSF from patients who have multiple sclerosis have multiple, distinct bands in the γ zone. This is called oligoclonal banding. More than 90% of patients with multiple sclerosis have oligoclonal bands, although the bands also have been found in inflammatory and infectious neurologic disease. The identification of discrete bands in the γ region that are present in the CSF but not in the serum is associated with production of IgG in the CSF, a finding characteristic of demyelinating diseases, such as multiple sclerosis. These bands cannot be seen on routine cellulose acetate electrophoresis but require a high-resolution technique in which agarose is usually used.

The elevated level of IgG in the CSF is not unique to multiple sclerosis. Because the increase in CSF IgG may result from either intrathecal synthesis or increased permeability of the blood-brain barrier, IgG concentrations can also increase in the conditions listed above, such as meningitis. To identify the source of the elevated CSF IgG levels, the IgG-albumin index can be calculated as follows:

$$\text{CSF IgG Index} = \frac{\text{CSF IgG (mg/dL)} \times \text{serum albumin (g/dL)}}{\text{serum IgG (g/dL)} \times \text{CSF albumin (mg/dL)}}$$

(Eq. 8–2)

The CSF albumin concentration corrects for increased permeability. The reference range for the index is 0.25–0.80. The index is elevated when there is increased CNS IgG production such as occurs in multiple sclerosis. IgG production is also increased in some bacterial infections and CNS inflammatory diseases. The IgG index is decreased when the integrity of the blood-brain barrier is compromised, as in some forms of meningitis and tumors. Another index to aid in discriminating the source of the IgG in the CSF is the IgG synthesis rate calculation using the formula of Tourtellotte.[41] The reference interval for the synthesis rate is –9.9 to +3.3 mg/day.

In the investigation of multiple sclerosis, myelin basic proteins present in the CSF are also assayed because these proteins can provide an index of active demyelination. Myelin basic proteins are constituents of myelin, the sheath that surrounds many of the CNS axons. In very active demyelination, concentrations of myelin basic proteins of 17–100 ng/mL were found by radioimmunoassay. In slow demyelination, values of 6–16 ng/mL occurred and, in remission, the values were less than 4 ng/mL. In addition to multiple sclerosis, other conditions that induce CNS demyelination and therefore elevated levels of myelin basic protein include meningoencephalitis, systemic lupus erythematosus of CNS, diabetes mellitus, and chronic renal failure.

SUMMARY

Amino acids are the building blocks of proteins. Inherited abnormalities in amino acid metabolism result in various conditions, most of which are associated with mental retardation. The synthesis of most proteins occurs in the liver, with the exception of the immunoglobulins, which are produced in the plasma cells. The linear sequence of amino acids in the protein, which composes the primary structure, is defined by the genetic code in cellular DNA. Proteins may be simple, comprised only of amino acids, or conjugated, in which the peptide chain is attached to a nonprotein moiety. With the large number of proteins in the plasma (more than 500 identified), the functions are varied. For example, albumin is primarily responsible for the colloid osmotic pressure; haptoglobin

---

CASE STUDY 8-8

A 36-year-old woman complained of intermittent blurred vision and numbness and weakness in her left leg that had persisted for more than three weeks. On examination, vertical nystagmus (involuntary back-and-forth or circular movements of eyes) was noted on upward gaze. CSF was drawn and the specimen was clear and colorless with normal cell count. The CSF total protein level was 49 mg/dL with an IgG of 8.1 mg/dL. Electrophoresis of the patient's serum and CSF revealed the following pattern:

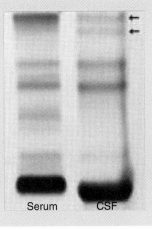

Serum   CSF

Questions

1. What is the significance of the protein bands indicated by the arrows?

2. What conditions would produce this type of protein electrophoresis pattern?

3. What other tests would be helpful in the investigation of this patient's diagnosis?

4. What laboratory test can be useful for monitoring the course of this patient's condition?

and transferrin are transport proteins, binding free hemoglobin and iron, respectively; immunoglobulins and components of the complement system help protect the body against infection; and other proteins, such as fibrinogen, aid in the maintenance of hemostasis. Low levels of total protein may be a result of excessive loss, decreased synthesis, or accelerated catabolism, whereas elevated levels are associated with dehydration or excessive production.

The most widely used method for measuring total serum protein levels is the biuret reaction, in which cupric ions complex with two or more peptide bonds. To determine the albumin fraction, dye-binding techniques are usually used with either BCG or BCP. The dye, when bound to albumin, is a different color than the free dye. Further fractionation of the serum proteins can be accomplished by electrophoresis, which uses the charge characteristics of the protein for separation. Routine SPE arranges the proteins in five bands: albumin travels farthest to the anode, followed by α_1-globulins, α_2-globulins, β-globulins, and γ-globulins. HRE separates protein into 12 zones. Capillary electrophoresis allows for faster separation.

Protein can also be measured in other body fluids. Either glomerular damage or tubular dysfunction will result in elevated urinary proteins. Abnormally increased CSF protein is found in conditions where there is an increased permeability of the capillary endothelial barrier or increased intrathecal synthesis.

REVIEW QUESTIONS

1. The Guthrie screening test for increased serum phenylalanine is based on:
   a. a fluorometric method, in which phenylalanine is reacted with ninhydrin.
   b. the microbiologic procedure, in which phenylalanine counteracts the effects of a metabolic antagonist on the growth of *B. subtilis*.
   c. the thin layer chromatography method, in which identification is made by comparison of the unknown Rf value to Rf values of the known.
   d. a dipstick procedure, in which phenylalanine is converted to phenylpyruvic acid and then reacted with ferric chloride.

2. The three dimensional spatial configuration of a single polypeptide chain as determined by disulfide linkages, hydrogen bonds, electrostatic attractions, and van der Waals forces is referred to as the:
   a. primary structure.
   b. secondary structure.
   c. tertiary structure.
   d. quaternary structure.

3. The plasma protein mainly responsible for maintaining colloidal osmotic pressure in vivo is:
   a. hemoglobin.
   b. fibrinogen.
   c. α_2-macroglobulin.
   d. albumin.

4. Intraindividual differences in total serum protein concentrations attributable to erect versus recumbent postures are:
   a. 0–0.5 g/dL (virtually no difference).
   b. approximately 0.5 g/dL.
   c. approximately 2 g/dL.
   d. approximately 5 g/dL.

5. Poor protein-caloric nutritional status is associated with:
   a. a low level of γ-globulins.
   b. an elevated haptoglobin concentration.
   c. a decreased level of prealbumin.
   d. an increased level of α_1-fetoprotein.

6. In which of the following conditions would a normal level of myoglobin be expected?
   a. Multiple myeloma
   b. Acute myocardial infarction
   c. Renal failure
   d. Crushing trauma received in a car accident

7. A total protein as assayed on serum from a patient with multiple myeloma. The result using the biuret method was lower than the result given by the Kjeldahl method. The discrepancy was a result of the fact that:
   a. the Kjeldahl total protein method measures all nitrogen containing compounds, including proteins and nonprotein nitrogens, and, therefore, overestimates the protein level.
   b. the two methods are based on different principles, a comparable result is not expected.
   c. in the biuret method, abnormally small proteins produce a complex that has a different shade of color than normal proteins, underestimating the protein level.
   d. hemolysis falsely elevates the Kjeldahl method but has no effect on the protein level determined by the biuret method.

8. The protein electrophoretic pattern of plasma, as compared with serum, reveals a:
   a. broad increase in the γ-globulins.
   b. fibrinogen peak with the α_2-globulins.
   c. a decreased albumin peak.
   d. fibrinogen peak between the β- and γ-globulins.

9. The following pattern of serum protein electrophoresis is obtained:

   albumin: decreased

   α_1- and α_2-globulins: increased

   γ-globulins: normal

   This pattern is characteristic of which of the following conditions?
   a. Cirrhosis
   b. Acute inflammation (primary response)
   c. Nephrotic syndrome
   d. Gammopathy

10. One advantage of high-resolution agarose electrophoresis over lower current electrophoresis is:
    a. high-resolution procedures detect monoclonal and oligoclonal bands at lower concentrations.
    b. a smaller sample volume is required.
    c. results are obtained more rapidly.
    d. more sample can be applied to the support medium.

11. When a protein is dissolved in a buffer solution, the pH of which is more alkaline than the pI, and an electric current is passed through the solution, the protein will act as:
    a. an anion and migrate to the anode.
    b. a cation and migrate to the cathode.
    c. an anion and migrate to the cathode.
    d. an uncharged particle and will not move.

12. High serum total protein with high levels of both albumin and globulins is usually seen in:
    a. Waldenström's macroglobulinemia.
    b. glomerulonephritis.
    c. cirrhosis.
    d. dehydration.

Match the serum protein in column A with its specific function in Column B:

Column A	Column B
13. Transferrin _____	a. transports copper
14. Haptoglobin _____	b. inhibits proteolytic enzymes
15. α-Antitrypsin _____	c. factor in the formation of a clot in vivo
	d. transports iron
	e. binds free hemoglobin
	f. regulates muscle contraction
	g. combines with specific antigens
	h. catalyst in the urea cycle

REFERENCES

1. Natelson S, Natelson E. Principles of Applied Clinical Chemistry Plasma Proteins in Nutrition and Transport. Vol. 3. New York: Plenum, 1980.
2. Phenylketonuria (PKU): Screening and management. NIH Consensus Statement 2000;17(3):1–33.
3. Levy HL, Albers S. Genetic screening of newborns. Annu Rev Genomics Hum Genet 2000;1:139–177.
4. Yamaguchi A, Mizushima Y, Fukushi M, et al. Microassay system for newborn screening for phenylketonuria, maple syrup urine disease, homocystinuria, histidinemia and galactosemia with use of a fluorometric microplate reader. Screening 1992;1:49.
5. Chace DH, Kalas TA, Naylor EW. The application of tandem mass spectrometry to neonatal screening for inherited disorders of intermediary metabolism. Annu Rev Genomics Hum Genet 2002;3:17–45.
6. Lidsky A, Guttler F, Woo S. Prenatal diagnosis of classic phenylketonuria by DNA analysis. Lancet 1985;1:549.
7. Kayaalp E, Treacy E, Waters PJ, Byck S, Nowacki P, Scriver CR. Human phenylalanine hydroxylase mutations and hyperphenylalaninemia phenotypes: a metanalysis of genotype-phenotype correlations. Am J Hum Genet 1997;61:1309–1317.
8. Brattström L, Wilcken DEL. Homocysteine and cardiovascular disease: cause or effect? Am J Clin Nutr 2000;72(2):315–323.
9. Ueland PM, Refsum H, Beresford SAA, Vollset SE. The controversy over homocysteine and cardiovascular risk. Am J Clin Nutr 2000;72(2):324–332.
10. Stephens AD. Cystinuria and its treatment: 25 years experience at St. Bartholomew's Hospital. J Inherit Metab Dis 1989;12:197.
11. Deyl Z, Hyanek J, Horokova M. Profiling of amino acids in body fluids and tissues by means of liquid chromatography. J Chromatogr 1986;379:177.
12. Hitzig WH, Joller PW. Developmental aspects of plasma proteins. In: Ritzmann SE, Killingsworth LM, eds. Body Fluids, Amino Acids, and Tumor Markers: Diagnostic and Clinical Aspects, 3rd ed. New York: Alan Liss, 1983:1.
13. Haferkamp O, Schlettwein-Gsell D, Schwick HG, et al. Serum protein in an aging population with particular reference to evaluation of immune globulins and antibodies. Gerontologia 1966;12:30.
14. Keyser JW. Human Plasma Proteins. New York: Wiley, 1979:280.
15. Gabant P, Forrester L, Nichols J, et al. Alpha-fetoprotein, the major fetal serum protein, is not essential for embryonic development but is required for female fertility. Proc Natl Acad Sci USA 2002;99(20):12865–12870.
16. Rubin H. The biology and biochemistry of antichymotrypsin and its potential role as a therapeutic agent. Biol Chem Hoppe Seyler 1992;373(7):497.
17. Balduyck M, Mizo J. Inter-alpha-trypsin inhibitor and its plasma and urine derivatives. Ann Biol Clin 1991;49(5):273.
18. Levy AP, Hochberg I, Jablonski K, et al. Haptoglobin phenotype is an individual risk factor for cardiovascular disease in individuals with diabetes: the strong heart study. J Am Coll Cardiol 2002;40(11):1984–1990.

19. Lyngbye J, Kroll J. Quantitative immunoelectrophoresis of proteins in serum from a normal population: season, age and sex-related variations. Clin Chem 1971;17:495.

20. Ridker PM. Clinical application of C-reactive protein for cardiovascular disease detection and prevention. Circulation 2003;107: 363–372.

21. LeGrys VA. The use of high sensitivity C-reactive protein in assessing the risk for coronary heart disease. Clin Lab Sci 2001; 14(4):243–246.

22. Wong SS. Strategic utilization of cardiac markers for the diagnosis of acute myocardial infarction. Ann Clin Lab Sci 1996;26(4): 301.

23. Mair J, Dienstl F, Puschendorf B. Cardiac troponin T in the diagnosis of myocardial injury. Crit Rev Clin Lab Sci 1992;29(1):31.

24. Christenson RH. Cardiac troponin T in the risk assessment of acute coronary syndromes. Am Clin Lab June 1997:18.

25. Ohman EM, et al. Cardiac troponin T levels for risk stratification in acute myocardial ischemia. N Engl J Med 1996;335(18):1333.

26. Li D, Keffer J, Corry K, et al. Nonspecific elevation of troponin T levels in patients with chronic renal failure. Clin Biochem 1995; 28(4):474.

27. Antman EM, et al. Cardiac-specific troponin I levels to predict the risk of mortality in patients with acute coronary syndromes. N Engl J Med 1996;335(18):1342.

28. Katrukha AG, et al. Troponin I is released in bloodstream of patients with acute myocardial infarction not in free form but as complex. Clin Chem 1997;43:1379.

29. Pankov R, Yamada KM. Fibronectin at a glance. J Cell Sci 2002; 115:3861–3863.

30. Koenn ME. Fetal fibronectin. Clin Lab Sci 2002;15(2):96–98.

31. Peters T Jr, Biamonte ET, Doumas BT. Protein (total) in serum, urine, cerebrospinal fluid, albumin in serum. In: Faulkner WR, Meites S, eds. Selected Methods in Clinical Chemistry. Vol. 9. Washington, D.C.: American Association for Clinical Chemistry, 1982:317.

32. Lines JG, Raines DN. Refractometric determination of serum concentration: 2. Comparison with biuret and Kjeldahl determination. Ann Clin Biochem 1970;7:6.

33. Chromy V, Fischer J. Photometric determination of total protein in lipemic serum. Clin Chem 1977;23:754.

34. Doumas BT, Watson WA, Biggs HG. Albumin standards and the measurement of serum albumin with bromcresol green. Clin Chem Acta 1971;31:87.

35. Speicher CE, Widish JR, Gaudot FJ, et al. An evaluation of the overestimation of serum albumin by bromcresol green. Am J Clin Pathol 1978;69:347.

36. Gustafsson JEC. Improved specificity of serum albumin determination and estimation of "acute phase reactants" by use of the bromocresol green reaction. Clin Chem 1976;22:616.

37. Maguire G, Price C. Bromcresol purple method for serum albumin gives falsely low values in patients with renal insufficiency. Clin Chem Acta 1986;155(1):83.

38. Keren D. High resolution electrophoresis aids detection of gammopathies. Clin Chem News 1989;14.

39. McElderry LA, Tarbit IF, Cassells-Smith AJ. Six methods for urinary protein compared. Clin Chem 1982;28:356.

40. Cembrowski G. Testing for microalbuminuria: promises and pitfalls. Lab Med 1990;21 (8):491.

41. Tourtellotte WW, Staugaitis SM, Walsh MJ, et al. The basis of intra-blood-brain-barrier IgG synthesis. Ann Neurol 1985;17(1): 21–27.

Nonprotein Nitrogen Compounds

Elizabeth L. Frank

CHAPTER OUTLINE

OBJECTIVES

Upon completion of this chapter, the clinical laboratorian should be able to:

• List the nonprotein nitrogen substances in the blood and recognize their chemical structures and relative physiologic concentrations.

• Describe the biosynthesis and excretion of urea, creatinine, creatine, uric acid, and ammonia.

• Describe the major clinical and metabolic conditions associated with increased and decreased plasma concentrations of urea, creatinine, creatine, uric acid, and ammonia.

• Describe the use of the urea nitrogen/creatinine ratio in distinguishing between prerenal, renal, and postrenal causes of uremia.

• Relate the solubility of uric acid to the pathologic consequences of increased plasma uric acid.

• Describe the toxic effects related to an increased plasma ammonia concentration.

• State the specimen collection, transport, and storage requirements necessary for determinations of urea, creatinine, creatine, uric acid, and ammonia.

• Discuss commonly used methods for the determination of urea, creatinine, creatine, uric acid, and ammonia in plasma and urine. Identify sources of error and variability in these methods and describe the effects on the clinical utility of the laboratory measurements.

• Recognize the reference intervals for urea, creatinine, uric acid, and ammonia in plasma and urine. State the effects of age and gender on these values.

• Suggest possible clinical conditions associated with the results, given patient values for urea, creatinine, uric acid, and ammonia and supporting clinical history.

KEY TERMS

Ammonia
Azotemia
Coupled enzymatic
  method
Creatine
Creatinine
Creatinine clearance

Glomerular filtration rate
  (GFR)
Gout
Hyperuricemia
Hypouricemia
Kinetic method of
  measurement

Nonprotein nitrogen
  (NPN)
Postrenal
Prerenal
Protein-free filtrate
Reabsorption
Secretion

Urea
Urea nitrogen/creatinine
  ratio
Uremia or uremic
  syndrome
Uric acid

The determination of nonprotein nitrogenous substances in the blood has traditionally been used to monitor renal function. The term *nonprotein nitrogen (NPN)* originated in the early days of clinical chemistry when analytic methodology required removal of protein from the sample before analysis. The concentration of nitrogen-containing compounds in this *protein-free filtrate* was quantified spectrophotometrically by converting nitrogen to ammonia and subsequent reaction with Nessler's reagent (HgI_2/KI) to produce a yellow color.[1] This technique is technically difficult, but is regarded as the most accurate method for the determination of total NPN concentration. However, more useful clinical information is obtained by analyzing a patient's specimen for individual components of the NPN fraction. Determination of total urinary nitrogen is of value in the assessment of nitrogen balance for nutritional management.[2,3]

The NPN fraction comprises about 15 compounds of clinical interest (Table 9-1). The majority of these compounds arise from the catabolism of proteins and nucleic acids.

UREA

Biochemistry

The NPN compound present in highest concentration in the blood is *urea* (Fig. 9-1). It is synthesized in the liver from CO_2 and the ammonia that arises from the deamination of amino acids in the reactions of the urea cycle. Urea is the major excretory product of protein metabolism.[4] Following synthesis in the liver, urea is carried in the blood to the kidney, where it is readily filtered from the plasma by the glomerulus. Most of the urea in the glomerular filtrate is excreted in the urine, although up to 40% is *reabsorbed* by passive diffusion during passage of the filtrate through the renal tubules. The amount reabsorbed depends on urine flow rate and degree of hydration. Small amounts of urea (<10% of the total) are excreted through the gastrointestinal (GI) tract and skin. The concentration of urea in the plasma is determined by renal function and perfusion, the protein content of the diet, and the amount of protein catabolism. The term *blood urea nitrogen (BUN)* has been used to refer to urea determination because historic assays for urea were based on nitrogen measurement. *Urea nitrogen (urea N)* is a more appropriate term.

Disease Correlations

An elevated concentration of urea in the blood is called *azotemia*. Very high plasma urea concentration accompanied by renal failure is called *uremia*, or the *uremic syndrome*. It is eventually fatal if not treated by dialysis or transplantation. Conditions causing elevations of plasma urea are classified according to cause into three main categories: prerenal, renal, and postrenal.

TABLE 9-1. CLINICALLY SIGNIFICANT NONPROTEIN NITROGEN COMPOUNDS

COMPOUND	APPROXIMATE PLASMA CONCENTRATION (% OF TOTAL NPN)
Urea	45
Amino acids	20
Uric acid	20
Creatinine	5
Creatine	1–2
Ammonia	0.2

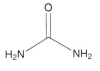
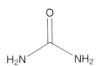

FIGURE 9-1. Structure of urea.

Prerenal azotemia is caused by reduced renal blood flow. Less blood and, therefore, less urea are delivered to the kidney; and, therefore, less urea is filtered. Causative factors include congestive heart failure, shock, hemorrhage, dehydration, and other factors resulting in a significant decrease in blood volume. The amount of protein metabolism also causes prerenal changes in blood urea concentration. A high-protein diet or increased protein catabolism, such as occurs in fever, major illness, stress, corticosteroid therapy, and gastrointestinal hemorrhage, may increase urea concentration. Plasma urea concentration is decreased during periods of low protein intake or increased protein synthesis, such as during late pregnancy and infancy.

Decreased renal function causes an increase in plasma urea concentration as a result of compromised urea excretion. Renal causes of elevated urea include acute and chronic renal failure, glomerular nephritis, tubular necrosis, and other intrinsic renal disease (see Chapter 24, *Renal Function*).

Postrenal azotemia can be due to obstruction of the urine flow anywhere in the urinary tract by renal calculi, tumors of the bladder or prostate, or severe infection.

The major causes of decreased plasma urea concentration include decreased protein intake and severe liver disease. The conditions affecting plasma urea concentration are summarized in Table 9-2.

Differentiation of the cause of abnormal urea concentration is aided by calculation of the *urea nitrogen/creatinine ratio*, which is normally 10:1 to 20:1. Prerenal conditions tend to elevate plasma urea, whereas plasma creatinine remains normal, causing a high urea N/creatinine ratio. A high urea N/creatinine ratio with an elevated creatinine is usually seen in postrenal conditions. A low urea N/creatinine ratio is observed in conditions associated with decreased urea production, such as low protein intake, acute tubular necrosis, and severe liver disease.

Analytic Methods

Measurements of urea were originally performed on a protein-free filtrate of whole blood and based on measuring the amount of nitrogen. Current analytic methods have retained this custom and urea often is reported in terms of nitrogen concentration rather than urea concentration. Urea nitrogen concentration can be converted to urea concentration by multiplying by 2.14, as shown in Equation 9-1.

$$\frac{1 \text{ mg urea N}}{dL} \times \frac{1 \text{ mmol N}}{14 \text{ mg N}} \times \frac{1 \text{ mmol urea}}{2 \text{ mmol N}}$$

$$\times \frac{60 \text{ mg urea}}{1 \text{ mmol urea}} = \frac{2.14 \text{ mg urea}}{dL} \qquad \text{(Eq. 9–1)}$$

Urea nitrogen concentration in milligrams per deciliter may be converted to urea concentration in millimoles per liter by multiplying by 0.36.

Two analytic approaches have been used to assay for urea. The oldest and most often used involves the hydrolysis of urea by the enzyme urease (urea amidohydrolase, EC 3.5.1.5), followed by quantification of ammonium ion (NH_4^+) produced in the reaction. Early colorimetric methods used Nessler's reagent or the Berthelot reaction with nitroprusside to detect NH_4^+.[5] The most common clinically used kinetic method couples the urease reaction with L-glutamate dehydrogenase (GLDH, EC 1.4.1.3) and measures the rate of disappearance of nicotinamide adenine dinucleotide (reduced, NADH) at 340 nm (Fig. 9-2).[6] A modification of this method using bacterial urease has been described for measuring urea in urine specimens.[7]

Ammonium from the urease reaction can also be measured by the color change associated with a pH indicator. This approach has been incorporated into instru-

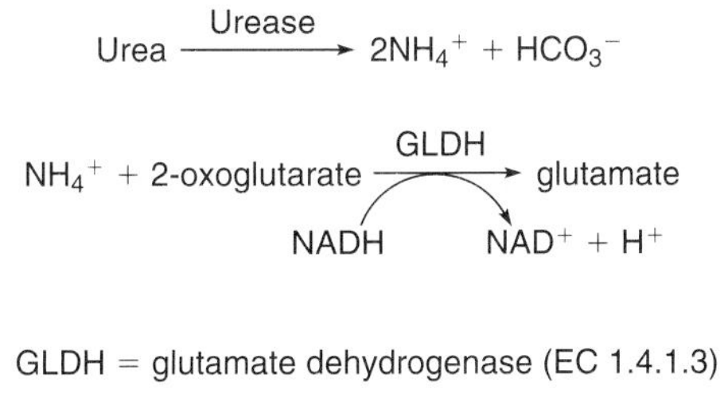

TABLE 9-2. CAUSES OF ABNORMAL PLASMA UREA CONCENTRATION

Increased Concentration

Prerenal	Congestive heart failure
	Shock, hemorrhage
	Dehydration
	Increased protein catabolism
	Corticosteroid therapy
Renal	Acute and chronic renal failure
	Glomerular nephritis
Postrenal	Urinary tract obstruction
Decreased Concentration	Decreased protein intake
	Severe liver disease
	Severe vomiting and diarrhea
	Pregnancy

$$\text{Urea} \xrightarrow{\text{Urease}} 2NH_4^+ + HCO_3^-$$

$$NH_4^+ + 2\text{-oxoglutarate} \xrightarrow[\text{NADH} \quad \text{NAD}^+ + H^+]{\text{GLDH}} \text{glutamate}$$

GLDH = glutamate dehydrogenase (EC 1.4.1.3)

FIGURE 9-2. Enzymatic assay for urea.

ments using liquid reagents, a multilayer film format, reagent strips.[8–10]

An electrode can be used to measure the rate of increase in conductivity as ammonium ions are produced from urea.[11] Because the rate of change in conductivity is measured, ammonia contamination is not a problem as it is in other methods. Potentiometric methods using an ammonia ion-selective electrode have been developed.[12]

Urea may be measured by condensation with diacetyl monoxime in the presence of strong acid and an oxidizing agent to form a yellow diazine derivative.[13] Iron (III) and thiosemicarbazide are added to the reaction mixture to stabilize the color.[14] The major advantage of this direct method of urea measurement is that ammonia does not interfere. Another direct approach reacts urea with o-phthalaldehyde and naphthylethylenediamine to form a chromogen that can be measured.[15]

Isotope-dilution mass spectrometry has been proposed as a definitive method for urea.[16] The coupled urease/GLDH enzymatic assay performed on a protein-free filtrate has been used as a reference method.[17] Analytic methods are summarized in Table 9-3.

Specimen Requirements and Interfering Substances

Urea concentration may be measured in plasma, serum, or urine. If plasma is collected, ammonium ions and high concentrations of sodium citrate and sodium fluoride must be avoided. Citrate and fluoride inhibit urease. Although the protein content of the diet influences urea concentration, the effect of a single protein-containing meal is minimal and a fasting sample is not required usually. A nonhemolyzed sample is recommended. Urea is susceptible to bacterial decomposition, so samples (particularly urine) that cannot be analyzed within a few hours should be refrigerated. Timed urine samples should be refrigerated during the collection period. Methods for plasma or serum may require modification for use with urine specimens because of high

---

CASE STUDY 9-1

A 65-year-old man was first admitted for treatment of chronic obstructive lung disease, renal insufficiency, and significant cardiomegaly. Pertinent laboratory data on admission (5/31) are shown in Case Study Table 9-1.1.

Because of severe respiratory distress, the patient was transferred to the intensive care unit, placed on a respirator, and given diuretics and intravenous (IV) fluids to promote diuresis. This treatment brought about a significant improvement in both cardiac output and renal function, as shown by laboratory results several days later (6/3). After 2 additional days on a respirator with IV therapy, the patient's renal function had returned to normal and, at discharge, his laboratory results were normal (6/7).

The patient was readmitted 6 months later because of the increasing inability of his family to arouse him. On admission, he was shown to have a tremendously enlarged heart with severe pulmonary disease, heart failure, and probable renal failure. Laboratory studies on admission were as shown in Case Study Table 9-1.2. Numerous attempts were made to improve the patient's cardiac and pulmonary function, all to no avail, and the patient died 4 days later.

Question

1. What is the most likely cause of the patient's elevated urea nitrogen? Which data support your conclusion?

CASE STUDY TABLE 9-1.1. LABORATORY RESULTS—FIRST ADMISSION

TEST	5/31	6/3	6/7
Urea N, mg/dL	45	24	11
Creatinine, mg/dL	1.8	1.3	0.9
Urea N/creatinine	25	18.5	12.2
pH	7.22	7.5	
PCO_2, mm Hg	74.4	48.7	
PO_2, mm Hg	32.8	57.6	
O_2 sat, %	51.3	91.0	

CASE STUDY TABLE 9-1.2. LABORATORY RESULTS—SECOND ADMISSION

Urea N, mg/dL	90
Creatinine, mg/dL	3.9
Uric acid, mg/dL	12.0
Urea N/creatinine	23
pH	7.35
PCO_2, mm Hg	59.9
PO_2, mm Hg	34.6
O_2 sat, %	63.7

TABLE 9-3. SUMMARY OF ANALYTIC METHODS—UREA

Enzymatic Methods

Methods use similar first step	Urea + H_2O $\xrightarrow{\text{Urease}}$ $2NH_4^+ + CO_3^{-2}$	
GLDH coupled enzymatic	NH_4^+ + 2-oxoglutarate + NADH $\xrightarrow{\text{GLDH}}$ NAD^+ + glutamate + H_2O	Used on common automated instruments; best as kinetic measurement; candidate reference method
Indicator dye	NH_3^+ + pH indicator $\longrightarrow$ color change	Used in multilayer film reagents, dry reagent strips, and automated systems
Conductimetric	Conversion of unionized urea to NH_4^+ and HCO_3^{2-} results in increased conductivity	Specific and rapid
Berthelot	$NH_4^+ + 5NaOCl + 2phenol \xrightarrow{\text{Nitroprusside/OH}^-}$ indophenol $+ 5NaCl + 5H_2O$	Nonspecific; very sensitive to interference from endogenous NH_3

Chemical Methods

Diacetyl monoxime	Diacetyl monoxime + H_2O $\xrightarrow[\text{heat}]{H^+}$ diacetyl + $HONH_2$ Urea + diacetyl $\xrightarrow{H^+}$ diazine (yellow) + $2H_2O$	Nonspecific; uses toxic reagents
o-Phthaldehyde	Urea + o-phthalaldehyde $\xrightarrow{H^+}$ isoindoline Isoindoline + N-(1-naphthyl)ethyienediamine $\xrightarrow{H^+}$ colored product	Used on some automated instruments; no NH_3 interference, sulfa drugs interfere

urea concentration and the presence of endogenous ammonia.

Reference Interval[18]

Urea nitrogen

Adult	Serum or plasma	6–20 mg/dL	(2.1–7.1 mmol/L urea)
	Urine, 24-hour	12–20 g/day	(0.43–0.71 mol/day urea)

CREATININE/CREATINE

Biochemistry

Creatine is synthesized primarily in the liver from arginine, glycine, and methionine.[4] It is then transported to other tissue, such as muscle, where it is converted to phosphocreatine, which serves as a high-energy source. Creatine phosphate loses phosphoric acid and creatine loses water to form *creatinine,* which passes into the plasma. The structures of these compounds are shown in Figure 9-3.

Creatinine is released into the circulation at a relatively constant rate that has been shown to be proportional to an individual's muscle mass. It is removed from the circulation by glomerular filtration and excreted in the urine. Additional amounts of creatinine are *secreted* by the *proximal tubule*. Small amounts may also be reabsorbed by the renal tubules.[19]

Plasma creatinine concentration is a function of relative muscle mass, the rate of creatine turnover, and renal function. The amount of creatinine in the bloodstream is reasonably stable, although the protein content of the diet does influence the plasma concentration. Because of the observed constancy of endogenous production, determination of creatinine excretion has been used as a measure of the completeness of 24-hour urine collections in a given individual, although this method may be unreliable.[20]

Disease Correlations

Creatinine

Elevated creatinine concentration is associated with abnormal renal function, especially as it relates to glomeru-

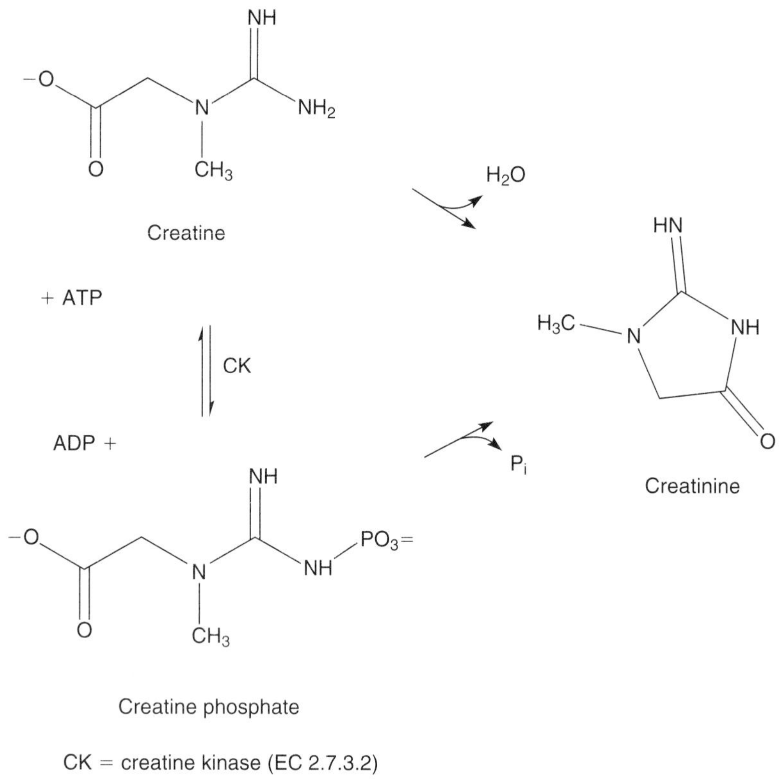

FIGURE 9-3. Interconversion of creatine, creatine phosphate, and creatinine.

CK = creatine kinase (EC 2.7.3.2)

lar function. The *glomerular filtration rate (GFR)* is the volume of plasma filtered (*V*) by the glomerulus per unit of time (*t*).

$$GFR = \frac{V}{t} \qquad \text{(Eq. 9–2)}$$

Assuming a substance, *S*, can be measured and is freely filtered at the glomerulus and neither secreted nor reabsorbed by the tubules, the volume of plasma filtered would be equal to the mass of S filtered (M_S) divided by its plasma concentration (P_S).

$$V = \frac{M_S}{P_S} \qquad \text{(Eq. 9–3)}$$

The mass of S filtered is equal to the product of its urine concentration (U_S) and the urine volume (V_U).

$$M_S = U_S V_U \qquad \text{(Eq. 9–4)}$$

If the urine and plasma concentrations of S, the volume of urine collected, and the time over which the sample was collected are known, the GFR can be calculated.

$$GFR = \frac{U_S V_U}{P_S t} \qquad \text{(Eq. 9–5)}$$

The *clearance* of a substance is the volume of plasma from which that substance is removed per unit time. The formula for *creatinine clearance (CrCl)* is given as fol-

lows, where U_{Cr} is urine creatinine concentration and P_{Cr} is plasma creatinine concentration.

$$CrCl = \frac{U_{Cr} V_U}{P_{Cr} t} \qquad \text{(Eq. 9–6)}$$

Creatinine clearance is usually reported in units of mL/minute and can be corrected for body surface area (see Chapter 24, *Renal Function*). Creatinine clearance overestimates GFR because a small amount of creatinine is reabsorbed by the renal tubules and up to 10% of urine creatinine is secreted by the tubules. However, CrCl provides a reasonable approximation of GFR.[21]

From Equation 9-6, it can be seen that the plasma concentration of creatinine is inversely proportional to clearance of creatinine. Therefore, when plasma creatinine concentration is elevated, GFR is decreased, indicating renal damage. Unfortunately, plasma creatinine is a relatively insensitive marker and may not be measurably increased until renal function has deteriorated more than 50%.[4] The observed relationship between plasma creatinine and GFR and the observation that plasma creatinine concentrations are relatively constant and unaffected by diet should make creatinine a good analyte for the assessment of renal function. However, because of the difficulties encountered in analyzing the small amount of creatinine normally present (see discussion under *Analytic Methods*), measurement of plasma creatinine may not provide sufficient sensitivity for the detection of mild renal

CASE STUDY 9-2

An 80-year-old woman was admitted with a diagnosis of hypertension, congestive heart failure, anemia, possible diabetes, and chronic renal failure. She was treated with diuretics and IV fluids and released 4 days later. Her laboratory results are shown in Case Study Table 9-2.1.

Five months later, she was readmitted for treatment of repeated bouts of dyspnea. She was placed on a special diet and medication to control her hypertension and was discharged. Medical staff believed that she had not been taking her medication as prescribed, and she was counseled regarding the importance of regular doses.

Questions

1. What is the most probable cause of the patient's elevated urea nitrogen? Which data support your conclusion?

2. Note that this patient's admitting diagnosis is "possible diabetes." If the patient had truly been a diabetic, with an elevated blood glucose and a positive acetone, what effect would this have had on the measured values of creatinine? Explain.

CASE STUDY TABLE 9-2.1. LABORATORY RESULTS

	FIRST ADMISSION		SECOND ADMISSION	
	2/11	2/15	7/26	7/28
Urea N, mg/dL	58	*	*	61.0
Creatinine, mg/dL	6.2	6.2	6.4	6.0
Uric acid, mg/dL	10.0	*	*	9.2
Urea N/creatinine	9.4	*	*	10.1
Glucose, mg/dL	86	80	113	*

* indicates test not performed.

dysfunction. Several other analytes, including cystatin C, have been proposed to monitor GFR.[22]

Creatine

In muscle disease such as muscular dystrophy, poliomyelitis, hyperthyroidism, and trauma, both plasma creatine and urinary creatinine are often elevated. Plasma creatinine concentrations usually are normal in these patients. Measurement of creatine kinase is used typically for the diagnosis of muscle disease because analytic methods for creatine are not readily available in most clinical laboratories. Plasma creatine concentration is not elevated in renal disease.[19]

Analytic Methods for Creatinine

The methods most frequently used to measure creatinine are based on the Jaffe reaction first described in 1886.[23] In this reaction, creatinine reacts with picric acid in alkaline solution to form a red-orange chromogen. The reaction was adopted for the measurement of blood creatinine by Folin and Wu in 1919.[24] The reaction is nonspecific and subject to positive interference by a large number of compounds, including acetoacetate, acetone, ascorbate, glucose, and pyruvate. More accurate results are obtained when creatinine in a protein-free filtrate is adsorbed onto Fuller's earth (aluminum magnesium silicate) or Lloyd's reagent (sodium aluminum silicate) then eluted and reacted with alkaline picrate.[25] Because this method is time consuming and not readily automated, it is not routinely used.

Two approaches have been used to increase the specificity of assay methods for creatinine: a *kinetic* Jaffe method and reaction with various enzymes. In the kinetic Jaffe method, serum is mixed with alkaline picrate and the rate of change in absorbance is measured.[26] Although this method eliminates some of the nonspecific reactants, it is subject to interference by α-keto acids and cephalosporins.[27] Bilirubin and hemoglobin may cause a negative bias, probably a result of their destruction in the strong base used. A study of both the kinetic Jaffe method and several enzymatic methods indicated elimination of interference in the measurement of serum creatinine has yet to be achieved.[28] The kinetic Jaffe method is used routinely despite these problems because it is inexpensive, rapid, and easy to perform.

In an effort to enhance the specificity of the Jaffe reaction, several *coupled enzymatic methods* have been developed.[29,30] The method using creatininase (creatinine amidohydrolase [EC 3.5.2.10]), creatinase (creatine amidinohydrolase [EC 3.5.3.3]), sarcosine oxidase (EC 1.5.3.1), and peroxidase (EC 1.11.1.7) has been adapted for use on a dry slide analyzer.[31]

Another approach to the analysis of creatinine has been the measurement of the color formed when creatinine reacts with 3,5-dinitrobenzoate.[32] This method has been successfully adapted to a reagent strip. However, the color produced is less stable than that of the Jaffe chromogen.[15]

High-performance liquid chromatography (HPLC) methods have been developed. One method uses pretreatment of the sample with trichloroacetic acid to remove protein, ion-exchange chromatography, and ultraviolet (UV) detection of creatinine.[33] Another method

TABLE 9-4. SUMMARY OF ANALYTIC METHODS—CREATININE

Chemical Methods Based on Jaffe Reaction

Jaffe-kinetic	Jaffe reaction performed directly on sample; detection of color formation timed to avoid interference of noncreatinine chromogens $$\text{Creatinine} + \text{picrate} \xrightarrow{\text{-OH}} \text{red-orange complex}$$	Positive bias from α-keto acids and cephalosporins; requires automated equipment for precision
Jaffe with adsorbent	Creatinine in protein-free filtrate adsorbed onto Fuller's earth (aluminum magnesium silicate); then reacted with alkaline picrate to form colored complex	Adsorbent improves specificity; previously considered reference method
Jaffe without adsorbent	Creatinine in protein-free filtrate reacts with alkaline picrate to form colored complex	Positive bias from ascorbic acid, glucose, glutathione, α-keto acids, uric acid, and cephalosporins

Enzymatic Methods

Creatininase-CK	$$\text{Creatinine} + H_2O \xrightarrow{\text{Creatininase}} \text{creatine}$$ $$\text{Creatine} + \text{ATP} \xrightarrow{\text{CK}} \text{creatine phosphate} + \text{ADP}$$ $$\text{ADP} + \text{phosphoenolpyruvate} \xrightarrow{\text{PK}} \text{pyruvate} + \text{ATP}$$ $$\text{Pyruvate} + \text{NADH} + H^+ \xrightarrow{\text{LD}} \text{lactate} + \text{NAD}^+$$	Requires large sample; not used widely
Creatininase-H_2O_2	$$\text{Creatinine} + H_2O \xrightarrow{\text{Creatininase}} \text{creatine}$$ $$\text{Creatine} + H_2O \xrightarrow{\text{Creatinase}} \text{sarcosine} + \text{urea}$$ $$\text{Sarcosine} + O_2 + H_2O \xrightarrow{\text{Sarcosine oxidase}} \text{glycine} + CH_2O + H_2O_2$$ $$H_2O_2 + \text{colorless substrate} \xrightarrow{\text{Peroxidase}} \text{colored product} + H_2O$$	Adapted for use as dry slide method; potential to replace Jaffe; no interference from acetoacetate or cephalosporins; some positive bias due to lidocaine

Other Methods

3,5-Dinitrobenzoic acid (DNBA)	$$\text{Creatinine} + \text{DNBA} \xrightarrow{\text{-OH}} \text{purple product}$$	Used on reagent strips; colored product unstable
HPLC	Reversed-phase or cation-exchange chromatography	Highly specific; proposed reference method

combines separation by HPLC with enzymatic determination of creatinine concentration.[34] Both methods have been recommended as reference methods for serum creatinine. Isotope dilution mass spectrometry has been proposed as a definitive method.[35]

The development and use of more accurate methods for plasma creatinine that tend to give lower values will have a significant effect on results obtained for creatinine clearance because results for urinary creatinine are not subject to as many interferences as plasma creatinine. Use of more specific methods for measurement of plasma creatinine may result in apparently higher clearance rates. These results will require careful interpretation.[21] Analytic methods for creatinine are summarized in Table 9-4.

Specimen Requirements and Interfering Substances

Creatinine may be measured in plasma, serum, or urine. Hemolyzed and icteric samples should be avoided particularly if a Jaffe method is used. Lipemic samples may produce erroneous results in some methods. A fasting sample is not required, although high protein ingestion may transiently elevate serum concentrations. Urine should be refrigerated after collection or frozen if longer storage than 4 days is required.[18]

Sources of Error

Ascorbate, glucose, α-keto acids, and uric acid may increase creatinine concentration measured by the Jaffe reaction, especially at temperatures above 30°C. This interference is significantly decreased when kinetic measurement is applied. Depending on the concentration of reactants and measuring time, interference from α-keto acids may persist in kinetic Jaffe methods. Some of these substances interfere in enzymatic methods for creatinine measurement. Bilirubin causes a negative bias in both Jaffe and enzymatic methods. Ascorbate will interfere in enzymatic methods that use peroxidase as a reagent.[28]

Patients taking cephalosporin antibiotics may have falsely elevated results when the Jaffe reaction is used. Other drugs have been shown to increase creatinine results. Dopamine, in particular, is known to affect both enzymatic and Jaffe methods. Lidocaine causes a positive bias in some enzymatic methods.[36]

A study of both the kinetic Jaffe method and several enzymatic methods indicated elimination of interference in the measurement of serum creatinine has yet to be achieved.[28] The use of a multipoint curve-fitting technique rather than the traditional two-point fixed time determination to calculate creatinine concentration is one proposed solution.[37]

TABLE 9-5. REFERENCE INTERVALS FOR CREATININE IN PLASMA OR SERUM, mg/dL (μmol/L)

POPULATION	JAFFE	ENZYMATIC
Adult		
Female	0.6–1.1 (53–97)	0.5–0.8 (44–71)
Male	0.9–1.3 (80–115)	0.6–1.1 (53–97)
Child	0.3–0.7 (27–62)	0–0.6 (0–53)

Reference Interval[18]

Reference intervals vary with assay type, age, and gender.[18] Creatinine concentration decreases with age beginning in the 5th decade of life. Serum reference intervals are listed in Table 9-5.

Creatinine			
Adult, female	Urine, 24-hour	600–1800 mg/day	(5.3–15.9 mmol/day)
Adult, male		800–2000 mg/day	(7.1–17.7 mmol/day)

Analytic Methods for Creatine

The traditional method for creatine measurement relies on analysis of the sample using an endpoint Jaffe method for creatinine before and after it is heated in acid solution. Heating converts creatine to creatinine and the difference between the two samples is the creatine concentration. High temperatures may result in the formation of additional chromogens and the precision of this method is poor. Several enzymatic methods have been developed; one is the creatininase assay. The initial enzyme is omitted and creatine kinase (EC 2.7.3.2), pyruvate kinase (EC 2.1.7.40), and lactate dehydrogenase (EC 1.1.1.27) are coupled to produce a measurable colored product.[38] Creatine can be measured by HPLC.[39,40]

URIC ACID

Biochemistry

In higher primates, such as humans and apes, *uric acid* is the final breakdown product of purine metabolism.[4] Most other mammals have the ability to catabolize purines to allantoin, a more water-soluble end product. This reaction is shown in Figure 9-4.

Purines, such as adenosine and guanine from the breakdown of ingested nucleic acids or from tissue destruction, are converted into uric acid, primarily in the liver. Uric acid is transported in the plasma from the liver to the kidney, where it is filtered by the glomerulus. *Reabsorption* of 98–100% of the uric acid in the glomerular filtrate occurs in the proximal tubules. Small amounts of

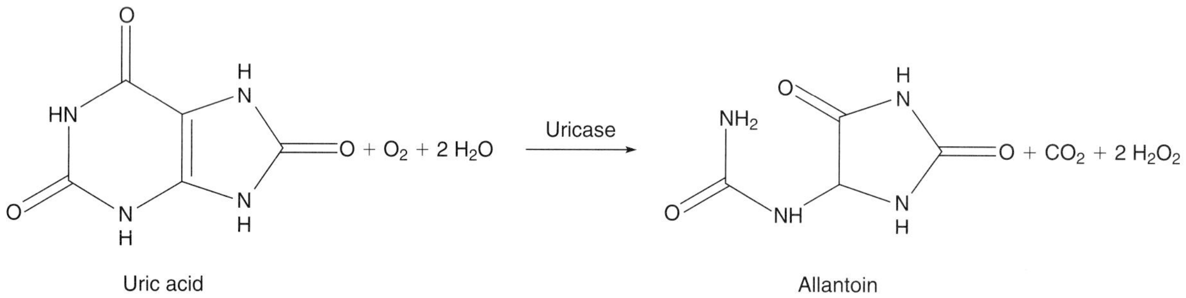

FIGURE 9-4. Conversion of uric acid to allantoin.

uric acid are secreted by the *distal tubules* into the urine. This route accounts for about 70% of the daily uric acid excretion. The remainder is excreted into the GI tract and degraded by bacterial enzymes.

Nearly all of the uric acid in plasma is present as monosodium urate. At the pH of plasma, urate is relatively insoluble; at concentrations greater than 6.4 mg/dL, the plasma is saturated. As a result, urate crystals may form and precipitate in the tissue. In the urine at pH <5.75, uric acid is the predominant species and uric acid crystals may form.

Disease Correlations

Three major disease states are associated with elevated plasma uric acid concentration: gout, increased catabolism of nucleic acids, and renal disease. *Gout* is a disease found primarily in men and usually is first diagnosed between 30 and 50 years of age. Patients have pain and inflammation of the joints caused by precipitation of sodium urates. In 25–30% of these patients, *hyperuricemia* is a result of overproduction of uric acid, although hyperuricemia may be exacerbated by a purine rich diet, drugs, or alcohol. Plasma uric acid concentration in these patients is usually greater than 6.0 mg/dL. Patients with gout are highly susceptible to the development of renal calculi, although not all patients with elevated serum urate levels develop this complication. In women, urate concentration rises after menopause. Postmenopausal women may develop hyperuricemia and gout. In severe cases, deposits of urates called tophi form in tissue, causing deformities.

Another common cause of elevated plasma uric acid concentration is increased metabolism of cell nuclei, as occurs in patients on chemotherapy for such proliferative diseases as leukemia, lymphoma, multiple myeloma, and polycythemia. Monitoring uric acid concentration in these patients is important to avoid nephrotoxicity. Allopurinol, which inhibits xanthine oxidase (EC 1.1.3.22), an enzyme in the uric acid synthesis pathway, is used as treatment.

Patients with hemolytic or megaloblastic anemia may exhibit elevated uric acid concentration. Chronic renal disease causes elevated uric acid concentration because filtration and secretion are impaired. However, uric acid is not useful as an indicator of renal function because many other factors affect its plasma concentration. Plasma urate levels above 6 mg/dL are associated with the development of gouty complications (Table 9-6). Elevated uric acid is found secondary to glycogen storage disease (glucose-6-phosphatase deficiency, EC 3.1.3.9) and other congenital enzyme deficiencies. Excess amounts of metabolites, such as lactate and triglycerides, are produced and compete with urate for renal excretion in these diseases.[19]

Lesch-Nyhan syndrome is an X-linked genetic disorder (seen only in males) caused by the complete deficiency of hypoxanthine guanine phosphoribosyltransferase (HGPRT, EC 2.4.2.8), an important enzyme in the biosynthesis of purines. Lack of this enzyme prevents the reutilization of purine bases in the nucleotide salvage pathway. Increased synthesis of purine nucleotides and

TABLE 9-6. CAUSES OF INCREASED PLASMA URIC ACID

Increased dietary intake
Increased urate production
Gout
Treatment of myeloproliferative disease with cytotoxic drugs
Decreased excretion
Lactic acidosis
Toxemia of pregnancy
Glycogen storage disease type I (glucose-6-phosphatase deficiency)
Drug therapy
Poisons: lead, alcohol
Renal disease
Catabolic pathway enzyme defects
Lesch-Nyhan syndrome

of the degradation product, uric acid, results in high plasma and urine concentrations of uric acid.[41] Neurologic symptoms, mental retardation, and self-mutilation characterize this extremely rare disease. Mutations in phosphoribosylpyrophosphate synthetase (EC 2.7.6.1) also cause elevated uric acid concentration.[19]

Hyperuricemia is a common feature of toxemia of pregnancy and lactic acidosis presumably a result of competition for binding sites in the renal tubules. Elevated levels may be found following ingestion of a diet rich in purines (*eg,* liver, kidney, sweetbreads, shellfish) or a significant decrease in total dietary intake as a result of increased tissue catabolism or starvation.

Hypouricemia is less common than hyperuricemia and is usually secondary to severe liver disease or defective tubular reabsorption, as in Fanconi's syndrome. Hypouricemia can be caused by chemotherapy with 6-mercaptopurine or azathioprine, inhibitors of de novo purine synthesis, as well as overtreatment with allopurinol.[19]

Analytic Methods

As shown in Figure 9-4, uric acid is readily oxidized to allantoin and, therefore, can function as a reducing agent in chemical reactions. This property was exploited in early analytic procedures for the determination of uric acid. The most common method of this type is the Caraway method, which is based on the oxidation of uric acid in a protein-free filtrate, with subsequent reduction of phosphotungstic acid to tungsten blue.[42] Sodium carbonate provides the alkaline pH necessary for color development. This method lacks specificity.

Methods using uricase (urate oxidase, EC 1.7.3.3), the enzyme that catalyzes the oxidation of uric acid to allantoin, are more specific. The simplest of these methods measures the differential absorption of uric acid and allantoin at 293 nm.[43] The difference in absorbance before and after incubation with uricase is proportional to the uric acid concentration. A modification of this method has been proposed as a candidate reference method.[44] Proteins can cause high background absorbance in this method, reducing sensitivity. Negative interference can occur caused by hemoglobin and xanthine.[45]

Methods have been developed using coupled enzymatic reactions to measure the hydrogen peroxide produced as *uric acid* is converted to allantoin.[46,47] Peroxidase or catalase (EC 1.11.1.6) is used to catalyze a chemical indicator reaction. The color produced is proportional to the quantity of uric acid in the specimen. Enzymatic methods of this kind have been adapted for

CASE STUDY 9-3

A 3-year-old girl was admitted with a diagnosis of acute lymphocytic leukemia. Her admitting laboratory data are shown in Case Study Table 9-3.1. After admission, she was treated with packed cells, 2 units of platelets, IV fluids, and allopurinol. On the 2nd hospital day, chemotherapy was begun, using IV vincristine and prednisone and intrathecal injections of methotrexate, prednisone, and cytosine arabinoside. She was discharged for home care 5 days later. She was continued on prednisone and allopurinol at home. She received additional chemotherapy 1 month later (11/1) and again on 11/14. On 12/6, she was readmitted because she had painful sores in her mouth and was unable to eat.

Questions

1. How would you explain the significant elevations of uric acid on admission?

2. What two factors are responsible for the normal levels of uric acid seen in subsequent admissions?

3. What is the most likely cause of the abnormally low level of urea nitrogen observed on 12/6? What other laboratory result would be useful to confirm your suspicions?

CASE STUDY TABLE 9-3.1. LABORATORY RESULTS

	10/1	10/2	10/3	10/4	11/14	12/6	6/20
Urea N, mg/dL	12.0	*	*	15	4.0	2.0	*
Creatinine, mg/dL	0.7	*	*	1.0	0.7	*	0.7
Uric acid, mg/dL	12.0	9.2	4.0	1.9	2.3	*	3.1
WBC, mm³	56,300			3,700	2,800		3,700

* indicates test not performed.

use on traditional wet chemistry analyzers and for dry chemistry slide analyzers. Bilirubin and ascorbic acid, which destroy peroxide, can interfere. Commercial reagent preparations often include potassium ferricyanide and ascorbate oxidase to minimize these interferences.

HPLC methods have been developed using several types of columns.[48,49] These methods are sensitive and specific; pretreatment of the sample to remove protein may be necessary. Isotope dilution mass spectrometry has been proposed as a candidate definitive method.[50] Analytic methods are summarized in Table 9-7.

Specimen Requirements and Interfering Substances

Uric acid may be measured in heparinized plasma, serum, or urine. Serum should be removed from cells as quickly as possible to prevent dilution by intracellular contents. Diet may affect uric acid concentration overall, but a recent meal has no significant effect and a fasting specimen is unnecessary. Gross lipemia should be avoided. High bilirubin concentration may falsely de-

crease results obtained by peroxidase methods. Significant hemolysis, with concomitant glutathione release, may result in low values. Drugs such as salicylates and thiazides have been shown to increase values for uric acid.[36]

Uric acid is stable in plasma or serum after red blood cells have been removed. Serum samples may be stored refrigerated for 3–5 days.[18]

Reference Interval[18]

Values are slightly lower in children and premenopausal females.

Uric acid (Uricase method)			
Adult, female	Plasma or serum	2.6–6.0 mg/dL	(0.16–0.36 mmol/L)
Adult, male		0.5–7.2 mg/dL	(0.21–0.43 mmol/L)
	Urine, 24-hour	250–750 mg/day	(1.48–4.43 mmol/day)
Child	Plasma or serum	2.0–5.5 mg/dL	(0.12–0.33 mmol/L)

TABLE 9-7. SUMMARY OF ANALYTIC METHODS—URIC ACID

Chemical methods

Phosphotungstic acid	Uric acid + $H_3PW_{12}O_{40}$ + O_2 $\xrightarrow{Na_2CO_3/OH^-}$ allantoin + tungsten blue + CO_2	Nonspecific; requires protein removal

Enzymatic methods

Very specific

Similar first step	Uric acid + O_2 + 2 H_2O $\xrightarrow{Uricase}$ allantoin + CO_2 + H_2O_2	
Spectrophotometric	Decrease in absorbance at 293 nm measured	Candidate reference method; hemoglobin and xanthine interfere
Coupled enzymatic (I)	H_2O_2 + CH_3OH $\xrightarrow{Catalase}$ H_2CO + 2 H_2O CH_2O + 3 $C_5H_8O_2$ + NH_3 $\longrightarrow$ 3 H_2O + colored compound	Commonly automated method; negative bias with reducing agents
Coupled enzymatic (II)	H_2O_2 + indicator dye $\xrightarrow{Peroxidase}$ colored compound + 2 H_2O	Readily automated; reducing agents interfere

Other methods

HPLC	Ion exchange, gel permeation, reverse-phase columns	Specific; usually requires sample extraction
Isotope dilution/MS	Sample diluted with known amount of isotope; ratio of two isotopes detected by mass spectrometer	Proposed definitive method

AMMONIA

Biochemistry

Ammonia (NH_3) arises from the deamination of amino acids, which occurs mainly through the action of digestive and bacterial enzymes on proteins in the intestinal tract.[19] Ammonia also is released from metabolic reactions that occur in skeletal muscle during exercise. It is consumed by the parenchymal cells of the liver in the production of urea. In severe liver disease in which there is significant collateral circulation or if parenchymal liver cell function is severely impaired, ammonia is not removed from the circulation and blood concentration increases. At normal physiologic pH, most ammonia in the blood exists as ammonium ion. Figure 9-5 shows the pH-dependent equilibrium between NH_3 and NH_4^+. Unlike other NPN substances, plasma ammonia concentration is not dependent on renal function. Measurement of urine ammonia can be used to confirm the ability of the kidneys to produce ammonia.

High concentrations of NH_3 are neurotoxic and often associated with *encephalopathy*. Toxicity may be partly a result of increased extracellular glutamate concentration and subsequent depletion of adenosine triphosphate (ATP) in the brain.[51] Ammonia is used to monitor the progress of several severe clinical conditions and a quantitative assay should be available in the laboratories of all tertiary care facilities.

Disease Correlations

Clinical conditions in which blood ammonia concentration provides useful information are hepatic failure, Reye's syndrome, and inherited deficiencies of urea cycle enzymes. Severe liver disease is the most common cause of disturbed ammonia metabolism. The monitoring of blood ammonia may be used to determine prognosis, although correlation between the extent of hepatic encephalopathy and plasma NH_3 may not be consistent. A recent study indicates ammonia concentration does correspond to severity of hepatic encephalopathy.[52]

Reye's syndrome, occurring most commonly in children, is a serious disease that can be fatal. Frequently, the disease is preceded by a viral infection, often treated with aspirin. Reye's syndrome is an acute metabolic disorder of the liver, and autopsy findings show severe fatty infiltration of that organ.[41] Blood ammonia concentration can be correlated with both the severity of the disease and prognosis. Survival reaches 100% if plasma NH_3 concentration remains below 5 times normal.[53]

Blood ammonia concentration is increased in the inherited deficiency of all of the urea cycle enzymes except

$$NH_4^+ + H_2O \rightleftharpoons NH_3 + H_3O^+$$

FIGURE 9-5. Interconversion of ammonium ion and ammonia.

argininosuccinase (EC 4.3.2.1). Measurement of plasma ammonia is important in the diagnosis and monitoring of these inherited metabolic disorders.

Analytic Methods

The accurate laboratory measurement of ammonia in plasma is complicated by its low concentration, instability, and pervasive contamination. Two approaches have been used for the measurement of plasma ammonia. One is a two-step approach in which ammonia is isolated from the sample and then assayed. The second involves direct measurement of ammonia by an enzymatic method or ion-selective electrode. Assays detect NH_3 or NH_4^+.

One of the first analytic methods for ammonia, developed by Conway in 1935, exploited the volatility of ammonia to separate the compound in a microdiffusion chamber.[54] Ammonia gas from the sample diffuses into a separate compartment and is absorbed in a solution containing a pH indicator. The amount of ammonia was determined by titration.

A second, more successful approach for isolating NH_3 is the use of a cation-exchange resin (Dowex 50) followed by elution of NH_3 with sodium chloride and quantification by the Berthelot reaction.[55] These isolation methods are time consuming and not readily automated.

An enzymatic assay using glutamate dehydrogenase is convenient and the most common method used currently.[56] The decrease in absorbance at 340 nm as nicotinamide adenine dinucleotide phosphate (reduced, NADPH) is consumed in the reaction is proportional to the ammonia concentration in the specimen. NADPH is the preferred coenzyme because it is used specifically by glutamate dehydrogenase; NADH will participate in reactions of other endogenous substrates, such as pyruvate. Adenosine diphosphate (ADP) is added to the reaction mixture to increase the rate of the reaction and to stabilize GLDH.[57] This method is used on many automated systems and is available as a prepared kit from numerous manufacturers.

Direct measurement using an ion-selective electrode has been developed.[58] The electrode measures the change in pH of a solution of ammonium chloride as ammonia diffuses across a semipermeable membrane. A thin film colorimetric assay is available.[59] In this method, ammonia reacts with an indicator to produce a colored compound that is detected spectrophotometrically. Analytic methods for ammonia are summarized in Table 9-8.

Specimen Requirements and Interfering Substances

Careful specimen handling is extremely important for plasma ammonia assays. Whole blood ammonia concentration rises rapidly following specimen collection be-

TABLE 9-8. SUMMARY OF ANALYTIC METHODS—AMMONIA

Enzymatic methods

GLDH

$$NH_4^+ + \text{2-oxoglutarate} + NADPH \xrightarrow{\text{GLDH}} \text{glutamate} + H_2O + NADP^+$$

Most common on automated instruments; accurate and precise

Chemical methods		
Ion exchange	NH_3 absorbed onto Dowex 50 resin, eluted, and quantitated with Berthelot reaction	Time-consuming manual method; accurate
Ion-selective electrode	Diffusion of NH_3 through selective membrane into NH_4Cl causing pH change, which is measured potentiometrically	Good accuracy and precision; membrane stability may be a problem
Spectrophotometric	NH_3 + bromophenol blue $\longrightarrow$ blue dye	

cause of in vitro amino acid deamination. Venous blood should be obtained without trauma and placed on ice immediately. Heparin and ethylenediaminetetraacetic acid (EDTA) are suitable anticoagulants. Commercial collection containers should be evaluated for ammonia interference before a new lot is put into use. Samples should be centrifuged at 0°–4°C within 20 minutes of collection and the plasma or serum removed. Specimens should be assayed as soon as possible or frozen. Frozen plasma is stable for several days at −20°C. Erythrocytes contain 2–3 times as much ammonia as plasma; hemolysis should be avoided.

Cigarette smoking by the patient is a significant source of ammonia contamination. It is recommended that patients do not smoke for several hours before the sample is drawn.[19]

Sources of Error

Ammonia contamination is a potential problem in the laboratory measurement of ammonia. Precautions must be taken to minimize contamination in the laboratory in which the assay is performed. Elimination of sources of ammonia contamination can significantly improve the accuracy of ammonia assay results. Sources of contamination include tobacco smoke, urine, and ammonia in detergents, glassware, reagents, and water.

The ammonia content of serum-based control material is unstable. Frozen aliquots of human serum albumin containing known amounts of ammonium chloride or ammonium sulfate may be used. Solutions containing known amounts of ammonium sulfate are commercially available.

Many substances influence the in vivo ammonia concentration.[18,45] Ammonium salts, asparaginase, barbiturates, diuretics, ethanol, hyperalimentation, narcotic anal-

gesics, and some other drugs may increase ammonia in plasma. Diphenhydramine, *Lactobacillus acidophilus*, lactulose, levodopa, and several antibiotics decrease values. Glucose at concentrations greater than 600 mg/dL (33 mmol/L) interferes in dry slide methods.

Reference Interval[18]

Values obtained vary somewhat with the method used. Higher concentrations are seen in newborns.

AMMONIA			
Adult	Plasma	19–60 μg/dL	(11–35 μmol/L)
	Urine, 24-hour	140–1500 mg N/day	(10–107 mmol N/day)
Child (10 days– 2 years)		68–136 μg/dL	(40–80 μmol/L)

SUMMARY

Clinically important NPN compounds found in the plasma include urea, creatinine, creatine, uric acid, ammonia, and amino acids. Urea, the primary excretory product of protein metabolism, comprises the major portion of the NPN fraction. Its plasma concentration is related to the protein content of the diet, renal blood flow, amount of protein catabolism, and renal function. Clinical conditions that cause elevated urea levels are classified according to cause as prerenal, renal, and postrenal. The urea nitrogen/creatinine ratio can be used to differentiate these conditions. Urea is usually measured by a coupled enzymatic method that quantifies the amount of ammonium produced by urease hydrolysis of the urea in the sample.

Creatinine is formed as creatine and phosphocreatine in muscle spontaneously lose water or phosphoric acid, respectively. Creatinine is excreted into the plasma at a constant rate related to muscle mass. GFR can be estimated by calculating creatinine clearance, which requires measurement of creatinine in both plasma and urine. Plasma creatinine is inversely related to GFR and, although an imperfect measure, it is commonly used to monitor renal filtration function. Measurement of creatinine in plasma and urine has traditionally been performed using the Jaffe reaction. This reaction is relatively nonspecific and subject to interference from many substances, including glucose, α-keto acids, and protein. Reaction specificity can be improved by using a kinetic rather than an endpoint method; however, the kinetic Jaffe method is subject to interference from bilirubin, α-keto acids, and some drugs. Enzymatic methods have been developed but have not been accepted widely. Use of a more specific method for measurement of creatinine may require readjustment of reference intervals for both plasma creatinine and creatinine clearance. Without such adjustment, mild renal dysfunction may not be discovered.

Uric acid is the breakdown product of the purines from nucleic acid catabolism. It is filtered by the glomerulus, reabsorbed in the proximal tubules, and secreted by the distal tubules into the urine. Additional uric acid is excreted into the GI tract and degraded by bacterial enzymes. Uric acid is relatively insoluble in plasma and, at high concentrations, can be deposited in the joints and tissue, causing painful inflammation. Increased plasma urate is seen in gout, increased nucleic acid catabolism, and renal disease. Increased uric acid is observed secondary to conditions that result in excess production of metabolites, such as lactate and triglycerides, which compete with urate for secretion in the distal tubule. Uric acid is usually quantified by a coupled enzymatic method in which uric acid is oxidized by uricase to allantoin and peroxide. The peroxide produced is detected by reaction with one of a variety of dyes. Bilirubin in sufficient quantity and other substances that destroy peroxide in the sample can falsely decrease results.

Ammonia is present in the plasma in low concentrations. It arises from the deamination of amino acids during protein metabolism and is normally removed from the circulation and converted to urea in the liver. High concentrations of ammonia are neurotoxic. Elevated plasma ammonia is associated with hepatic failure, Reye's syndrome, or an inherited deficiency in urea metabolism. Ammonia can be measured by an enzymatic method using glutamate dehydrogenase. The change in absorbance as NADPH is converted to $NADP^+$ is measured. Careful sample collection and handling is necessary to control measurement errors. The ammonia concentration of freshly drawn blood rises rapidly on standing. Specimens should be placed on ice after collection to avoid an increase in NH_3 as a result of deamination of amino acids. Plasma should be separated and analyzed as quickly as possible. Ammonia contamination in the laboratory and cigarette smoke are potential sources of sample contamination.

REVIEW QUESTIONS

1. Which of the following is not a NPN substance?
   a. Urea
   b. Ammonia
   c. Creatinine
   d. Troponin T

2. Which NPN fraction constitutes nearly half of the NPN substances in the blood?
   a. Urea
   b. Creatine
   c. Ammonia
   d. Uric acid

3. Prerenal azotemia is caused by:
   a. congestive heart failure.
   b. chronic renal failure.
   c. renal tumors.
   d. glomerular nephritis.

4. A high urea N/creatinine ratio with an elevated creatinine is usually seen in:
   a. liver disease.
   b. low protein intake.
   c. tubular necrosis.
   d. postrenal conditions.

5. Ammonia levels are usually measured to evaluate:
   a. renal failure.
   b. acid-base status.
   c. hepatic encephalopathy.
   d. glomerular filtration.

6. A technologist obtains a urea N value of 61 mg/dL and a serum creatinine value of 3.1 mg/dL on a patient. These results indicate:
   a. renal failure.
   b. kidney failure.
   c. gout.
   d. prerenal failure.

7. In the Jaffe reaction, a red-orange chromogen is formed when creatinine reacts with:
   a. picric acid.
   b. naphthylethylenediamine.
   c. diacetyl monoxime.
   d. nitroferricyanide

8. Substances known to increase results when measuring creatinine by the Jaffe reaction include all of the following EXCEPT:
   a. glucose.
   b. ascorbate.
   c. α-keto acids.
   d. bilirubin.

9. A urea N of 9 mg/dL is obtained by a technologist. What is the urea concentration?
   a. 18.3 mg/dL
   b. 19.3 mg/dL
   c. 10.3 mg/dL
   d. 9.3 mg/dL

10. Uric acid is the final breakdown product of:
    a. urea metabolism.
    b. purine metabolism.
    c. glucose metabolism.
    d. bilirubin metabolism.

REFERENCES

1. Gentzkow CJ. An accurate method for determination of blood urea nitrogen by direct nesslerization. J Biol Chem 1942;143:531.
2. Skogerboe KJ, Labbe RF, Rettmer RL, et al. Chemiluminescent measurement of total urinary nitrogen for accurate calculation of nitrogen balance. Clin Chem 1990;36:752.
3. Konstantinides FN, Konstantinides NN, Li JC, et al. Urinary urea nitrogen: too insensitive for calculating nitrogen balance studies in surgical clinical nutrition. JPEN J Parenter Enteral Nutr 1991;15:189.
4. Hristova EN, Henry JB. Metabolic intermediates, inorganic ions and biochemical markers of bone metabolism. In: Henry JB, ed. Clinical Diagnosis and Management by Laboratory Methods, 20th ed. Philadelphia: WB Saunders, 2001:180.
5. Berthelot MPE. Report Chim Appl 1859,1:282.
6. Talke H, Schubert GE. Enzymatische hamstoffbestimmung im blut und serum im optischen test nach warburg. Klin Wochenschr 1965;43:174.
7. Scott P, Maguire GA. A kinetic assay for urea in undiluted urine specimens. Clin Chem 1990;36:1830.
8. Orsonneau J, Massoubre C, Cabanes M, et al. Simple and sensitive determination of urea in serum and urine. Clin Chem 1992;38:619.
9. Ohkubo A, Kamei S, Yamanaka M, et al. Multilayer-film analysis for urea nitrogen in blood, serum, or plasma. Clin Chem 1984;30:1222.
10. Akai T, Naka K, Yoshikawa C, et al. Salivary urea nitrogen as an index to renal function: a test-strip method. Clin Chem 1983;29:1825.
11. Paulson G, Ray R, Sternberg J. A rate sensing approach to urea measurement. Clin Chem 1971;17:644.
12. Georges J. Determination of ammonia and urea in urine and of urea in blood by use of an ammonia-selective electrode. Clin Chem 1979;25:1888.
13. Veniamin MP, Vakirtzi-Lemonias C. Chemical basis of the carbamidodiacetyl micromethod for estimation of urea, citrulline, and carbamyl derivatives. Clin Chem 1970;16:3.
14. Marsh WH, Fingerhut B, Miller H. Automated and manual direct methods for determination of blood urea. Clin Chem 1965;11:624.
15. Pesce AJ, Kaplan LA. Methods in Clinical Chemistry. St. Louis: CV Mosby, 1987.
16. Kessler A, Siekmann L. Measurement of urea in human serum by isotope dilution mass spectrometry: a reference procedure. Clin Chem 1999;45:1523.
17. Sampson EJ, Baird MA, Burtis CA, et al. A coupled-enzyme equilibrium method for measuring urea in serum: optimization and evaluation of the AACC Study Group on urea candidate reference method. Clin Chem 1980;26:816.
18. Tietz N. Clinical Guide to Laboratory Tests. Philadelphia: WB Saunders, 1995.
19. Newman DJ, Price CP. Renal function and nitrogen metabolites. In: Burtis CA, Ashwood ER, eds. Tietz Textbook of Clinical Chemistry, 3rd ed. Philadelphia: WB Saunders, 1999:1204.
20. Narayanan S, Appelton H. Creatinine: a review. Clin Chem 1980;26:1119.
21. Perrone RD, Madias NE, Levey AS. Serum creatinine as an index of renal function: new insight into old concepts. Clin Chem 1992;38:1933.
22. Laterza OF, Price CP, Scott MG. Cystatin C: an improved estimator of glomerular filtration rate? Clin Chem 2002;48:699.
23. Jaffe M. Uber den niederschlag welchen pikrinsaure in normalen harn erzeugt und uber eine neue reaktion des kreatinins. Z Physiol Chem 1886;10:391.
24. Folin O, Wu H. System of blood analysis. J Biol Chem 1919;31:81.
25. Haeckel R. Assay of creatinine in serum with use of Fuller's earth to remove interferents. Clin Chem 1981;27:179.
26. Larsen K. Creatinine assay by a reaction kinetic principle. Clin Chem Acta 1972;41:209.
27. Bowers LD, Wong ET. Kinetic serum creatinine assays. II. A critical evaluation and review. Clin Chem 1980;26:555.
28. Weber JA, van Zanten AP. Interferences in current methods for measurements of creatinine. Clin Chem 1991;37:695.
29. Moss GA, Bondar RJL, Buzzelli DM. Kinetic enzymatic method for determining serum creatinine. Clin Chem 1975;21:1422.
30. Fossati P, Prencipe L, Berti G. Enzymic creatinine assay: a new colorimetric method based on hydrogen peroxide measurement. Clin Chem 1983;29:1494.
31. Creatinine test methodology. Kodak Ektachem clinical chemistry products. Rochester, NY: Eastman Kodak Company, 1992;Pub No MP2-49.
32. Langley WD, Evans M. The determination of creatinine with sodium 3,5-dinitrobenzoate. J Biol Chem 1936;115:333.
33. Rosano TG, Ambrose RT, Wu AHB, et al. Candidate reference method for determining creatinine in serum: method development and interlaboratory validation. Clin Chem 1990;36:1951.
34. Linnet K, Bruunshuus I. HPLC with enzymatic detection as a candidate reference method for serum creatinine. Clin Chem 1991;37:1669.

35. Welch MJ, Cohen A, Hertz HS, et al. Determination of serum creatinine by isotope dilution mass spectrometry as a candidate definitive method. Anal Chem 1986;58:1681.

36. Young DS. Effects of Drugs on Clinical Laboratory Tests, 5th ed. Washington, D.C.: American Association for Clinical Chemistry Press, 2000.

37. Bacon BL, Pardue Hl. Kinetic study of the Jaffe reaction for quantifying creatinine in serum: evaluation of buffered reagent and comparison of different data processing options. Clin Chem 1989;35:360.

38. Beyer, C. Creatine measurement in serum and urine with an automated enzymatic method. Clin Chem 1993;39:1613.

39. Murakita H. Simultaneous determination of creatine and creatinine in serum by high-performance liquid chromatography. J Chromatogr 1988;431:471.

40. Yang YD. Simultaneous determination of creatine, uric acid, creatinine and hippuric acid in urine by high performance liquid chromatography. Biomed Chromatogr 1998;12:47.

41. Harrison's Online. Available at: http://harrisons.accessmedicine.com. Accessed Winter 2003.

42. Caraway WT. Uric acid. In: Seligson, D, ed. Standard Methods of Clinical Chemistry. New York: Academic Press, 1965:239.

43. Feichtmeier TV, Wrenn HT. Direct determination of uric acid using uricase. Am J Clin Pathol 1955;25:833.

44. Duncan PH, Gochman N, Cooper T, et al. A candidate reference method for uric acid in serum: I. Optimization and evaluation. Clin Chem 1982;28:284.

45. Young DS. Effects of Preanalytical Variables on Clinical Laboratory Tests, 2nd ed. Washington, D.C.: American Association for Clinical Chemistry Press, 1997.

46. Gochman N, Schmitz JM. Automated determination of uric acid with use of a uricase-peroxidase system. Clin Chem 1971;17:1154.

47. Kageyama N. A direct colorimetric determination of uric acid in serum and urine with uricase-catalase system. Clin Chim Acta 1971;31:421.

48. Ingebretsen OC, Borgen J, Farstad M. Uric acid determinations: reversed-phase liquid chromatography with ultraviolet detection compared with kinetic and equilibrium adaptations of the uricase method. Clin Chem 1982;28:496.

49. Tanaka M, Hama M. Improved rapid assay of uric acid in serum by liquid chromatography. Clin Chem 1988;34:2567.

50. Ellerbe P, Cohen A, Welch MJ, et al. Determination of serum uric acid by isotope dilution mass spectrometry as a new candidate reference method. Anal Chem 1990;62:2173.

51. Monfort P, Kosenko E, Erceg S, et al. Molecular mechanism of acute ammonia toxicity: role of NMDA receptors. Neurochem Int 2002;41:95.

52. Ong JP, Aggarwal A, Krieger D, et al. Correlation between ammonia levels and the severity of hepatic encephalopathy. Am J Med 2003;114:188.

53. Fitzgerald JF, Clark JH, Angelides AG, et al. The prognostic significance of peak ammonia levels in Reye's syndrome. Pediatrics 1982;70:997.

54. Green A. When and how should we measure plasma ammonia? Ann Clin Biochem 1988;25:199.

55. Routh JI. Liver Function. In: Tietz NW, ed. Fundamentals of Clinical Chemistry. Philadelphia: WB Saunders, 1976:1052.

56. Mondzac A, Ehrlich GE, Seegmiller JE. An enzymatic determination of ammonia in biological fluids. J Lab Clin Med 1965;66:526.

57. Ammonia test methodology. Roche/Hitachi products. Indianapolis, IN: Roche Diagnostics Corporation, 2001.

58. Willems D, Steenssens W. Ammonia determined in plasma with a selective electrode. Clin Chem 1988;34:2372.

59. VITROS AMON Slides. Instructions for use. VITROS Chemistry Products. Rochester, NY: Ortho-Clinical Diagnostics, 2002;Pub No MP2-90.

Enzymes

Robin Gaynor Krefetz, Gwen A. McMillin

OBJECTIVES

Upon completion of this chapter, the clinical laboratorian should be able to:

- Define the term enzyme, including physical composition and structure.
- Classify enzymes according to the International Union of Biochemistry (IUB).
- Discuss the different factors affecting the rate of an enzymatic reaction.
- Explain enzyme kinetics including zero-order and first-order kinetics.
- Explain why the measurement of serum enzyme levels is clinically useful.

- Discuss which enzymes are useful in the diagnosis of various disorders, including cardiac, hepatic, bone, muscle, malignancies, and acute pancreatitis.
- Discuss the tissue sources, diagnostic significance, and assays, including sources of error, for the following enzymes: CK, LD, AST, ALT, ALP, ACP, GGT, amylase, lipase, cholinesterase, and G-6-PD.
- Evaluate patient serum enzyme levels in relation to disease states.

KEY TERMS

Activation energy
Activators
Apoenzyme
Coenzyme
Cofactor
Enzyme

Enzyme–substrate (ES)
  complex
First-order kinetics
Holoenzyme
Hydrolase
International unit (IU)

Isoenzyme
Isoforms
Kinetic assay
LD flipped pattern
Michaelis-Menten
  constant

Oxidoreductase
Transferase
Zero-order kinetics
Zymogen

Enzymes are specific biologic proteins that catalyze biochemical reactions without altering the equilibrium point of the reaction or being consumed or changed in composition. The other substances in the reaction are converted to products. The catalyzed reactions are frequently specific and essential to physiologic functions, such as the hydration of carbon dioxide, nerve conduction, muscle contraction, nutrient degradation, and energy use. Found in all body tissue, enzymes frequently appear in the serum following cellular injury or, sometimes, in smaller amounts, from degraded cells. Certain enzymes, such as those that facilitate coagulation, are specific to plasma and, therefore, are present in significant concentrations in plasma. Therefore, plasma or serum enzyme levels are often useful in the diagnosis of particular diseases or physiologic abnormalities. This chapter discusses the general properties and principles of enzymes, aspects relating to the clinical diagnostic significance of specific physiologic enzymes, and assay methods for those enzymes.

GENERAL PROPERTIES AND DEFINITIONS

Enzymes catalyze many specific physiologic reactions. These reactions are facilitated by the enzyme structure and several other factors. As a protein, each enzyme comprises a specific amino acid sequence (*primary structure*), with the resultant polypeptide chains twisting (*secondary structure*), which then folds (*tertiary structure*) and results in structural cavities. If an enzyme contains more than one polypeptide unit, the *quaternary structure* refers to the spatial relationships between the subunits. Each enzyme contains an *active site,* often a water-free cavity, where the substance on which the enzyme acts (the *substrate*) interacts with particular charged amino acid residues. An *allosteric site*—a cavity other than the active site—may bind regulator molecules and, thereby, be significant to the basic enzyme structure.

Even though a particular enzyme maintains the same catalytic function throughout the body, that enzyme may exist in different forms within the same individual. The different forms may be differentiated from each other based on certain physical properties, such as electrophoretic mobility, solubility, or resistance to inactivation. The term *isoenzyme* is generally used when discussing such enzymes; however, the International Union of Biochemistry (IUB) suggests restricting this term to multiple forms of genetic origin. An *isoform* results when an enzyme is subject to posttranslational modifications. Isoenzymes and isoforms contribute to heterogeneity in properties and function of enzymes.

In addition to the basic enzyme structure, a nonprotein molecule, called a *cofactor,* may be necessary for enzyme activity. Inorganic cofactors, such as chloride or magnesium ions, are called *activators.* A *coenzyme* is an organic cofactor, such as nicotinamide adenine dinucleotide (NAD). When bound tightly to the enzyme, the coenzyme is called a *prosthetic group.* The enzyme portion (*apoenzyme*), with its respective coenzyme, forms a complete and active system, a *holoenzyme.*

Some enzymes, mostly digestive enzymes, are originally secreted from the organ of production in a structurally inactive form, called a *proenzyme* or *zymogen.* Other enzymes later alter the structure of the proenzyme to make active sites available by hydrolyzing specific amino acid residues. This mechanism prevents digestive enzymes from digesting their place of synthesis.

ENZYME CLASSIFICATION AND NOMENCLATURE

To standardize enzyme nomenclature, the Enzyme Commission (EC) of the IUB adopted a classification system in 1961; the standards were revised in 1972 and 1978. The IUB system assigns a *systematic name* to each enzyme, defining the substrate acted on, the reaction catalyzed, and, possibly, the name of any coenzyme involved in the reaction. Because many systematic names are lengthy, a more usable, trivial, *recommended name* is also assigned by the IUB system.[1]

In addition to naming enzymes, the IUB system identifies each enzyme by an EC numerical code containing four digits separated by decimal points. The first digit places the enzyme in one of the following six classes:

1. Oxidoreductases: Catalyze an oxidation–reduction reaction between two substrates.
2. Transferases: Catalyze the transfer of a group other than hydrogen from one substrate to another.
3. Hydrolases: Catalyze hydrolysis of various bonds.
4. Lyases: Catalyze removal of groups from substrates without hydrolysis. The product contains double bonds.
5. Isomerases: Catalyze the interconversion of geometric, optical, or positional isomers.
6. Ligases: Catalyze the joining of two substrate molecules, coupled with breaking of the pyrophosphate bond in adenosine triphosphate (ATP) or a similar compound.

The second and third digits of the EC code number represent the subclass and sub-subclass of the enzyme, respectively, divisions that are made according to criteria specific to the enzymes in the class. The final number is the serial number specific to each enzyme in a sub-subclass. Table 10-1 provides the EC code numbers, as well as the systematic and recommended names, for enzymes frequently measured in the clinical laboratory.

Table 10-1 also lists common and standard abbreviations for commonly analyzed enzymes. Without IUB recommendation, capital letters have been used as a con-

TABLE 10-1. CLASSIFICATION OF FREQUENTLY QUANTITATED ENZYMES

CLASS	RECOMMENDED NAME	COMMON ABBREVIATION	STANDARD ABBREVIATION	EC CODE NO.	SYSTEMATIC NAME
Oxidoreductases	Lactate dehydrogenase	LDH	LD	1.1.1.27	L-Lactate: NAD$^+$ oxidoreductase
	Glucose-6-phosphate dehydrogenase	G-6-PDH	G-6-PD	1.1.1.49	D-Glucose-6-phosphate: NADP$^+$ 1-oxidoreductase
Transferases	Aspartate amino-transferase	GOT (glutamate oxaloacetate transaminase)	AST	2.6.1.1	L-Aspartate: 2-oxaloglutarate aminotransferase
	Alanine amino-transferase	GPT (glutamate transaminase)	ALT	2.6.1.2	L-Alanine: 2-oxaloglutarate aminotransferase
	Creatine kinase	CPK (creatine phosphokinase)	CK	2.7.3.2	ATP: creatine N-phospho-transferase
	γ-Glutamyltransferase	GGTP	GGT	2.3.2.2	(5-Glutamyl) peptide: amino acid-5-glutamyl-transferase
Hydrolases	Alkaline phosphatase	ALP	ALP	3.1.3.1	Orthophosphoric monoester phosphohydrolase (alkaline optimum)
	Acid phosphatase	ACP	ACP	3.1.3.2	Orthophosphoric monoester phosphohydrolase (acid optimum)
	α-Amylase	AMY	AMS	3.2.1.1	1,4-D-Glucan glucanohydrolase
	Triacylglycerol lipase		LPS	3.1.1.3	Triacylglycerol acyl-hydrolase
	Cholinesterase	CHS	CHS	3.1.1.8	Acylcholine acylhydrolase

Adapted from Competence Assurance, ASMT. Enzymology, An Educational Program. Bethesda, MD: RMI Corporation, 1980.

venience to identify enzymes. The common abbreviations, sometimes developed from previously accepted names for the enzymes, were used until the standard abbreviations listed in the table were developed.[2,3] These standard abbreviations are used in the United States and are used later in this chapter to indicate specific enzymes.

ENZYME KINETICS

Catalytic Mechanism of Enzymes

A chemical reaction may occur spontaneously if the free energy or available kinetic energy is higher for the reactants than for the products. The reaction then proceeds toward the lower energy if a sufficient number of the reactant molecules possess enough excess energy to break their chemical bonds and collide to form new bonds. The excess energy, called *activation energy,* is the energy required to raise all molecules in 1 mole of a compound at a certain temperature to the transition state at the peak of the energy barrier. At the transition state, each molecule is equally likely to either participate in product formation or to remain an unreacted molecule. Reactants possessing enough energy to overcome the energy barrier participate in product formation.

One way to provide more energy for a reaction is to increase the temperature and thus increase intermolecular collisions; however, this does not normally occur physiologically. Enzymes catalyze physiologic reactions by lowering the activation energy level that the reactants (*substrates*) must reach for the reaction to occur (Fig. 10-1). The reaction may then occur more readily to a state of equilibrium in which there is no net forward or reverse reaction, even though the equilibrium constant of the reaction is not altered. The extent to which the reaction progresses depends on the number of substrate molecules that pass the energy barrier.

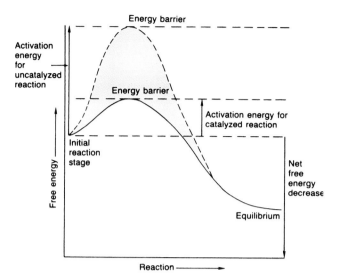

FIGURE 10-1. Energy versus progression of reaction, indicating the energy barrier that the substrate must surpass to react with and without enzyme catalysis. The enzyme considerably reduces the free energy needed to activate the reaction.

The general relationship among enzyme, substrate, and product may be represented as follows:

$$E + S \rightleftharpoons ES \rightleftharpoons E + P \qquad \text{(Eq. 10–1)}$$

where

E = enzyme
S = substrate
ES = enzyme–substrate complex
P = product

The ES complex is a physical binding of a substrate to the active site of an enzyme. The structural arrangement of amino acid residues within the enzyme makes the three-dimensional active site available. At times, the binding of ligand drives a rearrangement to make the active site. The transition state for the ES complex has a lower energy of activation than the transition state of S alone, so that the reaction proceeds after the complex is formed. An actual reaction may involve several substrates and products.

Different enzymes are specific to substrates in different extents or respects. Certain enzymes exhibit *absolute specificity,* meaning that the enzyme combines with only one substrate and catalyzes only the one corresponding reaction. Other enzymes are *group-specific* because they combine with all substrates containing a particular chemical group, such as a phosphate ester. Still other enzymes are specific to chemical bonds and thereby exhibit *bond specificity.*

Stereoisometric specificity refers to enzymes that predominantly combine with only one optical isomer of a certain compound. In addition, an enzyme may bind more than one molecule of substrate and this may occur in a cooperative fashion. Binding of one substrate molecule, therefore, may facilitate binding of additional substrate molecules.

Factors That Influence Enzymatic Reactions

Substrate Concentration

The rate at which an enzymatic reaction proceeds and whether the forward or reverse reaction occurs depend on several reaction conditions. One major influence on enzymatic reactions is substrate concentration. In 1913, Michaelis and Menten hypothesized the role of substrate concentration in formation of the *enzyme–substrate (ES) complex.* According to their hypothesis, represented in Figure 10-2, the substrate readily binds to free enzyme at a low-substrate concentration. With the amount of enzyme exceeding the amount of substrate, the reaction rate steadily increases as more substrate is added. The reaction is following *first-order kinetics* because the reaction rate is directly proportional to substrate concentration. Eventually, however, the substrate concentration is high enough to saturate all available enzyme, and the reaction velocity reaches its maximum. When product is formed, the resultant free enzyme immediately combines with excess free substrate. The reaction is in *zero-order kinetics,* and the reaction rate depends only on enzyme concentration.

The *Michaelis-Menten constant* (K_m), derived from Michaelis and Menten's theory, is a constant for a specific enzyme and substrate under defined reaction conditions and is an expression of the relationship between the velocity of an enzymatic reaction and substrate concentration. The assumptions are made that equilibrium among E, S, ES, and P is established rapidly and that the E + P → ES reaction is negligible. The rate-limiting step is the formation of product and enzyme from the ES complex.

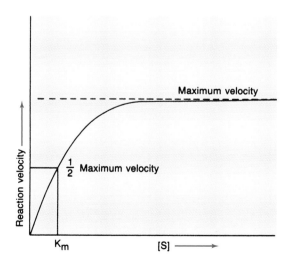

FIGURE 10-2. Michaelis-Menten curve of velocity versus substrate concentration for enzymatic reaction. K_m is the substrate concentration at which the reaction velocity is half of the maximum level.

Then, maximum velocity is fixed, and the reaction rate is a function of only the enzyme concentration. As designated in Figure 10-2, K_m is specifically the substrate concentration at which the enzyme yields half the possible maximum velocity. Therefore, K_m indicates the amount of substrate needed for a particular enzymatic reaction.

The Michaelis-Menten hypothesis of the relationship between reaction velocity and substrate concentration can be represented mathematically as follows:

$$V = \frac{V_{max}\,[S]}{K_m + [S]} \qquad \textbf{(Eq. 10–2)}$$

where

$\qquad V$ = measured velocity of reaction
$\qquad V_{max}$ = maximum velocity
$\qquad [S]$ = substrate concentration
$\qquad K_m$ = Michaelis-Menten constant of enzyme for specific substrate

Theoretically, V_{max} and then K_m could be determined from the plot in Figure 10-2. However, V_{max} is difficult to determine from the hyperbolic plot and often not actually achieved in enzymatic reactions because enzymes may not function optimally in the presence of excessive substrate. A more accurate and convenient determination of V_{max} and K_m may be made through a Lineweaver-Burk plot, a double-reciprocal plot of the Michaelis-Menten constant, which yields a straight line (Fig. 10-3). The reciprocal is taken of both the substrate concentration and the velocity of an enzymatic reaction. The equation becomes

$$\frac{1}{V} = \frac{K_m}{V_{max}}\,\frac{1}{[S]} + \frac{1}{V_{max}} \qquad \textbf{(Eq. 10–3)}$$

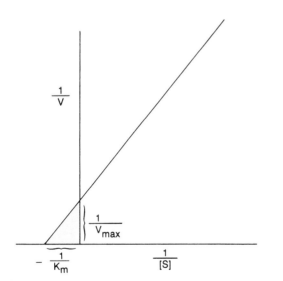

FIGURE 10-3. Lineweaver-Burk transformation of Michaelis-Menten curve. V_{max} is the reciprocal of the x intercept of the straight line. K_m is the negative reciprocal of the x intercept of the same line.

Enzyme Concentration

Because enzymes catalyze physiologic reactions, the enzyme concentration affects the rate of the catalyzed reaction. As long as the substrate concentration exceeds the enzyme concentration, the velocity of the reaction is proportional to the enzyme concentration. The higher the enzyme level, the faster the reaction will proceed because more enzyme is present to bind with the substrate.

pH

Enzymes are proteins that carry net molecular charges. Changes in pH may denature an enzyme or influence its ionic state, resulting in structural changes or a change in the charge on an amino acid residue in the active site. Hence, each enzyme operates within a specific pH range and maximally at a specific pH. Most physiologic enzymatic reactions occur in the pH range of 7.0–8.0, but some enzymes are active in wider pH ranges than others. In the laboratory, the pH for a reaction is carefully controlled at the optimal pH by means of appropriate buffer solutions.

Temperature

Increasing temperature usually increases the rate of a chemical reaction by increasing the movement of molecules, the rate at which intermolecular collisions occur, and the energy available for the reaction. This is the case with enzymatic reactions until the temperature is high enough to denature the protein composition of the enzyme. For each 10-degree increase in temperature, the rate of the reaction will approximately double until, of course, the protein is denatured.

Each enzyme functions optimally at a particular temperature, which is influenced by other reaction variables, especially the total time for the reaction. The optimal temperature is usually close to that of the physiologic environment of the enzyme; however, some denaturation may occur at the human physiologic temperature of 37°C. The rate of denaturation increases as the temperature increases and is usually significant at 40°–50°C.

Because low temperatures render enzymes reversibly inactive, many serum or plasma specimens for enzyme measurement are refrigerated or frozen to prevent activity loss until analysis. Storage procedures may vary from enzyme to enzyme because of individual stability characteristics. Repeated freezing and thawing, however, tends to denature protein and should be avoided.

Because of their temperature sensitivity, enzymes should be analyzed under strictly controlled temperature conditions. Incubation temperatures should be accurate within ± 0.1°C. Laboratories usually attempt to establish an analysis temperature for routine enzyme measurement of 25°C, 30°C, or 37°C. Attempts to establish a universal temperature for enzyme analysis have been futile and, therefore, reference ranges for enzyme levels may vary significantly among laboratories. In the United States, however, 37°C is most commonly used.

Cofactors

Cofactors are nonprotein entities that must bind to particular enzymes before a reaction occurs. Common *activators* (inorganic cofactors) are metallic (Ca^{2+}, Fe^{2+}, Mg^{2+}, Mn^{2}, Zn^{2+}, and K^{+}) and nonmetallic (Br^{-} and Cl^{-}). The activator may be essential for the reaction or may only enhance the reaction rate in proportion with concentration to the point at which the excess activator begins to inhibit the reaction. Activators function by alternating the spatial configuration of the enzyme for proper substrate binding, linking substrate to the enzyme or coenzyme, or undergoing oxidation or reduction.

Some common coenzymes (organic cofactors) are nucleotide phosphates and vitamins. Coenzymes serve as second substrates for enzymatic reactions. When bound tightly to the enzyme, coenzymes are called *prosthetic groups*. For example, NAD as a cofactor may be reduced to nicotinamide adenine dinucleotide phosphate (NADP) in a reaction in which the primary substrate is oxidized. Increasing coenzyme concentration will increase the velocity of an enzymatic reaction in a manner synonymous with increasing substrate concentration. When quantitating an enzyme that requires a particular cofactor, that cofactor should always be provided in excess so that the extent of the reaction does not depend on the concentration of the cofactor.

Inhibitors

Enzymatic reactions may not progress normally if a particular substance, an *inhibitor*, interferes with the reaction. *Competitive inhibitors* physically bind to the active site of an enzyme and compete with the substrate for the active site. With a substrate concentration significantly higher than the concentration of the inhibitor, the inhibition is reversible because the substrate is more likely than the inhibitor to bind the active site and the enzyme has not been destroyed.

A *noncompetitive inhibitor* binds an enzyme at a place other than the active site and may be reversible in the respect that some naturally present metabolic substances combine reversibly with certain enzymes. Noncompetitive inhibition also may be *irreversible* if the inhibitor destroys part of the enzyme involved in catalytic activity. Because the inhibitor binds the enzyme independently from the substrate, increasing substrate concentration does not reverse the inhibition.

Uncompetitive inhibition is another kind of inhibition in which the inhibitor binds to the ES complex—increasing substrate concentration results in more ES complexes to which the inhibitor binds and, thereby, increases the inhibition. The enzyme–substrate–inhibitor complex does not yield product.

Each of the three kinds of inhibition is unique with respect to effects on the V_{max} and K_{m} of enzymatic reactions (Fig. 10-4). In competitive inhibition, the effect of the inhibitor can be counteracted by adding excess substrate to bind the enzyme. The amount of the inhibitor is then negligible by comparison, and the reaction will proceed at a slower rate but to the same maximum velocity as an uninhibited reaction. The K_{m} is a constant for each enzyme and cannot be altered. However, because the amount of substrate needed to achieve a particular velocity is higher in the presence of a competing inhibitor,

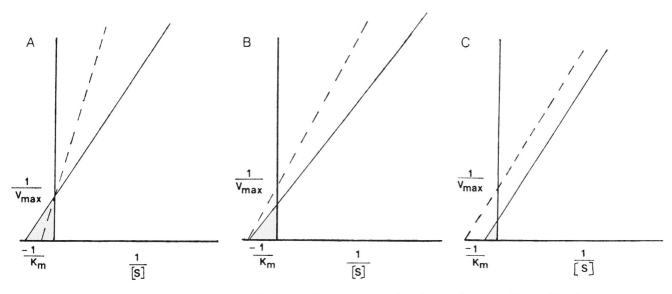

FIGURE 10-4. Normal Lineweaver-Burk plot (*solid line*) compared with each type of enzyme inhibition (*dotted line*). (**A**) Competitive inhibition V_{max} unaltered; K_{m} appears increased. (**B**) Noncompetitive inhibition V_{max} decreased; K_{m} unchanged. (**C**) Uncompetitive inhibition V_{max} decreased; K_{m} appears decreased.

the K_m appears to increase when exhibiting the effect of the inhibitor.

The substrate and inhibitor, commonly a metallic ion, may bind an enzyme simultaneously in noncompetitive inhibition. The inhibitor may inactivate either an ES complex or just the enzyme by causing structural changes in the enzyme. Even if the inhibitor binds reversibly and does not inactivate the enzyme, the presence of the inhibitor when it is bound to the enzyme slows the rate of the reaction. Thus, for noncompetitive inhibition, the maximum reaction velocity cannot be achieved. Increasing substrate levels has no influence on the binding of a noncompetitive inhibitor, so the K_m is unchanged.

Because uncompetitive inhibition requires the formation of an ES complex, increasing substrate concentration increases inhibition. Therefore, maximum velocity equal to that of an uninhibited reaction cannot be achieved, and the K_m appears to be decreased.

Measurement of Enzyme Activity

Because enzymes are usually present in very small quantities in biologic fluids and often difficult to isolate from similar compounds, a convenient method of enzyme quantitation is measurement of catalytic activity. Activity is then related to concentration. Common methods might photometrically measure an increase in product concentration, a decrease in substrate concentration, a decrease in coenzyme concentration, or an increase in the concentration of an altered coenzyme.

If the amount of substrate and any coenzyme is in excess in an enzymatic reaction, the amount of substrate or coenzyme used, or product or altered coenzyme formed, will depend only on the amount of enzyme present to catalyze the reaction. Enzyme concentrations, therefore, are always performed in zero-order kinetics, with the substrate in sufficient excess to ensure that not more than 20% of the available substrate is converted to product. Any coenzymes also must be in excess. NADH is a coenzyme frequently measured in the laboratory. NADH absorbs light at 340 nm, whereas NAD does not, and a change in absorbance at 340 nm is easily measured.

In specific laboratory methodologies, substances other than substrate or coenzyme are necessary and must be present in excess. NAD or NADH is often convenient as a reagent for a *coupled-enzyme* assay when neither NAD nor NADH is a coenzyme for the reaction. In other coupled-enzyme assays, more than one enzyme is added in excess as a reagent and multiple reactions are catalyzed. After the enzyme under analysis catalyzes its specific reaction, a product of that reaction becomes the substrate on which an intermediate *auxiliary enzyme* acts. A product of the intermediate reaction becomes the substrate for the final reaction, which is catalyzed by an *in-dicator enzyme* and commonly involves the conversion of NAD to NADH or vice versa.

When performing an enzyme quantitation in zero-order kinetics, inhibitors must be lacking and other variables that may influence the rate of the reaction must be carefully controlled. A constant pH should be maintained by means of an appropriate buffer solution. The temperature should be constant within $\pm 0.1°C$ throughout the assay at a temperature at which the enzyme is active (usually, 25°C, 30°C, or 37°C).

During the progress of the reaction, the period for the analysis also must be carefully selected. When the enzyme is initially introduced to the reactants and the excess substrate is steadily combining with available enzyme, the reaction rate rises. After the enzyme is saturated, the rates of product formation, release of enzyme, and recombination with more substrate proceed linearly. After a time, usually 6 to 8 minutes after reaction initiation, the reaction rate decreases as the substrate is depleted, the reverse reaction is occurring appreciably, and the product begins to inhibit the reaction. Hence, enzyme quantitations must be performed during the linear phase of the reaction.

One of two general methods may be used to measure the extent of an enzymatic reaction: (1) fixed-time, and (2) continuous-monitoring or kinetic assay. In the *fixed-time method,* the reactants are combined, the reaction proceeds for a designated time, the reaction is stopped (usually by inactivating the enzyme with a weak acid), and a measurement is made of the amount of reaction that has occurred. The reaction is assumed to be linear over the reaction time; the larger the reaction, the more enzyme is present.

In *continuous-monitoring or kinetic assays,* multiple measurements, usually of absorbance change, are made during the reaction, either at specific time intervals (usually every 30 or 60 seconds) or continuously by a continuous-recording spectrophotometer. These assays are advantageous over fixed-time methods because the linearity of the reaction may be more adequately verified. If absorbance is measured at intervals, several data points are necessary to increase the accuracy of linearity assessment. Continuous measurements are preferred because any deviation from linearity is readily observable.

The most common cause of deviation from linearity occurs when the enzyme is so elevated that all substrate is used early in the reaction time. For the remainder of the reaction, the rate change is minimal, with the implication that the coenzyme concentration is very low. With continuous monitoring, the laboratorian may observe a sudden decrease in the reaction rate (deviation from zero-order kinetics) of a particular determination and may repeat the determination using less patient sample. The decrease in the amount of patient sample operates as a dilution, and the answer obtained may be multiplied by the dilution factor to obtain the final answer. The sample itself is not diluted so that the diluent cannot interfere with the reaction. (Sample dilution with saline may be necessary to minimize negative effects in analysis caused by hemolysis or lipemia.) Enzyme activity measurements may not be accurate if storage conditions compromise integrity of the protein, if enzyme inhibitors are present, or if necessary cofactors are not present.

Calculation of Enzyme Activity

When enzymes are quantitated relative to their activity rather than a direct measurement of concentration, the units used to report enzyme levels are *activity units*. The definition for the activity unit must consider variables that may alter results (*eg,* pH, temperature, substrate). Historically, specific method developers frequently established their own units for reporting results and often named the units after themselves (*ie,* Bodansky and King units). To standardize the system of reporting quantitative results, the EC defined the *international unit (IU)* as the amount of enzyme that will catalyze the reaction of 1 μmol of substrate per minute under specified conditions of temperature, pH, substrates, and activators. Because the specified conditions may vary among laboratories, reference values are still often laboratory specific. Enzyme concentration is usually expressed in units per liter (IU/L). The unit of enzyme activity recognized by the International System of Units (Système Internationale d'Unités [SI]) is the katal (mol/s). The mole is the unit for substrate concentration, and the unit of time is the second. Enzyme concentration is then expressed as katals per liter (kat/L). 1.0 IU = 17 nkat.

When enzymes are quantitated by measuring the increase or decrease of NADH at 340 nm, the molar absorptivity (6.22×10^3 mol/L) of NADH is used to calculate enzyme activity.

Measurement of Enzyme Mass

Immunoassay methodologies that quantify enzyme concentration by mass are also available and are routinely used for quantification of some enzymes, such as CK-MB. Immunoassays may overestimate active enzyme as a result of possible cross-reactivity with inactive enzymes, such as zymogens, inactive isoenzymes, macroenzymes, or partially digested enzyme. The relationship between enzyme activity and enzyme quantity is generally linear but should be determined for each enzyme. Enzymes may also be determined and quantified by electrophoretic techniques, which provide resolution of isoenzymes and isoforms.

Ensuring the accuracy of enzyme measurements has long been a concern of laboratorians. The Clinical Laboratory Improvement Amendments Act of 1988 (CLIA 88) has established guidelines for quality control and proficiency testing for all laboratories. Problems with quality control materials for enzyme testing have been a significant issue. Differences between clinical specimens and control sera include species of origin of the enzyme, integrity of the molecular species, isoenzyme forms, matrix of the solution, addition of preservatives, and lyophilization processes. Many studies have been conducted to ensure accurate enzyme measurements and good quality control materials.[4]

Enzymes as Reagents

Enzymes may be used as reagents to measure many nonenzymatic constituents in serum. For example, glucose, cholesterol, and uric acid are frequently quantitated by means of enzymatic reactions, which measure the concentration of the analyte due to the specificity of the enzyme. Enzymes are also used as reagents for methods of quantitating analytes that are substrates for corresponding enzyme quantitations. One example, lactate dehydrogenase, may be a reagent when lactate or pyruvate concentrations are evaluated. For such methods, the enzyme is added in excess in a quantity sufficient to provide a complete reaction in a short period.

Immobilized enzymes are chemically bonded to adsorbents, such as agarose or certain types of cellulose, by azide groups, diazo, and triazine. The enzymes act as recoverable reagents. When substrate is passed through the preparation, the product is retrieved and analyzed, and the enzyme is present and free to react with more substrate. Immobilized enzymes are convenient for batch analyses and are more stable than enzymes in a solution. Enzymes are also commonly used as reagents in competitive and noncompetitive immunoassays, such as those used to measure HIV antibodies, therapeutic drugs, and cancer antigens. Commonly used enzymes include horseradish peroxidase, alkaline phosphatase, glucose-6-phosphate dehydrogenase, and β-galactosidase. The enzyme in these assays functions as an indicator that reflects either the presence or absence of the analyte.

ENZYMES OF CLINICAL SIGNIFICANCE

Table 10-2 lists the commonly analyzed enzymes, including their systematic names and clinical significance. Each enzyme is discussed in this chapter with respect to tissue source, diagnostic significance, assay method, source of error, and reference range.

Creatine Kinase

Creatine kinase (CK) is an enzyme with a molecular weight of approximately 82,000 that is generally associated with ATP regeneration in contractile or transport systems. Its predominant physiologic function occurs in muscle cells, where it is involved in the storage of high-

TABLE 10-2. MAJOR ENZYMES OF CLINICAL SIGNIFICANCE

ENZYME	CLINICAL SIGNIFICANCE
Acid phosphatase (ACP)	Prostatic carcinoma
Alanine amino-transferase (ALT)	Hepatic disorder
Alkaline phosphatase (ALP)	Hepatic disorder Bone disorder
Amylase (AMS)	Acute pancreatitis
Aspartate amino-transferase (AST)	Myocardial infarction Hepatic disorder Skeletal muscle disorder
Creatine kinase (CK)	Myocardial infarction Skeletal muscle disorder
γ-Glutamyltransferase (GGT)	Hepatic disorder
Glucose-6-phosphate dehydrogenase (G-6-PD)	Drug-induced hemolytic anemia
Lactate dehydrogenase (LD)	Myocardial infarction Hepatic disorder Carcinoma
Lipase (LPS)	Acute pancreatitis
Pseudocholinesterase (PChE)	Organophosphate poisoning Genetic variants

energy creatine phosphate. Every contraction cycle of muscle results in creatine phosphate use, with the production of ATP. This results in relatively constant levels of muscle ATP. The reversible reaction catalyzed by CK is shown in Equation 10-4.

$$\text{Creatine} + \text{ATP} \xrightleftharpoons{\text{CK}} \text{creatine phosphate} + \text{ADP}$$

(Eq. 10–4)

Tissue Source

CK is widely distributed in tissue, with highest activities found in skeletal muscle, heart muscle, and brain tissue. CK is present in much smaller quantities in other tissue sources, including the bladder, placenta, gastrointestinal tract, thyroid, uterus, kidney, lung, prostate, spleen, liver, and pancreas.

Diagnostic Significance

Because of the high concentrations of CK in muscle tissue, CK levels are frequently elevated in disorders of cardiac and skeletal muscle. The CK level is considered a sensitive indicator of acute myocardial infarction (AMI) and muscular dystrophy, particularly the Duchenne type. Striking elevations of CK occur in Duchenne-type muscular dystrophy, with values reaching 50–100 times the upper limit of normal (ULN). Although total CK levels are sensitive indicators of these disorders, they are not entirely specific indicators inasmuch as CK elevation is found in various other abnormalities of cardiac and skeletal muscle. Levels of CK also vary with muscle mass and, therefore, may depend on gender, race, degree of physical conditioning, and age.

Elevated CK levels are also occasionally seen in central nervous system disorders such as cerebral vascular accident, seizures, nerve degeneration, and central nervous system shock. Damage to the blood-brain barrier must occur to allow enzyme release to the peripheral circulation.

Other pathophysiologic conditions in which elevated CK levels occur are hypothyroidism, malignant hyperpyrexia, and Reye's syndrome. Table 10-3 lists the major disorders associated with abnormal CK levels. Serum CK levels and CK/progesterone ratio have been useful in the diagnosis of ectopic pregnancies.[5] Total serum CK levels have also been used as an early diagnostic tool to identify patients with *Vibrio vulnificus* infections.[6]

CASE STUDY 10-1

A 51-year-old, overweight Caucasian man visits his family doctor complaining of "indigestion" of 5 days' duration. He has also had bouts of sweating, malaise, and headache. His blood pressure is 140/105; his family history includes a father with diabetes who died at age 62 of AMI secondary to diabetes mellitus. An electrocardiogram revealed changes from one performed 6 months earlier. The results of the patient's blood work are as follows:

CK	129 U/L	(30–60)
CK-MB	4%	(<6%)
LD	280 U/L	(100–225)
LD	Isoenzymes	LD-1>LD-2
AST	35 U/L	(5–30)

Questions

1. Can a diagnosis of AMI be ruled out in this patient?

2. What further cardiac markers should be run on this patient?

3. Should this patient be admitted to the hospital?

TABLE 10-3. CREATINE KINASE ISOENZYMES—TISSUE LOCALIZATION AND SOURCES OF ELEVATION

ISOENZYME	TISSUE	CONDITION
CK-MM	Heart Skeletal muscle	Myocardial infarction Skeletal muscle disorder Muscular dystrophy Polymyositis Hypothyroidism Malignant hyperthermia Physical activity Intramuscular injection
CK-MB	Heart Skeletal muscle	Myocardial infarction Myocardial injury Ischemia Angina Inflammatory heart disease Cardiac surgery Duchenne-type muscular dystrophy Polymyositis Malignant hyperthermia Reye's syndrome Rocky Mountain spotted fever Carbon monoxide poisoning
CK-BB	Brain Bladder Lung Prostate Uterus Colon Stomach Thyroid	Central nervous system shock Anoxic encephalopathy Cerebrovascular accident Seizure Placental or uterine trauma Carcinoma Reye's syndrome Carbon monoxide poisoning Malignant hyperthermia Acute and chronic renal failure

Because enzyme elevation is found in numerous disorders, the separation of total CK into its various isoenzyme fractions is considered a more specific indicator of various disorders than total levels. Typically, the clinical relevance of CK activity depends more on isoenzyme fractionation than on total levels.

CK occurs as a dimer consisting of two subunits that can be separated readily into three distinct molecular forms. The three isoenzymes have been designated as CK-BB (brain type), CK-MB (hybrid type), and CK-MM (muscle type). On electrophoretic separation, CK-BB will migrate fastest toward the anode and is therefore called *CK-1*. CK-BB is followed by CK-MB (*CK-2*), and, finally, by CK-

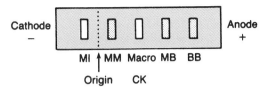

FIGURE 10-5. Electrophoretic migration pattern of normal and atypical CK isoenzymes.

MM (*CK-3*), exhibiting the slowest mobility (Fig. 10-5). Table 10-3 indicates the tissue localization of the isoenzymes and the major conditions associated with elevated levels. Separation of CK isoforms may also by visualized by high voltage electrophoretic separation. Isoforms occur following cleavage of the c-terminal amino acid from the M subunit by serum carboxypeptidase N. Three isoforms have been described for CK-MM and two isoforms for CK-MB; the clinical significance is not well established.

The major isoenzyme in the sera of healthy people is the MM form. Values for the MB isoenzyme range from undetectable to trace (<6% of total CK). It also appears that CK-BB is present in small quantities in the sera of healthy people; however, the presence of CK-BB in serum depends on the method of detection. Most techniques cannot detect CK-BB in normal serum.

CK-MM is the major isoenzyme fraction found in striated muscle and normal serum. Skeletal muscle contains almost entirely CK-MM, with a small amount of CK-MB. The majority of CK activity in heart muscle is also attributed to CK-MM, with approximately 20% a result of CK-MB.[7] Normal serum consists of approximately 94–100% CK-MM. Injury to both cardiac and skeletal muscle accounts for the majority of cases of CK-MM elevations (Table 10-3). Hypothyroidism results in CK-MM elevations because of the involvement of muscle tissue (increased membrane permeability), the effect of thyroid hormone on enzyme activity and, possibly, the slower clearance of CK as a result of slower metabolism.

Mild to strenuous activity may contribute to elevated CK levels, as may intramuscular injections. In physical activity, the extent of elevation is variable. However, the degree of exercise in relation to the exercise capacity of the individual is the most important factor in determining the degree of elevation.[8] Patients who are physically well conditioned show lesser degrees of elevation than patients who are less conditioned. Levels may be elevated for as long as 48 hours following exercise.

CK elevations are generally less than 5 × ULN following intramuscular injections and usually not apparent after 48 hours, although elevations may persist for 1 week. The predominant isoenzyme is CK-MM.

The quantity of CK-BB in the tissue (Table 10-3) is usually small. The small quantity, coupled with its relatively short half-life (1–5 hours), results in CK-BB activities that are generally low and transient and not usually measurable when tissue damage occurs. Highest concentrations are found in the central nervous system, the gastrointestinal tract, and the uterus during pregnancy.

Although brain tissue has high concentrations of CK, serum rarely contains CK-BB of brain origin. Because of its molecular size (80,000), its passage across the blood-brain barrier is hindered. However, when extensive damage to the brain has occurred, significant amounts of CK-BB can sometimes be detected in the serum.

It has been observed that CK-BB may be significantly elevated in patients with carcinoma of various organs. It has been found in association with untreated prostatic carcinoma and other adenocarcinomas. These findings indicate that CK-BB may be a useful tumor-associated marker.[9]

The most common causes of CK-BB elevations are central nervous system damage, tumors, childbirth, and the presence of macro-CK, an enzyme–immunoglobulin complex. In most of these cases, the CK-BB level is greater than 5 U/L, usually in the range of 10–50 U/L. Other conditions listed in Table 10-3 usually show CK-BB activity below 10 U/L.[10]

The value of CK isoenzyme separation can be found principally in detection of myocardial damage. Cardiac tissue contains significant quantities of CK-MB, approximately 20% of all CK-MB. Whereas CK-MB is found in small quantities in other tissue, myocardium is essentially the only tissue from which CK-MB enters the serum in significant quantities. Demonstration of elevated levels of CK-MB, greater than or equal to 6% of the total CK, is considered a good indicator of myocardial damage, particularly AMI. Other nonenzyme proteins, called troponins, have been found to be even more spe-cific and may elevate in the absence of CK-MB elevations. Following myocardial infarction, the CK-MB levels begin to rise within 4–8 hours, peak at 12–24 hours, and return to normal levels within 48–72 hours. This time frame must be considered when interpreting CK-MB levels.

CK-MB activity has been observed in other cardiac disorders (Table 10-3). Therefore, increased quantities are not entirely specific for AMI but probably reflect some degree of ischemic heart damage. The specificity of CK-MB levels in the diagnosis of AMI can be increased if interpreted in conjunction with lactate dehydrogenase (LD) isoenzymes and/or troponins and if measured sequentially over a 48-hour period to detect the typical rise and fall of enzyme activity seen in AMI (Fig. 10-6).

The MB isoenzyme also has been detected in the sera of patients with noncardiac disorders. CK-MB levels found in these conditions probably represent leakage from skeletal muscle, although in Duchenne-type muscular dystrophy, there may be some cardiac involvement as well. CK-MB levels in Reye's syndrome also may reflect myocardial damage.

Despite the findings of CK-MB levels in disorders other than myocardial infarction, its presence still remains a significant indicator of AMI.[11] The typical time course of CK-MB elevation following AMI is not found in other conditions.

Nonenzyme proteins (troponin I and troponin T) have been used as a more sensitive and specific marker of myocardial damage. These proteins are released into the bloodstream earlier and persist longer than CK and its isoenzyme CK-MB. More information on these protein markers of AMI can be found in Chapter 8, *Amino Acids and Proteins.*

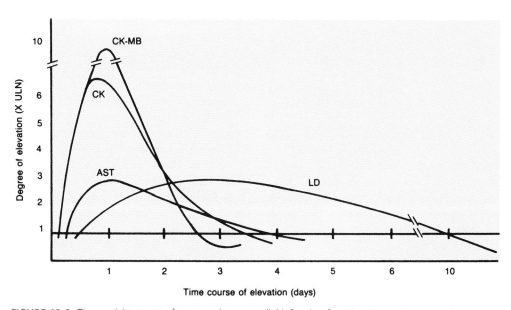

FIGURE 10-6. Time activity curves of enzymes in myocardial infarction for AST, CK, CK-MB, and LD. CK, specifically the MB fraction, increases initially, followed by AST and LD. LD is elevated the longest. All enzymes usually return to normal within 10 days.

Numerous reports have been made describing the appearance of unusual CK isoenzyme bands displaying electrophoretic properties that differ from the three major isoenzyme fractions (Fig. 10-5).[12–16] These atypical forms are generally of two types and are referred to as macro-CK and mitochondrial CK.

Macro-CK appears to migrate to a position midway between CK-MM and CK-MB. This type of macro-CK largely comprises CK-BB complexed with immunoglobulin. In most instances, the associated immunoglobulin is IgG, although a complex with IgA also has been described. The term *macro-CK* has also been used to describe complexes of lipoproteins with CK-MM.

The incidence of macro-CK in sera ranges from 0.8% to 1.6%. Currently, no specific disorder is associated with its presence, although it appears to be age- and sex-related, occurring most frequently in women older than age 50.

Mitochondrial CK (CK-Mi) is bound to the exterior surface of the inner mitochondrial membranes of muscle, brain, and liver. It migrates to a point cathodal to CK-MM and exists as a dimeric molecule of two identical subunits. It occurs in serum in both the dimeric state and in the form of oligomeric aggregates of high molecular weight (350,000). CK-Mi is not present in normal serum and is typically not present following myocardial infarct. The incidence of CK-Mi ranges from 0.8% to 1.7%. For it to be detected in serum, extensive tissue damage must occur, causing breakdown of the mitochondrion and cell wall. Its presence does not correlate with any specific disease state but appears to be an indicator of severe illness. CK-Mi has been detected in cases of malignant tumor and cardiac abnormalities.

In view of the indefinite correlation between these atypical CK forms and a specific disease state, it appears that their significance relates primarily to the methods used for detecting CK-MB. In certain analytic procedures, these atypical forms may be measured as CK-MB, resulting in erroneously high CK-MB levels.

Methods used for measurement of CK isoenzymes include electrophoresis; ion-exchange chromatography; and several immunoassays, including radioimmunoassay (RIA) and immunoinhibition methods. Although mass methods are more sensitive and preferred for quantitation of CK-MB, electrophoresis has been the reference method. The electrophoretic properties of the CK isoenzymes are shown in Figure 10-5. Generally, the technique consists of performing electrophoresis on the sample, measuring the reaction using an overlay technique and then visualizing the bands under ultraviolet light. With electrophoresis, the atypical bands can be separated, allowing their detection apart from the three major bands. Often a strongly fluorescent band appears, which migrates in close proximity to the CK-BB form. The exact nature of this fluorescence is unknown, but it has been attributed to the binding of fluorescent drugs or bilirubin by albumin.

In addition to visualizing atypical CK bands, other advantages of electrophoresis methods include detecting an unsatisfactory separation and allowing visualization of adenylate kinase (AK). AK is an enzyme released from erythrocytes in hemolyzed samples and appearing as a band cathodal to CK-MM. AK may interfere with chemical or immunoinhibition methods, causing a falsely elevated CK or CK-MB value.

Ion-exchange chromatography has the potential for being more sensitive and precise than electrophoretic procedures performed with good technique. On an unsatisfactory column, however, CK-MM may merge into CK-MB and CK-BB may be eluted with CK-MB. Also, macro-CK may elute with CK-MB.

Antibodies against both the M and B subunits have been used to determine CK-MB activity. Anti-M inhibits all M activity but not B activity. CK activity is measured before and after inhibition. Activity remaining after M inhibition is a result of the B subunit of both MB and BB activity. The residual activity after inhibition is multiplied by 2 to account for MB activity (50% inhibited). The major disadvantage of this method is that it detects BB activity, which, although not normally detectable, will cause falsely elevated MB results when BB is present. In addition, the atypical forms of CK-Mi and macro-CK are not inhibited by anti-M antibodies and also may cause erroneous results for MB activity.

Immunoassays detect CK-MB reliably with minimal cross-reactivity. Immunoassays measure the concentration of enzyme protein rather than enzymatic activity and can, therefore, detect enzymatically inactive CK-MB. This leads to the possibility of permitting detection of infarction earlier than other methods. A double-antibody immunoinhibition assay is also available. This technique allows differentiation of MB activity due to adenylate kinase and the atypical isoenzymes, resulting in a more specific analytic procedure for CK-MB.[17] Point-of-care assay systems for CM-MB are available but not as widely used as those for troponins.

Assay Enzyme Activity

As indicated by Equation 10-4, CK catalyzes both forward and reverse reactions involving phosphorylation of creatine or ADP. Typically, for analysis of CK activity, this reaction is coupled with other enzyme systems and a change in absorbance at 340 nm is determined. The forward reaction is coupled with the pyruvate kinase-lactate dehydrogenase-NADH system and proceeds according to Equation 10-5:

$$\text{Creatine} + \text{ATP} \underset{}{\overset{\text{CK}}{\rightleftharpoons}} \text{creatine phosphate} + \text{ADP}$$

$$\text{ADP} + \text{phosphoenolpyruvate} \underset{}{\overset{\text{PK}}{\rightleftharpoons}} \text{pyruvate} + \text{ATP}$$

$$\text{Pyruvate} + \text{NADH} + \text{H}^+ \underset{}{\overset{\text{LD}}{\rightleftharpoons}} \text{lactate} + \text{NAD}^+$$

(Eq. 10–5)

The reverse reaction is coupled with the hexokinase-glucose-6-phosphate dehydrogenase-NADP system, as indicated in Equation 10-6:

$$Creatine\ phosphate + ADP \underset{}{\overset{CK}{\rightleftharpoons}} creatine + ADP$$

$$ATP + glucose \underset{}{\overset{HK}{\rightleftharpoons}} ADP + glucose\text{-}6\text{-}phosphate$$

$$Glucose\ 6\text{-}phosphate + NADP^+ \underset{}{\overset{G\text{-}6\text{-}PD}{\rightleftharpoons}}$$
$$6\text{-}phosphogluconate + NADPH$$

(Eq. 10–6)

The reverse reaction proposed by Oliver and modified by Rosalki is the most commonly performed method in the clinical laboratory.[13] The reaction proceeds 2–6 times faster than the forward reaction, depending on the assay conditions and there is less interference from side reactions. The optimal pH for the reverse reaction is 6.8; for the forward reaction, it is 9.0.

CK activity in serum is unstable, being rapidly inactivated because of oxidation of sulfhydryl groups. Inactivation can be partially reversed by the addition of sulfhydryl compounds to the assay reagent. Compounds such as N-acetylcysteine, mercaptoethanol, thioglycerol, and dithiothreitol are among those used.

Source of Error

Hemolysis of serum samples may be a source of elevated CK activity. Erythrocytes are virtually devoid of CK; however, they are rich in AK activity. AK reacts with ADP to produce ATP, which is then available to participate in the assay reaction, causing falsely elevated CK levels. This interference can occur with hemolysis of greater than 320 mg/L of hemoglobin, which releases sufficient AK to exhaust the AK inhibitors in the reagent. Trace hemolysis causes little, if any, CK elevation. Serum should be stored in a dark place because CK is inactivated by daylight. Activity can be restored after storage in the dark at 4°C for 7 days or at –20°C for 1 month when the assay is conducted using a sulfhydryl activator.[18] Because of the effect of muscular activity and muscle mass on CK levels, it should be noted that people who are physically well-trained tend to have elevated baseline levels and that patients who are bedridden for prolonged periods may have decreased CK activity.

Reference Range

Total CK:

    Male, 15–160 U/L (37°C)

    Female, 15–130 U/L (37°C)

CK-MB: <6% total CK

The higher values in males are attributed to increased muscle mass. Note that enzyme reference ranges are subject to variation, depending on the method used and the assay conditions.

Lactate Dehydrogenase

Lactate dehydrogenase (LD) is an enzyme that catalyzes the interconversion of lactic and pyruvic acids. It is a hydrogen-transfer enzyme that uses the coenzyme NAD^+ according to Equation 10-7:

$$\begin{array}{ccc}
CH_3 & & CH_3 \\
| & & | \\
HC\text{—}OH + NAD^+ \underset{}{\overset{LD}{\rightleftharpoons}} & C=O + NADH + H^+ \\
| & & | \\
COOH & & COOH \\
Lactate & & Pyruvate
\end{array}$$

(Eq. 10–7)

Tissue Source

LD is widely distributed in the body. High activities are found in the heart, liver, skeletal muscle, kidney, and erythrocytes; lesser amounts are found in the lung, smooth muscle, and brain.

Diagnostic Significance

Because of its widespread activity in numerous body tissue, LD is elevated in a variety of disorders. Increased levels are found in cardiac, hepatic, skeletal muscle, and renal diseases, as well as in several hematologic and neoplastic disorders. The highest levels of total LD are seen in pernicious anemia and hemolytic disorders. Intramedullary destruction of erythroblasts causes elevation as a result of the high concentration of LD in erythrocytes. Liver disorders, such as viral hepatitis and cirrhosis, show slight elevations of 2–3 times ULN. AMI and pulmonary infarct also show slight elevations of approximately the same degree (2–3 × ULN). In AMI, LD levels begin to rise within 12–24 hours, reach peak levels within 48–72 hours, and may remain elevated for 10 days. Skeletal muscle disorders and some leukemias contribute to increased LD levels. Marked elevations can be observed in most patients with acute lymphoblastic leukemia in particular.

Because of the many conditions that contribute to increased activity, an elevated total LD value is a rather nonspecific finding. LD assays, therefore, assume more clinical significance when separated into isoenzyme fractions. The enzyme can be separated into five major fractions, each comprising four subunits. It has a molecular weight of 128,000 daltons. Each isoenzyme comprises four polypeptide chains with a molecular weight of 32,000 daltons each. Two different polypeptide chains, designated H (heart) and M (muscle), combine in five arrangements to yield the five major isoenzyme fractions.

Table 10-4 indicates the tissue localization of the LD isoenzymes and the major disorders associated with elevated levels. LD-1 migrates most quickly toward the anode, followed in sequence by the other fractions, with LD-5 migrating the slowest.

TABLE 10-4. LACTATE DEHYDROGENASE ISOENZYMES—TISSUE LOCALIZATION AND SOURCES OF ELEVATION

ISOENZYME	TISSUE	DISORDER
LD-1 (HHHH) and LD-2 (HHHM)	Heart Red blood cells Renal cortex	Myocardial infarct Hemolytic anemia Megaloblastic anemia Acute renal infarct Hemolyzed specimen
LD-3 (HHMM)	Lung Lymphocytes Spleen Pancreas	Pulmonary embolism Extensive pulmonary pneumonia Lymphocytosis Acute pancreatitis Carcinoma
LD-4 (HMMM) and LD-5 (MMMM)	Liver Skeletal muscle	Hepatic injury or inflammation Skeletal muscle injury

TABLE 10-5. LD ISOENZYMES AS A PERCENTAGE OF TOTAL LD[19]

ISOENZYME	%
LD-1	14–26
LD-2	29–39
LD-3	20–26
LD-4	8–16
LD-5	6–16

In the sera of healthy individuals, the major isoenzyme fraction is LD-2, followed by LD-1, LD-3, LD-4, and LD-5 (for the isoenzyme ranges, see Table 10-5). LD-1 and LD-2 are present to approximately the same extent in the tissues listed in Table 10-4. However, cardiac tissue and red blood cells contain a higher concentration of LD-1. Therefore, in conditions involving cardiac necrosis (AMI) and intravascular hemolysis, the serum levels of LD-1 will increase to a point at which they are present in greater concentration than LD-2, resulting in a condition known as the *LD flipped pattern* (LD-1 > LD-2).[19] This flipped pattern is suggestive of AMI. However, LD is not specific to cardiac tissue and is not a preferred marker of diagnosis of AMI. LD-1/LD-2 ratios greater than 1 also may be observed in hemolyzed serum samples.[20] Elevations of LD-3 occur most frequently with pulmonary involvement and are also observed in patients with various carcinomas. The LD-4 and LD-5 isoenzymes are found primarily in liver and skeletal muscle tissue, with LD-5 being the predominant fraction in these tissues. LD-5 levels have greatest clinical significance in the detection of hepatic disorders, particularly intrahepatic disorders. Disorders of skeletal muscle will reveal elevated LD-5 levels, as depicted in the muscular dystrophies.

A sixth LD isoenzyme has been identified, which migrates cathodic to LD-5.[21–23] LD-6 is alcohol dehydrogenase. In reporting studies, LD-6 has been present in patients with arteriosclerotic cardiovascular failure. It is believed that its appearance signifies a grave prognosis and impending death. LD-5 is elevated concurrently with the appearance of LD-6, probably representing hepatic congestion due to cardiovascular disease. It is suggested, therefore, that LD-6 may reflect liver injury secondary to severe circulatory insufficiency.

LD has been shown to complex with immunoglobulins and to reveal atypical bands on electrophoresis. LD complexed with IgA and IgG usually migrates between LD-3 and LD-4. This macromolecular complex is not associated with any specific clinical abnormality.

Analysis of LD isoenzymes can be accomplished by electrophoresis, by immunoinhibition or chemical inhibition methods, or by differences in substrate affinity. Because of limited clinical utility, such tests are not commonly used. The electrophoretic procedure has been widely used historically. After electrophoretic separation, the isoenzymes can be detected either fluorometrically or colorimetrically. LD can use other substrates in addition to lactate, such as α-hydroxybutyrate. The H subunits have a greater affinity for α-hydroxybutyrate than to the M subunits. This has led to the use of this substrate in an attempt to measure the LD-1 activity, which consists entirely of H subunits. The chemical assay, known as the measurement of α-hydroxybutyrate dehydrogenase activity (α-HBD), is outlined in Equation 10-8.

$$
\begin{array}{ccc}
\text{CH}_3 & & \text{CH}_3 \\
| & & | \\
\text{CH}_2 + \text{NADH} + \text{H}^+ \xrightleftharpoons{\ \alpha\text{-HBD}\ } & & \text{CH}_2 + \text{NAD}^+ \\
| & & | \\
\text{HC}{=}\text{O} & & \text{HC}{-}\text{OH} \\
| & & | \\
\text{COOH} & & \text{COOH} \\
\alpha\text{-Ketobutyrate} & & \alpha\text{-Hydroxybutyrate}
\end{array}
$$

(Eq. 10–8)

α-HBD is not a separate and distinct enzyme but is considered to represent the LD-1 activity of total LD. However, α-HBD activity is not entirely specific for the LD-1 fraction because LD-2, LD-3, and LD-4 also contain varying amounts of the H subunit. HBD activity is increased in those conditions in which the LD-1 and LD-2 fractions are increased.

LD is commonly used to measure lactic and pyruvic acids or as a coupled reaction.

Assay for Enzyme Activity

LD catalyzes the interconversion of lactic and pyruvic acids using the coenzyme NAD^+. The reaction sequence is outlined in Equation 10-9:

$$\text{Lactate} + NAD^+ \rightleftharpoons \text{pyruvate} + NADH + H^+$$

(Eq. 10–9)

The reaction can proceed in either a forward (lactate [L]) or reverse (pyruvate [P]) direction. Both reactions have been used in clinical assays. The rate of the reverse reaction is approximately 3 times faster, allowing smaller sample volumes and shorter reaction times. However, the reverse reaction is more susceptible to substrate exhaustion and loss of linearity. The optimal pH for the forward reaction is 8.3–8.9; for the reverse reaction, it is 7.1–7.4.

Source of Error

Erythrocytes contain an LD concentration approximately 100–150 times that found in serum. Therefore, any degree of hemolysis should render a sample unacceptable for analysis. LD activity is unstable in serum regardless of the temperature at which it is stored. If the sample cannot be analyzed immediately, it should be stored at 25°C and analyzed within 48 hours. LD-5 is the most labile isoenzyme. Loss of activity occurs more quickly at 4°C than at 25°C. Serum samples for LD isoenzyme analysis should be stored at 25°C and analyzed within 24 hours of collection.

Reference Range

LD, 100–225 U/L (37°C)

Aspartate Aminotransferase

Aspartate aminotransferase (AST) is an enzyme belonging to the class of *transferases*. It is commonly referred to as a *transaminase* and is involved in the transfer of an amino group between aspartate and α-keto acids. The older terminology, *serum glutamic-oxaloacetic transaminase (SGOT, or GOT)*, may also be used. Pyridoxal phosphate functions as a coenzyme. The reaction proceeds according to Equation 10-10:

(Eq. 10–10)

The transamination reaction is important in intermediary metabolism because of its function in the synthesis and degradation of amino acids. The ketoacids formed by the reaction are ultimately oxidized by the tricarboxylic acid cycle to provide a source of energy.

Tissue Source

AST is widely distributed in human tissue. The highest concentrations are found in cardiac tissue, liver, and skeletal muscle, with smaller amounts found in the kidney, pancreas, and erythrocytes.

Diagnostic Significance

The clinical use of AST is limited mainly to the evaluation of hepatocellular disorders and skeletal muscle involvement. In AMI, AST levels begin to rise within 6–8 hours, peak at 24 hours, and generally return to normal within 5 days. However, because of the wide tissue distribution, AST levels are not useful in the diagnosis of AMI.

AST elevations are frequently seen in pulmonary embolism. Following congestive heart failure, AST levels also may be increased, probably reflecting liver involvement as a result of inadequate blood supply to that organ. AST levels are highest in acute hepatocellular disorders. In viral hepatitis, levels may reach 100 times ULN. In cirrhosis, only moderate levels—approximately 4 times ULN—are detected (see Chapter 22, *Liver Function*). Skeletal muscle disorders, such as the muscular dystrophies, and inflammatory conditions also cause increases in AST levels (4–8 × ULN).

AST exists as two isoenzyme fractions located in the cell cytoplasm and mitochondria. The intracellular concentration of AST may be 7,000 times higher than the extracellular concentration. The cytoplasmic isoenzyme is the predominant form occurring in serum. In disorders producing cellular necrosis, such as liver cirrhosis, the mitochondrial form may be significantly increased. Isoenzyme analysis of AST is not routinely performed in the clinical laboratory.

Assay for Enzyme Activity

Assay methods for AST are generally based on the principle of the Karmen method, which incorporates a coupled enzymatic reaction using malate dehydrogenase (MD) as the indicator reaction and monitors the change in absorbance at 340 nm continuously as NADH is oxidized to NAD^+ (Eq. 10-11). The optimal pH is 7.3–7.8.

$$\text{Aspartate} + \alpha\text{-ketoglutarate} \xrightarrow{\text{AST}} \\ \text{oxaloacetate} + \text{glutamate}$$

$$\text{Oxaloacetate} + NADH + H^+ \rightleftharpoons \text{malate} + NAD^+$$

(Eq. 10–11)

Source of Error

Hemolysis should be avoided because it can dramatically increase serum AST concentration. AST activity is stable in serum for 3–4 days at refrigerated temperatures.

Reference Range

AST, 5–30 U/L (37°C).

Alanine Aminotransferase

Alanine aminotransferase (ALT) is a transferase with enzymatic activity similar to AST. Specifically, it catalyzes the transfer of an amino group from alanine to α-ketoglutarate with the formation of glutamate and pyruvate. The older terminology was serum *glutamic-pyruvic transaminase (SGPT, or GPT)*. Equation 10-12 indicates the transferase reaction. Pyridoxal phosphate acts as the coenzyme.

$$
\begin{array}{c}
\underset{\text{Alanine}}{
\begin{array}{c}
\text{CH}_3 \\
| \\
\text{HC}-\text{NH}_2 \\
| \\
\text{COOH}
\end{array}} +
\underset{\substack{\alpha\text{-keto-}\\\text{glutarate}}}{
\begin{array}{c}
\text{COOH} \\
| \\
\text{C}=\text{O} \\
| \\
\text{CH}_2 \\
| \\
\text{CH}_2 \\
| \\
\text{COOH}
\end{array}}
\underset{}{\overset{\text{ALT}}{\rightleftharpoons}}
\underset{\text{Pyruvate}}{
\begin{array}{c}
\text{CH}_3 \\
| \\
\text{C}=\text{O} \\
| \\
\text{COOH}
\end{array}} +
\underset{\text{Glutamate}}{
\begin{array}{c}
\text{COOH} \\
| \\
\text{HC}-\text{NH}_2 \\
| \\
\text{CH}_2 \\
| \\
\text{CH}_2 \\
| \\
\text{COOH}
\end{array}}
\end{array}
$$

(Eq. 10–12)

Tissue Source

ALT is distributed in many tissues, with comparatively high concentrations in the liver. It is considered the more liver-specific enzyme of the transferases.

Diagnostic Significance

Clinical applications of ALT assays are confined mainly to evaluation of hepatic disorders. Higher elevations are found in hepatocellular disorders than in extrahepatic or intrahepatic obstructive disorders. In acute inflammatory conditions of the liver, ALT elevations are frequently higher than those of AST and tend to remain elevated longer as a result of the longer half-life of ALT in serum (16 hours and 24 hours, respectfully).

Cardiac tissue contains a small amount of ALT activity, but the serum level usually remains normal in AMI unless subsequent liver damage has occurred. ALT levels have historically been compared with levels of AST to help determine the source of an elevated AST level and to detect liver involvement concurrent with myocardial injury.

Assay for Enzyme Activity

The typical assay procedure for ALT consists of a coupled enzymatic reaction using LD as the indicator enzyme, which catalyzes the reduction of pyruvate to lactate with the simultaneous oxidation of NADH. The change in absorbance at 340 nm measured continuously is directly proportional to ALT activity. The reaction proceeds according to Equation 10-13. The optimal pH is 7.3–7.8.

$$\text{Alanine} + \alpha\text{-ketoglutarate} \overset{\text{ALT}}{\rightleftharpoons} \text{pyruvate} + \text{glutamate}$$

$$\text{Pyruvate} + \text{NADH} + \text{H}^+ \overset{\text{LD}}{\rightleftharpoons} \text{lactate} + \text{NAD}^+$$

(Eq. 10–13)

Source of Error

ALT is stable for 3–4 days at 4°C. It is relatively unaffected by hemolysis.

Reference Range

ALT, 6–37 U/L (37°C).

CASE STUDY 10-2

While a 71-year-old woman is walking home from a shopping center, she faints and falls. She is driven home by a friend. When home, she realizes that she is bleeding from her mouth and is slightly disoriented. She appears injured from the fall, but she does not remember tripping or falling. The woman is taken to a local emergency department. The examining physician determines that there was a loss of consciousness; to determine the reason, he orders a head CT and ECG and the following lab tests: CBC, PT, APTT, CK, LD, AST, and troponin T and troponin I. All tests are within normal limits. The woman is sutured for the mouth injuries and admitted to a 24-hour observation unit.

Questions

1. What possible diagnoses is the physician considering?

2. What lab tests would be elevated at 6, 12, and 24 hours if this patient had an AMI?

3. What isoenzyme tests would be useful with this patient?

Alkaline Phosphatase

Alkaline phosphatase (ALP) belongs to a group of enzymes that catalyze the hydrolysis of various phosphomonoesters at an alkaline pH. Consequently, ALP is a nonspecific enzyme capable of reacting with many different substrates. Specifically, ALP functions to liberate inorganic phosphate from an organic phosphate ester with the concomitant production of an alcohol. The reaction proceeds according to Equation 10-14:

$$R—\overset{\overset{\displaystyle O}{\|}}{\underset{\underset{\displaystyle O^-}{|}}{P}}—O^- + H_2O \underset{\text{pH 9–10}}{\overset{\text{ALP}}{\rightleftharpoons}} R—OH + HO—\overset{\overset{\displaystyle O}{\|}}{\underset{\underset{\displaystyle O^-}{|}}{P}}—O^-$$

Phosophomonoester   Alcohol   Phosphate ion

(Eq. 10–14)

The optimal pH for the reaction is 9.0–10.0, but optimal pH varies with the substrate used. The enzyme requires Mg^+ as an activator.

Tissue Source

ALP activity is present on cell surfaces in most human tissue. The highest concentrations are found in the intestine, liver, bone, spleen, placenta, and kidney. In the liver, the enzyme is located on both sinusoidal and bile canalicular membranes; activity in bone is confined to the osteoblasts, those cells involved in production of bone matrix. The specific location of the enzyme within this tissue accounts for the more predominant elevations in certain disorders.

Diagnostic Significance

Elevations of ALP are of most diagnostic significance in the evaluation of hepatobiliary and bone disorders. In hepatobiliary disorders, elevations are more predominant in obstructive conditions than in hepatocellular disorders; in bone disorders, elevations are observed when there is involvement of osteoblasts.

In biliary tract obstruction, ALP levels range from 3 to 10 times the upper limits of normal (ULN). Increases are primarily a result of increased synthesis of the enzyme induced by cholestasis. In contrast, hepatocellular disorders, such as hepatitis and cirrhosis, show only slight increases, usually less than 3 times ULN. Because of the degree of overlap of ALP elevations that occurs in the various liver disorders, a single elevated ALP level is difficult to interpret. It assumes more diagnostic significance when evaluated along with other tests of hepatic function (see Chapter 22, *Liver Function*).

Elevated ALP levels may be observed in various bone disorders. Perhaps the highest elevations of ALP activity occur in Paget's disease (osteitis deformans). Other bone disorders include osteomalacia, rickets, hyperparathyroidism, and osteogenic sarcoma. In addition, increased levels are observed in healing bone fractures and during periods of physiologic bone growth.

In normal pregnancy, increased ALP activity, averaging approximately $1\frac{1}{2}$ times ULN, can be detected between weeks 16 and 20. ALP activity increases and persists until the onset of labor. Activity then returns to normal within 3–6 days.[24] Elevations also may be seen in complications of pregnancy such as hypertension, preeclampsia, and eclampsia, as well as in threatened abortion.

ALP levels are significantly decreased in the inherited condition of hypophosphatasia. Subnormal activity is a result of the absence of the bone isoenzyme and results in inadequate bone calcification.

ALP exists as a number of isoenzymes, which have been studied by a variety of techniques. The major isoenzymes, which are found in the serum and have been most extensively studied, are those derived from the liver, bone, intestine, and placenta.[25]

Electrophoresis is considered the most useful single technique for ALP isoenzyme analysis. However, because there may still be some degree of overlap between the fractions, electrophoresis in combination with another separation technique may provide the most reliable information. A direct immunochemical method for the measurement of bone-related ALP is now available; this has made ALP electrophoresis unnecessary in most cases.

The liver fraction migrates the fastest, followed by bone, placental, and intestinal fractions. Because of the similarity between liver and bone phosphatases, there is often not a clear separation between them. Quantitation by a densitometer is sometimes difficult because of the overlap between the two peaks. The liver isoenzyme can actually be divided into two fractions, the major liver band and a smaller fraction called *fast liver*, or α_1 liver, which migrates anodal to the major band and corresponds to the α_1 fraction of protein electrophoresis. When total ALP levels are increased, the major liver fraction is the most frequently elevated. Many hepatobiliary conditions cause elevations of this fraction, usually early in the course of the disease. The fast-liver fraction has been reported in metastatic carcinoma of the liver, as well as in other hepatobiliary diseases. Its presence is regarded as a valuable indicator of obstructive liver disease. However, it is occasionally present in the absence of any detectable disease state.

The bone isoenzyme increases due to osteoblastic activity and is normally elevated in children during periods of growth and in adults older than age 50. In these cases, an elevated ALP level may be difficult to interpret.[26]

The presence of intestinal ALP isoenzyme in serum depends on the blood group and secretor status of the individual. Individuals who have B or O blood group and are secretors are more likely to have this fraction. Apparently, intestinal ALP is bound by erythrocytes of group A.

Furthermore, in these individuals, increases in intestinal ALP occur after consumption of a fatty meal. Intestinal ALP may increase in several disorders, such as diseases of the digestive tract and cirrhosis. Increased levels are also found in patients undergoing chronic hemodialysis.

Difference in heat stability is the basis of a second approach used to identify the isoenzyme source of an elevated ALP. Typically, ALP activity is measured before and after heating the serum at 56°C for 10 minutes. If the residual activity after heating is less than 20% of the total activity before heating, then the ALP elevation is assumed to be a result of bone phosphatase. If greater than 20% of the activity remains, the elevation is probably a result of liver phosphatase. These results are based on the finding that placental ALP is the most heat stable of the four major fractions, followed by intestinal, liver, and bone fractions in decreasing order of heat stability. Placental ALP will resist heat denaturation at 65°C for 30 minutes.

Heat inactivation is an imprecise method for differentiation because inactivation depends on many factors, such as correct temperature control, timing, and analytic methods sensitive enough to detect small amounts of residual ALP activity. In addition, there is some degree of overlap between heat inactivation of liver and bone fractions in both liver and bone diseases.

A third approach to identification of ALP isoenzymes is based on selective chemical inhibition. Phenylalanine is one of several inhibitors that have been used. Phenylalanine inhibits intestinal and placental ALP to a much greater extent than liver and bone ALP. With phenylalanine use, however, it is impossible to differentiate placental from intestinal ALP or liver from bone ALP.

In addition to the four major ALP isoenzyme fractions, certain abnormal fractions are associated with neoplasms. The most frequently seen are the Regan and Nagao isoenzymes. They have been referred to as *carcinoplacental alkaline phosphatases* because of their similarities to the placental isoenzyme. The frequency of occurrence ranges from 3% to 15% in cancer patients. The Regan isoenzyme has been characterized as an example of an ectopic production of an enzyme by malignant tissue. It has been detected in various carcinomas, such as lung, breast, ovarian, and colon, with the highest incidences in ovarian and gynecologic cancers. Because of its low incidence in cancer patients, diagnosis of malignancy is rarely based on its presence. It is, however, useful in monitoring the effects of therapy because it will disappear on successful treatment.

The Regan isoenzyme migrates to the same position as the bone fraction and is the most heat stable of all ALP isoenzymes, resisting denaturation at 65°C for 30 minutes. Its activity is inhibited by phenylalanine.

The Nagao isoenzyme may be considered a variant of the Regan isoenzyme. Its electrophoretic, heat-stability,

and phenylalanine-inhibition properties are identical to the Regan fraction. However, Nagao also can be inhibited by L-leucine. Its presence has been detected in metastatic carcinoma of pleural surfaces and in adenocarcinoma of the pancreas and bile duct.

Assay for Enzyme Activity

Because of the relative nonspecificity of ALP with regard to substrates, a variety of methodologies for its analysis have been proposed and are still in use today. The major differences between these relate to the concentration and types of substrate and buffer used and the pH of the reaction. A continuous-monitoring technique based on a method devised by Bowers and McComb allows calculation of ALP activity based on the molar absorptivity of *p*-nitrophenol. The reaction proceeds according to Equation 10-15:

| *p*-Nitrophenyl-phosphate | *p*-Nitro-phenol | Phosphate ion |

(Eq. 10–15)

p-Nitrophenylphosphate (colorless) is hydrolyzed to *p*-nitrophenol (yellow) and the increase in absorbance at 405 nm, which is directly proportional to ALP activity, is measured.

Source of Error

Hemolysis may cause slight elevations because ALP is approximately 6 times more concentrated in erythrocytes than in serum. ALP assays should be run as soon as possible after collection. Activity in serum increases approximately 3–10% on standing at 25°C or 4°C for several hours. Diet may induce elevations in ALP activity of blood group B and O individuals who are secretors. Values may be 25% higher following ingestion of a high-fat meal.

Reference Range

ALP, 30–90 U/L (30°C).

Acid Phosphatase

Acid phosphatase (ACP) belongs to the same group of phosphatase enzymes as ALP and is a *hydrolase* that catalyzes the same type of reactions. The major difference between ACP and ALP is the pH of the reaction. ACP functions at an optimal pH of approximately 5.0. Equation 10-16 outlines the reaction sequence:

$$R\overset{\underset{\displaystyle |}{\overset{\displaystyle O}{\|}}}{-}P-O^- + H_2O \underset{pH\ 5}{\overset{ACP}{\rightleftharpoons}} R-OH + HO\overset{\underset{\displaystyle |}{\overset{\displaystyle O}{\|}}}{-}P-O^-$$

Phosphomonoester   Alcohol   Phosphate ion

(Eq. 10–16)

Tissue Source

ACP activity is found in the prostate, bone, liver, spleen, kidney, erythrocytes, and platelets. The prostate is the richest source, with many times the activity found in other tissue.

Diagnostic Significance

Historically, ACP measurement has been used as an aid in the detection of prostatic carcinoma, particularly metastatic carcinoma of the prostate. Total ACP determinations are relatively insensitive techniques, detecting elevated ACP levels resulting from prostatic carcinoma in the majority of cases only when the tumor has metastasized. Newer markers, such as prostate-specific antigen (PSA), are more useful screening and diagnostic tools (see Chapter 30, *Circulating Tumor Markers*).

One of the most specific substrates for prostatic ACP is thymolphthalein monophosphate. Chemical-inhibition methods used to differentiate the prostatic portion most frequently use tartrate as the inhibitor. The prostatic fraction is inhibited by tartrate. Serum and substrate are incubated both with and without the addition of L-tartrate. ACP activity remaining after inhibition with L-tartrate is subtracted from total ACP activity determined without inhibition, and the difference represents the prostatic portion:

Total ACP – ACP after tartrate inhibition
            = prostatic ACP   (Eq. 10–17)

The reaction is not entirely specific for prostatic ACP, but other tissue sources are largely uninhibited.

Neither of these methods of ACP determination is sensitive to prostatic carcinoma that has not metastasized. Values are usually normal in the majority of cases and, in fact, may be elevated only in about 50% of cases of prostatic carcinoma that have metastasized.

One technique with much improved sensitivity over conventional ACP assays is the immunologic approach using antibodies that are specific for the prostatic portion. Immunochemical techniques, however, are not of value as screening tests for prostatic carcinoma.

PSA is more likely than ACP to be elevated at each stage of prostatic carcinoma, even though a normal PSA

level may be found in stage D tumors. PSA is particularly useful to monitor the success of treatment; however, PSA is controversial as a screening test for prostatic malignancy because PSA elevation may occur in conditions other than prostatic carcinoma, such as benign prostatic hypertrophy and prostatitis.[27–29]

Other prostatic conditions in which ACP elevations have been reported include hyperplasia of the prostate and prostatic surgery. There are conflicting reports of elevations following rectal examination and prostate massage. Certain studies have reported ACP elevations, others have indicated no detectable change. When elevations are found, levels usually return to normal within 24 hours.[30]

ACP assays have proven useful in forensic clinical chemistry, particularly in the investigation of rape. Vaginal washings are examined for seminal fluid–ACP activity, which can persist for up to 4 days.[31] Elevated activity is presumptive evidence of rape in such cases.

Serum ACP activity may frequently be elevated in bone disease. Activity has been shown to be associated with the osteoclasts.[32] Elevations have been noted in Paget's disease; breast cancer with bone metastases; and Gaucher's disease, in which there is an infiltration of bone marrow and other tissue by Gaucher cells rich in ACP activity. Because of ACP activity in platelets, elevations are observed when platelet damage occurs, as in the thrombocytopenia resulting from excessive platelet destruction from idiopathic thrombocytopenic purpura.

Assay for Enzyme Activity

Assay procedures for total ACP use the same techniques as in ALP assays but are performed at an acid pH:

$$p\text{-Nitrophenolphosphate} \underset{pH\ 5}{\overset{ACP}{\rightleftharpoons}}$$

$$p\text{-nitrophenol} + \text{phosphate ion} \text{(Eq. 10–18)}$$

The reaction products are colorless at the acid pH of the reaction, but the addition of alkali stops the reaction and transforms the products into chromogens, which can be measured spectrophotometrically.

Some substrate specificities and chemical inhibitors for prostatic ACP measurements have been discussed previously. Thymolphthalein monophosphate is the substrate of choice for quantitative endpoint reactions. For continuous monitoring methods, α-naphthyl phosphate is preferred.

Immunochemical techniques for prostatic ACP use several approaches, including RIA, counterimmunoelectrophoresis, and immunoprecipitation. Also, an immunoenzymatic assay (Tandem E) includes incubation with an antibody to prostatic ACP followed by washing and incubation with p-NPP. The p-NP formed, measured photometrically, is proportional to the prostatic ACP in the sample.

Source of Error

Serum should be separated from the red cells as soon as the blood has clotted to prevent leakage of erythrocyte and platelet ACP. Serum activity decreases within 1–2 hours if the sample is left at room temperature without the addition of a preservative. Decreased activity is a result of a loss of carbon dioxide from the serum, with a resultant increase in pH. If not assayed immediately, serum should be frozen or acidified to a pH lower than 6.5. With acidification, ACP is stable for 2 days at room temperature. Hemolysis should be avoided because of contamination from erythrocyte ACP.

RIA procedures for measurement of prostatic ACP require nonacidified serum samples. Activity is stable for 2 days at 4°C.

Reference Range

Prostatic ACP, 0–3.5 ng/mL

γ-Glutamyltransferase

γ-Glutamyltransferase (GGT) is an enzyme involved in the transfer of the γ-glutamyl residue from γ-glutamyl peptides to amino acids, H_2O, and other small peptides. In most biologic systems, glutathione serves as the γ-glutamyl donor. Equation 10-19 outlines the reaction sequence:

$$\text{Glutathione} + \text{amino acid} \rightleftharpoons$$
$$\text{glutamyl} - \text{peptide} + \text{L-cysteinylglycine}$$

(Eq. 10–19)

The specific physiologic function of GGT has not been clearly established, but it is suggested that GGT is involved in peptide and protein synthesis, regulation of tissue glutathione levels, and the transport of amino acids across cell membranes.[33]

Tissue Source

GGT activity is found primarily in tissue of the kidney, brain, prostate, pancreas, and liver. Clinical applications of assay, however, are confined mainly to evaluation of liver and biliary system disorders.

Diagnostic Significance

In the liver, GGT is located in the canaliculi of the hepatic cells and particularly in the epithelial cells lining the biliary ductules. Because of these locations, GGT is elevated in virtually all hepatobiliary disorders, making it one of the most sensitive of enzyme assays in these conditions (see Chapter 22, *Liver Function*). Higher elevations are generally observed in biliary tract obstruction.

Within the hepatic parenchyma, GGT exists to a large extent in the smooth endoplasmic reticulum and is, therefore, subject to hepatic microsomal induction. Therefore, GGT levels will be increased in patients receiving enzyme-inducing drugs such as warfarin, pheno-

barbital, and phenytoin. Enzyme elevations may reach levels 4 times ULN.

Because of the effects of alcohol on GGT activity, elevated GGT levels may indicate alcoholism, particularly chronic alcoholism. Generally, enzyme elevations in persons who are alcoholics or heavy drinkers range from 2 to 3 times ULN, although higher levels have been observed. GGT assays are useful in monitoring the effects of abstention from alcohol and are used as such by alcohol treatment centers. Levels usually return to normal within 2–3 weeks after cessation but can rise again if alcohol consumption is resumed. Because of the susceptibility to enzyme induction, any interpretation of GGT levels must be done with consideration of the consequent effects of drugs and alcohol.

GGT levels are also elevated in other conditions, such as acute pancreatitis, diabetes mellitus, and myocardial infarction. The source of elevation in pancreatitis and diabetes is probably the pancreas, but the source of GGT in myocardial infarction is unknown. GGT assays are of limited value in the diagnosis of these conditions and not routinely requested.

GGT activity is useful in differentiating the source of an elevated ALP level because GGT levels are normal in skeletal disorders and during pregnancy. It is particularly useful in evaluating hepatobiliary involvement in adolescents because ALP activity will invariably be elevated as a result of bone growth.

Assay for Enzyme Activity

The most widely accepted substrate for use in GGT analysis is γ-glutamyl-*p*-nitroanilide. The γ-glutamyl residue is transferred to glycylglycine, releasing *p*-nitroaniline, a chromogenic product with a strong absorbance at 405–420 nm. The reaction, which can be used as a continuous-monitoring or fixed-point method, is outlined in Equation 10-20:

$$\text{HOOC}-\text{CHNH}_2-\text{CH}_2-\text{CH}_2-\text{CO}$$

γ-Glutamyl-*p*-nitroanilide

$$+ \text{H}_2\text{N}-\text{CH}_2-\text{CONH}-\text{CH}_2-\text{COOH}$$
Glycylglycine

$$\text{HOOC}-\text{CHNH}_2-\text{CH}_2-\text{CH}_2-\text{CO}$$
γ-Glutamyl-glycylglycine

$$+$$

$$\text{H}_2\text{N}-\text{NO}_2$$
p-Nitroaniline

(with GGT, pH 8.2 over the reaction arrow)

(Eq. 10–20)

Source of Error

GGT activity is stable, with no loss of activity for 1 week at 4°C. Hemolysis does not interfere with GGT levels because the enzyme is lacking in erythrocytes.

Reference Range

GGT: male, 6–45 U/L (37°C); female, 5–30 U/L (37°C)

Values are lower in females, presumably because of suppression of enzyme activity resulting from estrogenic or progestational hormones.

Amylase

Amylase (AMS) is an enzyme belonging to the class of hydrolases that catalyze the breakdown of starch and glycogen. Starch consists of both amylose and amylopectin. Amylose is a long, unbranched chain of glucose molecules, linked by α, 1–4 glycosidic bonds; amylopectin is a branched-chain polysaccharide with α, 1–6 linkages at the branch points. The structure of glycogen is similar to that of amylopectin but is more highly branched. α-AMS attacks only the α, 1–4 glycosidic bonds to produce degradation products consisting of glucose; maltose; and intermediate chains, called *dextrins*, which contain α, 1–6 branching linkages. Cellulose and other structural polysaccharides consisting of linkages are not attacked by α-AMS. AMS is therefore an important enzyme in the physiologic digestion of starches. The reaction proceeds according to Equation 10-21:

(Eq. 10–21)

AMS requires calcium and chloride ions for its activation.

Tissue Source

The acinar cells of the pancreas and the salivary glands are the major tissue sources of serum AMS. Lesser concentrations are found in skeletal muscle and the small intestine and fallopian tubes. AMS is the smallest enzyme, with a molecular weight of 50,000–55,000. Because of its small size, it is readily filtered by the renal glomerulus and also appears in the urine.

Digestion of starches begins in the mouth with the hydrolytic action of salivary AMS. Salivary AMS activity, however, is of short duration because, on swallowing, it is inactivated by the acidity of the gastric contents. Pancreatic AMS then performs the major digestive action of starches once the polysaccharides reach the intestine.

Diagnostic Significance

The diagnostic significance of serum and urine AMS measurements is in the diagnosis of acute pancreatitis.[34]

Disorders of tissue other than the pancreas can also produce elevations in AMS levels. Therefore, an elevated AMS level is a nonspecific finding. However, the degree of elevation of AMS is helpful, to some extent, in the differential diagnosis of acute pancreatitis. In addition, other laboratory tests (*eg,* measurements of urinary AMS levels, AMS clearance studies, AMS isoenzyme studies, and measurements of serum lipase (LPS) levels), when used in conjunction with serum AMS measurement, increase the specificity of AMS measurements in the diagnosis of acute pancreatitis.

In acute pancreatitis, serum AMS levels begin to rise 2–12 hours after onset of an attack, peak at 24 hours, and return to normal levels within 3–5 days. Values generally range from 250 to 1000 Somogyi units/dL ($2.55 \times$ ULN). Values can reach much higher levels.

Other disorders causing an elevated serum AMS level include salivary gland lesions, such as mumps and parotitis, and other intraabdominal diseases, such as perforated peptic ulcer, intestinal obstruction, cholecystitis, ruptured ectopic pregnancy, mesenteric infarction, and acute appendicitis. In addition, elevations have been reported in renal insufficiency and diabetic ketoacidosis. Serum AMS levels in intra-abdominal conditions other than acute pancreatitis are usually less than 500 Somogyi units/dL.

An apparently asymptomatic condition of hyperamylasemia has been noted in approximately 1–2% of the population. This condition, called *macroamylasemia*, results when the AMS molecule combines with immunoglobulins to form a complex that is too large to be filtered across the glomerulus. Serum AMS levels increase because of the reduction in normal renal clearance of the enzyme and, consequently, the urinary excretion of AMS is abnormally low. The diagnostic significance of macroamylasemia lies in the need to differentiate it from other causes of hyperamylasemia.

Much interest has been focused recently on the possible diagnostic use of AMS isoenzyme measurements.[34,35] Serum AMS is a mixture of a number of isoenzymes that can be separated by differences in physical properties, most notably electrophoresis, although chromatography and isoelectric focusing also have been applied. In normal human serum, two major bands and as many as four minor bands may be seen. The bands are designated as P-type and S-type isoamylase. P isoamylase is derived from pancreatic tissue; S isoamylase is derived from salivary gland tissue, as well as the fallopian tube and lung. The isoenzymes of salivary origin migrate most quickly (S1, S2, S3), whereas those of pancreatic origin are slower (P1, P2, P3). In normal human serum, the isoamylases migrate in regions corresponding to the β- to α-globulin regions of protein electrophoresis. The most commonly observed fractions are P2, S1, and S2.

In acute pancreatitis, there is typically an increase in P-type activity, with P3 being the most predominant isoenzyme. However, P3 also has been detected in cases of renal failure and, therefore, is not entirely specific for acute pancreatitis. S-Type isoamylase represents approximately two-thirds of AMS activity of normal serum, whereas P-type predominates in normal urine.

Assay for Enzyme Activity

AMS can be assayed by a variety of different methods, which are summarized in Table 10-6. The four main approaches are categorized as amyloclast, saccharogenic, chromogenic, and continuous monitoring.

In the amyloclastic method, AMS is allowed to act on a starch substrate to which iodine has been attached. As AMS hydrolyzes the starch molecule into smaller units, the iodine is released and a decrease in the initial dark-blue color intensity of the starch–iodine complex occurs. The decrease in color is proportional to the AMS concentration.

The saccharogenic method uses a starch substrate that is hydrolyzed by the action of AMS to its constituent carbohydrate molecules that have reducing properties. The amount of reducing sugars is then measured where the concentration is proportional to AMS activity. The saccharogenic method, the classic reference method for determining AMS activity, is reported in Somogyi units. Somogyi units are an expression of the number of milligrams of glucose released in 30 minutes at 37°C under specific assay conditions.

Chromogenic methods use a starch substrate to which a chromogenic dye has been attached, forming an insoluble dye–substrate complex. As AMS hydrolyzes the starch substrate, smaller dye-substrate fragments are produced, and these are water-soluble. The increase in color intensity of the soluble dye-substrate solution is proportional to AMS activity.

Recently, coupled-enzyme systems have been used to determine AMS activity by a continuous-monitoring technique in which the change in absorbance of NAD$^+$ at 340 nm is measured. Equation 10-22 is an example of a continuous-monitoring method. For AMS activity, the optimal pH is 6.9.

$$\text{Maltopentose} \overset{\text{AMS}}{\rightleftharpoons} \text{maltotriose} + \text{maltose}$$

$$\text{Maltotriose} + \text{maltose} \overset{\alpha\text{-glucosidase}}{\rightleftharpoons} \text{5-glucose}$$

TABLE 10-6. AMYLASE METHODOLOGIES

Amyloclastic	Measures the disappearance of starch substrate
Saccharogenic	Measures the appearance of the product
Chromogenic	Measures the increasing color from production of product coupled with a chromogenic dye
Continuous monitoring	Coupling of several enzyme systems to monitor amylase activity

$$\text{5-Glucose} + \text{5 ATP} \overset{\text{Hexokinase}}{\rightleftharpoons}$$

$$\text{5-glucose-6-phosphate} + \text{5 ADP}$$

$$\text{5-Glucose-6-phosphate} + \text{5 NAD} + \overset{\text{G-6-PD}}{\rightleftharpoons}$$

$$\text{5,6-phosphogluconolactone} + \text{5 NADH}$$

(Eq. 10–22)

Because salivary AMS is preferentially inhibited by wheat germ lectin, salivary and pancreatic AMS can be estimated by measuring total AMS in the presence and absence of lectin. Specific immunoassays are also available for measuring isoenzymes of AMS.

Source of Error

AMS in serum and urine is stable. Little loss of activity occurs at room temperature for 1 week or at 4°C for 2 months. Because plasma triglycerides suppress or inhibit serum AMS activity, AMS values may be normal in acute pancreatitis with hyperlipemia.

The administration of morphine and other opiates for pain relief before blood sampling will lead to falsely elevated serum AMS levels. The drugs presumably cause constriction of Oddi's sphincter and pancreatic ducts, with consequent elevation of inarticulate pressure causing regurgitation of AMS into the serum.

Reference Range

AMS: serum, 25–130 U/L; urine, 1–15 U/hour

Because of the various AMS procedures currently in use, activity is expressed according to each procedure. There is no uniform expression of AMS activity, although Somogyi units are frequently used. The approximate conversion factor between Somogyi units and International Units is 1.85.

Lipase

Lipase (LPS) is an enzyme that hydrolyzes the ester linkages of fats to produce alcohols and fatty acids. Specifically, LPS catalyzes the partial hydrolysis of dietary triglycerides in the intestine to the 2-monoglyceride intermediate, with the production of long-chain fatty acids. The reaction proceeds according to Equation 10-23:

$$
\begin{array}{l}
\quad\quad\quad\quad\text{O} \\
\quad\quad\quad\quad\|\\
\text{CH}_2\!-\!\text{O}\!-\!\text{C}\!-\!\text{R}_1 \quad\quad\quad \text{CH}_2\text{OH} \\
\quad | \\
\quad\quad\quad\quad \text{O} \quad\quad\quad\quad\quad\quad\quad\quad \text{O} \\
\quad\quad\quad\quad \| \quad\quad\quad\quad \text{LPS} \quad\quad\quad\quad \| \\
\text{CH}\!-\!\text{O}\!-\!\text{C}\!-\!\text{R}_2 + 2\text{H}_2\text{O} \rightleftharpoons \text{CH}\!-\!\text{O}\!-\!\text{C}\!-\!\text{R}_2 + 2 \text{ fatty} \\
\quad | \quad\quad\quad\quad\quad\quad\quad\quad\quad\quad\quad | \quad\quad\quad\quad\quad\quad\quad\quad \text{acids} \\
\quad\quad\quad\quad \text{O} \quad\quad\quad\quad\quad\quad\quad\quad \text{CH}_2\text{OH} \\
\quad\quad\quad\quad \| \\
\text{CH}_2\!-\!\text{O}\!-\!\text{C}\!-\!\text{R}_3 \\
\text{Triacylglycerol} \quad\quad\quad\quad \text{2-Monoglyceride}
\end{array}
$$

(Eq. 10–23)

The enzymatic activity of pancreatic LPS is specific for the fatty acid residues at positions 1 and 3 of the triglyceride molecule, but substrate must be an emulsion for activity to occur. The reaction rate is accelerated by the presence of colipase and a bile salt.

Tissue Source

LPS concentration is found primarily in the pancreas, although it is also present in the stomach and small intestine.

Diagnostic Significance

Clinical assays of serum LPS measurements are confined almost exclusively to the diagnosis of acute pancreatitis. It is similar in this respect to AMS measurements but is considered more specific for pancreatic disorders than AMS measurement. Both AMS and LPS levels rise quickly, but LPS elevations persist for approximately 5 days in acute pancreatitis, whereas AMS elevations persist for only 2–3 days. The extent of elevations does not correlate with severity of disease. Elevated LPS levels also may be found in other intra-abdominal conditions but with less frequency than elevations of serum AMS. Elevations have been reported in cases of penetrating duodenal ulcers and perforated peptic ulcers, intestinal obstruction, and acute cholecystitis. In contrast to AMS levels, LPS levels are normal in conditions of salivary gland involvement. Therefore, LPS levels are useful in differentiating serum AMS elevation as a result of pancreatic versus salivary involvement. Of the three lipase isoenzymes, L2 is thought to be the most clinically specific and sensitive.

Assay for Enzyme Activity

Procedures used to measure LPS activity include estimation of liberated fatty acids and turbidimetric methods. The reaction is outlined in Equation 10-24:

$$\text{Triglyceride} + 2\,H_2O \xrightleftharpoons[\text{(pH, 8.6-9.0)}]{\text{LPS}}$$
$$\text{2-monoglyceride} + 2 \text{ fatty acids}$$

(Eq. 10–24)

Early methods for LPS were historically poor. The classic Cherry-Crandall method used an olive oil substrate and measured the liberated fatty acids by titration after a 24-hour incubation. Modifications of the Cherry-Crandall method have been complicated by the lack of stable and uniform substrates. However, triolein is one substrate now used as a more pure form of triglyceride.

Turbidimetric methods are simpler and more rapid than titrimetric assays. Fats in solution create a cloudy emulsion. As the fats are hydrolyzed by LPS, the particles disperse, and the rate of clearing can be measured as an estimation of LPS activity. Colorimetric methods are also available and are based on coupled reactions with enzymes such as peroxidase or glycerol kinase.

Source of Error

LPS is stable in serum, with negligible loss in activity at room temperature for 1 week or for 3 weeks at 4°C. Hemolysis should be avoided because hemoglobin inhibits the activity of serum LPS, causing falsely low values.

Reference Range

LPS, 0–1.0 U/mL.

Glucose-6-Phosphate Dehydrogenase

Glucose-6-phosphate dehydrogenase (G-6-PD) is an *oxidoreductase* that catalyzes the oxidation of glucose 6-phosphate to 6-phosphogluconate or the corresponding lactone. The reaction is important as the first step in the pentose-phosphate shunt of glucose metabolism with the ultimate production of NADPH. The reaction is outlined in Equation 10-25:

Glucose-6-phosphate

6-Phosphogluconate

(Eq. 10–25)

Tissue Source

Sources of G-6-PD include the adrenal cortex, spleen, thymus, lymph nodes, lactating mammary gland, and erythrocytes. Little activity is found in normal serum.

CASE STUDY 10-3

A 36-year-old Hispanic woman presents to the emergency department with abdominal pain, weakness, and loss of appetite. She had not traveled in recent months. She has not been well for several days.

Questions

1. What lab tests should be ordered to help diagnose this patient?

2. What enzyme tests will be useful in diagnosing this patient?

3. What two diagnoses are most likely for this patient?

Diagnostic Significance

Most of the interest of G-6-PD focuses on its role in the erythrocyte. Here, it functions to maintain NADPH in reduced form. An adequate concentration of NADPH is required to regenerate sulfhydryl-containing proteins, such as glutathione, from the oxidized to the reduced state. Glutathione in the reduced form, in turn, protects hemoglobin from oxidation by agents that may be present in the cell. A deficiency of G-6-PD results in an inadequate supply of NADPH and, ultimately, in the inability to maintain reduced glutathione levels. When erythrocytes are exposed to oxidizing agents, hemolysis occurs because of oxidation of hemoglobin and damage of the cell membrane.

G-6-PD deficiency is an inherited sex-linked trait. The disorder can result in several different clinical manifestations, one of which is drug-induced hemolytic anemia. When exposed to an oxidant drug such as primaquine, an antimalarial drug, affected individuals experience a hemolytic episode. The severity of the hemolysis is related to the drug concentration. G-6-PD deficiency is most common in African Americans, but has been reported in virtually every ethnic group.

Increased levels of G-6-PD in the serum have been reported in myocardial infarction and megaloblastic anemias. No elevations are seen in hepatic disorders. G-6-PD levels, however, are not routinely performed as diagnostic aids in these conditions.

Assay for Enzyme Activity

The assay procedure for G-6-PD activity is outlined in Equation 10-26:

$$\text{Glucose 6-phosphate} + \text{NADP}^+ \xrightleftharpoons{\text{G-6-PD}}$$

$$\text{6-phosphogluconate} + \text{NADPH} + \text{H}^+$$

(Eq. 10–26)

A red cell hemolysate is used to assay for deficiency of the enzyme; serum is used for evaluation of enzyme elevations.

Reference Range

G-6-PD, 10–15 U/g Hgb

SUMMARY

Found in all body tissues, enzymes are proteins that catalyze biochemical reactions. The catalyzed reactions are specific and essential to physiologic well-being. In injury or in many disease states, certain enzymes are released from their normal locations and appear in increased amounts in the general circulation. An understanding of biologically significant enzymes and the reactions they catalyze, therefore, is useful in the diagnosis and treatment of certain disease states.

This chapter reviewed the general properties of enzymes and their classification and catalytic mechanisms. Several factors that affect the rate of enzymatic reactions and general methods for measuring enzyme activity were also discussed.

Many enzymes are clinically important. Quantitating serum levels of certain enzymes or isoenzymes can assist in the diagnosis and prognosis of hepatic disorders, skeletal muscle disorders, bone disorders, cardiac disorders, malignancy, or acute pancreatitis. This chapter discussed tissue source, diagnostic significance, preferred assay methodologies, and reference ranges of several clinically significant enzymes.

REVIEW QUESTIONS

1. When a reaction is performed in zero-order kinetics:
   a. the substrate concentration is very low.
   b. the rate of reaction is directly proportional to the substrate concentration.
   c. the rate of the reaction is independent of the substrate concentration.
   d. the enzyme level is always high.

2. Activation energy is:
   a. the energy needed for an enzyme reaction to stop.
   b. increased by enzymes.
   c. very high in catalyzed reactions.
   d. decreased by enzymes.

3. Enzyme reaction rates are increased by increasing temperatures until they reach the point of denaturation at:
   a. 40°–60°C.
   b. 25°–35°C.
   c. 100°C.
   d. 37°C.

4. An example of using enzymes as reagents in the clinical laboratory is:
   a. the diacetyl monoxime blood urea nitrogen (BUN) method.
   b. the hexokinase glucose method.
   c. the alkaline picrate creatinine method.
   d. the biuret total protein method.

5. Activity of enzymes in serum may be determined rather than concentration because:
   a. the temperature is too high.
   b. the amount of enzyme is too low to measure.
   c. there is not enough substrate.
   d. the amount of enzyme is too high to measure.

6. The isoenzymes LD-4 and LD-5 are elevated in:
   a. pulmonary embolism.
   b. liver disease.
   c. renal disease.
   d. myocardial infarction.

7. Which CK isoenzyme is elevated in muscle diseases?
   a. CK-BB
   b. CK-MB
   c. CK-MM
   d. CK-NN

8. Elevation of serum amylase and lipase is commonly seen in:
   a. acute appendicitis.
   b. acute pancreatitis.
   c. gallbladder disease.
   d. acid reflux disease.

9. The saccharogenic method for amylase determinations measures:
   a. the amount of product produced.
   b. the amount of substrate consumed.
   c. the amount of iodine present.
   d. the amount of starch present.

10. Elevation of tissue enzymes in serum may be used to detect:
    a. presence of toxins.
    b. infectious diseases.
    c. tissue necrosis or damage.
    d. diabetes mellitus.

REFERENCES

1. Enzyme Nomenclature 1978, Recommendations of the Nomenclature Committee of the International Union of Biochemistry on the Nomenclature and Classification of Enzymes. New York: Academic Press, 1979.
2. Baron DN, Moss DW, Walker PG, et al. Abbreviations for names of enzymes of diagnostic importance. J Clin Pathol 1971;24:656.
3. Baron DN, Moss DW, Walker PG, et al. Revised list of abbreviations for names of enzymes of diagnostic importance. J Clin Pathol 1975;28:592.
4. Rej R. Accurate enzyme measurements. Arch Pathol Lab Med 1998;117:352.
5. Spitzer M, Pinto A. Early diagnosis of ectopic pregnancy: can we do it accurately using a chemical profile? J Women's Health Gender Based Med 2000;9:537.
6. Na Kafusa J, et. al. The importance of serum creatine phosphokinase levels in the early diagnosis, and as a prognostic factor, of *Vibrio vulnificus* infection. Br Med J 2001;145:2.
7. Galen RS. The enzyme diagnosis of myocardial infarction. Human Pathol 1975;6:141.
8. Wilkinson JH. The Principles and Practice of Diagnostic Enzymology. Chicago, IL: Year Book Medical Publishers, 1976:395.
9. Silverman LM, Dermer GB, Zweig MH, et al. Creatine kinase BB: a new tumor-associated marker. Clin Chem 1979;25:1432.
10. Lang H, ed. Creatine Kinase Isoenzymes: Pathophysiology and Clinical Application. Berlin: Springer-Verlag, 1981.
11. Irvin RG, Cobb FR, Roe CR. Acute myocardial infarction and MB creatine phosphokinase: relationship between onset of symptoms of infarction and appearance and disappearance of enzyme. Arch Intern Med 1980;140:329.
12. Bark CJ. Mitochondrial creatine kinase—a poor prognostic sign. J Am Med Assoc 1980;243:2058.
13. Batsakis J, Savory J, eds. Creatine kinase. Crit Rev Clin Lab Sci 1982;16:291.
14. Lang H, Wurzburg U. Creatine kinase, an enzyme of many forms. Clin Chem 1982;28:1439.
15. Lott JA. Electrophoretic CK and LD isoenzyme assays in myocardial infarction. Lab Management 1983;Feb:23.
16. Pesce MA. The CK isoenzymes: findings and their meaning. Lab Management 1982;Oct:25.
17. Roche Diagnostics. Isomune-CK package insert. Nutley, NJ: Hoffman-La Roche, 1979.
18. Faulkner WR, Meites S, eds. Selected Methods for the Small Clinical Chemistry Laboratory: Selected Methods of Clinical Chemistry. Vol. 9. Washington, D.C.: American Association for Clinical Chemistry, 1982:475.
19. Lott JA, Stang JM. Serum enzymes and isoenzymes in the diagnosis and differential diagnosis of myocardial ischemia and necrosis. Clin Chem 1980;26:1241.
20. Leung FY, Henderson AR. Influence of hemolysis on the serum lactate dehydrogenase1/lactate dehydrogenase-2 ratio as determined by an accurate thin-layer agarose electrophoresis procedure. Clin Chem 1981;27:1708.

21. Bhagavan NV, Darm JR, Scottolini AG. A sixth lactate dehydrogenase isoenzyme (LD-6) and its significance. Arch Pathol Lab Med 1982; 106:521.

22. Cabello B, Lubin J, Rywlin AM, et al. Significance of a sixth lactate dehydrogenase isoenzyme (LDH₆). Am J Clin Pathol 1980; 73:253.

23. Goldberg DM, Werner M, eds. LD-6, A Sign of Impending Death From Heart Failure, Selected Topics in Clinical Enzymology. New York: Walter de Gruyter, 1983:347.

24. Posen S, Doherty E. The measurement of serum alkaline phosphatase in clinical medicine. Adv Clin Chem 1981;22:165.

25. Warren BM. The isoenzymes of alkaline phosphatase. Beaumont, TX: Helena Laboratories, 1981.

26. Fleisher GA, Eickelberg ES, Elveback LR. Alkaline phosphatase activity in the plasma of children and adolescents. Clin Chem 1977;23:469.

27. Gittes RF. Carcinoma of the prostate. N Engl J Med 1991;324:236.

28. Gittes RF. Prostate specific antigen. N Engl J Med 1987;318:954.

29. Oesterling JE. Prostate specific antigen: a critical assessment of the most useful tumor marker for adenocarcinoma of the prostate. J Urol 1991;145:907.

30. Griffiths JC. The laboratory diagnosis of prostatic adenocarcinoma. Crit Rev Clin Lab Sci 1983;19:187.

31. Lantz RK, Berg MJ. From clinic to court: acid phosphatase testing. Diagn Med 1981;Mar/Apr:55.

32. Yam LT. Clinical significance of the human acid phosphatases. A review. Am J Med 1974;56:604.

33. Rosalki SB. Gamma-glutamyl transpeptidase. Adv Clin Chem 1975;17:53.

34. Salt WB II, Schenker S. Amylase: its clinical significance. A review of the literature. Medicine 1976;4:269.

35. Murthy U, et al. Hyperamylasemia in patients with acquired immunodeficiency syndrome. Am J Gastroenterol 1992;87(3):332.

Carbohydrates

Vicki S. Freeman

OBJECTIVES

Upon completion of this chapter, the clinical laboratorian will be able to:
- Classify carbohydrates into their respective groups.
- Discuss the metabolism of carbohydrates in the body and the mode of action of hormones in carbohydrate metabolism.
- Differentiate the types of diabetes by clinical symptoms and laboratory findings according to the American Diabetes Association (ADA)
- Explain the clinical significance of the three ketone bodies.
- Relate expected laboratory results and clinical symptoms to the following metabolic complications of diabetes:
    - ketoacidosis
    - hyperosmolar coma

- Distinguish between reactive and spontaneous hypoglycemia.
- Describe the principle, specimen of choice, and the advantages and disadvantages of the glucose analysis methods.
- Describe the three commonly encountered methods for glycated hemoglobin, specimen of choice, and source of error.
- Describe the use of glycosylated hemoglobin in the long-term monitoring of diabetes.
- Discuss the methods of analysis and the advantages and disadvantages for ketone bodies.

KEY TERMS

Carbohydrates
Diabetes mellitus
Disaccharide
Embden-Myerhof
   pathway
Fisher projection

Glucagon
Gluconeogenesis
Glycogen
Glycogenolysis
Glycolysis

Glycosylated hemoglobin
Haworth projection
Hyperglycemic
Hypoglycemic
Insulin

Ketone
Microalbuminuria
Monosaccharide
Polysaccharide
Triose

Organisms rely on the oxidation of complex organic compounds to obtain energy. Three general types of such compounds are carbohydrates, amino acids, and lipids. Although all three are used as a source of energy, carbohydrates are the primary source for brain, erythrocytes, and retinal cells in humans. Carbohydrates are the major food source and energy supply of the body and are stored primarily as liver and muscle glycogen. Disease states involving carbohydrates are split into groups—hyperglycemia and hypoglycemia. Early detection of diabetes mellitus is the aim of the American Diabetes Association guidelines established in 1997. Acute and chronic complications may be avoided with proper diagnosis, monitoring, and treatment. The laboratory plays an important role through periodic measurements of glycosylated hemoglobin and microalbumin.

GENERAL DESCRIPTION OF CARBOHYDRATES

Carbohydrates are compounds containing C, H, and O. The general formula for a carbohydrate is $C_x(H_2O)_y$. All carbohydrates contain C=O and –OH functional groups. There are some derivatives from this basic formula because carbohydrate derivatives can be formed by the addition of other chemical groups, such as phosphates, sulfates, and amines. The classification of carbohydrates is based on four different properties: (1) the size of the base carbon chain, (2) the location of the CO function group, (3) the number of sugar units, and (4) the stereochemistry of the compound.

Classification of Carbohydrates

Carbohydrates can be grouped into generic classifications based on the number of carbons in the molecule. For example, *trioses* contain three carbons, tetroses contain four, pentoses contain five, and hexoses contain six. In actual practice, the smallest carbohydrate is glyceraldehyde, a three-carbon compound.

Carbohydrates are hydrates of aldehyde or ketone derivatives based on the location of the CO functional group (Fig. 11-1). The two forms of carbohydrates are aldose and ketose (Fig. 11-2). The aldose form has an aldehyde as its functional group, whereas the ketose form has a ketone as the functional group. The carbon in the functional group is called the anomeric carbon.

Several models are used to represent carbohydrates. The *Fisher projection* of a carbohydrate has the aldehyde or ketone at the top of the drawing. The carbons are numbered starting at the aldehyde or ketone end. The compound can be represented as a straight chain or might be linked to show a representation of the cyclic, hemiacetal form (Fig. 11-3). The *Haworth projection* represents the compound in the cyclic form that is more representative of the actual structure. This structure is formed when the functional group (ketone or aldehyde) reacts with an alcohol group on the same sugar to form a ring called the *hemiacetal ring* (Fig. 11-4).

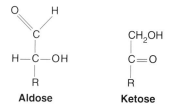

Aldose   **Ketose**

FIGURE 11-2. Two forms of carbohydrates.

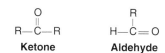

Ketone   **Aldehyde**

FIGURE 11-1. Aldehyde and ketone structure.

H—C=O   H—C—OH
H—C—OH   H—C—OH
HO—C—H   HO—C—H
H—C—OH   H—C—OH   O
H—C—OH   H—C—
CH₂OH   CH₂OH

FIGURE 11-3. Fisher projection of glucose. The *figure on the left* is the open chain Fisher projections, and the *figure on the right* is a cyclic Fisher projection.

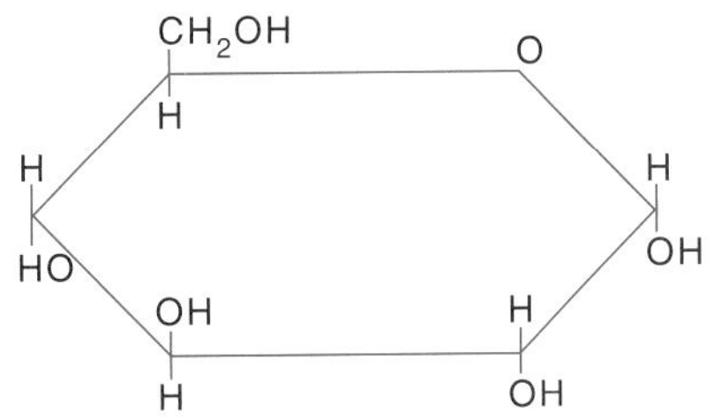

FIGURE 11-4. Haworth projection of glucose.

Stereoisomers

The central carbons of a carbohydrate are asymmetric—four different groups are attached to the carbon atoms. This allows for various spatial arrangements of carbohydrate molecules called *stereoisomers*. Stereoisomers have the same order and types of bonds but different spatial arrangements and different properties. For each asymmetric carbon, there are 2^n possible isomers; therefore, there are 2^1, or two, forms of glyceraldehyde. These isomers are mirror images. Because an aldohexose contains four asymmetric carbons, there are 2^4 or 16 possible isomers, two of which are paired stereoisomers named D-glucose and L-glucose. The D and L are terms used to describe some of the possible optical isomers of glucose and other compounds that exist as stereoisomers. They are mirror images that cannot be overlapped. The D-configuration has the –OH on the lowest asymmetric carbon on the right; the L-form has the –OH on the left. In Figure 11-5, D-glucose is represented in the Fisher projection with the hydroxy group on carbon number five positioned on the right. L-Glucose has the hydroxy group of carbon number five positioned on the left. Most sugars in humans are in the D-form.

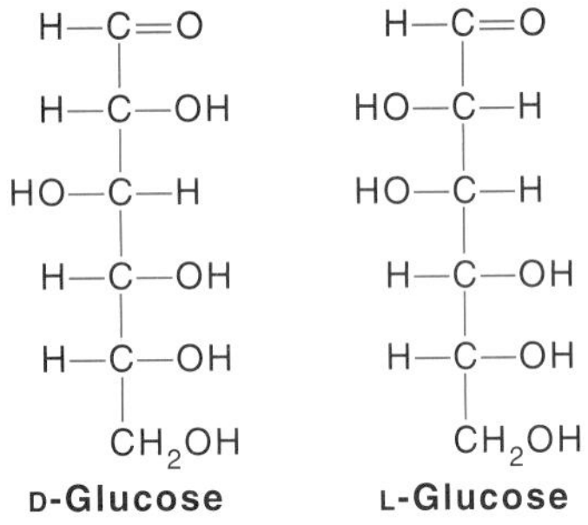

FIGURE 11-5. Stereoisomers of glucose.

Monosaccharides, Disaccharides, and Polysaccharides

Another classification of carbohydrates is based on number of sugar units in the chain: monosaccharides, disaccharides, oligosaccharides, and polysaccharides. This chaining of sugars relies on the formation of glycoside bonds that are bridges of oxygen atoms. When two carbohydrate molecules join, a water molecule is produced. When they split, one molecule of water is used to form the individual compounds. This reaction is called *hydrolysis*. The glycoside linkages of carbohydrate can involve any number of carbons; however, certain carbons are favored, depending on the carbohydrate.

Monosaccharides are simple sugars that cannot be hydrolyzed to a simpler form. These sugars can contain three, four, five, and six or more carbon atoms (known as trioses, tetroses, pentoses, and hexoses, respectively). The most common include glucose, fructose, and galactose.

Disaccharides are formed on the interaction of groups between two monosaccharides with the production of a molecule of water. On hydrolysis, disaccharides will be split into two monosaccharides by disaccharide enzymes (eg, lactase) located on the microvilli of the intestine. These monosaccharides are then actively absorbed. The most common disaccharides are maltose (comprising 2-β-D-glucose molecules in a 1→4 linkage), lactose, and sucrose.

Oligosaccharides are the chaining of two to ten sugar units, whereas *polysaccharides* are formed by the linkage of many monosaccharide units. On hydrolysis, polysaccharides will yield more than ten monosaccharides. Amylase hydrolyzes starch to disaccharides in the duodenum. The most common polysaccharides are starch (glucose molecules) and glycogen (Fig. 11-6).

Chemical Properties of Carbohydrates

Some carbohydrates are reducing substances; these carbohydrates can oxidize or reduce other compounds. To be a reducing substance, the carbohydrate must contain a ketone or aldehyde group. Examples of reducing substances include glucose, maltose, fructose, lactose, and galactose. This property was used in many laboratory methods in the past in the determination of carbohydrates.

Carbohydrates can form glycosidic bonds with other carbohydrates and with noncarbohydrates. The aldose or

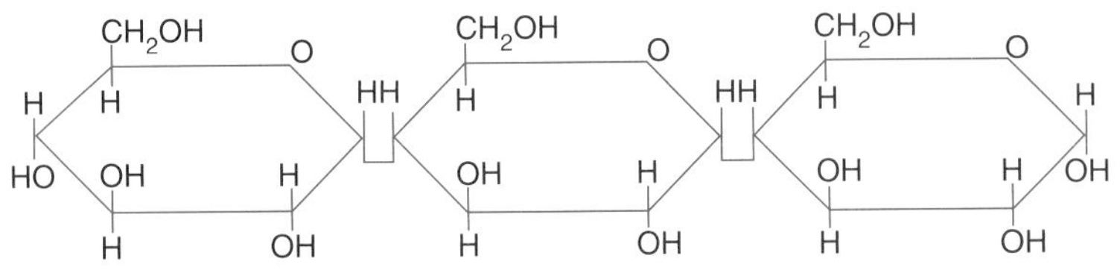

FIGURE 11-6. Linkage of monosaccharides.

ketone group on the carbohydrate forms an oxygen bond. If the bond forms with one of the other carbons on the carbohydrate other than the anomeric carbon, the anomeric carbon (functional group) is unaltered and the resulting compound remains a reducing substance.

If the bond is formed with the anomeric carbon on the other carbohydrate, the resulting compound is *no longer a reducing substance*. Nonreducing carbohydrates *do not have an active ketone or aldehyde group. They will not oxidize or reduce other compounds. The most common nonreducing sugar is sucrose—table sugar (Fig. 11-7).

All monosaccharides and many disaccharides are reducing agents. This is because a free aldehyde or ketone (the open chain form) can be oxidized under the proper conditions. As a disaccharide, one of the aldehydes or ketones is usually alpha to the glycosidic linkage. The other aldehyde or ketone is still free to function as a reducing agent. However, when both aldehydes or ketones are alpha to the glycosidic linkage, such as in sucrose, then the disaccharide is incapable of undergoing mutarotation and is, therefore, incapable of functioning as a reducing agent. Both maltose and lactose are reducing agents, whereas sucrose is not.

Glucose Metabolism

Glucose is a primary source of energy for humans. The nervous system, including the brain, totally depends on glucose from the surrounding extracellular fluid (ECF) for energy. Nervous tissue cannot concentrate or store carbohydrates; therefore, it is critical to maintain a steady supply of glucose to the tissue. For this reason, the concentration of glucose in the ECF must be maintained in a narrow range. When the concentration falls below a certain level, the nervous tissue lose the primary energy source and are incapable of maintaining normal function.

Fate of Glucose

Most of our ingested carbohydrates are polymers, such as starch and *glycogen*. Salivary amylase and pancreatic amylase are responsible for the digestion of these nonabsorbable polymers to dextrins and disaccharides, which are further hydrolyzed to monosaccharides by maltase, an enzyme released by the intestinal mucosa. Sucrase and lactase are two other important gut-derived enzymes that hydrolyze sucrose to glucose and fructose and lactose to glucose and galactose.

When disaccharides are converted to monosaccharides, they are absorbed by the gut and transported to the liver by the hepatic portal venous blood supply. Glucose is the only carbohydrate to be directly used for energy or stored as glycogen. Galactose and fructose must be converted to glucose before they can be used. After glucose enters the cell, it is quickly shunted into one of three possible metabolic pathways, depending on the availability of substrates or the nutritional status of the cell. The ultimate goal of the cell is to convert glucose to carbon dioxide and water. During this process, the cell obtains the high-energy molecule adenosine triphosphate (ATP) from inorganic phosphate and adenosine diphosphate (ADP). The cell requires oxygen for the final steps in the electron transport chain (ETC). Nicotinamide adenine dinucleotide (NAD) in its reduced form (NADH) will act as an intermediate to couple glucose oxidation to the ETC in the mitochondria where much of the ATP is gained.

The first step for all three pathways requires glucose to be converted to glucose 6-phosphate using the high-energy molecule, ATP. This reaction is catalyzed by the enzyme hexokinase (Fig. 11-8). Glucose 6-phosphate can enter the *Embden-Meyerhof pathway* or *the hexose monophosphate pathway* or can be converted to glycogen (Fig. 11-8). The first two pathways are important for the generation of energy from glucose; the conversion to glycogen pathway is important for the storage of glucose.

In the Embden-Meyerhof pathway, glucose is broken down into two, three-carbon molecules of pyruvic acid that can enter the *tricarboxylic acid cycle* (TCA cycle) on conversion to acetyl-coenzyme A (acetyl-CoA). This pathway requires oxygen and is called the *aerobic pathway* (Fig. 11-8). Other substrates have the opportunity to enter the pathway at several points. Glycerol released from the hydrolysis of triglycerides can enter at 3-phosphoglycerate, and fatty acids and ketones and some amino acids are converted or catabolized to acetyl-CoA, which is part of the TCA cycle. Other amino acids enter the pathway as pyruvate or as deaminated α-ketoacids and α-oxoacids. The conversion of amino acids by the liver and other specialized tissue, such as the kidney, to substrates that can be converted to glucose is called *gluconeogenesis*. Gluconeogenesis also encompasses the conversion of glycerol, lactate, and pyruvate to glucose.

Anaerobic *glycolysis* is important for tissue such as muscle, which often have important energy requirements without an adequate oxygen supply. These tissues can derive ATP from glucose in an oxygen-deficient environment by converting pyruvic acid into lactic acid. The lactic acid diffuses from the muscle cell, enters the systemic circulation, and is then taken up and used by the liver (Fig. 11-8). For anaerobic glycolysis to occur, 2 moles of

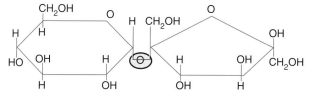

FIGURE 11-7. Haworth projection of sucrose.

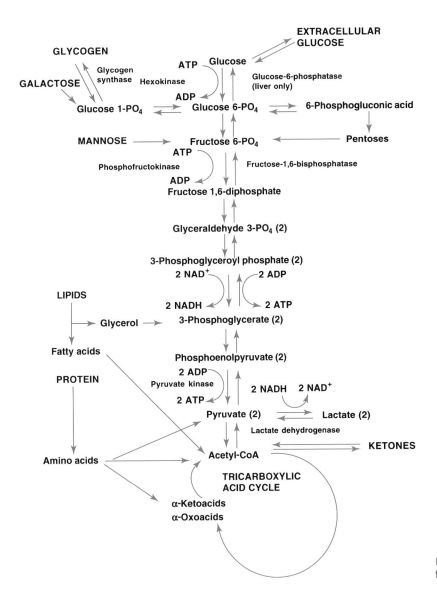

FIGURE 11-8. The Embden-Meyerhof pathway for anaerobic glycolysis.

ATP must be consumed for each mole of glucose; however, 4 moles of ATP are directly produced, resulting in a net gain of 2 moles of ATP. Further gains of ATP result from the introduction of pyruvate into the TCA cycle and NADH into the ETC.

The second energy pathway is the *hexose monophosphate shunt* (HMP shunt), which is actually a detour of glucose 6-phosphate from the glycolytic pathway to become 6-phosphogluconic acid. This oxidized product permits the formation of ribose 5-phosphate and NDP in its reduced form (NADPH). NADPH is important to erythrocytes that lack mitochondria and are therefore incapable of the TCA cycle. The reducing power of NADPH is required for the protection of the cell from oxidative and free radical damage. Without NADPH, the lipid bilayer membrane of the cell and critical enzymes would eventually be destroyed, resulting in cell death. The HMP shunt also permits pentoses, such as ribose, to enter the glycolytic pathway.

When the cell's energy requirements are being met, glucose can be stored as glycogen. This third pathway, which is called *glycogenesis,* is relatively straightforward. Glucose 6-phosphate is converted to glucose 1-phosphate, which is then converted to uridine diphosphoglucose and then to glycogen by glycogen synthase. Several tissues are capable of the synthesis of glycogen, especially the liver and muscles. Hepatocytes are capable of releasing glucose from glycogen or other sources to maintain the blood glucose concentration. This is because the liver synthesizes the enzyme glucose-6-phosphatase. Without this enzyme, glucose is trapped in the glycolytic pathway. Muscle cells do not synthesize glucose-6-phosphatase and, therefore, they are incapable of dephosphorylating glucose. Once glucose enters a muscle cell, it remains as glycogen unless it is catabolized. *Glycogenolysis* is the process by which glycogen is converted back to glucose 6-phosphate for entry into the glycolytic pathway. Table 11-1 outlines the major energy pathways involved either directly or indirectly with glucose metabolism.

Overall, dietary glucose and other carbohydrates can either be used by the liver and other cells for energy or can be stored as glycogen for later use. When the supply of glucose is low, the liver will use glycogen and other substrates to elevate the blood glucose concentration. These substrates include glycerol from triglycerides, lactic acid from skin and muscles, and amino acids. If the lipolysis of triglycerides is unregulated, it results in the formation of ketone bodies, which the brain can use as a source of energy through the TCA cycle. The synthesis of glucose from amino acids is gluconeogenesis. This process is used in conjunction with the formation of ketone bodies when glycogen stores are depleted—conditions normally associated with starvation. The principle pathway for glucose oxidation is through the Embden-Myerhof pathway. NADPH can be synthesized through the HMP shunt, which is a side pathway from the anaerobic glycolytic pathway (Fig. 11-8).

Regulation of Carbohydrate Metabolism

The liver, pancreas, and other endocrine glands are all involved in controlling the blood glucose concentrations within a narrow range. During a brief fast, glucose is supplied to the ECF from the liver through glycogenolysis. When the fasting period is longer than 1 day, glucose is synthesized from other sources through gluconeogenesis. Control of blood glucose is under two major hormones: insulin and glucagon, both produced by the pancreas. Their actions oppose each other. Other hormones and neuroendocrine substances also exert some

control over blood glucose concentrations, permitting the body to respond to increased demands for glucose or to survive prolonged fasts. It also permits the conservation of energy as lipids when excess substrates are ingested.

Insulin is the primary hormone responsible for the entry of glucose into the cell. It is synthesized by the β cells of islets of Langerhans in the pancreas. When these cells detect an increase in body glucose, they release insulin. The release of insulin causes an increased movement of glucose into the cells and increased glucose metabolism. Insulin is normally released when glucose levels are high and is *not* released when glucose levels are decreased. It decreases plasma glucose levels by increasing the transport entry of glucose in muscle and adipose tissue by way of nonspecific receptors. It also regulates glucose by increasing glycogenesis, lipogenesis, and glycolysis and inhibiting glycogenolysis. Insulin is the only hormone that decreases glucose levels and can be referred to as a *hypoglycemic* agent (Table 11-2).

Glucagon is the primary hormone responsible for increasing glucose levels. It is synthesized by the α cells of islets of Langerhans in the pancreas and released during stress and fasting states. When these cells detect a decrease in body glucose, they release glucagon. Glucagon acts by increasing plasma glucose levels by glycogenolysis in the liver and an increase in gluconeogenesis. It can be referred to as a *hyperglycemic* agent (Table 11-2).

Two hormones produced by the adrenal gland affect carbohydrate metabolism. *Epinephrine,* produced by the adrenal medulla, increases plasma glucose by inhibiting insulin secretion, increasing glycogenolysis, and promoting lipolysis. Epinephrine is released during times of stress. *Glucocorticoids,* primarily cortisol, are released from the adrenal cortex on stimulation by adrenocorticotropic hormone (ACTH). Cortisol increases plasma glucose by decreasing intestinal entry into the cell and increasing gluconeogenesis, liver glycogen, and lipolysis.

Two anterior pituitary hormones, growth hormone and ACTH, promote increased plasma glucose. *Growth hormone* increases plasma glucose by decreasing the entry of glucose into the cells and increasing glycolysis. Its release from the pituitary is stimulated by decreased glucose levels and inhibited by increased glucose. Decreased levels of cortisol stimulate the anterior pituitary to release ACTH. ACTH, in turn, stimulates the adrenal cortex to release cortisol and increases plasma glucose levels by converting liver glycogen to glucose and promoting gluconeogenesis.

Two other hormones affect glucose levels: thyroxine and somatostatin. The thyroid gland is stimulated by the production of thyroid-stimulating hormone (TSH) to release *thyroxine* that increases plasma glucose levels by increasing glycogenolysis, gluconeogenesis, and intestinal absorption of glucose. *Somatostatin,* produced by the δ

TABLE 11-1. PATHWAYS IN GLUCOSE METABOLISM

Glycolysis	Metabolism of glucose molecule to pyruvate or lactate for production of energy
Gluconeogenesis	Formation of glucose 6-phosphate from noncarbohydrate sources
Glycogenolysis	Breakdown of glycogen to glucose for use as energy
Glycogenesis	Conversion of glucose to glycogen for storage
Lipogenesis	Conversion of carbohydrates to fatty acids
Lipolysis	Decomposition of fat

TABLE 11-2. THE ACTION OF HORMONES

Action of Insulin

Increases glycogenesis and glycolysis: Glucose ———→ glycogen ———→ pyruvate ———→ acetyl-CoA

Increases lipogenesis

Decreases glycogenolysis

Action of Glucagon

Increases glycogenolysis:
   Glycogen ———→ glucose

Increases gluconeogenesis:
   Fatty acids ———→ acetyl-CoA ———→ ketone
   Proteins ———→ amino acids

cells of the islets of Langerhans of the pancreas, increases plasma glucose levels by the inhibition of insulin, glucagon, growth hormone, and other endocrine hormones.

HYPERGLYCEMIA

Hyperglycemia is an increase in plasma glucose levels. In healthy patients, during a hyperglycemia state, insulin is secreted by the β cells of the pancreatic islets of Langerhans. Insulin enhances membrane permeability to cells in the liver, muscle, and adipose tissue. It also alters the glucose metabolic pathways. Hyperglycemia, or increased plasma glucose levels, is caused by an imbalance of hormones.

Diabetes Mellitus

Diabetes mellitus is actually a group of metabolic diseases characterized by hyperglycemia resulting from defects in insulin secretion, insulin action, or both. In 1979, the National Diabetes Data Group developed a classification and diagnosis scheme for diabetes mellitus.[1] This scheme included dividing diabetes into two broad categories:

CASE STUDY 11-1

An 18-year-old, male high school student who had a 4-year history of diabetes mellitus was brought to the emergency department because of excessive drowsiness, vomiting, and diarrhea. His diabetes had been well controlled with 40 units of NPH insulin daily until several days ago when he developed excessive thirst and polyuria. For the past 3 days, he has also had headaches, myalgia, and a low-grade fever. Diarrhea and vomiting began 1 day ago.

URINALYSIS		CHEMISTRY TEST RESULTS	
Specific gravity	1.012	Sodium	126 mEq/L
pH	5.0	Potassium	6.1 mEq/L
Glucose	4+	Chloride	87 mEq/L
Ketone	Large	Bicarbonate	6 mEq/L
		Plasma glucose	600 mg/dL
		BUN	48 mg/dL
		Creatinine	2.0 mg/dL
		Serum ketones	4+

Questions

1. What is the probable diagnosis of this patient based on the data presented?

2. What laboratory test(s) should be performed to follow this patient and aid in adjusting insulin levels?

3. Why are the urine ketones positive?

4. What methods are used to quantitate urine ketones? Which ketone(s) do they detect?

type 1, insulin-dependent diabetes mellitus (IDDM); and type 2, non–insulin-dependent diabetes mellitus (NIDDM).

Established in 1995, the International Expert Committee on the Diagnosis and Classification of Diabetes Mellitus, working under the sponsorship of the ADA, was given the task of updating the 1979 classification system. The proposed changes included eliminating the older terms of IDDM and NIDDM. The categories of type 1 and type 2 were retained, with the adoption of Arabic numerals instead of Roman numerals (Table 11-3).[2]

Therefore, the ADA/World Health Organization (WHO) guidelines recommend the following categories of diabetes:

- Type 1 diabetes
- Type 2 diabetes
- Other specific types of diabetes
- Gestational diabetes mellitus (GDM).

Type 1 diabetes is characterized by inappropriate hyperglycemia primarily a result of pancreatic islet β-cell destruction and a tendency to ketoacidosis. Type 2 diabetes, in contrast, includes hyperglycemia cases that result from insulin resistance with an insulin secretory defect. An intermediate stage, in which the fasting glucose

in increased above-normal limits but not to the level of diabetes, has been named *impaired fasting glucose*. The term *impaired glucose tolerance* to indicate glucose tolerance values above normal but below diabetes levels was retained. Also, the term *gestational diabetes mellitus* was retained for women who develop glucose intolerance during pregnancy.

Type 1 diabetes mellitus is a result of cellular-mediated autoimmune destruction of the β cells of the pancreas, causing an absolute deficiency of insulin secretion. Upper limit of 110 mg/dL on the fasting plasma glucose is designated as the upper limit of normal blood glucose. Type 1 constitutes only 10–20% of all diabetes and commonly occurs in childhood and adolescence. This disease is usually initiated by an environmental factor or infection (usually a virus) in individuals with a genetic predisposition and causes the immune destruction of the β cells of the pancreas and, therefore, a decreased production of insulin. Characteristics of type 1 diabetes include abrupt onset, insulin dependence, and ketosis tendency. This diabetic type is genetically related. One or more of the following markers are found in 85–90% of individuals with fasting hyperglycemia: islet cell autoantibodies, insulin autoantibodies, glutamic acid decarboxylase autoantibodies, and tyrosine phosphatase IA-2 and IA-2B autoantibodies.

Signs and symptoms include polydipsia (excessive thirst), polyphagia (increased food intake), polyuria (excessive urine production), rapid weight loss, hyperventilation, mental confusion, and possible loss of consciousness (due to increased glucose to brain). Complications include microvascular problems such as nephropathy, neuropathy, and retinopathy. Increased heart disease is also found in patients with diabetes. Table 11-4 lists the laboratory findings in hyperglycemia. *Idiopathic type 1 diabetes* is a form of type 1 diabetes that has no known etiology, is strongly inherited, and does not have β-cell autoimmunity. Individuals with this form of diabetes have episodic requirements for insulin replacement.

Type 2 diabetes mellitus is characterized by hyperglycemia as a result of an individual's resistance to insulin with an insulin secretory defect. This resistance results in a relative, not an absolute, insulin deficiency. Type 2 con-

TABLE 11-3. CLASSIFICATION OF DIABETES MELLITUS

	PATHOGENESIS
Type 1	β-Cell destruction Absolute insulin deficiency Autoantibodies • Islet cell autoantibodies • Insulin autoantibodies • Glutamic acid decarboxylase autoantibodies • Tyrosine phosphatase IA-2 and IA-2B autoantibodies
Type 2	Insulin resistance with an insulin secretory defect Relative insulin deficiency
Other	Associated with secondary conditions • Genetic defects of β-cell function • Pancreatic disease • Endocrine disease • Drug or chemical induced • Insulin receptor abnormalities • Other genetic syndromes
Gestational	Glucose intolerance during pregnancy Due to metabolic and hormonal changes

TABLE 11-4. LABORATORY FINDINGS IN HYPERGLYCEMIA

Increased glucose in plasma and urine
Increased urine specific gravity
Increased serum and urine osmolality
Ketones in serum and urine (ketonemia and ketonuria)
Decreased blood and urine pH (acidosis)
Electrolyte imbalance

stitutes the majority of the diabetes cases. Most patients in this type are obese or have an increased percentage of body fat distribution in the abdominal region. This type of diabetes often goes undiagnosed for many years and is associated with a strong genetic predisposition, with patients at increased risk with an increase in age, obesity, and lack of physical exercise. Characteristics usually include adult onset of the disease and milder symptoms than in type 1, with ketoacidosis seldom occurring. However, these patients are more likely to go into a hyperosmolar coma and are at an increased risk of developing macrovascular and microvascular complications.

Other specific types of diabetes are associated with certain conditions (secondary), including genetic defects of β-cell function or insulin action, pancreatic disease, diseases of endocrine origin, drug or chemical induced insulin receptor abnormalities, and certain genetic syndromes. The characteristics and prognosis of this form of diabetes depends on the primary disorder. Maturity-onset diabetes of youth (MODY) is a rare form of diabetes that is inherited in an autosomal dominant fashion.[3]

Gestational diabetes mellitus (GDM) is "any degree of glucose intolerance with onset or first recognition during pregnancy."[4] Causes of GDM include metabolic and hor-

---

CASE STUDY 11-2

A 58-year-old, obese man with frequent urination is seen by his primary care physician. The following laboratory work was performed, and the following results were obtained:

Casual plasma glucose	225 mg/dL		
Urinalysis			
Color and appearance	Pale/clear	Blood	Negative
pH	6.0	Bilirubin	Negative
Specific gravity	1.025	Urobilinogen	Negative
Glucose	2+	Nitrites	Negative
Ketones	Negative	Leukocyte esterase	Negative

Questions

1. What is the probable diagnosis of this patient?

2. What other test(s) should be performed to confirm this? Which is the preferred test?

3. After diagnosis, what test(s) should be performed to monitor his condition?

CASE STUDY 11-3

A 14-year-old, male student was seen by his physician. His chief complaints were fatigue; weight loss; and increases in appetite, thirst, and frequency of urination. For the past 3–4 weeks, he had been excessively thirsty and had to urinate every few hours. He began to get up 3–4 times a night to urinate. Patient has a family history of diabetes mellitus.

Laboratory Data

Fasting plasma glucose	160 mg/dL	
Urinalysis	Specific gravity	1.040
	Glucose	4+
	Ketones	Moderate

Questions

1. Based on the preceding information, can this patient be diagnosed with diabetes?

2. What further tests might be performed to confirm the diagnosis?

3. According the American Diabetes Association, what criteria are required for the diagnosis of diabetes?

4. Assuming this patient has diabetes, which type would be diagnosed?

monal changes. Patients with GDM frequently return to normal postpartum. However, this disease is associated with increased perinatal complications and an increased risk for development of diabetes in later years. Infants born to mothers with diabetes are at increased risk for respiratory distress syndrome, hypocalcemia, and hyperbilirubinemia. Fetal insulin secretion is stimulated in the neonate of a mother with diabetes. However, when the infant is born and the umbilical cord is severed, the infant's oversupply of glucose is abruptly terminated, causing severe hypoglycemia.

Pathophysiology of Diabetes Mellitus

In both type 1 and type 2 diabetes, the individual will be hyperglycemic, which can be severe. Glucosuria can also occur after the renal tubular transporter system for glucose becomes saturated. This happens when the glucose concentration of plasma exceeds roughly 180 mg/dL in an individual with normal renal function and urine output. As hepatic glucose overproduction continues, the plasma glucose concentration reaches a plateau around 300–500 mg/dL (17–28 mmol/L). Provided renal output is maintained, glucose excretion will match the overproduction, causing the plateau.

The individual with type 1 diabetes has a higher tendency to produce ketones. Patients with type 2 diabetes seldom generate ketones, but instead have a greater tendency to develop hyperosmolar nonketotic states. The difference in glucagon and insulin concentrations in these two groups appears to be responsible for the generation of ketones through increased β-oxidation. In type 1, there is an absence of insulin with an excess of glucagon. This permits gluconeogenesis and lipolysis to occur. In type 2, insulin is present as is (at times) hyperinsulinemia; therefore, glucagon is attenuated. Fatty acid oxidation is inhibited in type 2. This causes fatty acids to be incorporated into triglycerides for release as very-low-density lipoproteins.

The laboratory findings of a patient with diabetes with ketoacidosis tend to reflect dehydration, electrolyte disturbances, and acidosis. Acetoacetate, β-hydroxybutyrate, and acetone are produced from the oxidation of fatty acids. The two former ketone bodies contribute to the acidosis. Lactate, fatty acids, and other organic acids can also contribute to a lesser degree. Bicarbonate and total carbon dioxide are usually decreased due to Kussmaul-Kien respiration (deep respirations). This is a compensatory mechanism to blow off carbon dioxide and remove hydrogen ions in the process. The anion gap in this acidosis can exceed 16 mmol/L. Serum osmolality is high as a result of hyperglycemia; sodium concentrations tend to be lower due in part to losses (polyuria) and in part to a shift of water from cells because of the hyperglycemia. The sodium value should not be falsely underestimated because of hypertriglyceridemia. Grossly elevated triglycerides will displace plasma volume and give the appearance of decreased electrolytes when flame photometry or prediluted, ion-specific electrodes are used for sodium determinations. Hyperkalemia is almost always present as a result of the displacement of potassium from cells in acidosis. This is somewhat misleading because the patient's total body potassium is usually decreased.

More typical of the untreated patient with type 2 diabetes is the nonketotic hyperosmolar state. The individual presenting with this syndrome has an overproduction of glucose; however, there appears to be an imbalance between production and elimination in urine. Often, this state is precipitated by heart disease, stroke, or pancreatitis. Glucose concentrations exceed 300–500 mg/dL (17–28 mmol/L) and severe dehydration is present. The severe dehydration contributes to the inability to excrete glucose in the urine. Mortality is high with this condition. Ketones are not observed because the severe hyperosmolar state inhibits the ability of glucagon to stimulate lipolysis. The laboratory findings of nonketotic hyperosmolar coma include plasma glucose values exceeding 1000 mg/dL (55 mmol/L), normal or elevated plasma sodium and potassium, slightly decreased bicarbonate, elevated blood urea nitrogen (BUN) and creatinine, and an elevated osmolality. The gross elevation in glucose and osmolality, the elevation in BUN, and the absence of ketones distinguish this condition from diabetic ketoacidosis.

Other forms of impaired glucose metabolism that does not meet the criteria for diabetes mellitus include impaired fasting glucose and impaired glucose tolerance. These forms are discussed in the following section.

Criteria for the Diagnosis of Diabetes Mellitus

The diagnostic criteria for diabetes mellitus were modified by the Expert Committee to allow for earlier detection of the disease. According to ADA recommendations, all adults older than age 45 years should have a measurement of fasting blood glucose every 3 years unless the individual is otherwise diagnosed with diabetes. Testing should be carried out at an earlier age or more frequently in individuals who display:

- Obesity (120% of desirable body weight or body mass index [BMI] of 27 kg/M^2).
- Family history of diabetes in a first-degree relative.
- Membership in a high-risk minority population (*eg,* African American, Hispanic American, Native American, or Asian American).
- History of GDM or delivering a baby >9 lb (>4.1 kg).
- Hypertension (>140/90)
- Low high-density lipoprotein (HDL) cholesterol concentrations (*eg,* <35 mg/dL)

TABLE 11-5. DIAGNOSTIC CRITERIA FOR DIABETES MELLITUS

1. Random plasma glucose ≥200 mg/dL (11.1 mmol/L) + symptoms of diabetes
2. Fasting plasma glucose ≥126 mg/dL (7.0 mmol/L)
3. Two-hour plasma glucose ≥200 mg/dL (11.1 mmol/L) during an OGTT

Any three criteria must be confirmed on a subsequent day by any of the three methods.

TABLE 11-6. CATEGORIES OF FASTING PLASMA GLUCOSE

Normal fasting glucose	FPG <110 mg/dL
Impaired fasting glucose	FPG ≥110 mg/dL and 126 mg/dL
Provisional diabetes diagnosis	FPG ≥126 mg/dL

TABLE 11-7. CATEGORIES OF ORAL GLUCOSE TOLERANCE

Normal glucose tolerance	2-hour PG <140 mg/dL
Impaired glucose tolerance	2-hour PG ≥140 mg/dL and <200 mg/dL
Provisional diabetes diagnosis	2-hour PG ≥200 mg/dL

- Elevated triglyceride concentrations (eg, >250 mg/dL)
- A history of impaired fasting glucose/impaired glucose tolerance.

The criteria listed in Tables 11-5, 11-6, and 11-7 suggest three methods of diagnosis, each of which must be confirmed on a subsequent day by any one of the three methods. These methods are (1) symptoms of diabetes plus a random plasma glucose level of ≥200 mg/dL, (2) a fasting plasma glucose of ≥126 mg/dL, or (3) an oral glucose tolerance test (OGTT) with a 2-hour postload (75-g glucose load) level ≥200 mg/dL. The preferred test for diagnosing diabetes is the measurement of the fasting plasma glucose level.

An intermediate group who did not meet the criteria of diabetes mellitus but who had glucose levels above normal was defined by two methods. First, those patients with fasting glucose levels ≥110 mg/dL but <126 mg/dL were called the impaired fasting glucose group. Another set of patients who had 2-hour OGTT levels of ≥140

mg/dL but <200 mg/dL was defined as impaired glucose tolerance.

The diagnostic criteria for gestational diabetes follows the guidelines established by the American College of Obstetrics and Gynecology. Only high-risk patients should be screened for GDM. The criteria for women at high risk include any of the following: age older than 25 years; overweight; family history of diabetes; or African American, Hispanic American, or Native American ethnicity. The screening tests include the measurement of plasma glucose at 1-hour postload (50-g glucose load). If the value is ≥140 mg/dL (7.8 mmol/L), then the need to perform a 3-hour OGTT using a 100-g glucose

CASE STUDY 11-4

A 13-year-old girl collapsed on a playground at school. When her mother was contacted, she mentioned that her daughter had been losing weight and making frequent trips to the bathroom in the night. The emergency squad noticed a fruity breath. On entrance to the emergency department, her vital signs were as follows:

Blood pressure	98/50
Respirations	Rapid
Temperature	99°F

Stat lab results included:

RANDOM URINE		SERUM CHEMISTRIES	
pH	5.5	Glucose	500 mg/dL
Protein	Negative	Ketones	Positive
Glucose	4+	BUN	6 mg/dL
Ketones	Moderate	Creatinine	0.4 mg/dL
Blood	Negative		

Questions

1. Identify this patient's most likely type of diabetes.

2. Based on your identification, circle the common characteristics associated with that type of diabetes in the case study above.

3. What is the cause of the fruity breath?

load is indicated. GDM is diagnosed when any two of the following four values are met or exceeded: fasting, >105 mg/dL; 1 hour, <190 mg/dL; 2 hours, ≥165 mg/dL; or 3 hours, ≥145 mg/dL.

HYPOGLYCEMIA

Hypoglycemia involves decreased plasma glucose levels and can have many causes—some are transient and relatively insignificant; others can be life threatening. The plasma glucose concentration at which glucagon and other glycemic factors are released is between 65 and 70 mg/dL (3.6–3.9 mmol/L); at about 50–55 mg/dL (2.8–3.0 mmol/L), observable symptoms of hypoglycemia appear. The warning signs and symptoms of hypoglycemia are all related to the central nervous system. The release of epinephrine into systemic circulation and norepinephrine at nerve endings of specific neurons act in unison with glucagon to increase plasma glucose. Glucagon is released from the islet cells of the pancreas and inhibits insulin. Epinephrine is released from the adrenal gland and increases glucose metabolism and inhibits insulin. In addition, cortisol and growth hormone are released and increase glucose metabolism.

Historically, hypoglycemia was classified as postabsorptive (fasting) and postprandial (reactive) hypoglycemia. However, the reactive hypoglycemia only described the timing of hypoglycemia, not the etiology. Current approaches suggest classification based on clinical characteristics. This classification separates patients into those who appear healthy and those who are sick (Table 11-8).[5]

Among healthy-appearing patients, are those with and without a compensated coexistent disease. This category includes individuals in which medications may be the cause of hypoglycemia through accidental ingestion by dispensing error. Sick persons may have an illness, which predisposes to hypoglycemia or may experience drug and illness interaction leading to hypoglycemia. Hypoglycemia in hospitalized patients can often be ascribed to iatrogenic factors. Symptoms of hypoglycemia are increased hunger, sweating, nausea and vomiting, dizziness, nervousness and shaking, blurring of speech and sight, and mental confusion. Laboratory findings include decreased plasma glu-

TABLE 11-8. CAUSES OF HYPOGLYCEMIA

Patient Appears Healthy

No coexisting disease	Drugs Insulinoma Islet hyperplasia/nesidioblastosis Factitial hypoglycemia from insulin or sulfonylurea Severe exercise Ketotic hypoglycemia
Compensated coexistent disease	Drugs

Patient Appears Ill

Drugs
Predisposing illness
Hospitalized patient

CASE STUDY 11-5

A 28-year-old woman delivered a 9.5-lb infant. The infant was above the 95th percentile for weight and length. The mother's history was incomplete; she claimed to have had no medical care through her pregnancy. Shortly after birth, the infant became lethargic and flaccid. A whole blood glucose and ionized calcium were performed in the nursery with the following results:

Whole blood glucose	25 mg/dL
Ionized calcium	4.9 mg/dL

Plasma glucose was drawn and analyzed in the main laboratory to confirm the whole blood findings.

Plasma glucose	33 mg/dL

An intravenous glucose solution was started, and whole blood glucose was measured hourly.

Questions

1. Give the possible explanation for the infant's large birth weight and size.

2. If the mother was a gestational diabetic, why was her baby hypoglycemic?

3. Why was there a discrepancy between the whole blood glucose concentration and the plasma glucose concentration?

4. If the mother had been monitored during pregnancy, what laboratory tests should have been performed and what criteria would have indicated that she had gestational diabetes?

Laboratory tests were performed on a 50-year-old, lean, Caucasian woman during an annual physical examination. She has no family history of diabetes or any history of elevated glucose levels during pregnancy.

Laboratory Results

Fasting blood glucose (FBG)	90 mg/dL
Cholesterol	140 mg/dL
HDL	40 mg/dL
Triglycerides	90 mg/dL

Questions

1. What is the probable diagnosis of this patient?

2. Describe the proper follow-up for this patient?

3. What is the preferred screening test for diabetes in nonpregnant adults?

4. What are the risk factors that would indicate a potential of this patient's developing diabetes?

cose levels during hypoglycemic episode and extremely elevated insulin levels in patients with pancreatic β-cell tumors (insulinoma). To investigate an insulinoma, the patient is required to fast under controlled conditions. Men and women have different metabolic patterns in prolonged fasts. The healthy male will maintain plasma glucose of 55–60 mg/dL (3.1–3.3 mmol/L) for several days. Healthy females will produce ketones more readily and permit plasma glucose to decrease to 40 mg/dL (2.2 mmol/L) or lower. Diagnostic criteria for an insulinoma includes a change in glucose level of $\geq$25 mg/dL (1.4 mmol/L) coincident with an insulin level of $\geq$6 μU/mL (36 pmol/L), C peptide levels of $\geq$0.2 nmol/L; proinsulin levels of $\geq$5 pmol/L; and/or β-hydroxybutyrate levels of $\leq$2.7 mmol/L.[6]

Genetic Defects in Carbohydrate Metabolism

Glycogen storage diseases are result of the deficiency of a specific enzyme that causes an alternation of glycogen metabolism. The most common congenital form of glycogen storage disease is glucose-6-phosphatase deficiency type 1, which is also called von Gierke disease, an autosomal recessive disease. This disease is characterized by severe hypoglycemia that coincides with metabolic acidosis, ketonemia, and elevated lactate and alanine. Hypoglycemia occurs because glycogen cannot be converted back to glucose by way of hepatic glycogenolysis. A glycogen buildup is found in the liver, causing hepatomegaly. The patients usually have severe hypoglycemia, hyperlipidemia, uricemia, and growth retardation. A liver biopsy will show a positive glycogen stain. Although the glycogen accumulation is irreversible, the disease can be kept under control by avoiding the development of hypoglycemia. Liver transplantation corrects the hypoglycemic condition. Other enzyme defects or deficiencies that cause hypoglycemia include glycogen synthase, fructose-1,6-bisphosphatase, phosphoenolpyru-

vate carboxykinase, and pyruvate carboxylase. Glycogen debrancher enzyme deficiency does not cause hypoglycemia but does cause hepatomegaly.

Galactosemia, a cause of failure to thrive syndrome in infants, is a congenital deficiency of one of three enzymes involved in galactose metabolism, resulting in increased levels of galactose in plasma. The most common enzyme deficiency is galactose-1-phosphate uridyl transferase. Galactosemia occurs because of the inhibition of glycogenolysis and is accompanied by diarrhea and vomiting. Galactose must be removed from the diet to prevent the development of irreversible complications. If left untreated, the patient will develop mental retardation and cataracts. The disorder can be identified by measuring erythrocyte galactose-1-phosphate uridyltransferase activity. Laboratory findings include hypoglycemia, hyperbilirubinemia, and galactose accumulation in the blood, tissue, and urine following milk ingestion. Another enzyme deficiency, fructose-1-phosphate aldolase deficiency, causes nausea and hypoglycemia after fructose ingestion.

Specific inborn errors of amino acid metabolism and long-chain fatty acid oxidation are also responsible for hypoglycemia. There are also alimentary and idiopathic hypoglycemias. Alimentary hypoglycemia appears to be caused by an increase in the release of insulin in response to rapid absorption of nutrients after a meal or the rapid secretion of insulin-releasing gastric factors. Idiopathic postprandial hypoglycemia is a controversial diagnosis that may be overused.[7]

ROLE OF LABORATORY IN DIFFERENTIAL DIAGNOSIS AND MANAGEMENT OF PATIENTS WITH GLUCOSE METABOLIC ALTERATIONS

The demonstration of hyperglycemia or hypoglycemia under specific conditions is used to diagnose diabetes

For 3 consecutive months, a fasting glucose and glycosylated hemoglobin was performed on a patient. The results are as follows:

	QUARTER 1	QUARTER 2	QUARTER 3
Glucose, fasting (FPG)	280 mg/dL	85 mg/dL	91 mg/dL
Glycosylated Hgb	7.8%	15.3%	8.5%

Hgb = hemoglobin.

Questions

1. In which quarter was the patient's glucose the best controlled? The least controlled?

2. Does the FPG and glycosylated Hgb match? Why or why not?

3. What methods are used to measure glycosylated hemoglobin?

4. What potential conditions might cause erroneous results?

mellitus and hypoglycemic conditions. Other laboratory tests have been developed to identify insulinomas and to monitor glycemic control and the development of renal complications.

Methods of Glucose Measurement

Glucose can be measured from serum, plasma, or whole blood. Today, most glucose measurements are performed on serum or plasma. The glucose concentration in whole blood is approximately 15% lower than the glucose concentration in serum or plasma. Serum or plasma must be refrigerated and separated from the cells within 1 hour to prevent substantial loss of glucose by the cellular fraction, particularly if the white blood cell count is elevated. Sodium fluoride ions (gray-top tubes) are often used as an anticoagulant and preservative of whole blood, particularly if analysis is delayed. Fluoride inhibits glycolytic enzymes. Fasting blood glucose (FBG) should be obtained after an approximately 10-hour fast (not >16 hours). Cerebrospinal fluid and urine can also be analyzed. Urine glucose measurement is not used in diabetes diagnosis; however, some patients use this measurement for monitoring purposes.

The ability of glucose to function as a reducing agent has been useful in the detection and quantitation of carbohydrates in body fluids. Glucose and other carbohydrates are capable of converting cupric ions in alkaline solution to cuprous ions. The solution loses its deep-blue color and a red precipitate of cuprous oxide forms. Benedict's and Fehling's reagents, which contain an alkaline solution of cupric ions stabilized by citrate or tartrate, respectively, have been used to detect reducing agents in urine and other body fluids. Another chemical characteristic that used to be exploited to quantitate carbohydrates is the ability of these molecules to form Schiff bases with aromatic amines. O-Toluidine in a hot acidic solution will yield a colored compound with an ab-

sorbance maxima at 630 nm. Galactose, an aldohexose, and mannose, an aldopentose, will also react with O-toluidine and produce a colored compound that can interfere with the reaction. The Schiff base reaction with O-toluidine is of historical interest only and has been replaced by more specific enzymatic methods, which are discussed in the following section.

The most used methods of glucose analysis use the enzymes glucose oxidase or hexokinase (Table 11-9). Glucose oxidase is the most specific enzyme reacting with only β-D-glucose. Glucose oxidase converts β-D-glucose to gluconic acid. Mutarotase may be added to the reaction to facilitate the conversion of α-D-glucose to β-D-glucose. Oxygen is consumed and hydrogen peroxide is produced. The reaction can be monitored polarographically either by measuring the rate of disappearance of oxygen using an oxygen electrode or by consuming hydrogen peroxide in a side reaction. Horseradish peroxidase is used to catalyze the second reaction, and the hydrogen peroxide is used to oxidize a dye compound. Two commonly used chromogens are 3-methyl-2-benzothiazolinone hydrazone and N,N-dimethylaniline. The shift in absorbance can be monitored spectrophotometrically and is proportional to the amount of glucose present in the specimen. This coupled reaction is known as the *Trinder reaction*. However, the peroxidase coupling reaction used in the glucose oxidase method is subject to positive and negative interference. Increased levels of uric acid, bilirubin, and ascorbic acid can cause falsely decreased values as a result of these substances being oxidized by peroxidase, which then prevents the oxidation and detection of the chromogen. Strong oxidizing substances, such as bleach, can cause falsely increased values. An oxygen consumption electrode can be used to perform the direct measurement of oxygen by the polarographic technique, which avoids this interference. Oxygen depletion is measured and is proportional to the amount of glucose present. Polarographic glucose analyzers measure the rate of oxygen consumption because glu-

TABLE 11-9. METHODS OF GLUCOSE MEASUREMENT

Glucose oxidate	Glucose + O_2 + H_2O $\xrightarrow{\text{glucose oxidase}}$ gluconic acid + H_2O_2
	H_2O_2 + reduced chromogen $\xrightarrow{\text{peroxidase}}$ oxidized chromogen + H_2O
Hexokinase	Glucose + ATP $\xrightarrow{\text{hexokinase}}$ glucose 6-PO_4 + ADP
	Glucose 6-PO_4 + NADP $\xrightarrow{\text{G-6-PD}}$ NADPH + H^+ + 6-phosphogluconate
Clinitest	Reducing substance + Cu^{+2} $\xrightarrow{\hspace{2cm}}$ $Cu^{+1}O$

cose is oxidized under first-order conditions using glucose oxidase reagent. The H_2O_2 formed must be eliminated in a side reaction to prevent the reaction from reversing. Molybdate can be used to catalyze the oxidation of iodide to iodine by H_2O_2 or catalase can be used to catalyze oxidation of ethanol by H_2O_2, forming acetaldehyde and H_2O.

The hexokinase method is considered more accurate than glucose oxidase methods because the coupling reaction using glucose-6-phosphate dehydrogenase is highly specific; therefore, it has less interference than the coupled glucose oxidase procedure. Hexokinase in the presence of ATP converts glucose to glucose 6-phosphate. Glucose 6-phosphate and the cofactor $NADP^+$ are converted to 6-phosphogluconate and NADPH by glucose-6-phosphate dehydrogenase. NADPH has a strong absorbance maxima at 340 nm, and the rate of appearance of NADPH can be monitored spectrophotometrically and is proportional to the amount of glucose present in the sample. Generally accepted as the reference method, this method is not affected by ascorbic acid or uric acid. Gross hemolysis and extremely elevated bilirubin may cause a false decrease in results. The hexokinase method may be performed on serum or plasma collected using heparin, ethylenediaminetetraacetic acid (EDTA), fluoride, oxalate, or citrate. The method can also be used for urine, cerebrospinal fluid, and serous fluids.

Nonspecific methods of measuring glucose are still used in the urinalysis section of the laboratory primarily to detect reducing substances other than glucose. The method below is the Benedict's modification, also called the Clinitest reaction.

Self-Monitoring of Blood Glucose (SMBG)

The ADA has recommended that individuals with diabetes should monitor their blood glucose levels in an effort to maintain levels as close to normal as possible. For persons with type 1 diabetes, the recommendation is 3–4 times/day; for persons with type 2, the optimal frequency is unknown. It is important that patients be taught how to use control solutions and calibrators to ensure the accuracy of their results.[9] Urine glucose testing should be replaced by SMBG; however, urine ketone testing will remain for type 1 and gestational diabetes.

Glucose Tolerance and 2-Hour Postprandial Tests

Guidelines for the performance and interpretation of the *2-hour postprandial test* were set by the Expert Committee. A variation of this test is to use a standardized load of glucose. A solution containing 75 g of glucose is administered, and a specimen for plasma glucose measure-

---

CASE STUDY 11-8

A 25-year-old, healthy, female patient complains of dizziness and shaking 1 hour after eating a large, heavy-carbohydrate meal. The result of a random glucose performed via fingerstick was 60 mg/dL.

Questions

1. Identify the characteristics of hypoglycemia in this case study.

2. What test(s) should be performed next to determine this young woman's problem?

3. To which category of hypoglycemia would this individual belong?

4. What criteria would be used to diagnose a potential insulinoma?

ment is drawn 2 hours later. Under this criteria, the patient drinks a standardized (75 g) glucose load and a glucose measurement is taken 2 hours later. If that level is ≥200 mg/dL and is confirmed on a subsequent day by either an increased random or fasting glucose level, the patient is diagnosed with diabetes (see earlier discussion).

The *oral glucose tolerance test (OGTT)* is not recommended for routine use under the ADA guidelines. This procedure is inconvenient to patients and is not being used by physicians for diagnosing diabetes. However, if the OGTT is used, WHO recommends the criteria listed in Table 11-7. It is important that proper patient preparation be given before this test is performed. The patient should be ambulatory and on a normal-to-high carbohydrate intake for 3 days before the test. The patient should be fasting for at least 10 hours and not more than 16 hours, and the test should be performed in the morning because of the hormonal diurnal effect on glucose. Just before tolerance and while the test is in progress, patients should refrain from exercise, eating, drinking (except that the patient may drink water), and smoking. Factors that affect the tolerance results include medications such as large doses of salicylates, diuretics, anticonvulsants, oral contraceptives, and corticosteroids. Also gastrointestinal problems including malabsorption problems, gastrointestinal surgery, and vomiting and endocrine dysfunctions can affect the OGTT results. The guidelines recommend that only the fasting and the 2-hour sample be measured, except when the patient is pregnant. The adult dose of glucose solution (glucola) is 75 g; children receive 1.75 g/kg of glucose to a maximum dose of 75 g.

Glycosylated Hemoglobin

The aim of diabetic management is to maintain the blood glucose concentration within or near the nondiabetic range with a minimal number of fluctuations. Serum or plasma glucose concentrations can be measured by laboratories in addition to patient self-monitoring of whole blood glucose concentrations. Long-term blood glucose regulation can be followed by measurement of glycosylated hemoglobins.

Glycosylated hemoglobin is the term used to describe the formation of a hemoglobin compound formed when glucose (a reducing sugar) reacts with the amino group of hemoglobin (a protein). The glucose molecule attaches nonenzymatically to the hemoglobin molecule in a ketoamine structure to form a ketoamine. The rate of formation is directly proportional to the plasma glucose concentrations. Because the average red blood cell lives approximately 120 days, the glycosylated hemoglobin level at any one time reflects the average blood glucose level over the previous 2–3 months. Therefore, measuring the glycosylated hemoglobin provides the clinician with a time-averaged picture of the patient's blood glu-

cose concentration over the past 3 months. Hemoglobin A_{1c} (HbA_{1c}), the most commonly detected glycosylated hemoglobin, is a glucose molecule attached to one or both N-terminus valines of the β-polypeptide chains of normal adult hemoglobin.[10] HbA_{1c} is a reliable method of monitoring long-term diabetes control rather than random plasma glucose (FBS). Normal values range from 4.5 to 8.0. Using a linear regression model, Rohlfing et al, determined that for every 1% change in the HbA_{1c} value, there is a 35 mg/dL (2 mmol/L) change in the mean plasma glucose (Table 11-10).[11] Remember that two factors determine the glycosylated hemoglobin levels: the average glucose concentration and the red blood cell life span. If the red blood cell life span is decreased because of another disease state such as hemoglobinopathies, the hemoglobin will have less time to become glycosylated and the glycosylated hemoglobin level will be lower.

The specimen requirement for HbA_{1c} measurement is an EDTA whole blood sample. Before analysis, a hemolysate must be prepared. The methods of measurement are grouped into two major categories: (1) based on charge differences between glycosylated and nonglycosylated hemoglobin (cation-exchange chromatography, electrophoresis, and isoelectric focusing), and (2) structural characteristics of glycogroups on hemoglobin (affinity chromatography and immunoassay). There is no consensus on the reference method and no single standard available to be used in the assays. Because of this, HbA_{1c} values vary with the method and laboratory performing them (Table 11-11).

Affinity chromatography is the preferred method of measurement. In this method, the glycosylated hemoglobin attaches to the boronate group of the resin and is selectively eluted from the resin bed using a buffer. This method is not temperature dependent and not affected by hemoglobin F, S, or C. Another method of measurement

TABLE 11-10. ESTIMATED CORRELATION BETWEEN MEAN PLASMA GLUCOSE LEVELS AND A_{1c} LEVELS[10]

MEAN PLASMA GLUCOSE	A_{1c} (%)
65 mg/dL (3.5 mmol/L)	4
100 mg/dL (5.5 mmol/L)	5
135 mg/dL (7.5 mmol/L)	6
170 mg/dL (9.5 mmol/L)	7
205 mg/dL (11.5 mmol/L)	8
240 mg/dL (13.5 mmol/L)	9
275 mg/dL (15.5 mmol/L)	10
310 mg/dL (17.5 mmol/L)	11
345 mg/dL (19.5 mmol/L)	12

TABLE 11-11. METHODS OF GLYCATED HEMOGLOBIN MEASUREMENT

Methods Based on Structural Differences

Immunoassays	Polyclonal or monoclonal antibodies toward the glycated N-terminal group of the β chain of Hgb	
Affinity chromatography	Separates based on chemical structure using borate to bind glycosylated proteins	Not temperature dependent Not affected by other hemoglobins

Methods Based on Charge Differences

Ion-exchange chromatography	Positive-charge resin bed	Highly temperature dependent Affected by hemoglobinopathies
Electrophoresis	Separation is based on differences in charge	Hgb F values >7% interferes
Isoelectric focusing	Type of electrophoresis using isoelectric point to separate	Pre-Hgb A_{1c} interferes
High-pressure liquid chromatography (HPLC)	A form of ion-exchange chromatography	Separates of all forms of glyco Hgb: A_{1a}, A_{1b}, A_{1c}

Hgb = hemoglobin.

uses cation exchange chromatography in which the negatively charged hemoglobins attach to the positively charged resin bed. The glycosylated hemoglobin is selectively eluted from the resin bed using a buffer of specific pH in which the glycohemoglobins are the most negatively charged and elute first from the column. However, this method is highly temperature dependent and affected by hemoglobinopathies. The presence of hemoglobin F yields false increased levels, and the presence of hemoglobins S and C yields false decreased levels. High-performance liquid chromatography and electrophoresis methods are also used to separate the various forms of hemoglobin. With high-performance liquid chromatography, all forms of glycosylated hemoglobin, A_{1a}, A_{1b}, A_{1c}, can be separated.

Ketones

The *ketone* bodies are produced by the liver through metabolism of fatty acids to provide a ready energy source from stored lipids at times of low carbohydrate availability. The three ketone bodies are acetone (2%), acetoacetic acid (20%), and 3-β-hydroxybutyric acid (78%). A low level of ketone bodies are present in the body at all times. However, in cases of carbohydrate deprivation or decreased carbohydrate use such as diabetes mellitus, star-

vation/fasting, high-fat diets, prolonged vomiting, and glycogen storage disease, blood levels increase to meet energy needs. The term *ketonemia* refers to the accumulation of ketones in blood, and the term *ketonuria* refers to accumulation of ketones in urine (Fig. 11-9). The measurement of ketones is recommended for patients with type I diabetes during acute illness, stress, pregnancy, elevated blood glucose levels above 300 mg/dL, or when the patient has signs of ketoacidosis.

The specimen requirement is *fresh* serum or urine; the sample should be tightly stoppered and analyzed immediately. No method used for determination of ketones reacts with all three ketone bodies. The historical test (Gerhardt's) that used ferric chloride reacted with acetoacetic acid to produce a red color. The procedure had many interfering substances, including salicylates. A more common method using sodium nitroprusside $(NaFe[CN]_5NO)$ reacts with acetoacetic acid in an alkaline pH to form a purple color. If the reagent contains glycerin, then acetone is also detected. This method is used with the urine reagent strip test and Acetest tablets. A newer enzymatic method adapted to some automated instruments uses the enzyme β-hydroxybutyrate dehydrogenase to detect either β-hydroxybutyric acid or acetoacetic acid, depending on the pH of the solution. A pH of 7.0 causes the reaction to proceed to the right (decreasing absorbance); a pH of 8.5–9.5 causes the

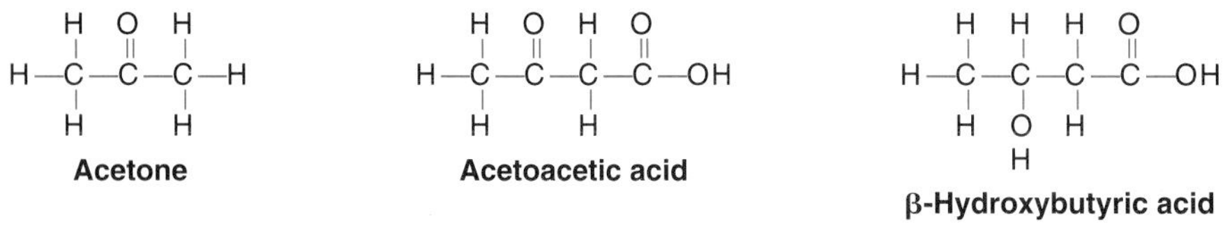

FIGURE 11-9. The three ketone bodies.

TABLE 11-12. METHODS OF KETONE MEASUREMENT

Nitroprusside	Acetoacetic acid + nitroprusside $\xrightarrow{\text{alkaline pH}}$ purple color
Enzymatic	NADH + H$^+$ + acetoacetic acid $\xleftrightarrow{\beta\text{-HBD}}$ NAD + β-hydroxybutyric acid

reaction to proceed to left (increasing absorbance, Table 11-12).

Microalbuminuria

Diabetes mellitus causes progressive changes to the kidneys and ultimately results in diabetic renal nephropathy. This complication progresses over years and may be delayed by aggressive glycemic control. An early sign that nephropathy is occurring is an increase in urinary albumin. Microalbumin measurements are useful to assist in diagnosis at an early stage and before the development of proteinuria. Microalbumin concentrations are between 20 and 300 mg/day. Proteinuria is typically greater than 0.5 g/day.[12] Although 3 methods for *microalbuminuria* screening are available, the use of a random spot collection for the measurement of the albumin-to-creatinine ratio is strongly recommended. The two other alternatives, a 24-hour collection or a timed, 4-hour overnight collection, are seldom required. A patient is determined to have microalbuminuria when 2 of 3 specimens collected within a 6-month period are abnormal.[13]

Islet Autoantibody and Insulin Testing

The presence of autoantibodies to the β islet cells of the pancreas is characteristic of type 1 diabetes. However, islet autoantibody testing is not currently recommended for routine screening for diabetes diagnosis. In the future, this testing might identify at-risk, prediabetic patients. Insulin measurements are not required for the diagnosis of diabetes mellitus. However, in certain hypoglycemic states, it is important to know the concentration of insulin in relation to the plasma glucose concentration.

SUMMARY

Carbohydrates have the general formula $C_x(H_2O)_n$. Glucose is a six-carbon aldohexose. There are 32 different possible isomers of aldohexoses with the glucose chemical formula. Glucose and other sugars can exist in the open chain or ring form. The open chain form permits free carbonyl to reduce Benedict's or Fehling's reagents. β-D-Glucose is a primary source of energy for humans. Energy in the form of ATP can be obtained from glucose through the anaerobic pathway. Additional energy is then obtained from the product pyruvate as it passes through the TCA cycle. The nervous system relies solely on glucose for energy in normal circumstances. Therefore, it is important to maintain the glucose concentration within a narrow range.

Insulin, produced in the β cells of the pancreas, is responsible for the uptake of glucose into cells and the reduction of plasma glucose postprandially. Insulin also promotes glycogenolysis and triglyceride synthesis. Glucagon, also produced in the β cells of the pancreas, opposes the action of insulin. Both glucagon and epinephrine increase plasma glucose by activating gluconeogenesis and glycogenolysis in the liver. Gluconeogenesis is the formation of glucose from lactate, amino acids, pyruvate, and glycerol.

Diabetes mellitus can be classified as type 1 or type 2. The development of type 1 appears to be partly related to an individual's human leukocyte antigen (HLA) genotype. Type 1 may also have an environmental component that is thought to trigger an immune reaction, which leads to an autoimmune response and causes β-cell destruction. Untreated hyperglycemia in diabetes is usually no greater than 500 mg/dL (28 mmol/L) when healthy renal function is present. Ketoacidosis is more common in type 1; osmolality is increased, plasma potassium is increased, and plasma sodium is slightly decreased. Bicarbonate is decreased in response to the acidosis.

Type 2 is also thought to have a genetic factor. Individuals with type 2 have no β-cell destruction and may have decreased, normal, or increased insulin concentrations—

CASE STUDY 11-9

A nurse caring for patients with diabetes performed a fingerstick glucose on the Accu-Chek glucose monitor and obtained a value of 200 mg/dL. A plasma sample, collected at the same time by a phlebotomist and performed by the laboratory, resulted in a glucose value of 225 mg/dL.

Questions

1. Are these two results significantly different?

2. Explain.

but they are insulin resistant at the tissue. There is a greater tendency in type 2 toward hyperosmolar nonketotic coma. Type 2 is characterized by a glucose concentration of greater than 600 mg/dL (33 mmol/L) and an absence of ketones. BUN and osmolality are increased and urine output is decreased. GDM may be related to type 2. The three definitive tests for diabetes are (1) symptoms of diabetes plus a random plasma glucose level of ≥200 mg/dL, (2) a fasting plasma glucose of ≥126 mg/dL, or (3) an OGTT with a 2-hour postload (75-glucose load) level ≥200 mg/dL. Any of the three criteria must be confirmed on a subsequent day by any of the three methods. Long-term monitoring of the patient with diabetes includes self-monitoring blood glucose, periodic glycosylated hemoglobin, and annual microalbumin levels.

Hypoglycemia is currently classified based on clinical symptoms, with categories split between patients who appear healthy and those that appear ill. Neonatal, congenital, and ketotic hypoglycemia occur in children. Congenital forms of hypoglycemia include von Gierke disease. Galactosemia is another relatively common congenital variety of hypoglycemia.

REVIEW QUESTIONS

1. Which of the following hormones promotes gluconeogenesis?
   a. Growth hormone
   b. Hydrocortisone
   c. Insulin
   d. Thyroxine

2. Glucose oxidase oxidizes glucose to gluconic acid and:
   a. H_2O_2.
   b. CO_2.
   c. HCO_3.
   d. H_2O.

3. From glucose and ATP, hexokinase catalyzes formation of:
   a. acetyl-CoA.
   b. fructose 6-phosphate.
   c. glucose 6-phosphate.
   d. lactose.

4. What is the preferred specimen for glucose analysis?
   a. EDTA plasma
   b. Fluoride oxalate plasma
   c. Heparinized plasma
   d. Serum

5. Hyperglycemic factor produced by the pancreas is:
   a. follicle-stimulating hormone (FSH).
   b. glucagon.
   c. insulin.
   d. luteinizing hormone (LH).

6. Polarographic methods of glucose assay are based on which principle?
   a. Nonenzymatic oxidation of glucose
   b. Rate of oxygen depletion measured
   c. Chemiluminescence caused by formation of ATP
   d. Change in electrical potential as glucose is oxidized

7. Select the enzyme that is most specific for β-D-glucose.
   a. Glucose oxidase
   b. Glucose-6-phosphate dehydrogenase
   c. Hexokinase
   d. Phosphohexisomerase

8. Select the coupling enzyme used in the hexokinase method for glucose.
   a. Glucose dehydrogenase
   b. Glucose-6-phosphatase
   c. Glucose-6-phosphate dehydrogenase
   d. Peroxidase

9. All of the following are characteristic of von Gierke disease EXCEPT:
   a. hypoglycemia.
   b. hypolipidemia.
   c. increased plasma lactate.
   d. subnormal response to epinephrine.

10. The preferred screening test for diabetes in nonpregnant adults is measurement of:
    a. fasting plasma glucose.
    b. random plasma glucose.
    c. glycohemoglobin.
    d. plasma glucose 1 hour after 50-g carbohydrate load.

11. Following the 2003 ADA guidelines, the times of measurement for plasma glucose levels during an OGTT in nonpregnant patients are:
    a. fasting and 2 hours.
    b. fasting and 60 minutes.
    c. 30, 60, 90, and 120 minutes.
    d. fasting, 30, 60, 90, and 120 minutes.

12. Monitoring levels of ketone bodies in the urine via nitroprusside reagents provides a semi-quantitative measure of:
    a. acetoacetate.
    b. 3-β-hydroxybutyrate.
    c. acetone.
    d. all three ketone bodies.

13. A factor, other than average plasma glucose values, that determines the glycosylated hemoglobin level is:
    a. serum ketone bodies level.
    b. red blood cell life span.
    c. ascorbic acid intake.
    d. increased triglyceride levels.

14. Monitoring levels of ketone bodies in the urine is:
    a. considered essential on a daily basis for all diabetic patients.
    b. a reliable method of assessing long-term glycemic control.
    c. recommended for patients with type 1 diabetes on sick days.
    d. not recommended by the ADA.

REFERENCES

1. National Diabetes Data Group. Classification and diagnosis of diabetes mellitus and other categories of glucose tolerance. Diabetes 1979;28:1039–1057.
2. Expert Committee on the Diagnosis and Classification of Diabetes Mellitus. Report of the Expert Committee on the Diagnosis and Classification of Diabetes Mellitus. Diabetes Care 2003; 26(Suppl 1):S7.
3. Malchoff CD. Diagnosis and classification of diabetes mellitus. Conn Med 1991;55(11):625.
4. Expert Committee on the Diagnosis and Classification of Diabetes Mellitus. Report of the Expert Committee on the Diagnosis and Classification of Diabetes Mellitus. Diabetes Care 2003; 26(Suppl 1):S10.
5. Service FJ. Classification of hypoglycemic disorders. Endocrinol Metab Clin 1999;28(3):501–517.
6. Service FJ. Medical progress: hypoglycemic disorders. N Engl J Med 1995;332(17):1144–1152.
7. Cryer PE. Glucose homeostasis and hypoglycemia. In: Wilson JD, Foster DW, eds. Williams Textbook of Endocrinology. Philadelphia: WB Saunders, 1992.
8. American Diabetes Association. Tests of glycemia in diabetes. Diabetes Care 2003;26(Suppl 1):S106.
9. Higgis PJ, Bunn HF. Kinetic analysis of the nonenzymatic glycosylation of hemoglobin. J Biol Chem 1981;256:5204–5208.
10. Eckfeldt JH, Bruns DE. Another step towards standardization of methods for measuring hemoglobin A_{1c}. Clin Chem 1997;43(10):1811–1813.
11. Rohlfing CL, Wiedmeyer HM, Little RR, et al. Defining the relationship between plasma glucose and HbA_{1c}. Diabetes Care 2002;25(2):275–278.
12. Stehouwer CDA, Donker AJM. Clinical usefulness of measurement of urinary albumin excretion in diabetes mellitus. Neth J Med 1993;42:175.
13. American Diabetes Association. Standards of medical care for patients with diabetes mellitus. Diabetes Care 2003;26(Suppl 1):S42–43.

CHAPTER 12

Lipids and Lipoproteins

Alan T. Remaley, Judith R. McNamara,
G. Russell Warnick

CHAPTER OUTLINE

OBJECTIVES

Upon completion of this chapter, the clinical laboratorian should be able to:
- Explain lipid/lipoprotein physiology and metabolism.
- Define lipoprotein, exogenous, endogenous, chylomicrons, fatty acids, phospholipids, triglycerides, cholesterol, VLDL, LDL, HDL, and Lp(a).
- Describe the clinical tests used to assess lipids and lipoproteins, including principles and procedures.
- Evaluate the patient's lipid or lipoprotein status, given clinical data.

- Identify the reference ranges for the major lipids discussed.
- Discuss the interaction in the body between the lipids and lipoproteins and various hormones.
- Relate the clinical significance of lipid and lipoprotein values in the assessment of coronary heart disease.
- Discuss the incidence and types of lipid and lipoprotein abnormalities.

KEY TERMS

Arteriosclerosis	Endogenous	HDL	Phospholipids
Cholesterol	Exogenous	LDL	Triglycerides
Chylomicrons	Fatty acids	Lipoprotein	VLDL
Dyslipidemias	Friedewald calculation	Lp(a)	

Lipoproteins constitute the body's "petroleum industry." Like great tankers that travel the oceans of the world transporting petroleum for fuel needs, the large chylomicrons carry dietary triglycerides throughout the circulatory system to cells, finally docking at the liver to deposit the chylomicron remnants. The *very-low-density lipoproteins (VLDL)* are like tanker trucks, carrying triglycerides assembled in the liver out to cells for energy needs or storage as fat. The *low-density lipoproteins (LDL)*, rich in cholesterol, are the almost empty tankers that deliver cholesterol to the peripheral cells after the triglycerides have been off-loaded. The *high-density lipoproteins (HDL)* are the cleanup crew, gathering up extra cholesterol for transport back to the liver. Cholesterol, which in excess contributes to heart disease, is used by the body for such useful functions as facilitating triglyceride transport in serving the fuel needs of the body and maintaining cell membranes and as a precursor for hormone synthesis.

The lipids and lipoproteins, which are central to the metabolism of the body, have become increasingly important in clinical practice, primarily because of their association with coronary heart disease (CHD). Many national and international epidemiologic studies have demonstrated that, especially in affluent countries with high fat consumption, there is a clear association between the blood lipid levels and the development of atherosclerosis. Decades of basic research have contributed to knowledge about the nature of the lipoproteins and their lipid and protein constituents, as well as their role in the pathogenesis of the atherosclerotic process.

The accurate measurement of the various lipid and lipoprotein parameters is critical in the diagnosis and treatment of patients with *dyslipidemia*. International efforts to reduce the impact of CHD on public health have focused attention on improving the reliability and convenience of the lipid and lipoprotein assays. Expert panels have developed guidelines for detection and treatment of high cholesterol, as well as laboratory performance goals and detailed recommendations for reliable measurement of the lipid and lipoprotein analytes. This chapter begins with a review of lipid chemistry and lipoprotein metabolism, followed by the diagnosis and treatment of dyslipidemia. Finally, the clinical laboratory measurement of lipids and lipoproteins will be discussed in the context of the guidelines from the National Cholesterol Education Program (NCEP).

LIPID CHEMISTRY

Lipids, commonly referred to as fats, have a dual role. First, because they are composed of mostly carbon-hydrogen (C-H) bonds, they are a rich source of energy and an efficient way for the body to store excess calories. Because of their unique physical properties, lipids are also an integral part of cell membranes and, therefore, also play an important structural role in cells. The lipids transported by lipoproteins, namely fatty acids, phospholipids, cholesterol, and cholesteryl esters, are the principal lipids found in cells and the main focus of this section.

Fatty Acids[1]

Fatty acids, as seen in the structure shown in Figure 12-1, are simply linear chains of carbon-hydrogen (C-H) bonds that terminate with a carboxyl group (-COOH). In plasma, only a relatively small amount of fatty acids exist in the free unesterified form, most of which is bound to albumin. The majority of plasma fatty acids are instead found as a constituent of triglycerides or phospholipids (Fig. 12-1). Fatty acids are covalently attached to the glycerol backbone of triglycerides and phospholipids by an ester bond that forms between the carboxyl group on the fatty acid and the hydroxyl group (-OH) on glycerol (Fig. 12-1). Fatty acids are variable in length and can be classified as short-chain (4–6 carbon atoms), medium-chain (8–12 carbon atoms), or long-chain (>12 carbon atoms) fatty acids. Most fatty acids in our diet are of the long-chain variety and contain an even number of carbon atoms. Not all of the carbon atoms on fatty acids are fully saturated or bonded with hydrogen atoms; some of them may instead form carbon-carbon (C=C) double-bonds. Depending on the number of C=C double-bonds, fatty acids can be classified as being saturated (no double-bonds), monounsaturated (one double-bond), or polyunsaturated (two or more double-bonds). The C=C double-bonds of unsaturated fatty acids are typically arranged in the *cis* form, with both hydrogen atoms on the same side of the C=C double-bond, which causes a bend in their structure (Fig. 12-1). These bends increase the space that unsaturated fatty acids require when packed in a lipid layer and, as a result, these fatty acids are more fluid because they do not as readily self-associate. Fatty acid C=C double-bonds can also occur in the *trans* configuration, with both hydrogen atoms on

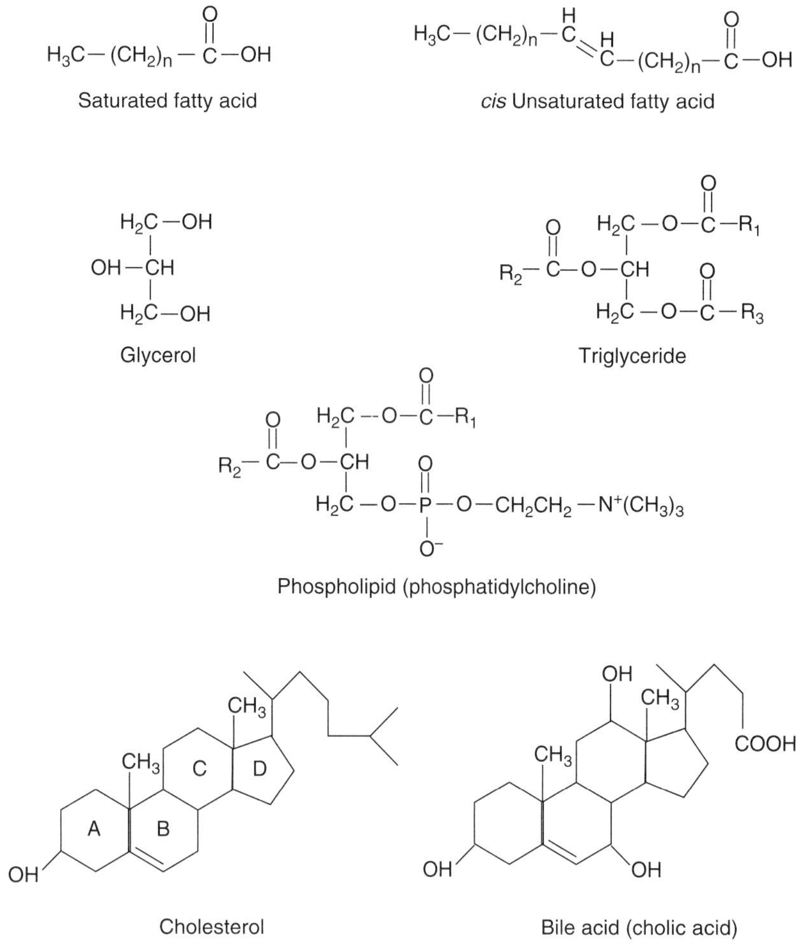

FIGURE 12-1. Chemical structures of lipids. Fatty acids are abbreviated as (R) for triglycerides and phospholipids.

opposite side of the C=C double-bond. Because of the spatial orientation of their double bonds, *trans* fatty acids do not bend and have physical properties similar to saturated fatty acids. *Trans* fatty acids are not commonly found in nature; however, they are present in our diet because the chemical hydrogenation used in the process of converting polyunsaturated plant oils into solid margarine introduces *trans* double bonds.

Triglycerides[2]

As can be inferred from the name, *triglycerides* contain three fatty acid molecules attached to one molecule of glycerol by ester bonds (Fig. 12-1). Because of the large number of possible forms of fatty acids, each fatty acid in the triglyceride molecule can potentially be different in structure, producing many possible structural forms of triglycerides. Triglycerides containing saturated fatty acids, which do not have kinks in their structure (Fig. 12-1), pack together more closely and tend to be solid at room temperature. In contrast, triglycerides, containing *cis* unsaturated fatty acids, with bends in their structure (Fig. 12-1), typically form oils at room temper-

ature. Most triglycerides from plant sources, such as corn, sunflower seeds, and safflower seeds, are rich in polyunsaturated fatty acids and are oils, whereas triglycerides from animal sources contain mostly saturated fatty acids and are usually solid at room temperature. As can be seen by inspecting the structure of triglyceride (Fig. 12-1), there are no charged groups or polar hydrophilic groups, making it very hydrophobic and virtually water insoluble.

Phospholipids[3–5]

Phospholipids are similar in structure to triglycerides except that they only have two esterified fatty acids (Fig. 12-1). The third position on the glycerol backbone contains a phospholipid head group. There are several types of phospholipid head groups, such as choline, inositol, serine, and ethanolamine, which are all hydrophilic in nature. Phospholipids are named based on the type of phospholipid head group present. Phosphatidylcholine (Fig. 12-1), for example, has a choline head group and is the most common phospholipid found on lipoproteins and in cell membranes. The two fatty acids in phospholipids are normally 14–24 carbon atoms long, with one fatty acid commonly saturated and the other unsaturated.

Because phospholipids contain both hydrophobic fatty acid C-H chains and a hydrophilic head group, they are by definition amphipathic lipid molecules and, as such, are found on the surface of lipid layers. The polar hydrophilic head group faces outward toward the aqueous environment, whereas the fatty acid chains face inward away from the water in a perpendicular orientation with respect to the lipid surface.

Cholesterol[6–8]

Cholesterol is an unsaturated steroid alcohol containing 4 rings (A, B, C, and D), and it has a single C-H side chain tail similar to a fatty acid in its physical properties (Fig. 12-1). The only hydrophilic part of cholesterol is the hydroxyl group in the A-ring. Cholesterol is, therefore, also an amphipathic lipid and is found on the surface of lipid layers along with phospholipids. Cholesterol is oriented in lipid layers so that the 4 rings and the side chain tail are buried in the membrane in a parallel orientation to the fatty acid acyl chains on adjacent phospholipid molecules. The polar hydroxyl group on the cholesterol A-ring faces outward, away from the lipid layer, allowing it to interact with water by noncovalent hydrogen bonding.

Cholesterol can also exist in an esterified form called *cholesteryl ester,* with the hydroxyl group conjugated by an ester bond to a fatty acid, in the same way as in triglycerides. In contrast to free cholesterol, there are no polar groups on cholesteryl esters, making them very hydrophobic. Because of their hydrophobic nature, cholesteryl esters are not found on the surface of lipid layers but are instead in the center of lipid drops, along with triglycerides.

Cholesterol is almost exclusively synthesized by animals, but plants do contain other sterols similar in structure to cholesterol. Cholesterol is also unique in that unlike other lipids, it is not readily catabolized by most cells and, therefore, does not serve as a source of fuel. Cholesterol can, however, be converted in the liver to primary bile acids, such as cholic acid (Fig. 12-1) and chenodeoxycholic acid, which promote fat absorption in the intestine by acting as detergents. A small amount of cholesterol can also be converted by some tissue, such as the adrenal gland, testis, and ovary, to steroid hormones, such as glucocorticoids, mineralocorticoids, and estrogens. Finally, a small amount of cholesterol, after first being converted to 7-dehydrocholesterol, can also be transformed to vitamin D_3 on irradiation of the skin by sunlight.

GENERAL LIPOPROTEIN STRUCTURE[9–12]

The prototypical structure of a lipoprotein particle is shown in Figure 12-2. Lipoproteins are typically spherical

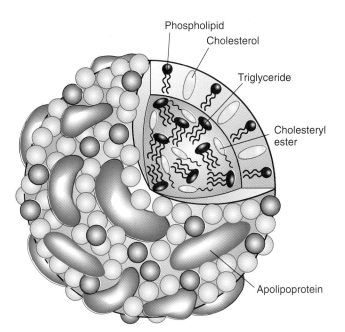

FIGURE 12-2. Model of lipoprotein structure.

in shape and range in size from 10 to 1200 nm (Table 12-1). As the name implies, lipoproteins are composed of both lipids and proteins, called *apolipoproteins.*[13] The amphipathic cholesterol and phospholipid molecules are primarily found on the surface of lipoproteins as a single monolayer, whereas the hydrophobic triglyceride and cholesteryl ester molecules are found in the central or core region (Fig. 12-2). Because a main role of lipoproteins is the delivery of fuel to peripheral cells, the core of the lipoprotein particle essentially represents the cargo that is being transported by lipoproteins. The size of the lipoprotein particle correlates with its lipid content. The larger lipoprotein particles have correspondingly larger core regions and, therefore, contain relatively more triglyceride and cholesteryl ester. The larger lipoprotein particles also contain more lipid relative to protein and are, therefore, lighter in density. The various lipoprotein particles were originally separated by ultracentrifugation into different density fractions (chylomicrons [chylos]; very-low-density lipoproteins [VLDL]; low-density lipoproteins [LDL]; and high-density lipoproteins [HDL]), which still form the basis for the most commonly used lipoprotein classification system (Table 12-1).

Apolipoproteins are primarily located on the surface of lipoprotein particles (Table 12-2). They help maintain the structural integrity of lipoproteins and also serve as ligands for cell receptors and as activators and inhibitors of the various enzymes that modify lipoprotein particles (Table 12-2). Apolipoproteins contain a structural motif called an amphipathic helix,[14] which accounts for the ability of these proteins to bind to lipids. Amphipathic helices are protein segments arranged in coils so that the

TABLE 12-1. CHARACTERISTICS OF THE MAJOR HUMAN LIPOPROTEINS

CHARACTERISTICS	CHYLOS	VLDL	LDL	HDL
Density (g/mL)	<0.93	0.93–1.006	1.019–1.063	1.063–1.21
Molecular weight (kD)	$(0.4–30) \times 10^9$	$(10–80) \times 10^6$	2.75×10^6	$(1.75–3.6) \times 10^5$
Diameter (nm)	80–1200	30–80	18–30	5–12
Total lipid (% by weight)	98	89–96	77	50
Triglyceride (% by weight)	84	44–60	11	3
Total cholesterol (% by weight)	7	16–22	62	19

hydrophobic amino acids residues interact with lipids, whereas the part of the helix containing hydrophilic amino acids faces away from the lipids and toward the aqueous environment.

Apo A-I, the major protein on HDL, is frequently used as an index of the amount of the antiatherogenic HDL present in plasma.[15] Apo B is a large protein with a molecular weight of approximately 500 kD and the principal protein on LDL, VLDL, and chylomicrons.[16] Apo B exists in two forms, apo B-100 and apo B-48. Apo B-100 is found on LDL and VLDL and is a ligand for the LDL receptor,[17] and it is, therefore, critical in the uptake of LDL by cells. Apo B-48, exclusively found in chylomicrons, is essentially the first 48% or first half of the apo B molecule and is produced by posttranscriptional editing of the apo B-100 mRNA. Apo B-100 can also be found covalently linked to apo (a),[18] a plasminogen-like protein that is found in a proatherogenic lipoprotein particle called lipoprotein (a) [Lp(a)]. Apo E, another important apolipoprotein found on many types of lipoproteins (LDL, VLDL, and HDL), also serves as a ligand for the LDL receptor and the chylomicron remnant receptor.[19]

There are three major isoforms of apo E: apo E2, E3, and E4. The apo E isoforms affect lipoprotein metabolism because they differ in their ability to interact with the LDL receptor.[20,21] For example, patients who are homozygous for the apo E2 isoform are at an increased risk for developing type III hyperlipoproteinemia. The relationship with lipid metabolism is not completely understood, but individuals with the apo E4 isoform have been shown to have an increased risk for developing Alzheimer's disease.[22]

Chylomicrons[19–24]

Chylomicrons, which contain apo B-48, are the largest and the least dense of the lipoprotein particles, having diameters as large as 1200 nm (Table 12-1). Because of their large size, they reflect light and account for the turbidity of postprandial plasma. Because they are so light, they also readily float to the top of stored plasma and form a creamy layer, which is characteristic for the presence of chylomicrons. Chylomicrons are produced by the intestine, where they are packaged with absorbed dietary

TABLE 12-2. CHARACTERISTICS OF THE MAJOR HUMAN APOLIPOPROTEINS

APOLIPOPROTEIN	MOLECULAR WEIGHT (kD)	PLASMA CONCENTRATION (mg/dL)	MAJOR LIPOPROTEIN LOCATION	FUNCTION
Apo A-I	28,000	100–200	HDL	Structural, LCAT activator, ABCA1 lipid acceptor
Apo A-II	17,400	20–50	HDL	Structural
Apo A-IV	44,000	10–20	Chylos, VLDL, HDL	Structural
Apo B-100	5.4×10^5	70–125	LDL, VLDL	Structural, LDL receptor ligand
Apo B-48	2.6×10^5	<5	Chylos	Structural, remnant receptor ligand
Apo C-I	6,630	5–8	Chylos, VLDL, HDL	Structural
Apo C-II	8,900	3–7	Chylos, VLDL, HDL	Structural, LPL cofactor
Apo C-III	9,400	10–12	Chylos, VLDL, HDL	Structural, LPL inhibitor
Apo E	34,400	3–15	VLDL, HDL	Structural, LDL receptor ligand
Apo(a)	$(3–7) \times 10^5$	<30	Lp(a)	Structural, Plasminogen inhibitor

lipids. Once they enter the circulation, triglycerides and cholesteryl esters in chylomicrons are rapidly hydrolyzed by lipases and, within a few hours, they are transformed into chylomicron remnant particles, which are taken up by remnant receptors in the liver.[19] Thus, the principal role of chylomicrons is the delivery of dietary lipids to hepatic and peripheral cells.

Very-Low-Density Lipoproteins[25,26]

VLDL is produced by the liver and contain apo B-100, apo E, and apo Cs; like chylomicrons, they are also rich in triglycerides. They are the major carriers of *endogenous* (hepatic derived) triglycerides and transfer triglycerides from the liver to peripheral tissue. Like chylomicrons, they readily reflect light and account for most of the turbidity observed in fasting hyperlipidemic plasma specimens, although they do not form a top, creamy layer like chylomicrons because they are more dense (Table 12-1). Excess dietary intake of carbohydrate, saturated fatty acids, and *trans* fatty acids enhances the hepatic synthesis of triglycerides that, in turn, increases VLDL production.

Low-Density Lipoproteins[27,28]

LDL contains apo B-100 and apo E and is more cholesterol-rich than other apo B-containing lipoproteins (Table 12-1). They primarily form as a consequence of the lipolysis of VLDL. LDL is readily taken up by cells via the LDL receptor and this, in part, accounts for the reason that elevated LDL levels promote atherosclerosis.[29] In addition, because LDL are significantly smaller than VLDL and chylomicrons, they can infiltrate into the extracellular space of the vessel wall, where they can be oxidized and taken up by macrophages by various scavenger receptors.[30] Macrophages that take up too much lipid become filled up with intracellular lipid drops and turn into foam cells,[30] which is the predominant cell type of fatty streaks, an early precursor of atherosclerotic plaques.

LDL particles can exist in various sizes and compositions and have been separated into as many as eight subclasses by density ultracentrifugation or gradient gel electrophoresis.[31,32] The LDL subclasses differ largely in their content of core lipids; the smaller particles are more dense and have relatively more triglyceride than cholesteryl esters. Recently, there has been great interest in quantitating the LDL subfractions because the small, dense, LDL particles have been shown to be more proatherogenic and may be a better marker for coronary heart disease risk.[31,32]

Lipoprotein (a)[18,33,34]

Lp(a) are LDL-like particles that each contain a molecule of apo (a) linked to apo B-100 by a disulfide bond. Lp(a) particles are heterogeneous in both size and density as a result of a differing number of peptide sequences, called

kringles, in the apo (a) portion of the molecule. The concentration of Lp(a) is inversely related to the size of the isoform. Plasma levels of Lp(a) vary widely among individuals in a population, but remain relatively constant within an individual.

Elevated levels of Lp(a) are thought to confer increased risk for premature coronary heart disease and stroke. Because the kringle domains of Lp(a) have a high level of homology with plasminogen, a protein that promotes clot lysis, it has been proposed that Lp(a) may compete with plasminogen for binding sites, thereby promoting clotting, a key contributor to both myocardial infarction and stroke.[29,30]

High-Density Lipoproteins[35,36]

HDL, the smallest and most dense lipoprotein particle, is synthesized by both the liver and intestine (Table 12-1). HDL can exist either as disk-shaped particles or as spherical-shaped particles.[15] Discoidal HDL typically contain two molecules of apo A-I, which form a ring around a central lipid bilayer of phospholipid and cholesterol. Discoidal HDL is believed to represent nascent or newly secreted HDL and is the most active form in removing excess cholesterol from peripheral cells. The ability of HDL to remove cholesterol from cells is one of the main mechanisms that has been proposed for the antiatherogenic property of HDL. When discoidal HDL has acquired additional lipid, cholesteryl esters and triglycerides form a core region between the central lipid bilayer, which transforms discoidal HDL into spherical HDL, the predominant form in plasma. Based on density differences, there are two major types of spherical HDL: HDL_2 and HDL_3. HDL_2 is larger in size and richer in lipid than HDL_3 and may be more efficient in delivering lipids to the liver.[37]

LIPOPROTEIN PHYSIOLOGY AND METABOLISM

The four major pathways involved in lipoprotein metabolism are shown in Figure 12-3. The lipid absorption pathway, the exogenous pathway, and the endogenous pathway, which all depend on apo B-containing lipoprotein particles, can be viewed as means to transport dietary lipid and hepatic-derived lipid to peripheral cells. In terms of energy metabolism, these three pathways are critical in the transport of fatty acids to peripheral cells, which are generated during the lipolysis of triglycerides and, to a lesser degree, cholesteryl esters on lipoproteins. In regard to the pathogenesis of atherosclerosis, the net result of these three pathways is also the net delivery or forward transport of cholesterol to peripheral cells, which can lead to atherosclerosis when the cells in the vessel wall accumulate too much cholesterol.[29,30] Peripheral cells are prone to accumulating cholesterol because

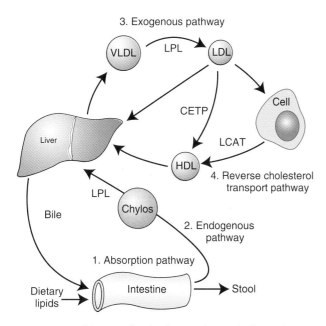

FIGURE 12-3. Diagram of major lipoprotein metabolism pathways.

they also synthesize their own cholesterol, and, unlike liver cells, they do not have the enzymatic pathways to further catabolize cholesterol. Furthermore, cholesterol is relatively water insoluble and cannot readily diffuse away from its site of deposition or synthesis.

One principal way that peripheral cells maintain their cholesterol equilibrium is the reverse cholesterol transport pathway (Fig. 12-3), which is mediated by HDL. In this pathway, excess cholesterol from peripheral cells is transported back to the liver, where it can be excreted into the bile as free cholesterol or it can be excreted after first being converted to bile acids. The liver is, therefore, involved in both the forward and reverse cholesterol transport pathways and, in many ways, acts as a buffer in helping the body maintain its overall cholesterol balance. There are several genetic defects in the genes that encode for proteins in the forward and reverse cholesterol transport pathways that result in a predisposition for atherosclerosis.[38,39] The majority of individuals with coronary artery disease, however, do not have a clear, single, genetic defect but instead have multiple genetic variations or gene polymorphisms that most likely interact with various lifestyle factors,[40] such as exercise frequency, diet, and smoking, to cause a predisposition for disease.

Lipid Absorption[41,42]

An average person ingests, absorbs, and transports about 60–130 g of fat daily, mostly in the form of triglycerides. Because fats are water insoluble, special mechanisms are required to facilitate their absorption in the intestine. During the process of digestion, pancreatic lipase, by cleaving off fatty acids, first converts dietary lipids into

more polar compounds with amphipathic properties. Thus, triglycerides are transformed into monoglycerides and diglycerides; cholesterol esters are transformed into free cholesterol; and phospholipids are transformed into lysophospholipids. These amphipathic lipids in the intestinal lumen form large aggregates with bile acids called *micelles*. Lipid absorption occurs when the micelles come in contact with the microvillus membranes of the intestinal mucosal cells. Absorption of some of these lipids may occur by a passive transfer process; however, recent evidence suggests that, in some cases, it might also be facilitated by specific transporters.[41,42] The smaller free fatty acids, with ten or fewer carbon atoms, can readily pass directly into the portal circulation and are carried by albumin to the liver. The absorbed long-chain fatty acids, monoglycerides, and diglycerides are reesterified in intestinal cells to form triglycerides and cholesteryl esters. The newly formed triglycerides and cholesteryl esters are then packaged into chylomicrons, along with apo B-48.

Triglyceride absorption is efficient; greater than 90% of dietary triglycerides are taken up by the intestine. In contrast, only about half of the 500 milligrams of cholesterol in the typical diet is absorbed each day. Even a smaller fraction of plant sterols are absorbed by the intestine. Recently, a specific transport system, involving the ABCG5 and ABCG8 transporters, has been described that prevents excess absorption of dietary cholesterol and plant sterols.[43] Individuals with defective ABCG5 or ABCG8 transporters have a disease called *sitosterolemia* and have a predisposition for atherosclerosis because of increased cholesterol and plant sterol absorption.[43]

Exogenous Pathway[19,23,24]

The newly synthesized chylomicrons in the intestine (Fig. 12-3) are initially secreted into the lymphatic ducts and eventually enter the circulation by way of the thoracic duct. Immediately after entering the circulation, chylomicrons interact with proteoglycans, such as heparan sulfate, on the surface of capillaries in various tissue, such as skeletal muscle, heart, and adipose tissue. The proteoglycans on capillaries also promote the binding of lipoprotein lipase (LPL),[44] which hydrolyzes triglycerides on chylomicrons. The free fatty acids and glycerol generated by the hydrolysis of triglycerides by LPL can then be taken up by cells and used as a source of energy. Excess fatty acids, particularly in fat cells (adipocytes), are reesterified into triglycerides for long-term storage in intracellular lipid drops. Hormone-sensitive lipase inside adipose cells can release free fatty acids from triglycerides in stored fat when energy sources from carbohydrates are insufficient for the body's energy needs. The hormones epinephrine and cortisol play a key role in the mobilization and hydrolysis of triglycerides from adipocytes, whereas insulin prevents lipolysis by adipocytes and promotes fat storage and glucose use.

During the lipolysis of chylomicrons, there is transfer of lipid and apolipoproteins onto HDL, and chlyomicrons are converted within a few hours after a meal into chylomicron remnant particles. Chylomicron remnants are rapidly taken up by the liver through interaction of apo E with specific remnant receptors on the surface of liver cells. Once in the liver, lysosomal enzymes break down the remnant particles to release free fatty acids, free cholesterol, and amino acids. Some cholesterol is converted to bile acids. Both bile acids and free cholesterol are directly excreted into the bile but not all of the excreted cholesterol and bile salt exits the body. As previously described, approximately half of the excreted biliary cholesterol is reabsorbed by the intestine, with the remainder appearing in the stool, as fecal neutral steroids. In the case of bile acids, almost all of the bile acids are reabsorbed and reused by the liver for bile production.

Endogenous Pathway[25–28]

Most triglycerides in the liver that are packaged into VLDL are derived from the diet after recirculation from adipose tissue. Only a small fraction is synthesized de novo in the liver from dietary carbohydrate. VLDL particles, once secreted into the circulation, undergo a lipolytic process similar to that of chylomicrons (Fig. 12-3). Primarily by the action of LPL, VLDL loses core lipids, which causes the dissociation and transfer of apolipoproteins and phospholipids to other lipoprotein particles. During this process, VLDL is converted to VLDL remnants, which can be further transformed by lipolysis into LDL. About half of VLDL are eventually completely converted to LDL, and the remainder are taken up as VLDL remnants by the liver remnant receptors.

Because of the efficient uptake of LDL by the LDL receptors,[17] LDL are the major lipoproteins responsible for the delivery of exogenous cholesterol to peripheral cells. Once bound to LDL receptors, they are endocytosed by cells and transported to the lysosome, where they are degraded. The triglycerides in LDL are converted by acid lipase into free fatty acids and glycerol and further metabolized by the cell for energy or are reesterified and stored in lipid drops for later use. Free cholesterol derived from degraded LDL can be used for membrane biosynthesis, and excess cholesterol is converted by acyl-CoA:acyl-cholesterol acyltransferase (ACAT) into cholesteryl esters and stored in lipid drops.[45] The regulation of cellular cholesterol biosynthesis is, in part, coordinated by the availability of cholesterol delivered by the LDL receptor.[17] Many enzymes in the cholesterol biosynthetic pathway (eg, HMG-CoA reductase, the main target for the cholesterol-lowering statin-type drugs) are down-regulated (along with the LDL receptor) when there is excess cellular cholesterol by a complex mechanism involving both gene regulation and posttranscriptional gene regulation.[46]

Abnormalities in LDL receptor function result in elevation of LDL in the circulation and lead to hypercholesterolemia and premature atherosclerosis.[17,47] Patients who are heterozygous for a disease called familial hypercholesterolemia (incidence, approximately 1 of 500) have only half the normal LDL receptors, which results in decreased hepatic uptake of LDL by the liver and increased hepatic cholesterol biosynthesis. The LDL that accumulates in the plasma of these individuals often leads to the development of coronary heart disease by midadulthood in heterozygotes and even earlier for homozygotes.[17,47]

Reverse Cholesterol Transport Pathway[48–51]

As previously described, one of the major roles of HDL is to maintain the equilibrium of cholesterol in peripheral cells by the reverse cholesterol transport pathway (Fig. 12-3). HDL is believed to remove excess cholesterol from cells by two different pathways, the aqueous diffusion pathway[51] and the ABCA1 transporter pathway.[49] In the aqueous diffusion pathway, HDL acts as a sink for the small amount of cholesterol that can diffuse away from the cells. Although cholesterol is relatively water insoluble, because it is an amphipathic lipid, it is soluble in plasma in micromolar amounts and can spontaneously dissociate from the surface of cell membranes and enter the extracellular fluid. Some free cholesterol will then bind to HDL in the extracellular space, and, once bound, it becomes trapped in lipoproteins after it is converted to cholesteryl ester by lecithin-cholesterol acyltransferase (LCAT),[52] which resides on HDL. HDL can then directly deliver cholesterol to the liver by the SR-BI receptor[53] and, possibly, other receptors.[9,36] Approximately one half of the cholesterol on HDL is returned to the liver by the LDL receptor, after first being transferred from HDL to LDL by the cholesteryl ester transfer protein (CETP),[54] which connects the forward and reverse cholesterol transport pathways (Fig. 12-3). Cholesterol that reaches the liver is then directly excreted into the bile or first converted to a bile acid before excretion.

The other pathway in which HDL mediates the removal of cholesterol from cells, involves the ABCA1 transporter. The ABCA1 transporter is a member of the ATP-binding cassette transporter family[55] that pumps various ligands across the plasma membrane. Defects in the gene for the ABCA1 transporter lead to Tangier disease,[49] a disorder associated with low HDL and a predisposition to premature coronary heart disease. The exact mechanism of the ABCA1 transporter is not known, but it is believed that the transporter modifies the plasma membrane by transporting a lipid, which then enables

CASE STUDY 12-1

A 52-year-old man went to his physician for a physical. The patient had been a district manager for an automobile insurance company for the last 10 years and was 24 pounds overweight. He had missed his last two appointments with the physician because of business. The urinalysis dipstick was not remarkable. His blood pressure was elevated. The blood chemistry results listed in Case Study Table 12-1.1 were obtained.

Questions

1. Given the abnormal tests, what additional information would you like to have?

2. If this patient had triglycerides of 100 mg/dL (1.1 mmol/L) and an HDL cholesterol of 23 mg/dL (0.6 mmol/L), what would be his calculated LDL-cholesterol value?

3. If, however, his triglycerides were 476 mg/dL (5.4 mmol/L), with an HDL cholesterol of 23 mg/dL (0.6 mmol/L), what would be his calculated LDL-cholesterol value?

CASE STUDY TABLE 12-1.1. LABORATORY RESULTS

ANALYTE	PATIENT VALUE	REFERENCE RANGE
Na$^+$	151	135–143 mEq/L
K$^+$	4.5	3.0–5.0 mEq/L
Cl$^-$	106	98–103 mEq/L
CO$_2$ content	13	22–27 mmol/L
Total protein	5.7	6.5–8.0 g/dL
Albumin	1.6	3.5–5.0 g/dL
Calcium	7.9	9.0–10.5 mg/dL
Cholesterol	210	140–200 mg/dL
Uric acid	6.2	3.5–7.9 mg/dL
Creatinine	2.5	0.5–1.2 mg/dL
BUN	95	7–25 mg/dL
Glucose	88	75–105 mg/dL
Total bilirubin	1.2	0.2–1.0 mg/dL
Alkaline phosphatase	27	7–59 IU/L
Lactate dehydrogenase	202	90–190 IU/L
Aspartate transaminase	39	8–40 IU/L
Amylase	152	76–375 IU/L

apo A-I that has dissociated from HDL to bind to the cell membrane. In a detergent-like extraction mechanism, apo A-I then removes excess cholesterol and phospholipid from the plasma membrane of cells to form a discoidal-shaped HDL particle. The newly formed HDL is then competent to accept additional cholesterol by the aqueous diffusion pathway and is eventually converted into spherical HDL by the action of LCAT (Fig. 12-3).

LIPID AND LIPOPROTEIN DISTRIBUTIONS IN THE POPULATION

Serum lipoprotein concentrations differ between adult men and women, primarily as a result of differences in sex hormone levels, with women having higher HDL cholesterol levels and lower total cholesterol and triglyceride levels than men.[56] The difference in total cholesterol, however, disappears after menopause as estrogen decreases.[57,58] Men and women both show a tendency toward increased total cholesterol, LDL cholesterol, and

triglyceride concentrations with age.[56,59,60] HDL cholesterol concentrations generally remain stable after the onset of puberty and do not drop in women with the onset of menopause.[61] General adult reference ranges are shown in Table 12-3.

Circulating levels of total cholesterol, LDL cholesterol, and triglycerides in young children are generally much lower than those seen in adults.[62,63] In addition, concentrations do not differ significantly between boys

TABLE 12-3. ADULT REFERENCE RANGES FOR LIPIDS

ANALYTE	REFERENCE RANGE
Total cholesterol	140–200 mg/dL
HDL cholesterol	40–75 mg/dL
LDL cholesterol	50–130 mg/dL
Triglyceride	60–150 mg/dL

and girls. HDL cholesterol levels for both boys and girls are comparable to those of adult women. At the onset of puberty, however, HDL cholesterol concentrations in boys fall to adult male levels, a drop of approximately 20%, whereas those of girls do not change. It is the lower concentration of HDL cholesterol in men, combined with their higher LDL cholesterol and triglyceride levels that account for much of the observed association with increased risk of premature heart disease.

The incidence of heart disease is strongly associated with serum cholesterol concentration,[64,65] and comparisons have been performed in various societies showing that individuals in societies who traditionally eat less animal fat and more grains, fruits, and vegetables, such as many Asian populations, have lower levels of LDL cholesterol and lower rates of heart disease than societies that ingest more fat, particularly animal fat, in their diet and are more sedentary.[66,67] These differences can be attributed to both genetic and lifestyle factors. The importance of dietary factors was clearly shown in a study that compared the dietary patterns and heart disease rates in Japanese men living in Japan, Hawaii, and California.[68] In this study, as dietary intake became more westernized, with increased consumption of fat and cholesterol, the LDL cholesterol concentrations increased significantly, as did the rates of heart disease, so that Japanese men living in California had much higher rates of heart disease than Japanese men living in Japan; those in Hawaii were intermediate. Within societies in which diet tends to be more homogeneous, LDL cholesterol levels become somewhat less discriminatory as a risk factor, and HDL cholesterol levels become more important because of the ability of HDL to remove excess cholesterol from the circulation.[69]

The National Cholesterol Education Program (NCEP) was formed to alert the American population to the risk factors associated with heart disease. NCEP has used panels of experts, including Adult Treatment Panels, the Children and Adolescents Treatment Panel, and the Laboratory Standardization Panel, to produce recommendations within the scope of each panel's activities.[62,70–73]

In 1988, the first NCEP Adult Treatment Panel (ATP) developed a list of heart disease risk factors. These guidelines were most recently updated by ATP III in 2002.[73] The current list of risk factors is shown in Table 12-4. ATP III also has recommended that all adults (≥20 years) have a fasting lipoprotein profile performed (total, LDL, and HDL cholesterol and triglycerides), once every 5 years and has developed guidelines for the diagnosis and follow-up treatment of individuals with abnormal levels (Table 12-5). The Children and Adolescents Treatment Panel has developed similar criteria for the pediatric population.[62]

The NCEP Laboratory Standardization Panel and its successor, the Lipoprotein Measurement Working

TABLE 12-4. CORONARY HEART DISEASE RISK FACTORS DETERMINED BY THE NCEP ADULT TREATMENT PANELS

Positive Risk Factors

- Age: ≥45 years for men; ≥55 years or premature menopause for women
- Family history of premature CHD
- Current cigarette smoking
- Hypertension (BP ≥140/90 mm Hg or taking antihypertensive medication)
- LDL cholesterol concentration ≥160 mg/dL (≥4.1 mmol/L), with ≤1 risk factor
- LDL cholesterol concentration ≥130 mg/dL (3.4 mmol/L), with ≥2 risk factors
- LDL cholesterol concentration ≥100 mg/dL (2.6 mmol/L), with CHD or risk equivalent
- HDL cholesterol concentration >40 mg/dL (<1.0 mmol/L)
- Diabetes mellitus = CHD risk equivalent
- Metabolic syndrome (multiple metabolic risk factors)

Negative Risk Factors

- HDL cholesterol concentration ≥60 mg/dL (≥1.6 mmol/L)
- LDL cholesterol <100 mg/dL (<2.6 mmol/L)

Group,[70–72] set laboratory guidelines for acceptable precision and accuracy when measuring total cholesterol, triglycerides, and lipoprotein cholesterol (HDL and LDL cholesterol) (Table 12-6).

Obviously, the best way to reduce the prevalence of heart disease is through prevention. Learning and practicing good dietary and exercise patterns early in life, maintaining these patterns throughout life,[56] refraining from smoking, and controlling blood pressure are important means for reducing the incidence of CHD and stroke.[74–76] Lipoprotein profile measurements provide a method of identifying individuals who may have levels that put them at risk, so that they can receive treatment to reduce the level of risk. Treatment of other diseases that may affect lipoproteins, such as diabetes mellitus, hypothyroidism, and renal disease, is also important.

A prudent diet, low in fat and cholesterol, with a caloric intake adjusted to meet and maintain ideal body weight, along with regular exercise, can reduce the risk of heart disease, stroke, diabetes, and cancer.[77–80] Dietary intake of fat and cholesterol have been shown to have a synergistic effect, such that dietary cholesterol is more efficiently absorbed when in the presence of fat.[81] Additionally, saturated fat is more atherogenic than unsaturated fat.[56,82,83] The American Heart Association has recommended dietary guidelines for the intake of fat and cholesterol for most adult Americans (Table 12-7).

TABLE 12-5. TREATMENT GUIDELINES ESTABLISHED BY THE NCEP ADULT TREATMENT PANELS (INITIAL TESTING SHOULD CONSIST OF FASTING FOR ≥12 HOURS)

RISK CATEGORY AND ACTION

TC, <200 mg/dL (5.2 mmol/L); TG, <150 mg/dL (<1.7 mmol/L); LDLC, <130 mg/dL (<3.4 mmol/L); HDLC, ≥40 mg/dL (≥1.0 mmol/L)
   Repeat within 5 years
   Provide risk reduction information

TC, 200–239 mg/dL (5.2–6.2 mmol/L); TG, 150–199 mg/dL (1.7–2.2 mmol/L); LDLC, 130–159 mg/dL (3.4–4.1 mmol/L); HDLC, ≥40 mg/dL (1.0 mmol/L); and 0–1 risk factors
   Provide TLC diet and physical activity information and reevaluate in 1 year
   Provide risk reduction information

TC, ≥200 mg/dL (5.2–6.2 mmol/L); TG, ≥200 mg/dL (≥2.2 mmol/L); LDLC, 130–159 mg/dL (3.4–4.1 mmol/L); HDLC, <40 mg/dL (1.0 mmol/L); and ≥2 risk factors
   Do clinical evaluation, including family history
   Start dietary therapy (see below)

TC, ≥240 mg/dL (6.2 mmol/L)   Perform lipoprotein analysis (see below)

TREATMENT DECISIONS		
RISK CATEGORY	ACTION LEVEL	GOAL
Dietary Therapy		
No CHD; 0–1 risk factors	≥160 mg/dL (4.1 mmol/L)	<160 mg/dL (4.1 mmol/L)
No CHD; ≥2 risk factors (10-year risk, ≥20%)	≥130 mg/dL (3.4 mmol/L)	<130 mg/dL (3.4 mmol/L)
CHD; CHD risk equivalent (10-year risk, >20%)	>100 mg/dL (2.6 mmol/L)	<100 mg/dL (2.6 mmol/L)
Drug Therapy		
No CHD; 0–1 risk factors	≥190 mg/dL (4.9 mmol/L)	<160 mg/dL (4.1 mmol/L)
No CHD; ≤2 risk factors (10-year risk, ≤10%)	≥160 mg/dL (4.1 mmol/L)	<130 mg/dL (3.4 mmol/L)
No CHD; ≥2 risk factors (10-year risk, 10–20%)	≥130 mg/dL (4.1 mmol/L)	<100 mg/dL (3.4 mmol/L)
CHD; CHD risk equivalent	≥130 mg/dL (3.4 mmol/L)	<100 mg/dL (2.6 mmol/L)

TABLE 12-6. NCEP ANALYTIC PERFORMANCE GOALS

	PRECISION	BIAS	TOTAL ERROR
Total cholesterol	3% CV	±3%	±8.9%
HDL cholesterol ≥42 mg/dL <42 mg/dL	4% CV SD <1.7 mg/dL	±5%	±12.8%
LDL cholesterol	4% CV	±4%	±11.8%
Triglycerides	5% CV	±5%	±14.8%

TABLE 12-7. COMPOSITION OF THE THERAPEUTIC LIFESTYLE CHANGES (TLC) DIET RECOMMENDED BY THE NCEP ADULT TREATMENT PANEL III (AS COMPARED WITH THE AVERAGE AMERICAN DIET)

DIETARY NUTRIENT	TLC DIET	AVERAGE AMERICAN DIET
Total fat (% total calories)	25–35%	36%
Saturated	<7%	15%
Monounsaturated	≤20%	15%
Polyunsaturated	≤10%	6%
Cholesterol		>400 mg/day
Carbohydrate	50–60%	
Fiber	20–30 g/day	
Protein	~15%	

A 30-year-old man with chest pain was brought to the emergency department after a softball game. He was placed in the coronary care unit when his ECG showed erratic waves in the ST region. A family history revealed that his father died of a heart attack at the age of 45 years. The patient had always been athletic in high school and college, so he had not concerned himself with a routine physical. The laboratory tests listed in Case Study Table 12-2.1 were run.

Questions

1. Given the symptoms and the family history, what additional tests should be recommended?

2. If his follow-up total cholesterol remains in the same range after he is released from the hospital, and his triglycerides and HDL cholesterol are within the normal range, what course of treatment should be recommended?

CASE STUDY TABLE 12-2.1. LABORATORY RESULTS

ANALYTE	PATIENT VALUES	REFERENCE RANGE
Sodium	139	135–143 mEq/L
Potassium	4.1	3.0–5.0 mEq/L
Chloride	101	98–103 mEq/L
CO_2 content	29	22–27 mmol/L
Total protein	6.9	6.5–8.0 g/dL
Albumin	3.2	3.5–5.0 g/dL
Calcium	9.3	9.0–10.5 mg/dL
Cholesterol	278	140–200 mg/dL
Uric acid	5.9	3.5–7.9 mg/dL
Creatinine	1.1	0.5–1.2 mg/dL
BUN	20	7–25 mg/dL
Glucose	97	75–105 mg/dL
Total bilirubin	0.8	0.2–1.0 mg/dL
Alkaline phosphatase	20	7–59 IU/L
Lactate dehydrogenase	175	90–190 IU/L
Aspartate transaminase	35	8–40 IU/L
Amylase	98	76–375 IU/L

DISEASE PREVENTION, DIAGNOSIS, AND TREATMENT

Diseases associated with abnormal lipid concentrations are referred to as *dyslipidemias*. They can be caused directly by genetic abnormalities or through environmental/lifestyle imbalances, or they can develop secondarily, as a consequence of other diseases.[84–86] Dyslipidemias are generally defined by the clinical characteristics of patients and the results of blood tests, and are not necessarily defined by the specific defect associated with the abnormality. Many dyslipidemias, regardless of etiology, are associated with CHD, or arteriosclerosis.

Arteriosclerosis

In the United States and many other developed countries, *arteriosclerosis* is the single leading cause of death and disability. The mortality rate has decreased in the United States in the past few years, partly a result of advances in diagnosis and treatment, but also a result of changes in lifestyle in the American population, resulting from increased awareness of the relationship between cholesterol and heart disease. This increased awareness has resulted in an overall decrease in the average serum cholesterol concentration and in a lower prevalence of heart disease; however, it still exceeds all other causes of death combined. As many women as men develop arteriosclerosis; however, on average, women develop it 10 years later than men.

The relationship between heart disease and lipid abnormalities stems from the deposition of lipids, mainly in the form of esterified cholesterol, in artery walls. This lipid deposition starts with thin layers called *fatty streaks*. In studies examining blood vessels at autopsy, fatty streaks have been seen in almost everyone older than age 15, regardless of cause of death.[87,88] Fatty streaks can develop over time into plaques that partially block (occlude) blood flow. When plaque develops in arteries of the arms or legs, it is called peripheral vascular disease (PVD); when it develops in the heart, it is referred to as coronary artery disease (CAD); and, when it develops in the vessels of the brain, it is called cerebrovascular disease (CVD). CAD is associated with angina and myocardial infarction, and CVD is associated with stroke. Many genetic and acquired abnormalities may also lead to lipid deposits in the liver and kidney, resulting in impaired function of these vital organs. Lipid deposits in skin form nodules called *xanthomas,* which are a clue to genetic abnormalities.

Plaque formation involves cell injury, followed by infiltration and cell proliferation to repair the site. As blood travels through blood vessels, small injuries occur that signal macrophages and platelets to heal the injury. LDL brings cholesterol to the site so that new cell membranes can be formed and macrophages can repair the area. LDL that has been modified by oxidative processes and chemical alterations can be taken up by the macrophages, producing foam cells.[89–92] These foam cells accumulate beneath the endothelial layer of the arterial wall. Future injury leads to more deposits and, eventually, plaque is formed. Continual injury and repair lead to additional narrowing of the vessel opening, or lumen, causing the blood to circulate under greater and greater pressure.

Deposits in the vessel walls are frequently associated with increased serum concentrations of LDL cholesterol or decreased HDL cholesterol.[65,93–95] Lowering the LDL cholesterol concentration is an important step in preventing and treating CHD.[95–100] It is estimated that for every 1% decrease in LDL cholesterol concentration there is a 2% decrease in a person's of risk of developing arteriosclerosis.[101] For patients with established heart disease, studies have shown that aggressive treatment to reduce LDL cholesterol levels below 100 mg/dL (2.6 mmol/L) is effective in the stabilization and sometimes regression of plaques.[102–105] Stabilization of plaque is thought to be at least as important as plaque regression in terms of rupture potential.[103,104,106]

In some individuals, high levels of blood cholesterol or triglycerides are caused by genetic abnormalities in which either too much is synthesized or too little is removed.[86,107–112] High levels of cholesterol and/or triglycerides in most people, however, are a result of increased consumption of foods rich in fat and cholesterol, smoking, and lack of exercise, or to other disorders or disease states that affect lipid metabolism, such as diabetes, hypertension, hypothyroidism, obesity, other hormonal imbalances, liver and kidney diseases, and alcoholism. Low levels of HDL cholesterol are also associated with increased risk of heart disease,[65,110,111] but few therapies significantly raise HDL cholesterol levels. Statin and fibrate therapies are well tolerated and produce small increases (5–10%) in HDL cholesterol levels, while also reducing LDL cholesterol and triglyceride concentrations, all of which are beneficial for CHD risk reduction.[113–117] The use of gemfibrozil in the Veterans' Affairs HDL Intervention Trial to raise HDL cholesterol levels in CHD patients with low levels at baseline, showed significant, direct benefit from the 7% rise in the on-trial HDL cholesterol levels.[114]

Laboratory analyses can aid in the diagnosis of arteriosclerosis. Accurate determinations of total, HDL, and LDL cholesterol levels can indicate the need for diet or diet and drug therapy. As shown in Table 12-5, individuals on a low fat diet who continue to have LDL cholesterol levels ≥190 mg/dL (≥4.9 mmol/L) on repeated measurement will benefit from drug intervention. If they have ≥2 CAD risk factors and continue to have LDL cholesterol levels of ≥160 mg/dL (≥4.1 mmol/L), they also would benefit from drug therapy. And, if they have already been diagnosed with heart disease, drug therapy should be considered when the LDL cholesterol level is ≥130 mg/dL (≥3.4 mmol/L). The average of at least two measurements, taken 1–8 weeks apart, should be used to determine treatment.[73]

Classic bile-acid sequestrant drug treatments, such as cholestyramine, work by sequestering cholesterol in the gut so that it is not absorbed and, until recently, were considered to be the only safe drugs for use in children.[101] Bile-acid sequestrants have uncomfortable adverse effects, however, such as bloating and constipation, and are poorly tolerated. The newest class of drugs includes the HMG-CoA reductase inhibitors lovastatin, simvastatin, pravastatin, fluvastatin, atorvastatin, and rosuvastatin. These drugs, known as statins, block intracellular cholesterol synthesis by inhibiting the enzyme HMG-CoA reductase. The major safety issues are myositis hepatotoxic effects; however, patient monitoring in clinical trials has shown that fewer than 2% of patients have sustained increases in liver enzymes. These drugs are effective in reducing LDL cholesterol 20–40% and are generally well tolerated.[97–100,102,115–117] Recent studies of statin therapy in children with familial hypercholesterolemia indicate that this therapy is also effective, well tolerated, and appears to be safe for them as well.[118–120] Niacin is also a potent drug for reducing LDL cholesterol and raising HDL cholesterol levels; however, it causes flushing and diarrhea in many patients and can be hepatotoxic and can aggravate glucose intolerance and hyperuricemia.[121] Other drugs include probucol, which prevents lipid oxidation and macrophage uptake,[122] and fibric acid derivatives, such as clofibrate, gemfibrozil, fenofibrate, and etiofibrate, which reduce triglyceride and VLDL cholesterol levels and increase HDL cholesterol.[113,121]

Hyperlipoproteinemia

Lipoproteins are complex transport vehicles for moving cholesterol, cholesteryl esters, and triglycerides in the blood. Disease states associated with abnormal serum lipids are generally caused by malfunctions in the synthesis, transport, or catabolism of lipoproteins.[110,121] Dyslipidemias can be subdivided into two major categories: *hyper*lipoproteinemias, which are diseases associated with elevated lipoprotein levels, and *hypo*lipoproteinemias, which are associated with decreased lipoprotein levels. The hyperlipoproteinemias can be subdivided into hypercholesterolemia, hypertriglyceridemia, and combined hyperlipidemia with elevations of both cholesterol and triglycerides.

Hypercholesterolemia

Hypercholesterolemia is the lipid abnormality most closely linked to heart disease.[65] One form of the disease, which is associated with genetic abnormalities that predispose affected individuals to elevated cholesterol levels, is called familial hypercholesterolemia (FH). Homozygotes for FH are fortunately rare (1:1,000,000 in the population), but can have total cholesterol concentrations as high as 800–1000 mg/dL (20–26 mmol/L). These patients frequently have their first heart attack when still in their teenage years.[123] Heterozygotes for the disease are seen much more frequently because the disease is caused by an autosomal codominant disorder. Heterozygotes tend to have total cholesterol concentrations in the range of 300–600 mg/dL (8–15 mmol/L) and, if not treated, become symptomatic for heart disease in their 20s–50s. Approximately 5% of patients younger than age 50 with CAD are FH heterozygotes. Other symptoms associated with FH include tendinous and tuberous xanthomas, which are cholesterol deposits under the skin, and arcus, which is cholesterol deposits in the cornea.[110]

In both homozygotes and heterozygotes, the cholesterol elevation is primarily associated with an increase in LDL cholesterol. These individuals synthesize intracellular cholesterol normally, but lack, or are deficient in, active LDL receptors. Consequently, cholesterol derived through absorption and incorporated into LDL builds up in the circulation because there are no receptors to bind the LDL and transfer the cholesterol into the cells. The cells, however, which require cholesterol for use in cell membrane and hormone production, synthesize cholesterol intracellularly at an increased rate to compensate for the lack of cholesterol from the receptor mediated mechanism.

In FH heterozygotes and other forms of hypercholesterolemia in which there is insufficient LDL receptor activity, reduction in the rate of internal cholesterol synthesis, through inhibition of HMG-CoA reductase activity by use of HMG-CoA reductase inhibitors (statins), stimulates the production of additional receptors, increasing cell internalization of cholesterol from LDL that, in turn, lowers the serum levels. Homozygotes, however, cannot significantly benefit from this type of therapy because they have no functional receptors to stimulate. Homozygotes rely primarily on a technique called *LDL pheresis*, a method similar to the dialysis treatment used for kidney patients, in which blood is periodically drawn from the patient, processed to remove LDL, and returned to the patient.[123,124]

Most individuals with elevated LDL cholesterol levels do not have FH, but are still at increased risk for premature CHD[56,65,69,73,101] and should be maintained on a low fat, low-cholesterol diet, with the caloric intake adjusted to attain or maintain ideal body weight.[56,125–127] Regular physical activity should also be incorporated, with drug therapy added when necessary (Table 12-5).

Hypertriglyceridemia

The NCEP Adult Treatment Panel has identified borderline high triglycerides as levels of 150–200 mg/dL (1.7–2.3 mmol/L), high as 200–500 mg/dL (2.3–5.6 mmol/L), and very high as >500 mg/dL (5.6 mmol/L).[73] *Hypertriglyceridemia* can derive from genetic abnormalities, called *familial hypertriglyceridemia,* or from secondary causes, such as hormonal abnormalities associated with the pancreas, adrenal glands, and pituitary or from diabetes mellitus or nephrosis. Diabetes mellitus leads to increased shunting of glucose into the pentose pathway, causing increased fatty acid synthesis. Nephrosis depresses the removal of large molecular weight constituents like triglycerides, causing increased serum levels. Hypertriglyceridemia is generally a result of an imbalance between synthesis and clearance of VLDL in the circulation.[128–131] In most studies, hypertriglyceridemia has not been statistically implicated as an independent risk factor for CHD, but many CHD patients have moderately elevated triglycerides in conjunction with decreased HDL cholesterol levels.[132,133] It is difficult to separate the risk associated with increased triglycerides from that of decreased HDL cholesterol because the two are linked and serum concentrations are usually inversely related.

Triglycerides are influenced by a number of hormones, such as pancreatic insulin and glucagon, pituitary growth hormone, adrenocorticotropic hormone (ACTH), and thyrotropin and adrenal medulla epinephrine and norepinephrine from the nervous system. Epinephrine and norepinephrine influence serum triglyceride levels by triggering production of hormone sensitive lipase, which is located in adipose tissue.[134] Other body processes that trigger hormone sensitive lipase activity are cell growth (growth hormone), adrenal stimulation (ACTH), thyroid stimulation (thyrotropin), and fasting (glucagon). Each process, through its action on hormone sensitive lipase, results in an increase in serum triglyceride values.

Although severe hypertriglyceridemia (>500 mg/dL [5.6 mmol/L]) is not associated with high risk for CHD, it is a potentially life-threatening abnormality because it can cause acute and recurrent *pancreatitis* (inflammation of the pancreas).[121,134,135] It is, therefore, imperative that these patients be diagnosed and treated with triglyceride-lowering medication and that they be closely monitored.

Severe hypertriglyceridemia is generally caused by a deficiency of LPL or by a deficiency in apolipoprotein C-II, which is a necessary cofactor for LPL activity.[136] Normally, LPL hydrolyzes triglycerides carried in chylomicrons and VLDL to provide cells with free fatty acids for energy from exogenous and endogenous triglyceride sources. A deficiency in LPL or apo C-II activity keeps chylomicrons from being cleared and serum triglycerides remain extremely elevated, even when the patient has fasted for 12–14 hours.

Treatment of hypertriglyceridemia consists of dietary modifications, fish oil, triglyceride-lowering drugs (primarily, fibric acid derivatives) in cases of severe hypertriglyceridemia or when an accompanying low HDL cholesterol value indicates risk of CHD and sometimes oils with specific fatty acid compositions.[137,138] It is possible that only certain subspecies of chylomicrons and VLDL are atherogenic. *Remnants* of chylomicrons and VLDL represent subspecies that have been partially hydrolyzed by lipases and are thought to be particularly atherogenic.[139–143] New methodology to isolate chylomicron and VLDL remnants now makes it possible to study the potential atherogenicity of these particles.[144–146]

Combined Hyperlipoproteinemia

Combined hyperlipoproteinemia is generally defined as the presence of elevated levels of serum total cholesterol and triglycerides. Individuals presenting with this syndrome are considered at increased risk for CHD. In the genetically derived form, called *familial combined hyperlipoproteinemia (FCH),* some individuals of affected kindred may have only elevated cholesterol; others, only elevated triglycerides; and yet others, elevations of both.

Another rare genetic form of combined hyperlipoproteinemia is called *familial dysbetalipoproteinemia,* or type III hyperlipoproteinemia. The name type III hyperlipoproteinemia is a holdover from a lipoprotein typing system developed by Fredrickson et al[147] that is otherwise generally no longer used. The disease results from an accumulation of cholesterol-rich VLDL and chylomicron remnants as a result of defective catabolism of those particles. The disease is also associated with the presence of a relatively rare form of apo E, called apo E2/2. Individuals with type III will frequently have total cholesterol values of 200–300 mg/dL (5–8 mmol/L) and triglycerides of 300–600 mg/dL (3–7 mmol/L). To distinguish them from other combined hyperlipoproteinemics, it is first necessary to isolate the VLDL fraction of their serum by ultracentrifugation. A ratio derived from the cholesterol concentration in VLDL to total serum triglycerides will be >0.30 in the presence of type III hyperlipoproteinemia. If the VLDL fraction is subjected to agarose electrophoresis, the particles will migrate in a broad β region, rather than in the normal pre-β region. Definitive diagnosis requires a determination of apo E isoforms by isoelectric focusing or DNA typing, resulting in either apo E2/2 homozygosity or, rarely, apo E deficiency. Treatment does not totally rely on a diagnosis, however, because these patients can be treated with a standard therapy of diet, niacin, gemfibrozil, and HMG-CoA reductase inhibitors, as the clinical lipoprotein results dictate. Because of the cholesterol-enriched composition of these particles, use of the Friedewald equation[148] to calculate LDL cholesterol levels will result in an underestimation of VLDL cholesterol and, therefore, an overestimation of LDL cholesterol, as compared with beta-quantification.[149,150]

Lp(a) Elevation

Elevations in the serum concentration of Lp(a) are currently thought to confer increased risk of CHD and CVD.[151–155] Higher Lp(a) levels have been observed in patients with CHD than in normal control subjects, although prospective studies have not conclusively determined the positive association.[156,157] Lp(a) are variants of LDL with an extra apolipoprotein, called apo (a); the size and serum concentrations of Lp(a) are genetically determined.[158] Because apo (a) has a high degree of homology with the coagulation factor, plasminogen,[159] the general atherogenic hypothesis involves competition between plasminogen and apo (a) for fibrin binding sites.[160–162] Under this hypothesis, successful competition by apo (a) will block plasminogen, forming clots along the arterial wall that will not be dissolved. Most LDL-lowering drugs have no effect on Lp(a) concentration, even when LDL cholesterol becomes significantly lowered. The two drugs shown to have some effect are niacin and replacement estrogen in postmenopausal women. Until prospective studies confirm Lp(a) atherogenicity, however, treatment with niacin is not advised except in conjunction with other dyslipidemic conditions in which niacin is also indicated.

Hypolipoproteinemia

Hypolipoproteinemias are abnormalities marked by decreased lipoprotein concentrations. There are two major categories: hypo*alpha*lipoproteinemia and hypo*beta*lipoproteinemia. Hypobetalipoproteinemia is associated with isolated low levels of LDL cholesterol (ie, without other accompanying lipoprotein disorders), but because it is not generally associated with CHD, it is not discussed further.

Hypoalphalipoproteinemia

Hypoalphalipoproteinemia indicates an isolated decrease in circulating HDL, currently defined by the NCEP as an HDL cholesterol concentration <40 mg/dL (1.0 mmol/L),[73]

CASE STUDY 12-3

A 43-year-old white man was diagnosed with hyper-lipidemia at age 13 years when his father died of a myocardial infarction at age 34 years. The man's grandfather had died at age 43 years, also of a myocar-dial infarction. Currently, the man is active and asymptomatic with regard to CHD. He is taking 40 mg of lovastatin (Mevacor), 2 times/day (maximum dose). He had previously taken niacin, but could not tolerate it because of flushing and gastrointestinal distress, nor could he tolerate cholestyramine resin (Questran). His physical exam is remarkable for bilateral Achilles ten-don thickening/xanthomas and a right carotid bruit.

Questions

1. What is his diagnosis?

2. Does he need further workup?

3. What other laboratory tests should be done?

4. Does he need further drug treatment? If so, what?

CASE STUDY TABLE 12-3.1. LABORATORY RESULTS

Triglycerides	91 mg/dL
Total cholesterol	269 mg/dL
HDL cholesterol	47 mg/dL
LDL cholesterol	204 mg/dL
Aspartate aminotransferase (AST)	34 U/L
Alanine aminotransferase (ALT)	36 U/L
Alkaline phosphatase (ACP)	53 U/L
Electrolytes and fasting glucose	normal

CASE STUDY 12-4

A 60-year-old woman came to her physician because she was having problems with urination. Her previ-ous history included hypertension and episodes of edema. The physician ordered various laboratory tests on blood drawn in his office. The results are shown in Case Study Table 12-4.1.

Questions

1. What are the abnormal results in this case?

2. Why do you think the triglycerides are abnormal?

3. What is the primary disease exhibited by this pa-tient's laboratory data?

CASE STUDY TABLE 12-4.1. LABORATORY RESULTS

ANALYTE	PATIENT VALUES	REFERENCE RANGE
Na^+	149	135–143 mEq/L
K^+	4.5	3.0–5.0 mEq/L
Cl^-	120	98–103 mEq/L
CO_2 content	12	22–27 mmol/L
Total protein	5.7	6.5–8.0 g/dL
Albumin	2.3	3.5–5.0 g/dL
Calcium	7.6	9.0–10.5 mg/dL
Cholesterol	201	140–200 mg/dL
Uric acid	15.4	3.5–7.9 mg/dL
Creatinine	4.5	0.5–1.2 mg/dL
BUN	87	7–25 mg/dL
Glucose	88	75–105 mg/dL
Total bilirubin	1.3	0.2–1.0 mg/dL
Triglycerides	327	65–157 mg/dL
Lactate dehydrogenase	200	90–190 IU/L
Aspartate transaminase	45	8–40 IU/L
Amylase	380	76–375 IU/L

without the presence of hypertriglyceridemia. The term *alpha* denotes the region in which HDL migrate on agarose electrophoresis. There are several defects, often genetically determined, that are associated with hypoalphalipoproteinemia.[163–168] Virtually all of these defects are associated with increased risk of premature CHD. An extreme form of hypoalphalipoproteinemia, *Tangier disease,* is associated with HDL cholesterol concentrations as low as 1–2 mg/dL (0.03–0.05 mmol/L) in homozygotes, accompanied by total cholesterol concentrations of 50–80 mg/dL (1.3–2.1 mmol/L).

Treatment of individuals with isolated decreases of HDL cholesterol is limited. Niacin is somewhat effective but has adverse effects, such as hepatotoxicity, that sometimes precludes its use, although newer, timed-release preparations may ameliorate those effects; estrogen replacement in postmenopausal women is also effective.[110,121,169,170]

Acute, transitory hypoalphalipoproteinemia can be seen in cases of severe physiologic stress, such as acute infections (primarily viral), other acute illnesses, and surgical procedures.[171] HDL cholesterol, as well as total cholesterol concentrations, can be significantly reduced under these conditions but will return to normal levels as recovery proceeds. For this reason, lipoprotein concentrations drawn during hospitalization or with a known disease state should be reassessed in the healthy, nonhospitalized state before intervention is considered.

LIPID AND LIPOPROTEIN ANALYSES

Lipid Measurement

Lipids and lipoproteins are important indicators of CHD risk, which is a major reason for their measurement in research as well as in clinical practice. For individual laboratories or diagnostic manufacturers to establish their own cut-points as is commonly done for other analytes is impractical with the lipids. Rather, decision cut-points used to characterize CHD risk have been developed by the NCEP based on consideration of population distributions from large epidemiologic studies, intervention studies that demonstrated the efficacy of treatment regimens and cost-effectiveness.[73] To improve the reliability of the analytic measurements, standardization programs were implemented for the research laboratories performing the population and intervention studies, which helped to make results comparable among laboratories and over time.[172] More recently, standardization programs have been extended to diagnostic manufacturers and routine clinical laboratories to facilitate reliable classification of patients using the national decision cut-points. Thus, accuracy and standardization of results is especially important with the lipid and lipoprotein analytes.

Cholesterol Measurement

The lipid work-up traditionally has begun with measurement of total serum cholesterol. The lipoproteins are also generally quantified based on their cholesterol content. Early analytic methods used strong acids (*eg,* sulfuric and acetic) sometimes together with other chemicals (*eg,* acetic anhydride or ferric chloride) to produce a measurable color with cholesterol.[173] Because the strong acid reactions are relatively nonspecific, partial or full extraction by organic solvents was sometimes used to improve specificity. The current reference method for cholesterol uses hexane extraction after hydrolysis with alcoholic KOH followed by reaction with Liebermann-Burchard color reagent, which comprises sulfuric and acetic acids and acetic anhydride.[174,175] This multistep manual method is complicated but gives good agreement with the gold standard method developed and applied at the U.S. National Institute for Standards and Technology, the so-called Definitive Method, using isotope dilution mass spectrometry.[176]

In recent years, enzymatic reagents have generally replaced strong acid chemistries. Enzymes, selected for specificity to the analyte of interest, provide reasonably accurate quantitation without the necessity for extraction or other pretreatment. Enzymic reagents are mild compared with the earlier acid reagents and better suited for the modern generation of automated microprocessor-controlled robotic instruments. The lipoproteins, HDL, and sometimes LDL, are generally quantified based on their cholesterol content using the same enzymatic reagents. Thus, measurements of total, LDL, and HDL cholesterol, together with triglycerides, can be completed routinely in panels on automated batch and discrete chemistry analyzers.

Although several enzymatic reaction sequences have been described, one sequence (Fig. 12-4) is most common for measuring cholesterol.[177–179] The enzyme cholesteryl ester hydrolase is used to cleave the fatty acid residue from the cholesteryl esters, which comprise about two thirds of circulating cholesterol, converting cholesteryl esters to unesterified or free cholesterol. The free cholesterol is reacted by the second enzyme, cholesterol oxidase, producing hydrogen peroxide, which is the substrate for a common enzymatic color reaction using horseradish peroxidase to couple two colorless chemicals into a colored compound. The intensity of the resulting color, proportional to the amount of cholesterol, can be measured by a spectrophotometer, usually at a wavelength around 500 nm. Enzymes and reagents have improved so that most appropriately calibrated commercial reagents can be expected to give reliable results. This reaction sequence is generally used on serum without an extraction step but can be subject to interference. For example, vitamin C and bilirubin are reducing agents that

1. Cholesteryl ester + H_2O $\xrightarrow{\text{Cholesteryl esterase}}$ Cholesterol + Fatty acid

2. Cholesterol + O_2 $\xrightarrow{\text{Cholesterol oxidase}}$ Cholestenone + H_2O_2

3. H_2O_2 + Dye $\xrightarrow{\text{Peroxidase}}$ Color

FIGURE 12-4. Enzymic assay sequence—cholesterol.

can interfere with the peroxidase-catalyzed color reaction.[180]

Triglyceride Measurement

Measurement of serum triglycerides in conjunction with cholesterol is useful in detecting certain genetic and other types of metabolic disorders, as well as in characterizing risk of developing coronary disease. The triglyceride value is also commonly used in the estimation of LDL cholesterol by the Friedewald equation. Several enzymatic reaction sequences are available for triglyceride measurement, all having the use of lipases to cleave fatty acids from glycerol.[181] The freed glycerol participates in any one of several enzymatic sequences. One of the more common earlier reactions, ending in a product measured in the ultraviolet (UV) region, used glycerol kinase and pyruvate kinase, culminating in the conversion of NADH to NAD$^+$ with an associated decrease in absorbance.[182] This reaction is susceptible to interference and side reactions. The UV end point is also less convenient for modern analyzers, so this and other UV sequences have gradually been replaced by a second sequence (Fig. 12-5) involving glycerol kinase and glycerol-phosphate oxidase, coupled to the same peroxidase color reaction described for cholesterol.[183]

The enzymatic triglyceride reaction sequences also react with any endogenous free glycerol, which is universally present in serum and constitutes a significant source of interference.[184,185] In most specimens, the endogenous free glycerol contributes to a 10–20 mg/dL overestimation of triglycerides. About 20% of specimens will have higher glycerol, with levels increased in certain conditions such as diabetes and liver disease or from glycerol-based medications. Most research laboratories incorporate a correction for endogenous free glycerol, but this

practice is uncommon in clinical laboratories. The most common correction, designated "double-cuvet blank," is accomplished with a second parallel measurement using the triglyceride reagent without the lipase enzyme to quantify only the free glycerol blank. The glycerol blank measurement is subtracted from the total glycerol measurement obtained with the complete reagent to determine a net or blank-corrected triglyceride result.[186] Another approach, designated "single-cuvet blank," begins with the lipase-free reagent. After a brief incubation, a blank reading is taken to measure only endogenous free glycerol. The lipase enzyme is then added as a second separate reagent and, after additional incubation, a final reading is taken that, after correcting for the blank by the instrument, gives a net or glycerol-blanked triglyceride value.[187] Commercial reagents with glycerol blanking are available, but their increased cost is not readily justified by the accuracy requirements in routine clinical practice. A convenient and easily implemented alternative that does not increase cost—designated calibration blanking—can be done by simply adjusting the calibrator set points to net or blank corrected values, compensating for the average free glycerol content of specimens. This approach, employed by some diagnostic reagent companies, is usually reasonably accurate because free glycerol levels are generally relatively low and fairly consistent in most specimens. Most specimens will be blank-corrected reasonably well and only a few specimens will be under corrected but still better than without the calibration adjustment.

The triglyceride reference method involves alkaline hydrolysis, solvent extraction, and a color reaction with chromotropic acid,[188] an assay that is tedious, poorly characterized, and only applied in the lipid standardization laboratory at the Centers for Disease Control and Prevention (CDC). A more suitable designated compari-

1. Triglyceride + H_2O $\xrightarrow{\text{Bacterial lipase}}$ Fatty acid + Glycerol

2. Glycerol + ATP $\xrightarrow{\text{Glycerokinase}}$ Glycerophosphate + ADP

3. Glycerophosphate + O_2 $\xrightarrow{\text{Glycerophosphate oxidase}}$ Dihydroxyacetone + H_2O_2

4. H_2O_2 + Dye $\xrightarrow{\text{Peroxidase}}$ Color

FIGURE 12-5. Enzymic assay sequence—triglycerides.

son method with solvent extraction followed by an optimized enzymatic assay has been developed and recently adopted by a few standardization laboratories.

However, note that accuracy in triglyceride measurements for clinical purposes might be considered less relevant than that for cholesterol because the physiologic variation is so large, with coefficient of variation (CV) in the range of 25–30%, making the contribution of analytic variation relatively insignificant.

Lipoprotein Methods

Various methods have been used for the separation and quantitation of the serum lipoproteins, taking advantage of physical properties such as density, size, charge, and apolipoprotein content. The range in density observed among the lipoprotein classes is a function of the relative lipid and protein content and enables fractionation by ultracentrifugation. Electrophoretic separations take advantage of differences in charge and size. Chemical precipitation methods, which are most common in clinical laboratories, depend on particle size, charge, and differences in the apolipoprotein content. Antibodies specific to apolipoproteins can be used to bind and separate lipoprotein classes. Chromatographic methods take advantage of size differences in molecular sieving methods or composition in affinity methods using, for example, heparin sepharose.

Many ultracentrifugation methods have been used in the research laboratory, but ultracentrifugation is uncommon in the clinical laboratory.[189] The most common approach, called *preparative ultracentrifugation,* uses sequential density adjustments of serum to fractionate major and minor lipoprotein classes.[190] Density gradient methods, either nonequilibrium techniques in which separations are based on the rate of flotation, or equilibrium techniques in which the lipoproteins separate based on their density, permit fractionation of several or all classes in a single run.[191–195] The available methods use different types of ultracentrifuge rotors: swinging bucket, fixed angle, vertical, and zonal. Newer methods have trended toward smaller scale separations in small rotors using tabletop ultracentrifuges.[196,197] Ultracentrifugation, although tedious, expensive, and technically demanding, remains a workhorse for separation of lipoproteins for quantitative purposes and preparative isolations. Ultracentrifugation is also used in the reference methods for lipoprotein quantitation, which is appropriate because the lipoproteins are classically defined in terms of hydrated density.

Electrophoretic methods allow separation and quantitation of major lipoprotein classes and provide a visual display useful in detecting unusual or variant patterns.[198,199] Agarose gel has been the most common medium for separation of intact lipoproteins, providing a clear background and convenient use.[200–203] Electrophoretic methods, in general, have been considered useful for qualitative analysis but less than desirable for lipoprotein quantitation because of poor precision and large systematic biases compared with other methods.[204] Evaluations of newer commercial automated electrophoretic systems, however, demonstrate that electrophoresis can be precise and accurate.[205]

Electrophoresis in polyacrylamide gels is used for separation of lipoprotein classes,[206] subclasses, and the apolipoproteins.[207,208] Of particular interest are methods that fractionate LDL subclasses to characterize the more atherogenic, heavier, lipid depleted, and smaller fractions versus the larger, lighter subclasses.[209]

Chemical precipitation, usually with polyanions, such as heparin, and divalent cations, such as manganese, can be used to separate the lipoproteins, but are most common for HDL.[210–212] Apo B in VLDL and LDL is rich in positively charged amino acids, which preferentially form complexes with polyanions. Addition of divalent cations neutralizes the charged groups on the lipoproteins, making them aggregate and become insoluble, resulting in their precipitation leaving HDL in solution. At appropriate concentrations of polyanion and divalent cation, the separation is reasonably specific.

Immunochemical methods, using antibodies specific to epitopes on the apolipoproteins, have been useful in both research and routine methods.[213,214] Antibodies have been immobilized on solid supports, such as a column matrix or latex beads. For example, the apo B–containing lipoproteins as a group can be bound by antibodies to apo B. Selectivity within the apo B–containing lipoproteins, such as removing VLDL while retaining LDL, can be obtained by including antibodies to minor apolipoproteins. HDL can be selectively bound using antibodies to apo A-I, the major protein of HDL. As an example, immobilized monoclonal antibodies have been used to separate a fraction of remnant lipoproteins designated RLP (remnant-like particles).[144–146]

HDL Methods

The measurement of HDL cholesterol has assumed progressively greater importance in the NCEP ATP III treatment guidelines, released in 2001. In the earliest guidelines, HDL cholesterol was measured as a risk factor but otherwise was not considered in treatment decisions. Following recommendations of a National Institutes of Health–sponsored consensus panel,[96] the 1993 NCEP ATP II guidelines included HDL cholesterol measurement with total cholesterol in the first medical workup, which was reinforced by the 2001 ATP III guidelines.[73] Because the risk associated with HDL cholesterol is expressed over a relatively small concentration range, accuracy in the measurement is especially important.

CASE STUDY 12-5

A 49-year-old woman was referred for a lipid evaluation by her dermatologist after developing a papular rash over her trunk and arms. The rash consisted of multiple, red, raised lesions with yellow centers. She had no previous history of such a rash and no family history of lipid disorders or CHD. She is postmenopausal, on standard estrogen replacement therapy, and otherwise healthy.

CASE STUDY TABLE 12-5.1. LABORATORY RESULTS

SERUM	GROSSLY LIPEMIC
Triglycerides	6200 mg/dL
Total cholesterol	458 mg/dL
Fasting glucose	160 mg/dL
Liver function tests and electrolytes	normal

Questions

1. What is the rash? What is the cause of her rash?

2. Is her oral estrogen contributing?

3. Is her glucose contributing?

4. What treatments are warranted and what is her most acute risk?

For routine diagnostic purposes, HDL has been separated almost exclusively by chemical precipitation and, for many years, HDL cholesterol measurement has required a two-step procedure with manual pretreatment. A precipitation reagent added to serum or plasma aggregates non-HDL lipoproteins, which are sedimented by centrifugation. Early methods used centrifugation forces of approximately 1500 × gravity, requiring lengthy centrifugation times of 10–30 minutes. Newer methods went to higher-speed centrifugation with forces of 10,000–15,000 × gravity, decreasing centrifugation times to 3 minutes. HDL is then quantified as cholesterol in the supernate usually by one of the enzymatic assays modified for the lower HDL cholesterol range.

The earliest common precipitation method used heparin in combination with manganese to precipitate the apo B–containing lipoproteins.[215–218] Because manganese interfered with enzymatic assays, alternative reagents were developed.[219] Sodium phosphotungstate[220,221] with magnesium became common in routine use but, because of its sensitivity to reaction conditions and greater variability, was largely replaced by dextran sulfate (a synthetic heparin) with magnesium.[222] The earliest dextran sulfate methods used material of 500 kD, which was replaced by a 50 kD material, considered more specific.[212] Polyethylene glycol also precipitates lipoproteins, but requires 100-fold higher reagent concentrations with highly viscous reagents, difficult to pipet precisely.[223–225] Numerous commercial versions of these precipitation reagents became available but often gave quite different results in the early years as a result of a lack of standardization. However, with a standardization process available to reagent manufacturers for certification of accuracy, differences have tended to decrease.

A significant problem with HDL precipitation methods is interference from elevated triglyceride levels.[226] When triglyceride-rich VLDL and chylomicrons are present, the low density of the aggregated lipoproteins may prevent them from sedimenting or may even cause floating during centrifugation. This incomplete sedimentation, indicated by cloudiness, turbidity, or particulate matter floating in the supernate, results in overestimation of HDL cholesterol. High-speed centrifugation will reduce the proportion of turbid supernates. Predilution of the specimen also promotes clearing but may lead to errors in the cholesterol analysis. Turbid supernates may also be cleared by ultrafiltration, a method that is reliable but tedious and inefficient. Because of these drawbacks and the lack of full automation, precipitation methods became increasingly out of step with the modern automated clinical laboratory.

The result has been development of a new class of direct, sometimes termed *homogeneous,* methods, which streamline the HDL quantification. Specific polymers, detergents, and even modified enzymes are used to suppress the enzymatic cholesterol reaction in lipoproteins other than HDL.[227] The reagents are capable of full automation with most chemistry analyzers and are well suited to the modern laboratory. In general, a first reagent is added to "block" non-HDL lipoproteins, followed by a second reagent with the enzymes to quantify the accessible (HDL) cholesterol. Homogeneous assays, which appear to be highly precise and reasonably accurate, were rapidly adopted and generally replaced pretreatment methods in the routine laboratory.[228] However, the methods have been shown to lack specificity for HDL in unusual specimens, for example, from patients with liver or kidney conditions.[229] Also, the reagents have been subject to frequent modifications by the manufacturers in an effort to improve performance, which can affect results in long-term studies. For these reasons, the methods have not been recommended for use in research laboratories.

The accepted reference method for HDL cholesterol is a three-step procedure developed at the CDC. This method involves ultracentrifugation to remove VLDL, heparin manganese precipitation from the 1.006 g/mL infranate to remove LDL, and analysis of supernatant cholesterol by the Abell-Kendall assay.[175] Because this method is tedious and expensive, a simpler, direct precipitation method has been validated by the CDC Network Laboratory Group as a designated comparison method, using direct dextran sulfate (50 kD) precipitation of serum with Abell-Kendall cholesterol analysis.[172]

LDL Methods

LDL cholesterol, well validated as a treatable risk factor for CHD, is the primary basis for treatment decisions in the NCEP clinical guidelines.[73] The most common research method for LDL cholesterol quantitation and the basis for the reference method has been designated *beta-quantification*, in which beta refers to the electrophoretic term for LDL. Beta-quantification combines ultracentrifugation and chemical precipitation.[218,230] Ultracentrifugation of serum at the native density of 1.006 g/L is used to float VLDL and any chylomicrons for separation. The fractions are recovered by pipetting after separating the fractions by slicing the tube. Ultracentrifugation has been preferred for VLDL separation because other methods, such as precipitation, are not as specific for VLDL and may be subject to interference from chylomicrons. In general, ultracentrifugation is a robust but tedious technique that can give reliable results provided the technique is meticulous.

In a separate step, chemical precipitation is used to separate HDL from either the whole serum or the infranate obtained from ultracentrifugation. Cholesterol is quantified in serum, in the 1.006 g/mL infranate, and in the HDL supernate by enzymatic or other assay methods. LDL cholesterol is calculated as the difference between cholesterol measured in the infranate and in the HDL fraction. VLDL cholesterol is usually calculated as the difference between that in whole serum and the amount in the infranate fraction. The requirement for the need of an ultracentrifuge has generally limited beta-quantification to lipid specialty laboratories. Beta-quantification is also the basis for the accepted reference method for LDL. The

method is the same as that described for HDL above with the measured HDL cholesterol subtracted from that in the bottom fraction to obtain LDL cholesterol.

A more common approach that bypasses ultracentrifugation, which is used in both routine and research laboratories, is the *Friedewald calculation,* or *derived beta-quantification.*[148] HDL cholesterol is quantified either after precipitation or using one of the direct methods, and total cholesterol and triglycerides are measured in the serum. VLDL cholesterol is estimated as triglycerides divided by 5 (when using mg/dL units), an approximation that works reasonably well in most normolipemic specimens. The presence of elevated triglycerides (400 mg/dL is the accepted limit), chylomicrons, and β-VLDL characteristic of the rare type III hyperlipoproteinemia preclude this estimation. The estimated VLDL cholesterol and measured HDL cholesterol are subtracted from total serum cholesterol to estimate or derive LDL cholesterol.

LDL = Total Cholesterol − LDL − Trig/5. This method, commonly referred to as a lipid panel and used almost universally in estimating LDL cholesterol in routine clinical practice, has been recommended by the NCEP ATP III guidelines. Investigations in lipid specialty laboratories have suggested the method is reliable for patient classification, provided the underlying measurements are made with appropriate accuracy and precision.[231,232] There has been concern about the reliability in routine laboratories, however, because the error in calculating LDL cholesterol combines the error in the underlying measurements: total cholesterol, triglycerides, and HDL cholesterol. The NCEP laboratory expert panel reviewed performance data and concluded that the level of analytic performance required to derive LDL cholesterol accurately enough to meet clinical needs was beyond the capability of most routine laboratories. To meet the requisite NCEP precision goal of 4% CV for LDL cholesterol (Table 12-6), a laboratory would be required to achieve half the NCEP goals for each of the underlying measurements. The NCEP panel concluded that better methods are needed for routine diagnostic use, preferably methods that directly separate LDL for cholesterol quantitation.[71]

In response to the NCEP request, direct LDL cholesterol methods have been developed or refined for general use, which are similar to the homogeneous assays for HDL cholesterol.[230,233] Besides achieving full automation of the challenging LDL cholesterol separation, these assays have the potential to streamline the measurement while improving precision. However, separating LDL with adequate specificity from other lipoproteins in this manner is more challenging even than that for HDL, and the few evaluations of the direct methods have not been encouraging.[234] More experience will be required, especially with specimens of unusual composition, to judge the adequacy of the homogeneous separations.[235]

Compact Analyzers

The common lipids and lipoproteins can be measured with compact analysis systems designed for use in point-of-care testing at the patient's bedside, in the physician's office, in wellness centers, and even in the home.[236] The earliest systems, introduced in the 1980s, were relatively large and measured cholesterol and triglycerides as well as other common analytes, usually separately and sequentially. HDL separations involving offline pretreatment steps were subsequently developed. Subsequent systems became smaller and more sophisticated, offering integrated separation of HDL and analysis of cholesterol and triglycerides simultaneously from fingerstick blood. Now one system can measure cholesterol, triglycerides, HDL cholesterol, and glucose simultaneously from a fingerstick sample. Noninstrumented systems are also available for total cholesterol. These new technologies offer the capability of measuring lipids and lipoproteins with reasonable reliability outside the conventional laboratory.

Apolipoprotein Methods

Lipids by nature tend to be insoluble in the aqueous environment of the circulation; hence, the lipoproteins include various protein constituents, designated apolipoproteins, which enhance solubility as well as play other functional roles (Table 12-2). Apolipoproteins are commonly measured in research, and some specialty laboratories supporting cardiovascular practices or clinical studies measure them routinely in addition to the lipoproteins. For clinical diagnostic purposes, three apolipoproteins in particular have been of interest. Apo B, the major protein of LDL and VLDL, is an indicator of combined LDL and VLDL concentration that can be measured directly in serum by immunoassay.[237] Some researchers have suggested apo B as an alternative to the separation and measurement of LDL cholesterol.[238] Apo A-I, as the major protein of HDL, could be measured directly in serum in place of separation and analysis of HDL cholesterol; however, because quantification in terms of cholesterol content is more common, the latter practice has prevailed. Lp(a), the variant of LDL, shown to be an independent indicator of CHD risk, is sometimes determined in managing patients. Measurement of these three apolipoprotein can be useful in patient management by skilled practitioners, but they have not yet been accepted or recommended in any of the consensus guidelines for use in routine practice. Results from prospective studies have been inconsistent in demonstrating them to be independent predictors of CHD risk.

Lp(a) has pre-β mobility on agarose electrophoresis and can be quantified by this technique. However, the apolipoproteins are commonly measured by immunoassays of various types, with several commercial kit methods available.[237] Most common in routine laboratories are turbidimetric assays for chemistry analyzers or nephelometric assays for dedicated nephelometers. Especially for apo B and Lp(a), these light-scattering assays may be subject to interference from the larger triglyceride-rich lipoproteins (chylomicrons) and VLDL. Enzyme-linked immunosorbent assay (ELISA), radial immunodiffusion (RID), and radioimmunoassay (RIA) methods have also been available, but the latter two methods are becoming less common. Antibodies used in the immunoassays may be polyclonal or monoclonal. International efforts to develop reference materials and standardization programs for the assays are in progress. Because Lp(a) is genetically heterogeneous and the levels and CHD risk correlate with the isoform size, qualitative assessment of isoform distribution may also be important.[158]

Phospholipid Measurement

Quantitative measurement of phospholipids is rare in routine clinical practice. Phospholipids are sometimes measured in research (*eg*, in studies of dietary influences). The choline-containing phospholipids lecithin, lysolecithin, and sphingomyelin, which account for at least 95% of total phospholipids in serum, can be measured by an enzymic reaction sequence using phospholipase D, choline-oxidase, and horseradish peroxidase.[239,240] Kit methods with this enzymic sequence are available commercially. Before the availability of enzymic reagents, the common quantitative method involved extraction and acid digestion with analysis of the total lipid-bound phosphorus.[241]

Certain choline-containing phospholipids and, in some applications, their ratios, have been determined in the clinical laboratory. For example, fetal lung maturity has been evaluated from characteristic patterns of phospholipids in amniotic fluid. In this instance, phospholipids may be recovered by solvent extraction, applied to a silica gel plate for separation by thin-layer chromatography, and quantified after visualization by treating with iodine vapor. The ratio of lecithin to sphingomyelin has been used to predict fetal lung maturity.

Fatty Acid Measurement

Although studies suggest that fatty acids have potential in assessing CHD risk, analysis is primarily used in research laboratories for studies of diet.[82] Less common is their measurement in the diagnosis of rare genetic conditions. Fatty acids are commonly analyzed by gas-liquid chromatography, after extraction, alkaline hydrolysis, and conversion to methyl esters of diazomethane. A reference standard typically contains laurate, myristate, palmitate, palmitoleate, phytanate, stearate, oleate, linoleate, arachidate, and arachidonate.[242]

CASE STUDY 12-6

Three patients are seen in clinic:

- Patient one is a 40-year-old man with hypertension, who also smokes, but has not been previously diagnosed with CHD. His father developed CHD at age 53 years. He is fasting, and the results of his lipids include a total cholesterol concentration of 210 mg/dL, triglycerides of 150 mg/dL, and an HDL cholesterol value of 45 mg/dL. He has a fasting glucose level of 98 mg/dL.
- Patient two is a 60-year-old woman with no family history of CHD, who is normotensive and does not smoke, with a total cholesterol concentration of 220 mg/dL, triglycerides of 85 mg/dL, and an HDL cholesterol value of 80 mg/dL. Her fasting glucose level is 85 mg/dL.
- Patient three is a 49-year-old man with no personal or family history of CHD, and who is not hypertensive and does not smoke. His fasting total cholesterol level is 260 mg/dL, his triglycerides are 505 mg/dL, his HDL cholesterol is 25 mg/dL, and his glucose level is 134 mg/dL.

Questions

For each patient seen in clinic:

1. What is the LDL cholesterol level, as calculated using the Friedewald calculation?

2. Which patient, if any, should have their LDL cholesterol measured, rather than calculated? Why?

3. How many known CHD risk factors does each patient have?

4. Based on what is known, are these patients recommended for lipid therapy (diet or drug) and, if so, on what basis?

STANDARDIZATION OF LIPID AND LIPOPROTEIN ASSAYS

Precision

Precision is a prerequisite for accuracy; a method may have no overall systematic error or bias; however, if it is imprecise, it will still be inaccurate on individual measurements. With the shift to modern automated analyzers, analytic variation has generally become less of a concern than biologic and other sources of preanalytic variation. Cholesterol levels are affected by many factors that can be categorized into biologic, clinical, and sampling sources.[243,244] Changes in lifestyle that affect usual diet, exercise, weight, and smoking patterns can result in fluctuations in the observed cholesterol and triglyceride values and the distribution of the lipoproteins. Similarly, the presence of clinical conditions, various diseases, or the medications used in their treatment, affect the circulating lipoproteins. Conditions during blood collection, such as fasting status, posture, the choice of anticoagulant in the collection tube, and storage conditions, can alter the measurements. Typical observed biologic variation for more than 1 year for total cholesterol averages approximately 6.1% CV. In the average patient, measurements made over the course of a year would fall 66% of the time within ±6.1% of the mean cholesterol concentration and 95% of the time within twice this range.

Some patients may exhibit substantially more biologic variation. Thus, preanalytic variation generally is relatively large in relation to the usual analytic variation, which is typically less than 3% CV, and must be considered in interpreting cholesterol results. Some factors, such as posture and blood collection, can be standardized to minimize the variation. The NCEP guidelines recommend averaging at least two successive measurements to reduce the effects of both preanalytic and analytic sources.[73] The use of stepped cut-points also reduces the practical effect of variation.

Accuracy

Accuracy or trueness is assured by demonstrating traceability or agreement through calibration to the respective reference method. With cholesterol, the reference system is advanced and complete, having served as a model for standardization of other laboratory analytes.[172,177] The definitive method at the National Institute for Standards and Technology provides the ultimate accuracy target but is too expensive and complicated for frequent use.[176] The reference method developed and applied at the CDC, and calibrated by an approved primary reference standard to the definitive method, provides a transferable, practical reference link.[175] The reference method has been made conveniently accessible through a network of standardized laboratories, the Cholesterol Reference Method Laboratory Network. This network was established in the United States and some of the European and Asian countries to extend standardization to manufacturers and clinical laboratories.[172] The network provides accuracy comparisons using fresh native serum specimens, necessary for reliable accuracy transfer because of analyte–matrix interaction problems on processed reference materials.[245–247]

Matrix Interactions

In the early stages of cholesterol standardization, which were directed toward diagnostic manufacturers and routine laboratories, commercial lyophilized or freeze-dried materials were used. These materials, made in large quantities, often with spiking or artificial addition of analytes, were assayed by the definitive and/or reference methods and distributed widely for accuracy transfer. Subsequently, biases were observed in enzymic assays on fresh patient specimens. Although such manufactured reference materials are convenient, stable, and amenable to shipment at ambient temperatures, the manufacturing process, especially spiking and lyophilization, altered the measurement properties in enzymic assays such that results were not representative of those on patient specimens. To achieve reliable feedback on accuracy and facilitate transfer of the accuracy base, direct comparisons with the reference methods on actual patient specimens were determined to be necessary.[172]

CDC Cholesterol Reference Method Laboratory Network

In response, the CDC cholesterol network program was organized. (Information available at: http://www.cdc.gov/nceh/dls/crmln/crmln.htm) The network offers formal certification programs for total, HDL and LDL cholesterol, whereby laboratories and manufacturers can document traceability to the national reference systems.[172] Through this program, clinical laboratories are able to identify certified commercial methods. Certification does not ensure all aspects of quality in a reagent system but primarily ensures that the accuracy is traceable to reference methods within accepted limits and that precision can meet the NCEP targets. The certification process is somewhat tedious and, thus, most efficient through manufacturers, but individual laboratories desiring to confirm the performance of their systems can complete a scaled-down certification protocol for cholesterol.

Analytic Performance Goals

The NCEP laboratory panels have established requisite analytic performance goals based on clinical needs for routine measurements (Table 12-6).[70–72,177] For analysis

of total cholesterol, the performance goal for total error is 8.9%. That is, the overall error should be such that each individual cholesterol measurement falls within ±8.9% of the Reference Method value. Actually, because the goals are based on 95% certainty, 95 of 100 measurements should fall within the total error limit. One can assay a specimen many times and calculate the mean to determine the usual value or the central tendency. The scatter or random variation around the mean is described by the standard deviation, an interval around the mean that includes, by definition, two thirds of the observations. In the laboratory, because the scatter or imprecision is often proportional to the concentration, random variation is usually specified in relative terms as CV, the coefficient of variation or relative standard deviation, calculated as the standard deviation divided by the mean. Overall accuracy or systematic error is described as bias or trueness, the difference between the mean and the true value. Bias is primarily a function of the method's calibration and may vary by concentration. Of greatest concern in this context is bias at the NCEP decision cut-points. The bias and CV targets presented in Table 12-6 are representative of performance that will meet the NCEP goals for total error.

Quality Control

Achieving acceptable analytic performance requires the use of reliable quality control materials, which should preferably closely emulate actual patient specimens. Currently, the best materials are prepared from freshly collected patient serum, aliquoted into securely sealed vials, quick frozen, and stored at −70°C. Such pools of fresh, frozen serum are less subject to matrix interactions than the usual commercial materials, most important in monitoring accuracy in lipoprotein separation and analysis, and preferable for monitoring cholesterol and other lipid measurements. At least two pools should be analyzed, preferably with levels at or near decision points for each analyte.

Specimen Collection

Serum, usually collected in serum separator vacuum tubes with clotting enhancers, has been the fluid of choice for lipoprotein measurement in the routine clinical laboratory. Ethylenediaminetetraacetic acid (EDTA) plasma was the traditional choice in lipid research laboratories, especially for lipoprotein separations, because the anticoagulant enhances stability by chelating metal ions. EDTA has potential disadvantages that discourage routine use. Microclots, which form in plasma during storage, plug the sampling probes on the modern chemistry analyzers. EDTA osmotically draws water from red cells, diluting the plasma constituents, and the dilution effect can vary depending on such factors as fill volume, the analyte being measured, and the extent of mixing. Because the NCEP cut-points are based on serum values, cholesterol measurements made on EDTA plasma require correction by the factor of 1.03.

SUMMARY

Lipoproteins are complex particles that interact with many other metabolic pathways of the body. Their homeostasis can be affected by imbalances of other pathways, such as hormone imbalances and diabetes and, likewise, abnormal lipoprotein metabolism can disrupt the body's system and cause disease, as seen in pancreatitis and coronary disease. Some aspects of lipoprotein balance are genetically determined (*ie*, gender, enzyme, or receptor defects), whereas others can be controlled through diet, decreased smoking, exercise, and the monitoring of blood pressure. Precise and accurate measurements of lipid and lipoproteins are essential for the proper diagnosis and treatment of dyslipidemias. Finally, public health measures to educate the population on risk factors is important in the prevention of diseases that develop as a consequence of dyslipidemia, such as coronary artery disease.

REVIEW QUESTIONS

1. Which of the following methods for lipoprotein electrophoresis depend on charge *and* molecular size?
   a. Paper
   b. Polyacrylamide gel
   c. Cellulose acetate
   d. Agarose

2. Which of the following statements concerning chylomicrons is FALSE?
   a. This lipoprotein is produced in the intestinal mucosa.
   b. The primary function is to carry dietary (exogenous) lipids to the liver.
   c. The major lipid transported by this lipoprotein is cholesterol.
   d. It remains at the origin (point of application) during lipoprotein electrophoresis.

3. The lipoprotein that contains the greatest amount of protein is called:
   a. chylomicrons.
   b. VLDL.
   c. HDL.
   d. LDL.

4. Pre-β (VLDL) lipoproteins migrate further toward the anode on polyacrylamide gel than they do on cellulose acetate or agarose.
   a. True
   b. False

5. Several enzymatic triglycerides methods measure the production or consumption of:
   a. fatty acids.
   b. glycerol.
   c. diacetyl lutidine.
   d. NADH.

6. The most likely cause for serum/plasma to appear "milky" is the presence of:
   a. VLDL.
   b. LDL.
   c. HDL.
   d. chylomicrons.

7. In the colorimetric determination of cholesterol, using the enzyme cholesterol oxidase, the agent that oxidizes the colorless organic compound 4-aminoantipyrine to a pink complex is:
   a. cholest-4-ene-3-one.
   b. NAD.
   c. hydrogen peroxide.
   d. phenol.

8. Which lipoprotein is the major carrier of cholesterol *to* peripheral tissue?
   a. Chylomicrons
   b. VLDL
   c. LDL
   d. HDL

9. Increased levels of apolipoprotein A-I are associated with increased risk of coronary artery disease.
   a. True
   b. False

10-11. A patient is admitted to the hospital with intense chest pains. The patient's primary care physician requests the emergency department doctor to order several tests, including a lipid profile with cholesterol fractionation. Given the patient's results provided below, answer the next two questions.

   Total cholesterol = 400 mg/dL; Triglycerides = 300 mg/dL; HDL cholesterol = 100 mg/dL; LP electrophoresis, pending

10. The LDL cholesterol for this patient, given the above results, would be:
    a. 160 mg/dL.
    b. 200 mg/dL.
    c. 240 mg/dL.
    d. 300 mg/dL.

11. This patient's LDL cholesterol is:
    a. optimal.
    b. desirable.
    c. borderline.
    d. high.

12. As part of a lipoprotein phenotyping, it is necessary to perform total cholesterol and triglyceride determinations, as well as lipoprotein electrophoresis. The test results obtained from such studies were:

    • triglyceride, 340 mg/dL (reference range, <150 mg/dL).
    • total cholesterol, 180 mg/dL (reference range, <200 mg/dL).
    • pre-β-lipoprotein fraction increased.
    • β-lipoprotein fraction normal.
    • no chylomicrons present.
    • serum appearance turbid.

    The best explanation for these results would be that the patient exhibits a phenotype indicative of:
    a. type I hyperlipoproteinemia.
    b. type II hyperlipoproteinemia.
    c. type III hyperlipoproteinemia.
    d. type IV hyperlipoproteinemia.
    e. type V hyperlipoproteinemia.

13. Which of the following results are the most consistent with high risk for coronary heart disease?
    a. 20 mg/dL HDL cholesterol and 250 mg/dL total cholesterol
    b. 35 mg/dL HDL cholesterol and 200 mg/dL total cholesterol
    c. 50 mg/dL HDL cholesterol and 190 mg/dL total cholesterol
    d. 55 mg/dL HDL cholesterol and 180 mg/dL total cholesterol
    e. 60 mg/dL HDL cholesterol and 170 mg/dL total cholesterol

14. What is the presumed defect in most cases of familial type IIa hyperlipoproteinemia?
    a. Deficiency of hydroxymethylglutaryl (HMG)-CoA reductase
    b. Deficiency of cholesterol esterase
    c. Deficiency of lipoprotein lipase
    d. Defective receptors for LDL
    e. Defective esterifying enzymes LCAT and ACAT

15. Hyperchylomicronemia (type I) in childhood has been associated with which of the following:
    1. A deficiency of apolipoprotein CII?
    2. A deficiency of LCAT?
    3. A deficiency of lipoprotein lipase?
    4. A deficiency of apolipoprotein Al?
       a. 1 and 3
       b. 3 and 4
       c. 1, 3 and 4
       d. 1, 2 and 4
       e. 2 only

REFERENCES

1. Laposata M. Fatty acids. Biochemistry to clinical significance. Am J Clin Pathol 1995;104:172.
2. Kritchevsky D. Effects of triglyceride structure on lipid metabolism. Nutr Rev 1988;46:177.
3. Ridgway ND, Byers DM, Cook HW, Storey MK. Integration of phospholipid and sterol metabolism in mammalian cells. Prog Lipid Res 1999;38:337.
4. Alb JG Jr, Kearns MA, Bankaitis VA. Phospholipid metabolism and membrane dynamics. Curr Opin Cell Biol 1996;8:534
5. Kent C. Eukaryotic phospholipid biosynthesis. Annu Rev Biochem 1995;64:315.
6. Nwokoro NA, Wassif CA, Porter FD. Genetic disorders of cholesterol biosynthesis in mice and humans. Mol Genet Metab 2001; 74:105.
7. Libby P, Aikawa M, Schonbeck U. Cholesterol and atherosclerosis. Biochim Biophys Acta 2000;1529:299.
8. Barenholz Y. Cholesterol and other membrane active sterols: from membrane evolution to "rafts." Prog Lipid Res 2002;41:1.
9. Pauciullo P. Lipoprotein transport and metabolism: a brief update. Nutr Metab Cardiovasc Dis 2002;12:90.
10. Mahley RW, Innerarity TL, Rall SC Jr, Weisgraber KH. Plasma lipoproteins: apolipoprotein structure and function. J Lipid Res 1984;25:1277.
11. Hevonoja T, Pentikainen MO, Hyvonen MT, et al. Structure of low density lipoprotein (LDL) particles: basis for understanding molecular changes in modified LDL. Biochim Biophys Acta 2000;1488:189.
12. Jackson RL, Morrisett JD, Gotto AM Jr. Lipoprotein structure and metabolism. Physiol Rev 1976;56:259.
13. Li WH, Tanimura M, Luo CC, et al. The apolipoprotein multigene family: biosynthesis, structure, structure-function relationships, and evolution. J Lipid Res 1988;29:245.
14. Anantharamaiah GM, Brouillette CG, Engler JA, et al. Role of amphipathic helixes in HDL structure/function. Adv Exp Med Biol 1991;285:131.
15. Segrest JP, Li L, Anantharamaiah GM, et al. Structure and function of apolipoprotein A-I and high-density lipoprotein. Curr Opin Lipidol 2000;11:105.
16. Burnett JR, Barrett PH. Apolipoprotein B metabolism: tracer kinetics, models, and metabolic studies. Crit Rev Clin Lab Sci 2002;39:89.

17. Javitt NB. Cholesterol homeostasis: role of the LDL receptor. FASEB J 1995;9:1378.

18. Marcovina SM, Morrisett JD. Structure and metabolism of lipoprotein (a). Curr Opin Lipidol 1995;6:136.

19. Cooper AD. Hepatic uptake of chylomicron remnants. J Lipid Res 1997;38:2173.

20. Mahley RW. Apolipoprotein E: cholesterol transport protein with expanding role in cell biology. Science 1988;240:622.

21. Walden CC, Hegele RA. Apolipoprotein E in hyperlipidemia. Ann Intern Med 1994;120:1026.

22. Corder EH, Lannfelt L, Bogdanovic N, et al. The role of APOE polymorphisms in late-onset dementias. Cell Mol Life Sci 1998; 54:928.

23. Harris WS. Chylomicron metabolism and omega 3 and omega 6 fatty acids. World Rev Nutr Diet 1994;76:23.

24. van Greevenbroek MM, de Bruin TW. Chylomicron synthesis by intestinal cells in vitro and in vivo. Atherosclerosis 1998; 141(Suppl 1):S9.

25. Gruffat D, Durand D, Graulet B, Bauchart D. Regulation of VLDL synthesis and secretion in the liver. Reprod Nutr Dev 1996;36:375.

26. Griffin BA, Packard CJ. Metabolism of VLDL and LDL subclasses. Curr Opin Lipidol 1994;5:200.

27. Havel RJ. Genetic underpinnings of LDL size and density: a role for hepatic lipase? Am J Clin Nutr 2000;71:1390.

28. Rosendorff C. Effects of LDL cholesterol on vascular function. J Hum Hypertens 2002;16(Suppl 1):S26.

29. Ginsberg HN. Lipoprotein metabolism and its relationship to atherosclerosis. Med Clin North Am 1994;78:1.

30. Plenz G, Robenek H. Monocytes/macrophages in atherosclerosis. Eur Cytokine Net 1998;9:701.

31. McNamara JR, Small DM, Li Z, Schaefer EJ. Differences in LDL subspecies involve alterations in lipid composition and conformational changes in apolipoprotein B. J Lipid Res 1996;37:1924.

32. Lamarche B, Lemieux I, Despres JP. The small, dense LDL phenotype and the risk of coronary heart disease: epidemiology, pathophysiology and therapeutic aspects. Diabetes Metab 1999;25:199.

33. Erbagci AB, Tarakcioglu M, Aksoy M, et al. Diagnostic value of CRP and Lp(a) in coronary heart disease. Acta Cardiol 2002;57:197.

34. Karmansky I, Gruener N. Structure and possible biological roles of Lp(a). Clin Biochem 1994;27:151.

35. Barrans A, Jaspard B, Barbaras R, et al. Pre-beta HDL: structure and metabolism. Biochim Biophys Acta 1996;1300:73.

36. Silver DL, Jiang XC, Arai T, et al. Receptors and lipid transfer proteins in HDL metabolism. Ann NY Acad Sci 2000;902:103.

37. Patsch JR, Prasad S, Gotto AM, et al. Postprandial lipemia: A key for the conversion of HDL2 into HDL3 by hepatic lipase. J Clin Inves 1984;74:2017.

38. Sing CF, Moll PP. Genetics of atherosclerosis. Annu Rev Genet 1990;24:171.

39. Drash AL. Genetic forms of dyslipidemia in children. Ann NY Acad Sci 1991;623:222.

40. Frohlich J, Lear SA. Old and new risk factors for atherosclerosis and development of treatment recommendations. Clin Exp Pharmacol Physiol 2002;29:838.

41. Phan CT, Tso P. Intestinal lipid absorption and transport. Front Biosci 2001;6:D299.

42. Carey MC, Small DM, Bliss CM. Lipid digestion and absorption. Annu Rev Physiol 1983;45:651.

43. Lee MH, Lu K, Patel SB. Genetic basis of sitosterolemia. Curr Opin Lipidol 2001;12:141.

44. Goldberg IJ, Merkel M. Lipoprotein lipase: physiology, biochemistry, and molecular biology. Front Biosci 2001;6:D388.

45. Schmitz G, Becker A, Aslanidis C. ACAT/CEH and ACEH/LAL: two key enzymes in hepatic cellular cholesterol homeostasis and their involvement in genetic disorders. Z Gastroenterol 1996; 34(Suppl 3):68.

46. Osborne TF. Cholesterol homeostasis: clipping out a slippery regulator. Curr Biol 1997;7:R172.

47. Aalto-Setala K, Kontula K. Molecular genetics of familial hypercholesterolemia. Adv Exp Med Biol 1991;285:33.

48. Sviridov D, Nestel P. Dynamics of reverse cholesterol transport: protection against atherosclerosis. Atherosclerosis 2002;161:245.

49. Attie AD, Kastelein JP, Hayden MR. Pivotal role of ABCA1 in reverse cholesterol transport influencing HDL levels and susceptibility to atherosclerosis. J Lipid Res 2001;42:1717.

50. Tall AR, Costet P, Wang N. Regulation and mechanisms of macrophage cholesterol efflux. J Clin Invest 2002;110:899.

51. Rothblat GH, de la Llera-Moya M, Atger V, et al. Cell cholesterol efflux: integration of old and new observations provides new insights. J Lipid Res 1999;40:781.

52. Dobiasova M, Frohlich JJ. Advances in understanding of the role of lecithin cholesterol acyltransferase (LCAT) in cholesterol transport. Clin Chim Acta 1999;286:257.

53. Arrese MA, Crawford JM. Of plaques and stones: the SR-B1 (scavenger receptor class B, type 1). Hepatology 1997;26:1072.

54. Lagrost L. Regulation of cholesteryl ester transfer protein (CETP) activity: review of in vitro and in vivo studies. Biochim Biophys Acta 1994;1215:209.

55. Dean M, Hamon Y, Chimini G. The human ATP-binding cassette (ABC) transporter superfamily. J Lipid Res 2001;42:1007.

56. Schaefer EJ, Lichtenstein AH, Lamon-Fava S, et al. Lipoproteins, nutrition, aging, and atherosclerosis. Am J Clin Nutr 1995; 61(Suppl):7265.

57. Hall G, Collins A, Csemiczky G, Landgren BM. Lipoproteins and BMI: A comparison between women during transition to menopause and regularly menstruating healthy women. Maturitas 2002;41:177.

58. Campos H, McNamara JR, Wilson PWF, et al. Differences in low-density lipoprotein subfractions and apolipoproteins in premenopausal and postmenopausal women. J Clin Endocrinol Metab 1988;67:30.

59. Cohn JS, McNamara JR, Cohn SD, et al. Postprandial plasma lipoprotein changes in human subjects of different ages. J Lipid Res 1988;29:469.

60. McNamara JR, Campos H, Ordovas JM, et al. Effect of gender, age, and lipid status on low-density lipoprotein subfraction distribution: results of the Framingham Offspring Study. Arteriosclerosis 1987;7:483.

61. Gardner CD, Tribble DL, Young DR, et al. Population frequency distributions of HDL, HDL(2), and HDL(3) cholesterol and apolipoproteins A-I and B in healthy men and women and associations with age, gender, hormonal status, and sex hormone use: The Stanford Five City Project. Prev Med 2000;31:335.

62. National Cholesterol Education Program (NCEP). Highlights of the report of the Expert Panel on blood cholesterol levels in children and adolescents. Pediatrics 1992;89:495.

63. Garcia RE, Moodie DS. Routine cholesterol surveillance in childhood. Pediatrics 1989;84:751.

64. Keys A, ed. Coronary heart disease in seven countries. Circulation 1970;41(Suppl I):1.

65. Castelli WP, Garrison RJ, Wilson PWF, et al. Incidence of coronary heart disease and lipoprotein cholesterol levels: the Framingham Study. JAMA 1986;256:2835.

66. Stamler J, Stamler R, Shekelle RB. Regional differences in prevalence, incidence, and mortality from atherosclerotic coronary heart disease. In: deHaas JH, Hemker HC, Snellen HA, eds. Ischaemic Heart Disease. Leiden, The Netherlands: Leiden University Press, 1970:84.

67. Thom TJ, Epstein FH, Feldman JJ, et al. Total mortality and mortality from heart disease, cancer, and stroke from 1950 to 1987 in 27 countries. NIH Pub. No. 923088. Washington, D.C.: 1992.

68. Kato H, Tillotson J, Nichaman MZ, et al. Epidemiologic studies of coronary heart disease and stroke in Japanese men living in Japan, Hawaii, and California. Am J Epidemiol 1973;97:372.

69. Wilson PW, D'Agostino RB, Levy D, et al. Prediction of coronary heart disease using risk factor categories. Circulation 1998;97:1837.

70. Warnick GR, Wood PD, for the National Cholesterol Education Program Working Group on Lipoprotein Measurement. National Cholesterol Education Program recommendations for measurement of high-density lipoprotein cholesterol: executive summary. Clin Chem 1995;41:1427.

71. Bachorik PS, Ross JW, for the National Cholesterol Education Program Working Group on Lipoprotein Measurement. National Cholesterol Education Program recommendations for measurement of low-density lipoprotein cholesterol: executive summary. Clin Chem 1995;41:1414.

72. Stein EA, Myers GL, for the National Cholesterol Education Program Working Group on Lipoprotein Measurement. National Cholesterol Education Program recommendations for triglyceride measurement: executive summary. Clin Chem 1995;41:1421.

73. National Cholesterol Education Program (NCEP) Expert Panel on Detection, Evaluation, and Treatment of High Blood Cholesterol in Adults (Adult Treatment Panel III). Third Report of the National Cholesterol Education Program (NCEP) Expert Panel on Detection, Evaluation, and Treatment of High Blood Cholesterol in Adults (Adult Treatment Panel III) final report. Circulation 2002;106:3143.

74. Rea TD, Heckbert SR, Kaplan RC, et al. Smoking status and risk for recurrent coronary events after myocardial infarction. Ann Intern Med 2002;137:494.

75. Holme I, Hjermann I, Helgelend A, et al. The Oslo Study: diet and antismoking advice. Additional results from a 5-year primary preventive trial in middle-aged men. Prev Med 1985;14:279.

76. Njolstad I, Arnesen E, Lund-Larsen PG. Smoking, serum lipids, blood pressure, and sex differences in myocardial infarction. A 12-year follow-up of the Finnmark Study. Circulation 1996;93:450.

77. Hegsted DM, Ausman LM, Johnson JA, et al. Dietary fat and serum lipids: An evaluation of the experimental data. Am J Clin Nutr 1993;57:875.

78. Ornish D, Brown SE, Scherwitz LW, et al. Can lifestyle changes reverse coronary heart disease? The lifestyle heart trial. Lancet 1990;336:129.

79. Niebauer J, Hambrecht R, Velich T, et al. Attenuated progression of coronary artery disease after 6 years of multifactorial risk intervention: role of physical exercise. Circulation 1997;96:2534.

80. Kromhout D, Menotti A, Bloemberg B, et al. Dietary saturated and trans fatty acids and cholesterol and 25-year mortality from coronary heart disease: The Seven Countries Study. Prev Med 1995;24:308.

81. Connor WE, Stone DB, Hodges RE. The interrelated effects of dietary cholesterol and fat upon human serum lipid levels. J Clin Invest 1964;43:1691.

82. Lichtenstein AH, Ausman LM, Carrasco W, et al. Hydrogenation impairs the hypolipidemic effect of corn oil in humans: hydrogenation, trans fatty acids, and plasma lipids. Arterioscler Thromb 1993;13:154.

83. Nicolosi RJ, Stucchi AF, Kowala MC, et al. Effect of dietary fat saturation and cholesterol on LDL composition and metabolism. In vivo studies of receptor and nonreceptor-mediated catabolism of LDL in cebus monkeys. Arteriosclerosis 1990;10:119.

84. Coleman MP, Key TJ, Wang DY, et al. A prospective study of obesity, lipids, apolipoproteins, and ischaemic heart disease in women. Atherosclerosis 1992;92:177.

85. Genest JJ Jr, Martin-Munley SS, McNamara JR, et al. Familial lipoprotein disorders in patients with premature coronary artery disease. Circulation 1992;85:2025.

86. Genest JJ Jr, Ordovas JM, McNamara JR, et al. DNA polymorphisms of the apolipoprotein B gene in patients with premature coronary artery disease. Atherosclerosis 1990;82:7.

87. Stary HC. Evolution and progression of atherosclerotic lesions in coronary arteries of children and young adults. Arteriosclerosis 1989;9(Suppl 1):I19.

88. Stary HC. Macrophages, macrophage foam cells, and eccentric intimal thickening in the coronary arteries of young children. Atherosclerosis 1987;64:91.

89. Catapano AL, Maggi FM, Tragni E. Low-density lipoprotein oxidation, antioxidants, and atherosclerosis. Curr Opin Cardiol 2000;15:355.

90. Craig WY, Rawstron MW, Rundell CA, et al. Relationship between lipoprotein- and oxidation-related variables and atheroma lipid composition in subjects undergoing coronary artery bypass graft surgery. Arterioscler Thromb Vasc Biol 1999;19:1512.

91. Jialal I, Chait A. Differences in the metabolism of oxidatively modified low density lipoprotein and acetylated low density lipoprotein by human endothelial cells: inhibition of cholesterol esterification by oxidatively modified low density lipoprotein. J Lipid Res 1989;30:1561.

92. Steinberg D, Parthasarathy S, Carew TE, et al. Beyond cholesterol. Modifications of low-density lipoprotein that increase its atherogenicity. N Engl J Med 1989;320:915.

93. Genest JJ, McNamara JR, Salem DN, et al. Prevalence of risk factors in men with premature coronary artery disease. Am J Cardiol 1991;67:1185.

94. Rackley CE. Cardiovascular basis for cholesterol therapy. Cardiol Rev 2000;8:124.

95. Domanski MJ, Borkowf CB, Campeau L, et al. Prognostic factors for atherosclerosis progression in saphenous vein grafts: The postcoronary artery bypass graft (Post-CABG) trial. Post-CABG Trial Investigators. J Am Coll Cardiol 2000;36:1877.

96. National Institutes of Health Consensus Conference. Triglyceride, HDL cholesterol and coronary heart disease. JAMA 1993;269:505.

97. Randomized trial of cholesterol lowering in 4444 patients with coronary heart disease: the Scandinavian Simvastatin Survival Study. Lancet 1994;344:1383.

98. Shepherd J, Cobbe SM, Ford I, et al. Prevention of coronary heart disease with pravastatin in men with hypercholesterolemia: the West of Scotland Coronary Prevention Study. N Engl J Med 1995;333:1301.

99. Jukema JW, Bruschke AV, van Boven AJ, et al. Effects of lipid lowering by pravastatin on progression and regression of coronary artery disease in symptomatic men with normal to moderately elevated serum cholesterol levels. The Regression Growth Evaluation Statin Study (*REGRESS*). Circulation 1995;91:2528.

100. Sacks FM, Pfeiffer MA, Moye LA, et al. The effect of pravastatin on coronary events after myocardial infarction in patients with average cholesterol levels. N Engl J Med 1996;335:1001.

101. Lipid Research Clinics program: the Lipid Research Clinics Coronary Primary Prevention Trial. I. Reduction in incidence of coronary heart disease. JAMA 1984;251:351.

102. Blankenhorn DH, Azen SP, Kramsch DM, et al. Coronary angiographic changes with lovastatin therapy. The monitored atherosclerosis regression study (MARS). Ann Intern Med 1993;119:969.

103. Brown BG, Zhao XQ, Sacco DE, et al. Lipid lowering and plaque regression. New insights into prevention of plaque disruption and clinical events in coronary disease. Circulation 1993;87:1781.

104. Zhao XQ, Yuan C, Hatsukami TS, et al. Effects of prolonged intensive lipid-lowering therapy on the characteristics of carotid atherosclerotic plaques in vivo by MRI: a case-control study. Arterioscler Thromb Vasc Biol 2001;21:1623.

105. Matthan NR, Giovanni A, Schaefer EJ, et al. Impact of simvastatin and niacin with and without antioxidants on plasma cholesterol absorption and synthesis markers in coronary artery disease patients with low HDL. J Lipid Res 2003;44:800.

106. Yamagishi M, Terashima M, Awano K, et al. Morphology of vulnerable coronary plaque: insights from follow-up of patients examined by intravascular ultrasound before an acute coronary syndrome. J Am Coll Cardiol 2000;35:106.

107. Regis-Bailly A, Visvikis S, Steinmetz J, et al. Frequencies of five genetic polymorphisms in coronarographed patients and effects on lipid levels in a supposedly healthy population. Clin Genet 1996;50:339.

108. Gylling H, Kontula K, Koivisto UM, et al. Polymorphisms of the genes encoding apoproteins A-I, B, C-III, and E and LDL receptor, and cholesterol and LDL metabolism during increased cholesterol intake. Common alleles of the apoprotein E gene show the greatest regulatory impact. Arterioscler Thromb Vasc Biol 1997;17:38.

109. Welty FK, Lichtenstein AH, Barrett PHR, et al. Decreased production and increased catabolism of apolipoprotein B-100 in apolipoprotein B67/B-100 heterozygotes. Arterioscler Thromb Vasc Biol 1997;17:881.

110. Schaefer EJ, McNamara JR. Overview of the diagnosis and treatment of lipid disorders. In: Rifai N, Warnick GR, eds. Handbook of Lipoprotein Testing. Washington, D.C.: AACC Press, 1997:25.

111. Clee SM, Zwinderman AH, Engert JC, et al. Common genetic variation in ABCA1 is associated with altered lipoprotein levels and a modified risk for coronary artery disease. Circulation 2001;103:1198.

112. Russo GT, Meigs JB, Cupples LA, et al. Association of the Sst-I polymorphism at the APOC3 gene locus with variations in lipid levels, lipoprotein subclass profiles and coronary heart disease risk: the Framingham offspring study. Atherosclerosis 2001;158:173.

113. Rubins HB, Robins SJ, Collins D, et al. Gemfibrozil for the secondary prevention of coronary heart disease in men with low levels of high-density lipoprotein cholesterol. Veterans Affairs High-Density Lipoprotein Cholesterol Intervention Trial Study Group. N Engl J Med 1999;341:410.

114. Robins SJ, Collins D, Wittes JT, et al. Veterans Affairs High-Density Lipoprotein Intervention Trial. Relation of gemfibrozil treatment and lipid levels with major coronary events: VA-HIT: a randomized controlled trial. JAMA 2001;285:1585.

115. Downs JR, Clearfield M, Weis S, et al. Primary prevention of acute coronary events with lovastatin in men and women with average cholesterol levels. Results of AFCAPS/TexCAPS. JAMA 1998;279: 1615.

116. Schaefer EJ, McNamara JR, Taylor T, et al. Effects of atorvastatin on fasting and postprandial lipoprotein subclasses in coronary heart disease patients versus control subjects. Am J Cardiol 2002;90:689.

117. Asztalos BF, Horvath KV, McNamara JR, et al. Comparing the effects of five different statins on the HDL subpopulation profiles of coronary heart disease patients. Atherosclerosis 2002;164: 361.

118. Stein EA, Illingworth DR, Kwiterovich PO Jr, et al. Efficacy and safety of lovastatin in adolescent males with heterozygous familial hypercholesterolemia: a randomized controlled trial. JAMA 1999;281:137.

119. de Jongh S, Ose L, Szamosi T, et al. Efficacy and safety of statin therapy in children with familial hypercholesterolemia: a randomized, double-blind, placebo-controlled trial with simvastatin. Circulation 2002;106:2231.

120. Kwiterovich PO Jr. Safety and efficacy of treatment of children and adolescents with elevated low density lipoprotein levels with a step two diet or with lovastatin. Nutr Metab Cardiovasc Dis 2001;11(Suppl 5):30.

121. Batiste MC, Schaefer EJ. Diagnosis and management of lipoprotein abnormalities. Nutr Clin Care 2002;5:115.

122. Sawayama Y, Shimizu C, Maeda N, et al. Effects of probucol and pravastatin on common carotid atherosclerosis in patients with asymptomatic hypercholesterolemia. Fukuoka Atherosclerosis Trial (FAST). J Am Coll Cardiol 2002;39:610.

123. Sprecher DL, Schaefer EJ, Kent KM, et al. Cardiovascular features of homozygous familial hypercholesterolemia: analysis of 16 patients. Am J Cardiol 1984;54:20.

124. Palcoux JB, Meyer M, Jouanel P, et al. Comparison of different treatment regimens in a case of homozygous familial hypercholesterolemia. Ther Apher 2002;6:136.

125. Grundy SM, Denke MA. Dietary influences on serum lipids and lipoproteins. J Lipid Res 1990;31:1149.

126. Hunninghake DB, Stein EA, Dujovne CA, et al. The efficacy of intensive dietary therapy alone or combined with lovastatin in outpatients with hypercholesterolemia. N Engl J Med 1993;328:1213.

127. Kris-Etherton P, Daniels SR, Eckel RH, et al. AHA scientific statement: summary of the Scientific Conference on Dietary Fatty Acids and Cardiovascular Health. Conference summary from the Nutrition Committee of the American Heart Association. J Nutr 2001;131:1322.

128. Cohn JS, McNamara JR, Krasinski SD, et al. Role of triglyceride-rich lipoproteins from the liver and intestine in the etiology of postprandial peaks in plasma triglyceride concentration. Metabolism 1989;38:484.

129. Karpe F, Hellenius ML, Hamsten A. Differences in postprandial concentrations of very-low-density lipoprotein and chylomicron remnants between normotriglyceridemic and hypertriglyceridemic men with and without coronary heart disease. Metabolism 1999;48:301.

130. Kovar J, Havel RJ. Sources and properties of triglyceride-rich lipoproteins containing apoB-48 and apoB-100 in postprandial blood plasma of patients with primary combined hyperlipidemia. J Lipid Res 2002;43:1026.

131. Couillard C, Bergeron N, Pascot A, et al. Evidence for impaired lipolysis in abdominally obese men: postprandial study of apolipoprotein B-48- and B-100-containing lipoproteins. Am J Clin Nutr 2002;76:311.

132. Schaefer EJ, McNamara JR, Genest J Jr, et al. Clinical significance of hypertriglyceridemia. Semin Thromb Hemost 1988;14:142.

133. Genest J Jr, Cohn J. Plasma triglyceride-rich lipoprotein and high density lipoprotein disorders associated with atherosclerosis. J Invest Med 1998;46:31.

134. Reynisdottir S, Eriksson M, Angelin B, Arner P. Impaired activation of adipocyte lipolysis in familial combined hyperlipidemia. J Clin Invest 1995;95:2161.

135. Yadav D, Pitchumoni CS. Issues in hyperlipidemic pancreatitis. J Clin Gastroenterol 2003;36:54.

136. Jackson RL, McLean LR, Ponce E, et al. Mechanism of action on LPL and hepatic triglyceride lipase. In: Malmendier CL, Alaupovic P, eds. Advances in Experimental Medicine and Biology. Vol. 210: Lipoproteins and Atherosclerosis. New York: Plenum Press, 1987:73.

137. Pschierer V, Richter WO, Schwandt P. Primary chylomicronemia in patients with severe familial hypertriglyceridemia responds to long-term treatment with (n-3) fatty acids. J Nutr 1995;125: 1490.

138. Santamarina-Fojo S. The familial chylomicronemia syndrome. Endocrinol Metab Clin North Am 1998;27:551.

139. Zilversmit DB. Atherogenic nature of triglycerides, postprandial lipemia, and triglyceride-rich remnant lipoproteins. Clin Chem 1995;41:153.

140. Packard CJ. Understanding coronary heart disease as a consequence of defective regulation of apolipoprotein B metabolism. Curr Opin Lipidol 1999;10:237.

141. Masuoka H, Kamei S, Wagayama H, et al. Association of remnant-like particle cholesterol with coronary artery disease in patients with normal total cholesterol levels. Am Heart J 2000;139:305.

142. Bjorkegren J, Boquist S, Samnegard A, et al. Accumulation of apolipoprotein C-I-rich and cholesterol-rich VLDL remnants during exaggerated postprandial triglyceridemia in normolipidemic patients with coronary artery disease. Circulation 2000;101:227.

143. McNamara JR, Shah PK, Nakajima K, et al. Remnant-like particle (RLP) cholesterol is an independent cardiovascular disease risk factor in women: results from the Framingham Heart Study. Atherosclerosis 2001;154:229.

144. Campos E, Nakajima K, Tanaka A, et al. Properties of an apolipoprotein E-enriched fraction of triglyceride-rich lipoproteins isolated from human blood plasma with a monoclonal antibody to apolipoprotein B-100. J Lipid Res 1992;33:369.

145. Nakajima K, Saito T, Tamura A, et al. Cholesterol in remnant-like lipoproteins in human serum using monoclonal anti apo B-100 and anti apo A-I immunoaffinity mixed gels. Clin Chim Acta 1993;223:53.

146. McNamara JR, Shah PK, Nakajima K, et al. Remnant lipoprotein cholesterol and triglyceride: reference ranges from the Framingham Heart Study. Clin Chem 1998;44:1224.

147. Fredrickson DS, Levy RI, Lees RS. Fat transport in lipoproteins: An integrated approach to mechanisms and disorders. N Engl J Med 1967;276:34, 94, 148, 215, 273.

148. Friedewald WT, Levy RI, Fredrickson DS. Estimation of the concentration of low-density lipoprotein cholesterol in plasma, without use of the preparative ultracentrifuge. Clin Chem 1972;18:499.

149. McNamara JR, Cole TG, Contois JH, et al. Immunoseparation method for measuring low-density lipoprotein cholesterol directly from serum evaluated. Clin Chem 1995;41:232.

150. Jialal I, Hirany SV, Devaraj S, et al. Comparison of an immunoseparation method for direct measurement of LDL cholesterol with beta-quantification (ultracentrifugation). Am J Clin Path 1995;104:76.

151. Genest J Jr, Jenner JL, McNamara JR, et al. Prevalence of lipoprotein (a) [Lp(a)] excess in coronary artery disease. Am J Cardiol 1991;67:1039.

152. Schaefer EJ, Lamon-Fava S, Jenner JL, et al. Lipoprotein(a) levels and risk of coronary heart disease in men. The Lipid Research Clinics Coronary Primary Prevention Trial. JAMA 1994;271:999.

153. Schwartzman RA, Cox ID, Poloniecki J, et al. Elevated plasma lipoprotein(a) is associated with coronary artery disease in patients with chronic stable angina pectoris. J Am Coll Cardiol 1998;31:1260.

154. Hopkins PN, Hunt SC, Schreiner PJ, et al. Lipoprotein(a) interactions with lipid and non-lipid risk factors in patients with early onset coronary artery disease: results from the NHLBI Family Heart Study. Atherosclerosis 1998;141:333.

155. Dahlen GH, Stenlund H. Lp(a) lipoprotein is a major risk factor for cardiovascular disease: pathogenic mechanisms and clinical significance. Clin Genet 1997;52:272.

156. Ridker PM, Hennekens CH, Stampfer MJ. A prospective study of lipoprotein(a) and the risk of myocardial infarction. JAMA 1993;270:2195.

157. Berg K, Dahlen G, Christophersen B, et al. Lp(a) lipoprotein level predicts survival and major coronary events in the Scandinavian Simvastatin Survival Study. Clin Genet 1997;52:254.

158. Marcovina SM, Koschinsky ML. Lipoprotein (a): structure, measurement, and clinical significance. In: Rifai N, Warnick GR, Dominczak MH, eds. Handbook of Lipoprotein Testing, 2nd ed. Washington, D.C.: AACC Press, 2000:345.

159. McLean JW, Tomlinson JE, Kuang WJ, et al. cDNA sequence of human apolipoprotein(a) is homologous to plasminogen. Nature 1987;330:132.

160. Hajjar KA, Gavish D, Breslow JL, et al. Lipoprotein (a) modulation of endothelial cell surface fibrinolysis and its potential role in atherosclerosis. Nature 1989;339:303.

161. Loscalzo J, Weinfield M, Fless GM, et al. Lipoprotein (a), fibrin binding, and plasminogen activation. Arteriosclerosis 1990; 10:240.

162. Miles LA, Fless GM, Levin EG, et al. A potential basis for the thrombotic risks associated with lipoprotein(a). Nature 1989; 339:301.

163. Genest JJ Jr, Bard JM, Fruchart JC, et al. Familial hypoalphalipoproteinemia in premature coronary artery disease. Arterioscler Thromb 1993;13:1728.

164. Schaefer EJ, Heaton WH, Wetzel MG, et al. Plasma apolipoprotein A-I absence associated with a marked reduction of high density lipoproteins and premature coronary artery disease. Arteriosclerosis 1982;2:16.

165. Schaefer EJ, Ordovas JM, Law SW, et al. Familial apolipoprotein A-I and C-III deficiency, variant II. J Lipid Res 1985;26:1089.

166. Third JL, Montag J, Flynn M, et al. Primary and familial hypoalphalipoproteinemia. Metabolism 1984;33:136.

167. Mott S, Yu L, Marcil M, et al. Decreased cellular cholesterol efflux is a common cause of familial hypoalphalipoproteinemia: role of the ABCA1 gene mutations. Atherosclerosis 2000;152: 457.

168. Baldassarre D, Amato M, Pustina L, et al. Increased carotid artery intima-media thickness in subjects with primary hypoalphalipoproteinemia. Arterioscler Thromb Vasc Biol 2002;22: 317.

169. Granfone A, Campos H, McNamara JR, et al. Effects of estrogen replacement on plasma lipoproteins and apolipoproteins in postmenopausal dyslipidemic women. Metabolism 1992;41: 1193.

170. Stampfer MJ, Colditz GA. Estrogen replacement therapy and coronary heart disease: a quantitative assessment of the epidemiologic evidence. Prev Med 1991;20:47.

171. Genest JJ, Corbett H, McNamara JR, et al. Effect of hospitalization on high-density lipoprotein cholesterol in patients undergoing elective coronary angiography. Am J Cardiol 1988;61:998.

172. Myers GL, Cooper GR, Greenberg N, et al. Standardization of lipid and lipoprotein measurements. In: Rifai N, Warnick GR, Dominczak MH, eds. Handbook of Lipoprotein Testing, 2nd ed. Washington, D.C.: AACC Press, 2000:717.

173. Zak B. Cholesterol methodologies: a review. Clin Chem 1977; 23:1201.

174. Abell LL, Levy BB, Brody BB, Kendall FC. A simplified method for the estimation of total cholesterol in serum and demonstration of its specificity. J Biol Chem 1952;195:357.

175. Duncan IW, Mather A, Cooper GR. The procedure for the proposed cholesterol reference method. Atlanta, GA: Division of Environmental Health Laboratory Sciences, Center for Environmental Health, Centers for Disease Control, 1982:75.

176. Cohen A, Hertz HS, Mandel J, et al. Total serum cholesterol by isotope dilution/mass spectrometry: a candidate definitive method. Clin Chem 1980;26:854.

177. Report from the Laboratory Standardization Panel of the National Cholesterol Education Program. Recommendations for improving cholesterol measurement. NIH Publication No. 902964. Bethesda, MD: National Institutes of Health, 1990.

178. Allain CC, Poon LS, Chan CS, et al. Enzymatic determination of total serum cholesterol. Clin Chem 1974;20:470.

179. Richmond W. Preparation and properties of a cholesterol oxidase from *Nocardia* sp. and its application to the enzymatic assay of total cholesterol in serum. Clin Chem 1973;19:1350.

180. McGowan MW, Artiss JD, Zak B. Spectrophotometric study on minimizing bilirubin interference in an enzyme reagent mediated cholesterol reaction. Microchem J 1983;27:564.

181. Klotzsch SG, McNamara JR. Triglyceride measurements: a review of methods and interferences. Clin Chem 1990;36:1605.

182. Bucolo G, Yabut J, Chang TY. Mechanized enzymatic determination of triglycerides in serum. Clin Chem 1975;21:420.

183. McGowan M, Artiss J, Strandbergh DR, et al. A peroxidase-coupled method for the colorimetric determination of serum triglycerides. Clin Chem 1983;29:538.

184. Cole TG. Glycerol blanking in triglyceride assays: is it necessary? Clin Chem 1990;36:1267.

185. Stinshoff K, Weisshaar D, Staehler F, et al. Relation between concentrations of free glycerol and triglycerides in human sera. Clin Chem 1977;23:1029.

186. Warnick GR. Enzymatic methods for quantification of lipoprotein lipids. In: Albers JJ, Segrest JP, eds. Methods in Enzymology. Vol. 129. Orlando, FL: Academic Press, 1986:101.

187. Sullivan DR, Kruijswijk Z, West CE, et al. Determination of serum triglycerides by an accurate enzymatic method not affected by free glycerol. Clin Chem 1985;31:1227.

188. Lofland HB Jr. A semiautomated procedure for the determination of triglycerides in serum. Anal Biochem 1964;9:393.

189. Hatch FT, Lees RS. Practical methods for plasma lipoprotein analysis. In: Pachetti R, ed. Advances in Lipid Research. Orlando, FL: Academic Press, 1968;6:1.

190. Havel RJ, Eder HA, Bragdon JH. The distribution and chemical composition of ultracentrifugally separated lipoproteins in human serum. J Clin Invest 1955;34:1345.

191. Chapman MJ, Goldstein S, Lagrange D, et al. A density gradient ultracentrifugal procedure for the isolation of the major lipoprotein classes from human serum. J Lipid Res 1981;22:339.

192. Kulkarni KR, Garber DW, Schmidt CF, et al. Analysis of cholesterol in all lipoprotein classes by single vertical ultracentrifugation of fingerstick blood and controlled-dispersion flow analysis. Clin Chem 1992;38:1898.

193. Patsch JR, Patsch W. Zonal ultracentrifugation. In: Albers JJ, Segrest JP, eds. Methods of Enzymology. Orlando, FL: Academic Press, 1986;129:3.

194. Redgrave TG, Roberts DCK, West CE. Separation of plasma lipoproteins by density-gradient ultracentrifugation. Anal Biochem 1975;65:42.

195. Rosseneu M, Van Diervliet JP, Bury J, et al. Isolation and characterization of lipoprotein profiles in newborns by density gradient ultracentrifugation. Pediatr Res 1983;17(10):788.

196. Brousseau T, Clavey V, Bard JM, et al. Sequential ultracentrifugation micromethod for separation of serum lipoproteins and assays of lipids, apolipoproteins, and lipoprotein particles. Clin Chem 1993;39:960.

197. Wu LL, Warnick GR, Wu JT, et al. A rapid micro-scale procedure for determination of the total lipid profile. Clin Chem 1989;35(7):1486.

198. Lewis LA, Opplt JJ. CRC Handbook of Electrophoresis. Vols. 1 and 2. Boca Raton, FL: CRC Press, 1980.

199. Schmitz G, Boettcher A, Barlage S. New approaches to the use of lipoprotein electrophoresis in the clinical laboratory. In: Rifai N, Warnick GR, Dominczak MH, eds. Handbook of Lipoprotein Testing, 2nd ed. Washington, D.C.: AACC Press, 2000:593.

200. Conlon D, Blankstein LA, Pasakarnis PA, et al. Quantitative determination of high-density lipoprotein cholesterol by agarose gel electrophoresis updated. Clin Chem 1979;24:227.

201. Lindgren FT, Silvers A, Jutaglr R, et al. A comparison of simplified methods for lipoprotein quantitation using the analytic ultracentrifuge as a standard. Lipids 1977;12:278.

202. Noble RP. Electrophoretic separation of plasma lipoproteins in agarose gel. J Lipid Res 1968;9:963.

203. Warnick GR, Nguyen T, Bergelin RO, et al. Lipoprotein quantification: an electrophoretic method compared with the Lipid Research Clinics method. Clin Chem 1982;28:2116.

204. Rifai N, Warnick GR, McNamara JR, et al. Measurement of low-density-lipoprotein cholesterol in serum: a status report. Clin Chem 1992;38:150.

205. Warnick GR, Leary ET, Goetsch J. Electrophoretic quantification of LDL-cholesterol using the Helena REP [Abstract]. Clin Chem 1993;39:1122.

206. Muniz N. Measurement of plasma lipoproteins by electrophoresis on polyacrylamide gel. Clin Chem 1977;23:1826.

207. Blanche PJ, Gong EL, Forte TM, et al. Characterization of human high-density lipoproteins by gradient gel electrophoresis. Biochem Biophys Acta 1981;665:408.

208. Li Z, McNamara JR, Ordovas JM, et al. Analysis of high-density lipoproteins by a modified gradient gel electrophoresis method. J Lipid Res 1994;35:1698.

209. Krauss RM, Lindgren FT, Ray RM. Interrelationships among subgroups of serum lipoproteins in normal human subjects. Clin Chem Acta 1980;104:275.

210. Burstein M, Legmann P. Lipoprotein precipitation. In: Clarkson TB, Kritchevsky D, Pollak OJ, eds. Monographs on Atherosclerosis. Vol. 2. New York: Karger, 1982:1.

211. Levin SJ. High-density lipoprotein cholesterol: review of methods. The American Society of Clinical Pathologists. Check Sample, Core Chemistry, No. PTS 892(PTS36), 1989;5(2).

212. Warnick GR, Benderson J, Albers JJ, et al. Dextran sulfate-Mg^{2+} precipitation procedure for quantitation of high-density-lipoprotein cholesterol. Clin Chem 1982;28:1379.

213. Kerscher L, Schiefer S, Draeger B, et al. Precipitation methods for the determination of LDL-cholesterol. Clin Biochem 1985; 18:118.

214. Schumaker VN, Robinson MT, Curtiss LK, et al. Anti-apoprotein B monoclonal antibodies detect human low density lipoprotein polymorphism. J Biol Chem 1984;259:6423.

215. Burstein M, Samaille J. Sur un dosage rapide du cholesterol lie aux α- et aux β-lipoproteines du serum. Clin Chim Acta 1960;5:609.

216. Fredrickson DS, Levy RI, Lindgren FT. A comparison of heritable abnormal lipoprotein patterns as defined by two different techniques. J Clin Invest 1968;47:2446.

217. Bachorik PS. Measurement of total cholesterol, HDL-cholesterol, and LDL-cholesterol. Clin Lab Med 1989;9:61.

218. Manual of Laboratory Operations, Lipid Research Clinics Program, Lipid and Lipoprotein Analysis. Washington, D.C.: U.S. Department of Health and Human Services, National Institutes of Health, revised 1983.

219. Steele BW, Koehler DF, Azar MM, et al. Enzymatic determinations of cholesterol in high-density-lipoprotein fractions prepared by a precipitation technique. Clin Chem 1976; 22:98.

220. Burstein M, Scholnick HR. Lipoprotein–polyanion–metal interactions. Adv Lipid Res 1973;11:68.

221. Lopes-Virella MF, Stone P, Ellis S, et al. Cholesterol determination in high-density lipoproteins separated by three different methods. Clin Chem 1977;23:882.

222. Warnick GR, Cheung MC, Albers JJ. Comparison of current methods for high-density lipoprotein cholesterol quantitation. Clin Chem 1979;25:596.

223. Allen JK, Hensley WJ, Nichols AV, et al. An enzymic and centrifugal method for estimating high-density lipoprotein cholesterol. Clin Chem 1979;25:325.

224. Demacker PNM, Vos-Janssen HE, Hijmans AGM, et al. Measurement of high-density lipoprotein cholesterol in serum: comparison of six isolation methods combined with enzymic cholesterol analysis. Clin Chem 1980;26:1780.

225. Viikari J. Precipitation of plasma lipoproteins by PEG6000 and its evaluation with electrophoresis and ultracentrifugation. Scand J Clin Lab Invest 1976;36:265.

226. Warnick GR, Albers JJ, Bachorik PS, et al. Multi-laboratory evaluation of an ultrafiltration procedure for high-density lipoprotein cholesterol quantification in turbid heparin-manganese supernates. J Lipid Res 1981;22:1015.

227. Sugiuchi H, Uji Y, Okabe H, et al. Direct measurement of high-density lipoprotein cholesterol in serum with polyethylene glycol-modified enzymes and sulfated a-cyclodextrin. Clin Chem 1995;41:717.

228. Harris N, Galpchian V, Rifai N. Three routine methods for measuring high-density lipoprotein cholesterol compared with the reference method. Clin Chem 1996;42:738.

229. Warnick GR, Nauck M, Rifai N. Evolution of methods for measurement of HDL-cholesterol: from ultracentrifugation to homogeneous assays. Clin Chem 2001;47:1579–1596.

230. Bachorik PS. Measurement of low-density lipoprotein cholesterol. In: Rifai N, Warnick GR, Dominczak MH, eds. Handbook of Lipoprotein Testing, 2nd ed. Washington, D.C.. AACC Press 2000:245.

231. McNamara JR, Cohn JS, Wilson PWF, et al. Calculated values for low-density lipoprotein cholesterol in the assessment of lipid abnormalities and coronary disease risk. Clin Chem 1990;36:36.

232. Warnick GR, Knopp RH, Fitzpatrick V, et al. Estimating low-density lipoprotein cholesterol by the Friedewald equation is adequate for classifying patients on the basis of nationally recommended cutpoints. Clin Chem 1990;36:15.

233. Sugiuchi H, Irie T, Uji Y, et al. Homogeneous assay for measuring low-density lipoprotein cholesterol in serum with triblock copolymer and a-cyclodextrin sulfate. Clin Chem 1998;44:522.

234. Rifai N, Iannotti E, DeAngelis K, et al. Analytical and clinical performance of a homogeneous enzymatic LDL-cholesterol assay compared with the ultracentrifugation-dextran sulfate-Mg^{2+} method. Clin Chem 1998;44:1242.

235. Nauck M, Warnick GR, Rifai N. Methods for measurement of LDL-cholesterol: a critical assessment of direct measurement by homogeneous assays versus calculation. Clin Chem 2002;48:236.

236. Bachorik PS. Lipid and lipoprotein analysis with desktop analyzers. In: Rifai N, Warnick GR, Dominczak MH, eds. Handbook of Lipoprotein Testing, 2nd ed. Washington, D.C.: AACC Press, 2000:265.

237. Bhatnagar D, Durrington PN. Measurement and clinical significance of apolipoproteins A-1 and B. In: Rifai N, Warnick GR, Dominczak MH, eds. Handbook of Lipoprotein Testing, 2nd ed. Washington, D.C.: AACC Press, 2000:287.

238. Miremadi S, Sniderman A, Frohlich J. Can measurement of serum apolipoprotein B replace the lipid profile monitoring of patients with lipoprotein disorders? Clin Chem 2002;48:484.

239. Takayama M, Itoh S, Nagasaki T, et al. A new enzymatic method for determination of serum choline-containing phospholipids. Clin Chim Acta 1977;79:93.

240. McGowan, MW, Artiss JD, Zak B. A procedure for the determination of high-density lipoprotein choline-containing phospholipids. J Clin Chem Clin Biochem 1982;20:807.

241. Bartlett GR. Phosphorus assay in column chromatography. J Biol Chem 1959;234:466.

242. LePage G, Roy C. Direct transesterification of all classes of lipids in a one-step reaction. J Lipid Res 1986;27:114.

243. Cooper GR, Myers GL, Smith SJ, et al. Blood lipid measurements. Variations and practical utility. JAMA 1992;267:1652.

244. Cooper GR, Smith SJ, Myers GL, et al. Estimating and minimizing effects of biologic sources of variation by relative range when measuring the mean of serum lipids and lipoproteins. Clin Chem 1994;40:227.

245. Eckfeldt JH, Copeland KR. Accuracy verification and identification of matrix effects. The College of American Pathologist's protocol. Arch Pathol Lab Med 1993;117:381.

246. Greenberg N, Li ZM, Bower GN. National Reference System for Cholesterol (NRS-CHOL): problems with transfer of accuracy with matrix materials. Clin Chem 1988;24:1230.

247. Kroll MH, Chesler R, Elin RJ. Effect of lyophilization on results of five enzymatic methods for cholesterol. Clin Chem 1989;35:1523.

Electrolytes

Joan E. Polancic

OBJECTIVES

Upon completion of this chapter, the clinical laboratorian should be able to:

- Define electrolyte, osmolality, anion gap, anion, and cation.
- Discuss the physiology of each electrolyte described in the chapter.
- State the clinical significance of each of the electrolytes mentioned in the chapter.
- Calculate osmolality, osmolal gap, and anion gap and discuss the clinical usefulness of each.
- Discuss the analytic techniques used to assess electrolyte concentrations.
- Correlate the information with disease state, given patient data.
- Identify the reference ranges for sodium, potassium, chloride, bicarbonate, magnesium, and calcium.
- State the specimen of choice for the major electrolytes.
- Discuss the role of the kidney in electrolyte excretion and conservation in a healthy individual.
- Discuss the usefulness of urine electrolyte results: sodium, potassium, calcium, and osmolality.

KEY TERMS

Active transport
Anion
Anion gap
Cation
Diffusion
Electrolyte
Extracellular fluid (ECF)
Hypercalcemia
Hyperchloremia
Hyperkalemia
Hypermagnesemia
Hypernatremia
Hyperphosphatemia
Hypocalcemia
Hypochloremia
Hypokalemia
Hypomagnesemia
Hyponatremia
Hypophosphatemia
Hypovolemia
Intracellular fluid (ICF)
Osmolal gap
Osmolality
Osmolarity
Osmometer
Polydipsia
Tetany

Electrolytes are ions capable of carrying an electric charge. They are classified as anions or cations based on the type of charge they carry. These names were determined years ago based on how the ion migrates in an electric field. *Anions* have a negative charge and move toward the anode, whereas *cations* migrate in the direction of the cathode because of their positive charge.

Electrolytes are an essential component in numerous processes, including volume and osmotic regulation (Na, Cl, K); myocardial rhythm and contractility (K, Mg, Ca); cofactors in enzyme activation (*eg*, Mg, Ca, Zn); regulation of adenosine triphosphatase (ATPase) ion pumps (Mg); acid-base balance (HCO_3, K, Cl); blood coagulation (Ca, Mg); neuromuscular excitability (K, Ca, Mg); and the production and use of ATP from glucose (*eg*, Mg, PO_4). Because many of these functions require electrolyte concentrations to be held within narrow ranges, the body has complex systems for monitoring and maintaining electrolyte concentrations.

This chapter explores both the metabolic physiology and regulation of each electrolyte and relates these factors to the clinical significance of electrolyte measurements. In addition, methodologies used in determining concentrations of the individual analytes are discussed.

WATER

The average water content of the human body varies 40–75% of total body weight, with values declining with age and especially with obesity. Women have lower average water content than men as a result of a higher fat content. Water is the solvent for all processes in the human body. It transports nutrients to cells, determines cell volume by its transport into and out of cells, removes waste products by way of urine, and acts as the body's coolant by way of sweating. Water is located in intracellular and extracellular compartments. *Intracellular fluid (ICF)* is the fluid inside the cells and accounts for about two thirds of total body water. *Extracellular fluid (ECF)* accounts for the other one third of total body water and can be subdivided in the *intravascular extracellular fluid (plasma)* and the *interstitial cell fluid* that surrounds the cells in the tissue. Normal plasma is about 93% water, with the remaining volume occupied by lipids and proteins. The concentrations of ions within cells and in plasma are maintained both by energy-consuming active transport processes and by diffusion or passive transport processes.

Active transport is a mechanism that requires energy to move ions across cellular membranes. For example, maintaining a high intracellular concentration of potassium and a high extracellular (plasma) concentration of sodium requires use of energy from ATP in ATPase-dependent ion pumps. *Diffusion* is the passive movement of ions across a membrane. It depends on the size and charge of the ion being transported and on the nature of the membrane through which it is passing. The rate of diffusion of various ions also may be altered by physiologic and hormonal processes.

By maintaining the concentration of proteins and electrolytes in a controlled yet somewhat flexible environment, the distribution of water in these compartments also can be controlled. Because most biologic membranes are freely permeable to water but not to ions or proteins, the concentration of ions and proteins on one side of the membrane or the other will influence the flow of water across a membrane (an osmoregulator). In addition to the osmotic effects of sodium, other ions, proteins, and blood pressure influence the flow of water across a membrane.

Osmolality

Osmolality is a physical property of a solution that is based on the concentration of solutes (expressed as millimoles) per kilogram of solvent (w/w). Osmolality is related to several changes in the properties of a solution relative to pure water, such as freezing point depression and vapor pressure decrease. These colligative properties (see Chapter 1, *Basic Principles and Practice*) are the basis for routine measurements of osmolality in the laboratory. The term *osmolarity* is still occasionally used, with results reported in milliosmoles per liter (w/v), but it is inaccurate in cases of hyperlipidemia or hyperproteinemia; for urine specimens; or in the presence of certain osmotically active substances, such as alcohol or mannitol. Both the sensation of thirst and antidiuretic hormone (ADH) secretion are stimulated by the hypothalamus in response to an increased osmolality of blood. The natural response to the thirst sensation is to consume more fluids, increasing the water content of the ECF, diluting the elevated solute (sodium) levels, and decreasing the osmolality of the plasma. Thirst, therefore, is important in mediating fluid intake. The other means of controlling osmolality is by secretion of ADH (vasopressin). This hormone is secreted by the posterior pituitary gland and acts on the cells of the collecting ducts in the kidneys to increase water reabsorption. As water is conserved, osmolality decreases, turning off ADH secretion.[1]

Clinical Significance of Osmolality

Osmolality in plasma is important because it is the parameter to which the hypothalamus responds. The regulation of osmolality also affects the sodium concentration in plasma, largely because sodium and its associated anions account for approximately 90% of the osmotic activity in plasma. Another important process affecting the sodium concentration in blood is the regulation of blood volume. As discussed later, although osmolality and volume are regulated by separate mechanisms (except for ADH and thirst), they are related because osmolality (sodium) is regulated by changes in water balance, whereas volume is regulated by changes in sodium balance.[1]

To maintain a normal plasma osmolality (~275–295 mOsm/kg of plasma H_2O), osmoreceptors in the hypothalamus respond quickly to small changes in osmolality. A 1–2% increase in osmolality causes a 4-fold increase in the circulating concentration of ADH, and a 1–2% decrease in osmolality shuts off ADH production. ADH acts by increasing the reabsorption of water in the cortical and medullary collecting tubules. ADH has a half-life in the circulation of only 15–20 minutes.

Renal water regulation by ADH and thirst play important roles in regulating plasma osmolality. Renal water excretion is more important in controlling water excess, whereas thirst is more important in preventing water deficit or dehydration. Consider what happens in several conditions.

Water Load. As excess intake of water (*eg*, in polydipsia) begins to lower plasma osmolality, both ADH and thirst are suppressed. In the absence of ADH, water is not reabsorbed, causing a large volume of dilute urine to be excreted, as much as 10–20 L daily, well above any normal intake of water. Therefore, hypoosmolality and hyponatremia usually occur only in patients with impaired renal excretion of water.[1]

Water Deficit. As a deficit of water begins to increase plasma osmolality, both ADH secretion and thirst are activated. Although ADH contributes by minimizing renal water loss, thirst is the major defense against hyperosmolality and hypernatremia. Although hypernatremia rarely occurs in a person with a normal thirst mechanism and access to water, it becomes a concern in infants, unconscious patients, or anyone who is unable to either drink or ask for water. Osmotic stimulation of thirst progressively diminishes in people who are older than age 60. In the older patient with illness and diminished mental status, dehydration becomes increasingly likely. As an example of the effectiveness of thirst in preventing dehydration, a patient with diabetes insipidus (no ADH) may excrete 10 L of urine per day; however, because thirst persists, water intake matches output and plasma sodium remains normal.[1]

Regulation of Blood Volume

Adequate blood volume is essential to maintain blood pressure and ensure good perfusion to all tissue and organs. Regulation of both sodium and water are interrelated in controlling blood volume. The renin-angiotensin-aldosterone system responds primarily to a decreased blood volume. Renin is secreted near the renal glomeruli in response to decreased renal blood flow (decreased blood volume or blood pressure). Renin converts angiotensinogen to angiotensin I, which then becomes angiotensin II. Angiotensin II causes vasoconstriction, which quickly increases blood pressure, and secretion of aldosterone, which increases retention of sodium and the water that accompanies the sodium. The effects of blood volume and osmolality on sodium and water metabolism are shown in Figure 13-1. Changes in blood volume (actually pressure) are initially detected by a series of stretch receptors located in areas such as the cardiopulmonary

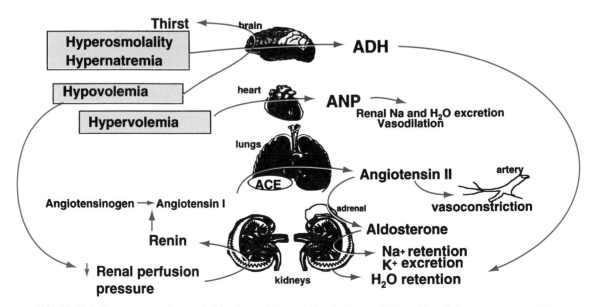

FIGURE 13-1. Responses to changes in blood osmolality and blood volume. *ADH*, antidiuretic hormone; *ANP*, atrial natriuretic peptide. The primary stimuli are shown in *boxes* (*eg*, hypovolemia).

circulation, carotid sinus, aortic arch, and glomerular arterioles. These receptors then activate a series of responses (effectors) that restore volume by appropriately varying vascular resistance, cardiac output, and renal sodium and water retention.[1]

Four other factors affect blood volume: (1) atrial natriuretic peptide (ANP), released from the myocardial atria in response to volume expansion, promotes sodium excretion in the kidney (B-type natriuretic peptide [BNP] and ANP act together in regulating blood pressure and fluid balance); (2) volume receptors independent of osmolality stimulate the release of ADH, which conserves water by renal reabsorption; (3) glomerular filtration rate (GFR) increases with volume expansion and decreases with volume depletion; and (4) all other things equal, an increased plasma sodium will increase urinary sodium excretion and vice versa. The normal reabsorption of 98–99% of filtered sodium by the tubules conserves nearly all of the 150 L of glomerular filtrate produced daily. A 1–2% reduction in tubular reabsorption of sodium can increase water loss by several liters per day.

Urine osmolality values may vary widely depending on water intake and the circumstances of collection. However, it is generally decreased in diabetes insipidus (inadequate ADH) and *polydipsia* (excessive H_2O intake) and increased in conditions such as the syndrome of inappropriate ADH secretion (SIADH) and *hypovolemia* (although urinary Na is usually decreased).

Determination of Osmolality

Specimen. Osmolality may be measured in serum or urine. Plasma use is not recommended because osmotically active substances may be introduced into the specimen from the anticoagulant.

Discussion. The methods for determining osmolality are based on properties of a solution that are related to the number of molecules of solute per kilogram of solvent (colligative properties), such as changes in freezing point and vapor pressure. An increase in osmolality decreases the freezing point temperature and the vapor pressure. Measurement of freezing point depression and vapor pressure decrease (actually, the dew point) are the two most frequently used methods of analysis. For detailed information on theory and methodology, consult Chapter 4, *Analytic Techniques and Instrumentation,* or the operator's manual of the instrument being used.

Samples must be free of particulate matter to obtain accurate results. Turbid serum and urine samples should be centrifuged before analysis to remove any extraneous particles. If reusable sample cups are used, they should be thoroughly cleaned and dried between each use to prevent contamination.

Osmometers that operate by freezing point depression are standardized using sodium chloride reference solutions. After calibration, the appropriate amount of sample is pipetted into the required cuvet or sample cup and placed in the analyzer. The sample is then supercooled to –7°C and seeded to initiate the freezing process. When temperature equilibrium has been reached, the freezing point is measured, with results for serum and urine osmolality reported as milliosmoles per kilogram.

Calculation of osmolality has some usefulness either as an estimate of the true osmolality or to determine the *osmolal gap,* which is the difference between the measured osmolality and the calculated osmolality. The osmolal gap indirectly indicates the presence of osmotically active substances other than sodium, urea, or glucose, such as ethanol, methanol, ethylene glycol, lactate, or β-hydroxybutyrate.

Two formulas are presented, each having theoretic advantages and disadvantages. Both are adequate for the purpose previously described. For more discussion, the reader may consult other references.[2]

$$2\,Na + \frac{glucose(mg/dL)}{20} + \frac{BUN(mg/dL)}{3}$$

$$1.86\,Na + \frac{glucose}{18} + \frac{BUN}{2.8} + 9 \quad \textbf{(Eq. 13–1)}$$

Reference Ranges[3]
See Table 13-1.

THE ELECTROLYTES

Sodium

Sodium is the most abundant cation in the ECF, representing 90% of all extracellular cations, and largely determines the osmolality of the plasma. A normal plasma osmolality is approximately 295 mmol/L, with 270 mmol/L being the result of sodium and associated anions.

Sodium concentration in the ECF is much larger than inside the cells. Because a small amount of sodium can diffuse through the cell membrane, the two sides would eventually reach equilibrium. To prevent equilibrium from occurring, active transport systems, such as ATPase

TABLE 13-1. REFERENCE RANGES FOR OSMOLALITY

Serum	275–295 mOsm/kg
Urine (24-hour)	300–900 mOsm/kg
Urine/serum ratio	1.0–3.0
Osmolal gap	<15

CASE STUDY 13-1

A 32-year-old woman was admitted to the hospital following 2½ days of severe vomiting. Before this episode, she was reportedly well. Physical findings revealed decreased skin turgor and dry mucous membranes. Admission study results were as follows:

Serum
- Na^+: 129 mmol/L
- K^+: 5.0 mmol/L
- Cl^-: 77 mmol/L
- HCO_3^-: 9 mmol/L
- Osmolality: 265 mOsm/kg

Urine
- Na^+: 8 mmol/day
- Ketones: trace

Questions

1. What is the cause for each abnormal plasma electrolyte result?

2. What is the significance of the urine sodium and serum osmolality results?

ion pumps, are present in all cells. Potassium (see *Potassium*) is the major intracellular cation. Like sodium, potassium would eventually diffuse across the cell membrane until equilibrium is reached. The NaK ATPase ion pump moves three sodium ions out of the cell in exchange for two potassium ions moving into the cell as ATP is converted to ADP. Because water follows electrolytes across cell membranes, the continual removal of sodium from the cell prevents osmotic rupture of the cell by also drawing water from the cell.

Regulation

The plasma sodium concentration depends greatly on the intake and excretion of water and, to a somewhat lesser degree, the renal regulation of Na. Three processes are of primary importance: (1) the intake of water in response to thirst, as stimulated or suppressed by plasma osmolality; (2) the excretion of water, largely affected by ADH release in response to changes in either blood volume or osmolality; and (3) the blood volume status, which affects sodium excretion through aldosterone, angiotensin II, and ANP (atrial natriuretic peptide). The kidneys have the ability to conserve or excrete large amounts of sodium, depending on the sodium content of the ECF and the blood volume. Normally, 60–75% of filtered sodium is reabsorbed in the proximal tubule; electroneutrality is maintained by either Cl reabsorption or H ion secretion. Some sodium is also reabsorbed in the loop and distal tubule and (controlled by aldosterone) exchanged for K in the connecting segment and cortical collecting tubule. The regulation of osmolality and volume has been summarized in Figure 13-1.

Clinical Applications

Hyponatremia. Hyponatremia is defined as a serum/plasma level <135 mmol/L.[4] Levels below 130 mmol/L are clinically significant. Hyponatremia can be assessed by the cause for the decrease or with the osmolality level.

Decreased levels may be caused by increased sodium loss, increased water retention, or water imbalance (Table 13-2). *Increased sodium loss* in the urine can occur with decreased aldosterone production, certain diuretics (thiazides), with ketonuria (sodium lost with ketones), or a salt-losing nephropathy (with some renal tubular disorders). Potassium deficiency also causes Na loss because of the inverse relationship of the two ions in the renal tubules. When serum K levels are low, the tubules will conserve K and excrete Na in exchange for the loss of the monovalent cation. Each disorder results in an increased urine sodium level (>20 mmol/day), which exceeds the amount of water loss.[5]

Prolonged vomiting or diarrhea or severe burns can result in sodium loss. Urine sodium levels are usually

TABLE 13-2. CAUSES OF HYPERNATREMIA

Increased Sodium Loss
Hypoadrenalism
Potassium deficiency
Diuretic use
Ketonuria
Salt-losing nephropathy
Prolonged vomiting or diarrhea
Severe burns

Increased Water Retention
Renal failure
Nephrotic syndrome
Hepatic cirrhosis
Congestive heart failure

Water Imbalance
Excess water intake
SIADH
Pseudohyponatremia

<20 mmol/day in these disorders, which can be used to differentiate among causes for urinary loss.

Increased water retention causes dilution of serum/plasma sodium as with acute or chronic renal failure. In nephrotic syndrome and hepatic cirrhosis, plasma proteins are decreased, resulting in a decreased colloid osmotic pressure (COP) in which intravascular fluid migrates to the tissue (edema results). The low plasma volume causes ADH to be produced, causing fluid retention and resulting dilution of Na. This compensatory mechanism is also seen with CHF as a result of increased venous pressure. Urine sodium levels can be used to differentiate the cause for increased water retention. When urine sodium is >20 mmol/day, acute or chronic renal failure is the likely cause. When urine levels are <20 mmol/day, water retention may be a result of nephrotic syndrome, hepatic cirrhosis, or congestive heart failure (CHF).[5]

Water imbalance can occur as a result of excess water intake, as with polydipsia (increased thirst). The increased intake must be chronic before water imbalance occurs, which may cause mild or severe hyponatremia. In a normal individual, excess intake will not affect Na levels. Syndrome of inappropriate ADH secretion (SIADH) causes an increase in water retention because of increased ADH production. A defect in ADH regulation has been associated with pulmonary disease, malignancies, CNS disorders, infections (eg, *Pneumocystis carinii* pneumonia), or trauma.[5] Pseudohyponatremia can occur when Na is measured using indirect ISE in a patient who is hyperproteinemic or hyperlipidemic. An indirect ISE dilutes the sample prior to analysis and as a result of plasma/serum water displacement; the ion levels are falsely decreased. (For detailed information on the theory of water displacement with indirect ISEs, consult Chapter 4, *Analytic Techniques and Instrumentation*.)

Hyponatremia can also be *classified according to plasma/serum osmolality* (Table 13-3). Because Na is a major contributor to osmolality, both levels can assist in identifying the cause of hyponatremia. There are three categories of hyponatremia—low osmolality, normal osmolality, or high osmolality.[4] Most instances of *hyponatremia* occur *with decreased osmolality*. This may be a result of Na loss or water retention, as previously mentioned.

Hyponatremia with a normal osmolality may be a result of a high increase in nonsodium cations as listed in Table 13-4. In multiple myeloma, the cationic γ-globulins replace some Na to maintain the electroneutrality; however, because it is a multivalent cation, it has little affect on osmolality.

Pseudohyponatremia, as mentioned earlier, may also be seen with in vitro hemolysis, considered the most common cause for a false decrease.[4] When red blood cells (RBC) lyse, Na, K, and water are released. Na concentration is lower in RBC, resulting in a false decrease. *Hyponatremia with a high osmolality* is associated with hyperglycemia. This high solute causes a shift of water from the cells to the blood, resulting in a dilution of sodium.

Symptoms of hyponatremia. Symptoms depend on the serum level. Between 125 and 130 mmol/L, symptoms are primarily gastrointestinal (GI). More severe neuropsychiatric symptoms are seen below 125 mmol/L, including nausea and vomiting, muscular weakness, headache, lethargy, and ataxia. More severe symptoms also include seizures, coma, and respiratory depression.[5] Serum and urine electrolytes are monitored as treatment to return sodium levels to normal occurs.[6]

Treatment of hyponatremia. Treatment is directed at correction of the condition that caused either water loss or sodium loss in excess of water loss. Correcting severe hyponatremia too rapidly can cause cerebral myelinolysis; too slowly can cause cerebral edema.[6] Appropriate

TABLE 13-3. CLASSIFICATION OF HYPONATREMIA BY OSMOLALITY

With Low Osmolality
Increased sodium loss
Increased water retention

With Normal Osmolality
Increased nonsodium cations
  Lithium excess
  Increased γ-globulins—cationic (multiple myeloma)
  Severe hyperkalemia
  Severe hypermagnesemia
  Severe hypercalcemia
Pseudohyponatremia
  Hyperlipidemia
  Hyperproteinemia
  Pseudohyperkalemia as a result of in vitro hemolysis

With High Osmolality
Hyperglycemia
Mannitol infusion

TABLE 13-4. CAUSES OF HYPERNATREMIA

Excess Water Loss
Diabetes insipidus
Renal tubular disorder
Prolonged diarrhea
Profuse sweating
Severe burns

Decreased Water Intake
Older persons
Infants
Mental impairment

Increased Intake or Retention
Hyperaldosteronism
Sodium bicarbonate excess
Dialysis fluid excess

management of fluid administration is critical. Fluid administration and monitoring is required during treatment of the underlying cause of the hyponatremia.

Hypernatremia. *Hypernatremia* (increased serum sodium concentration) results from excess loss of water relative to sodium loss, decreased water intake, or increased sodium intake or retention. Hypernatremia is less commonly seen in hospitalized patients than hyponatremia.[5]

Loss of hypotonic fluid may occur either by the kidney or through profuse sweating, diarrhea, or severe burns.

Hypernatremia may result from loss of water in diabetes insipidus, either because the kidney cannot respond to ADH (nephrogenic diabetes insipidus) or ADH secretion is impaired (central diabetes insipidus). Diabetes insipidus is characterized by copious production of dilute urine (3–20 L/day). Because people with diabetes insipidus drink large volumes of water, hypernatremia usually does not occur unless the thirst mechanism is also impaired. Partial defects of either ADH release or the response to ADH may also occur. In such cases, urine is concentrated to a lesser extent than appropriate to correct the hypernatremia. Excess water loss may also occur in renal tubular disease, such as acute tubular necrosis, in which the tubules become unable to fully concentrate the urine.

The measurement of urine osmolality is necessary to evaluate the cause of hypernatremia. With renal loss of water, the urine osmolality is low or normal. With extrarenal fluid losses, the urine osmolality is increased. Interpretation of the urine osmolality in hypernatremia is shown in Table 13-5.

Water loss through the skin and by breathing (insensible loss) accounts for about 1 L of water loss per day in adults. Any condition that increases water loss, such as fever, burns, diarrhea, or exposure to heat, will increase the likelihood of developing hypernatremia. Commonly, hypernatremia occurs in those persons who may be thirsty but who are unable to ask for or obtain water, such as adults with altered mental status and infants. When urine cannot be fully concentrated (eg, in neonates, young children, older persons, and certain patients with renal insufficiency), a relatively lower urine osmolality may occur.

Chronic hypernatremia in an alert patient is indicative of hypothalamic disease, usually with a defect in the osmoreceptors rather than from a true resetting of the osmostat. A reset osmostat may occur in primary hyperaldosteronism, in which excess aldosterone induces mild hypervolemia that retards ADH release, shifting plasma sodium upward by ~3–5 mmol/L.[1]

Hypernatremia may be from excess ingestion of salt or administration of hypertonic solutions of sodium, such as sodium bicarbonate or hypertonic dialysis solutions. Neonates are especially susceptible to hypernatremia from this cause. In these cases, ADH response is appropriate, resulting in urine osmolality more than 800 mOsm/kg (Table 13-5).

TABLE 13-5. HYPERNATREMIA (150 mmol/L) RELATED TO URINE OSMOLALITY

Urine Osmolality <300 mOsm/kg
Diabetes insipidus (impaired secretion of ADH or kidneys cannot respond to ADH)

Urine Osmolality 300–700 mOsm/kg
Partial defect in ADH release or response to ADH
Osmotic diuresis

Urine Osmolality >700 mOsm/kg
Loss of thirst
Insensible loss of water (breathing, skin)
GI loss of hypotonic fluid
Excess intake of sodium

Symptoms of hypernatremia. Symptoms most commonly involve the central nervous system (CNS) as a result of the hyperosmolar state. These symptoms include altered mental status, lethargy, irritability, restlessness, seizures, muscle twitching, hyperreflexes, fever, nausea or vomiting, difficult respiration, and increased thirst. Serum sodium of more than 160 mmol/L is associated with a mortality rate of 60–75%.[5]

Treatment of hypernatremia. Treatment is directed at correction of the underlying condition that caused the water depletion or sodium retention. The speed of correction depends on the rate with which the condition developed. Hypernatremia must be corrected gradually because too rapid a correction of serious hypernatremia (>160 mmol/L) can induce cerebral edema and death, the maximal rate should be 0.5 mmol/L per hour.[1]

Determination of Sodium

Specimen. Serum, plasma, and urine are all acceptable for sodium measurements. When plasma is used, lithium heparin, ammonium heparin, and lithium oxalate are suitable anticoagulants. Hemolysis does not cause a significant change in serum or plasma values as a result of decreased levels of intracellular sodium. However, with marked hemolysis, levels may be decreased as a result of a dilutional effect.

Whole blood samples may be used with some analyzers. Consult the instrument operation manual for acceptability. The specimen of choice in urine sodium analyses is a 24-hour collection. Sweat is also suitable for analysis. Sweat collection and analysis is discussed in Chapter 27, *Body Fluid Analysis.*

Methods. Through the years, sodium has been measured in various ways, including chemical methods, flame emission spectrophotometry (FES), atomic absorption spectrophotometry (AAS), and ion specific electrodes (ISE). Chemical methods are outdated because of large sample volume requirements and lack of precision. ISE is the most routinely used method in clinical laboratories.

Na⁺ Electrode

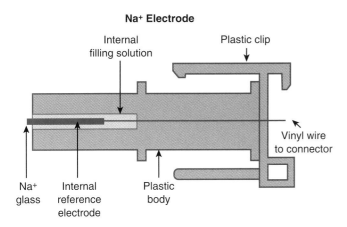

FIGURE 13-2. Diagram of sodium ISE with glass capillary membrane. (Courtesy of Nova Biomedical, Waltham, MA.)

ISE uses a semipermeable membrane to develop a potential produced by having different ion concentrations on either side of the membrane. In this type system, two electrodes are used. One electrode has a constant potential, making it the reference electrode. The difference in potential between the reference and measuring electrodes can be used to calculate the "concentration" of the ion in solution. However, it is the activity of the ion, not the concentration that is being measured (see Chapter 4, *Analytic Techniques and Instrumentation*).

Most analyzers use a glass ion-exchange membrane in its ISE system for sodium measurement (Fig. 13-2). There are two types of ISE measurement, based on sample preparation: direct and indirect. Direct measurement provides an undiluted sample to interact with the ISE membrane. With the indirect method, a diluted sample is used for measurement. There is no significant difference in results, except when samples are hyperlipidemic or hyperproteinemic. Excess lipids or proteins displace plasma water, which leads to a falsely decreased measurement of ionic activity in mmol/L of plasma, whereas the direct method measures in plasma water only. In these cases, direct ISE is more accurate.

One source of error with ISEs is protein buildup on the membrane through continuous use. The protein-coated membranes cause poor selectivity, which results in poor reproducibility of results.

Vitros analyzers (Ortho-Clinical Diagnostics) use a single-use direct ISE system. Each disposable slide contains a reference and measuring electrode (Fig. 13-3). A drop of sample fluid and a drop of reference fluid are si-

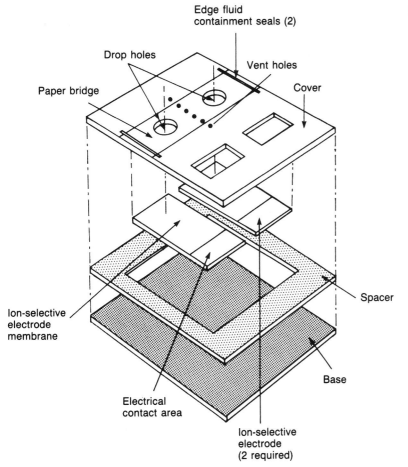

FIGURE 13-3. Schematic diagram of the ISE system for the potentiometric slide on the Vitros. (Courtesy of OCD, a Johnson & Johnson company, Rochester, NY.)

TABLE 13-6. REFERENCE RANGES FOR SODIUM

Serum, plasma	136–145 mmol/L
Urine (24-hour)	40–220 mmol/day, varies with diet
CSF	136–150 mmol/L

multaneously applied to the slide, and the potential difference between the two is measured.[7]

Reference Ranges[3]
See Table 13-6.

Potassium

Potassium is the major intracellular cation in the body, with a concentration 20 times greater inside the cells than outside. Many cellular functions require that the body maintain a low ECF concentration of K^+. As a result, only 2% of the body's total potassium circulates in the plasma. Functions of potassium in the body include regulation of neuromuscular excitability, contraction of the heart, ICF volume, and hydrogen ion concentration.[1]

The potassium ion concentration has a major effect on the contraction of skeletal and cardiac muscles. An elevated plasma potassium decreases the resting membrane potential (RMP) of the cell (the RMP is closer to zero), which decreases the net difference between the cell's resting potential and threshold (action) potential. A lower than normal difference increases cell excitability, leading to muscle weakness. Severe hyperkalemia can ultimately cause a lack of muscle excitability (as a result of a higher RMP than action potential), which may lead to paralysis or a fatal cardiac arrhythmia.[1] Hypokalemia decreases cell excitability by increasing the RMP, often resulting in an arrhythmia or paralysis.[1] The heart may cease to contract in extreme cases of either hyperkalemia or hypokalemia.

Potassium concentration also affects the hydrogen ion concentration in the blood. For example, in hypokalemia (low serum potassium), as potassium ions are lost from the body, sodium and hydrogen ions move into the cell. The hydrogen ion concentration is, therefore, decreased in the ECF, resulting in alkalosis.

Regulation

The kidneys are important in the regulation of potassium balance. Initially, the proximal tubules reabsorb nearly all the potassium. Then, under the influence of aldosterone, additional potassium is secreted into the urine in exchange for sodium in both the distal tubules and the collecting ducts. Thus, the distal nephron is the principal determinant of urinary potassium excretion. Most individuals consume far more potassium than needed; the excess is excreted in the urine but may accumulate to toxic levels if renal failure occurs.

Potassium uptake from the ECF into the cells is important in normalizing an acute rise in plasma K concentration due to an increased K intake. Excess plasma K rapidly enters the cells to normalize plasma K. As the cellular K gradually returns to the plasma, it is removed by urinary excretion. Note that chronic loss of cellular K may result in cellular depletion before there is an appreciable change in the plasma K concentration because excess K is normally excreted in the urine.

Three factors that influence the distribution of potassium between cells and ECF are: (1) potassium loss frequently occurs whenever the NaK ATPase pump is inhibited by conditions such as hypoxia, hypomagnesemia, or digoxin overdose; (2) insulin promotes acute entry of K ions into skeletal muscle and liver by increasing NaK ATPase activity; and (3) catecholamines, such as epinephrine ($\beta2$-stimulator), promote cellular entry of K, whereas propranolol (β-blocker) impairs cellular entry of K. Dietary deficiency or excess is rarely a primary cause of hypokalemia or hyperkalemia. However, with a preexisting condition, dietary deficiency (or excess) can enhance the degree of hypokalemia (or hyperkalemia).

Exercise. Potassium is released from cells during exercise, which may increase plasma K by 0.3–1.2 mmol/L with mild to moderate exercise and by as much as 2–3 mmol/L with exhaustive exercise. These changes are usually reversed after several minutes of rest. Forearm exercise during venipuncture can cause erroneously high plasma K concentrations.[8]

Hyperosmolality. Hyperosmolality, as with uncontrolled diabetes mellitus, causes water to diffuse from the cells, carrying K ions with the water, which leads to gradual depletion of potassium if kidney function is normal.

Cellular Breakdown. Cellular breakdown releases K into the ECF. Examples are severe trauma, tumor lysis syndrome, and massive blood transfusions.

Clinical Applications

Hypokalemia. *Hypokalemia* is a plasma potassium concentration below the lower limit of the reference range. Hypokalemia can occur with GI or urinary loss of potassium or with increased cellular uptake of potassium. Common causes of hypokalemia are shown in Table 13-7. Of these, therapy with thiazide-type diuretics is the most common.[9] GI loss occurs when GI fluid is lost through vomiting, diarrhea, gastric suction, or discharge from an intestinal fistula. Increased K loss in the stool also occurs with certain tumors, malabsorption, cancer therapy (chemotherapy or radiation therapy), and large doses of laxatives.

Renal loss of potassium can result from kidney disorders such as potassium-losing nephritis and renal tubular acidosis (RTA). In RTA, as tubular excretion of H^+ de-

TABLE 13-7. CAUSES OF HYPOKALEMIA

GI Loss
Vomiting
Diarrhea
Gastric suction
Intestinal tumor
Malabsorption
Cancer therapy—chemotherapy, radiation therapy
Large doses of laxatives

Renal Loss
Diuretics—thiazides, mineralocorticoids
Nephritis
Renal tubular acidosis (RTA)
Hyperaldosteronism
Cushing's syndrome
Hypomagnesemia
Acute leukemia

Cellular Shift
Alkalosis
Insulin overdose

Decreased Intake

creases, K excretion increases. Because aldosterone promotes Na retention and K loss, hyperaldosteronism can lead to hypokalemia and metabolic alkalosis.[1] Hypomagnesemia can lead to hypokalemia by promoting urinary loss of potassium. Magnesium deficiency also diminishes the activity of NaK ATPase and enhances the secretion of aldosterone. Effective treatment requires supplementation with both Mg and K.[1] Renal K loss also occurs with acute myelogenous leukemia, acute myelomonocytic leukemia, and acute lymphocytic leukemia.[9] Although reduced dietary intake of K rarely causes hypokalemia in healthy persons, decreased intake may intensify hypokalemia caused by use of diuretics, for example.

Both alkalemia and insulin increase the cellular uptake of potassium. Because alkalemia promotes intracellular loss of H^+ to minimize elevation of intracellular pH, both K and sodium enter cells to preserve electroneutrality. Plasma K decreases by about 0.4 mmol/L per 0.1 unit rise in pH.[1] Insulin promotes the entry of K into skeletal muscle and liver cells. Because insulin therapy can sometimes uncover an underlying hypokalemic state, plasma K should be monitored carefully whenever insulin is administered to susceptible patients.[1] A rare cause of hypokalemia is associated with a blood sample from a leukemic patient with a significantly elevated white blood cell count. The K present in the sample is taken up by the white cells if the sample is left at room temperature for several hours.[9]

Symptoms of hypokalemia. Symptoms (*eg*, weakness, fatigue, and constipation) often become apparent as plasma potassium decreases below 3 mmol/L. Hypokalemia can lead to muscle weakness or paralysis, which can interfere with breathing. The dangers of hypokalemia concern all patients, but especially those with cardiovascular disorders because of an increased risk of arrhythmia, which may cause sudden death in certain patients. Mild hypokalemia (3.0–3.4 mmol/L) is usually asymptomatic.

Treatment of hypokalemia. Treatment typically includes oral KCl replacement of potassium over several days. In some instances, intravenous (IV) replacement may be indicated. In some cases, chronic mild hypokalemia may be corrected simply by including food in the diet with high potassium content, such as dried fruits, nuts, bran cereals, bananas, and orange juice. Plasma electrolytes are monitored as treatment to return K levels to normal occurs.

Hyperkalemia. The most common causes of hyperkalemia are shown in Table 13-8. Patients with *hyperkalemia* often have an underlying disorder, such as renal insufficiency, diabetes mellitus, or metabolic acidosis, that contributes to hyperkalemia.[8] For example, during administration of KCl, a person with renal insufficiency is far more likely to develop hyperkalemia than a person with normal renal function. The most common cause of hyperkalemia in hospitalized patients is due to therapeutic K administration. The risk is greatest with intravenous K replacement.[8]

In healthy persons, an acute oral load of potassium will briefly increase plasma K because most of the absorbed K rapidly moves intracellularly. Normal cellular processes gradually release this excess K back into the plasma, where it is normally removed by renal excretion. Impairment of urinary K excretion is usually associated with chronic hyperkalemia.[1]

If a shift of K from cells into plasma occurs too rapidly to be removed by renal excretion, acute hyperkalemia de-

TABLE 13-8. CAUSES OF HYPERKALEMIA

Decreased Renal Excretion
Acute or chronic renal failure (GFR, <20 mL/minute)
Hypoaldosteronism
Addison's disease
Diuretics

Cellular Shift
Acidosis
Muscle/cellular injury
Chemotherapy
Leukemia
Hemolysis

Increased Intake
Oral or IV potassium replacement therapy

Artifactual
Sample hemolysis
Thrombocytosis
Prolonged tourniquet use or excessive fist clenching

velops. In diabetes mellitus, insulin deficiency promotes cellular loss of K. Hyperglycemia also contributes by producing a hyperosmolar plasma that pulls water and K from cells, promoting further loss of K into the plasma.[1]

In metabolic acidosis, as excess H^+ moves intracellularly to be buffered, K leaves the cell to maintain electroneutrality. Plasma K increases by 0.2–1.7 mmol/L for each 0.1 unit reduction of pH.[1] Because cellular K often becomes depleted in cases of acidosis with hyperkalemia (including diabetic ketoacidosis), treatment with agents such as insulin and bicarbonate can cause a rapid intracellular movement of K, producing severe hypokalemia.

Various drugs may cause hyperkalemia, especially in patients with either renal insufficiency or diabetes mellitus. These drugs include captopril (inhibits angiotensin converting enzyme), nonsteroidal anti-inflammatory agents (inhibit aldosterone), spironolactone (K-sparing diuretic), digoxin (inhibits NaK pump), cyclosporine (inhibits renal response to aldosterone), and heparin therapy (inhibits aldosterone secretion).

Hyperkalemia may result when potassium is released into the ECF during enhanced tissue breakdown or catabolism, especially if renal insufficiency is present. Increased cellular breakdown may be caused by trauma, administration of cytotoxic agents, massive hemolysis, tumor lysis syndrome, and blood transfusions. In banked blood, K is gradually released from erythrocytes during storage, often causing elevated K concentration in plasma supernatant.

Patients on cardiac bypass may develop mild elevations in plasma potassium during warming after surgery because warming causes cellular release of potassium. Hypothermia causes movement of potassium into cells.

Symptoms of hyperkalemia. Hyperkalemia can cause muscle weakness, tingling, numbness, or mental confusion by altering neuromuscular conduction. Muscle weakness does not usually develop until plasma potassium reaches 8 mmol/L.[1]

Hyperkalemia disturbs cardiac conduction, which can lead to cardiac arrhythmias and possible cardiac arrest. Plasma potassium concentrations of 6–7 mmol/L may alter the electrocardiogram, and concentrations more than 10 mmol/L may cause fatal cardiac arrest.[1]

Treatment of hyperkalemia. Treatment should be immediately initiated when serum K is ≥6.0–6.5 mmol/L or if there are ECG changes.[8] To offset the effect of potassium, which lowers the resting potential of myocardial cells, calcium may be given to reduce the threshold potential of myocardial cells. Therefore, calcium provides immediate but short-lived protection to the myocardium against the effects of hyperkalemia. Substances that acutely shift potassium back into cells, such as sodium bicarbonate, glucose, or insulin, may also be administered. Potassium may be quickly removed from the body by use of diuretics (loop), if renal function is adequate, or sodium poly-styrene sulfonate (Kayexalate) enemas, which binds to K secreted in the colon. Hemodialysis can be used if other measures fail.[8] Patients treated with these agents must be monitored carefully to prevent hypokalemia as K moves back into cells or is removed from the body.

Collection of Samples

Proper collection and handling of samples for K analysis is extremely important because there are many causes of artifactual hyperkalemia. First, the coagulation process releases K from platelets, so that serum K may be 0.1–0.5 mmol/L higher than plasma K concentrations.[2] If the patient's platelet count is elevated (thrombocytosis), serum potassium may be further elevated. Second, if a tourniquet is left on the arm too long during blood collection or if patients excessively clench their fists or otherwise exercise their forearms before venipuncture, cells may release potassium into the plasma. The first situation may be avoided by using a heparinized tube to prevent clotting of the specimen and the second by using proper care in the drawing of blood. Third, because storing blood on ice promotes the release of potassium from cells,[10] whole blood samples for potassium determinations should be stored at room temperature (never iced) and analyzed promptly or centrifuged to remove the cells. Fourth, if hemolysis occurs after the blood is drawn, potassium may be falsely elevated—the most common cause of artifactual hyperkalemia.

Determination of Potassium

Specimen. Serum, plasma, and urine may be acceptable for analysis. Hemolysis must be avoided because of the high K^+ content of erythrocytes. Heparin is the anticoagulant of choice. Whereas serum and plasma generally give similar potassium levels, serum reference intervals tend to be slightly higher. Significantly elevated platelet counts may result in the release of potassium during clotting from rupture of these cells, causing a spurious hyperkalemia. In this case, plasma is preferred. Whole blood samples may be used with some analyzers. Consult the instrument's operations manual for acceptability. Urine specimens should be collected over a 24-hour period to eliminate the influence of diurnal variation.

Methods. As with sodium, the current method of choice is ISE. For ISE measurements, a valinomycin membrane is used to selectively bind K^+, causing an impedance change that can be correlated to K^+ concentration. KCl is the inner electrolyte solution.

Reference Ranges[3]
See Table 13-9.

Chloride

Chloride (Cl^-) is the major extracellular anion. Its precise function in the body is not well understood; how-

TABLE 13-9. REFERENCE RANGES FOR POTASSIUM

Plasma, serum	3.4–5.0 mmol/L
Urine (24-hour)	25–125 mmol/day

ever, it is involved in maintaining osmolality, blood volume, and electric neutrality. In most processes, chloride ions shift secondarily to a movement of sodium or bicarbonate ions.

Chloride ingested in the diet is almost completely absorbed by the intestinal tract. Chloride ions are then filtered out by the glomerulus and passively reabsorbed, in conjunction with sodium, by the proximal tubules. Excess chloride is excreted in the urine and sweat. Excessive sweating stimulates aldosterone secretion, which acts on the sweat glands to conserve sodium and chloride.

Chloride maintains electrical neutrality in two ways. First, Na^+ is reabsorbed along with Cl^- in the proximal tubules. In effect, Cl^- acts as the rate-limiting component, in that Na^+ reabsorption is limited by the amount of Cl^- available. Electroneutrality is also maintained by chloride through the *chloride shift*. In this process, carbon dioxide (CO_2) generated by cellular metabolism within the tissue diffuses out into both the plasma and the red cell. In the red cell, CO_2 forms carbonic acid (H_2CO_3), which splits into H^+ and HCO_3^- (bicarbonate). Deoxyhemoglobin buffers H^+, whereas the HCO_3^- diffuses out into the plasma and Cl diffuses into the red cell to maintain the electric balance of the cell (Fig. 13-4).

Clinical Applications

Chloride disorders are often a result of the same causes that disturb Na levels because Cl passively follows Na. There are a few exceptions. *Hyperchloremia* may also occur when there is an excess loss of bicarbonate ion as a result of GI losses, RTA, or metabolic acidosis. *Hypochloremia* may also occur with excessive loss of chloride from prolonged vomiting, diabetic ketoacidosis, aldosterone deficiency, or salt-losing renal diseases such as pyelonephritis. A low serum level of chloride may also be encountered in conditions associated with high serum bicarbonate concentrations, such as compensated respiratory acidosis or metabolic alkalosis.

Determination of Chloride

Specimen. Serum or plasma may be used, with lithium heparin being the anticoagulant of choice. Hemolysis does not cause a significant change in serum or plasma values as a result of decreased levels of intracellular chloride. However, with marked hemolysis, levels may be decreased as a result of a dilutional effect.

Whole blood samples may be used with some analyzers. Consult the instrument's operation manual for acceptability. The specimen of choice in urine chloride analyses is 24-hour collection because of the large diurnal variation. Sweat is also suitable for analysis. Sweat collection and analysis is discussed in Chapter 27, *Body Fluid Analysis*.

Methods. There are several methodologies available for measuring chloride, including ISEs, amperometric-coulometric titration, mercurimetric titration, and colorimetry. The most commonly used is ISE. For ISE mea-

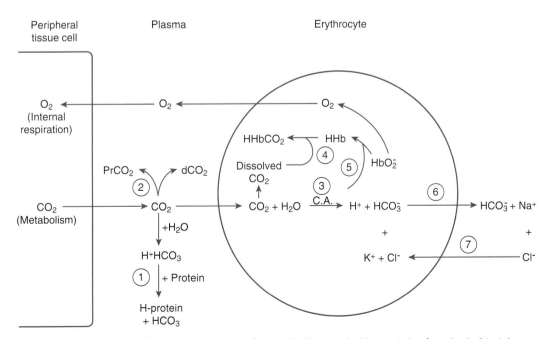

FIGURE 13-4. Chloride shift mechanism. See text for details. (Reprinted with permission from Burtis CA, Ashwood ER, eds. Tietz Textbook of Clinical Chemistry, 2nd ed. Philadelphia: WB Saunders, 1994.)

surement, an ion-exchange membrane is used to selectively bind Cl ions.

Amperometric-coulometric titration is a method using coulometric generation of silver ions (Ag^+), which combine with Cl^- to quantitate the Cl ion concentration.

$$Ag^{+2} + 2Cl^- \rightarrow AgCl_2 \qquad \text{(Eq. 13–2)}$$

When all patient Cl^- ions are bound to Ag^+ ions, excess or free Ag^+ ions are used to indicate the endpoint. As Ag^+ ions accumulate, the coulometric generator and timer are turned off. The elapsed time is used to calculate the concentration of Cl ions in the sample. The Cotlove Chloridometer (Buchler Instruments) uses this principle in chloride analysis.

Reference Ranges[3]
See Table 13-10.

Bicarbonate

Bicarbonate is the second most abundant anion in the ECF. Total CO_2 comprises the bicarbonate ion (HCO_3^-), carbonic acid (H_2CO_3), and dissolved CO_2, with bicarbonate accounting for more than 90% of the total CO_2 at physiologic pH. Because HCO_3^- composes the largest fraction of total CO_2, total CO_2 measurement is indicative of HCO_3^- measurement.

Bicarbonate is the major component of the buffering system in the blood. Carbonic anhydrase in RBC converts CO_2 and H_2O to carbonic acid, which dissociates into H^+ and HCO_3^-.

$$CO_2 + H_2O \xleftrightarrow{CA} H_2CO_3 \xleftrightarrow{CA} H^+ + HCO_3^-$$

$$\text{(Eq. 13–3)}$$

CA, carbonic anhydrase

Bicarbonate diffuses out of the cell in exchange for chloride to maintain ionic charge neutrality within the cell (chloride shift; see Fig. 13-4). This process converts potentially toxic CO_2 in the plasma to an effective buffer: bicarbonate. Bicarbonate buffers excess hydrogen ion by combining with acid, then eventually dissociating into H_2O and CO_2 in the lungs where the acidic gas CO_2 is eliminated.

Regulation

Most of the bicarbonate ion in the kidneys (85%), is reabsorbed by the proximal tubules, with 15% being reabsorbed by the distal tubules. Because tubules are only slightly permeable to bicarbonate, it is usually reab-

TABLE 13-10. REFERENCE RANGES FOR CHLORIDE

Plasma, serum	98–107 mmol/L
Urine (24-hour)	110–250 mmol/day, varies with diet

sorbed as CO_2. This happens as bicarbonate, after filtering into the tubules, combines with hydrogen ions to form carbonic acid, which then dissociates into H_2O and CO_2. The CO_2 readily diffuses back into the ECF. Normally, nearly all the bicarbonate ions are reabsorbed from the tubules, with little lost in the urine. When bicarbonate ions are filtered in excess of hydrogen ions available, almost all excess HCO_3^- flows into the urine.

In alkalosis, with a relative increase in bicarbonate ion compared to CO_2, the kidneys increase excretion of HCO_3^- into the urine, carrying along a cation such as sodium. This loss of HCO_3^- from the body helps correct pH.

Among the responses of the body to acidosis is an increased excretion of H^+ into the urine. In addition, HCO_3 reabsorption is virtually complete, with 90% of the filtered bicarbonate reabsorbed in the proximal tubule and the remainder in the distal tubule.[1]

Clinical Applications

Acid-base imbalances cause changes in bicarbonate and CO_2 levels. A decreased bicarbonate may occur from metabolic acidosis as bicarbonate combines with H^+ to produce CO_2, which is exhaled by the lungs. The typical response to metabolic acidosis is compensation by hyperventilation, which lowers PCO_2. Elevated total CO_2 concentrations occur in metabolic alkalosis as bicarbonate is retained, often with increased PCO_2 as a result of compensation by hypoventilation. Typical causes of metabolic alkalosis include severe vomiting, hypokalemia, and excessive alkali intake.

Determination of Carbon Dioxide

Specimen. This chapter deals specifically with venous serum or plasma determinations. For discussion of arterial and whole blood PCO_2 measurements, refer to Chapter 14, *Blood Gases, pH, and Buffer Systems.*

Serum or lithium heparin plasma is suitable for analysis. Although specimens should be anaerobic for the highest accuracy, many current analyzers (excluding blood gas analyzers) do not permit anaerobic sample handling. In most instances, the sample is capped until the serum or plasma is separated and the sample is analyzed immediately. If the sample is left uncapped before analysis, CO_2 escapes. Levels can decrease by 6 mmol/L per hour.[2]

Carbon dioxide measurements may be obtained in several ways; however, the actual portion of the total CO_2 being measured may vary with the method used. Two common methods are ISE and an enzymatic method.

One type of ISE for measuring total CO_2 uses an acid reagent to convert all the forms of CO_2 to CO_2 gas and is measured by a PCO_2 electrode (Chapter 14, *Blood Gases, pH, and Buffer Systems*).

The enzyme method alkalinizes the sample to convert all forms of CO_2 to HCO_3^-. HCO_3^- is used to carboxylate phosphoenolpyruvate (PEP) in the presence of phosphoenolpyruvate (PEP) carboxylase, which catalyzes the formation of oxaloacetate.

$$\text{Phosphoenolpyruvate} + HCO_3^- \xrightarrow{\text{PEP carboxylate}}$$

$$\text{Oxaloacetate} + H_2PO_4^- \qquad \textbf{(Eq. 13–4)}$$

This is coupled to the following reaction, in which NADH is consumed as a result of the action of malate dehydrogenase (MDH).

$$\text{Oxaloacetate} + NADH + H^+ \xrightarrow{\text{MDH}} \text{Malate} + NAD^+$$

$$\textbf{(Eq. 13–5)}$$

The rate of change in absorbance of NADH is proportional to the concentration of HCO_3^-.

Reference Ranges[3]
Carbon dioxide, venous 22–29 mmol/L (plasma, serum).

Magnesium

Magnesium Physiology
Magnesium (Mg) is the fourth most abundant cation in the body and second most abundant intracellular ion. The average human body (70 kg) contains 1 mole (24 g) of magnesium. Approximately 53% of magnesium in the body is found in bone, 46% in muscle and other organs and soft tissue, and less than 1% is present in serum and red blood cells.[11] Of the Mg present in serum, about one third is bound to protein, primarily albumin. Of the remaining two thirds, 61% exists in the free or ionized state and about 5% is complexed with other ions, such as phosphate and citrate. Similar to calcium, it is the free ion that is physiologically active in the body.[12]

The role of magnesium in the body is widespread. It is an essential cofactor of more than 300 enzymes, including those important in glycolysis, transcellular ion transport, neuromuscular transmission, synthesis of carbohydrates, proteins, lipids, and nucleic acids, and release of and response to certain hormones.

The clinical usefulness of serum magnesium levels has greatly increased in the past 10 years as more information about the analyte has been discovered. The most significant findings are the relationship between abnormal serum magnesium levels and cardiovascular, metabolic, and neuromuscular disorders. Although serum levels may not reflect total body stores of Mg, serum levels are useful in determining acute changes in the ion.

Regulation
Rich sources of Mg in the diet include raw nuts, dry cereal, and "hard" drinking water; other sources include vegetables, meats, fish, and fruit.[11] Processed foods, an ever-increasing part of the average U.S. diet, have low levels of magnesium that may cause an inadequate intake. This in turn may increase the likelihood of Mg deficiency. The small intestine may absorb 20–65% of the dietary magnesium, depending on the need and intake.

The overall regulation of body magnesium is controlled largely by the kidney, which can reabsorb magnesium in deficiency states or readily excrete excess magnesium in overload states. Of the nonprotein-bound Mg that gets filtered by the glomerulus, 25–30% is reabsorbed by the proximal convoluted tubule (PCT), unlike Na, in which 60–75% is absorbed in the PCT. Henle's loop is the major renal regulatory site, where 50–60% of filtered Mg is reabsorbed in the ascending limb. In addition, 2–5% is reabsorbed in the distal convoluted tubule.[13] The renal threshold for magnesium is approximately 0.60–0.85 mmol/L (~1.46–2.07 mg/dL). Because this is close to normal serum concentration, slight excesses of magnesium in serum are rapidly excreted by the kidneys. Normally, only about 6% of filtered Mg is excreted in the urine per day.[11]

Magnesium regulation appears to be related to that of calcium and sodium. Parathyroid hormone (PTH) increases the renal reabsorption of magnesium and enhances the absorption of magnesium in the intestine. However, changes in ionized calcium have a far greater effect on PTH secretion. Aldosterone and thyroxine apparently have the opposite effect of PTH in the kidney, increasing the renal excretion of magnesium.[12]

Clinical Applications
Hypomagnesemia. *Hypomagnesemia* is most frequently observed in hospitalized individuals in intensive care units or those receiving diuretic therapy or digitalis therapy. These patients most likely have an overall tissue depletion of magnesium as a result of severe illness or loss, which leads to low serum levels. Hypomagnesemia is rare in nonhospitalized individuals.[12]

There are many causes of hypomagnesemia; however, it can be grouped into general categories (Table 13-11). Reduced intake is least likely to cause severe deficiencies in the United States. A magnesium-deficient diet as a result of starvation, chronic alcoholism, or Mg-deficient IV therapy can cause a loss of the ion.

Various GI disorders may cause decreased absorption by the intestine, which can result in an excess loss of magnesium via the feces. Malabsorption syndromes; intestinal resection or bypass surgery; nasogastric suction; pancreatitis; and prolonged vomiting, diarrhea, or laxative use may lead to a magnesium deficiency. Neonatal hypomagnesemia has been reported as a result of various surgical procedures. A primary deficiency has also been reported in infants as a result of a selective malabsorption of the ion.[12] A chronic congenital hypomagnesemia with secondary hypocalcemia (autosomal recessive disorder) has also been reported; molecular studies have revealed a specific transport protein defect in the intestine.[14]

TABLE 13-11. CAUSES OF HYPOMAGNESEMIA

Reduced Intake
Poor diet/starvation
Prolonged magnesium-deficient IV therapy
Chronic alcoholism

Decreased Absorption
Malabsorption syndrome
Surgical resection of small intestine
Nasogastric suction
Pancreatitis
Vomiting
Diarrhea
Laxative abuse
Neonatal
Primary
Congenital

Increased Excretion—Renal
Tubular disorder
Glomerulonephritis
Pyelonephritis

Increased Excretion—Endocrine
Hyperparathyroidism
Hyperaldosteronism
Hyperthyroidism
Hypercalcemia
Diabetic ketoacidosis

Increased Excretion—Drug Induced
Diuretics
Antibiotics
Cyclosporin
Digitalis

Miscellaneous
Excess lactation
Pregnancy

Adapted from Polancic JE. Magnesium: metabolism, clinical importance, and analysis. Clin Lab Sci 1991;4(2).

Mg loss due to increased excretion by way of the urine can occur as a result of various renal and endocrine disorders or the effects of certain drugs on the kidneys. Renal tubular disorders and other select renal disorders may result in excess amounts of magnesium being lost through the urine because of decreased tubular reabsorption.

Several endocrine disorders can cause a loss of magnesium. Hyperparathyroidism and hypercalcemia may cause increased renal excretion of magnesium as a result of excess calcium ions. Excess serum sodium levels caused by hyperaldosteronism may also cause increased renal excretion of magnesium. A pseudohypomagnesemia may also be the result of hyperaldosteronism caused by increased water reabsorption. Hyperthyroidism may result in an increased renal excretion of magnesium and may also cause an intracellular shift of the ion. In persons with diabetes, excess urinary loss of

Mg is associated with glycosuria. Hypomagnesemia can aggravate the neuromuscular and vascular complications commonly found in this disease. Some studies have shown a relationship between Mg deficiency and insulin resistance; however, Mg is not thought to play a role in the pathophysiology of diabetes mellitus. The American Diabetes Association has issued a statement regarding dietary intake of magnesium and measurement of serum Mg in patients with diabetes.[15]

Several drugs, including diuretics, gentamicin, cisplatin, and cyclosporine, increase renal loss of magnesium and frequently result in hypomagnesemia. The loop diuretics, such as furosemide, are especially effective in increasing renal loss of Mg. Thiazide diuretics require a longer period of use to cause hypomagnesemia. Cisplatin has a nephrotoxic effect that inhibits the ability of the renal tubule to conserve magnesium. Cyclosporine, an immunosuppressant, severely inhibits the renal tubular reabsorption of magnesium and has many adverse effects, including nephrotoxicity, hypertension, hepatotoxicity, and neurologic symptoms such as seizures and tremors. Cardiac glycosides, such as digoxin and digitalis, can interfere with Mg reabsorption. The resulting hypomagnesemia is a significant finding because the decreased level of Mg can amplify the symptoms of digitalis toxicity.[12]

Excess lactation has been associated with hypomagnesemia as a result of increased use and loss through milk production. Mild deficiencies have been reported in pregnancy, which may cause a hyperexcitable uterus, anxiety, and insomnia.

Symptoms of hypomagnesemia. A patient who is hypomagnesemic may be asymptomatic until serum levels fall below 0.5 mmol/L.[12] A variety of symptoms can occur. The most frequent involve cardiovascular, neuromuscular, psychiatric, and metabolic abnormalities (Table 13-12). The cardiovascular and neuromuscular

TABLE 13-12. SYMPTOMS OF HYPOMAGNESEMIA

Cardiovascular	Psychiatric
Arrhythmia	Depression
Hypertension	Agitation
Digitalis toxicity	Psychosis
Neuromuscular	**Metabolic**
Weakness	Hypokalemia
Cramps	Hypocalcemia
Ataxia	Hypophosphatemia
Tremor	Hyponatremia
Seizure	
Tetany	
Paralysis	
Coma	

Adapted from Polancic JE. Magnesium: metabolism, clinical importance, and analysis. Clin Lab Sci 1991;4(2).

symptoms result primarily from the ATPase enzyme's requirement for Mg. Mg loss leads to decreased intracellular K levels because of a faulty NaK pump (ATPase). This change in cellular RMP causes increased excitability that may lead to cardiac arrhythmias. This condition may also lead to digitalis toxicity.

Muscle contraction also requires magnesium and ATPase for normal calcium uptake following contraction. Normal nerve and muscle cell stimulation requires magnesium to assist with the regulation of acetylcholine, a potent neurotransmitter. Hypomagnesemia can cause a variety of symptoms from weakness to tremors, tetany, paralysis, or coma. The CNS can also be affected, resulting in psychiatric disorders that range from subtle changes to depression or psychosis.

Metabolic disorders are associated with hypomagnesemia. Studies have indicated that approximately 40% of hospitalized patients with hypokalemia are also hypomagnesemic.[13] In addition, 20–30% of patients with hyponatremia, hypocalcemia, or hypophosphatemia are also hypomagnesemic.[13] Mg deficiency can impair PTH release and target tissue response, resulting in hypocalcemia. Replenishing any of these deficient ions alone, often does not remedy the disorder unless magnesium therapy is provided. Mg therapy alone may restore both ion levels to normal; serum levels of the ions must be monitored during treatment.

Treatment of hypomagnesemia. The preferred form of treatment is by oral intake using Mg-lactate, Mg-oxide, or Mg-Cl or an antacid that contains Mg. In severely ill patients, a $MgSO_4$ solution is given parenterally. Before initiation of therapy, renal function must be evaluated to avoid inducing hypermagnesemia during treatment.[13]

Hypermagnesemia. *Hypermagnesemia* is observed less frequently than hypomagnesemia.[12] Causes for elevated serum magnesium levels are summarized in Table 13-13; the most common is renal failure (GFR, <30 mL/min). The most severe elevations are usually a result of the combined effects of decreased renal function and increased intake of commonly prescribed magnesium-containing medications, such as antacids, enemas, or cathartics. Nursing home patients are at greatest risk for this occurrence.[12]

TABLE 13-13. CAUSES OF HYPERMAGNESEMIA

Decreased Excretion
Acute or chronic renal failure
Hypothyroidism
Hypoaldosteronism
Hypopituitarism ($\downarrow$GH)

Increased Intake
Antacids
Enemas
Cathartics
Therapeutic—eclampsia, cardiac arrhythmia

Miscellaneous
Dehydration
Bone carcinoma
Bone metastases

Adapted from Polancic JE. Magnesium: metabolism, clinical importance, and analysis. Clin Lab Sci 1991;4(2).

CASE STUDY 13-2

A 60-year-old man entered the emergency department after 2 days of "not feeling so well." History revealed a myocardial infarction 5 years ago, when he was prescribed digoxin. Two years ago, he was prescribed a diuretic after periodic bouts of edema. An electrocardiogram at time of admission indicated a cardiac arrhythmia. Admitting lab results are shown in Case Study Table 13-2.1.

Questions

1. Because the digoxin level is within the therapeutic range, what may be the cause for the arrhythmia?
2. What is the most likely cause for the hypomagnesemia?
3. What is the most likely cause for the decreased potassium and ionized calcium levels?
4. What type of treatment would be helpful?

CASE STUDY TABLE 13-2.1. LABORATORY RESULTS

Venous Blood

Digoxin: 1.4 ng/mL, therapeutic 0.5–2.2 (1.8 nmol/L, therapeutic 0.6–2.8)
Na^+: 137 mmol/L
K^+: 2.5 mmol/L
Cl^-: 100 mmol/L
HCO^-: 25 mmol/L
Mg^{+2}: 0.4 mmol/L
Ion/free Ca^{+2}: 1.0 mmol/L

Hypermagnesemia has been associated with several endocrine disorders. Thyroxine and growth hormone cause a decrease in tubular reabsorption of Mg, and a deficiency of either hormone may cause a moderate elevation in serum Mg. Adrenal insufficiency may cause a mild elevation as a result of decreased renal excretion of Mg.[12]

$MgSO_4$ may be used therapeutically with preeclampsia, cardiac arrhythmia, or myocardial infarction. Mg is a vasodilator, and can decrease uterine hyperactivity in eclampsic states and increase uterine blood flow. This therapy can lead to maternal hypermagnesemia, as well as neonatal hypermagnesemia due to the immature kidney of the newborn. Premature infants are at greater risk to develop actual symptoms.[12] Studies have shown that IV Mg therapy in myocardial infarction patients may reduce early mortality.[11]

Dehydration can cause a pseudohypermagnesemia, which can be corrected with rehydration. Because of increased bone loss, mild serum magnesium elevations can occur in individuals with multiple myeloma or bone metastases.

Symptoms of hypermagnesemia. Symptoms of hypermagnesemia typically do not occur until the serum level exceeds 1.5 mmol/L.[12] The most frequent symptoms involve cardiovascular, dermatologic, GI, neurologic, neuromuscular, metabolic, and hemostatic abnormalities (Table 13-14). Mild to moderate symptoms, such as hypotension, bradycardia, skin flushing, increased skin temperature, nausea, vomiting, and lethargy may occur when serum levels are 1.5–2.5 mmol/L.[12] Life-threatening symptoms, such as electrocardiogram changes, heart block, asystole, sedation, coma, respiratory depression or arrest, and paralysis, can occur when serum levels reach 5.0 mmol/L.[12]

Elevated Mg levels may inhibit PTH release and target tissue response. This may lead to hypocalcemia and hypercalcuria.[12] Normal hemostasis is a calcium-dependent process that may be inhibited as a result of competition between increased levels of magnesium and calcium ions. Thrombin generation and platelet adhesion are two processes in which interference may occur.[12]

Treatment of hypermagnesemia. Treatment of Mg excess associated with increased intake is to discontinue the source of Mg. Severe symptomatic hypermagnesemia requires immediate supportive therapy for cardiac, neuromuscular, respiratory, or neurologic abnormalities. Patients with renal failure require hemodialysis. Patients with normal renal function may be treated with a diuretic and IV fluid.

Determination of Magnesium

Specimen. Nonhemolyzed serum or lithium heparin plasma may be analyzed. Because the Mg^{2+} concentration inside erythrocytes is 10 times greater than that in the ECF, hemolysis should be avoided and the serum should be separated from the cells as soon as possible. Oxalate, citrate, and ethylenediaminetetraacetic acid (EDTA) anticoagulants are unacceptable because they will bind with magnesium. A 24-hour urine is preferred for analysis because of a diurnal variation in excretion. The urine must be acidified with HCl to avoid precipitation.

Methods. The three most common methods for measuring total serum Mg are colorimetric: calmagite, formazen dye, and methylthymol blue. In the calmagite method, Mg binds with calmagite to form a reddish-violet complex that may be read at 532 nm. In the formazen dye method, Mg binds with the dye to form a colored complex that may be read at 660 nm. In the methylthymol blue method, Mg binds with the chromogen to form a colored complex. Most methods use a calcium shelter to prohibit interference from this divalent cation. The reference method for measuring magnesium is AAS.

Although the measurement of total magnesium concentrations in serum remains the usual diagnostic test for detection of magnesium abnormalities, it has limitations. First, because approximately 25% of magnesium is protein bound, total magnesium may not reflect the physiologically active free ionized magnesium. Second, because magnesium is primarily an intracellular ion, serum concentrations will not necessarily reflect the status of intracellular magnesium. Even when tissue and cellular magnesium is depleted by as much as 20%, serum magnesium concentrations may remain normal.

Reference Ranges[3]
See Table 13-15.

TABLE 13-14. SYMPTOMS OF HYPERMAGNESEMIA

Cardiovascular	Neuromuscular
Hypotension	Decreased reflexes
Bradycardia	Dysarthria
Heart block	Respiratory depression
	Paralysis
Dermatologic	**Metabolic**
Flushing	Hypocalcemia
Warm skin	
GI	**Hemostatic**
Nausea	Decreased thrombin generation
Vomiting	Decreased platelet adhesion
Neurologic	
Lethargy	
Coma	

Adapted from Polancic JE. Magnesium: metabolism, clinical importance, and analysis. Clin Lab Sci 1991;4(2).

TABLE 13-15. REFERENCE RANGE FOR MAGNESIUM

Serum, plasma	0.63–1.0 mmol/L (1.2–2.1 mEq/L)

CASE STUDY 13-3

An 84-year-old nursing home resident was seen in the emergency department with the following symptoms: nausea, vomiting, decreased respiration, hypotension, and low pulse rate (46). Physical exam showed the skin was warm to the touch and flushed. Admission lab data are found in Case Study Table 13-3.1.

Questions

1. What is the most likely cause for the patient's symptoms?

2. What is the most likely cause for the hypermagnesemia?

3. What could be the cause for the hypocalcemia?

CASE STUDY TABLE 13-3.1. LABORATORY RESULTS

		RESULT	REFERENCE RANGE
Serum	Total protein	5.6 g/dL	6.0–8.0 g/dL
	Albumin	3.0 g/dL	3.5–5.0 g/dL
	Total calcium	8.2 g/dL	8.6–10.0 g/dL
	BUN	45 mg/dL	5–20 mg/dL
	Creatinine	2.3 mg/dL	0.7–1.5 mg/dL
	Magnesium	4.0 mmol/L	0.63–1.0 mmol/L
Plasma	Na$^+$	129 mmol/L	136–145 mmol/L
	K$^+$	5.3 mmol/L	3.4–5.0 mmol/L
	Cl$^-$	96 mmol/L	
	HCO$_3^-$	16 mmol/L	

Calcium

Calcium Physiology

In 1883, Ringer showed that calcium was essential for myocardial contraction.[16] While attempting to study how bound and free forms of calcium affected frog heart contraction, McLean and Hastings showed that the ionized/free calcium concentration was proportional to the amplitude of frog heart contraction, whereas protein-bound and citrate-bound calcium had no effect.[17] From this observation, they developed the first assay for ionized/free calcium using isolated frog hearts. Although the method had poor precision by today's standards, the investigators were able to show that blood-ionized calcium was closely regulated and had a mean concentration in humans of about 1.18 mmol/L. Because decreased ionized calcium impairs myocardial function, it is important to maintain ionized calcium at a near normal concentration during surgery and in critically ill patients. Decreased ionized calcium concentrations in blood can cause neuromuscular irritability, which may become clinically apparent as irregular muscle spasms, called *tetany*.

Regulation

Three hormones, PTH, vitamin D, and calcitonin, are known to regulate serum calcium by altering their secretion rate in response to changes in ionized calcium. The actions of these hormones are shown in Figure 13-5.

PTH secretion in blood is stimulated by a decrease in ionized calcium and, conversely, PTH secretion is stopped by an increase in ionized calcium. PTH exerts three major effects on both bone and kidney. In the bone, PTH activates a process known as *bone resorption,* in which activated osteoclasts break down bone and subsequently release calcium into the ECF. In the kidneys, PTH conserves calcium by increasing tubular reabsorption of calcium ions. PTH also stimulates renal production of active vitamin D.

Vitamin D$_3$, a cholecalciferol, is obtained from the diet or exposure of skin to sunlight. Vitamin D$_3$ is then converted in the liver to 25-hydroxycholecalciferol (25-OH-D$_3$), still an inactive form of vitamin D. In the kidney, 25-OH-D$_3$ is specifically hydroxylated to form 1,25-dihydroxycholecalciferol (1,25-[OH]$_2$-D$_3$), the biologically active form. This active form of vitamin D increases calcium absorption in the intestine and enhances the effect of PTH on bone resorption.

Calcitonin, which originates in the medullary cells of the thyroid gland, is secreted when the concentration of calcium in blood increases. Calcitonin exerts its calcium-lowering effect by inhibiting the actions of both PTH and vitamin D. Although calcitonin is apparently not secreted during normal regulation of the ionized calcium concentration in blood, it is secreted in response to a hypercalcemic stimulus.

Distribution

About 99% of calcium in the body is part of bone. The remaining 1% is mostly in the blood and other ECF. Little is in the cytosol of most cells. In fact, the concentration of ionized calcium in blood is 5,000–10,000 times higher than in the cytosol of cardiac or smooth muscle cells. Maintenance of this large gradient is vital to maintain the essential rapid inward flux of calcium ions.

Calcium in blood is distributed among several forms. About 45% circulates as free calcium ions (referred to as

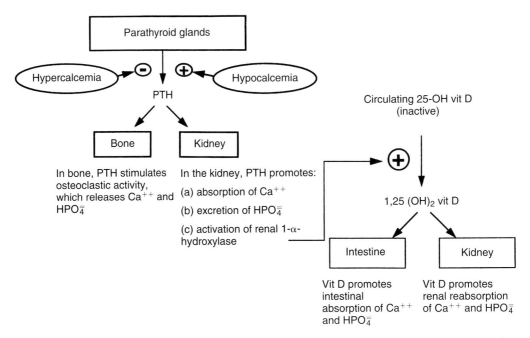

FIGURE 13-5. Hormonal response to hypercalcemia and hypocalcemia. *PTH,* parathyroid hormone; *25-OH vit D,* 25-hydroxy vitamin D; *1,25(OH)₂ vit D,* dihydroxy vitamin D.

ionized calcium), 40% is bound to protein, mostly albumin, and 15% is bound to anions, such as bicarbonate, citrate, phosphate, and lactate. Clearly, this distribution can change in disease. It is noteworthy that concentrations of citrate, bicarbonate, lactate, phosphate, and albumin can change dramatically during surgery or critical care. This why ionized calcium cannot be reliably calculated from total calcium measurements, especially in acutely ill individuals.

Clinical Applications

Tables 13-16 and 13-17 summarize causes of hypocalcemic and hypercalcemic disorders. Although both total

calcium and ionized calcium measurements are available in many laboratories, ionized calcium is usually a more sensitive and specific marker for calcium disorders.

Hypocalcemia. When PTH is not present, as with *primary hypoparathyroidism,* serum calcium levels are not properly regulated. Bone tends to "hang on" to its storage pool and the kidney increases excretion of calcium. Because PTH is also required for normal vitamin D metabolism, the lack of vitamin D's effects also leads to a decreased level of calcium. Parathyroid gland aplasia, destruction, or removal are obvious reasons for primary hypoparathyroidism.

Because hypomagnesemia has become more frequent in hospitalized patients, chronic hypomagnesemia has also become recognized as a frequent cause of *hypocalcemia.* Hypomagnesemia may cause hypocalcemia by

TABLE 13-16. CAUSES OF HYPOCALCEMIA

Primary hypoparathyroidism—glandular aplasia, destruction, or removal
Hypomagnesemia
Hypermagnesemia
Hypoalbuminemia (total calcium only, ionized not affected by)—chronic liver disease, nephrotic syndrome, malnutrition
Acute pancreatitis
Vitamin D deficiency
Renal disease
Rhabdomyolysis
Pseudohypoparathyroidism

TABLE 13-17. CAUSES OF HYPERCALCEMIA

Primary hyperparathyroidism—adenoma or glandular hyperplasia
Hyperthyroidism
Benign familial hypocalciuria
Malignancy
Multiple myeloma
Increased vitamin D
Thiazide diuretics
Prolonged immobilization

three mechanisms: (1) it inhibits the glandular secretion of PTH across the parathyroid gland membrane, (2) it impairs PTH action at its receptor site on bone, and (3) it causes vitamin D resistance.[11] Elevated Mg levels may inhibit PTH release and target tissue response, perhaps leading to hypocalcemia and hypercalciuria.[12]

When total calcium is the only result reported, hypocalcemia can appear with hypoalbuminemia. Common causes are associated with chronic liver disease, nephrotic syndrome, and malnutrition. In general, for each 1 g/dL decrease in serum albumin, there is a 0.2 mmol/L (0.8 mg/dL) decrease in total calcium levels.[18]

About one half of the patients with acute pancreatitis develop hypocalcemia. The most consistent cause appears to be a result of increased intestinal binding of calcium as increased intestinal lipase activity occurs.[18] Vitamin D deficiency and malabsorption can cause decreased absorption, which leads to increased PTH production or secondary hyperparathyroidism.

Patients with renal disease caused by glomerular failure often have altered concentrations of calcium, phosphate, albumin, magnesium, and hydrogen ion (pH). In chronic renal disease, secondary hyperparathyroidism frequently develops as the body tries to compensate for hypocalcemia caused either by hyperphosphatemia (phosphate binds and lowers ionized calcium) or altered vitamin D metabolism. Monitoring and controlling ionized calcium concentrations may avoid problems due to hypocalcemia, such as osteodystrophy, unstable cardiac output or blood pressure, or problems arising from hypercalcemia, such as renal stones and other calcifications. Rhabdomyolysis, as with major crush injury and muscle damage, may cause hypocalcemia as a result of increased phosphate release from cells, which bind to calcium ions.[18]

Pseudohypoparathyroidism is a rare hereditary disorder in which PTH target tissue response is decreased (end organ resistance). PTH production responds normally to loss of calcium; however, without normal response (decreased cAMP [adenosine 3':5'-cyclic phosphate] production), calcium is lost in the urine or remains in the bone storage pool. Patients often have common physical features, including short stature, obesity, shortened metacarpals and metatarsals, and abnormal calcification.

Surgery and intensive care. Because appropriate calcium concentrations promote good cardiac output and maintain adequate blood pressure, the maintenance of a normal ionized calcium concentration in blood is beneficial to patients in either surgery or intensive care. Controlling calcium concentrations may be critical in open heart surgery when the heart is restarted and during liver transplantation because large volumes of citrated blood are given.

Because these patients may receive large amounts of citrate, bicarbonate, calcium salts, or fluids, the greatest

discrepancies between total calcium and ionized calcium concentrations may be seen during major surgical operations. Consequently, ionized calcium measurements are the calcium measurement of greatest clinical value.

Hypocalcemia occurs commonly in critically ill patients, that is, those with sepsis, thermal burns, renal failure, or cardiopulmonary insufficiency. These patients frequently have abnormalities of acid-base regulation and losses of protein and albumin, which are best suited to monitoring calcium status by ionized calcium measurements. Normalization of ionized calcium may have beneficial effects on cardiac output and blood pressure.

Neonatal monitoring. Typically, blood-ionized calcium concentrations in neonates are high at birth and then rapidly decline by 10–20% after 1–3 days. After about 1 week, ionized calcium concentrations in the neonate stabilize at levels slightly higher than in adults.[19]

The concentration of ionized calcium may decrease rapidly in the early neonatal period because the infant may lose calcium rapidly and not readily reabsorb it. Several possible etiologies have been suggested: abnormal PTH and vitamin D metabolism, hypercholesterolemia, hyperphosphatemia, and hypomagnesemia.

Symptoms of hypocalcemia. Neuromuscular irritability and cardiac irregularities are the primary groups of symptoms that occur with hypocalcemia. Neuromuscular symptoms include parasethesia, muscle cramps, tetany, and seizures. Cardiac symptoms may include arrhythmia or heart block. Symptoms usually occur with severe hypocalcemia, in which total calcium levels are below 1.88 mmol/L (7.5 mg/dL).[18]

Treatment of hypocalcemia. Oral or parenteral calcium therapy may occur, depending on the severity of the decreased level and the cause. Vitamin D may sometimes be administered in addition to oral calcium to increase absorption. If hypomagnesemia is a concurrent disorder, magnesium therapy should also be provided.

Hypercalcemia. Primary hyperparathyroidism is the main cause of *hypercalcemia.*[18] *Hyperparathyroidism,* or excess secretion of PTH, may show obvious clinical signs or may be asymptomatic. The patient population seen most frequently with primary hyperparathyroidism is older women.[18] Although either total or ionized calcium measurements are elevated in serious cases, ionized calcium is more frequently elevated in subtle or asymptomatic hyperparathyroidism. In general, ionized calcium measurements are elevated in 90–95% of cases of hyperparathyroidism, whereas total calcium is elevated in 80–85% of cases.

The second leading cause of hypercalcemia is associated with various types of malignancy, with hypercalcemia sometimes being the sole biochemical marker for disease.[18] Many tumors produce PTH-related peptide (PTH-rP), which binds to normal PTH receptors and causes increased calcium levels. Assays to measure PTHrP are available because this abnormal protein is not detected by most PTH assays.

Because of the proximity of the parathyroid gland to the thyroid gland, hyperthyroidism can sometimes cause hyperparathyroidism. A rare, benign, familial hypocaluria has also been reported. Thiazide diuretics increase calcium reabsorption, leading to hypercalcemia. Prolonged immobilization may cause increased bone resorption. Hypercalcemia associated with immobilization is further compounded by renal insufficiency.

Symptoms of hypercalcemia. A mild hypercalcemia (2.62–3.00 mmol/L [10.5–12 mg/dL]) is often asymptomatic.[18] Moderate or severe calcium elevations include neurologic, GI, and renal symptoms. Neurologic symptoms may include mild drowsiness or weakness, depression, lethargy, and coma. GI symptoms may include constipation, nausea, vomiting, anorexia, and peptic ulcer disease. Hypercalcemia may cause renal symptoms of nephrolithiasis and nephrocalcinosis. Hypercalciuria can result in nephrogenic diabetes insipidus, which causes polyuria that results in hypovolemia, which further aggravates the hypercalcemia.[18] Hypercalcemia can also cause symptoms of digitalis toxicity.

Treatment of hypercalcemia. Treatment of hypercalcemia depends on the level of hypercalcemia and the cause. Often people with primary hyperparathyroidism are asymptomatic. Estrogen deficiency in postmenopausal women has been implicated in primary hyperparathyroidism in older women.[18] Often, estrogen replacement therapy reduces calcium levels. Parathyroidectomy may be necessary in some hyperparathyroidic patients. Patients with moderate to severe hypercalcemia are treated to reduce calcium levels. Salt and water intake is encouraged to increase calcium excretion and avoid dehydration, which can compound the hypercalcemia. Thiazide diuretics should be discontinued. Biphosphanates (a derivative of pyrophosphate) are the main drug class used to lower calcium levels, achieved by its binding action to bone, which prevents bone resorption.[18]

Determination of Calcium

Specimen. The preferred specimen for total calcium determinations is either serum or lithium heparin plasma collected without venous stasis. Because anticoagulants such as EDTA or oxalate bind calcium tightly and interfere with measurement, they are unacceptable for use.

The proper collection of samples for ionized calcium measurements requires greater care. Because loss of CO_2 will increase pH, samples must be collected anaerobically. Although heparinized whole blood is the preferred sample, serum from sealed evacuated blood-collection tubes may be used if clotting and centrifugation are done quickly (<30 minutes) and at room temperature. No liquid heparin products should be used. Most heparin anticoagulants (sodium, lithium) partially bind to calcium and lower ionized calcium concentrations. A heparin concentration of 25 IU/mL, for example, decreases ionized calcium by about 3%. Dry heparin products are available titrated with small amounts of Ca or Zn ions or with small amounts of heparin dispersed in an inert "puff" that essentially eliminates the interference by heparin.

For analysis of calcium in urine, an accurately timed urine collection is preferred. The urine should be acidified with 6 mol/L HCl, with approximately 1 mL of the acid added for each 100 mL of urine.

Methods. The two commonly used methods for total calcium analysis use either ortho-cresolphthalein complexone (CPC) or arsenzo III dye to form a complex with calcium. Prior to the dye-binding reaction, calcium is released from its protein carrier and complexes by acidification of the sample. The CPC method uses 8-hydroxyquinoline to prevent magnesium interference. AAS remains the reference method for total calcium, although is rarely used in the clinical setting.

Current commercial analyzers that measure ionized/free calcium use ISEs for this measurement. These systems may use membranes impregnated with special molecules that selectively, but reversibly, bind calcium ions. As calcium ions bind to these membranes, an electric potential develops across the membrane that is proportional to the ionized calcium concentration. A diagram of one such electrode is shown in Figure 13-6.

Reference Ranges[3]

For total calcium, the reference range varies slightly with age. In general, calcium concentrations are higher through adolescence when bone growth is most active. Ionized/free calcium concentrations can change rapidly from day 1 to day 3 of life. Following this, they stabilize at relatively high levels, with a gradual decline through adolescence; see Table 13-18.

Phosphate

Phosphate Physiology

Found everywhere in living cells, phosphate compounds participate in many of the most important biochemical processes. The genetic materials deoxyribonucleic acid (DNA) and ribonucleic acid (RNA) are complex phosphodiesters. Most coenzymes are esters of phosphoric or pyrophosphoric acid. The most important reservoirs of biochemical energy are ATP, creatine phosphate, and phosphoenolpyruvate. Phosphate deficiency can lead to ATP depletion, which is ultimately responsible for many of the clinical symptoms observed in hypophosphatemia.

Alterations in the concentration of 2,3-bisphosphoglycerate (2,3-BPG) in red blood cells affect the affinity of hemoglobin for oxygen, with an increase facilitating the release of oxygen in tissue and a decrease making oxygen bound to hemoglobin less available. By affecting

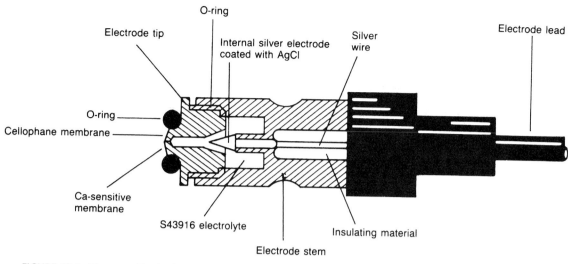

FIGURE 13-6. Diagram of ionized calcium electrode for the ICA ionized calcium analyzer. (Courtesy of Radiometer America, Westlake, OH.)

the formation of 2,3-BPG, the concentration of inorganic phosphate indirectly affects the release of oxygen from hemoglobin.

Understanding the cause of an altered phosphate concentration in the blood is often difficult because transcellular shifts of phosphate are a major cause of hypophosphatemia in blood. That is, an increased shift of phosphate into cells can deplete phosphate in the blood. Once phosphate is taken up by the cell, it remains there to be used in the synthesis of phosphorylated compounds. As these phosphate compounds are metabolized, inorganic phosphate slowly leaks out of the cell into the blood, where it is regulated principally by the kidney.

Regulation

Phosphate in blood may be absorbed in the intestine from dietary sources, released from cells into blood, and lost from bone. In healthy individuals, all these processes are relatively constant and easily regulated by renal excretion or reabsorption of phosphate.

Disturbances to any of these processes can alter phosphate concentrations in the blood; however, the loss of regulation by the kidneys will have the most profound effect. Although other factors, such as vitamin D, calcitonin, growth hormone, and acid-base status, can affect renal regulation of phosphate, the most important factor is PTH, which overall lowers blood concentrations by increasing renal excretion.

Vitamin D acts to increase phosphate in the blood. Vitamin D increases both phosphate absorption in the intestine and phosphate reabsorption in the kidney.

Growth hormone, which helps regulate skeletal growth, can affect circulating concentrations of phosphate. In cases of excessive secretion or administration of growth hormone, phosphate concentrations in the blood may increase because of decreased renal excretion of phosphate.

Distribution

Although the concentration of all phosphate compounds in blood is about 12 mg/dL (3.9 mmol/L), most of that is organic phosphate and only about 3–4 mg/dL is inorganic phosphate. Phosphate is the predominant intracellular anion, with intracellular concentrations varying, depending on the type of cell. About 80% of the total body pool of phosphate is contained in bone, 20% in soft tissues, and less than 1% is active in the serum/plasma.

Clinical Applications

Hypophosphatemia. *Hypophosphatemia* occurs in about 1–5% of hospitalized patients.[20] The incidence of hypophosphatemia increases to 20–40% in patients with the following disorders: diabetic ketoacidosis, chronic

TABLE 13-18. REFERENCE RANGES FOR CALCIUM

TOTAL CALCIUM (SERUM, PLASMA)	
Child	2.20–2.70 mmol/L (8.8–10.8 mg/dL)
Adult	2.15–2.50 mmol/L (8.6–10.0 mg/dL)
IONIZED CALCIUM (SERUM)	
Neonate	1.20–1.48 mmol/L (4.8–5.9 mg/dL)
Child	1.20–1.38 mmol/L (4.8–5.5 mg/dL)
Adult	1.16–1.32 mmol/L (4.6–5.3 mg/dL)
Urine (24-hour)	2.50–7.50 mmol/day (100–300 mg/day), varies with diet

obstructive pulmonary disease (COPD), asthma, malignancy, long-term treatment with total parenteral nutrition (TPN), inflammatory bowel disease, anorexia nervosa, and alcoholism. The incidence increases to 60–80% in ICU patients with sepsis. In addition, hypophosphatemia can also be caused by increased renal excretion, as with hyperparathyroidism, and decreased intestinal absorption, as with vitamin D deficiency or antacid use.[20]

Although most cases are moderate and seldom cause problems, severe hypophosphatemia (<1.0 g/dL or 0.3 mmol/L) requires monitoring and possible replacement therapy. There is a 30% mortality rate in those who are severely hypophosphatemic versus a 15% rate in those with normal or mild hypophosphatemia.[20]

Hyperphosphatemia. Patients at greatest risk for *hyperphosphatemia* are those with acute or chronic renal failure.[20] An increased intake of phosphate or increased release of cellular phosphate may also cause hyperphosphatemia. Because they may not yet have developed mature PTH and vitamin D metabolism, neonates are especially susceptible to hyperphosphatemia caused by increased intake, such as from cow's milk or laxatives. Increased breakdown of cells can sometimes lead to hyperphosphatemia, as with severe infections, intensive exercise, neoplastic disorders, or intravascular hemolysis. Because immature lymphoblasts have about 4 times the phosphate content of mature lymphocytes, patients with lymphoblastic leukemia are especially susceptible to hyperphosphatemia.

Determination of Inorganic Phosphorus

Specimen. Serum or lithium heparin plasma is acceptable for analysis. Oxalate, citrate, or EDTA anticoagulants should not be used because they interfere with the analytic method. Hemolysis should be avoided because of the higher concentrations inside the red cells. Circulating phosphate levels are subject to circadian rhythm, with highest levels in late morning and lowest in the evening. Urine analysis for phosphate requires a 24-hour sample collection because of significant diurnal variations.

Methods. Most of the current methods for phosphorus determination involve the formation of an ammonium phosphomolybdate complex. This colorless complex can be measured by ultraviolet absorption at 340 nm or can be reduced to form molybdenum blue, a stable blue chromophore, which is read between 600 and 700 nm.

Reference Ranges

Phosphate values vary with age. Divided into age groups, the ranges are shown in Table 13-19.

Lactate

Lactate Biochemistry and Physiology

Lactate is a by-product of an emergency mechanism that produces a small amount of ATP when oxygen delivery is

TABLE 13-19. REFERENCE RANGES FOR PHOSPHATE

SERUM, PLASMA	
Neonate	1.45–2.91 mmol/L (4.5–9.0 mg/dL)
Child	1.45–1.78 mmol/L (4.5–5.5 mg/dL)
Adult	0.87–1.45 mmol/L (2.7–4.5 mg/dL)
Urine (24-hour)	13–42 mmol/day (0.4–1.3 g/day)

severely diminished. Pyruvate is the normal end product of glucose metabolism (glycolysis). The conversion of pyruvate to lactate is activated when a deficiency of oxygen leads to an accumulation of excess NADH (Fig. 13-7). Normally, sufficient oxygen maintains a favorably high ratio of NAD to NADH. Under these conditions, pyruvate is converted to acetyl-coenzyme A (CoA), which enters the citric acid cycle and produces 38 moles of ATP for each mole of glucose oxidized. However, under hypoxic conditions, acetyl-CoA formation does not occur and NADH accumulates, favoring the conversion of pyruvate to lactate through anaerobic metabolism. As a result, only 2 moles ATP are produced for each mole of glucose metabolized to lactate, with the excess lactate released into the blood. This release of lactate into blood has clinical importance because the accumulation of excess lactate in blood is an early, sensitive, and quantitative indicator of the severity of oxygen deprivation (Fig. 13-8).

Regulation

Because lactate is a by-product of anaerobic metabolism, it is not specifically regulated, as with potassium or calcium, for example. As oxygen delivery decreases below a critical level, blood lactate concentrations rise rapidly and indicate tissue hypoxia earlier than pH. The liver is the major organ for removing lactate by converting lactate back to glucose by a process called *gluconeogenesis.*

Clinical Applications

Measurements of blood lactate are useful for metabolic monitoring in critically ill patients, for indicating the severity of the illness, and for objectively determining patient prognosis.

There are two types of lactic acidosis. Type A is associated with hypoxic conditions, such as shock, myocardial infarction, severe congestive heart failure, pulmonary edema, or severe blood loss. Type B is of metabolic origin, such as with diabetes mellitus, severe infection, leukemia, liver or renal disease, and toxins (ethanol, methanol, or salicylate poisoning).

Determination of Lactate

Specimen Handling. Special care should be practiced when collecting and handling specimens for lactate analysis. Ideally, a tourniquet should be not be used because venous stasis will increase lactate levels. If a tourniquet is

Aerobic Metabolism

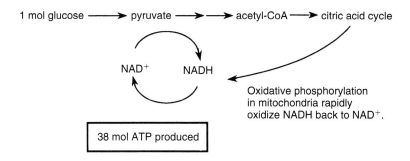

Anaerobic Metabolism

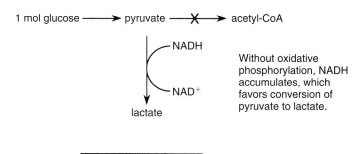

FIGURE 13-7. Aerobic versus anaerobic metabolism of glucose.

used, blood should be collected immediately and the patient should not exercise the hand before or during collection.[10] After sample collection, glucose is converted to lactose by way of anaerobic glycolysis and should be prevented. Heparinized blood may be used but must be delivered on ice and the plasma must be quickly separated. Iodoacetate or fluoride, which inhibit glycolysis without affecting coagulation, are usually satisfactory additives, but the specific method directions must be consulted.

Methods. Although lactate is a sensitive indicator of inadequate tissue oxygenation, the use of blood lactate measurements has been hindered because older methods were slow and laborious. Other means of following perfusion or oxygenation have been used, such as in-

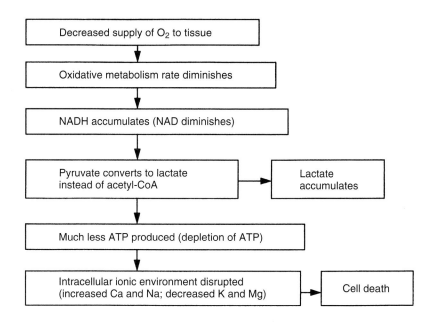

FIGURE 13-8. Metabolic effects of hypoxia, leading to cell death.

TABLE 13-20. REFERENCE RANGES FOR LACTATE

ENZYMATIC METHOD, PLASMA	
Venous	0.5–2.2 mmol/L (4.5–19.8 mg/dL)
Arterial	0.5–1.6 mmol/L (4.5–14.4 mg/dL)
CSF	1.1–2.4 mmol/L (10–22 mg/dL)

dwelling catheters that measure blood flow, pulse oximeters, base-excess determinations, and measurements of oxygen consumption (VO_2). Current enzymatic methods make lactate determination readily available.

The most commonly used enzymatic method uses lactate oxidase to produce pyruvate and H_2O_2.

$$\text{Lactate} + O_2 \xrightarrow{\text{Lactate oxidase}} \text{pyruvate} + H_2O_2 \quad \textbf{(Eq. 13–6)}$$

One of two couple reactions may then be used. Peroxidase may be used to produce a colored chromogen from H_2O_2.

$$H_2O_2 + \text{H donor} + \text{chromogen} \xrightarrow{\text{Peroxidase}}$$
$$\text{colored dye} + 2H_2O \quad \textbf{(Eq. 13–7)}$$

Reference Ranges[5]
See Table 13-20.

ANION GAP

Routine measurement of electrolytes usually involves only Na^+, K^+, Cl^-, and HCO_3^- (as total CO_2). These values may be used to approximate the *anion gap (AG)*, which is the difference between unmeasured anions and unmeasured cations. There is never a "gap" between total cationic charges and anionic charges. The AG is created by the concentration difference between commonly measured cations (Na + K) and commonly measured anions (Cl + HCO_3), as shown in Figure 13-9. AG is useful in indicating an increase in one or more of the unmeasured anions in the serum and also as a form of quality control for the analyzer used to measure these electrolytes. Consistently abnormal anion gaps in serum from healthy persons may indicate an instrument problem.

There are two commonly used methods for calculating the anion gap. The first equation is

$$AG = Na^+ - (Cl^- + HCO_3^-) \quad \textbf{(Eq. 13–8)}$$

It is equivalent to unmeasured anions minus the unmeasured cations in this way:

$$AG = (\text{protein} + \text{organic acids} +$$
$$PO_4^- + 2SO_4^{2-}) - (K^+ + 2Ca^{+2} + Mg^{+2}) \quad \textbf{(Eq. 13–9)}$$

The reference range for the AG using this calculation is 7–16 mmol/L.[3] The second calculation method is

$$AG = (Na^+ + K^+) - (Cl^- + HCO_3^-) \quad \textbf{(Eq. 13–10)}$$

It has a reference range of 10–20 mmol/L.[3]

An elevated anion gap may be caused by uremia/renal failure, which leads to PO_4^- and SO_4^{2-} retention; ketoacidosis, as seen in cases of starvation or diabetes; methanol, ethanol, ethylene glycol poisoning, or salicylate; lactic acidosis; hypernatremia; and instrument error.

CASE STUDY 13-4

Consider the following laboratory results from three adult patients:

Questions

1. Which set of laboratory results (Case A, B, or C) is most likely associated with each of the following diagnoses:
   - Primary hyperparathyroidism
   - Malignancy
   - Hypomagnesemic hypocalcemia

CASE STUDY TABLE 13-4.1. LABORATORY RESULTS

			REFERENCE RANGES		
CASE	ION Ca^{+2} 1.16–1.32 mmol/L	TOTAL Mg^{+2} 0.63–1.0 mmol/L	PO_4^- 0.87–1.45 mmol/L	HEMATOCRIT 35–45%	INTACT PARATHYROID HORMONE 13–64 ng/L
A	1.44	0.90	0.85	42	100
B	1.08	0.50	0.90	40	25
C	1.70	0.98	1.43	30	12

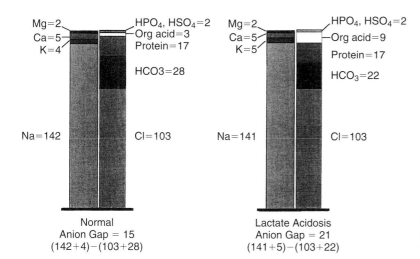

FIGURE 13-9. Demonstration of anion gap from concentrations of anions and cations in normal state and in lactate acidosis.

Low anion gap values are rare but may be seen with hypoalbuminemia (decrease in unmeasured anions) or severe hypercalcemia (increase in unmeasured cations).

ELECTROLYTES AND RENAL FUNCTION

The kidney is central to the regulation and conservation of electrolytes in the body. For a review of kidney structure, refer to Figure 13-10 and Chapter 24, *Renal Function*. The following is a summary of electrolyte excretion and conservation in a healthy individual:

1. Glomerulus: This portion of the nephron acts as a filter, retaining large proteins and protein-bound constituents while most other plasma constituents pass into the filtrate. The concentrations in the filtered plasma should be approximately equal to ECF without protein.
2. Renal tubules:
   a. Phosphate reabsorption is inhibited by PTH and increased by 1,25-dihydroxycholecalciferol. Excretion of PO_4 is stimulated by calcitonin.
   b. Calcium is reabsorbed under the influence of PTH and 1,25-dihydroxycholecalciferol. Calcitonin stimulates excretion of calcium.
   c. Magnesium reabsorption occurs largely in the thick ascending limb of Henle's loop.
   d. Sodium reabsorption can occur through three mechanisms:

   Approximately 70% of the sodium in the filtrate is reabsorbed in the proximal tubules by iso-osmotic reabsorption. It is limited, however, by the availability of chloride to maintain electrical neutrality.

   Sodium is reabsorbed in exchange for H^+. This reaction is linked with HCO_3^- and depends on carbonic anhydrase.

   Stimulated by aldosterone, Na^+ is reabsorbed in exchange for K^+ in the distal tubules. (H^+ competes with K^+ for this exchange.)

   e. Chloride is reabsorbed, in part, by passive transport in the proximal tubule along the concentration gradient created by Na^+.
   f. Potassium is reabsorbed by two mechanisms:
      • Active reabsorption in the proximal tubule almost completely conserves K^+.
      • Exchange with Na^+ is stimulated by aldosterone. H^+ competes with K^+ for this exchange.

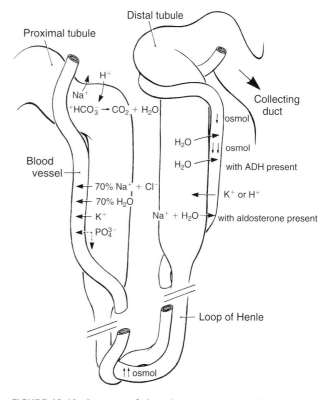

FIGURE 13-10. Summary of electrolyte movements in the renal tubules.

CASE STUDY 13-5

A 15-year-old girl in a coma was brought to the emergency department by her parents. She has diabetes and has been insulin-dependent for 7 years. Her parents stated that there have been several episodes of hypoglycemia and ketoacidosis in the past, and that their daughter has often been "too busy" to take her insulin injections. The laboratory results obtained on admission are shown in Case Study Table 13-5.1.

Questions

1. What is the diagnosis?

2. Calculate the anion gap. What is the cause of the anion gap result in this patient?

3. Why are chloride and bicarbonate decreased? What is the significance of the elevated potassium value?

4. What is the significance of the plasma osmolality?

CASE STUDY TABLE 13-5.1. LABORATORY RESULTS

		RESULT	REFERENCE RANGE
Venous blood	Sodium	145 mmol/L	136–145 mmol/L
	Potassium	5.8 mmol/L	3.4–5.0 mmol/L
	Chloride	87 mmol/L	98–107 mmol/L
	Bicarbonate	8 mmol/L	22–29 mmol/L
	Glucose	1050 mg/dL	70–110 mg/dL
	Urea nitrogen	35 mg/dL	7–18 mg/dL
	Creatinine	1.3 mg/dL	0.5–1.3 mg/dL
	Lactate	5 mmol/L	0.5–2.2 mmol/L
	Osmolality	385 mOsmol/kg	275–295 mOsmol/kg
Arterial blood	pH	7.11	7.35–7.45
	PO_2	98 mm Hg	83–100 mm Hg
	PCO_2	20 mm Hg	35–45 mm Hg
Urine		Normal	
	Glucose	4+	Negative
	Ketones	4+	Negative

g. Bicarbonate is recovered from the glomerular filtrate and converted to CO_2 when H^+ is excreted in the urine.

Henle's loop: With normal ADH function, it creates an osmotic gradient that enables water reabsorption to be increased or decreased in response to body fluid changes in osmolality.

Collecting ducts: Also under ADH influence, this is where final adjustment of water excretion is made.

SUMMARY

Electrolytes are ions capable of carrying an electric charge. They are classified as anions or cations based on the type of charge they carry. Anions have a negative charge and move toward the anode; cations have a positive charge and migrate toward the cathode. Electrolytes are essential for numerous processes in the body, including volume and osmotic regulation, myocardial rhythm and contractility, enzyme activation, regulation of ATPase ion pumps, acid-base balance, blood coagulation, neuromuscular excitability, and the production and use of ATP from glucose. The electrolytes discussed in this chapter were sodium, potassium, chloride, bicarbonate, magnesium, calcium, phosphate, and lactate. This chapter also discussed the metabolic physiology and regulation of each electrolyte, as well as the commonly used methods of assessment. Regulation of electrolyte concentrations in the narrow physiologic ranges is primarily accomplished by the kidneys.

REVIEW QUESTIONS

1. What is the major intracellular cation?
   a. Calcium
   b. Magnesium
   c. Sodium
   d. Potassium

2. What is the major extracellular cation?
   a. Chloride
   b. Sodium
   c. Magnesium
   d. Calcium

3. Osmolality can be defined as a measure of the concentration of a solution based on the:
   a. number of ionic particles present.
   b. number and size of the dissolved particles.
   c. number of dissolved particles.
   d. density of the dissolved particles.

4. Hyponatremia may be caused by each of the following EXCEPT:
   a. hypomagnesemia.
   b. aldosterone deficiency.
   c. prolonged vomiting or diarrhea.
   d. acute or chronic renal failure.

5. Hypokalemia may be caused by each of the following EXCEPT:
   a. acidosis.
   b. prolonged vomiting or diarrhea.
   c. hypomagnesemia.
   d. hyperaldosteronism.

6. Hyperkalemia may be caused by each of the following EXCEPT:
   a. acute or chronic renal failure.
   b. hypoaldosteronism.
   c. alkalosis.
   d. sample hemolysis.

7. The main difference between a direct and indirect ISE is:
   a. the type of membrane that is used.
   b. that direct ISEs use a reference electrode, whereas indirect ISEs do not.
   c. sample is diluted in the indirect method, not in the direct method.
   d. whole blood samples can be measured with the direct method and not with the indirect method.

8. Which method of analysis will provide the most accurate electrolyte results if a grossly lipemic sample is used?
   a. Indirect ISE
   b. Direct ISE
   c. Flame-emission photometry
   d. Atomic absorption

9. The most frequent cause of hypermagnesemia is due to:
   a. increased intake.
   b. hypoaldosteronism.
   c. acidosis.
   d. renal failure.

10. A hemolyzed sample will cause falsely increased levels of each of the following EXCEPT:
    a. potassium.
    b. sodium.
    c. phosphate.
    d. magnesium.

REFERENCES

1. Rose BD, ed. Clinical Physiology of Acid-Base and Electrolyte Disorders, 5th ed. New York: McGraw-Hill, 2001:163–228, 241–257, 372–402, 696–793, 836–930.
2. Burtis CA, Ashwood ER, eds. Tietz Textbook of Clinical Chemistry. Philadelphia: WB Saunders, 1999:1058, 1066–1068.
3. Tietz NW, ed. Clinical Guide to Laboratory Tests. Philadelphia: WB Saunders, 1995:56, 100–105, 110, 124–126, 418, 456–458, 486, 502–506, 562–564.
4. Oh MS. Pathogenesis and diagnosis of hyponatremia. Nephron 2002;92(Suppl. 1):2–8.
5. Kumar S, Tomas B. Sodium. Lancet 1998;352:220–228.
6. Crook M. The investigation and management of severe hyponatremia. J Clin Pathol 2002;55:883.
7. Vitros Na+ package insert, Version 2.0. Rochester, NY: Ortho-Clinical Diagnostics, 2003.
8. Gennari FJ. Disorders of potassium homeostasis: hypokalemia and hyperkalemia. Crit Care Clin 2002;18:273–288.
9. Gennari FJ. Hypokalemia. N Engl J Med 1998;339(7):451–458.
10. Burtis CA, Ashwood ER, eds. Tietz Fundamentals of Clinical Chemistry. Philadelphia: WB Saunders, 2001:496, 451.
11. Elin RJ. Magnesium: The fifth but forgotten electrolyte. Am J Clin Pathol 1994;102(5):616–622.
12. Polancic JE. Magnesium: metabolism, clinical importance, and analysis. Clin Lab Sci 1991;4(2):105–109.
13. Whang R. Clinical disorders of magnesium metabolism. Comp Ther 1997;23(3):168–173.

14. Schlingman KP, Weber S, et al. Hypomagnesemia with secondary hypocalcemia is caused by mutations in TRPM6, a new member of the TRPM gene family. Nat Genet 2002;31:166–170.

15. Whang R, Sims G. Magnesium and potassium supplementation in the prevention of diabetic vascular disease. Med Hypoth 2000;55:263–265.

16. Ringer S. A further contribution regarding the influence of different constituents of blood on contractions of the heart. J Physiol 1883;4:29.

17. McLean FC, Hastings AB. A biological method for estimation of calcium ion concentration. J Biol Chem 1934;107:337.

18. Bushinsky DA, Monk RD. Calcium. Lancet 1998;352:23.

19. Wandrup J. Critical analytical and clinical aspects of ionized calcium in neonates. Clin Chem 1989;35:2027.

20. Shiber JR, Mattu A. Serum phosphate abnormalities in the emergency department. J Emerg Med 2002;23:395–400.

Blood Gases, pH, and Buffer Systems

Sharon S. Ehrmeyer, Ronald H. Laessig, John J. Ancy

OBJECTIVES

Upon completion of this chapter, the clinical laboratorian should be able to:
- Describe the principles involved in the measurement of pH, PCO_2, PO_2, and the various hemoglobin species.
- Outline the interrelationship of the buffering mechanisms of bicarbonate, carbonic acid, and hemoglobin.
- Explain the clinical significance of the following pH and blood gas parameters: pH, PCO_2, PO_2, actual bicarbonate, carbonic acid, base excess, oxygen saturation, fractional oxyhemoglobin, hemoglobin oxygen (binding) capacity, oxygen content, and total CO_2.
- Determine whether data are normal or represent metabolic or respiratory acidosis or metabolic or respiratory alkalosis using the Henderson-Hasselbalch equation and blood gas data. Identify whether the data represent uncompensated or compensated conditions.
- Identify some common causes of nonrespiratory acidosis and alkalosis, respiratory acidosis and alkalosis, and mixed abnormalities. State how the body attempts to compensate (kidney and lungs) for the various conditions.

- Describe the significance of the hemoglobin–oxygen dissociation curve and the impact of pH, 2,3-diphosphoglycerate (2,3-DPG), temperature, pH, and PCO_2 on its shape and release of O_2 to the tissues.
- Discuss problems and precautions in collecting and handling samples for pH and blood gas analysis. Include syringes, anticoagulants, mixing, icing, and capillary and venous samples as well as arterial samples in the discussion.
- Describe approaches to quality assurance, including quality control (commercial liquid controls, tonometry, proficiency testing, and delta checks) to assess analytic quality.
- Discuss the reasons for possible discrepancies, given oxygen saturation data calculated by the blood gas analyzer and measured by the co-oximeter.
- Calculate partial pressures for PCO_2 and PO_2 for various percentages of carbon dioxide and oxygen. In doing these calculations, account for the barometric pressure and vapor pressure of water.

KEY TERMS

Acidemia	Analytic error	Fractional	Hypoxemia
Acidosis	Base excess	oxyhemoglobin	Oxygen saturation
Alkalemia	Compensation	Hypercarbia	Preanalytic error
Alkalosis	FiO_2	Hypocarbia	

An important aspect of clinical biochemistry is information on a patient's acid-base balance and blood gas homeostasis. These data often are used to assess patients in life-threatening situations. Because the test parameters are interrelated, test sites are expected to provide panels of tests frequently supplemented with calculated parameters. Focusing on only one test result can be misleading.

This chapter discusses exchange of gases, carbon dioxide and oxygen, together with the body's mechanisms to maintain acid-base balance. The interpretation of data, from measurement of pH and other blood gas parameters, and the techniques and instrumentation used in these measurements are also described. Preanalytic considerations—sample collection and handling—that greatly affect the quality of test results are addressed. Quality assurance approaches to blood gas analysis also are presented.

DEFINITIONS: ACID, BASE, BUFFER

A discussion of acid-base balance requires a review of several basic concepts: acid, base, buffer, pH, and pK, and the principles of equilibrium and the law of mass action.

An *acid* is a substance that can yield a hydrogen ion (H^+) or hydronium ion when dissolved in water. A *base* is a substance that can yield hydroxyl ions (OH^-). The relative strengths of acids and bases, their ability to dissociate in water, are described by their dissociation constant (also ionization constant K value). Tables can be found in most biochemistry texts. The pK, defined as the negative log of the ionization constant, is also the pH in which the protonated and unprotonated forms are present in equal concentrations. Strong acids have pK values of less than 3.0, whereas strong bases have pK values greater than 9.0. For acids, raising the pH above the pK will cause the acid to dissociate and yield a H^+. For bases, lowering the pH below the pK will cause the base to release OH^-. Many species have more than one pK, meaning they can accept or donate more than one H^+.

A *buffer,* the combination of a weak acid or weak base and its salt, is a system that resists changes in pH. The effectiveness of a buffer depends on the pK of the buffering system and the pH of the environment in which it is placed. In plasma, the bicarbonate–carbonic acid system, having a pK of 6.1, is one of the principal buffers.

$$H_2CO_3 \leftrightarrow HCO_3^- + H^+$$

Carbonic   Bicarbonate
acid

(Eq. 14–1)

The reference value for blood plasma pH is 7.40. Weisberg cited an example to demonstrate the effectiveness of the blood buffers.[1] If the pH of 100 mL of distilled water is 7.35 and one drop of 0.05 N HCl is added, the pH will change to 7.00. To change 100 mL of normal blood from a pH of 7.35 to a pH of 7.00, approximately 25 mL of 0.05 N HCl is needed. With 5.5 L of blood in the average body, more than 1300 mL of HCl would be required to make this same change in pH.

ACID-BASE BALANCE

Maintenance of H^+

The normal concentration of H^+ in the extracellular body fluid ranges from 36 to 44 nmol/L (pH 7.34 to pH 7.44); however, through metabolism, the body produces much greater quantities of H^+. Through exquisite mechanisms that involve the lungs and kidneys, the body controls and excretes H^+ in order to maintain pH homeostasis. Any H^+ value outside this range will cause alterations in the rates of chemical reactions within the cell and affect the many metabolic processes of the body and can lead to alterations in consciousness, neuromuscular irritability, tetany, coma, and death.

The logarithmic pH scale expresses H^+ concentration (c is concentration):

$$pH = \log\frac{1}{cH^+} = -\log cH^+ \qquad \text{(Eq. 14–2)}$$

The reference value for arterial blood pH is 7.40 and is equivalent to an H^+ concentration of 40 nmol/L. Because pH is the negative log of the cH^+, an increase in H^+ concentration decreases the pH, whereas a decrease in H^+ concentration increases the pH. A pH below the reference range (<7.34) is referred to as *acidosis,* whereas a pH above the reference range (>7.44) is referred to as *alkalosis.* Technically, the suffix *-osis* refers to a process in the body; the suffix *-emia* refers to the corresponding state in blood (*-osis* is the cause of the *-emia*).

The arterial pH is controlled by systems that regulate the production and retention of acids and bases. These include buffers, the respiratory center and lungs, and the kidneys.

Buffer Systems: Regulation of H^+

The body's first line of defense against extreme changes in H^+ concentration is the buffer systems present in all body fluids. All buffers consist of a weak acid, such as carbonic acid (H_2CO_3), and its salt or conjugate base, bicarbonate (HCO_3^-), for the bicarbonate–carbonic acid buffer system. H_2CO_3 is a weak acid because it does not completely dissociate into H^+ and HCO_3^-. (In contrast, a strong acid, such as HCl, completely dissociates into H^+ and Cl^- in solution.) When an acid is added to the bicarbonate–carbonic acid system, the HCO_3^- will combine with the H^+ from the acid to form H_2CO_3. When a base is added, H_2CO_3 will combine with the OH^- group to form H_2O and HCO_3^-. In both cases, there is a smaller change in pH than would result from adding the acid or base to an unbuffered solution.

Although the bicarbonate–carbonic acid system has low buffering capacity, it still is an important buffer for three reasons: (1) H_2CO_3 dissociates into CO_2 and H_2O, allowing CO_2 to be eliminated by the lungs and disposing of H^+ as water; (2) changes in CO_2 modify the ventilation (respiratory) rate; and (3) HCO_3^- concentration can be altered by the kidneys. In addition, this buffering system immediately counters the effects of fixed nonvolatile acids (H^+A^-) by binding the dissociated hydrogen ion ($H^+A^- + HCO_3^- = H_2CO_3 + A^-$). The resultant H_2CO_3 then dissociates, and the H^+ is neutralized by the buffering capacity of hemoglobin. Figure 14-1 shows the interrelationship of hemoglobin in the red blood cells and the H^+ from the bicarbonate buffering system.

Other buffers also are important. The phosphate buffer system ($HPO_4^{-2} - H_2PO_4^-$) plays a role in plasma and red blood cells and is involved in the exchange of sodium ion in the urine H^+ filtrate. Plasma protein, especially the imidazole groups of histidine, also forms an important buffer system in plasma. Most circulating proteins have a net negative charge and are capable of binding H^+.

The lungs and kidneys play important roles in regulating blood pH. The interrelationship of the lungs and kidneys in maintaining pH is depicted with the Henderson-Hasselbalch equation (Equation 14-4). The numerator (HCO_3^-) denotes kidney function, whereas the denominator (PCO_2, which represents H_2CO_3) denotes lung function. The lungs regulate pH through retention or elimination of CO_2 by changing the rate and volume of ventilation. The kidneys regulate pH by excreting acid, primarily in the ammonium ion, and by reclaiming HCO_3^- from the glomerular filtrate.

Regulation of Acid-Base Balance: Lungs and Kidneys

Carbon dioxide, the end product of most aerobic metabolic processes, easily diffuses out of the tissue where it is produced and into the plasma and red cells in the surrounding capillaries. In plasma, a small amount of CO_2 is physically dissolved or combined with proteins to form carbamino compounds. Most of the CO_2 combines with H_2O to form H_2CO_3, which quickly dissociates into H^+ and HCO_3^- (Fig. 14-1). The reaction is accelerated by the enzyme carbonic anhydrase found in the red cell membrane. The dissociation of H_2CO_3 causes the HCO_3^- concentration to increase in the red cells and diffuse into the plasma. To maintain electroneutrality (the same number of positively and negatively charged ions on each side of the red cell membrane), chloride diffuses into the cell. This is known as the *chloride shift*. Plasma proteins and plasma buffers combine with the freed H^+ to maintain a stable pH.

In the lungs, the process is reversed. Inspired O_2 diffuses from the alveoli into the blood and is bound to hemoglobin, forming oxyhemoglobin (O_2Hb). The H^+ that was carried on the (reduced) hemoglobin in the venous blood is released to recombine with HCO_3^- to form H_2CO_3, which dissociates into H_2O and CO_2. The CO_2 diffuses into the alveoli and is eliminated through ventilation. The net effect of the interaction of these two buffering systems is a minimal change in H^+ concentration between the venous and arterial circulation. When the lungs do not remove CO_2 at the rate of its production (as a result of decreased ventilation or disease), it accumulates in the blood, causing an increase in H^+ concentration. If, however, CO_2 removal is faster than production (hyperventilation), the H^+ concentration will be decreased. Consequently, ventilation affects the pH of the blood. A change in the H^+ concentration of blood that results from nonrespiratory disturbances causes the respiratory center to respond by altering the rate of ventilation in an effort to restore the blood pH to normal. The lungs, by responding within seconds, together with the buffer systems, provide the first of defense to changes in acid-base status.

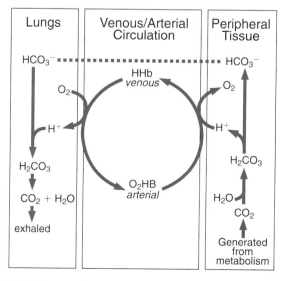

FIGURE 14-1. Interrelationship of the bicarbonate and hemoglobin buffering systems.

The kidneys are also able to excrete variable amounts of acid or base, making them an important player in the regulation of acid-base balance. The kidney's main role in maintaining acid-base homeostasis is to reclaim HCO_3^- from the glomerular filtrate. Without this reclamation, the loss of HCO_3^- in the urine would result in an excessive acid gain in the blood. The main site for HCO_3^- reclamation is the proximal tubules (Fig. 14-2). The glomerular filtrate contains essentially the same HCO_3^- levels as plasma. The process is not a direct transport of HCO_3^- across the tubule membrane into the blood. Instead, sodium (Na^+) in the glomerular filtrate is exchanged for H^+ in the tubular cell. The H^+ combines with HCO_3^- in the filtrate to form H_2CO_3, which is converted into H_2O and CO_2 by carbonic anhydrase. The CO_2 easily diffuses into the tubule and reacts with H_2O to reform H_2CO_3 and then HCO_3^-, which is reabsorbed into the blood along with sodium. With alkalotic conditions, the kidney excretes HCO_3^- to compensate for the elevated blood pH. The exchange between H^+ and Na^+ suggests, in part, why clinicians order pH and blood gases together, along with electrolytes (Na^+, K^+, and Cl^-), to assess the patient. (*Reabsorption* or *reclamation* refers to the process of reentering the blood. *Secretion* or *excretion* by the tubule cells concentrate or remove substances from the filtrate. These reactions determine the pH of the urine, as well as the pH of the blood.)

Under normal conditions, the body produces a net excess (50–100 mmol/L) of acid (H^+) each day that must be excreted by the kidney. Because the minimum urine pH is approximately 4.5, the kidney excretes little non-buffered H^+. The remainder of the urinary H^+ combines with dibasic phosphate ($HPO_4^=$) and ammonia (NH_3) and is excreted as dihydrogen phosphate ($H_2PO_4^=$) and ammonium (NH_4^+). The amount of $HPO_4^=$ available for combining with H^+ is fairly constant; therefore, the daily excretion of H^+ in urine largely depends on the amount of NH_4^+ formed. Because the renal tubular cells are able to generate NH_3 from glutamine and other amino acids,

the concentration of NH_3 will increase in response to a decreased blood pH.

Various factors affect the reabsorption of HCO_3^-. When the blood or plasma HCO_3^- level is higher than 26–30 mmol/L, HCO_3^- will be excreted. It is unlikely that the plasma will exceed an HCO_3^- value of 30 mmol/L unless these excretory capabilities fail (*eg*, kidney failure occurs). However, a frequent exception to this is compensatory retention of HCO_3^- for chronic *hypercarbia* as seen with chronic lung disease.

The HCO_3^- level may increase if an excessive amount of lactate, acetate, or HCO_3^- is intravenously infused. It also may increase if there is an excessive loss of chloride without replacement (as from sweating, vomiting, or prolonged nasogastric suction) because the HCO_3^- will be retained by the tubule to preserve electroneutrality.

Several factors may result in decreased HCO_3^- levels. Most diuretics, regardless of mechanism of action, favor the excretion of HCO_3^-. Reduced HCO_3^- reabsorption also occurs in conditions in which there is an excessive loss of cations. In kidney dysfunction (such as chronic nephritis or infections), HCO_3^- reabsorption may be impaired.

ASSESSMENT OF ACID-BASE HOMEOSTASIS

The Bicarbonate Buffering System and the Henderson-Hasselbalch Equation

In assessing acid-base homeostasis, components of the bicarbonate buffering system are measured and calculated. From the data, inferences can be made pertaining to the other buffers and the systems that regulate the production, retention, and excretion of acids and bases. For the bicarbonate buffering system, the dissolved CO_2 (dCO_2) is in equilibrium with CO_2 gas, which can be expelled by way of the lungs. Therefore, the bicarbonate buffering system is referred to as an *open* system, and the dCO_2, which is controlled by the lungs, is the *respiratory component*. The lungs participate rapidly in the regulation of blood pH through hypoventilation or hyperventi-

---

CASE STUDY 14-1

A 50-year-old man came to the emergency department after returning from foreign travel. His symptoms included persistent diarrhea (over the past 3 days) and rapid respiration (tachypnea). Blood gases were drawn:

pH   = 7.21
PCO_2 = 19 mm Hg
PO_2 = 96 mm Hg
HCO_3^- = 7 mmol/L
SO_2 = 96% (calculated) (reference range, >95%)

Questions

1. What is the patient's acid-base status?

2. Why is the HCO_3^- level so low?

3. Why does the patient have rapid respiration?

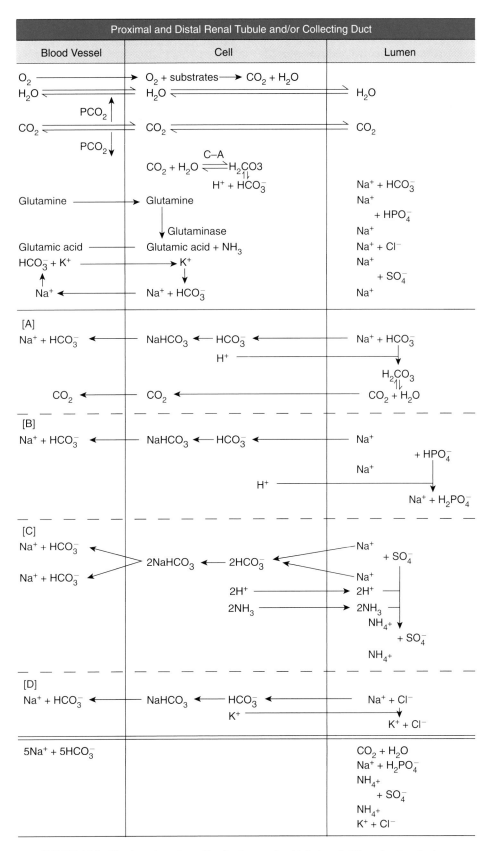

FIGURE 14-2. Bicarbonate reabsorption by the proximal tubule cell. *CA,* carbonic anhydrase.

lation. Mainly, the kidneys, the nonrespiratory or metabolic component, control the bicarbonate concentration.

The *Henderson-Hasselbalch equation* expresses acid-base relationships in a mathematical formula:

$$pH = PK' + \log\frac{cA^-}{cHA} \qquad \text{(Eq. 14–3)}$$

where A^- = proton acceptor (*eg*, HCO_3^-), HA = proton donor, or weak acid (*eg*, H_2CO_3), and pK' = pH at which there is an equal concentration of protonated and unprotonated species. Knowing any of the three variables allows for the calculation of the fourth.

In plasma and at body temperature (37° C), the pK' of the bicarbonate buffering system is 6.1. The equilibrium between H_2CO_3 and CO_2 in plasma is approximately 1:800. The concentration of H_2CO_3 is proportional to the partial pressure exerted by the dissolved CO_2. In plasma at 37°C, the value for the combination of the solubility constant for PCO_2 and the factor to convert mm Hg to millimoles per liter is 0.0307 mmol L^{-1} mm Hg^{-1}. Temperature and the solvent affect the constant. If either of these change, the solubility constant also will change. Both pH and PCO_2 are measured in blood gas analysis, and the pK' is a constant; therefore, HCO_3^- can be calculated:

$$pH = pK' + \log\frac{cHCO_3^-}{0.031 \times PCO_2} \qquad \text{(Eq. 14–4)}$$

In health, when the kidneys and lungs are functioning properly, a 20:1 ratio of HCO_3^- to H_2CO_3 will be maintained (resulting in a pH of 7.40). This is illustrated by substituting normal values (Table 14-1) for HCO_3^- and PCO_2 into the preceding equation:

$$\frac{24 \text{ mmol/L}}{(0.031 \text{ mmol/L} - \text{mm Hg}) \times 40 \text{ mm Hg}}$$

$$= \frac{24}{1.2} = \frac{20}{1} \qquad \text{(Eq. 14–5)}$$

TABLE 14-1. ARTERIAL BLOOD GAS REFERENCE RANGE AT 37°C

pH	7.35–7.45
PCO_2 (mm Hg)	35–45
HCO_3^- (mmol/L)	22–26
Total CO_2 content (mmol/L)	23–27
PO_2 (mmol/L)	80–110
SO_2 (%)	>95
O_2Hb (%)	>95

Adding the log of 20 (1.3) to the pK' of the bicarbonate system yields a normal pH of 7.40 (7.40 = 6.1 + 1.3).

Acid-Base Disorders: Acidosis and Alkalosis

Acid-base disorders result from a variety of pathologic conditions. When blood pH is less than the reference range, it is termed *acidemia*, which reflects excess acid or H^+ concentration. A pH greater than the reference range is termed *alkalemia*, or excess base. A disorder caused by ventilatory dysfunction (a change in the PCO_2, the respiratory component) is termed *primary respiratory acidosis* or *alkalosis*. A disorder resulting from a change in the bicarbonate level (a renal or metabolic function) is termed a *nonrespiratory (metabolic) disorder*. Mixed respiratory and nonrespiratory disorders occasionally arise from more than one pathologic process and represent the most serious of medical conditions as compensation for the primary disorder is failing.

Because the body's cellular and metabolic activities are pH dependent, the body tries to restore acid-base homeostasis whenever an imbalance occurs. This action by the body is termed *compensation*—the body accomplishes this by altering the factor not primarily affected by the pathologic process. For example, if the imbalance is of

---

CASE STUDY 14-2

An 80-year-old woman fell on the ice and fractured her femur. After several hours, when she arrived at the emergency department, she was anxious, panting, and complaining of severe chest pain and not being able to breathe. Her pulse was rapid (tachycardia) as was her respiration rate (tachypnea). Blood gases were drawn and yielded the following results:

pH	=	7.31
PCO_2	=	27 mm Hg
PO_2	=	62 mm Hg
HCO_3^-	=	12 mmol/L
SO_2	=	78% (calculated) (reference range, >95%)

Questions

1. What is the patient's acid-base status?

2. Why is the HCO_3^- level so low?

3. What clinically caused the acid-base imbalance?

nonrespiratory origin, the body compensates by altering ventilation. For disturbances of the respiratory component, the kidneys compensate by selectively excreting or reabsorbing anions and cations. The lungs can compensate immediately, but the response is short term and often incomplete. The kidneys are slower to respond (2–4 days), however, but the response is long term and potentially complete. *Fully compensated* implies that the pH has returned to the normal range (the 20:1 ratio has been restored); *partially compensated* implies that the pH is approaching normal. Compensation may successfully return the ratio to the normal 20:1, but the primary abnormality is not corrected.

Acidosis may be caused by a primary nonrespiratory (metabolic) abnormality or by a primary respiratory problem. In primary nonrespiratory acidosis, there is a decrease in bicarbonate (<24 mmol/L), resulting in a decreased pH as a result of the ratio for the nonrespiratory to respiratory component in the Henderson-Hasselbalch equation being less than 20:1:

$$pH \propto \frac{\downarrow cHCO_3^-}{N(0.0307 \times PCO_2)} < \frac{20}{1} \quad \textbf{(Eq. 14–6)}$$

where N = normal value, and < indicates a decreased level.

Nonrespiratory acidosis may be caused by the direct administration of an acid-producing substance, such as ammonium chloride or calcium chloride, or by excessive formation of organic acids as seen with diabetic ketoacidosis and starvation. Nonrespiratory acidosis is also seen with reduced excretion of acids, as in renal tubular acidosis, and with excessive loss of bicarbonate from diarrhea or drainage from a biliary, pancreatic, or intestinal fistula.

The body compensates for nonrespiratory acidosis through *hyperventilation,* which is an increase in the rate or depth of breathing. By "blowing off" CO_2, the base-to-acid ratio will return toward normal. Secondary compensation occurs when the "original" organ (the kidneys, in this case) begins to correct the ratio by retaining bicarbonate.

Primary *respiratory acidosis* results from a decrease in alveolar ventilation (*hypoventilation*), causing a decreased elimination of CO_2 by the lungs:

$$pH \propto \frac{NcHCO_3^-}{\uparrow(0.0307 \times PCO_2)} < \frac{20}{1} \quad \textbf{(Eq. 14–7)}$$

Respiration is regulated in the medulla of the brain. Chemoreceptors present in the aortic arch and the carotid sinus respond to levels of H^+ (pH), O_2, and CO_2 in the blood and cerebrospinal fluid. There are several situations, including many lung diseases, in which CO_2 is not effectively removed from the blood. In certain patients with chronic obstructive pulmonary disease (COPD), for example, destructive changes in the airways and alveolar walls increase the size of the alveolar air spaces, with the resultant reduction of the lung surface area available for

gas exchange. As a result, CO_2 is retained in the blood, causing chronic hypercarbia (elevated PCO_2). In bronchopneumonia, gas exchange is impeded because of the secretions, white blood cells, bacteria, and fibrin in the alveoli. Hypoventilation caused by drugs such as barbiturates, morphine, or alcohol will increase blood PCO_2 levels, as will mechanical obstruction or asphyxiation (strangulation or aspiration). Decreased cardiac output, such as that seen with congestive heart failure, also will result in less blood presented to the lungs for gas exchange and, therefore, an elevated PCO_2.

In primary respiratory acidosis, the compensation occurs through nonrespiratory processes. The kidneys increase the excretion of H^+ and increase the reclamation of HCO_3^-. Although the renal compensation begins immediately, it takes days to weeks for maximal compensation to occur. When the HCO_3^- in the blood increases as a result of the action of the kidneys, the base-to-acid ratio will be altered and the pH will return toward normal.

Primary *nonrespiratory alkalosis* results from a gain in HCO_3^-, causing an increase in the nonrespiratory component and an increase in the pH:

$$pH \propto \frac{\uparrow cHCO_3^-}{N(0.0307 \times PCO_2)} > \frac{20}{1} \quad \textbf{(Eq. 14–8)}$$

This condition may result from the excess administration of sodium bicarbonate or through ingestion of bicarbonate-producing salts, such as sodium lactate, citrate, or acetate. Excessive loss of acid through vomiting, nasogastric suctioning, or prolonged use of diuretics that augment renal excretion of H^+ can produce an apparent increase in HCO_3^-. The body responds by depressing the respiratory center. The resulting hypoventilation increases the retention of CO_2.

Primary *respiratory alkalosis* from an increased rate of alveolar ventilation causes excessive elimination of CO_2 by the lungs:

$$pH \propto \frac{Nc(HCO_3^-)}{\downarrow(0.0307 \times PCO_2)} > \frac{20}{1} \quad \textbf{(Eq. 14–9)}$$

The causes of respiratory alkalosis include *hypoxemia;* chemical stimulation of the respiratory center by drugs, such as salicylates; an increase in the environmental temperature; fever; hysteria (hyperventilation); pulmonary emboli; and pulmonary fibrosis. The kidneys compensate by excreting HCO_3^- in the urine and reclaiming H^+ to the blood. The popular treatment for hysterical hyperventilation, breathing into a paper bag, is self-explanatory.

OXYGEN AND GAS EXCHANGE

Oxygen and Carbon Dioxide

The role of oxygen in metabolism is crucial to all life. In cell mitochondria, electron pairs from the oxidation of NADH and $FADH_2$ are transferred to molecular oxygen,

CASE STUDY 14-3

A 24-year-old graduate student was brought to the emergency department in a comatose state after being found in his room unconscious. A bottle of secobarbital was on his bed stand. He did not respond to painful stimuli, his respiration was barely perceptible, and his pulse was weak. Blood gases were drawn, and yielded the following results:

pH	=	7.10
PCO_2	=	70 mm Hg
PO_2	=	58 mm Hg
HCO_3^-	=	20 mmol/L
O_2Hb	=	80% (reference range, >95%)

Questions

1. What is the patient's acid-base status?

2. What caused the profound hypoventilation?

3. Once the respiratory component returns to normal, what will be the patient's expected acid-base status?

causing release of the energy used to synthesize ATP from the phosphorylation of ADP. Although measurement of intracellular O_2 is not feasible with current technology, evaluation of a patient's oxygen status is possible using the partial pressure of oxygen (PO_2) measured with pH and PCO_2 in the blood gas analysis.

For adequate tissue oxygenation, the following seven conditions are necessary: (1) available atmospheric oxygen, (2) adequate ventilation, (3) gas exchange between the lungs and arterial blood, (4) loading of O_2 onto hemoglobin, (5) adequate hemoglobin, (6) adequate transport (cardiac output), and (7) release of O_2 to the tissue. Any disturbances in these conditions can result in poor tissue oxygenation.

The amount of O_2 available in atmospheric air depends on the barometric pressure (BP). At sea level, the BP is 760 mm Hg. (In the International System of Units, 1 mm Hg = 0.133 kPa, where 1 Pa = 1 N/m².) Dalton's law states that total atmospheric pressure is the sum of the individual gas pressures. One atmosphere exerts 760 mm Hg pressure and is made up of O_2 (20.93%), CO_2 (0.03%), nitrogen (78.1%), and inert gases (approximately 1%). The percentage for each gas is the same at all altitudes; the *partial pressure* for each gas in the atmosphere is equal to the BP at a particular altitude times the appropriate percentage for each gas. The vapor pressure of water (47 mm Hg at 37°C) must be accounted for in calculating the partial pressure for the individual gases (Fig. 14-3). In the body, these gases are always fully saturated with water. For example,

Partial pressure of O_2 at sea level (in the body) = (760 mm Hg − 47 mm Hg) × 20.93% = 149 mm Hg (at 37°C)

Partial pressure of CO_2 at sea level (in the body) = (760 mm Hg − 47 mm Hg) × 0.03% = 0.2 mm Hg (at 37°C)

CASE STUDY 14-4

A 24-year-old Himalayan man was accepted to graduate school in the United States. Before leaving home, he had an extensive physical exam that included various blood tests. When the medical staff at the U.S. university reviewed his medical records, it was noted that all test results were normal except the HCO_3^-, which was 15 mmol/L (reference range, 22–26 mmol/L). The HCO_3^- was done separately on a serum sample. It was not part of a blood gas panel. To rule out nonrespiratory acidosis, the university physician wanted the HCO_3^- repeated. The repeated value was 24 mmol/L.

Questions

1. Was the initial assumption of a nonrespiratory acidosis valid?

2. What would be a better description of the acid-base disturbance?

3. Why, on repeat testing, did the HCO_3^- return to normal?

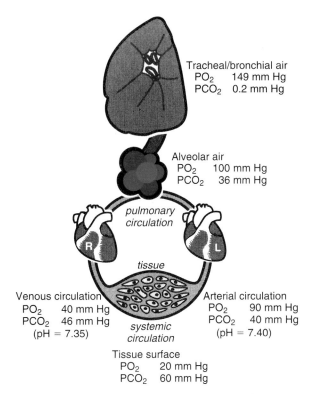

Tracheal/bronchial air
PO_2 149 mm Hg
PCO_2 0.2 mm Hg

Alveolar air
PO_2 100 mm Hg
PCO_2 36 mm Hg

pulmonary circulation

tissue

Venous circulation
PO_2 40 mm Hg
PCO_2 46 mm Hg
(pH = 7.35)

systemic circulation

Arterial circulation
PO_2 90 mm Hg
PCO_2 40 mm Hg
(pH = 7.40)

Tissue surface
PO_2 20 mm Hg
PCO_2 60 mm Hg

FIGURE 14-3. Gas content in lungs and pulmonary and systemic circulation.

Air is moved into the lungs by the expansion of the thoracic cavity, which creates a temporary negative pressure gradient, causing air to move into the numerous tracheal branches and the alveoli. At the beginning of inspiration, these airways still are filled with air (gas) retained from the previously expired breath. This air, termed *dead space air*, dilutes the air being inspired. The inspired air, in addition to being somewhat diluted, is warmed to 37°C and fully saturated with water vapor. The PO_2 in the alveoli averages about 110 mm Hg instead of the potential 150 mm Hg (expected with no dilution from dead space air and not accounting for the vapor pressure of water). Three other factors can influence PO_2 in the alveoli: (1) The percentage of O_2 in the inspired air can be increased by breathing gas mixtures up to 100% O_2, and the higher the supplemental O_2 concentration inspired, the higher the fraction of inspired oxygen (FiO_2); (2) the amount of PCO_2 in the expired air dilutes the inspired air so that a patient with increased metabolism (*eg,* hyperthermia) may produce more CO_2 than can be eliminated, increasing both the PCO_2 in the blood and the expired gas; and (3) the ratio of the volume of inspired air to the volume of the dead space air. The volume of dead space (in the airways) is usually constant because it is controlled by the person's anatomy; people with shallow breaths have less "fresh" air entering the lungs than those breathing deeply.

There are many factors that can influence the amount of O_2 that moves through the alveoli into the blood and then to the tissue. Among the more common are:

- Destruction of the alveoli. The normal surface area of the alveoli is as big as a tennis court. When the surface area is destroyed to a critically low value by diseases such as emphysema, inadequate O_2 will move into the blood.
- Pulmonary edema. Gas diffuses from the alveoli to the capillary through a small space. With pulmonary edema, fluid "leaks" into this space, increasing the distance between the alveoli and capillary walls and causing a barrier to diffusion.
- Airway blockage. Airways can be blocked, preventing the air from the atmosphere from reaching the alveoli. Asthma and bronchitis are more common causes of this type of problem.
- Inadequate blood supply. When the blood supply to the lung is inadequate, the amount of O_2 entering the blood is sufficient, but not enough blood is being carried away to the tissue where it is needed. This may be the consequence of a blockage in a pulmonary blood vessel (pulmonary embolism), pulmonary hypertension, or a failing heart.
- Diffusion of CO_2 and O_2. Because O_2 diffuses 20 times slower than CO_2, it is more sensitive to problems with diffusion. Structural or physiologic alterations to the alveolar-capillary bed impair O_2 uptake with minimal alteration of CO_2 excretion. This type of hypoxemia is generally treated with supplemental O_2. The percentage of O_2 can be increased temporarily when needed; however, 60% or higher O_2 concentrations must be used with caution because it can be toxic to the lungs.

Oxygen Transport

Most O_2 in arterial blood is transported to the tissue by hemoglobin. Each adult hemoglobin (A_1) molecule can combine reversibly with up to four molecules of O_2. The actual amount of O_2 loaded onto hemoglobin depends on the availability of O_2; the concentration and type(s) of hemoglobin present; the presence of interfering substances, such as carbon monoxide (CO); the pH; the temperature of the blood; and the levels of PCO_2 and 2,3-DPG. With adequate atmospheric and alveolar O_2 available, and with normal diffusion of O_2 to the arterial blood, more than 95% of "functional" hemoglobin (hemoglobin capable of *reversibly* binding O_2) will bind O_2. Increasing the availability of O_2 to the blood further saturates the hemoglobin. However, once the hemoglobin is 100% saturated, an increase in O_2 to the alveoli serves only to increase the concentration of dissolved (dO_2) in the arterial blood. This offers minimal increase in oxygen delivery. Prolonged administration of high concentrations of O_2 may cause oxygen toxicity and, in some cases, decreased ventilation that leads to hypercarbia. The ability of hemoglobin to carry O_2 can be affected significantly by other molecules. Normally, blood hemoglobin exists in one of four conditions:

1. Oxyhemoglobin (O_2Hb), which is O_2 reversibly bound to hemoglobin.
2. Deoxyhemoglobin (HHb; reduced hemoglobin), which is hemoglobin not bound to O_2 but capable of forming a bond when O_2 is available.
3. Carboxyhemoglobin (COHb), which is hemoglobin bound to CO. The bond between CO and Hb is reversible, but is greater than 200 times as strong as the bond between O_2 and Hb.
4. Methemoglobin (MetHb), which is hemoglobin unable to bind O_2 because iron (Fe) is in an oxidized rather than reduced state. The Fe^{3+} can be reduced by the enzyme methemoglobin reductase, which is found in red blood cells.

Dedicated spectrophotometers (co-oximeters), which are discussed later in this chapter, are used to determine the relative concentrations (relative to the total hemoglobin) of each of these species of hemoglobin.

Quantities Associated With Assessing a Patient's Oxygen Status

Four parameters commonly used to assess a patient's oxygen status are oxygen saturation (SO_2); measured fractional (percent) oxyhemoglobin (FO_2Hb); trends in oxygen saturation assessed by transcutaneous, pulse oximetry (SpO_2) assessments; and the amount of O_2 dissolved in plasma (PO_2).

Oxygen saturation (SO_2) represents the ratio of O_2 that is bound to the carrier protein, hemoglobin, compared with the total amount of hemoglobin capable of binding O_2.[2]

$$SO_2 = \frac{cO_2Hb}{(cO_2Hb + cHHb)} \times 100 \quad \textbf{(Eq. 14–10)}$$

The symbol c represents concentration. Software included with blood gas instruments can calculate SO_2 from PO_2, pH, and temperature of the sample. These calculated results, however, can differ significantly from those determined by direct measurement due to the assumption that only adult hemoglobin is present and the oxyhemoglobin dissociation curve has a specific shape and location. These algorithms for the calculation do not account for the other hemoglobin species, such as COHb and MetHb, that are incapable of reversibly binding O_2. Because of the potential for generating erroneous information, calculated SO_2 should not be used to assess oxygenation status.[2,3]

Fractional (or percent) oxyhemoglobin (FO_2Hb) is the ratio of the concentration of oxyhemoglobin to the concentration of total hemoglobin ($ctHb$),

$$FO_2Hb = \frac{cO_2Hb}{ctHb} = \frac{cO_2Hb}{cO_2Hb + cHHb + dysHb}$$

$$\textbf{(Eq. 14–11)}$$

where the $cdysHb$ represents hemoglobin derivatives, such as COHb, that cannot reversibly bind with O_2 but are still part of the "total" hemoglobin measurement.

These two terms, SO_2 and FO_2Hb, can be confused because, in most healthy individuals (and even those individuals with some disease states), the numeric values for SO_2 are close to those for FO_2Hb. However, the values for FO_2Hb and SO_2 will deviate when dyshemoglobins are present and even when the patient is a smoker, owing to the preferential binding of CO to hemoglobin and the resultant loss of hemoglobin to bind O_2.

Partial pressure of oxygen dissolved in plasma (PO_2) accounts for little of the body's O_2 stores. A healthy adult breathing room air will have a PO_2 of 90–95 mm Hg. For an adult blood volume of 5 L, only 13.5 mL of O_2 will be available from PO_2 in plasma, as compared with more than 1000 mL of O_2 carried as O_2Hb.

Noninvasive measurements for following "trends" in oxygenation are attained with *pulse oximetry* (SpO_2). These devices pass light of two or more wavelengths through the tissue of the toe, finger, or ear. The pulse oximeter differentiates between the absorption of light as a result of oxyhemoglobin and deoxyhemoglobin in the capillary bed and calculates oxyhemoglobin saturation. Because SpO_2 does not measure COHb or any other dyshemoglobins, it overestimates oxygenation when one or more are present. In addition, the accuracy of pulse oximetry can be compromised by many factors, including diminished pulse as a result of poor perfusion and severe anemia.

The maximum amount of O_2 that can be carried by hemoglobin in a given quantity of blood is the *hemoglobin oxygen (binding) capacity*. The molecular weight of tetramer hemoglobin is 64,458 g/mol. One mole of a perfect gas occupies 22,414 mL. Therefore, each gram of hemoglobin carries 1.39 mL of O_2:

$$\frac{22,414 \text{ mL/mol}_4}{64,458 \text{ g/mol}} = 1.39 \text{ mL/g} \quad \textbf{(Eq. 14–12)}$$

When the total hemoglobin (tHb) is 15 g/dL and the hemoglobin is 100% saturated with O_2, the O_2 capacity is:

$$15 \text{ g/100 mL} \times 1.39 \text{ mL/g}$$
$$= 20.8 \text{ mL } O_2/100 \text{ mL of blood}$$

$$\textbf{(Eq. 14–13)}$$

Oxygen content is the total O_2 in blood and is the sum of the O_2 bound to hemoglobin (O_2Hb) and the amount dissolved in the plasma (PO_2). (Because PO_2 and PCO_2 are only indices of gas-exchange efficiency in the lungs, they do not reveal the *content* of either gas in the blood.) For every mm Hg PO_2, 0.00314 mL of O_2 will be dissolved in 100 mL of plasma at 37°C. For example, if the PO_2 is 100 mm Hg, 0.3 mL of O_2 will be dissolved in every 100 mL of blood plasma. The amount of dissolved O_2 is usually not clinically significant. However, with low tHb or at hyperbaric conditions, it may become a significant source of O_2 to the tissue. Normally, 98–99% of the available hemoglobin is saturated with O_2. Assuming a tHb of 15 g/dL, the O_2 content for every 100 mL of blood plasma becomes

$$0.3 \text{ mL} + (20.8 \text{ mL} \times 0.97) = 20.5 \text{ mL}$$

(Eq. 14–14)

Hemoglobin–Oxygen Dissociation

In addition to adequate ventilation and gas exchange with the pulmonary circulation, O_2 must be released at the tissues. Hemoglobin transports O_2. The increased H^+ concentration and PCO_2 levels at the tissue from cellular metabolism change the molecular configuration of O_2Hb, facilitating O_2 release.

Oxygen dissociates from adult hemoglobin (A_1) in a characteristic fashion. If this dissociation is graphed (Fig. 14-4) with PO_2 on the *x*-axis and % SO_2 on the *y*-axis, the resulting curve is sigmoid, or slightly S-shaped. Hemoglobin "holds on" to O_2 until the O_2 tension in the tissue is reduced to about 60 mm Hg. Below this tension, the O_2 is released rapidly. The position of the oxygen dissociation curve reflects the *affinity* that hemoglobin has for O_2 and affects the rate of this dissociation.

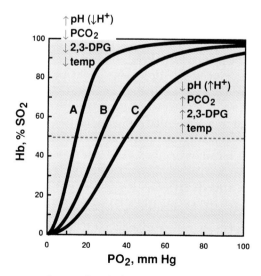

FIGURE 14-4. Oxygen-dissociation curves. Curve *B* is the normal human curve. Curves *A* and *C* are from blood with increased affinity and decreased affinity, respectively.

Hydrogen ion activity, PCO_2 and CO levels, body temperature, and 2,3-DPG can affect the position and shape of the oxygen-dissociation curve as well as the affinity of hemoglobin for O_2. In actively metabolizing tissue, the conditions in the microenvironment promote release of oxygen. Oxidative metabolism increases the temperature, H^+, CO_2, and 2,3-DPG concentrations in the tissue, which results in a right shift of the dissociation curve. This decreased affinity of hemoglobin for O_2 promotes release of oxygen to the tissue and allows patients, even those with low PO_2 and hemoglobin levels, to benefit from released O_2. In the lungs, temperature, H^+, PCO_2, and 2,3-DPG decrease relative to tissue levels, shifting the oxygen-dissociation curve slightly to the left. This enhances O_2 binding to hemoglobin and improves O_2 uptake. The metabolic by-product, 2,3-DPG, also is involved in two seemingly unrelated adaptations to potentially hypoxic conditions. When the β chains of the hemoglobin molecule bind 2,3-DPG, oxyhemoglobin dissociation shifts to the right, with subsequent enhancement of oxygen release. Many patients with slow onset of anemia demonstrate elevated levels of 2,3-DPG, which may partially explain why patients with extremely low hemoglobin values are able to function. In addition, 2,3-DPG levels increase as an adaptation to high altitude.

Hemoglobin is a remarkable molecule. Its unique structure allows it to act as both an acid-base buffer and O_2 buffer. As hemoglobin courses through the body, exposure to the various microenvironments promotes appropriate association and dissociation of O_2, CO_2, and H^+. In tissue, exposure to elevated CO_2 and H^+ results in enhanced O_2 release (oxygen buffering). This release of oxygen from hemoglobin accelerates the uptake of CO_2 and H^+ by hemoglobin (acid-base buffering). In the lungs, the microenvironment promotes uptake of O_2 and release of CO_2.

Dyshemoglobins, such as carboxyhemoglobin (COHb) or methemoglobin (MetHb), can also affect oxyhemoglobin dissociation. An elevation in CO from cigarette smoking or carbon monoxide exposure causes the curve to shift to the left. As the percentage of COHb increases, the shape of the curve loses some of its sigmoid characteristics and shifts to the left, making the release of O_2 bound to hemoglobin much more difficult.

The preceding discussion refers to normal adult (A_1) hemoglobin. In patients with hemoglobinopathies and in newborns, the pattern of dissociation may differ. For example, fetal hemoglobin causes a shift to the left, but with little change in the sigmoid shape.

MEASUREMENT

Spectrophotometric (Co-oximeter) Determination of Oxygen Saturation

The *actual percent oxyhemoglobin* (O_2Hb) can be determined spectrophotometrically using a co-oximeter designed to directly measure the various hemoglobin species. Each species of hemoglobin has a characteristic absorbance curve (Fig. 14-5). The number of hemoglobin species measured will depend on the number and specific wavelengths incorporated into the instrumentation. For example, two-wavelength instrument systems can measure only two hemoglobin species (ie, O_2Hb and HHb), which are expressed as a fraction or percentage of the total hemoglobin.

Instruments, at a minimum, should have four wavelengths for measurements of HHb, O_2Hb, and the two most common dyshemoglobins, COHb, and MetHb. Instruments with more than four wavelengths can recognize dyes and pigments, turbidity, other hemoglobin species, and abnormal proteins. Microprocessors control the sequencing of multiple wavelengths of light through the sample and apply the necessary matrix equations after absorbance readings are made to calculate the percentage of the hemoglobin species:

$$O_2HB = a_1A_1 + a_2A_2 + \ldots + a_nA_n$$
$$HHb = b_1A_1 + b_2A_2 + \ldots + b_nA_n$$
$$COHb = c_1A_1 + c_2A_2 + \ldots + c_nA_n$$
$$MetHb = d_1A_1 + d_2A_2 + \ldots + d_nA_n$$

(Eq. 14–15)

where a_1, a_n, b_n, etc., are coefficients that are analogues of the absorption constant a that are derived from established methods, and A_1, A_2, and so on are the absorbances of the sample. The matrix equations will change depending on the number of wavelengths of light (which is manufacturer specific) passed through the sample. (The "calculation" made by these instruments should not be confused with a calculated SO_2 from a blood gas analyzer, which, in reality, *estimates* the value from a measured PO_2 and an empirical equation for the location and shape of the oxygen-hemoglobin dissociation curve. Only O_2Hb values reflect the patient's true status because calculated SO_2 and O_2Hb values will be vastly different in the pres-

ence of dyshemoglobins. In CO poisoning, for example, SO_2 will likely be normal with a significantly decreased O_2Hb value.

As with any spectrophotometric measurement, potential sources of error exist, including faulty calibration of the instrument and spectral-interfering substances. The presence of any substances absorbing light at the wavelengths used in the measurement of any hemoglobin pigment has the potential of being a source of error. Product claims for specific instruments must be consulted for specific interferences.

Because the primary purpose of determining O_2Hb is to assess oxygen transport from the lungs, it is best to stabilize the patient's ventilation status before blood sample collection. An appropriate waiting period before the sample is redrawn should follow changes in supplemental O_2 or mechanical ventilation. All blood samples should be collected under anaerobic conditions and mixed immediately with heparin or other appropriate anticoagulant. If the blood gas analysis is not being done on the same sample, ethylenediaminetetraacetic acid (EDTA) can be used as an anticoagulant. All samples should be analyzed promptly to avoid changes in saturation resulting from the use of oxygen by metabolizing cells.[2,4]

Blood Gas Analyzers: pH, PCO_2, and PO_2

Blood gas analyzers use *electrodes* (macroelectrochemical or microelectrochemical sensors) as sensing devices to measure PO_2, PCO_2, and pH. The PO_2 measurement is amperometric, meaning that the amount of current flow is an indication of the oxygen present. The PCO_2 and pH measurements are potentiometric, in which a change in voltage indicates the activity of each analyte.

The *cathode* can be defined in at least three ways: (1) the negative electrode, (2) a site to which cations tend to travel, or (3) a site at which reduction occurs. *Reduction* is the gain of electrons by a particle (atom, molecule, or ion). The *anode* is the positive electrode, the site to which anions migrate or the site at which oxidation occurs. *Oxidation* is the loss of electrons by a particle. An *electrochemical cell* is formed when two opposite electrodes are immersed in a liquid that will conduct the current. The blood gas analyzer can calculate several additional parameters: bicarbonate, total CO_2, *base excess,* and SO_2.

Measurement of PO_2

PO_2 electrodes, called *Clarke electrodes,* measure the amount of current flow in a circuit that is related to the amount of O_2 being reduced at the cathode. A gas-permeable membrane covering the tip of the electrode selectively allows the O_2 to diffuse into an electrolyte and contact the cathode. Electrons are drawn from the anode surface to the cathode surface to reduce the O_2. A small,

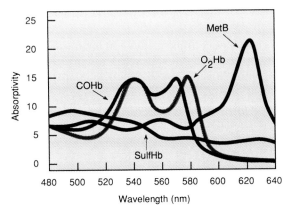

FIGURE 14-5. Optical absorption of hemoglobin fractions. (Reproduced with permission from Clin Chem News 1990(January).)

CASE STUDY 14-5

A 37-year-old man was admitted to the emergency department (ED). He was short of breath, dizzy, flushed (hyperemic), sweating (diaphoretic), and nauseous. Shortly after being admitted, blood gases were drawn:

pH	=	7.48
PCO_2	=	32 mm Hg
PO_2	=	96 mm Hg
HCO_3^-	=	24 mmol/L
SO_2	=	98% (calculated)
SpO_2	=	99% (pulse oximetry oxygen saturation)

After a few hours, the patient's symptoms receded and he was released. Two weeks later, the same patient was again admitted to the ED with the same symptoms. This time, arterial blood was drawn for both blood gases and co-oximetry measurements. The results were as follows:

pH	=	7.49
PCO_2	=	33 mm Hg
PO_2	=	95 mm Hg
HCO_3^-	=	23 mmol/L
SO_2	=	98% (calculated) (reference range, >95%)
SpO_2	=	99% (pulse oximetry oxygen saturation) (reference range, >95%)

Spectrophotometric (co-oximeter) measurement of hemoglobin species:

tHb	=	13.5 g/L
O_2Hb	=	73% (reference range, >95%)
$COHb$	=	22% (reference range, <2%; higher with smokers)
$MetHb$	=	1% (reference range, <1.5%)

Questions

1. Is the patient hypoxic on the first admission to the ED?

2. Considering the new laboratory data, is this patient hypoxic on the second admission to the ED?

3. Why is there a discrepancy between calculated SO_2, SpO_2, and O_2Hb?

4. What is a possible cause of this patient's shortness of breath and low O_2Hb?

---

constant polarizing potential (typically, –0.65V) is applied between the anode and cathode. A *microammeter* placed in the circuit between the anode and cathode measures the movement of electrons (current). Four electrons are drawn for every mole of O_2 reduced, making it possible to determine PO_2. The semipermeable membrane also will allow other gases to pass, such as CO_2 and N_2, but these gases will not be reduced at the cathode if the polarizing voltage is tightly controlled.

The primary source of error for PO_2 measurement is associated with the buildup of protein material on the surface of the membrane. This buildup retards diffusion and slows the electrode response. Bacterial contamination within the measuring chamber, although uncommon, will consume O_2 and cause low and drifting values. Other errors are mostly associated with a system malfunction, such as incorrect calibration.

Nonanalytic concerns, including sample collection and handling, are addressed later in this chapter. However, it is particularly important not to expose the sample to room air when collecting, transporting, and making O_2 measurements. Contamination of the sample with room air ($PO_2 \cong 150$ mm Hg) can result in significant error. Even after the sample is drawn, leukocytes continue to metabolize O_2. Unless the sample is analyzed immediately after being drawn, low PO_2 values may be seen with high white blood cell counts.

Continuous measurements for PO_2 also are possible using *transcutaneous* (TC) *electrodes* placed directly on the skin. Measurement depends on oxygen diffusing from the capillary bed through the tissue to the electrode. Although most commonly used with neonates and infants, this noninvasive approach is not without problems. Skin thickness and tissue perfusion with arterial blood can significantly affect the results. Heating the electrode placed on the skin can enhance diffusion of O_2 to the electrode; however, burns can result unless the electrodes are moved regularly. Although PO_2 measured by these electrodes may *reflect* the arterial PO_2, the two values are not equivalent. Oxygen consumption by tissue at the electrode site, the effects of heating the tissue, and possible hypoperfusion from cardiovascular instability can all contribute to the unpredictability of the arterial tissue O_2 gradient.

CASE STUDY 14-6

A 48-year-old man with diabetes with a history of alcohol abuse was admitted to the emergency department. He had an elevated heart rate (tachycardia) and was experiencing extreme shortness of breath. Blood was drawn for glucose and blood gases and urine collected for ketones:

Glucose	=	570 mg/dL
Urinary ketones	=	Large (reference range, negative)
pH	=	7.00
PCO_2	=	48 mm Hg
PO_2	=	68 mm Hg
HCO_3^-	=	12 mmol/L
SO_2	=	81% (calculated)
tHb	=	10 g/dL

Questions

1. Is the patient's acidemia a result of respiratory or nonrespiratory disturbances or a combination of both?

2. If the patient was not having respiratory problems, how would you classify the acid-base disturbance?

3. What is the significance of shortness of breath, tachycardia, and elevated PCO_2?

4. What is the significance of the urinary ketones result in terms of identifying the type of diabetes?

Measurement of pH and PCO_2

To understand potentiometric measurements, it is helpful to think of atoms and ions as having a chemical energy. An increased concentration or *activity* of the ions leads to an increase in force exerted by those ions.

To measure how much force—energy or potential—a given ion possesses, certain elements in the measuring device are required; namely, two electrodes (the measuring electrode responsive to the ion of interest and the reference electrode) and a voltmeter, which measures the potential difference (ΔE) between the two electrodes. The potential difference is related to the concentration of the ion of interest by the Nernst equation:

$$\Delta E = \Delta E° + \frac{0.05916}{n} \log a_i \qquad \text{at } 25°C$$

(Eq. 14–16)

where $\Delta E°$ = standard potential of the electrochemical cell, n = charge of the analyte ion i, and a_i = activity of the analyte ion i.

To measure pH, a glass membrane sensitive to H^+ is placed around an internal Ag–AgCl electrode to form a measuring electrode. The potential that develops at the glass membrane as a result of H^+ from the unknown solution diffusing into the membrane's surface is proportional to the difference in cH^+ between the unknown sample and the buffer solution inside the electrode. For the potential developed at the glass membrane to be measured, a reference electrode must be introduced into the solution and both electrodes must be connected to a pH (volt) meter. The reference electrode (commonly either a calomel [Hg–HgCl] or an Ag–AgCl half-cell) provides a steady reference voltage against which voltage changes from the measuring electrode are compared. The pH meter reflects the potential difference between the two electrodes.

For the cell described, the Nernst equation predicts that a change of + 59.16 mV, at 25°C, is the result of a 10-fold increase in H^+ activity or a decrease of an entire pH unit (eg, pH 7.0–6.0). Changing the temperature affects the response. At 37°C, a change of 1 pH unit elicits a 61.5 mV change. The glass membrane of the measuring electrode must be kept free from protein buildup because coating of the membrane causes sluggish or erratic responses.

PCO_2 is determined with a modified pH electrode, called a *Severinghaus electrode*. An outer semipermeable membrane that allows CO_2 to diffuse into a layer of electrolyte, usually a bicarbonate buffer, covers the glass pH electrode. The CO_2 that diffuses across the membrane reacts with the buffer, forming *carbonic acid,* which then dissociates into bicarbonate plus H^+. The change in activity of the H^+ is measured by the pH electrode and related to PCO_2.

As with the other electrodes, the buildup of protein material on the membrane will affect diffusion and cause errors. PCO_2 electrodes are the slowest to respond because of the chemical reaction that must be completed. Other error sources include erroneous calibration caused by incorrect or contaminated calibration materials.

Types of Electrochemical Sensors

Macroelectrode sensors have been used in blood gas instruments since the beginning of the clinical measurement of blood gases. These have been modified over time in an effort to simplify their use and minimize the re-

CASE STUDY 14-7

A 64-year-old woman with chronic obstructive pulmonary disease (COPD) was admitted to the emergency department with extreme shortness of breath. She had a bluish color that was particularly pronounced on her lips and nail beds and she displayed a weak and persistent cough with diminished, but rattling breath sounds. Home medications included bronchodilators, steroids, Lasix (a loop diuretic that does not conserve plasma potassium), and digitalis. Vital signs: heart rate, 148; blood pressure, 100/88; temperature, 37; and respiratory rate, 38. Initial blood gas results on room air were:

pH   =   7.289
PCO_2 =   91 mm Hg
PO_2 =   53 mm Hg
HCO_3^- =   43 mmol/L

Questions

1. What is the patient's acid-base status?

2. Would the pH be normal if the patient was able to decrease her PCO_2 to 50 mm Hg?

3. In addition to COPD, what condition likely contributed to her poor gas exchange (hypercarbia and hypoxemia)?

She was treated with a bolus of Lasix intravenously and two albuterol (bronchodilator) respiratory treatments. Her vital signs improved: heart rate, 124; blood pressure, 120/80; and respiratory rate, 22. Blood gases were repeated with the patient breathing 28% O_2 (FiO_2 = .28):

pH   =   7.306
PCO_2 =   75 mm Hg
PO_2 =   78 mm Hg
HCO_3^- =   36 mmol/L

Questions

1. Should more oxygen be administered to this patient?

2. How did Lasix administration and respiratory treatment benefit the patient?

3. Which critical electrolyte should be closely monitored in the management of this case?

quired sample volume and maintenance. *Microelectrodes* basically are miniaturized macroelectrodes. Miniaturization became possible with better manufacturing capabilities and with the development of the sophisticated electronics required to handle minute changes in signal.

Thick and thin film technology is a further modification of electrochemical sensors. Although the measurement principle is identical, the sensors are reduced to tiny wires embedded in a printed circuit card. The special card has etched grooves to separate components. A special paste material containing the required components (similar in function to the electrolytes of macroelectrodes) is spread over the sensors. To reduce the required sample volume, several sensors can be placed on a single small card. These sensors are disposable and less expensive to manufacture, which reduces maintenance.

Optical Sensors

Another technology for blood gas measurements is based on the fact that certain fluorescent dyes will react predictably with specific chemicals, such as O_2, CO_2, and H^+. The dye is separated from the sample by a membrane, as with electrodes, and the analyte diffuses into the dye, causing either an increase in or a quenching of fluorescence proportional to the amount of analyte. Calibration is used to establish the relationship between concentration and fluorescence. Normally, a single calibration will suffice for long periods because this technology is not subject to the drifts seen in electrochemical technology.

Optical technology has been applied to indwelling blood gas systems. Fiberoptic bundles carry light to sensors positioned in the tip of catheters and other bundles carry light back, allowing changes in fluorescence to be measured in a catheter within the patient's arterial system. The commercial development of indwelling systems has been limited by the increased probability of thrombogenesis and protein buildup on the membrane, separating the sample from the fluorescing dyes. This buildup impedes free sample diffusion into the measuring chamber.

Calibration

Temperature is an important factor in the measurement of pH and blood gases. The Nernst equation specifies the expected voltage output of an electrochemical cell at a given temperature. If the temperature of the measurement system changes, the output (voltage) will change. The solubility of gases in a liquid medium also depends on the temperature: as the temperature goes down, the solubility of the gas increases. Because pH and blood gas measurements are extremely sensitive to temperature, it is critical that the electrode sample chamber be maintained at constant temperature for all measurements. All blood gas analyzers have electrode chambers thermostatically controlled to 37°C ± 0.1°.

The pH electrode is usually calibrated with two buffer solutions traceable to standards prepared by the National Institute of Standards and Technology (NIST). *Traceable* usually means that the actual value of the calibrator has been determined using a NIST standard as a reference. Usually, one calibrator is near 6.8 and the other is near 7.38 because most pH electrodes produce "0" voltage at this point. The calibrators must be stored at the stated temperature and not exposed to room air because pH changes with the absorption of CO_2.

Calibration of any blood gas analyzer will vary depending on the manufacturer. Normally, two gas mixtures are used for PCO_2 and PO_2. One gas has no O_2 to set the zero point of the O_2 electrode (which is usually a stable point). The same gas has approximately 5% CO_2 because this is the null (zero potential and stable) point for the CO_2 electrode. The other gas sets the gain, that is, the amount of change in the electrode signal relative to the change for the analyte. The gas can have any value.

Most instruments are self-calibrating (calibrate automatically at specified time intervals) and are programmed to indicate a calibration error if the electronic signal from the electrode is inconsistent with the programmed expected value. For example, if the value(s) obtained during calibration exceed(s) a programmed tolerance limit, flagging of a *drift* error will occur at the time of calibration, and corrective action will need to be taken before patient samples can be analyzed.

Calculated Parameters

Several acid-base parameters can be calculated from measured pH and PCO_2 values. Manufacturers of blood gas instruments include algorithms to perform the calculations. No calculated parameter is universally used; many physicians have "favorite" parameters for identifying various pathologies.

The calculation of HCO_3^- is based on the Henderson-Hasselbalch equation. This can be calculated when pH and PCO_2 are known. One basic assumption is that the pK' of the bicarbonate buffer system in plasma at 37°C is 6.1.

Carbonic acid concentration can be calculated using the solubility coefficient of CO_2 in plasma at 37°C. The solubility constant to convert PCO_2 to millimoles per liter of H_2CO_3 is 0.0307. If the temperature or the composition of plasma changes (eg, an increase in lipids, in which gases are more soluble), the constant will change.

Total carbon dioxide content ($ctCO_2$) is the bicarbonate plus the dissolved CO_2 (carbonic acid) plus the associated CO_2 with proteins (carbamates). A blood gas analyzer approximates $ctCO_2$ by adding the bicarbonate and carbonic acid values ($ctCO_2 = cHCO_3^- + [0.0307 \times PCO_2]$).

Some clinicians use *base excess* to assess the nonrespiratory (metabolic) component of a patient's acid-base disorder. Base excess is calculated from an algorithm that uses the patient's pH, PCO_2, and hemoglobin. A positive value (base excess) indicates an excess of bicarbonate or relative deficit of noncarbonic acid and suggests *nonrespiratory (metabolic) alkalosis*. A negative value (base deficit) indicates a deficit of bicarbonate or relative excess of noncarbonic acids and suggests *nonrespiratory (metabolic) acidosis*. However, the indicated nonrespiratory alkalosis or acidosis may be a result of primary disturbances or compensatory mechanisms. Consequently, base excess values should not be used alone in assessing a patients' acid-base status.

Correction for Temperature

Values for pH, PCO_2, and PO_2 are temperature dependent. By convention, all of these measurements are made at 37°C. The question becomes, "When the patient's body temperature differs from 37°C, should the blood gas values be 'corrected' to the actual temperature of the patient?" Although the blood gas instrument software can easily perform the correction, the data may be confusing because appropriate reference ranges *for the patient's temperature* must be used for proper interpretation. For reference, usually results are reported at 37°C when values also are reported at actual patient temperature.

QUALITY ASSURANCE

Preanalytic Considerations

Blood gas measurements, like all laboratory measurements, are subject to preanalytic, analytic, and postanalytic errors. Few other measurements, however, are as affected by preanalytic errors—those introduced during the collection and transport of samples before analysis.[2,4]

Figure 14-6 depicts the quality assurance cycle. The steps included in the analytic area are under the direct control of the laboratory. Because much of the quality assurance cycle lies outside the laboratory, the laboratorian must take an active role in educating *all* people involved in developing policies and procedures for controlling all the processes in the cycle to ensure quality.

Only personnel who have experience with the drawing equipment and technique and have knowledge of the

CASE STUDY 14-8

A 23-year-old woman with a history of asthma was brought to the emergency department by ambulance. She was extremely short of breath. Her level of consciousness was diminished greatly, and she was only able to respond to questions with nods or one-word responses. She had a weak cough, with nearly inaudible breath sounds. After drawing blood gases, she was placed on supplemental oxygen. Vital signs: heart rate, 160; blood pressure, 120/84; temperature, 37; and respiratory rate, 36. Her initial blood gas and total hemoglobin results were:

pH   =   7.330
PCO_2 =   25 mm Hg
PO_2 =   58 mm Hg
HCO_3^- =   13 mmol/L
tHb =   12.4 g/L

Questions

1. What is the patient's acid-base and oxygenation status?

2. What is the cause of the acid-base disturbance?

3. Would the pH be normal if the patient's PCO_2 increased to 40 mm Hg?

4. Does asthma typically present in this manner?

5. What clinical findings are most indicative of this patient's impending failure?

possible sources of error should draw samples for pH and blood gas analyses. Because collection may be painful and result in patient hyperventilation, which lowers the PCO_2 and increases the pH, the ability to reassure the patient is essential. The choice of site—radial, brachial, femoral, or temporal artery—is usually customary within an institution, depending on the predominant patient population (eg, pediatric patients, burn patients, outpatients). The National Committee for Clinical Laboratory Standards (NCCLS) publication *Procedures for the Collection of Arterial Blood Specimens* is an excellent reference.[4]

The use of arterial samples for pH and blood gas studies is recommended. However, peripheral venous samples can be used if pulmonary function or O_2 transport is not being assessed. For venous samples, the source of the specimen must be clearly identified and the appropriate (venous) reference ranges included for data interpretation with the results. Depending on the patient, capillary blood may need to be used to measure pH and PCO_2. Although the correlation with arterial blood is good for pH and PCO_2, capillary PO_2 values, even with warming of the skin before drawing the sample, do not correlate well with arterial PO_2 values as a result of sample exposure to room air. Central venous (pulmonary artery) blood samples are obtained to assess O_2 consumption, which is calculated from the difference between the O_2 content of arterial blood and pulmonary artery blood times the cardiac output.

Sources of error in the collection and handling of blood gas specimens include the collection device, form and concentration of heparin, speed of syringe filling, maintenance of the anaerobic environment, mixing of the sample to ensure dissolution and distribution of the

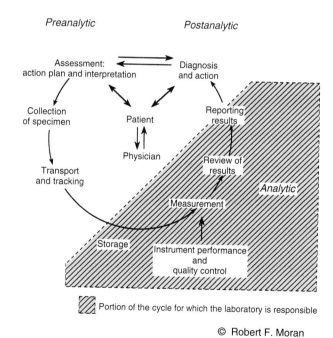

Blood Gas Analysis Quality Assurance Cycle

FIGURE 14-6. Blood gas analysis quality assurance cycle. (Reproduced with permission from Robert F. Moran.)

heparin anticoagulant, and transport and storage time before analysis. For proper interpretation of blood gas results, the patient's status at the time the sample is collected must be documented in terms of ventilation (on room air or supplemental O_2), temperature, and posture.

The recommended collection device for arterial blood samples is a preheparinized plastic syringe. Evacuated collection tubes are not appropriate for blood gases. Both dry and liquid forms of heparin are acceptable anticoagulants. However, because of the potential for dilution of the sample when excess amounts are used and possible contamination of the heparin with room air, liquid heparin is not recommended.[2,4] The blood in the syringe must be mixed with the dry heparin to prevent clots from forming. Adequate mixing is again important immediately before the sample is injected or aspirated into the blood gas analyzer. Although sodium and lithium salts of heparin are recommended for pH and blood gas analysis, other forms are available: ammonium, zinc, electrolyte balanced, and calcium-titrated. Selection of the proper type heparin is particularly important with instruments combining blood gas and electrolyte analyses. It is important to consult the manufacturer's product insert.

Slow filling of the syringe may be caused by a mismatch of syringe and needle sizes. Although too small a needle reduces the pain and, therefore, the likelihood of arteriospasm and hematoma, it may produce bubbles that affect PCO_2 and PO_2 values as well as hemolysis, which is important when potassium is measured along with pH and blood gases. Maintenance of an anaerobic environment is critical to correct results.

Transport time of the sample should be minimal. Because cooling samples in plastic syringes in ice water can cause significant changes in PO_2 values, the NCCLS guidelines advocate samples be kept at room temperature and analyzed in less than 30 minutes.[2] Because of the potential for preanalytic error, the best practice is to analyze the sample as quickly as possible.

Because sample procurement and handling are the source of many possible errors in blood gas analysis, it is necessary that procedures and policies are carefully constructed and adherence monitored to ensure quality. No QC product can monitor the preanalytic aspects of blood gas analysis.

Analytic Assessments: Quality Control and Proficiency Testing

Quality control (QC) for blood systems assesses only the analytic phase of the testing process. Although a laboratory tries to choose a control material that closely mimics actual patient samples, this is impossible for blood gases. Traditionally, QC for blood gases has included the analysis of commercial liquid controls, tonometered samples, and duplicate patient samples.[2] All these approaches have limitations. The ideal approach would encompass some combination of the three.

Commercial liquid control materials are the basis of most of today's QC practices.[5] Usually, these are sold in sealed glass ampules that contain solutions equilibrated with gases. These can be analyzed by the analyst or placed in a device for automatic analysis by the instrument at programmed intervals. Some manufacturers now pool the same levels of liquid control material into a sealed bag that resides on the analyzer for automatic analysis. Ideally, such materials are stable and have minimal variance.

Liquid controls are available in at least three levels, corresponding to values observed with low, expected or "normal," and elevated values for each of the measured analytes, which may include additional analytes, such as sodium, potassium, chloride, lactate, ionized calcium and magnesium, and glucose. The materials vary in stability and are susceptible to temperature variation in storage and handling. Each must be handled as described by the manufacturer to eliminate precision errors caused by improper handling of the material. Because liquid control materials have significantly different matrices than fresh whole blood, the laboratorian must be aware that they may not detect problems that affect patient samples, or they may detect errors induced by improper handling of the commercial controls. Aqueous-based controls, the most commonly used QC material, have low O_2 solubility, making them sensitive to factors that affect the determination of PO_2. Aqueous controls must be at room temperature for analysis. Manufacturer recommendations must be followed closely or PO_2 values may be unreliable. Hemoglobin-containing and emulsion-based controls have increased O_2 solubility and better resist O_2 changes.

Tonometry is the equilibration of a fluid with gases of known concentration and under controlled conditions, such as constant temperature, barometric pressure, humidification.[2] It is a relatively inexpensive way to check the precision and accuracy of PCO_2 and PO_2 (not pH) measurements when whole blood or aqueous materials are tonometered. When whole blood is used, it is considered the reference procedure to establish the accuracy for PCO_2 and PO_2. Many problems have been documented, however, causing laboratories to view tonometry as too cumbersome and time consuming.

Another approach is *duplicate assays* using two or more instruments for simultaneous analysis of a patient sample. *Delta checks*, or the difference in values obtained on the two instruments, often pick up problems that might be missed in routine QC. However, extreme care must be taken to expel air during replicate analyses to assure reliable PO_2 values. The allowable difference in duplicates run on split patient samples should be tighter than those observed with commercial liquid controls. Discrepancies between results provide no clue regarding which data point is wrong or which instrument is malfunctioning. Although two instruments are unlikely to have the same error simultaneously, this is not always true. Therefore, the duplicate-assay approach cannot be used as the sole method of QC. Used in conjunction with commercial liquid controls or tonometry, it can be a useful technique for detecting errors and also for troubleshooting instruments.

Still another approach, particularly for small testing devices used at point of care, is electronic QC, which involves substituting an electronic check to evaluate the instrument's readout and/or electronics in place of the analysis of a control sample. Although checking the instrument's electronics is essential, it is not sufficient to ensure that the entire analytic process is functioning correctly. Electronic QC needs to be used in conjunction with other QC procedures to monitor the quality of the total testing process.

An effective QC scheme also includes peer review and duplicate sample analysis (on the same instrument) to help minimize the inadequacies of commercial controls that do not mimic blood. Peer review is information obtained from the manufacturers of the controls. Accuracy is estimated by comparing the laboratory's mean value obtained on a lot of controls to the average value (the mean of the means) obtained by many laboratories on the same lot. The information is similar to proficiency testing but is done on a continual basis. In addition to the standard deviation and coefficient of variation calculated from accumulated QC data, imprecision can be estimated by duplicate analysis of patient samples done throughout the workday. Changes in instrument performance that will affect patient care are quickly ascertained using this scheme.

Whatever the QC approach, the QC needs of the blood gas laboratory contrast sharply with those of the general laboratory, which analyzes many patient samples as a group and includes multiple control specimens with each run. In the blood gas laboratory, the critical nature of the measurements or patient sample volume do not always allow for repeat analyses if problems exist. Consequently, the blood gas laboratory must perform *prospective* QC because instruments must be *prequalified* to ensure proper performance before the patient sample arrives for analysis.

Participating in external, interlaboratory surveys or proficiency testing programs assists in identifying and monitoring accuracy problems.[6] Ongoing comparisons of results through proficiency testing help ensure that systematic (accuracy) errors do not slowly increase and go undetected by internal QC procedures. A rigorous internal QC program ensures internal consistency. Good performance in a proficiency testing program ensures the absence of significant bias relative to other laboratories and confirms the validity of a laboratory's patient results. If an individual analyzer does not produce proficiency testing results consistent with its peer laboratories (those using the same method/instrument) or if the differences between values change over time, suspicion of the instrument's performance is warranted.

Interpretation of Results

Laboratory professionals need certain knowledge, attitudes, and skills for obtaining and analyzing specimens for pH and blood gases. Although the patient's physician assimilates all results—laboratory, radiology, nuclear medicine, surgical pathology findings, and so on, along with the patient's clinical history—laboratory personnel must immediately assess patient results and make preliminary judgments about the "fit," that is, do the results make sense? Simple evaluation of the data may reveal an instrument problem (possible bubble in the sample chamber or fibrin plug) or a possible sample handling problem (PO_2 out of line with previous results and current inspired FiO_2 levels). The application of knowledge saves time. The ability to correlate data quickly reduces turnaround time and prevents mistakes.

SUMMARY

Arterial pH and blood gas measurements are ordered to facilitate the care and treatment of critically ill patients. The body maintains acid-base balance through various buffering systems. In the laboratory, the bicarbonate–carbonic acid buffer system, which works in conjunction with and reflects the status of the body's other buffering systems, is used to evaluate acid-base status. pH and PCO_2 measurements assess the patient's acid-base status. To differentiate metabolic (nonrespiratory) from respiratory conditions, it often is helpful to evaluate calculated parameters, such as HCO_3^- and base excess.

The PO_2 measurement also is important. In arterial blood, it directly assesses the ability of the lungs to oxygenate the blood. It is used as an indirect measurement of the body's tissue oxygenation status. However, this measurement alone can be misleading. For example, an anemic patient will have a decreased O_2 content and capacity and a normal PO_2, provided the cardiovascular and pulmonary systems are intact. Consequently, other parameters are used in conjunction with PO_2. These include FO_2Hb, identification of dyshemoglobins, and the calculated parameters of O_2 content and capacity.

1. The presence of dyshemoglobins will cause a calculated % SO_2 result to be falsely (elevated, decreased) and a pulse oximeter % SpO_2 value to be falsely (elevated, decreased):
    a. elevated, elevated.
    b. decreased, decreased.
    c. elevated, decreased.
    d. decreased, elevated.

2. The anticoagulant of choice for arterial blood gas measurements is _____ in the _____ state.
    a. EDTA; dry
    b. potassium oxalate; liquid
    c. sodium citrate; dry
    d. lithium heparin; dry

3. At a pH of 7.10, the H^+ concentration is equal to:
    a. 20 nmol/L.
    b. 40 nmol/L.
    c. 60 nmol/L.
    d. 80 nmol/L.

4. The kidneys compensate for respiratory alkalosis by (excretion, retention) of bicarbonate and (increased, decreased) excretion of NaH_2PO_4.
    a. Excretion, increased
    b. Retention, increased
    c. Execution, decreased
    d. Retention, decreased

5. The normal ratio of carbonic acid to bicarbonate in arterial blood is:
    a. 7.4:6.1.
    b. 1:20.
    c. 0.003:1.39.
    d. 20:1.

6. When arterial blood from a normal patient is exposed to room air:
    a. PCO_2 decreases; PO_2 increases.
    b. PCO_2 increases; PO_2 decreases.
    c. PCO_2 decreases; PO_2 decreases.
    d. PCO_2 increases; PO_2 increases.

7. A patient's arterial blood gas results are: pH, 7.37; PCO_2, 75 mm Hg; HCO_3^-, 37 mmol/L. These values are consistent with:
    a. compensated respiratory acidosis.
    b. compensated nonrespiratory acidosis.
    c. uncompensated respiratory alkalosis.
    d. uncompensated nonrespiratory alkalosis.

8. A patient's arterial blood gas results are: pH, 7.48; PCO_2, 54 mm Hg; HCO_3^-, 38 mmol/L. These values are consistent with:
    a. compensated nonrespiratory alkalosis.
    b. compensated nonrespiratory alkalosis.
    c. uncompensated nonrespiratory alkalosis.
    d. uncompensated nonrespiratory alkalosis.

9. In the circulatory system, bicarbonate leaves the red blood cells and enters the plasma through an exchange mechanism with _____ to maintain electroneutrality.
    a. Carbonic acid
    b. Lactate
    c. Chloride
    d. Sodium

10. Hypoventilation can compensate for:
    a. mixed alkalosis.
    b. mixed acidosis.
    c. nonrespiratory acidosis.
    d. nonrespiratory alkalosis.

11. The hemoglobin oxygen binding capacity for a blood sample that is 100% saturated with O_2 and has a total hemoglobin value of 12 g/dL is approximately:
    a. 4 mL O_2/dL.
    b. 8 mL O_2/dL.
    c. 17 mL O_2/dL.
    d. 34 mL O_2/dL.

12. Carbonic acid concentration in blood plasma equals:
    a. apparent pK of carbonic acid, 6.1, plus the PCO_2 value in mm Hg.
    b. 0.0307 $mmoL^{-1}$ mm Hg^{-1} times the PCO_2 value in mm Hg.
    c. PCO_2 value in mm Hg plus HCO_3^- value in mm Hg.
    d. bicarbonate concentration divided by the PCO_2 value in mm Hg.

13. Oxygen content in blood reflects:
    a. O_2Hb only.
    b. O_2 dissolved in blood plasma only.
    c. PO_2 value.
    d. the patient's total hemoglobin value.
    e. all of the above.

REFERENCES

1. Weisberg HF. Water, Electrolyte, and Acid-Base Balance, 2nd ed. Baltimore: Williams & Wilkins, 1962.
2. Burnett RW, Ehrmeyer SS, Moran, RF, VanKessel AL. Blood Gas and pH Analysis and Related Measurements (C46A). Wayne, PA: National Committee for Clinical Laboratory Standards, 2001.
3. Ehrmeyer S, Ancy J, Laessig R. Oxygenation: measure the right thing. Respir Ther 1998;11(3):25–28.
4. Blonshine S, Alberti R, Olesinski RL. Procedures for the Collection of Arterial Blood Specimens (H11A3). Wayne, PA: National Committee for Clinical Laboratory Standards, 1999.
5. Westgard JO, et al. Statistical Quality Control for Quantitative Measurements: Principles and Definitions (C24A2). Wayne, PA: National Committee for Clinical Laboratory Standards, 1999.
6. Laessig RH, Ehrmeyer SS. Lab 2000: fundamental features—proficiency testing—then, now and the future. Clin Chem News 1999;25:18–20.

CHAPTER 15

Trace Elements

John G. Toffaletti

CHAPTER OUTLINE

OBJECTIVES

Upon completion of this chapter, the clinical laboratorian should be able to:

- **Define metalloprotein, metalloenzyme, cofactor, oxidation state, essential trace element, trace element, and ultratrace element.**
- **Describe the absorption, transport, and excretion of the essential trace elements.**
- **State the biologic functions of the essential trace elements.**
- **Discuss the clinical significance of the trace elements and the consequences of deficiency states.**
- **Discuss specimen collection considerations and laboratory determination.**

KEY TERMS

Chelator
Cofactor
Essential trace elements
Metalloenzyme
Metalloprotein
Prooxidant
Total iron-binding capacity (TIBC)
Trace elements
Transferrin
Ultratrace elements

The trace elements included in this chapter all have biochemical importance, whether minor or major. They are usually associated with an enzyme (*metalloenzyme*) or another protein (*metalloprotein*) as an essential component or *cofactor*. Deficiencies typically impair one or more biochemical functions and excess concentrations are associated with at least some degree of toxicity (Table 15-1). Although *trace elements,* such as iron, copper, and zinc, are found in mg/L concentrations, *ultratrace elements,* such as selenium, chromium, and manganese, are found in less than μg/L concentrations. An element is considered essential if a deficiency impairs a biochemical or functional process and replacement of the element corrects this impairment. Decreased intake, impaired absorption, increased excretion, and genetic abnormalities are examples of conditions that could result in deficiency of trace elements. The World Health Organization has established the dietary requirement for nutrients as the smallest amount of the nutrient needed to maintain optimal function and health.

This chapter presents information on the trace elements regarding absorption, transport, distribution, and removal. The biochemical functions will be described and related to the clinical significance of disease states or toxicity. Finally, the use and techniques for laboratory determination will be described. Table 15-2 summarizes some of this information for *essential trace elements.*

TABLE 15-1. ESSENTIAL TRACE ELEMENTS IN CLINICAL CHEMISTRY

	PROVEN ESSENTIAL	PROBABLY ESSENTIAL	NONESSENTIAL TO DATE
Trace	Iron Zinc Copper		
Ultratrace	Manganese Cobalt Selenium Molybdenum Chromium Iodine	Nickel Vanadium Tin	Aluminum Arsenic Cadmium Fluoride Gold Lead Mercury Silicon

TABLE 15-2. TRACE ELEMENT FUNCTION AND ABNORMALITIES

METALS	REFERENCE VALUES	BIOCHEMICAL FUNCTIONS	DEFICIENCY CHARACTERISTICS	TOXICITY CHARACTERISTICS
Iron	Serum 50–160 μg/dL, male 45–150 μg/dL, female	Oxygen transport Respiration (cytochromes) Oxidative processes	Anemia	Hepatic failure Cardiomyopathy Peripheral neuropathy
Zinc	Serum 66–110 μg/dL	Hemoglobin synthesis Collagen metabolism Bone development Growth and reproduction	Impaired wound healing Retarded growth Skeletal abnormalities Male impotence	Ataxia Pancreatitis Anemia, fever Nausea, vomiting
Copper	Serum 70–150 μg/dL, male 80–155 μg/dL, female	Pigmentation disorders Bone development Oxygen transport Nucleic acid synthesis Protein synthesis	Nausea, vomiting Retarded growth Anemia in children Wilson's disease Menkes' syndrome	Liver necrosis Hemolytic anemia Renal dysfunction Neurologic dysfunction
Manganese	Serum 0.4–0.8 μg/L	Growth and reproduction Oxidative phosphorylation Cholesterol metabolism	Disorders in spermatogenesis Bone abnormalities Bleeding disorders	Neurologic alterations Psychosis Speech disturbances
Cobalt	Serum 0.11–0.45 μg/L	Vitamin B_{12} function Methionine metabolism	Megaloblastic anemia	Gastrointestinal function Cardiomyopathy
Selenium	Whole blood 46–143 μg/L	Oxygen metabolism Free radical protection	Cardiovascular disease Muscle degeneration Carcinogenesis	Neurotoxicity Hepatotoxicity
Molybdenum	Serum 0.1–3.0 μg/L	Xanthine metabolism	Mental disturbances Esophageal cancer	Hyperuricemia
Chromium	Serum 0.05–0.15 μg/L	Insulin uptake Glucose metabolism	Reduced glucose tolerance	Renal failure Pulmonary cancer

GENERAL CONSIDERATIONS IN SAMPLE COLLECTION, PROCESSING, AND LABORATORY DETERMINATIONS OF TRACE ELEMENTS

Specimens for analysis of trace elements must be collected with scrupulous attention to details such as anticoagulant, collection apparatus, and specimen type (serum, plasma, or blood). By the low concentration in biologic specimens and the ubiquitous presence in the environment, extraordinary measures are required to prevent contamination of the specimen. This includes using special sampling and collection devices, specially cleaned glassware, and water and reagents of high purity. The selection of needles, evacuated blood collection tubes, anticoagulants and other additives, water and other reagents, pipettes, and sample cups must be carefully evaluated for use in trace and ultratrace analyses.

Methodology and instrumentation must have high analytic sensitivity and specificity because of the extremely low concentrations of trace elements found in body fluids and the physicochemical similarity of some elements. For many years, the most commonly used instrument for trace metal analysis has been the atomic absorption spectrometer, often with flameless atomization.

Reference ranges for trace and ultratrace elements are listed in Table 15-2.

IRON

Distribution of Iron

Of the 3–5 g of iron in the body, ~2–2.5 g of iron is in hemoglobin, which is contained mostly in red blood cells either in the blood or as precursors in the bone marrow. A moderate amount of iron (~130 mg) is in myoglobin, the oxygen-carrying protein of muscle. A small (8 mg), but extremely important, pool is in tissue where iron is bound to several enzymes that require iron for full activity. These include peroxidases, cytochromes, and many of the Krebs cycle enzymes. Iron is also stored as ferritin and hemosiderin, primarily in the bone marrow, spleen, and liver. This critical pool of iron may be the first to become diminished in iron deficiency states.[1] Only 3–5 mg of iron is found in plasma associated with transferrin, albumin, and free hemoglobin.[2]

Dietary Requirements of Iron

In an adult male, the average loss of 1 mg of iron per day must be replaced by dietary sources.[3] Pregnant or premenopausal women and children have greater iron requirements, often obtained by dietary supplementation. To address this concern, the U.S. Food and Drug Administration has raised its standards for supplementation of foods. However, because the general population includes both iron-deficient individuals and those with adequate iron status, there is debate about whether dietary iron supplements may contribute to iron overload in persons with adequate iron.[4–5]

Iron Absorption

Absorption of iron from the intestine is the primary means of regulating the amount of iron within the body. In fact, only about 10% of the 1 g/day of dietary iron is typically absorbed. Iron absorption is controlled at several locations. To be absorbed by intestinal cells, iron must be in the $+2$ (ferrous) oxidation state and bound to protein. Because Fe^{+3} is the predominant form of iron in foods, it must first be reduced to Fe^{+2} by agents such as vitamin C before it can be absorbed. In the intestinal mucosal cell, Fe^{+2} is bound by apoferritin, then oxidized by ceruloplasmin to Fe^{+3} bound to ferritin. From there, iron is absorbed into the blood by apotransferrin, which becomes transferrin as it binds two Fe^{+3} ions. In plasma, transferrin carries and releases Fe to the bone marrow, where it is incorporated into hemoglobin of red blood cells. After about 4 months in circulation, red cells are degraded by the spleen, liver, and macrophages, which return Fe the circulation where it is bound and carried by transferrin for reuse (Fig. 15-1).

Iron absorption can be adjusted to meet current needs. Iron absorption and transport capacity can be increased in conditions such as iron deficiency, anemia, or hypoxia. In the mucosal cell of an individual with adequate plasma iron concentration, iron is sequestered by ferritin. The short life of an intestinal mucosal cell results in loss of ferritin when the cell is shed.[3]

Iron Transport

When intracellular iron concentration is low, an iron regulatory protein inhibits the synthesis of apoferritin and promotes the synthesis of transferrin receptor.[6,7] Newly absorbed iron, or iron released from ferritin, is converted from Fe^{+2} to Fe^{+3} by ceruloplasmin, transferred to apotransferrin in the cell, and then released into the circulation as transferrin.[3] In normal states, both intracellular ferritin and circulating transferrin[8] are only partially saturated. The small amount of circulating ferritin is mostly apoferritin that contains little iron.[9] Transferrin delivers iron to tissue such as bone marrow for synthesis of heme for erythrocytes. At the tissue site, transferrin receptors provide recognition sites for attachment and transport into the cell.

Iron Excretion

Most of the small amount of iron normally lost each day is contained in epithelial and red cells excreted in the urine or lost in the feces. With each menstrual cycle, women lose approximately 20–40 mg of iron.

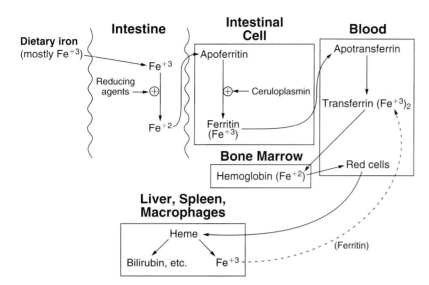

FIGURE 15-1. Pathways for iron transport and usage in tissues, cells, and blood. Note that (1) reducing agents promote conversion of Fe^{+3} to Fe^{+2} and ceruloplasmin promotes oxidation of Fe^{+2} to Fe^{+3} and (2) red cells gradually break down after about 4 months in blood circulation and are metabolized by macrophages, the spleen, and the liver.

Biochemical Functions of Iron

Fe^{+2} is an essential component of hemoglobin, allowing it to bind reversibly with oxygen in the lung and release oxygen to the tissue. As oxygen is released to the tissue, hemoglobin binds carbon dioxide, then releases it in the lung where it is removed by ventilation. Iron must remain in the Fe^{+2} state for hemoglobin to carry oxygen. If iron is oxidized to Fe^{+3}, hemoglobin becomes nonfunctional methemoglobin. Fe^{+3} may be converted back to Fe^{+2} by methemoglobin reductase. In addition to the tissue environment providing increased acid (H^+ ions) and PCO_2 to enhance release of oxygen from hemoglobin, myoglobin also facilitates diffusion of oxygen into tissue because it binds oxygen with greater affinity than hemoglobin. A decrease in myoglobin caused by iron deficiency can decrease oxygen diffusion into tissue.[3]

The cytochromes are essential for electron transport in the respiratory chain, with the reversible cycling of Fe^{+3} to Fe^{+2}, ultimately resulting in the production of energy as ATP.[3] Peroxidase and catalase are iron-containing enzymes that convert potentially harmful hydrogen peroxide to water. Thyroperoxidase incorporates iodide into hormone precursors in the thyroid gland.

Clinical Disorders of Iron Deficiency

Iron deficiency is one of the most prevalent disorders known, with 15% of the worldwide population affected. Those with a higher than average risk for iron deficiency anemia include pregnant women, both young children and adolescents, and women of reproductive age.[3,10] Increased blood loss, decreased dietary iron intake, or decreased release from ferritin may result in iron deficiency. Reduction in iron stores usually precedes both a reduction in circulating iron and anemia, as demonstrated by a decreased red blood cell count, mean corpuscular hemoglobin concentration, and microcytic red blood cells (Table 15-3).[3]

TABLE 15-3. LABORATORY MARKERS OF IRON STATUS IN SEVERAL DISEASE STATES

CONDITION	SERUM IRON (50–160 μg/dL)	TRANSFERRIN (200–400 mg/dL)	% SATURATION (20–55)	FERRITIN (20–250 μg/L)
Iron deficiency	Decreased	Increased	Decreased	Decreased
Iron poisoning/overdose	Increased	Decreased	Increased	Increased
Hematochromatosis	Increased	Decreased	Increased	Increased
Malnutrition	Decreased	Decreased	Variable	Decreased
Malignancy	Decreased	Decreased	Decreased	Increased
Chronic infection	Decreased	Decreased	Decreased	Increased
Viral hepatitis	Increased	Increased	Normal/increased	Increased
Anemia of chronic disease	Decreased	Normal/decreased	Decreased	Normal/increased
Sideroblastic anemia	Increased	Normal/decreased	Increased	Increased

A patient with thalassemia was under treatment with deferoxamine. The patient failed to follow the instructions regarding concurrent use of vitamin C, developed cardiac failure, and died 4 hours after ingesting a large amount of ascorbic acid.

Questions

1. What is the role of deferoxamine in treatment?

2. How does vitamin C interact with iron?

Although a decrease in serum iron and an increase in transferrin/TIBC are classic indices of iron deficiency, the serum ferritin concentration has evolved as a more sensitive and reliable test for confirming this condition.

Clinical Disorders of Iron Overload

Iron overload is usually caused by an abnormal excess absorption of iron from a normal diet. Iron overload states are collectively referred to as hemochromatosis, whether or not tissue damage is present. Hemosiderosis has been used to specifically designate a condition of iron overload as demonstrated by an increased serum iron and TIBC or transferrin, but without demonstrable tissue damage. Hereditary hemochromatosis is caused by a genetic defect that causes tissue accumulation of iron, affects liver function, and often leads to hyperpigmentation of the skin. Although elevated serum iron and transferrin are characteristic of early stages of hemochromatosis, the serum ferritin steadily increases with progression of the disease, often to very high levels as the condition becomes severe. Some conditions associated with severe hemochromatosis include diabetes mellitus, arthritis, cardiac arrhythmia or failure, cirrhosis, hypothyroidism, impotence, and liver cancer. Treatment may include therapeutic phlebotomy or administration of *chelators,* such as deferoxamine. Transferrin can be administered in the case of atransferrinemia.[11]

Role of Iron in Tissue Damage

Iron may play a role as a *prooxidant,* by contributing to lipid peroxidation,[12,13] atherosclerosis,[13,14] deoxyribonu-cleic acid (DNA) damage,[12,15] carcinogenesis,[16,17] and neurodegenerative diseases.[18-19] Fe^{+3}, released from binding proteins, can enhance production of free radicals to cause oxidative damage. In iron-loaded individuals with thalassemia who are treated with chelators to bind and mobilize iron, intake of ascorbic acid may actually promote the generation of free radicals.[20]

Laboratory Evaluation of Iron Status

Disorders of iron metabolism may be evaluated by the following measurements: packed cell volume, hemoglobin, red cell count and indices, total iron and TIBC, percent saturation, transferrin, and ferritin. Expected results are outlined in Tables 15-3 and 15-4.

A recent laboratory test for evaluation of iron status is the measurement of serum transferrin receptors (circulating TrfR). The number of these receptors increases in iron deficiency and decreases in iron overload.[21] Although some claim a high reliability of this test in detecting iron deficiency, others have found it to be less sensitive than serum ferritin.[1]

Total Iron Content (Serum Iron)

Measurement of serum iron concentration refers specifically to the Fe^{+3} bound to transferrin and not to the iron circulating as free hemoglobin in serum. The specimen may be collected as serum without anticoagulant or as plasma with heparin. Oxalate, citrate, or ethylenediaminetetraacetic acid bind Fe ions and are unacceptable anticoagulants. Early morning sampling is preferred because of the diurnal variation in iron

TABLE 15-4. REFERENCE RANGES FOR PARAMETERS USED TO ASSESS IRON STATUS[1,21]

PATIENT POPULATION	SERUM IRON (µg/dL)	TRANSFERRIN (mg/dL)	FERRITIN (µg/L)	% SATURATION	TIBC (µg/dL)
Adult, male	50–160	200–380	20–250	20–55	250–425
Female, 16–40 years	45–150	200–380	10–120	15–50	250–425
Female, >40 years					10–250
Newborn	100–250	130–275	25–200	12–50	100–400
Infant	40–100	200–360	200–600	12–50	100–400
Child	50–120	200–360	7–140	12–50	100–400

concentration. Specimens with visible hemolysis should be rejected.

Spectrophotometric determinations have been adapted to automated analysis. These procedures generally have the following steps: Fe^{+3} is released from binding proteins by acidification, reduced to Fe^{+2} by ascorbate or a similar reducing agent, and complexed with a color reagent such as ferrozine, ferene, or bathophenanthroline.

Total Iron-Binding Capacity

Total iron-binding capacity (TIBC) refers to the amount of iron that could be bound by saturating transferrin and other minor iron-binding proteins present in the serum or plasma sample. Typically, about one third of the iron-binding sites on transferrin are saturated. TIBC may be calculated from direct measurement of serum transferrin by the following equation:

$$TIBC\ (\mu g/dL) = serum\ transferrin\ (mg/dL) \times 1.25^{21}$$

(Eq. 15–1)

Because a small proportion of serum iron is bound by other proteins, this equation tends to slightly underestimate TIBC. This difference is of little or no clinical importance.

TIBC is determined by adding sufficient Fe^{+3} to saturate the binding sites on transferrin, with the excess iron removed by addition of $MgCO_3$ to precipitate any Fe^{+3} remaining in solution. After centrifugation to remove the precipitated Fe^{+3}, the supernatant solution containing the soluble iron bound to proteins is analyzed for total iron content. This is the TIBC, which ranges from around 250 to 425 μg/dL.

Percent Saturation

The percent saturation, also called the transferrin saturation, is the ratio of serum iron to TIBC, calculated as follows:

$$\%\ saturation = total\ iron\ (\mu g/dL)/TIBC\ (\mu g/dL) \times 100$$

(Eq. 15–2)

The normal range for this is approximately 20–50%, but varies with age and sex (Table 15-4).

Transferrin and Ferritin

Transferrin is measured by immunochemical methods such as nephelometry. Transferrin or TIBC is increased in iron deficiency and decreased in iron overload and hemochromatosis. Transferrin (TIBC) may also be decreased in chronic infections and malignancies (Table 15-3). Transferrin is primarily monitored as an indicator of nutritional status. As a negative acute phase protein, its concentration decreases in inflammatory conditions.

Ferritin is measured in serum by immunochemical methods, such as IRMA, ELISA, and chemiluminescent techniques. Several manufacturers provide kits for measuring serum ferritin by either manual or automated means. Ferritin is decreased in iron deficiency anemia and increased in iron overload and hemochromatosis. Ferritin is often increased in several other conditions, such as chronic infections, malignancy, and viral hepatitis.

COPPER

Dietary Requirements of Copper

Significant sources of copper include shellfish, liver, nuts, and legumes.[22] Although most diets contain less, an adequate intake of copper appears to be in the range of 1.5–3.0 mg/d for adults.[23]

Copper Absorption, Transport, and Excretion

The intestines play an important role in regulation of copper, with absorption modulated by need, resulting in a 55–75% rate of absorption. Both zinc and iron compete with copper for intestinal absorption.[22,24] Absorbed copper becomes bound to albumin or complexed to histidine residues as it is transported to the liver where it is stored in the form of cuproproteins. Although a small amount of circulating copper is bound to albumin and transcuprein, most is incorporated into ceruloplasmin. Ceruloplasmin is synthesized in the liver and has ferroxidase activity, converting Fe^{+2} to Fe^{+3} as it is incorporated into transferrin.[25,26] Ceruloplasmin is also an acute phase reactant, whereby increased concentrations scavenge oxygen radicals.[27]

Copper is mainly removed by fecal excretion as unabsorbed dietary copper and copper contained in biliary and intestinal secretions. Less than 3% of dietary copper is lost in urine and sweat.[23]

Biochemical Functions of Copper

A major function of copper is as a component of enzymes involved in redox reactions, with many involving reactions with oxygen. These metalloenzymes include ceruloplasmin, cytochrome *c* oxidase, superoxide dismutase, dopamine-β-hydroxylase, tyrosinase, and ascorbate oxidase. Ceruloplasmin, as mentioned earlier, has ferroxidase activity, as noted in Figure 15-1. Cytochrome *c* oxidase contains two heme groups and two copper atoms and catalyzes the reduction of oxygen to water in the last step of the electron transport chain. Superoxide dismutase (SOD), which contains both copper and zinc, plays a key role in antioxidant defense by converting highly reactive O_2^- radicals to O_2 and H_2O_2. Tyrosinase is involved in the production of melanin. Dopamine-β-hydroxylase is important in catecholamine metabolism.[22]

Copper Deficiency

Copper deficiency is uncommon; however, certain circumstances promote its occurrence, such as malnutrition and malabsorption. Zinc competes with copper for absorption from the intestine; therefore, increased intake of zinc could cause copper deficiency. Copper deficiency causes a microcytic, hypochromic anemia associated with low concentrations of ceruloplasmin. An early feature of copper deficiency is neutropenia, which may be related to decreased activity of the copper-containing antioxidant enzyme SOD, shortening the life of erythrocytes and neutrophils.[28,29]

Severe copper deficiency is associated with neurologic symptoms, decreased pigmentation, and other conditions (Table 15-2).[22] In addition, both coronary heart disease caused by arrhythmia and hyperlipidemia and aneurisms caused by blood vessel defects are more likely in severe copper deficiency.[22]

Menkes' syndrome is caused by a recessive X-linked genetic defect in copper transport and storage. Although copper is absorbed in a normal manner by intestinal mucosal cells, it accumulates because of defective transport from mucosal cells and results in a copper deficiency syndrome. Mental deterioration, failure to thrive, diminished activities of copper-containing enzymes, connective tissue abnormalities, kinky hair, and early death are features of this disease.[22] If started early enough, the condition may be treated with copper-histidine.[30]

Copper Excess

Copper excess occurs mostly by accidental ingestion of copper solutions, use of intrauterine devices containing copper, or exposure to copper-containing fungicides. Acute copper toxicity is associated with nausea, vomiting, and epigastric pain.[31] Excess copper, as with excess iron, can cause free radical production and damage.[32]

Wilson's disease, or hepatolenticular degeneration, is associated with copper accumulation in the liver, brain, kidney, and cornea. In Wilson's disease, copper is transported normally from the intestine to the liver, but cannot be transported out of the liver into the bile.[22] Patients develop copper overload in the brain and liver,[22,33] resulting in cirrhosis of the liver and brain lesions. Because the liver synthesizes less ceruloplasmin, less serum copper is transported by ceruloplasmin, which usually results in a low serum copper concentration. A low serum copper concentration (<20 µg/dL), decreased ceruloplasmin, and increased urinary copper excretion are characteristics of Wilson's disease.[22] In addition, copper deposits in the cornea (Kayser-Fleischer rings) may also be present. Treatment may include zinc administration to reduce copper absorption[22] or administration of dimercaprol (BAL), penicillamine, or ammonium tetrathiomolybdate to chelate copper and increase urinary excre-

tion. Although penicillamine and BAL treatment have harmful adverse effects, ammonium tetramolybdate blocks copper absorption while preserving neurologic function.[34] Early diagnosis of Wilson's disease is important because chelation therapy is effective in preventing complications.

Laboratory Evaluation of Copper Status

Although measurement of serum or plasma copper is usually available as a routine laboratory test, circulating copper levels are an insensitive index of overall copper status. If plasma copper is decreased, it typically indicates a severe depletion of copper. In addition, circulating copper concentrations have a diurnal variation, being highest in the morning; are increased by inflammation and pregnancy; and may be decreased by steroid hormones. The usual method for measuring serum or urine copper is by atomic absorption spectroscopy, although methods based on plasma emission spectroscopy are also used.

Associated with about 95% of serum copper, ceruloplasmin is also an index of copper status. Serum ceruloplasmin may be measured by either immunochemical methods or by measurement of enzyme oxidase activity. Although some suggest that enzymatic analysis may be preferred for assessing copper status, a recent study suggests that the ratio of enzymatically measured ceruloplasmin to immunochemically measured ceruloplasmin may be a more sensitive index of copper status than either test.[23]

ZINC

Dietary Requirements of Zinc

Rich sources of zinc include meat, fish, and dairy products.[24] Typical diets supply from 10 to 15 mg of zinc per day, which is close to the required dietary allowance (RDA) of 15 mg/day. Pregnant women and children should especially ensure adequate dietary zinc.

Zinc Absorption, Transport, and Excretion

Zinc absorption is mainly in the small intestine and is an active, energy dependent process that plays an important role in regulation of zinc. Approximately 65% of zinc is transported in the circulation by albumin and about 35% by α_2-macroglobulin.[24,35] The major route of excretion is by the feces; about 25% is by pancreatic secretions.[36] Urine and sweat account for a relatively small amount of zinc loss.

Biochemical Functions of Zinc

Next to iron, zinc is the most abundant trace element, with about 2 g being present in an adult body. Along with magnesium, zinc is the most frequently encountered metal cofactor for enzyme activity, being essential for more than 300 enzymes. It is usually an integral component of the active site of the enzyme. Alkaline phosphatase, alcohol dehydrogenase, and carbonic anhydrase require zinc. Because carbonic anhydrase activity is high in erythrocytes, zinc depletion often leads to both diminished activity of this enzyme and lowered zinc levels in erythrocytes. DNA and RNA polymerases require zinc and zinc ions are essential in maintaining the proper structural conformation of DNA. Among the other important functions, zinc enzymes are essential for growth, wound healing, integrity of connective tissue, reproductive function, the immune system, and protection from free radical damage.[24,37]

Zinc Deficiency and Toxicity

Insufficient dietary zinc appears to be the major cause of zinc deficiency throughout the world, although diets high in fiber or phosphate are also associated with zinc deficiency.[24] Administration of steroids or metal chelating agents can lead to zinc deficiency. GI malabsorption syndromes and urinary loss from a variety of conditions may also be causes. Concentrations of plasma zinc often do not change significantly until zinc deficiency is pronounced.[36] Symptoms of zinc deficiency include growth retardation, skin lesions, slow wound healing, diarrhea, impotence, dwarfism, sensory alterations, and susceptibility to infection by reduced immune T-cell function.[24,38] The clinical effects are often reversed by increasing dietary intake of zinc to 30–40 mg/d. Zinc is relatively nontoxic, and zinc excess is rare.

Laboratory Evaluation of Zinc Status

Consideration should be made for both the diurnal and postprandial variations of zinc, with values highest in the morning when fasting.[39] Also, serum values are about 10% higher than plasma values as a result of osmotic shifts caused by anticoagulants.[23] It is noteworthy that the concentration of zinc in erythrocytes is about 10 times higher than in plasma.

Although a decreased level of zinc in plasma or serum may indicate zinc deficiency, it may also be related to a decreased albumin level. Plasma zinc also has a diurnal variation and can decrease with inflammation. Measurement of zinc in red cells and functional activities of zinc-containing enzymes appear to correlate with zinc deficiency and may offer useful information in assessing overall zinc status. Urinary zinc also typically correlates with zinc deficiency.[23]

The most reliable method for measuring zinc in plasma, serum, or urine that is suitable for routine use in the clinical laboratory is atomic absorption spectroscopy. Other methods available include spectrophotometry and emission spectroscopy. Activities of the enzymes alkaline phosphatase and carbonic anhydrase may also be useful indicators of zinc status.

COBALT

The only known essential function of cobalt is as a constituent of vitamin B_{12}, which is involved in folate metabolism and erythropoiesis. Although cobalt salts may be absorbed by the same mechanism as iron, many questions remain about its metabolism and utilization. As with many other trace elements, cobalt has toxic effects at high doses.[24] The most common method of measurement is atomic absorption.

CHROMIUM

Because of its wide industrial use in metal alloys, metal plating, dyes, and leather tanning, chromium is common in the environment, occurring both naturally and as industrial waste. Although chromium can exist in an unusually large number of oxidation states, only the $^{+3}$ and $^{+6}$ ions are present in living systems. The $^{+6}$ ion is far more toxic than the $^{+3}$ ion.

Although meats and grains are relatively rich sources of chromium, the typical diet may be low in chromium.[40] From 50 to 200 μg/day appears to be an adequate intake of chromium. Chromium must be present at much higher concentrations to have toxic effects.[41] Once absorbed, chromium is transported to the tissue by transferrin, which has about an equal affinity for Cr^{+3} ion and for Fe^{+3} ion.[42]

Chromium is important in glucose metabolism as an essential activator of insulin. A low MW complex of Cr^{+3} with nicotinic acid and other organic compounds appears to be the factor that activates insulin. Chromium deficiency is associated with insulin resistance,[23] and chromium supplementation has demonstrated improved glucose tolerance, reduced insulin concentrations, and decreased total cholesterol in type 2 diabetes.[41]

The most common methods for measuring chromium are based on flameless atomic absorption.[23]

FLUORIDE

The importance of fluoride is well known for its role in preventing dental caries. Although excess intake is associated with mottling of teeth and calcifications in soft tissue,[24] fluoride may also minimize bone loss or even stimulate bone formation.[23] Fluoride is incorporated into bone crystal, increasing bone mass in the vertebrae. Administration of vitamin D_3, with cyclic administration of fluoride, may enhance bone formation, correct calcium deficiency, and lessen the occurrence of fracture.[43,44]

Fluoride is readily absorbed by the gut and distributed almost totally to the bone and teeth. Renal excretion is the major route for removal of fluoride from the body.

A 45-year-old woman, being treated for type 2 diabetes for 2 years, relayed to her physician a continued noncompliance with dietary restrictions and suggested exercise regimen. After obtaining a laboratory report (fasting blood glucose, 138 mg/dL; total cholesterol, 289 mg/dL), her physician prescribed a chromium picolinate supplement (500 μg, twice daily). After 4 months, her fasting blood glucose decreased to 102 mg/dL and her total cholesterol decreased to 243 mg/dL.

Questions

1. What effect does chromium have on carbohydrate and lipid metabolism?

2. Is the form and dose of chromium administered related to its biologic activity?

3. Is Cr^{+3} toxic? Is it more or less toxic than Cr^{+6}?

The concentration of fluoride is approximately 10–200 μg/L in serum, 450 μg/L in erythrocytes, and 0.2–3.2 μg/L in urine.[23] Ion-selective electrodes have been developed for measuring fluoride.[45]

MANGANESE

Both +2 and +3 manganese ions are present in biologic systems, largely as protein-bound ions. Manganese is an activator of several enzymes, including arginase, pyruvate carboxylase, and superoxide dismutase. It is noteworthy that several other metal ions (such as magnesium, copper, or iron) can substitute for magnesium as an activator of these enzymes, which can mask a manganese deficiency.

Manganese intake should be 2–5 mg/day for adults.[23] The rate of absorption of manganese is low and is decreased by phosphate, phytate, calcium, and iron. Manganese is transported in plasma by albumin, α_2-macroglobulin, and transferrin[46] and excreted in bile and pancreatic secretions.

Many enzymes require manganese for activity, including pyruvate carboxylase, mitochondrial superoxide dismutase, arginase, and glucokinase. The effect of manganese deficiency is minimized by substitution of other similar ions in enzymes; therefore, symptoms of manganese deficiency are rare. In children, manganese deficiency may be associated with seizures and possibly epilepsy. High dosages, except by inhalation, are not toxic.[24] Recent reports have associated manganese deposition in brain with neurologic symptoms in persons with exposure to manganese agents and patients with cholestatic liver disease.[46,47]

The concentration of manganese in whole blood, blood cells, or lymphocytes may be more reliable than concentration in serum or plasma for assessing the tissue stores of manganese. Although reported concentrations vary widely due to differences in sample collection, processing, and methodology, the reference ranges appear to be 0.4–0.8 μg/L for plasma and 7.7–12 μg/L for whole blood.[23] The most practical clinical laboratory method for measurement of manganese is flameless atomic absorption with selective chelation and extraction.[48]

MOLYBDENUM

Molybdenum is important as an essential cofactor for several oxidase enzymes: xanthine dehydrogenase/xanthine oxidase, aldehyde oxidase, and sulfite oxidase. Xanthine oxidase converts hypoxanthine to uric acid, aldehyde oxi-

A 74-year-old woman recently fractured her left femur. Treated for osteoporosis with estrogen, calcium, vitamin D, and fluoride for 2 years before the fracture, the patient's serial bone density measurements have showed a continuing increase in density. At the time of hospitalization, her urinary calcium output was 0.9 mg/day (decreased).

Questions

1. What is the role of fluoride in osteoporosis treatment?

2. Is the fluoride treatment associated with increased incidence of fractures?

3. Why was this patient's calcium output very low?

CASE STUDY 15-4

A 65-year-old woman with a history of diabetes was seen by her physician for weight loss, anorexia, and general fatigue. As part of the physical exam, both "bronze" skin pigmentation (hyperpigmentation) and enlarged liver were noted. Her initial chemistry panel showed the following relevant results:

Albumin	3.7 g/dL (3.8–5.0)
ALP	180 U/L (30–135)
ALT	200 U/L (10–60)
Total bilirubin	2.5 mg/dL (0.2–1.2)
Serum iron	180 µg/dL (45–150)

Further testing for the elevated iron showed the following:

Serum iron	170 µg/dL (45–150)
Transferrin	210 mg/dL (200–380)
Ferritin	300 µg/L (10–250)
% transferrin saturation	80

The patient was diagnosed with hemochromatosis that caused iron overload.

Questions

1. What happens to serum ferritin in this condition?

2. Are this patient's conditions and symptoms typical of hemochromatosis?

3. What is a treatment plan for iron overload and what is the main goal?

---

dase catalyzes the conversion of acetyl-CoA to acetate, and sulfite oxidase converts sulfite to sulfate.[24] Xanthine oxidase and aldehyde oxidase can also produce oxygen radicals, such as during reperfusion following ischemia.[49,50]

Dietary molybdenum is mostly absorbed in the stomach and small intestine. Both copper and iron may inhibit absorption of molybdenum. Although the liver takes up most molybdenum, it is released and excreted either in the urine or in the bile.

Although molybdenum is relatively nontoxic, excess exposure may cause inhibition of copper-dependent enzymes such as ceruloplasmin and cytochrome oxidase. The formation of a molybdenum–copper complex is the basis of a treatment for Wilson's disease, as discussed in the copper section of this chapter.[34] Elevated exposures to molybdenum have been linked to elevated uric acid and gout.[23]

Reference ranges for molybdenum in adults are approximately 0.1–3.0 µg/L for serum or plasma, about 0.8–33 µg/L for whole blood, and about 18 µg/L for red cells. Urinary excretion ranges from 8 to 34 µg/L.[23]

SELENIUM

Selenium has numerous essential functions in humans: it is a cofactor in glutathione peroxidase and iodothyronine diodinase; selenocysteine is an essential amino acids coded by DNA; selenomethionine can substitute for methionine as an essential amino acid in some proteins.

Selenium also has antioxidant properties and is involved in metabolism of thyroid hormones.[51]

Because selenium is incorporated into proteins such as glutathione peroxidase,[24] its activity may reflect sele-

nium status. Selenium deficiency has been associated with cardiomyopathy and skeletal muscle weakness, osteoarthritis, and increased incidence of cancer.[52] Although more work is needed, studies on the effects of micronutrients on cancer risk have demonstrated that selenium supplementation is associated with a decreased risk of cancer, especially in the stomach, lung, and prostate. Such risks may be reduced with concurrent intake of β-carotene and α-tocopherol.[53]

Selenium may be determined by atomic absorption. Because of the volatility of organoselenium compounds, generation of volatile selenium hydride with detection by atomic absorption has proven to be a useful technique. Reference ranges for selenium in adults are: 46–143 µg/L in plasma, 58–234 µg/L in whole blood, and 75–240 µg/L in red cells.[23]

SUMMARY

Trace elements are important or essential for many critical biochemical processes, and their concentrations are tightly regulated in the healthy individual. Deficiencies are often associated with decreased activities of the enzymes that require trace elements for optimal activity. Function can be usually be restored by dietary replacement, but care must be exercised not to induce toxicity. The laboratory evaluation of trace element status includes both determination of body fluid concentrations and activity of relevant enzymes. There is still much research needed to determine the function of trace element in health and disease and the most effective tests for accurate diagnosis.

CASE STUDY 15-5

A 36-year-old man had undergone multiple partial small bowel resections because of Crohn's disease. After recovery from surgery, he was placed on total parenteral nutrition (TPN). After adequate rehabilitation, he was discharged under the care of a home health care nurse who visited him 3 times a week to follow his overall progress and check his physical and vital conditions. Periodic routine laboratory tests were performed to assess nutritional status. Although his first few months after surgery were unremarkable, he eventually experienced symptoms of weakness, diarrhea, general malaise, and hair loss. He visited his physician, who did a complete workup and obtained the following laboratory values:

Na^+	147 mmol/L (135–145 mmol/L)
K^+	4.9 mmol/L (3.5–5.0 mmol/L)
Cl^-	118 mmol/L (98–106 mmol/L)
Glucose	102 mg/dL (80–100 mg/dL)
Creatinine	0.6 mg/dL (0.6–1.2 mg/dL)

Calcium	7.9 mg/dL (8.4–10.2 mg/dL)
Hemoglobin	10.4 g/dL (13.3–17.7 g/dL)
Hematocrit	31% (40–52%)
Albumin	2.5 g/dL (3.5–5.5 g/dL)
Transferrin	112 mg/dL (200–380 mg/dL)
Copper	38 µg/dL (70–150 µg/dL)
Zinc	46 µg/dL (66–110 µg/dL)

Questions

1. What do the laboratory studies suggest as a possible cause of this patient's problem?

2. What is the significance of the low copper and zinc levels? Could his diet be the underlying cause of these deficiencies?

3. What medical treatment should be instituted in this patient?

REVIEW QUESTIONS

1. Iron is physiologically active, only in the ferrous form in:
   a. cytochromes.
   b. ferritin.
   c. hemoglobin.
   d. transferrin.

2. Which pattern most likely represents iron deficiency?
   a. Decreased ferritin, increased transferrin, increased serum iron
   b. Increased ferritin, increased transferrin, increased serum iron
   c. Decreased ferritin, increased transferrin, decreased serum iron
   d. Decreased ferritin, decreased transferrin, decreased serum iron

3. The deficiency of what trace metal is associated with growth retardation, dermatitis, reduced taste acuity, and impaired wound healing?
   a. Copper
   b. Iron
   c. Selenium
   d. Zinc

4. Which of the following metals are required for optimal activity of superoxide dismutase?
   a. Iron and chromium
   b. Zinc and selenium
   c. Magnesium and manganese
   d. Copper and zinc

5. The deficiency of which of the following metals can cause a deficiency of iron?
   a. Copper
   b. Chromium
   c. Cobalt
   d. Zinc

6. A metal ion required for optimal enzyme activity is best termed a(an):
   a. accelerator.
   b. cofactor.
   c. coenzyme.
   d. catalyst.

7. Which statement about iron is NOT true?
   a. TIBC may be calculated from the transferrin concentration.
   b. Myoglobin has a higher affinity for iron than hemoglobin.
   c. Transferrin in serum is typically 99% saturated with iron.
   d. Serum iron is typically higher in males than females.

8. Which trace metal is contained in glucose tolerance factor?
   a. Copper
   b. Chromium
   c. Selenium
   d. Zinc

9. Menkes' syndrome is caused by an accumulation in the intestinal mucosal cells and associated low plasma concentrations of:
   a. iron.
   b. zinc.
   c. copper.
   d. manganese.

10. What metal may be used as a treatment for Wilson's disease?
   a. Copper
   b. Molybdenum
   c. Fluorine
   d. Zinc

11. The trace element that appears to be associated with enhanced bone formation is:
   a. iron.
   b. fluoride.
   c. copper.
   d. manganese

12. The metal ion essential for activity of xanthine oxidase and xanthine dehydrogenase is:
   a. iron.
   b. zinc.
   c. molybdenum.
   d. manganese.

REFERENCES

1. Fairbanks VF, Klee GG. Biochemical aspects of hematology. In: Burtis CA, Ashwood ER, eds. Tietz Textbook of Clinical Chemistry, 3rd ed. Philadelphia: WB Saunders, 1999:1642–1710.
2. Kratz A, Lee-Lewandrowski E, Lewandrowski K. The plasma proteins. In: Lewandrowski K, ed. Clinical Chemistry: Laboratory Management and Clinical Correlations. Philadelphia: Lippincott Williams & Wilkins, 2002:531–560.
3. Beard J, Dawson B, Pinero D. Iron metabolism: a comprehensive review. Nutr Rev 1996;54(10):295–317.
4. Sullivan JL. Stored iron and ischemic heart disease—empirical support for a new paradigm. Circulation 1992;86:1036–1037.
5. Lauffer R. Preventive measures for the maintenance of low but adequate iron stores. In: Lauffer R, ed. Iron and Human Disease. Boca Raton, FL: CRC Press, 1992.
6. Levine DS, Woods JW. Immunolocalization of transferrin-transferrin receptor in mouse small intestine absorptive cells. Histochem Cytochem 1996;38:851–858.
7. Pantopoulos K, Gray NK, Hentze MW. Differential regulation of two related RNA-binding proteins, iron regulatory protein (IRP) and IRP$_B$. RNA 1995;1:155–163.
8. Crichton R, Ward RJ. Iron metabolism—new perspectives in view. Biochemistry 1992;31:11255–11264.
9. Linder MC, Schaeffer KJ, Hazegh-Azam M, et al. Serum ferritin: does it differ from tissue ferritin? J Gastroenterol Hepatol 1996; 11:1033–1036.
10. DeMaeyer E, Adiels-Tegman M. The prevalence of anaemia in the world. World Health Stat Q 1985;38:302–316.
11. Bottomly S. Secondary iron overload disorders. Semin Hematol 1998;35(1):77–86.
12. Meneghini R. Iron homeostasis, oxidative stress, and DNA damage. Free Radic Biol Med 1997;23(5):783–792.
13. Smith C, Mitchinson MJ, Aruoma OI, et al. Stimulation of lipid peroxidation and hydroxyl-radical generation by the contents of human atherosclerotic lesions. Biochem J 1992;286:901–915.
14. Schwartz CJ, Valente AJ, Sprague EA, et al. The pathogenesis of atherosclerosis: an overview. Clin Cardiol 1991;14:I-1–I-16.
15. Halliwell B, Aruoma OI. DNA damage by oxygen-derived species: Its mechanism and measurement in mammalian system. FEBS Lett 1991;281:9–19.
16. Weinberg ED. Cellular iron metabolism in health and disease. Drug Metab Rev 1990;22:531–579.
17. Anghileri L. Iron, intracellular calcium ion, lipid peroxidation and carcinogenesis. Anticancer Res 1995;15:1395–1400.
18. Smith MA, Perry G. Free radical damage, iron, and Alzheimer's disease. J Neurol Sci 1995;134S:92–94.
19. McCord J. Iron, free radicals, and oxidative injury. Sem Hematol 1998;35(1):5–12.
20. Herbert V, Shaw S, Jayatilleke E. Vitamin C-driven free radical generation from iron. J Nutr 1996;126;1213S–1220S.
21. Jacobs DS, Oxley DK, DeMott WR. Jacobs & DeMott Laboratory Test Handbook, 5th ed. Cleveland: Lexi-Comp, 2001.
22. Linder MC. The Biochemistry of Copper. New York: Plenum, 1991.
23. Milne DB. Trace elements. In: Burtis CA, Ashwood ER, eds. Tietz Textbook of Clinical Chemistry, 3rd ed. Philadelphia: WB Saunders, 1999:1029–1055.
24. Linder MC. Nutrition and metabolism of trace elements. In: Linder MC, ed. Nutritional Biochemistry and Metabolism, 2nd ed. New York: Elsevier, 1991:215–276.
25. Sandstead H. Requirements and toxicity of essential trace elements, illustrated by zinc and copper. Am J Clin Nutr 1995; 61S:621S–624S.
26. Walshe JM. Copper: not too little, not too much, but just right. J R Coll Physicians Lond 1995;29(4):280–287.
27. Linder MC. Interactions between copper and iron in mammalian metabolism. In: Elsenhans BE, Forth W, Schumann K, eds. Metal–Metal Interactions. Gutersloh, Germany: Bertelsheim Foundation, 1994;11–41.
28. Percival, S. Neutropenia caused by copper deficiency: possible mechanisms of action. Nutr Rev 1995;53(3):59–66.
29. Hirase N, et al. Anemia and neutropenia in a case of copper deficiency: role of copper in normal hematopoiesis. Acta Haematol 1992;87:195–197.

30. Sakar B, Lingertat-Walsh K, Clarke JTR. Copper-histidine therapy for Menkes' disease. J Pediatr 1993;123:828–830.

31. Olivares, M. Limits of metabolic tolerance to copper and biological basis for present recommendations and regulations. Am J Clin Nutr 1996;63:846S–852S.

32. Halliwell B. Free radicals and antioxidants: a personal view. Nutr Rev 1994;52:253–265.

33. Brewer GJ, Yuzbasiyan-Gurkan V. Wilson's disease. Medicine 1992;71:139–164.

34. Brewer G, et al. Treatment of Wilson's disease with ammonium tetramolybdate. Arch Neurol 1996;53:1017–1025.

35. Parisi AF, Vallee BL. Isolation of a zinc alpha-2-macroglobulin from human serum. Biochemistry 1970;9:2421–2426.

36. King J. Assessment of zinc status. J Nutr 1990;120:1474–1479.

37. Cunningham-Rundles S. Zinc modulation of immune function: specificity and mechanism of interaction. J Lab Clin Med 1996; 128:9–11.

38. Prasad AS, et al. Zinc metabolism in normals and patients with the syndrome of iron deficiency anemia, hepatosplenomegaly, dwarfism, and hypogonadism. J Lab Clin Med 1963;61:531–537.

39. Pilch SM, Senti FR. Assessment of the zinc nutritional status of the US population based on data collected in the second national health and nutrition examination survey. FASEB FDA 223-223-83-2384. Bethesda, MD: Life Science Research Office, 1984.

40. Anderson RA, et al. Dietary chromium intake—freely chosen diets, institutional diets and individual foods. Biol Trace Elem Res 1992;117–121.

41. Anderson RA, et al. Elevated intakes of supplemental chromium improve glucose and insulin variables in individuals with type-2 diabetes. Diabetes 1997;46(11):1786–1791.

42. Anderson RA. Chromium as an essential nutrient for humans. Regul Toxicol Pharmacol 1997;26:S35–S41.

43. Dure-Smith BA, Farley SM, Linkhart SG, et al. Calcium deficiency in fluoride-treated osteoporotic patients despite calcium supplementation. J Clin Endocrinol Metab 1996;81:269–275.

44. Pak CYC, et al. Slow-release sodium fluoride in the management of postmenopausal osteoporosis. Ann Intern Med 1994;120: 625–632.

45. Blanke RV, Decker WJ. Analysis of toxic substances. In: Tietz NW, ed. Textbook of Clinical Chemistry. Philadelphia: WB Saunders, 1986:1717–1719.

46. Misselwitz B, Muhler A, Weinmann H-J. A toxicologic risk for using manganese complexes? A literature survey of existing data through several medical specialties. Invest Radiol 1995;30(10): 611–620.

47. Krieger D, et al. Manganese and chronic hepatic encephalopathy. Lancet 1995;346(8970):270–274.

48. Baruthio F, Guillard O, Arnaud J, et al. Determination of manganese in biological materials by electrothermal atomic absorption spectrometry: a review. Clin Chem 1988;34:227–234.

49. Repine JE. Oxidant—antioxidant balance: some observations from studies of ischemia-reperfusion in isolated perfused rat hearts. Am J Med 1991;91(3C):45S–53S.

50. Wright RM, Repine JE. The human molybdenum hydroxylase gene family: co-conspirators in metabolic free-radical generation and disease. Biochem Soc Trans 1997;25:799–804.

51. Gladyshev VN, Jeang KT, Stadtman TC. Selenocysteine, identified as the penultimate C-terminal residue in human T-cell thioredoxin reductase, corresponds to TGA in the human placental gene. Proc Natl Acad Sci USA 1996;93:6146-6151.

52. Mo DX. Pathology and selenium deficiency in Kashin-Beck disease. In: Combs GF, et al, eds. Selenium in Biology and Medicine. New York: Avi 1987:924–933.

53. Clark LC, et al. Effects of selenium supplementation for cancer prevention in patients with carcinoma of the skin. A randomized controlled trial. JAMA 1996;276:1957–1963.

Porphyrins and Hemoglobin

Louann W. Lawrence, Larry A. Broussard

OBJECTIVES

Upon completion of this chapter, the clinical laboratorian should be able to:

- Describe the chemical nature and structure of porphyrins and hemoglobin.
- Relate the role of porphyrins in the body.
- Outline the biochemical pathway of porphyrin and heme synthesis.
- Discuss the clinical significance of the porphyrias.
- Compare and contrast the porphyrias with regard to enzyme deficiency, clinical symptoms, and clinical laboratory data.
- Explain the principles of the basic qualitative and quantitative porphyrin tests, to include PBG,

ALA, uroporphyrin, coproporphyrin, and protoporphyrin.
- Describe the degradation of hemoglobin.
- Discuss the clinical significance and laboratory data associated with the hemoglobinopathies and thalassemias.
- Identify the tests used in the diagnosis of hemoglobinopathies and thalassemias.
- Discuss the structure and clinical significance of myoglobin in the body.

KEY TERMS

Cytochrome
Hemoglobinopathy
Myoglobin

Porphyria
Porphyrin

Porphyrinogen
Porphyrinuria

Pyrrole
Thalassemia

Because of chemical similarities, porphyrins, hemoglobin, and myoglobin are discussed together in this chapter. These compounds all contain the porphyrin ring, which comprises four pyrrole groups bonded by methene bridges (Fig. 16-1). Porphyrins are able to chelate metals to form the functional groups that participate in oxidative metabolism. The analysis of porphyrins in the laboratory aids in the diagnosis of a group of disorders resulting from disturbances in heme synthesis called the *porphyrias*. Each defective enzyme that causes porphyria may be assayed by various methods. Hemoglobin molecules are specially designed to bind, deliver, and release oxygen. Qualitative defects in the hemoglobin molecule result in a group of disorders called *hemoglobinopathies*, such as sickle cell anemia. Quantitative defects in production of normal hemoglobin molecules lead to another group of disorders called *thalassemias*. Analytic methods to diagnose these disorders are discussed. *Myoglobin* is a simple heme protein found only in skeletal and cardiac muscle, which may be analyzed to aid in diagnosis of acute myocardial infarction.

PORPHYRINS

Role in the Body

Porphyrins are chemical intermediates in the synthesis of hemoglobin, myoglobin, and other respiratory pigments called *cytochromes*. They also form part of the peroxidase and catalase enzymes, which contribute to the efficiency of internal respiration. Iron is chelated within porphyrins to form heme. Heme is then incorporated into proteins to become biologically functional hemoproteins. Porphyrins are analyzed in clinical chemistry to aid in the diagnosis of *porphyrias*, which result from disturbances in heme synthesis. Excess amounts of these intermediate compounds in urine, feces, or blood indicate a metabolic block in heme synthesis.

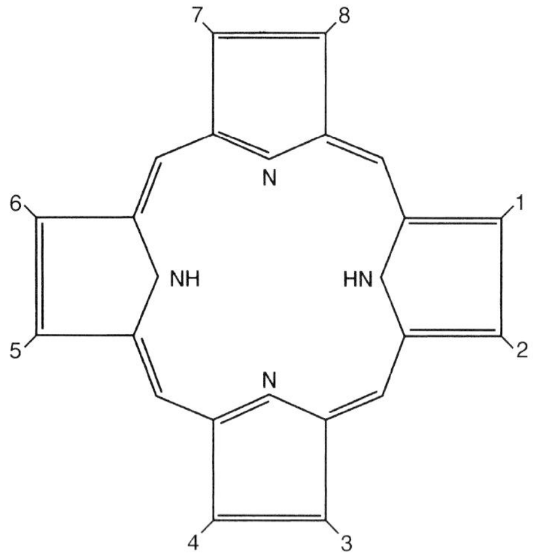

FIGURE 16-1. Basic structure of porphyrins.

Chemistry of Porphyrins

The porphyrins found in nature are all compounds in which side chains are substituted for the eight hydrogen atoms found in the four *pyrrole* rings that make up porphyrin (Fig. 16-1). Because of the wide variety of substitutions, many porphyrins have been described in nature. The pigment chlorophyll is a magnesium porphyrin and is essential for plants to use light energy to synthesize carbohydrates. Four basic isomers may exist for every porphyrin compound; however, only type I and type III occur in nature. The difference between types I and III isomers is in the arrangement of side chains. Only type III isomers form heme; however, in some disorders, the functionless type I isomers may be present in excess in the tissue. Porphyrins are stable compounds, red-violet to red-brown in color, that fluoresce red when excited by light near 400 nm. Only three porphyrin compounds are clinically significant in humans: protoporphyrin (PROTO), uroporphyrin (URO), and coproporphyrin (COPRO). Their presence in excess in biologic fluids is a clinical sign of abnormal heme synthesis. The three compounds have different solubility properties and different degrees of ionization determined by the addition of various carboxyl groups to the basic porphyrin structure. This allows for separate assays of each. URO is excreted primarily in urine, PROTO in the feces, and COPRO in either, depending on the rate of formation of the urine and its pH.

The reduced forms of porphyrins are termed *porphyrinogens*, the functional form of the compound that must be used in heme synthesis. Porphyrinogens are highly unstable, colorless, and do not fluoresce, which makes them more difficult to analyze. With light, oxygen, or oxidizing agents, porphyrinogens are readily oxidized to the corresponding porphyrin form. Therefore, the porphyrin form is routinely analyzed in clinical laboratories as a result of the increased stability and ease of detection by various common clinical laboratory systems.

Porphyrin Synthesis

All cells contain hemoproteins and can synthesize heme; however, the bone marrow and liver are the main sites. The series of irreversible reactions is outlined in Figure 16-2. Some steps occur in the mitochondria of the cell and some steps in the cytoplasm. The transport of substrates across the mitochondrion membrane is a complex process and a potential point for interruptions in heme synthesis.

Control of the rate of heme synthesis in the cells in the liver is achieved largely through regulation of the enzyme δ-aminolevulinic acid (ALA) synthase. The main mechanism is repression of synthesis of new enzyme. A negative feedback mechanism exists in which increases in the

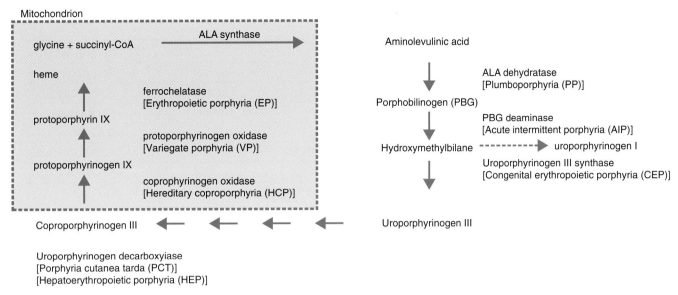

FIGURE 16-2. Synthesis of heme. *Brackets* indicate diseases associated with enzyme deficiencies.

pool of hepatic heme diminish the production of ALA synthase. Conversely, ALA synthase production is increased with a depletion of heme. The size of the regulatory heme pool may be affected by the requirement for hemoproteins in the liver. Drugs and other compounds appear to induce ALA synthase production by several different mechanisms, but all result in a depletion of the regulatory heme pool. Therefore, the rate of heme synthesis is flexible and can change rapidly in response to a wide variety of external stimuli. In bone marrow erythrocytes, other enzymes in the pathway and the rate of cellular iron uptake seem to control the rate of heme synthesis.[1]

Clinical Significance and Disease Correlation

The porphyrias are inherited or acquired enzyme deficiencies that result in overproduction of heme precursors in the bone marrow (erythropoietic porphyrias) or the liver (hepatic porphyrias). Disease states corresponding to enzyme deficiencies have been identified in every step of heme synthesis except for ALA synthase. Some patients demonstrate an enzyme deficiency but do not show clinical or biochemical manifestations of porphyria, indicating that other factors, such as demand for increased heme biosynthesis, are also important in causing disease expression. An excess of the early precursors in the pathway of heme synthesis (ALA, porphobilinogen, or both) causes neuropsychiatric symptoms, including abdominal pain, vomiting, constipation, tachycardia, hypertension, psychiatric symptoms, fever, leukocytosis, and paresthesia. Porphyrias in this category include ALA dehydratase (ALAD) deficiency porphyria (ADP) or plumboporphyria (PP) and acute intermittent porphyria

(AIP). Excesses of the later intermediates (UROs, COPROs, and PROTOs) may cause cutaneous symptoms, including photosensitivity, blisters, excess facial hair, and hyperpigmentation. Porphyria cutanea tarda (PCT), hepatoerythropoietic porphyria (HEP), erythropoietic porphyria (EP), and congenital erythropoietic porphyria (CEP) are associated with cutaneous symptoms. Porphyrin-induced photosensitivity manifests by increased fragility of light-exposed skin, as in PCT, or by burning of light-exposed skin, as in EP. The photosensitizing effects of the porphyrins are attributable to absorption of light. There may also be excesses of both early and late intermediates, causing neurocutaneous symptoms. Hereditary coproporphyria (HCP) and variegate porphyria (VP) fall into this category. All porphyrias are inherited as autosomal dominant traits producing about a 50% reduction in enzyme levels, except for ADP and CEP, which are autosomal recessive.[2]

The diagnosis of porphyrias is made by a combination of history and physical and laboratory findings. The cutaneous porphyrias are easier to diagnose because photosensitivity is usually the presenting symptom. Laboratory diagnosis, if necessary, is made by analysis of the appropriate sample for intermediates in heme synthesis (Table 16-1). The differentiation of neurologic porphyrias from other disorders is more difficult based on history and physical examination and must be verified by laboratory findings.

Inherited ADP is extremely rare, with only four cases reported.[3] Urinary ALA is significantly elevated with normal porphobilinogen (PBG) excretion. Increased urinary coproporphyrin III may provide supporting evidence for the diagnosis but this also occurs in lead poisoning, which is the most common cause of low ALAD activity

TABLE 16-1. METABOLITES FOUND IN EXCESS IN THE PORPHYRIAS

PORPHYRIA	URINE	FECES	ERYTHROCYTES	SYMPTOMS
ADP (PP)	ALA, COPRO III	Normal	ZPP	Neuropsychiatric
AIP	ALA, PBG, URO I	Normal	Normal	Neuropsychiatric
CEP	URO I, COPRO I	URO I, COPRO I	URO, ZPP	Cutaneous
PCT	URO I, ISOCOPRO	ISOCOPRO	Normal	Cutaneous
HEP	URO, COPRO	ISOCOPRO	ZPP	Cutaneous
HCP	*ALA, *PBG, *COPRO III	COPRO, HARDERO	Normal	Neurocutaneous
VP	*ALA, *PBG, *COPRO III	PROTO > COPRO	Normal	Neurocutaneous
EP	Normal	PROTO > COPRO	PROTO	Cutaneous

* indicates during acute attacks; PBG, porphobilinogen; HARDERO, harderoporphyrin.

and must be ruled out before making a diagnosis of ADP. ADP may be distinguished from lead poisoning by the in vitro addition of dithiothreitol or other sulfhydryl reagents. This results in restoration of erythrocyte ALAD activity to normal in patients with lead poisoning but no change in the reduced ALAD activity in ADP patients.[3]

AIP results from a deficiency of the enzyme PBG deaminase (PBGD). The estimated frequency of acute attacks of AIP in most developed countries is one to two per 100,000, with a higher prevalence in Scandinavian countries.[3] PBGD is encoded on chromosome 11q23, with more than 100 mutations of this gene described.[3] Although the inheritance is autosomal dominant, only about 10% of patients with the deficiency suffer attacks of the disease, so other etiologic factors are involved. Drugs are the most common precipitating cause of disease, especially barbiturates and sulfonamides; however, a wide variety of drugs are potentially hazardous. This disease is characterized by multiple neurologic symptoms with colicky stomach pain and, occasionally, fever and vomiting. The characteristic laboratory findings are a marked elevation of ALA and PBG in the urine, although these test results may be normal between attacks. A patient's urine with clinically manifest AIP may turn red or dark brown due to nonenzymatic conversion to uroporphyrin I, a process that may be delayed with refrigeration, protection from light, and alkaline adjustment to pH 8.0–9.0. Electrolyte abnormalities, including hyponatremia during acute attacks may help suggest the diagnosis.[3] Measurement of levels of erythrocyte or lymphoblast PBGD may be performed to confirm the diagnosis.[4]

CEP, a deficiency of uroprophyrinogen III cosynthase, is one of the rarest porphyrias (less than 200 cases reported) and usually appears shortly after birth, with the first signs often being red-brown urine staining of diapers and cutaneous photosensitivity.[4] It is also known as *Günther's disease*. The teeth will fluoresce red under ultraviolet light and exhibit a red or brownish discoloration un-

der normal light as a result of porphyrin deposits in the dentin. Urine and fecal porphyrins, URO I and COPRO I, are significantly elevated. The urine is often red because of the presence of URO and COPRO. Photosensitivity is a major clinical problem, resulting in lesions that may become infected and leave the patient scarred or with multiple occurrences that may lead to mutilation of the ears, nose, or digits. Abnormal hair growth is often seen in exposed areas. It is thought that the disfigurements of this disorder and the tendency to avoid daylight (hence, only coming outside at night) led to the legend of the werewolf.[5] Patients may also develop a hemolytic anemia and splenomegaly with hemolysis serving as a stimulus for increased porphyrin production in the bone marrow.[6] Allogenic bone marrow transplantation has proved curative in patients with CEP, and the use of stem cells for treatment of CEP patients is being investigated.[3]

Deficiency of uroporphyrinogen decarboxylase (UROD) occurs in PCT, the most common porphyria, and in the rarer HEP. PCT is subdivided into two types: sporadic type I, in which decreased UROD activity is restricted to the liver and there is no family history of the disease; and familial type II, characterized by UROD deficiency in all tissue and an autosomal dominant inheritance pattern. Genetic studies have shown that PCT is not a single monogenic disorder but rather a group of diseases characterized by different mutations to the gene (mapped on chromosome 1p34) coding for UROD and possibly to other genes outside the UROD locus.[7] PCT usually presents in adulthood with cutaneous blistering and fragility in light-exposed areas, typically the hands, along with some abnormal hair growth. Liver biopsy specimens from these patients show fluorescence, hemosiderosis, fatty infiltration, and variable degrees of necrosis and fibrosis. PCT is differentiated from all other porphyrias by three features: (1) association of skin lesions with severe deficiency of UROD, resulting in increased excretion of uroporphyrin, heptacarboxylic porphyrin, isocoproporphyrin, and other porphyrins; (2) remission following low-dose chloroquine or iron depletion; and (3) some degree of liver cell damage in almost all patients.[8] In genetically predisposed patients, PCT may be induced by multiple factors including alcohol, estrogen, halogenated aromatic hydrocarbons (hexachlorobenzene and 2,3,7,8-tetrachlorodibenzo-p-dioxin), infection by hepatitis C and human immunodeficiency virus (HIV), thalassemia, hepatic tumors, hemodialysis, and bone marrow transplantation.[7,9] In laboratory tests, PCT is characterized by increased levels of urinary URO, COPRO, and 7-carboxyl porphyrin III, plasma URO, and fecal isocoproporphyrins (ISOCOPROs)[4]. Other laboratory findings that may also be seen in this disease are elevated serum iron, ferritin, and liver enzymes.

HEP, a rare form of PCT, occurs in individuals who are homozygous or compound heterozygous for mutations that result in marked UROD deficiency.[3] Clinical features are similar to those of CEP, including photosensitivity beginning in childhood. Patients are severely affected and develop excess facial hair and scarring of the hands and face. The severity of photosensitivity improves somewhat with age, but hepatic disease follows. Urine and fecal porphyrin levels are similar to those found in PCT. Erythrocyte zinc protoporphyrin (ZPP) levels are increased in HEP and normal in PCT.[4]

HCP, a deficiency of coproporphyrinogen oxidase, is a fairly mild condition with primarily neurologic manifestations and cutaneous photosensitivity in about 30% of patients.[4] Attacks have been precipitated by exposure to certain drugs, hormones, and nutritional changes.[3] The hallmark of HCP is significantly increased excretion of COPRO III in urine and feces and the presence of harderoporphyrin, a three-carboxyl porphyrin in feces. Increased plasma COPRO also occurs. During acute attacks, urinary excretion of COPRO III, ALA, and PBG is increased. VP is prevalent in South Africa and can be traced to a single couple that emigrated from The Netherlands in 1688. The cause is a deficiency of protoporphyrinogen oxidase activity. Clinical manifestations include acute attacks of neurologic dysfunction (such as those in AIP), photodermatitis (as in HCP and PCT), or both. Hallmark laboratory findings are increased levels of COPRO and PROTO in feces, with levels of PROTO exceeding those of COPRO and COPRO III levels higher than COPRO I levels. Porphyrin-protein complexes specific for VP (X-porphyrins) are present in plasma.[4] During acute attacks, urinary ALA and PBG excretion is increased; however, in asymptomatic subjects, the excretion is often normal.

EPP, the second most common porphyria, results from a deficiency of ferrochelatase, the last enzyme in the heme pathway. The major clinical symptom is photosensitivity, which is usually present from infancy. Patients complain of burning, itching, or pain in the skin on exposure to sunlight. Some patients also have severe liver disease. The diagnosis of EPP is made by demonstrating increased levels of PROTO in erythrocytes, plasma, and stool, along with normal urinary porphyrins or increased COPRO I. High levels of free protoporphyrin (not bound to zinc) in erythrocytes and plasma occur in EPP. Clinical expression of the disease is highly variable. Some individuals have no clinical manifestations of the disease but have increased levels of erythrocyte PROTO. Coinheritance of a second weak mutation of the ferrochelatase gene (in addition to the primary mutations detected) may explain the significant individual differences in clinical expression.[3]

Treatment of the inherited porphyrias is aimed at modifying the biochemical abnormalities causing clinical symptoms. The cutaneous symptoms are treated by avoiding sunlight, using sun-blocking agents, and using oral β-carotene, which acts as a singlet oxygen trap, preventing skin damage. Reduction of the heme load can be accomplished by phlebotomy or by giving desferrioxamine to chelate iron. Intravenous hematin may be used to counteract acute attacks of neurologic dysfunction. Hematin, an enzyme inhibitor, limits synthesis of porphyrins in cells in the bone marrow. Cessation of precipitating factors, such as ingestion of alcohol or estrogens, should be the first line of PCT treatment.[10] Gene therapy (adding the normal gene to a patient's bone marrow stem cells, such as addition of the normal ferrochelatase gene to an EPP patient's cells) appears to be a feasible future treatment of porphyrias.[10]

The term *secondary porphyrias,* or *porphyrinurias,* is given to acquired conditions in which a mild to moderate increase in excretion of urinary porphyrins is seen. In this case, the disorders are not the result of an inherited biochemical defect in heme synthesis but a result of another disorder, toxin, or drug interfering with heme synthesis. Symptoms may be similar to the inherited porphyrias in some cases. Various anemias, liver diseases, and toxins, such as lead and alcohol, fit into this category. Lead is known to inhibit both the activity of PBG synthase and the incorporation of iron into heme. Secondary porphyrias can be distinguished from true porphyrias by measuring levels of urinary ALA and PBG. In secondary porphyria, ALA levels are increased in the urine, whereas PBG excretion usually remains normal. Lead poisoning also classically exhibits increased COPRO in the urine and erythrocyte ZPP, as well as increased ALA. However, determination of blood lead is the most accurate method to detect lead poisoning.

Methods of Analyzing Porphyrins

There are individual enzyme assays available for each defective enzyme that causes porphyria. These procedures typically include addition of substrate under conditions close to physiologic pH and temperature, cessation of the

CASE STUDY 16-1

A 58-year-old man with a history of alcoholism complained of increased skin fragility and skin lesion formation on his hands, forehead, neck, and ears on exposure to the sun. Also noted on physical exam was hyperpigmentation and hypertrichosis. Laboratory findings showed an increase in urinary uroporphyrin and a slight increase in coproporphyrin, with normal levels of ALA and porphobilinogen. Isocoproporphyrin was elevated in the feces. Serum ferritin and serum transaminase were increased. Erythrocyte ZPP and FEP levels were normal.

Questions

1. What is the most probable disorder?

2. What confirmatory test should be done?

3. What is the most probable precipitating factor?

4. What are other causes of acquired cases of this type of porphyria?

5. How is this case differentiated from the homozygous deficiency of this enzyme?

6. How is this type of porphyria differentiated from other porphyrias causing cutaneous symptoms?

reaction by addition of protein-precipitating agents, and separation (usually by HPLC), followed by fluorometric identification and quantitation of porphyrin products.[4] However, most are still limited to use in specialized laboratories and are not discussed here. Screening tests can be performed easily and may be beneficial in emergency situations, but care should be taken in interpretation because false-negatives and false-positives occur.[11,12] Quantitative assays should follow all screening tests. Quantitative assays of the three porphyrins (URO, PROTO, and COPRO) and two porphyrin precursors (ALA and PBG) will serve to classify most porphyrias.

Tests for Urinary PBG and ALA

The two most common screening tests for urinary PBG are the Watson-Schwartz and the Hoesch tests.[4,13] Both tests are based on the principle of PBG forming a red-orange color when mixed with Ehrlich's reagent (acidic p-dimethylaminobenzaldehyde). In the Watson-Schwartz test, an extraction with chloroform or butanol is performed to differentiate PBG from interfering substances such as urobilinogen or indole. If a cherry-red color remains in the aqueous phase after addition of chloroform or butanol, this indicates a positive test for PBG. The reagent in the Hoesch test does not react with urobilinogen; therefore, it is sometimes used to confirm the results of the Watson-Schwartz test. Porphobilinogen and ALA are determined quantitatively by successive separation on two ion-exchange columns.[4] An aliquot of urine is loaded on an anion-exchange or alumina column that retains PBG while ALA passes through. Following washes to remove interfering substances, PBG is eluted with acetic acid and measured spectrophotometrically using Ehrlich's reagent. The eluate from the first column is loaded on a cation-exchange column to retain ALA and then eluted with sodium acetate. The eluted ALA is re-

CASE STUDY 16-2

A few days after a laparotomy for "intestinal obstruction," a young nurse from South Africa became emotionally disturbed and appeared to be hysterical. For longer than 1 week before the operation, she had taken barbiturate capsules to help her sleep. When first seen, she complained of severe abdominal and muscle pain and general weakness, her tendon reflexes were absent, and she was vomiting and constipated. Her urine was dark in color on standing and gave a brilliant pink-fluorescence when viewed in ultraviolet light. Within 24 hours, she was totally paralyzed, and within 2 days she died.

Questions

1. What possible condition did this young woman have, and why did it manifest at this time?

2. Would any members of her family have a similar disease?

3. What enzyme defect did she have?

4. What other confirmatory tests, if any, could be done?

acted with Ehrlich's reagent after first being condensed with acetylacetone to form a pyrrole and then measured spectrophotometrically.[4]

Tests for Porphyrins

Screening and quantitative tests for porphyrins in urine, blood (erythrocytes and plasma), and feces are based on the enhanced fluorescence of these compounds in acidic solution. Typically, an aliquot of specimen is extracted into an organic solvent and then back-extracted into an acidified aqueous layer. For screening procedures, samples containing porphyrins will exhibit a pink or red fluorescence in the aqueous layer when viewed under a Wood's (ultraviolet) lamp. Quantitative procedures include fluorometric measurements usually at an excitation wavelength of 400–405 nm and an emission wavelength of 594–598 nm. Standard solutions of coproporphyrin, uroporphyrin and, possibly, protoporphyrin are used to calculate the porphyrin concentrations in the samples. Each porphyrin exhibits different excitation and emission wavelengths (solvent dependent) and some procedures use average wavelengths whereas other procedures include multiple measurements and calculation of levels of each porphyrin. To verify positive results and eliminate possible interferences, fluorescence scan with comparison to scans of standards is recommended. Fluorometric procedures are more sensitive than those measuring the absorbance of porphyrins.

Other tests for porphyrins use chromatographic separation and quantitation of the individual porphyrins with spectrophotometry or fluorometry. Reversed-phase high-performance liquid chromatography (HPLC) separates porphyrins, including isomers. Capillary zone electrophoresis (CZE), which separates compounds based on charge/mass ratio (modified by pH adjustment), is another chromatographic technique used for quantitation of porphyrins. This technique is as sensitive as HPLC with fluorescence detection and has the advantages of simpler instrumentation, minimum usage of organic solvent, and lower reagent consumption.[4]

Zinc protoporphyrin, a normal metabolite formed by the chelation of zinc instead of iron with protoporphyrin during heme biosynthesis, is another porphyrin that may be measured. Increased zinc protoporphyrin formation occurs during periods of iron insufficiency or impaired iron use. Clinically ZPP has been advocated as a valuable test for evaluating iron nutrition and metabolism in various settings, including pediatrics, obstetrics, and blood banking, as well as a screening test for iron deficiency anemia and lead exposure in adults.[14] A rapid screening method for determination of ZPP includes measurement of the fluorescence of whole blood and washed erythrocytes using a hematofluorometer. It is recommended that ZPP concentrations be reported as a ratio to the heme concentration (per mole of heme).[14]

Molecular diagnostic techniques are becoming useful in the diagnosis of porphyrias.[3,15] Most of the genes that encode the enzymes of heme synthesis have been identified and mutations, which cause various porphyrias, have been discovered. The use of these techniques to aid in the diagnosis of porphyrias has certain advantages over traditional biochemical assays. The interpretation of the traditional tests is complicated by the fact that analytes being measured may be normal except during an acute attack and the amount of porphyrin excreted in the various disorders is highly variable, causing significant overlap between affected and normal patients. By testing for the disease-causing mutation, these problems of biologic variability and disease activity can be overcome. However, perhaps the most important application of molecular testing is its use in detecting asymptomatic gene carriers, which are not easily identified by standard laboratory testing.[15]

HEMOGLOBIN

Role in the Body

Hemoglobin has many important functions in the body. Its major role is oxygen transport to the tissue and CO_2 transport back to the lungs. The hemoglobin molecule is designed to take up oxygen in areas of high oxygen tension and release oxygen in areas of low oxygen tension. Hemoglobin is carried to all tissues of the body by erythrocytes. Hemoglobin is also one of the major buffering systems of the body.

Structure of Hemoglobin

Hemoglobin is a large, complex protein molecule with a molecular weight of approximately 64,000. It is roughly spherical in shape and comprises two major parts: heme, which makes up 3% of the molecule, and globin proteins, which make up the remaining 97%. The heme portion comprises a porphyrin ring with iron chelated in the center. The iron atom is the site of reversible oxygen attachment. The protein portion comprises two pairs of globin chains that are twisted together so that the heme groups are exposed on the exterior of the molecule (Fig. 16-3). The complete hemoglobin molecule contains four heme groups attached to each of four globin chains and may carry up to four molecules of oxygen. Each globin chain contains 141 or more amino acids.

The structure of each chain is 4-fold. The primary structure consists of the individual amino acids and their sequences. Their sequences vary and are the basis of chain nomenclature: α, β, δ, and γ. The secondary structure is the three-dimensional arrangement of the amino acids making up the polypeptide chain. Regions of amino

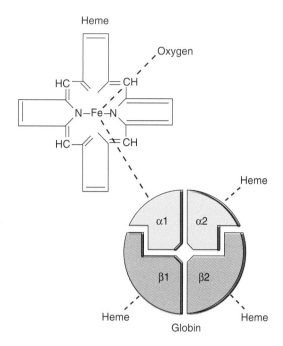

FIGURE 16-3. Hemoglobin A: structure of the hemoglobin molecule.

acids may form helixes or a pleated structure. The tertiary structure is a larger fold superimposed on the helical or pleated forms. It represents the position taken by each chain or subunit in three-dimensional space. The quaternary structure represents the relationship of the four subunits to one another, particularly at the points of contact. Mutations at particular points of contact result in altered specific functional properties of the molecule, such as its oxygen affinity.

The majority of hemoglobin in normal adults is designated as hemoglobin A, or A_1, which contains two α and two β chains (Fig. 16-3). Hemoglobin A_2, which comprises two α and two δ chains, makes up less than 3% of normal adult hemoglobin. The remainder is composed of hemoglobin F, which contains two α and two γ chains. Hemoglobin F is the main hemoglobin during fetal life and is about 60% of normal hemoglobin at birth. There is a gradual switch from production of δ chains to β chains, and, by about age 9 months, hemoglobin F usually constitutes less than 1% of total hemoglobin. Hemoglobin F has a greater affinity for oxygen than hemoglobin A; therefore, it is a more efficient oxygen carrier for the fetus. Hemoglobin F is more resistant to alkali than hemoglobin A, and this is the basis of one laboratory test to differentiate these two types of hemoglobin.

Two other hemoglobin chains, designated ζ and ε, are present only in embryonic life. Production of these chains stops by week 8 of gestation, and γ-chain production takes over. The three embryonic hemoglobins are identified as Gower I, two ζ chains and two ε chains;

Gower II, two α chains and two ε chains; and Portland I, two ζ chains and two γ chains.

Genetic control of hemoglobin synthesis occurs in two areas: control of structure and control of rate and quantity of production. Defects in structure produce a group of diseases called the *hemoglobinopathies*. Defects in rate and quantity of production lead to disorders called the *thalassemias*. Structurally, each globin chain has its own genetic locus; therefore, it is the individual chains, not the whole hemoglobin molecule, that are under genetic control. The genes for the globin chains can be divided into two major groups: the α genes, located on chromosome 16, and the non-α genes, on chromosome 11. In most persons, the α-gene locus is duplicated—there are two α-chain genes per haploid set of chromosomes. The α gene and, hence, its polypeptide chains are identical in hemoglobins A, A_2, and F. The non-α genes for the β, δ, and γ chains are sufficiently close in genetic terms to be subjected to nonhomologous crossover, with the resulting production of fused or hybrid globin chains, such as hemoglobin Lepore (δ-β-globin chain) and Kenya (γ-β-globin chain).

Based on the genetics of the globin chain production, the structural abnormalities can be divided into four groups:

1. Amino acid substitutions (*eg*, hemoglobins S, C, D, E, O, and G)
2. Amino acid deletion—deletions of three or multiples of three nucleotides in deoxyribonucleic acid (DNA; *eg*, hemoglobin Gun Hill)
3. Elongated globin chains resulting from chain termination, frame shift, or other mutations (*eg*, hemoglobin Constant Spring)
4. Fused or hybrid chains resulting from nonhomologous crossover (*eg*, hemoglobins Lepore and Kenya)

The amino acid substitutions are the most common abnormalities, with several hundred described so far. Approximately two thirds of the hemoglobinopathies have an affected β chain. They may be clinically silent or they may cause severe damage, as with hemoglobin S. Amino acid substitutions, for the majority of defects, result from a single-base nucleotide substitution in DNA.

Absent or diminished synthesis of one of the polypeptide chains of human hemoglobin characterizes the thalassemias, a heterogeneous group of inherited disorders. In α-thalassemia, α-globin chain synthesis is absent or reduced; in β-thalassemia, β-globin chain synthesis is absent ($β^0$-thal) or partially reduced ($β^1$-thal).

Synthesis and Degradation of Hemoglobin

Hemoglobin synthesis occurs in the immature RBCs in the bone marrow: 65% in the nucleated cells and 35% in reticulocytes. Normal synthesis depends on adequate iron supply as well as normal synthesis of heme and protein synthesis to form the globin portion. Heme is synthesized in the mitochondria of the cells. Iron is transported to the developing RBCs by transferrin, a plasma protein. Iron traverses the cell membrane and the mitochondria, where it is inserted into the PROTO ring to form heme. Protein synthesis of the globin chains occurs in the cytoplasmic polyribosomes. Heme leaves the mitochondria and is joined to the globin chains in the cytoplasm in the final step.

Two possible pathways degrade hemoglobin. The normal pathway is called extravascular because it occurs outside of the circulatory system in the reticuloendothelial, or mononuclear phagocyte, system. Within the splenic phagocytic cells, or macrophages, hemoglobin loses its iron to transferrin, its α carbon is expired as CO, the globin chains return to the amino acid pool, and the rest of the molecule is converted to bilirubin, which undergoes further metabolism. Normally, 90% of all hemoglobin is degraded in this manner (Fig. 16-4).

Normally, less than 10% hemoglobin is released directly into the blood stream and dissociated into α and β dimers. Greater amounts are released during hemolytic episodes. The dimers are bound to haptoglobin, which prevents renal excretion of plasma hemoglobin and stabilizes the heme–globin bond. This complex is then removed from the circulation by the liver and processed in a fashion similar to extravascular degradation. If the amount of circulating haptoglobin is decreased, as during a hemolytic episode, the unbound dimers go through the kidneys, are reabsorbed, and the iron is stored as hemosiderin. Some hemoglobin dimers may be excreted in the urine, resulting in hemoglobinuria. If the storage limit of the kidneys is exceeded, cells lining the renal tubules may be shed and free hemoglobin, methemoglobin, and/or hemosiderin will appear in the urine.[16]

Hemoglobin that is not entirely bound by haptoglobin or processed by the kidneys is oxidized to methemoglobin. Heme groups are released and taken up by the protein hemopexin. The heme–hemopexin complex is cleared by the liver and catabolized. Then, heme groups present in excess of the binding capacity of hemopexin complex combine with albumin to form methemalbumin and are held by this protein until additional hemopexin becomes available for shuttle to the liver (Fig. 16-5). Laboratory measurement of any of these hemoglobin degradation products can help to determine increased RBC destruction, such as in a hemolytic anemia.

Clinical Significance and Disease Correlation

Hemoglobin Qualitative Defects: The Hemoglobinopathies

Hemoglobin S. The amino acid defect in hemoglobin S is at the sixth position on the β chain, where glutamic acid is substituted by valine, giving the hemoglobin a less negative charge than hemoglobin A. This is the most common hemoglobinopathy in the United States.

Individuals have either sickle cell trait (HbAS, the heterozygous state) or sickle cell disease (HbSS, the homozygous state). Black Africans and African Americans have the highest incidence: 1 of 500 infants have sickle cell anemia and 8–10% carry the HbAS trait. It is also

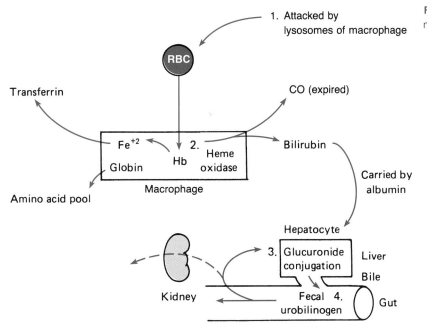

FIGURE 16-4. Extravascular degradation of hemoglobin.

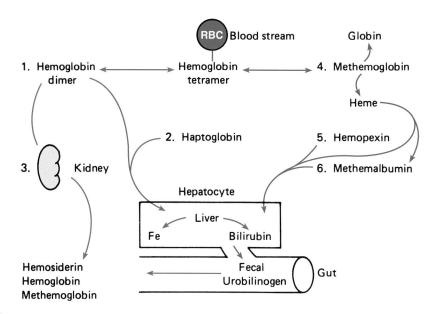

FIGURE 16-5. Intravascular breakdown of hemoglobin.

Intravascular Breakdown of Hemoglobin <10%

found in Mediterranean countries, such as Greece, Italy, and Israel, as well as in Saudi Arabia and India.

Because of the high mortality and morbidity associated with homozygous expression of the gene, the frequency of the mutant gene would be expected to decline in the gene pool. However, a phenomenon known as balanced polymorphism exists, which indicates that the heterozygous state (HbAS) has a selective advantage over either of the homozygous states (HbAA or HbSS). It appears that the heterozygous condition offers protection from parasites, particularly *Plasmodium falciparum*, especially in children. When infected with *P. falciparum*, children with sickle cell trait have a lower parasite count, the infection is shorter in duration, and the incidence of death is low. It is thought that the infected RBCs are pref-

erentially sickled and, therefore, efficiently destroyed by phagocytic cells.[17]

When hemoglobin S is deoxygenated in vitro under near-physiologic conditions, it becomes relatively insoluble as compared with hemoglobin A and aggregates into long, rigid polymers called *tactoids*. These cells appear as sickle- or crescent-shaped forms on stained blood films. Sickled cells may return to their original shape when oxygenated; however, after several sickling episodes, irreversible membrane damage occurs and cells are phagocytized by macrophages in the spleen, liver, or bone marrow, causing anemia. The severity of the hemolytic process is directly related to the number of damaged cells in circulation. The rigid sickled cells are unable to deform and circulate through small capillaries, resulting in

---

CASE STUDY 16-3

A 32-year-old African American woman came to the obstetrics and gynecology clinic of her local hospital because she was feeling a little weak. A CBC showed hemoglobin of 9.9 g/dL, with an MCV of 87 fL. The physician ordered a hemoglobin electrophoresis as a follow-up. The cellulose-acetate pattern showed a peak of 58% at the hemoglobin A position, a peak of 35% at the hemoglobin S position, and a peak of 5% at the A_2 position. Further studies indicated a positive dithionite solubility test result and a hemoglobin F value of 1%.

Questions

1. What is the best possible diagnosis for this woman?

2. Does this condition require further follow-up and treatment?

3. What implications does this disease have for her unborn child?

4. Are the values for hemoglobins A_2 and F normal for this condition?

blockage. Tissue hypoxia results, causing extreme pain and leading to tissue death. Infarctions in the spleen are common, causing excessive necrosis and scarring, leading to a nonfunctional spleen in most adults with sickle cell anemia. This is referred to as *autosplenectomy*. The amount of sickling is related to the amount of hemoglobin S in the cells. The reported inhibitory effect of hemoglobins A and F is due to a dilutional effect. There is also a lower tendency for hemoglobin F to copolymerize with hemoglobin S than with hemoglobin A. This is considered responsible for the observed protective effect of elevated hemoglobin F levels in individuals with sickle cell anemia.

Laboratory findings in the homozygous disease include a normocytic, normochromic anemia, increased reticulocyte count, and variation in size and shape of RBCs with target cells and sickle cells present. Polychromatophilia and nucleated RBCs are common. The heterozygous disease is clinically asymptomatic and usually has a normal blood film. The solubility test for hemoglobin S will be positive in both homozygous and heterozygous forms, but should always be confirmed with hemoglobin electrophoresis. On cellulose acetate electrophoresis at an alkaline pH, hemoglobin S moves in a position between hemoglobin A and A_2. Of total hemoglobin, 85–100% will be hemoglobin S in the homozygous state and usually less than 50% in the heterozygous state. Hemoglobins D and G migrate in the same position as hemoglobin S, but both would be negative with the solubility test. Electrophoresis on citrate agar at an acid pH is necessary to separate these hemoglobins from hemoglobin S (see Fig. 16-7).

Hemoglobin C. The glutamic acid in the sixth position of the β chain is replaced by lysine, resulting in a net positive charge. Hemoglobin C is found in West Africa in the vicinity of North Ghana in 17–28% of the population and in 2–3% of African Americans.

The heterozygous form, hemoglobin AC, is asymptomatic. The homozygous form usually causes a mild, well-compensated anemia characterized by abdominal pain and splenomegaly. The most prominent laboratory feature is the presence of target cells. There is a tendency to form large, oblong, hexagonal crystalloid structures within the red cell. These structures are most prominent in patients who have undergone splenectomy.

A differential diagnosis is obtained by cellulose acetate electrophoresis. Hemoglobin C moves with hemoglobin A_2 and is negative with the solubility test. In the heterozygous form, hemoglobin C falls in the range of 35–48%. Hemoglobins E, O, and C_{Harlem} migrate with hemoglobin C. These hemoglobin variants can be readily distinguished from hemoglobin C by citrate agar electrophoresis at an acid pH.

Hemoglobin SC. Hemoglobin SC disease is the most common mixed *hemoglobinopathy*. One β-gene codes for β-S chains and the other β-gene codes for β-C chains, leaving no normal β chains to produce hemoglobin A. Clinically, this disease is less severe than homozygous sickle cell anemia but has similar clinical symptoms. The blood film characteristically shows many target cells and occasional abnormal shapes resembling the sickle cell, the hexagonal hemoglobin C crystal, and a combination of the two. The solubility test is positive, and electrophoresis on cellulose acetate shows about equal amounts of hemoglobin S and hemoglobin C.

Hemoglobin E. Hemoglobin E is an amino acid substitution of lysine for glutamic acid in the 26th position of the β chain, resulting in a net positive charge. Hemoglobin E is somewhat unstable when subjected to oxidizing agents.

Found in Asia, it is estimated to occur in about 20 million individuals, 80% of whom live in Southeast Asia. In the homozygous form, there is a mild anemia with microcytosis and target cells. In the heterozygous form, the patient is asymptomatic. The differential diagnosis is obtained by electrophoresis. On cellulose acetate, hemoglobin E moves with A_2, C, and O. It is present in the heterozygous form in amounts varying from 30% to 45%, which is somewhat lower than the percentage for hemoglobin C. This is probably a result of the somewhat unstable nature of hemoglobin E. On citrate agar, hemoglobin E migrates with A. It is more common to find this defect in association with both α- and β-thalassemia. ∈-β-Thalassemia is a more severe disorder, with moderate anemia and splenomegaly.

Hemoglobin D. The letter *D* is given to any hemoglobin variant with an electrophoretic mobility on cellulose acetate similar to that of hemoglobin S but that has a negative solubility test. Hemoglobin $D_{Los Angeles}$ and its identical variant, Hemoglobin D_{Punjab}, are the most common, with glycine substituted for glutamic acid at the 121st position of the β chain. Hemoglobin D_{Punjab} is found in Northwest India but occasionally can be seen in English, Portuguese, and French individuals because of the close historical connection of these countries with East India. Hemoglobin $D_{Los Angeles}$ is found in 0.02% of African Americans.

The homozygous state is rare. There is a mild anemia and/or splenomegaly and only a slight anisocytosis. The oxygen affinity is higher than in normal blood. Heterozygous individuals are asymptomatic. Differential diagnosis is accomplished with electrophoresis. On cellulose acetate, hemoglobin D migrates with hemoglobin S in proportions of 35–50%. On citrate agar, hemoglobin D migrates with A.

Hemoglobin Quantitative Defects: The Thalassemias

The thalassemias are a group of diseases in which a defect occurs in the rate of synthesis of one or more of the hemoglobin chains, but the chains are structurally normal.

CASE STUDY 16-4

A 54-year-old African American woman was admitted to the hospital with the chief complaint of left hip pain and lethargy. She had a long history of multiple emergency department visits for hip pain requiring medication. She previously had been found to have a positive solubility test for hemoglobin S, but denied a history of sickle cell disease. There was family history of sickle cell trait. She had a mastectomy for breast cancer 10 years before. Admission laboratory values were as follows:

Hemoglobin	5.3 g/dL
Hematocrit	17%
MCV	82 fL
MCHC	31 g/dL
WBC	12,000/μL
Platelet count	53,000/μL
Differential	Normal
Reticulocyte count	6.4% (corrected, 2.4%)
RBC morphology	Target cells; spherocytes; schistocytes; basophilic stippling; and bizarre forms, including elongated, block-shaped, and more densely stained cells

A hemoglobin electrophoresis was ordered. Patterns from the cellulose acetate and citrate agar electrophoresis are shown in Case Study Figure 16-4.1. Chest x-ray showed a right lower lobe infiltrate with pulmonary vascular congestion and an enlarged spleen. Fluid aspirated from the nasogastric tube was positive for blood.

The patient was given medication for an aspiration pneumonia, gastrointestinal bleeding, and congestive heart failure. She was given packed RBCs, fresh-frozen plasma, and platelets, but her condition continued to worsen. Six hours later, laboratory tests confirmed disseminated intravascular coagulation (DIC). A bone marrow biopsy was performed and revealed extensive necrosis of marrow elements. Three hours later, the patient died of cardiac arrest.

Questions

1. What hemoglobinopathy is indicated by the hemoglobin electrophoresis patterns?

2. What clinical feature of this disease differs from the typical picture in sickle cell anemia?

3. What other hemoglobins interact with hemoglobin S, and how can these be differentiated from hemoglobin C?

4. Was this patient's death due to the hemoglobinopathy? Is it unusual for hemoglobin SC to be life shortening?

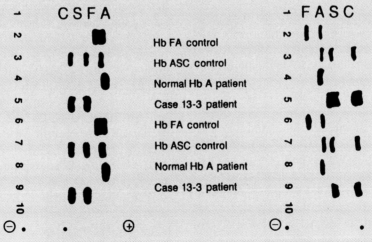

CASE STUDY FIGURE 16-4.1. Hemoglobin electrophoretic patterns. (**A**) Cellulose acetate at pH 8.4. (**B**) Citrate agar at pH 6.2. (Case study data courtesy of Margaret Uthman, MD, University of Texas Medical School at Houston.)

Gene deletions or point mutations are the cause for decreased or absent chain synthesis.[18] The two most common types are α-thalassemia, resulting from defective production of α chains, and β-thalassemia, resulting from a defect in production in β chains. Defects in production of the δ and γ chains have been described, but these are not involved in production of hemoglobin A and, therefore, not clinically significant. Rarely, combinations of gene deletions, such as δ and β, may lead to clinical disease. Any form of unbalanced production of globin chains causes the erythrocytes to be small, hypochromic, and sometimes deformed. Intracellular accumulation of unmatched chains in the developing erythrocytes causes precipitation of the proteins, which leads to cell destruction in the bone marrow. Although erythropoiesis is occurring, it is ineffective because mature cells do not reach the peripheral blood to carry oxygen.

Thalassemia is inherited as an autosomal dominant disorder with heterogeneous expression of the disease. One of the most common hereditary disorders, it is distributed worldwide. The prevalence of the thalassemia gene has been attributed to the protection it offers against falciparum malaria. The heterozygous state produces a disorder called *thalassemia minor,* which is clinically asymptomatic and resembles iron deficiency. The homozygous state, *thalassemia major,* is either lethal before birth or in childhood.

α-Thalassemias. α-Thalassemia occurs with high frequency in Asian populations but is also seen in the Black African, African American, Indian, and Middle Eastern populations. There are four principal clinical types of different severity known to occur in the population, and these four types can be explained, respectively, by deletions of 4, 3, 2, or 1 of the α-globin gene loci (Fig. 16-6). The type of α-thalassemia found in Black Africans and African Americans is also associated with deletion of the α-globin genes but in a different pattern than is found in the Asian population (Fig. 16-6). The four clinical types of α-thalassemia in order of most deletions to least deletions are the following:

1. Hydrops fetalis is the most clinically severe form of α-thalassemia because of the total absence of α-chain synthesis. Hemoglobin Bart's, which is a tetramer of γ chains, is the main hemoglobin found in the red cells of affected infants. Hemoglobin Bart's has an extremely high O_2 affinity and allows almost no oxygen transport to the tissue. These infants are either stillborn or die of hypoxia shortly after birth.

2. Hemoglobin H disease has α-chain synthesis at about one third the amount of β-chain synthesis. As a result, β chains accumulate and form tetramers, which are called *hemoglobin H.* β-Chain precipitates (hemoglobin H inclusions) alter the shape and ability of the cell to deform, significantly shortening the life span of the

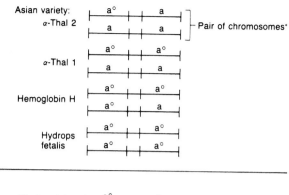

a   is normal α chain (normal gene loci).
a° is deleted α chain (deleted α gene loci).
+   note that a loci is duplicated on each chromosome.

FIGURE 16-6. Deletions of α-globin gene loci in α-thalassemia.

cells. These individuals have a moderate hemolytic anemia, with 5–30% hemoglobin H, 1% hemoglobin A_2, and the remainder hemoglobin A. Hemoglobin H inclusions can be seen in the red cells with a supravital stain. Cord blood contains 10–20% hemoglobin Bart's.

3. α-Thalassemia trait (or α-thalassemia minor) results from two gene deletions, either on the same or on different chromosomes. The deletion on two separate chromosomes is more common in Black Africans and African Americans (Fig. 16-6). These individuals have a mild, microcytic, hypochromic anemia. Occasionally, excess β chains may form hemoglobin H inclusions. Cord blood contains 2–10% hemoglobin Bart's; however, after age 3 months, electrophoresis is normal.

4. Silent carriers are missing only one α gene, and the remaining genes direct production of sufficient α chains for normal hemoglobin production. This state can only be detected by expression of 1–2% of hemoglobin Bart's in a neonate. After age 3 months, it can only be detected by more specialized testing, such as gene mapping, α:β-globin messenger ribonucleic acid (mRNA) ratio, or other polymerase chain reaction (PCR)-based methods.[18,19] It has been estimated that the frequency of this genetic disorder may be as high as 27% in the African American population.[18]

β-Thalassemias. In contrast to α-thalassemia, gene deletions usually do not cause β-thalassemia. One of several types of mutations in the β gene results in failure to produce normal amounts of β-globin chains. In general, they may involve faulty transcription, processing, or translation of the mRNA from the gene directing β-chain production.[18] The β-thalassemias are classically divided into homozygous disease, called thalassemia major or Cooley's anemia, and heterozygous disease, called thalassemia minor. However, the clinical expression of the disease is heterogeneous, depending on the type of genetic defect and involvement with other gene loci. The disease may be broadly divided into two major subtypes according to genetic expression: β[1], in which β chains are produced in reduced amounts, and β[0], which is complete absence of β chains.

β[1]-Thalassemia is the most common type. There is some synthesis of β-globin chains but in significantly reduced amounts (5–30%) of normal. The biochemical defect shows a quantitative deficiency of β-globin mRNA. The hemoglobin electrophoresis pattern and hemoglobin F and A_2 quantitation show about 2–8% hemoglobin A_2, an elevated but varying amount of hemoglobin F, and the remainder hemoglobin A. The mean cell volume (MCV) is low, with severe anemia, reticulocytes, nucleated RBCs, basophilic stippling, target cells, extreme poikilocytosis, and anisocytosis.

β[0]-Thalassemia accounts for 10% of homozygous β-thalassemia, with a total absence of β-chain synthesis but intact synthesis of γ chains. In the homozygous form, there is 1–6% hemoglobin A_2 and 95% hemoglobin F. The hemoglobin concentration is low, with a severe anemia. The heterozygous form appears clinically the same as homozygous β[1]-thalassemia.

Homozygous β-thalassemia—β-thalassemia major—either β[1] or β[0], is a crippling disease of childhood. This is unlike α-thalassemia, in which the child either dies shortly after birth or leads a normal life. The hypochromic, microcytic anemia is a result of both the defect of functional hemoglobin tetramer synthesis and the premature destruction of RBCs, both intramedullary and extramedullary, due to increased α chains. The bone marrow compensates by enormously expanding in size, sometimes causing structural bone abnormalities. Treatment of severe forms of the disease include regular transfusion therapy, iron chelation drugs to remove excess iron, and folic acid supplements.[20] Bone marrow transplantation has been successful if an HLA-identical donor is available.[18] Gene therapy is being studied as an alternative treatment of the future.[21,22]

Heterozygous β-thalassemia—thalassemia minor—may be caused by inheritance of one thalassemia gene, either β[1] or β[0]. The other gene directing β-chain production is normal and RBC survival is not shortened. About 1% of African Americans are affected and it also commonly occurs in individuals of Mediterranean and Arabic descent. Clinically, the condition is usually asymptomatic but may sometimes cause a mild microcytic anemia. The hematologic laboratory values resemble those of iron deficiency anemia, and it is important to distinguish the two because quite different treatments are required. The RBC count in thalassemia minor is usually higher than would be expected with the accompanying hemoglobin concentration and a few target cells or occasional basophilic stippling may be seen on a stained smear. The red cell distribution width (RDW) parameter on automated instruments, which is a quantitative measure of RBC variation in size, may be helpful to distinguish the two disorders. It is typically normal in thalassemia and increased in iron deficiency as a result of the heterogeneity of the RBCs. Hemoglobin electrophoresis of thalassemia minor characteristically shows an increase in hemoglobin A_2. Quantitation of hemoglobin A_2 by column chromatography usually reveals values between 3.5% and 7%.

δ-β-Thalassemia is a rare type characterized by total absence of both β-chain synthesis of hemoglobin A and δ-chain synthesis of hemoglobin A_2. Homozygous patients have 100% hemoglobin F. The heterozygous individuals have 93% hemoglobin A, 2–3% hemoglobin A_2, and 3–10% hemoglobin F.

Patients are anemic and show a thalassemic phenotype because the γ-chain synthesis of hemoglobin F is not equal to α-chain synthesis. There is approximately one third as much γ chain produced as α chain. Hemoglobin F is heterogeneously distributed among the erythrocytes, as revealed by the acid elution stain procedure.

Hereditary persistence of fetal hemoglobin (HPFH) is genetically and hematologically heterogeneous. In African Blacks and African Americans, there is a total absence of β- as well as δ-chain synthesis because of deletions in chromosome 11. γ-Chain synthesis is present in the adult at a high level and, in contrast to synthesis of hemoglobin F in β-thalassemia or δ-β-thalassemia, is uniformly distributed. In heterozygotes, there is no imbalance of globin-chain synthesis. There is 17–33% hemoglobin F. The patients are clinically normal. In homozygotes, there is 100% hemoglobin F, with no synthesis of hemoglobin A or A_2. There are no significant hematologic abnormalities, other than erythrocytosis, and these patients are also asymptomatic.

Methodology

Most hemoglobinopathies and thalassemias can be diagnosed by use of the complete blood count (CBC), blood film evaluation, solubility test, and cellulose acetate electrophoresis. Citrate agar electrophoresis may be necessary for confirmation of some abnormal hemoglobins. Thalassemias may require quantitation of hemoglobin A_2 or F by more definitive methods. A serum ferritin may be helpful to distinguish thalassemia minor from iron deficiency anemia. The more complicated cases may require more specialized procedures, such as α/β-globin chain

CASE STUDY 16-5

A 5-year-old Caucasian boy was seen by a physician for an upper respiratory tract infection and splenomegaly was noted. A CBC was ordered and, subsequently, a hemoglobin electrophoresis. The following were the results:

		REFERENCE RANGE
Hemoglobin	8.5 g/dL	11.7–15.7 g/dL
Hematocrit	27%	35–47%
RBC	4.3×10^{12}/L	$3.8–5.2 \times 10^{12}$/L
MCV	62.3 fL	80–100 fL
MCHC	32.0%	32–26%
RDW	18.5%	11.5–14.5%
Platelet	538×10^9/L	$150–440 \times 10^9$/L
WBC	10.7×10^9/L	$3.5–11.0 \times 10^9$/L
Reticulocyte count	5.6%	0.5–1.5%
WBC differential	Normal except for 1 nucleated RBC/100 WBC	
RBC morphology	Moderate anisocytosis, moderate microcytosis, slight polychromasia, slight target cells, slight schistocytes	
Hemoglobin electrophoresis (cellulose acetate)		
Hemoglobin C	89%	
Hemoglobin F	11%	

A hemoglobin electrophoresis by citrate agar method confirmed hemoglobins C and F. Hemoglobin F was determined by the alkali denaturation method to be 7.5%. Hemoglobin A_2 could not be quantitated due to the presence of hemoglobin C. The patient's father had been previously told that he was slightly anemic due to a blood disorder called thalassemia. The patient's mother and four older siblings were healthy and unaware of any abnormal hemoglobin.

Questions

1. What combination of disorders did the patient most probably inherit?

2. Why were the mother and other siblings unaware of an abnormality?

3. Why was the patient unable to produce hemoglobin A?

4. What caused the discrepancy in values for hemoglobin F from electrophoresis and the alkali denaturation test?

5. Why was it unusual to find hemoglobin C in a Caucasian family?

analysis,[23,24] cation exchange high-performance liquid chromatography,[24,25] or DNA technology testing.[24–26]

Solubility Test (Screening Test for Sickling Hemoglobins)[27,28]

The solubility test is based on the principle that sickling hemoglobin, in the deoxygenated state, is relatively insoluble and forms a precipitate when placed in a high-molarity phosphate buffer solution. The precipitate appears because the deoxygenated hemoglobin molecules form tactoids that refract and deflect light rays, producing a turbid solution. A small amount of packed red blood cells (RBCs) is placed in a buffered solution of sodium dithionite with saponin to lyse the RBCs in a 12×75 mm glass tube. After mixing well and incubating at room temperature for 5 minutes, the tube containing the solution is placed approximately 1 inch in front of a heavy, black-lined index card. If there is no sickling hemoglobin present, the lines on the card will be easily seen. If sickling hemoglobin is present, the lines will be indistinct or impossible to read. The test is reported as positive or negative for sickling hemoglobin. A positive and a negative control should be run with each test batch.

Outdated reagents and reagents not at room temperature interfere with the test. False-negative tests may be due to anemia or recent transfusions or may occur in infants younger than age 6 months because of high concentrations of hemoglobin F. If whole blood is used instead of packed RBCs, false-positive results may occur due to erythrocytosis, hyperglobulinemia, extreme leukocytosis, or hyperlipidemia and false-negative results may occur in anemia. This test does not differentiate between the homozygous and heterozygous presence of hemoglobin S, and other rare sickling variants, such as hemoglobin C_{Harlem}, may give a positive test. Commonly used as a screening test for sickling hemoglobin in adults, this test may also be used as a confirmatory test for sickling hemoglobin after initial evaluation with cellulose acetate electrophoresis.

Cellulose Acetate Hemoglobin Electrophoresis[28–30]

A fresh hemolysate made from a packed RBC sample is applied to a cellulose acetate plate using a buffer of alkaline pH (8.4–8.6) and electrophoresis is performed. After electrophoresis, the membrane is stained and cleared. The patient's hemoglobin migration is compared with that of a control for test interpretation. A rough estimate of proportions of different hemoglobins may be made using a densitometer.

The order of electrophoretic mobility, from slowest to fastest, is hemoglobins C, S, F, and A (Fig. 16-7). (There are several mnemonic devices for remembering the migration pattern, such as **A**ccelerated, **F**ast, **S**low, and **C**rawl.) Hemoglobin that migrates beyond hemoglobin A is termed *fast hemoglobin*. Hemoglobin Bart's and hemoglobin H both migrate here. Any abnormal hemoglobin or any normal hemoglobin present in increased amounts, such as hemoglobin A_2 and F, should be confirmed. If there is abnormal hemoglobin, confirm with citrate agar electrophoresis and solubility test if hemoglobin S is suspected. If an increased amount of A_2 or F occurs, then quantify the amount. Hemoglobin D and G comigrate with hemoglobin S in this method.

Citrate Agar Electrophoresis

Citrate agar electrophoresis is performed at an acid pH (6.0–6.2) after abnormal hemoglobin is detected on cellulose-acetate electrophoresis.[28,31] In this method, an important factor in determining the mobility of hemoglobin is solubility. Hemoglobin F, with the fastest cathodal mobility, is also the most soluble, probably because it is most resistant to denaturation at pH 6.0. Adult hemoglobins with solubility similar to that of hemoglobin A, such as D, E, G, O, I, and so forth, move with hemoglo-

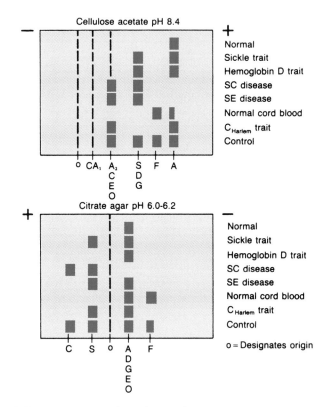

FIGURE 16-7. Comparison of various hemoglobin samples on cellulose acetate and citrate agar.

bin A. The relatively insoluble hemoglobin S moves behind hemoglobin A, and the even more insoluble hemoglobin C moves behind hemoglobin S (Fig. 16-7).

Hemoglobin A_2 Quantitation

The quantity of hemoglobin A_2 may be estimated by hemoglobin electrophoresis; however, this yields only a rough estimate. Quantitation is best accomplished by microcolumn chromatography[23,32] or high-performance liquid chromatography.[24,25]

Acid Elution Stain for Hemoglobin F[28,33]

Erythrocytes containing an increased amount of hemoglobin F can be distinguished from normal adult cells by the acid-elution technique. This method may be helpful in the diagnosis of hereditary persistence of fetal hemoglobin or to detect fetal cells in maternal circulation during problem pregnancies. In the microscopic method, adult hemoglobin, hemoglobin A, is eluted from the erythrocytes by incubation in an acid buffer. Hemoglobin F remains behind and is stained with eosin. Adult cells are negative and have no staining because they contain no hemoglobin F. Fetal RBCs may also be detected by flow cytometric assay methods.[34]

Hemoglobin F Quantitation

Fetal hemoglobin may be quantitated based on the principle that it is resistant to alkali denaturation in 1.25 mol/L NaOH for 2 minutes. Denatured hemoglobin A is precipitated out with ammonium sulfate and removed by filtration. The optical density of the clear supernatant solution is read at 540 nm, and the percentage of fetal hemoglobin is calculated against the optical density of the total hemoglobin solutions.[28] High-performance liquid chromatography has been recommended as the method of choice for quantitation of fetal hemoglobin.[25]

The average adult has less than 1.5% fetal hemoglobin. However, elevated levels may be found in several inherited and acquired diseases. The hereditary persistence of fetal hemoglobin should be suspected in individuals who possess 10% or more fetal hemoglobin with no other apparent clinical abnormalities.

DNA Technology

The definitive diagnosis of some hemoglobinopathies and thalassemias that involve combinations of genetic defects may require DNA analysis. With increased use and efficiency of the polymerase chain reaction technique, the DNA sequence of interest may be easily analyzed from whole blood or spots of dried blood on filter paper. With currently available automated sequencing methods, the time required to perform this type of analysis is not significantly greater than standard methodology. Disadvantages of these methods are higher cost and lack of availability in most routine laboratories. The advantages are that it provides definitive information on the genotype of individuals tested and, in some cases, direct detection of the molecular lesions is possible. Specific techniques are discussed elsewhere.[24,26]

A special strength of the DNA technology is in the prenatal diagnosis of thalassemia major. Because the globin genes are represented in all tissue, including those in which they are not active, prenatal diagnosis of thalassemic states may be made by sampling tissue that is relatively easy to obtain, such as chorionic villi or amniotic fluid cells, rather than fetal blood, which is obtained with much greater difficulty and at a much greater risk to the fetus.[26]

DNA technology also has been used in the prenatal diagnosis of sickle cell anemia. Fetal cells obtained by amniocentesis or chorionic villus sampling may be analyzed using similar techniques as in the thalassemias. Hemoglobin electrophoresis on a hemolysate of fetal blood cells also can be used in cases in which DNA probe technology is unavailable or when rapid results are needed, owing to a patient's advanced gestational age.[28]

MYOGLOBIN

Structure and Role in the Body

Myoglobin is a heme protein found only in the skeletal and cardiac muscle of humans. It can reversibly bind oxygen in a manner similar to the hemoglobin molecule; however, myoglobin is unable to release oxygen, except under low oxygen tension. Myoglobin is a simple heme protein containing one polypeptide chain and one heme group per molecule. The polypeptide chain contains 153 amino acids, making it slightly larger than one chain in the hemoglobin molecule. Therefore, its size is slightly larger than one fourth that of a hemoglobin molecule,

---

CASE STUDY 16-6

A 22-year-old Caucasian woman of Italian heritage had been told that she was slightly anemic and had been treated with iron periodically throughout her life. She was a student in a clinical laboratory science program and had a CBC performed as a part of a hematology class.
Laboratory values were as follows:

		Reference Range
Hemoglobin	11.0 g/dL	11.7–15.7 g/dL
Hematocrit	34%	35–47%
RBC	5.8×10^{12}/L	3.8–5.2×10^{12}/L
MCV	59.4 fL	80–100 fL
MCHC	31.9%	32–36%
RDW	14.2%	11.5–14.5%

From these values, the hematology instructor suspected an inherited disorder instead of iron deficiency and suggested that the student contact her doctor for further testing. A hemoglobin electrophoresis revealed slightly increased amounts of hemoglobin F and A_2, which were subsequently quantitated to reveal hemoglobin F of 3.2% and hemoglobin A_2 of 4.2%. Iron studies were normal.

Questions

1. What is the most probable disorder?

2. What CBC values caused the instructor to suggest further testing?

3. Why is it important for this disorder to be correctly diagnosed?

with a molecular weight of approximately 17,000. The iron atom in the center of the heme group is the site of reversible oxygen binding, identical to the hemoglobin molecule. In the body, myoglobin acts as an oxygen carrier in the cytoplasm of the muscle cell. Transport of oxygen from the muscle cell membrane to the mitochondria is its main role. Myoglobin serves as an extra reserve of oxygen to help exercising muscle maintain activity longer.

Clinical Significance

Damage to muscles often results in elevated levels of serum and urine myoglobin (Table 16-2). Renal clearance is rapid, and myoglobinemia following a single injury tends to be transient. High concentrations of myoglobin may cause acute renal failure (ARF). Measurement of myoglobin in serum and urine can be used to calculate a myoglobin clearance rate. The combination of a high serum myoglobin (≥400 ng/mL) and a low clearance rate (≤4 mL/min) indicates a high risk for ARF.[35] Myoglobin in urine will cross-react with the hemoglobin test on the dipstick and cause a positive reaction. Confirmation of myoglobinuria by a more specific assay, such as an immunoassay, allows differentiation from hemoglobinuria. Myoglobin measurement in urine or serum may be performed when rhabdomyolysis or any disease/injury resulting in muscle damage is suspected.

Currently the primary use of serum myoglobin testing is in the investigation of chest pain to diagnose or rule out acute myocardial infarction (AMI). Myoglobin is recommended as the marker of choice for the early detection of AMI.[36] Damaged heart muscle cells release myoglobin within the first few hours of onset of myocardial infarction, and peak values are reached within 2–3 hours and as early as 30 minutes. Myoglobin, therefore, is the first cardiac marker to rise, sooner than the MB isoenzyme of creatine kinase (CKMB) or troponin (T or I). Al-though an increase of myoglobin in the circulation provides an early indicator of myocardial infarction, false-positive results may occur from any injury to skeletal muscle that also contains myoglobin. The use of myoglobin as an early marker should be followed by use of a definitive marker, such as troponin (T or I), that is more cardiac-specific but does not appear in the blood as early. Despite the poor specificity of myoglobin for myocardium, skeletal muscle damage can be ruled out in many cases. Negative myoglobin results within the first few hours after chest pain can be used to rule out myocardial infarction. In cases in which thrombolytic therapy is used in the treatment of myocardial infarction, myoglobin levels combined with CKMB and clinical indications may be used as monitors of reperfusion of the occluded artery.[37] Myoglobin also has been investigated to aid in the diagnosis and differentiation of the different types of hereditary progressive muscular dystrophy.[38] Myoglobin is discussed in greater detail in Chapter 8, *Amino Acids and Proteins.*

Methodology

There are several immunoassay methods for measurement and identification of myoglobin. These procedures incorporate the binding of specific antibodies to myoglobin, with a resulting chemical or physical change (*eg,* fluorescence, chemiluminescence, immunochromic) that can be measured and correlated to myoglobin concentration. These methods have been adapted to point-of-care devices for rapid assessment of chest pain, as well as conventional methods for multianalyte analyzer platforms.[39,40] Although plasma is the specimen of choice for cardiac marker analysis, there is evidence that different anticoagulants have different effects on particular commercial assays for myoglobin.[39] It has also been shown that there are precision and reference range differences between the different myoglobin assays.[39]

SUMMARY

Porphyrins are the intermediates in the multistep synthesis of heme, an iron-chelating group that binds oxygen. The synthesis of heme is started in the mitochondrion by combination of glycine and succinyl-CoA to form ALA. PBG is formed from ALA in the cytoplasm. ALA and PBG are precursors to the formation of porphyrins. Uroporphyrinogen and coproporphyrinogen are formed in the cytoplasm, and protoporphyrinogen is synthesized in the mitochondrion. PROTO is then formed, which incorporates iron to form heme. ALA synthase is the rate-controlling enzyme of heme synthesis and is regulated by the amount of heme. Enzyme deficiencies can occur at almost every step of heme synthesis, resulting in a group of inherited disorders called the porphyrias. A buildup of intermediates occurs, which can cause cutaneous symp-

TABLE 16-2. CAUSES OF MYOGLOBIN ELEVATIONS

Acute myocardial infarction	Angina without infarction
Rhabdomyolysis	Multiple fractures; muscle trauma
Renal failure	Myopathies
Vigorous exercise	Intramuscular injections
Open heart surgery	Tonic–clonic seizures
Electric shock	Arterial thrombosis
Certain toxins	Malignant hyperthermia
Muscular dystrophy	Systemic lupus erythematosus

toms, neuropsychiatric symptoms, or both. Blocks in the early steps of heme synthesis tend to produce cutaneous symptoms, whereas buildups of later intermediates cause neuropsychiatric symptoms. Most porphyrias can be differentiated by laboratory analysis of ALA, PBG, URO, COPRO, and PROTO.

Hemoglobin is synthesized in immature erythroid cells in the bone marrow and functions in carrying oxygen to the tissue. Hemoglobin comprises two pairs of globin proteins, each containing a heme molecule capable of carrying oxygen. There are six types of globin chains: α, β, γ, δ, ϵ, and ζ, with ϵ and ζ being present only in the embryo. In the healthy adult, three types of hemoglobin are present: A ($\alpha_2\beta_2$), A_2 ($\alpha_2\delta_2$), and F ($\alpha_2\lambda_2$). Hemoglobinopathies result when defects are present in the structure of hemoglobin. The most common hemoglobinopathy is hemoglobin S, which can be inherited as heterozygous (AS, sickle cell trait) or homozygous (SS, sickle cell disease). Heterozygotes are asymptomatic, whereas homozygotes may have anemia and compromised microcirculation. This and most other hemoglobinopathies can be detected by a combination of alkaline and acid electrophoresis. Thalassemias are inherited disorders in the rate of synthesis of one or more globin chains, usually a result of gene deletions or point mutations. Defects in the rate of α-globin synthesis are termed α-thalassemias, and β-thalassemia denotes defective β-globin production. The heterozygous state is termed *thalassemia minor* and the homozygous state is called *thalassemia major*. These disorders are common in Asian, Black African, African American, Indian, and Middle Eastern populations and cause anemias of varying degrees.

Myoglobin is a heme-containing protein present in skeletal and cardiac muscle. Its presence in serum or urine indicates skeletal or cardiac muscle damage. Because of its relatively small molecular weight, it is exuded into the plasma within a few hours after muscle damage. In this respect, it is useful as a marker of myocardial infarction or as a marker of reperfusion after thrombolytic therapy.

REVIEW QUESTIONS

1. The main purpose of porphyrins in the body is to:
   a. carry oxygen to the tissue.
   b. transport iron.
   c. combine with free hemoglobin.
   d. contribute to the synthesis of heme.

2. The two main sites in the body for accumulation of excess porphyrins are:
   a. liver and bone marrow.
   b. heart and lung.
   c. muscle and blood.
   d. liver and spleen.

3. The two main classes of porphyrias, according to symptoms, are:
   a. erythropoietic and hepatic.
   b. neurologic and cutaneous.
   c. congenital and acquired.
   d. hematologic and muscular.

4. Porphobilinogen is most commonly quantitated in the urine by:
   a. the Watson-Schwartz method.
   b. thin-layer chromatography.
   c. ion-exchange column.
   d. electrophoresis.

5. Extremely high levels of ALA and PBG in the urine with normal porphyrin levels in the feces and blood most likely indicates:
   a. acute intermittent porphyria (AIP).
   b. erythropoietic porphyria (EP).
   c. hereditary coproporphyria (HCP).
   d. porphyria cutanea tarda (PCT).

6. Inherited disorders in which a genetic defect causes abnormalities in rate and quantity of synthesis of structurally normal polypeptide chains of the hemoglobin molecule are called:
   a. hemoglobinopathies.
   b. porphyrias.
   c. molecular dyscrasias.
   d. thalassemias.

7. Increased intravascular hemolysis is indicated by a *decrease* in:
   a. methemoglobin.
   b. methemalbumin.
   c. haptoglobin.
   d. hemopexin.

8. Which of the following abnormal hemoglobins, found frequently in individuals from Southeast Asia, migrates with hemoglobin A_2 on cellulose acetate electrophoresis?
   a. Hemoglobin D
   b. Hemoglobin E
   c. Hemoglobin C
   d. Hemoglobin Lepore

9. Which type of α-thalassemia results from deletion of three genes and produces a moderate hemolytic anemia?
   a. Hemoglobin H disease
   b. Hemoglobin Bart's
   c. Hydrops fetalis
   d. Thalassemia trait

10. The most effective way to quantitate hemoglobin A_2 is by:
    a. densitometry.
    b. citrate agar electrophoresis.
    c. alkali denaturation test.
    d. column chromatography.

11. Serum or plasma myoglobin levels are used as:
    a. liver function tests.
    b. an early marker of acute myocardial infarction.
    c. lead poisoning indicator.
    d. indicator of congestive heart failure.

12. Which of the following is the best test to differentiate β-thalassemia minor from iron deficiency anemia?
    a. Hemoglobin electrophoresis (cellulose acetate, alkaline pH)
    b. Solubility test
    c. Complete blood count
    d. Hemoglobin A_2 quantitation

13. Which is the correct sequence of electrophoretic migration of hemoglobins from slowest to fastest on cellulose acetate at an alkaline pH?
    a. C, S, F, A
    b. C, A, S, F
    c. C, S, A, F
    d. A, F, S, C

REFERENCES

1. Schreiber WE. Iron, porphyrin, and bilirubin metabolism. In: Kaplan LA, Pesce AJ, eds. Clinical Chemistry—Theory, Analysis, Correlation, 3rd ed. St. Louis: CV Mosby, 1996:696.
2. Deacon AC, Elder GH. Front line tests for the investigation of suspected porphyria. J Clin Pathol 2000;54:500.
3. Sassa S, Kappas A. Molecular aspects of the inherited porphyrias. J Int Med 2000;247:169.
4. Zaider E, Bickers DR. Clinical laboratory methods for diagnosis of the porphyrias. Clin Dermatol 1998;16:277.
5. Nuttall KL. Porphyrins and disorders of porphyrin metabolism. In: Burtis CA, Ashwood ER, eds. Tietz Fundamentals of Clinical Chemistry, 4th ed. Philadelphia: WB Saunders, 1996:731.
6. Kappas A, Sassa S, Galbraith RA, et al. The porphyrias. In: Scriver CR, Beaudet AL, Sly WS, et al, eds. The Metabolic and Molecular Bases of Inherited Disease, 7th ed. New York: McGraw-Hill, 1995:2103.
7. Elder GH. Porphyria cutanea tarda. Semin Liver Dis 1998; 18:67.
8. Elder GH. Alcohol intake and porphyria cutanea tarda. Clin Dermatol 1999;17:431.
9. Rich M. Porphyria cutanea tarda. Postgrad Med 1999;105:208.
10. Mathews-Roth MM. Treatment of the cutaneous porphyrias. Clin Dermatol 1998;16:295.
11. Nuttall KL. Porphyrins and disorders of porphyrin metabolism. In: Burtis CA, Ashwood ER, eds. Tietz Textbook of Clinical Chemistry, 2nd ed. Philadelphia: WB Saunders, 1994:2073.
12. Buttery JE, Chamberlain B, Beng CG. A sensitive method of screening for urinary porphobilinogen. Clin Chem 1989;35:2311.
13. Watson CJ, Schwartz S. A simple test for urinary porphobilinogen. Proc Soc Exp Biol Med 1941;47:393.
14. Labbe RF, Vreman HJ, Stevenson DK. Zinc protoporphyrin: a metabolite with a mission. Clin Chem 1999;45:2060.
15. Elder GH. Genetic defects in the porphyrias: types and significance. Clin Dermatol 1998;16:225.
16. Lee GR. Hemolytic disorders. In: Lee GR, Foerster J, Lukens J, et al, eds. Wintrobe's Clinical Hematology, 10th ed. Baltimore: Lippincott Williams & Wilkins, 1999:1119.
17. Wang WC, Lukens JN. Sickle cell anemia and other sickling syndromes. In: Lee GR, Foerster J, Lukens J, et al, eds. Wintrobe's Clinical Hematology, 10th ed. Baltimore: Lippincott Williams & Wilkins, 1999:1348.
18. Lukens JN. The thalassemias and related disorders: quantitative disorders of hemoglobin synthesis. In: Lee GR, Foerster J, Lukens J, et al, eds. Wintrobe's Clinical Hematology, 10th ed. Baltimore: Lippincott Williams & Wilkins, 1999:1407, 1420, 1434.
19. Galanello R, Sollaine C, Paglietti E, et al. α-Thalassemia carrier identification by DNA analysis in the screening for thalassemia. Am J Hematol 1998;59:273.
20. Harrison CR. Hemolytic anemias: intracorpuscular defects, IV Thalassemia. In: Harmening DM, ed. Clinical Hematology and Fundamentals of Hemostasis, 4th ed. Philadelphia: FA Davis, 2002:194.
21. Herzog RW, Hagstrom JN. Gene therapy for hereditary hematological disorders. Am J PharmacoGenomics 2001;1:137.
22. Tisdale J, Sadelain M. Toward gene therapy for disorders of globin synthesis. Semin Hematol 2001;38:382.
23. Williams JL. Anemias of abnormal globin development—thalassemias. In: Stiene-Martin EA, Lotspeich CA, Koepke JA, eds. Clinical Hematology—Principles, Procedures, Correlations, 2nd ed. Philadelphia: Lippincott Williams & Wilkins, 1998:220, 236.
24. Tuzmen S, Schecter AN. Genetic diseases of hemoglobin: diagnostic methods for elucidating β-thalassemia mutations. Blood Rev 2001;15:19.
25. Clarke GM, Higgins TN. Laboratory investigation of hemoglobinopathies and thalassemias: review and update. Clin Chem 2000;46:1284.
26. Arcasoy MO, Gallagher PG. Molecular diagnosis of hemoglobinopathies and other red blood cell disorders. Semin Hematol 1999;36:328.
27. Nalbandian RM, et al. Dithionite tube test—a rapid, inexpensive technique for the detection of hemoglobin. Clin Chem 1971;17:1028.
28. Safko R. Anemia of abnormal globin development–hemoglobinopathies. In: Stiene-Martin EA, Lotspeich CA, Koepke JA, eds. Clinical Hematology—Principles, Procedures, Correlations, 2nd ed. Philadelphia: Lippincott Williams & Wilkins, 1998:196.

29. Briere RO, Golias T, Gatsakis JG. Rapid qualitative and quantitative hemoglobin fractionation. Am J Clin Pathol 1965;44:695.

30. Graham JL, Grunbaum BW. A rapid method for microelectrophoresis and quantitation of hemoglobins on cellulose acetate. Am J Clin Pathol 1963;39:567.

31. Milner PF, Gooden H. Rapid citrate-agar electrophoresis in routine screening for hemoglobinopathies using a simple hemolysate. Am J Clin Pathol 1975;64:58.

32. Huisman THJ, Schroeder WA, Brodie AN, et al. Microchromatography of hemoglobins: II. A simplified procedure for the determination of hemoglobin A$_2$. J Lab Clin Med 1975;86:700.

33. Clayton E, Foster BE, Clayton EP. New stain for fetal erythrocytes in peripheral blood smears. Obstet Gynecol 1970;35:642.

34. National Committee for Clinical Laboratory Standards. Fetal Red Cell Detection; Approved Guideline. Document H52-A. Villanova, PA: National Committee for Clinical Laboratory Standards, 2001.

35. Wu AH, et al. Immunoassays for serum and urine myoglobin: myoglobin clearance assessed as a risk factor for acute renal failure. Clin Chem 1994;40:796.

36. Wu AH, et al. National Academy of Clinical Biochemistry Standards of Laboratory Practice: recommendations for the use of cardiac markers in coronary artery diseases. Clin Chem 1999;45:1104.

37. Christenson RH, Azzazy HME. Biochemical markers of the acute coronary syndromes. Clin Chem 1998;44:1855.

38. Poche H, et al. Hereditary progressive muscular dystrophies: serum myoglobin pattern in patients with different types of muscular dystrophies. Clin Physiol Biochem 1989;7:40.

39. Zaninotto M, et al. Multicenter evaluation of five assays for myoglobin determination. Clin Chem 2000;46:1631.

40. Apple FS, et al. Simultaneous rapid measurement of whole blood myoglobin, creatine kinase MB, and cardiac troponin I by the triage cardiac panel for detection of myocardial infarction. Clin Chem 1999;45:199.

Assessment of Organ System Functions

Introduction to Hormones and Pituitary Function

Robert E. Jones

OBJECTIVES

Upon completion of this chapter, the clinical laboratorian should be able to:

- Describe the functions of the anterior and posterior pituitary.
- Define the anatomic relationship between the pituitary and hypothalamus.
- Understand the concept of open-loop negative feedback and relate this to the function of the various hypothalamic-pituitary-endocrine target gland loops.
- Understand the effects of pulsatility and cyclicity on the results of hormone measurements.
- Differentiate between tropic and direct effector in relationship to pituitary hormones.

- Discuss the regulation of prolactin secretion.
- State the non-neoplastic causes of prolactin elevation.
- Understand the difference between primary and secondary endocrine deficiency states.
- Describe the clinical features of the excess and deficiency states for growth hormone, prolactin, and vasopressin.
- Relate the physiology underlying the strategies used for screening and definitive testing for suspected disorders of growth hormone.

KEY TERMS

Adenohypophysis
Adrenocorticotropin (ACTH)
Anterior pituitary
Corticotropin-releasing hormone (CRH)
Direct effector
Diurnal rhythms
Dopamine
Feedback loops

Follicle-stimulating hormone (FSH)
Gonadotropin-releasing hormone (GnRH)
Growth hormone
Growth hormone-releasing hormone (GHRH)
Hypothalamic–hypophysial portal system
Hypothalamus

Infundibulum
Insulin-like growth factor (IGF)
Luteinizing hormone (LH)
Median eminence
Neurohypophysis
Oxytocin
Pituitary stalk
Posterior pituitary
Prolactin

Prolactin inhibitory factor (PIF)
Pulsatile secretion
Sella turcica
Somatostatin (SS)
Thyroid-stimulating hormone (TSH)
Thyrotropin-releasing hormone (TRH)
Tropic hormone
Vasopressin (ADH)

The term *pituitary* (derived from both Latin and Greek) literally means to "spit mucus," reflecting the primitive notion of pituitary function. In one way, the ancient physiologists were correct—they believed that the brain was responsible for signaling the pituitary to secrete; however, instead of mucus, it was later discovered that the brain directs the pituitary to secrete hormones that regulate other endocrine glands. When this was recognized, the pituitary was designated the "master gland" because, without the pituitary, there was a cessation of growth, together with profound alterations in intermediary metabolism and failure of gonadal, thyroidal, and adrenal function. The pituitary is also referred to as the *hypophysis*, from Greek meaning *under growth*, attesting to its unique position under the hypothalamus.

Our concept of pituitary function and its role in regulating other endocrine glands has changed. Rather than viewed as the master gland, it is more appropriately recognized as a transponder that translates neural input into a hormonal or an endocrinologic product. Features that distinguish the function of the pituitary include *feedback loops, pulsatile secretions, diurnal rhythms,* and environmental or external modification of its performance. These characteristics of pituitary operation can vex the clinical evaluation of suspected endocrine disease or, alternatively, lend incredible insight into subtle defects in endocrinologic function.

EMBRYOLOGY AND ANATOMY

The three distinct parts of the pituitary are the *anterior pituitary,* or *adenohypophysis;* the intermediate lobe, or pars intermedialis; and the *posterior pituitary,* or *neurohypophysis*. The intermediate lobe is poorly developed in humans and has little functional capacity other than to confuse radiologists by forming nonfunctional, benign, cystic enlargements of the pituitary. The posterior pituitary, which arises from the diencephalon, is responsible for the storage and release of *oxytocin* and *vasopressin* (also called *antidiuretic hormone* [ADH]). The anterior pituitary, the largest portion of the gland, originates from Rathke's pouch, an evagination of buccal ectoderm that

progressively extends upward and is eventually enveloped by the sphenoid bone. The creation of the *median eminence,* the inferior portion of the hypothalamus, and the *pituitary stalk* are the other critical events in the formation of the hypothalamic–hypophysial unit. Pituitary function can be detected about the 9th week of gestation.

The pituitary resides in a pocket of the sphenoid (the *sella turcica,* meaning Turkish saddle) and is surrounded by dura mater. The reflection of dura that separates the superior portion of the pituitary from the hypothalamus, the diaphragma sella, is penetrated by the *infundibulum,* or pituitary stalk, that connects the adenohypophysis to the *median eminence* and *hypothalamus*. The pituitary stalk contains both neural and vascular structures that terminate in the hypophysis. The posterior pituitary is connected to the supraoptic and paraventricular hypothalamic nuclei (where vasopressin and oxytocin are produced) by way of two, distinct neurosecretory tracts that pass through the stalk. The anterior pituitary receives 80–90% of its blood supply and many hypothalamic factors via the *hypothalamic–hypophysial portal system,* also contained in the stalk. The primary plexus of this portal system is located in the median eminence and is composed of capillaries lacking a blood-brain barrier (fenestrated capillaries) where the hypothalamic nuclei that modulate pituitary function terminate their axons. In turn, the long portal vessels connect the primary plexus to the anterior pituitary and serve as a conduit for these hypothalamic–hypophysiotropic hormones. These anatomic relationships are illustrated in Figure 17-1.[1]

FUNCTIONAL ASPECTS OF THE HYPOTHALAMIC–HYPOPHYSIAL UNIT

Afferent pathways (inputs) to the hypothalamus are integrated in various specialized nuclei, processed, and then resolved into specific patterned responses. Because the hypothalamus has many efferent neural connections (outputs) to higher brain centers (the limbic system, the autonomic nervous system, and the pituitary), these responses appear to be rather diffuse but are actually

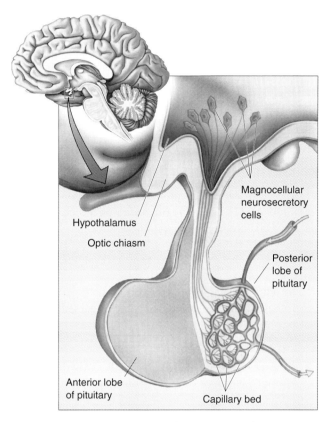

FIGURE 17-1. Relational anatomy of the pituitary and hypothalamus. (Reproduced with permission from Bear MF, Connors BW, Paradiso MA. Neuroscience: Exploring the Brain, 2nd ed. Baltimore: Lippincott Williams & Wilkins, 2001:501.)

stereotypical.[2] The hypothalamic response patterns are similar for each specific pituitary hormone and characterized by open-loop negative feedback mechanisms, pulsatility, and cyclicity. Negative feedback resembles a typical servomechanism and forms the basis of our understanding of hypothalamic–pituitary function. An example of negative feedback is the relationship between a thermostat and a home heating unit. The thermostat is set to a given temperature. As the temperature in the home falls below this set point, the thermostat sends an electrical impulse to the furnace and turns the furnace on. Heat is restored to the room and, when the temperature in the room exceeds the predetermined set point, the thermostat turns off the furnace. Because the thermostat set point can be adjusted for the comfort of the occupants, the furnace–thermostat functional relationship is termed an *open-loop negative feedback system*. Most endocrine feedback loops are of the open-loop variety, meaning that they are subject to external modulation and generally influenced or modified by higher neural input or other hormones.

A simple example of an endocrine feedback loop is the hypothalamic-pituitary-thyroidal axis. The hypothalamus produces the hypophysiotropic hormone, *thyrotropin-*

releasing hormone (TRH), and releases it into the portal system where it directs the thyrotrophs (or TSH-producing cells) in the anterior pituitary to secrete *thyroid-stimulating hormone (TSH)*. TSH circulates to the thyroid and stimulates several steps in the thyroid that are critical in the production and release of thyroid hormone (thyroxine). Thyroxine is released in the blood and circulates to the hypothalamus and pituitary to suppress further TRH and TSH production. This axis can be partially inhibited by adrenal steroids (glucocorticoids) and by cytokines; as a result, thyroid hormone production may decline during periods of severe physiologic stress.[3] The feedback of thyroxine at the level of the pituitary is called a *short feedback loop*, and feedback at the level of the hypothalamus is called a *long feedback loop*. Feedback between the pituitary and hypothalamus (when present) is called an *ultrashort feedback loop*. Figure 17-2 illustrates this simple feedback loop.

All anterior pituitary hormones are secreted in a pulsatile fashion. The pulse frequency of secretion is generally regulated by neural modulation and is specific for each hypothalamic-pituitary-end organ unit. Perhaps the best example of pituitary pulsatility is the secretion of the hormones that regulate gonadal function (*luteinizing hormone [LH]* and *follicle-stimulating hormone [FSH]*). In normal male subjects, the median interpulse interval for LH is 55 minutes, and the average LH peak duration is 40 minutes.[4] The pulse frequency of the regulatory hypothalamic hormone, *gonadotropin-releasing hormone (GnRH)*, has profound effects on LH secretion profiles—increasing the frequency of GnRH pulses reduces the gonadotrope secretory response and decreasing the GnRH pulse frequency increases the amplitude of the subsequent LH pulse.[5]

Another feature of the hypothalamic-pituitary unit is the cyclic nature of hormone secretion. The nervous system usually regulates this function through external signals, such as light-dark changes or the ratio of daylight to darkness. The term *zeitgeber* (time giver) refers to the

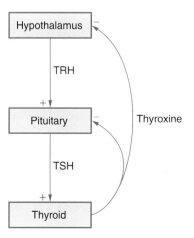

FIGURE 17-2. Simple feedback loop.

process of entraining or synchronizing these external cues into the function of internal biologic clocks. As a result, many pituitary hormones are secreted in different amounts, depending on the time of day. These circadian, or diurnal, rhythms are typified by *adrenocorticotropin (ACTH)*, or TSH secretion. With ACTH, the nadir of secretion is between 11:00 p.m. and 3:00 a.m., and the peak occurs on awakening or around 6:00 to 9:00 a.m.[6] The circadian rhythm of ACTH is a result of variations in pulse amplitude and not alterations in pulse frequency.[7] The nocturnal levels of TSH are approximately twice the daytime levels, and, in contrast to ACTH, the nocturnal rise in TSH is a result of increased pulse amplitude.[8]

HYPOPHYSIOTROPIC OR HYPOTHALAMIC HORMONES

The hypothalamus produces many different products; however, only those that have a direct effect on classical pituitary function will be discussed in this chapter. Most products are peptides; however, bioactive amines are also synthesized and transported from the hypothalamus. Hypothalamic hormones may have multiple actions. For example, TRH stimulates the secretion of both TSH and *prolactin;* GnRH stimulates both LH and FSH production; and *somatostatin (SS)* inhibits growth hormone (GH) and TSH release from the pituitary. In addition to its effects on water metabolism, vasopressin (ADH) can also stimulate *adrenocorticotropin (ACTH)* secretion. These hypophysiotropic hormones are found throughout the central nervous system and various other tissue, including the gut, pancreas, and other endocrine glands. Their function outside the hypothalamus and pituitary is poorly understood. The action of hypophysiotropic hormones on anterior pituitary function is summarized in Table 17-1.

ANTERIOR PITUITARY HORMONES

The hormones secreted from the anterior pituitary are larger and more complex than those synthesized in the hypothalamus. These pituitary hormones are either *tropic*, meaning their actions are specific for another endocrine gland, or they are *direct effectors* because they act directly on peripheral tissue. TSH and its unique role in regulating thyroid function is an example of tropic; an example of a direct effector is GH. GH has direct effects on substrate metabolism in numerous tissue and also stimulates the liver to produce growth factors that are critical in enhancing linear growth. The tropic hormones are LH, which directs testosterone production from Leydig cells in men and ovulation in women; FSH, which is responsible for ovarian recruitment and early folliculogenesis in women and spermatogenesis in men; TSH, which directs thyroid hormone production from the thyroid; and ACTH, which regulates adrenal steroidogenesis. Both GH and prolactin are direct effectors. A general summary of relationships among anterior pituitary hormones and their target organs and feedback effectors are listed in Table 17-2.

The actions of the trophic hormones are discussed in other chapters devoted to the specific target gland.

GROWTH HORMONE

The pituitary is vital for normal growth. Growth ceases if the pituitary is removed and, if the hormonal products from other endocrine glands that are acted on by the pituitary are replaced (thyroxine, adrenal steroids, and gonadal steroids), growth is not restored until growth hormone is administered. However, if growth hormone is given in isolation without the other hormones, growth is not promoted. Therefore, it takes complete functioning of the pituitary to establish conditions ripe for growth of the individual. It also takes adequate nutrition, normal levels of insulin, and overall good health to achieve a person's genetic growth potential.

Growth hormone, also called *somatotropin*, is structurally related to prolactin and human placental lactogen. A single peptide with two intramolecular disulfide bridges, it belongs to the direct effector class of anterior pituitary hormones. The somatotrophs, pituitary cells that produce growth hormone, comprise over one third of normal pituitary weight. Release of somatotropin from

TABLE 17-1. HYPOPHYSIOTROPIC HORMONES

HORMONE	STRUCTURE	ACTION
Thyrotropin-releasing hormone (TRH)	3 amino acids	Releases TSH and prolactin
Gonadotropin-releasing hormone (GnRH)	10 amino acids	Releases LH and FSH
Corticotropin-releasing hormone (CRH)	41 amino acids	Releases ACTH
Growth hormone-releasing hormone (GHRH)	44 amino acids	Releases GH
Somatostatin	14 and 28 amino acids	Inhibits GH and TSH release (additional effects on gut and pancreatic function)
Dopamine (prolactin inhibitory factor)	1 amino acid	Inhibits prolactin release

TABLE 17-2. ANTERIOR PITUITARY HORMONES

PITUITARY HORMONE	TARGET GLAND	STRUCTURE	FEEDBACK HORMONE
Luteinizing hormone (LH)	Gonad (tropic)	Dimeric glycoprotein	Sex steroids (E_2/T)
Follicle-stimulating hormone (FSH)	Gonad (tropic)	Dimeric glycoprotein	Inhibin
Thyroid-stimulating hormone (TSH)	Thyroid (tropic)	Dimeric glycoprotein	Thyroid hormones (T_4/T_3)
Adrenocorticotropin (ACTH)	Adrenal (tropic)	Single peptide derived from POMC	Cortisol
Growth hormone	Multiple (direct effector)	Single peptide	Insulin-like growth factor (IGF-I)
Prolactin	Breast (direct effector)	Single peptide	Unknown

T_4, thyroxine; T_3, triiodothyronine; E_2, estradiol; T, testosterone.

the pituitary is stimulated by the hypothalamic peptide *growth hormone-releasing hormone (GHRH)*; somatotropin's secretion is inhibited by somatostatin (SS).[9] Growth hormone is secreted in pulses, with an average interpulse interval of 2–3 hours, with the most reproducible peak occurring at the onset of sleep.[10] Between these pulses, the level of growth hormone may fall below the detectable limit, resulting in the clinical evaluation of growth hormone deficiency being based on a single, challenging measurement.

No other hypothalamic–hypophysial system more vividly illustrates the concept of an open-loop paradigm than that seen with growth hormone. The on-and-off functions of GHRH/SS and the basic pattern of secretory pulses of growth hormone are heavily modulated by other factors (Table 17-3).[11]

TABLE 17-3. OTHER MODIFIERS OF GROWTH HORMONE SECRETION

STIMULATE GROWTH HORMONE SECRETION	INHIBIT GROWTH HORMONE SECRETION
Sleep	Glucose loading
Exercise	β-Agonists (eg, epinephrine)
Physiologic stress	α-Blockers (eg, phentolamine)
Amino acids (eg, arginine)	Emotional/Psychogenic stress
Hypoglycemia	Nutritional deficiencies
Sex steroids (eg, estradiol)	Insulin deficiency
α-Agonists (eg, norepinephrine)	Thyroxine deficiency
β-Blockers (eg, propranolol)	

Actions of Growth Hormone

Growth hormone has many diverse effects on metabolism; it is considered an amphibolic hormone because it directly influences both anabolic and catabolic processes. One major effect of growth hormone is that it allows an individual to effectively transition from a fed state to a fasting state without experiencing a shortage of substrates required for normal intracellular oxidation. Growth hormone directly antagonizes the effect of insulin on glucose metabolism, promotes hepatic gluconeogenesis, and stimulates lipolysis.[9] From a teleologic viewpoint, this makes perfect sense—enhanced lipolysis provides oxidative substrate for peripheral tissue, such as skeletal muscle, and yet conserves glucose for the central nervous system by stimulating the hepatic delivery of glucose and opposing insulin-mediated glucose disposal. Indeed, growth hormone deficiency in children may be accompanied by hypoglycemia[12]; in adults, hypoglycemia may occur if both GH and ACTH are deficient.

The anabolic effects of growth hormone are reflected by enhanced protein synthesis in skeletal muscle and other tissue. This is translated into a positive nitrogen balance and phosphate retention.

Although growth hormone has direct effects on many tissues, it also has indirect effects that are mediated by factors that were initially called *somatomedins*. In early experiments, it became apparent that growth hormone supplementation in hypophysectomized animals induced the production of an additional factor that stimulated the incorporation of sulfate into cartilage. As this "protein" was purified, it was evident that there was more than one somatomedin, and, because of their structural homology to proinsulin, the nomenclature shifted to *insulin-like growth factor (IGF)*. For example, somatomedin C, the major growth factor induced by growth hormone, is now IGF-I. IGFs also have cell surface receptors that are distinct from insulin; however, supraphysiologic levels of IGF-II can "bleed" over on the insulin receptor and cause hypoglycemia,[13] and hyperinsulinemia can partially activate IGF-I receptors.[14] Growth hormone stimulates the production of IGF-I from the liver and, as a result, IGF-I becomes a biologic amplifier of growth hormone levels. IGFs are complexed to specific serum binding proteins that have been shown to affect the actions of IGFs in multifaceted ways.[15] IGF-binding protein III (IGFBP-III) is perhaps the best studied member of the IGFBP family. The levels of IGFBP III are positively correlated with IGF-I levels and, as a result, GH levels.[16] Because of this relationship, IGF-I has been used in the clinical evaluation of both GH deficiency and excess.[17]

Testing

As noted above, a single, random measurement of growth hormone is rarely diagnostic. The current testing paradigms for growth hormone are soundly based on the dynamic physiology of the growth hormone axis. For example, circulating levels of IGF-I and, perhaps, IGFBP-III reasonably integrate the peaks of growth hormone secretion, and elevated levels of both are consistent with a sustained excess of growth hormone.[18] Other conditions, however, notably hepatomas, can be associated with high levels of IGF-I, and levels of IGFBP-III may be inappropriately normal in some people with active acromegaly.[19] Conversely, low IGF-I levels may reflect inadequate production of growth hormone; however, low IGF levels are also seen in patients with poorly controlled diabetes, malnutrition, or other chronic illnesses.[20]

Definitive testing for determining the autonomous production of growth hormone relies upon the normal suppressibility of growth hormone by oral glucose loading.[21] The test is performed after an overnight fast, and the patient is given a 100-gram oral glucose load. Growth hormone is measured at time zero and at 60 and 120 minutes after glucose ingestion. Following oral glucose loading, growth hormone levels are undetectable in normal individuals; however, in patients with acromegaly, growth hormone levels fail to suppress and may even paradoxically rise.

Testing patients for suspected growth hormone deficiency is more complicated. There are several strategies to stimulate growth hormone, and new protocols are currently evolving.[22] Once considered the gold standard, insulin-induced hypoglycemia is being replaced by less uncomfortable testing schemes. Combination infusions of GHRH and the amino acid L-arginine or an infusion of L-arginine coupled with oral L-DOPA are the most widely used. If growth hormone levels rise above 3–5 ng/mL, it is unlikely that the patient is growth hormone deficient.[22]

Acromegaly

Acromegaly results from pathologic or autonomous growth hormone excess and, in the vast majority of pa-

tients, is a result of a pituitary tumor. There have been isolated case reports of tumors causing acromegaly as a result of the ectopic production of GHRH,[23] and, although exceedingly interesting or instructive, the ectopic production of GHRH or growth hormone (one case) remains rare.[24] If a growth hormone–producing tumor occurs before epiphyseal closure, the patient develops gigantism and may grow to an impressive height; otherwise, the patient develops classical, but insidious, features of bony and soft tissue overgrowth.[25] These features include progressive enlargement of the hands and feet as well as growth of facial bones, including the mandible and bones of the skull. In advanced cases, the patient may develop significant gaps between their teeth. Diffuse (not longitudinal if the condition occurred following puberty) overgrowth of the ends of long bones or the spine can produce a debilitating form of arthritis. Because growth hormone is an insulin antagonist, glucose intolerance or overt diabetes can occur. Hypertension; accelerated atherosclerosis; and proximal muscle weakness, resulting from acquired myopathy, may be seen late in the illness. Sleep apnea is common. Organomegaly, especially thyromegaly, is common, but hyperthroidism is exceedingly rare. Growth hormone excess is also a hypermetabolic condition and, as a result, acromegalic patients may complain of excessive sweating or heat intolerance. The features of acromegaly slowly develop over time, and the patient (or their family) may be oblivious that changes in physiognomy have occurred. In these cases, the patient's complaints may center on the local effects of the tumor (headache or visual complaints) or symptoms related to the loss of other anterior pituitary hormones (hypopituitarism). A careful, retrospective review of older photographs may be crucial in differentiating coarse features due to inheritance from the classical consequences of acromegaly. If left untreated, acromegaly shortens life expectancy because of increased risk of heart disease, resulting from the combination of hypertension, coronary artery disease, and diabetes/insulin resistance. Because patients with acromegaly also have a greater lifetime risk of developing cancer, cancer surveillance programs (especially regular colonoscopy) are recommended.

Cosecretion of prolactin can be seen in up to 40% of patients with acromegaly.[26] Only a few TSH/growth hormone–secreting tumors have also been reported.[27]

Confirming the diagnosis of acromegaly is relatively easy; however, some patients with acromegaly have normal random levels of growth hormone. An elevated level of growth hormone that does not suppress normally with glucose loading equates to an easy diagnosis. In those patients with normal, but inappropriately sustained, random levels of growth hormone, elevated levels of IGF-I are helpful; however, nonsuppressibility of growth hormone to glucose loading is the definitive test.[21]

Treatment of acromegaly can be challenging. The goal of treatment is tumor ablation, with continued function of the remainder of the pituitary. Transphenoidal adenomectomy is the procedure of choice.[28] If normal growth hormone levels and kinetics (normal suppressibility to glucose) are restored following surgery, the patient is likely cured. Unfortunately, growth hormone-producing tumors may be too large or may invade into local structures that preclude complete surgical extirpation, and the patient is left with a smaller, but hormonally active, tumor. External beam or focused irradiation is frequently used at this point, but it may take several years before growth hormone levels decline.[29] In the interim, efforts are made to suppress growth hormone. Two different classes of agents, somatostatin analogs and dopaminergic agonists, may be employed.[30]

Growth Hormone Deficiency

Growth hormone deficiency occurs in both children and adults. In children, it may be familial or it may be due to tumors, such as craniopharyngiomas. In adults, it is a result of structural or functional abnormalities of the pituitary (see, *Hypopituitarism* in this chapter); however, a decline in growth hormone production is an inevitable consequence of aging and the significance of this phenomenon is poorly understood.[31]

Although growth hormone deficiency in children is manifest by growth failure, not all patients with short stature have growth hormone deficiency (see above). There have been several genetic defects identified in the growth hormone axis. The more common type is a recessive mutation in the GHRH gene that causes a failure of growth hormone secretion. A rarer mutation, loss of the growth hormone gene itself, has also been observed. Mutations that cause GH insensitivity have also been reported. These mutations may involve the GH receptor, IGF-I biosynthesis, IGF-I receptors, or defects in GH signal transduction. Patients with GH insensitivity do not respond normally to exogenously administered growth hormone. Finally, structural lesions of the pituitary or hypothalamus may also cause GH deficiency and may be associated with other anterior pituitary hormone deficiencies.[32]

An adult growth hormone deficiency syndrome has been described in patients who have complete or even partial failure of the anterior pituitary. The symptoms of this syndrome are extremely vague and include social withdrawal, fatigue, loss of motivation, and a diminished feeling of well-being,[33] but several studies have documented increased mortality in adults who are GH deficient.[34] Osteoporosis and alterations in body composition (*ie*, reduced lean body mass) are frequent concomitants of adult growth hormone deficiency.[35]

Growth hormone replacement therapy has become relatively simple with the advent of recombinant human growth hormone. Currently, the cost of growth hormone is the major limiting factor for replacement.

PROLACTIN

Prolactin is structurally related to growth hormone and human placental lactogen. Considered a stress hormone, it has vital functions in relationship to reproduction. Prolactin is classified as a direct effector hormone (as opposed to a tropic hormone) because it has diffuse target tissue and lacks a single endocrine end organ.

Prolactin is unique among the anterior pituitary hormones because its major mode of hypothalamic regulation is tonic inhibition rather than intermittent stimulation. *Prolactin inhibitory factor* (PIF) was once considered a polypeptide hormone capable of inhibiting prolactin secretion; *dopamine*, however, is the only neuroendocrine signal that inhibits prolactin and is now considered to be the elusive PIF. Any compound that affects dopaminergic activity in the median eminence of the hypothalamus will also alter prolactin secretion.[36] Examples of medications that cause hyperprolactinemia include phenothiazines, butyrophenones, metoclopramide, reserpine, tricyclic antidepressants, and α-methyldopa. Any disruption of the pituitary stalk (*eg*, tumors, trauma, or inflammation) causes an elevation in prolactin as a result of interruption of the flow of dopamine from the hypothalamus to the lactotropes, the pituitary prolactin-secreting cells. TRH directly stimulates prolactin secretion, and increases in TRH (as seen in primary hypothyroidism) elevate prolactin levels.[37] Estrogens also directly stimulate lactotropes to synthesize prolactin. Pathologic stimulation of the neural suckling reflex is the likely explanation of hyperprolactinemia associated with chest wall injuries. Hyperprolactinemia may also be seen in renal failure and polycystic ovary syndrome. Physiologic stressors, such as exercise and seizures, also elevate prolactin. The feedback effector for prolactin is unknown.

As mentioned, the physiologic effect of prolactin is lactation. The usual consequence of prolactin excess is hypogonadism, either by suppression of gonadotropin secretion from the pituitary or by inhibition of gonadotropin action at the gonad.[38] The suppression of ovulation seen in lactating postpartum mothers is related to this phenomenon.

Prolactinoma

A prolactinoma is a pituitary tumor that directly secretes prolactin, and it represents the most common type of functional pituitary tumor. The clinical presentation of a patient with a prolactinoma depends on the age and gender of the patient and the size of the tumor. Premenopausal women most frequently complain of menstrual irregularity/amenorrhea, infertility, or galactorrhea; men or postmenopausal women generally present with symptoms of a pituitary mass, such as headaches or visual complaints. Occasionally, a man may present with reduced libido or complaints of erectile dysfunction. The reason(s) for the varied presentations of a prolactinoma are somewhat obscure but likely relate to the dramatic, noticeable alteration in menses or the abrupt onset of a breast discharge in younger women. By contrast, the decline in reproductive function in older patients may be overlooked as an inexorable consequence of "aging."

One recently recognized complication of prolactin-induced hypogonadism is osteoporosis.[39]

Other Causes of Hyperprolactinemia

There are many physiologic, pharmacologic, and pathologic causes of hyperprolactinemia, and a common error by clinicians is to ascribe any elevation in prolactin to a "prolactinoma." Generally, substantial elevations in prolactin (>150 ng/mL) indicate prolactinoma, and the degree of elevation in prolactin is correlated with tumor size.[40] Modest elevations in prolactin (25–100 ng/ml) may be seen with pituitary stalk interruption, use of dopaminergic antagonist medications, or to other medical conditions.

Clinical Evaluation of Hyperprolactinemia

A careful history and physical examination is usually sufficient to exclude most common, nonendocrine causes of hyperprolactinemia. It is essential to obtain TSH and free T_4 (or total thyroxine and T_3 resin uptake) to eliminate primary hypothyroidism as a cause for the elevated prolactin. If a pituitary tumor is suspected, a careful assessment of other anterior pituitary function (basal cortisol, LH, FSH, and gender-specific gonadal steroid [either estradiol or testosterone]) and an evaluation of sellar anatomy with a high-resolution MRI should be obtained.

Management of Prolactinoma

The therapeutic goals are correction of symptoms that result from local invasion or extension of the tumor by reducing tumor mass, restoration of normal gonadal function and fertility, prevention of osteoporosis, and preservation of normal anterior and posterior pituitary function. The different therapeutic options include simple observation, surgery, radiotherapy, or medical management with dopamine agonists.[36] However, the management of prolactinoma also depends on the size of the tumor (macroadenomas [tumor size >10 mm] are less likely to be "cured" than microadenomas [tumor size <10 mm])[41] and the preferences of the patient.

CASE STUDY 17-2

A 23-year-old woman has experienced recent onset of a spontaneous, bilateral breast discharge and gradual cessation of menses. She reports normal growth and development and has never been pregnant.

Questions

1. What conditions could be causing her symptoms?

2. What medical conditions (other than a prolactinoma) are associated with hyperprolactinemia?

3. Which medications raise prolactin?

4. How would your thinking change if she had galactorrhea but normal levels of prolactin?

Dopamine agonists are the most commonly employed therapy for microprolactinomas. Tumor shrinkage is noted in more than 90% of patients treated with bromocriptine mesylate (Parlodel) or the new dopamine agonist, cabergoline (Dostinex). Both drugs also shrink prolactin-secreting macroadenomas.[42] A resumption of menses and restoration of fertility is also frequently seen during medical therapy. The adverse effects of bromocriptine include orthostatic hypotension, dizziness, and nausea. The gastrointestinal adverse effects of bromocriptine can be ameliorated through intravaginal administration, and its efficacy is otherwise uncompromised.[43] Cabergoline has fewer adverse effects and may be administered biweekly because of its longer duration of action. Either agent should be discontinued during pregnancy unless tumor regrowth has been documented.

Neurosurgery is not a primary mode of prolactinoma management. The indications for neurosurgical intervention include pituitary apoplexy (hemorrhage), acute visual loss due to macroadenoma, cystic prolactinoma, or intolerance to medical therapy. Surgical cure rates are inversely proportional to tumor size and the degree of prolactin elevation. External beam radiotherapy is generally reserved for high surgical risk patients with locally aggressive macroadenomas who are unable to tolerate dopamine agonists.

Idiopathic Galactorrhea

Lactation occurring in women with normal prolactin levels is defined as *idiopathic galactorrhea*. This condition is usually seen in women who have been pregnant several times and has no pathologic implication.

HYPOPITUITARISM

The failure of either the pituitary or hypothalamus results in the loss of anterior pituitary function. Complete loss of function is termed panhypopituitarism; however, there may be a loss of only a single pituitary hormone, which is referred to as a monotropic hormone deficiency. The loss of a tropic hormone (ACTH, TSH, LH, and FSH) is reflected in function cessation of the affected en-

docrine gland. Loss of the direct effectors (growth hormone and prolactin) may not be readily apparent. This section will concentrate on the causes of hypopituitarism and certain subtleties involved in the therapy of panhypopituitarism; more detailed descriptions of various hormone deficiency states are covered in other chapters.

The laboratory diagnosis of hypopituitarism is relatively straightforward. In contrast to the primary failure of an endocrine gland that is accompanied by dramatic increases in circulating levels of the corresponding pituitary tropic hormone, secondary failure (hypopituitarism) is associated with low or normal levels of tropic hormone. In primary hypothyroidism, for example, the circulating levels of thyroxine are low and TSH levels may exceed 200 μU/mL (normal, 0.4–5.0). As a result of pituitary failure in hypothyroidism, TSH levels are inappropriately low and typically less than 1.0 μU/mL.

There are several important issues in distinguishing between primary and secondary hormone deficiency states. To differentiate between primary and secondary deficiencies, both tropic and target hormone levels should be measured when there is any suspicion of pituitary failure or as part of the routine evaluation of gonadal or adrenal function. If one secondary deficiency is documented, it is essential to search for other deficiency states and the cause for pituitary failure. For example, failure to recognize secondary hypoadrenalism may have catastrophic consequences if the patient is treated with thyroxine. Similarly, initially overlooking a pituitary or hypothalamic lesion could preclude early diagnosis and treatment of a potentially aggressive tumor.

Etiology of Hypopituitarism

The many causes of hypopituitarism are listed in Table 17-4. Direct effects of pituitary tumors, or the sequelae of treatment of tumors, are the most common causes of pituitary failure. Pituitary tumors may cause panhypopituitarism by compressing or replacing normal tissue or interrupting the flow of hypothalamic hormones by destroying the pituitary stalk. Large, nonsecretory pituitary tumors (chromophobe adenomas) or macroprolactinomas are most commonly associated with this phe-

---

CASE STUDY 17-3

A 60-year-old man presented with intractable headaches. An MRI was requested to evaluate this complaint, and a 2.5 cm pituitary tumor was discovered. In retrospect, he noted an unexplained 20-kg weight loss, cold intolerance, fatigue, and loss of sexual desire.

Questions

1. How would you approach the evaluation of his anterior pituitary function?

2. What additional testing may be required to confirm a loss in anterior pituitary function?

TABLE 17-4. CAUSES OF HYPOPITUITARISM

1. Pituitary tumors
2. Parapituitary/hypothalmic tumors
3. Trauma
4. Radiation therapy/surgery
5. Infarction
6. Infection
7. Infiltrative disease
8. Immunologic
9. Familial
10. Idiopathic

nomenon. Parasellar tumors (meningiomas and gliomas), metastatic tumors (breast and lung), and hypothalamic tumors (craniopharyngiomas or dysgerminomas) can also cause hypopituitarism through similar mechanisms. Hemorrhage into a pituitary tumor (pituitary apoplexy) is rare; however, when it occurs, it frequently causes complete pituitary failure. Postpartum ischemic necrosis of the pituitary following a complicated delivery (Sheehan's syndrome) typically presents as profound, unresponsive shock or as failure to lactate in the puerperium. Infiltrative diseases, such as hemachromatosis, sarcoidosis, or histiocytosis, can also affect pituitary function. Fungal infections, tuberculosis, and syphilis can involve the pituitary or hypothalamus and may cause impairment of function. Lymphocytic hypophysitis, an autoimmune disease of the pituitary, may only affect a single cell type in the pituitary, resulting in a monotropic hormone deficiency, or can involve all cell types, yielding total loss of function. Severe head trauma may shear the pituitary stalk or may interrupt the portal circulation. Similarly, surgery involving the pituitary may compromise the stalk and/or blood supply to the pituitary or may iatrogenically diminish the mass of functioning pituitary tissue. Panhypopituitarism can result from radiotherapy used to treat a primary pituitary tumor or a pituitary that was inadvertently included in the radiation port; loss of function, however, may be gradual and may occur over several years. There have been rare instances of familial panhypopituitarism or monotropic hormone deficiencies. In Kallmann's syndrome, for example, GnRH is deficient and the patient presents with secondary hypogonadism. Lastly, there may not be an apparent identified cause for the loss of pituitary function, and the patient is classified as having idiopathic hypopituitarism, although one recent case report emphasized the need to continue the search for an etiology.[44]

Treatment of Panhypopituitarism

In the average patient, replacement therapy for panhypopituitarism is the same as for primary target organ failure. Patients are treated with thyroxine, glucocorticoids, and gender-specific sex steroids. It is less clear about growth hormone replacement in adults, and additional studies are needed to clarify this issue.[45,46] Replacement becomes more complicated in panhypopituitary patients who desire fertility. Pulsatile GnRH infusions have induced puberty and restored fertility in patients with Kallmann's syndrome, and gonadotropin preparations have restored ovulation/spermatogenesis in people with gonadotropin deficiency.[47]

POSTERIOR PITUITARY HORMONES

The posterior pituitary is an extension of the forebrain and represents the storage region for vasopressin (also called *antidiuretic hormone* [ADH]) and oxytocin. Both of these small peptide hormones are synthesized in the supraoptic and paraventricular nuclei of the hypothalamus and transported to the neurohypophysis via their axons in the hypothalamoneurohypophysial tract. This tract transits the median eminence of the hypothalamus and continues into the posterior pituitary through the pituitary stalk. The synthesis of each of these hormones is tightly linked to the production of neurophysin, a larger protein whose function is poorly understood. Both hormones are synthesized outside of the hypothalamus in various tissue, and it is plausible they have an autocrine or paracrine function.

CASE STUDY 17-4

An 18-year-old woman was admitted to the neurologic intensive care unit following a severe closed head injury. Her course stabilized after 24 hours, but the nursing staff noticed a dramatic increase in the patient's urine output, which exceeded 1000 mL/hour.

Questions

1. What caused her increased urine production?

2. How could you prove your suspicions?

3. Could she have other possible endocrinologic problems?

Oxytocin

Oxytocin is a cyclic nonapeptide, with a disulfide bridge connecting amino acid residues 1 and 6. As a posttranslational modification, the C-terminus is amidated. Oxytocin has a critical role in lactation[48] and likely plays a major role in labor and parturition.[49] In addition to its reproductive effects, oxytocin has been shown to have effects on pituitary, renal, cardiac, and immune function.

Vasopressin

Structurally similar to oxytocin, vasopressin is a cyclic nonapeptide with an identical disulfide bridge; it differs from oxytocin by only two amino acids. Vasopressin's major action is to regulate renal free water excretion and, therefore, have a central role in water balance. The vasopressin receptors in the kidney (V_2) are concentrated in the renal collecting tubules and the ascending limb of the loop of Henle. They are coupled to adenylate cyclase and, once activated, they induce insertion of aquaporin-2, a water channel protein, into the tubular luminal membrane.[50] Vasopressin is also a potent pressor agent and effects blood clotting[51] by promoting factor VII release from hepatocytes and von Willebrand factor release from the endothelium. These vasopressin receptors (V_{1a} and V_{1b}) are coupled to phospholipase C.

Hypothalamic osmoreceptors and vascular baroreceptors regulate the release of vasopressin from the posterior pituitary. The osmoreceptors are extremely sensitive to even small changes in plasma osmolality, with an average osmotic threshold for vasopressin release in humans of 284 mOsm/kg. As plasma osmolality increases, vasopressin secretion increases. The consequence is a reduction in renal free water clearance, a lowering of plasma

osmolality, and a return to homeostasis. The vascular baroreceptors (located in the left atrium, aortic arch, and carotid arteries) initiate vasopressin release in response to a fall in blood volume or blood pressure. A 5–10% fall in arterial blood pressure in normal humans will trigger vasopressin release; however, in contrast to an osmotic stimulus, the vasopressin response to a baroreceptor-induced stimulus is exponential. In fact, baroreceptor-induced vasopressin secretion will override the normal osmotic suppression of vasopressin secretion.

Diabetes insipidus (DI), characterized by copious production of urine (polyuria) and intense thirst (polydipsia), is a consequence of vasopressin deficiency. However, total vasopressin deficiency is unusual, and the typical patient presents with a partial deficiency. The causes of hypothalamic DI include apparent autoimmunity to vasopressin-secreting neurons, trauma, diseases affecting pituitary stalk function, and various CNS or pituitary tumors. A sizable percentage of patients (up to 30%) will have idiopathic DI.[52]

Depending on the degree of vasopressin deficiency, diagnosis of DI can be readily apparent or may require extensive investigation. Documenting an inappropriately low vasopressin level with an elevated plasma osmolality would yield a reasonably secure diagnosis of DI. In less obvious cases, the patient may require a water deprivation test in which fluids are withheld from the patient and serial determinations of serum and urine osmolality are performed in an attempt to document the patient's ability to conserve water. Under selected circumstances, a health care provider may simply offer a therapeutic trial of vasopressin or a synthetic analog, such as dDAVP, and assess the patient's response. In this circumstance, amelioration of both polyuria and polydipsia would be considered a positive response, and a presumptive diagnosis of DI is made.

REVIEW QUESTIONS

1. Open-loop negative feedback refers to the phenomenon of:
    a. negative feedback with a modifiable set point.
    b. blood flow in the hypothalamic–hypophysial portal system.
    c. blood flow to the pituitary via dural-penetrating vessels.
    d. negative feedback involving an unvarying, fixed set point.

2. The specific feedback effector for FSH is:
    a. activin.
    b. inhibin.
    c. progesterone.
    d. estradiol.

3. Which anterior pituitary hormone lacks a stimulatory hypophysiotropic hormone?
    a. Growth hormone
    b. Prolactin
    c. Vasopressin
    d. ACTH

4. The definitive suppression test to prove autonomous production of growth hormone is:
    a. somatostatin infusion.
    b. estrogen priming.
    c. dexamethasone suppression.
    d. oral glucose loading.

5. Which of the following are influenced by growth hormone?
   a. IGF-I
   b. IGFBP-III
   c. Lipolysis
   d. All of the above

6. What statement concerning vasopressin secretion is NOT true?
   a. Vasopressin secretion is closely tied to plasma osmolality.
   b. Changes in blood volume also alter vasopressin secretion.
   c. A reduction in effective blood volume overrides the effects of plasma osmolality in regulating vasopressin secretion.
   d. All of the above.

7. What are the long-term sequelae of untreated or partially treated acromegaly?
   a. An increased risk of colon and lung cancer
   b. A reduced risk of heart disease
   c. Enhanced longevity
   d. Increased muscle strength

8. Thyrotropin-releasing hormone (TRH) stimulates the secretion of:
   a. prolactin.
   b. growth hormone.
   c. TSH.
   d. both A and C.

9. Estrogen influences the secretion of which of the following hormones?
   a. Growth hormone
   b. Prolactin
   c. Luteinizing hormone
   d. All of the above

REFERENCES

1. Frohman LA. Diseases of the anterior pituitary. In: Felig P, Baxter JD, Broadus AE, Frohman LA, eds. Endocrinology and Metabolism, 2nd ed. New York: McGraw-Hill, 1981:247–337.

2. Asa SL, Horvath E, Kovacs KT. Functional pituitary anatomy and histology. In: Melmed S, ed. Endocrinology, 4th ed. Philadelphia: WB Saunders, 2001:167–182.

3. Monig H, Arendt A, Meyer M, et al. Activation of the hypothalamo-pituitary-adrenal axis in response to septic or non-septic diseases—implications for the euthyroid sick syndrome. Intensive Care Med 1999;25:1402–1496.

4. Urban RJ, Evans WS, Rogol, AD, et al. Contemporary aspects of discrete pulse detection algorithms I. The paradigm of the LH pulse signal in men. Endocr Rev 1988;9:3–37.

5. Crowley WF Jr, Whitcomb RN, Jameson JL, et al. The neuroendocrine control of reproduction in the male. Recent Prog Horm Res 1991;47:27–62.

6. Follenius M, Brandenberger G: Plasma free cortisol during secretory episodes. J Clin Endocrinol Metab 1986;62:609–612.

7. Veldhuis JD, Iranmanesh A, Johnson ML, Lizarraldo G. Amplitude, but not frequency, modulation of adrenocorticotropin secretory bursts gives rise to the nyctohemeral rhythm of the corticotropic axis in man. J Clin Endocrinol Metab 1990;71:452–463.

8. Samuels MH, Veldhuis JD, Henry P, Ridgeway EC. Pathophysiology of pulsatile and copulsatile release of thyroid stimulating hormone, luteinizing hormone, follicle stimulating hormone and α-subunit. J Clin Endocrinol Metab 1990;71:425–432.

9. Casanueva FF. Physiology of growth hormone secretion and action. Endocrinol Metab Clin North Am 1992;21:483–517.

10. Van Cauter E, Plat L, Copinschi G. Interrelations between sleep and the somatotropic axis. Sleep 1998;21:553–566.

11. Herman-Bonert VS, Prager D, Melmed S. Growth hormone. In: Melmed S, ed. The Pituitary. Cambridge, MA: Blackwell Science, 1995:98–135.

12. Pinto G, Adan L, Souberbielle JC, et al. Idiopathic growth hormone deficiency: presentation, diagnosis and treatment. Ann Endocrinol (Paris) 1999;60:224–231.

13. Teale JD, Marks V. Inappropriately elevated plasma insulin-like growth factor II in relation to suppressed insulin-like growth factor I in the diagnosis of non-islet cell hypoglycemia. Clin Endocrinol (Oxf) 1990;33:87–98.

14. Blakesley VA, Scrimgeour A, Esposito D, LeRoith D. Signaling via the insulin-like growth factor ! receptor. Does it differ from insulin receptor signaling. Cytokine Growth Factor Rev 1996;7: 153–159.

15. Clemmons DR. Insulin-like growth factor-I and its binding proteins. In: Melmed S, ed. Endocrinology, 4th ed. Philadelphia: WB Saunders, 2001:439–460.

16. Binoux M, Roghani M, Hossenlopp P, et al. Molecular forms of IGF binding proteins: physiological implications. Acta Endocrinol (Copenh) 1991;124:41–47.

17. Span JP, Pieters GF, Sweep CG, et al. Plasma IGF-I is a useful marker of growth hormone deficiency in adults. J Endocrinol Invest 1999;22:446–450.

18. van der Lely AJ, de Herder WW, Janssen JA, et al. Acromegaly: the significance of serum total and free IGF-I and IGF-binding protein-3 in diagnosis. J Endocrinol 1997;155:9–16.

19. de Herder WW, van der Lely AJ, Janssen JA, et al. IGFBP-3 is a poor parameter for assessment of clinical activity in acromegaly. Clin Endocrinol (Oxf) 1995;43:501–505.

20. Clemmons DR. Insulin-like growth factor binging proteins. Trends Endocrinol Metab 1990;1:412–417.

21. Ezzat S. Acromegaly. Endocrinol Metab Clin North Am 1997; 26:703–723.

22. Biller BMK, Samuels MH, Zagar A, et al. Sensitivity and specificity of six tests for the diagnosis of adult GH deficiency. J Clin Endocrinol Metab 2002;87:2067–2079.

23. Faglia G, Arosio M, Bazzoni N. Ectopic acromegaly. Endocrinol Metab Clinics NA 1992;21:575–596.

24. Ezzat S, Ezrin C, Yamashita S, Melmed S. Recurrent acromegaly resulting from ectopic growth hormone gene expression by a metastatic pancreatic tumor. Cancer 1993;71:66–70.

25. Molitch ME. Clinical aspects of acromegaly. Endocrinol Metab Clin North Am 1992;597–614.

26. Lamberts SW, Klijn JGM, van Vroonhoven CCJ, et al. Different responses of growth hormone secretion to guanfacine, bromocriptine and thyrotropin-releasing hormone in acromegalic patients with pure growth hormone (GH)-containing and mixed GH/prolactin-containing pituitary adenomas. J Clin Endocrinol Metab 1985;60:1148–1153.

27. Beck-Peccoz P, Brucker-Davis F, Persani L, et al. Thyrotropin-secreting pituitary tumors. Endocr Rev 1996;17:610–638.

28. Fahlbusch R, Honegger J, Buchfelder M. Surgical management of acromegaly. Endocrinol Metab Clin North Am 1992;21:669–692.

29. Jackson IM, Norén G. Role of gamma knife therapy in the management of pituitary tumors. Endocrinol Metab Clin North Am 1999;28:133–142.

30. Newman C. Medical therapy for acromegaly. Endocrinol Metab Clin North Am 1999;28:171–190.

31. Rudman D, Kutner MH, Rogers CM, et al. Impaired growth hormone secretion in the adult population: relation to age and adiposity. J Clin Invest 1981;67:1361–1369.

32. Rosenfeld RG: Growth hormone deficiency in children. In: Melmed S, ed. Endocrinology, 4th ed. Philadelphia: WB Saunders, 2001:503–519.

33. Cuneo RC, Salomon F, McGauley GA, Sönksen PH. The growth hormone deficiency syndrome in adults. Clin Endocrinol (Oxf) 1992;37:387–397.

34. Rosén T, Bengtsson BA. Premature mortality due to cardiovascular disease in hypopituitarism. Lancet 1990;336:285–288.

35. Hansen TB, Vahl N, Jørgensen JO, et al. Whole body and regional soft tissue changes in growth hormone deficient adults after one year of growth hormone treatment: a double-blind, randomized, placebo-controlled study. Clin Endocrinol 1995;43:689–696.

36. Molitch M. Medical management of prolactinomas. Endocrinol Metab Clin North Am 1999;28:143–169.

37. Honbo KS, Herle AVJ, Kellett KA. Serum prolactin levels in untreated hypothyroidism. Am J Med 1978;64:782–787.

38. Odell WD. Prolactin-producing tumors. In: Odell WD, Nelson DH, eds. Pituitary Tumors. Mt Kisco, NY: Futura Publishing, 1984;159–179.

39. Wardlaw SL, Bilezikian JP. Hyperprolactinemia and osteopenia. J Clin Endocrinol Metab 1002;75:690–691.

40. Faglia G. Prolactinomas and hyperprolactinemic syndrome. In: Melmed S, ed. Endocrinology, 4th ed. Philadelphia: WB Saunders, 2001:329–342.

41. Molitch ME: Prolactinomas. In: Melmed S, ed. The Pituitary. Cambridge, MA: Blackwell Science, 1995:443–477.

42. Demura R, Kubo O, Demura H, et al. Changes in computed tomographic findings in microprolactinomas before and after bromocriptine. Acta Endocrinol 1985;110:308–312.

43. Vermesh M, Fossum GT, Kletzky OA. Vaginal bromocriptine: pharmacology and effect on serum prolactin in normal women. Obstet Gynecol 1988;72:693–698.

44. Katz BJ, Jones RE, Digre KB, et al. Panhypopituitarism as an initial manifestation of primary central nervous system non-Hodgkin's lymphoma. Endocr Pract 2003;9:296–300.

45. Isley WL. Growth hormone therapy for adults: not ready for prime time? Ann Intern Med 2002;137:190–196.

46. Cook DM. Shouldn't adults with growth hormone deficiency be offered growth hormone replacement therapy? Ann Intern Med 2002;137:197–201.

47. Hayes FJ, Seminara SB, Crowley WF Jr. Hypogonadotropic hypogonadism. Endocrinol Metab Clin North Am 1998;27:739–763.

48. Nishimori K, Young LJ, Guo Q, et al. Oxytocin is required for nursing but is not essential for parturition or reproductive behavior. Proc Natl Acad Sci USA 1996;93:11699–11704.

49. Goodwin TM, Zograbyan A. Oxytocin receptor antagonists—update. Clin Perinatol 1998;25:859–871.

50. Cheng A, van Hoek AN, Yeager M, et al. Three-dimensional organization of a human water channel. Nature 1997;387:627–630.

51. Mannucci PM, Ruggeri ZM, Pareti FI, Capitanio A. DDAVP: A new pharmacological approach to the management of hemophilia and von Willebrand disease. Lancet 1977;1:869–872.

52. Moses AM, Notman DD. Diabetes insipidus and syndrome of inappropriate antidiuretic hormone secretion (SIADH). Adv Int Med 1982;27:73–110.

Adrenal Function

LeAnne Swenson, Daniel H. Knodel

OBJECTIVES

Upon completion of this chapter, the clinical laboratorian should be able to:

• Explain how the adrenal gland functions to maintain blood pressure, potassium, and glucose homeostasis.
• Describe steroid biosynthesis, regulation, and actions according to anatomic location within the adrenal gland.
• Discuss the pathophysiology of adrenal cortex disorders, namely Cushing's syndrome and Addison's disease.
• Differentiate the adrenal enzyme deficiencies and their blocking pathways in establishing a diagnosis.

• Describe the synthesis, storage, and metabolism of catecholamines.
• State the most useful measurements in supporting the diagnosis of pheochromocytoma.
• List the clinical findings associated with hypertension that suggest an underlying adrenal etiology is causing high blood pressure.
• List the appropriate laboratory tests to differentially diagnose primary and secondary Cushing's syndrome and Addison's disease.

KEY TERMS

Abnormal aldosterone production

Adrenocorticotropic hormone (ACTH)

Aldosterone (Aldo)

Angiotensin-converting enzyme (ACE)

Antidiuretic hormone (ADH)

Atrial natriuretic peptide (ANP)

Cardiovascular disease (CVD)

Catechol methyltransferase (COMT)

Congenital Adrenal hyperplasia (CAH)

Corticotropin-releasing hormone (CRH)

Dehydroepiandrosterone (DHEA)

5-Dehydrotestosterone (5-DHT)

11-Deoxycortisol (11-DOC)

Epinephrine (EPI)

Headache (HA)

Homovanillic acid (HVA)

17-Hydroxycorticosteroid (17-OHCS)

Hypertension (HTN)

Monoamine oxidase (MAO)

Nonsteroidal anti-inflammatory drug (NSAID)

Norepinephrine (NE)

Phenylethanolamine *N*-methyltransferase (PNMT)

Pheochromocytoma (Pheo)

Plasma aldosterone (PA)

Plasma renin activity (PRA)

Renin-angiotensin system (RAS)

Squamous cell carcinoma (SSC)

Vasoactive inhibitory peptide (VIP)

Vesicle monoamine transporters (VMAT)

Zona fasciculata (F-zone)

Zona glomerulosa (G-zone)

Zona reticularis (R-zone)

THE ADRENAL GLAND: AN OVERVIEW

The adrenal gland is a multifunctional organ that produces the hormones and neuropeptides essential for life. Despite the complex effects of adrenal hormones, most pathologic conditions of the adrenal gland are linked by their impact on blood pressure.[1] As such, an adrenal etiology should be considered in the differential diagnosis of all patients with abnormal blood pressure, particularly when accompanied by electrolyte abnormalities, unexplained change in weight, inappropriate virilization, and periods of anxiety, weakness, orthostasis, palpitations, *headache,* and chest or abdominal pain.

In clinical practice, patients often present with states of diminished production or overproduction of one or more adrenal hormones. Hypofunction is generally treated with exogenous hormone replacement; hyperfunction with pharmacologic suppression or surgical excision.

EMBRYOLOGY AND ANATOMY

The adrenal gland is composed of two embryologically distinct, but conjoined, glands—the outer adrenal cortex and inner adrenal medulla. The cortex is derived from mesenchymal cells located near the urogenital ridge that differentiate into three structurally and functionally distinct zones (Fig. 18-1). The medulla arises from neural crest cells that invade the cortex during the second month of development. By adulthood, the medulla contributes 10% of total adrenal weight. To date, mechanisms involved in maintaining adrenal size and function are poorly understood.[2]

Adult adrenal glands are shaped like pyramids, located just above and medial to the kidneys in the retroperitoneal space (suprarenal glands). On gross sectioning, both regions remain distinct; the cortex appears yellow, the medulla is dark mahogany.

Adrenal arterial supply is symmetric. Small arterioles branch to form a dense subcapsular plexus that drains into the sinusoidal plexus of the cortex. There is no direct supply to zona fasciculata and zona reticularis. In contrast, venous drainage from the central vein displays laterality. After crossing the medulla, the right adrenal vein empties into the inferior vena cava, and the left adrenal vein drains into the left renal vein. There is a separate capillary sinusoidal network from the medullary arterioles that also drains into the central vein and limits the exposure of cortical cells to medullary venous blood. Glucocorticoids from the cortex are carried directly to the

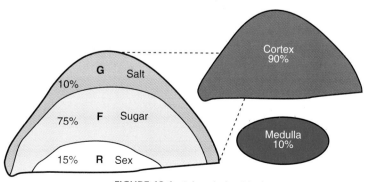

FIGURE 18-1. Adrenal gland by layer.

adrenal medulla via the portal system, where they stimulate production of *epinephrine (EPI)* (see Fig. 18-17).

Sympathetic and parasympathetic axons reach the medulla through the cortex. En route, these axons release neurotransmitters (*eg,* catecholamines, neuropeptide Y) that modulate cortex blood flow, cell growth, and function. Medullary projections into the cortex have been found to contain cells that also synthesize and release neuropeptides, such as *vasoactive inhibitory peptide (VIP)*, adrenomedullin, and *atrial natriuretic peptide (ANP)*, and potentially influence cortex function.

THE ADRENAL CORTEX BY ZONE

The major cortex hormones, aldosterone, cortisol, and *dehydroepiandrosterone sulfate (DHEAS)*, are uniquely synthesized from a common precursor by cells located in one of three functionally distinct zonal layers of the adrenal cortex: *zona glomerulosa, zona fasciculata, and zona reticularis*, respectively (Fig. 18-1).

G-zone. Zona glomerulosa cells (outer 10%) synthesize mineralocorticoids (aldosterone) critical for sodium (volume), potassium, and acid-base homeostasis. They have low cytoplasmic-to-nuclear ratios and small nuclei with dense chromatin with intermediate lipid inclusions.

F-zone. Zona fasciculata cells (middle 75%) synthesize glucocorticoids, such as cortisol, critical to blood glucose homeostasis. Fasciculata cells are cords of clear cells, with a high cytoplasmic-to-nuclear ratio and lipids laden with "foamy" cytoplasm. The fasciculata also generate androgen precursors such as *dehydroepiandrosterone (DHEA)*, which is sulfated in the innermost *zona reticularis (R-layer)*. Subcapsular adrenal remnants (cortex only) can regenerate into fasciculate adrenals, metastasize, and survive in ectopic locations such as the liver, gallbladder wall, broad ligaments, celiac plexus, ovaries, scrotum, and cranium.

R-zone. Zona reticularis cells (inner 10%) sulfate DHEA to *dehydroepiandrosterone sulfate (DHEAS)*, a precursor for adrenal sex hormones. The zone is sharply demarcated with lipid-deficient cords of irregular, dense cells with lipofuscin deposits.

Adrenal cell-types are presumed to arise from stem cells. A proposed tissue layer between the zona glomerulosa and fasciculata may serve as a site for progenitor cells to regenerate zonal cells.[3]

Cortex Steroidogenesis

Control of steroid hormone biosynthesis is complex. It occurs via substrate availability, enzyme activities, and inhibitory feedback loops that are layer-specific. Defining adrenal cortex biosynthesis and actions in terms of three layers simplifies its complexity.

All adrenal steroids are derived by sequential enzymatic conversion of a common substrate, cholesterol. Adrenal parenchymal cells accumulate and store approximately 80% of circulating low-density lipoproteins (LDL). The adrenal gland can also synthesize additional cholesterol using acetyl-CoA, assuring adrenal steroidogenesis remains normal in patients with variable lipid disorders and in patients on lipid lowering agents.

Only free cholesterol can enter steroidogenic pathways after transport to the inner mitochondrial membrane in response to *adrenocorticotropic hormone (ACTH)*. The availability of free intracellular cholesterol is metabolically regulated by LDL negatively and ACTH positively through multiple mechanisms. *Corticotropin-releasing hormone (CRH)* is secreted from the hypothalamus to circadian signals, serum cortisol, and stress, causing release of stored ACTH, which stimulates transport of free cholesterol into adrenal mitochondria, initiating steroid production.

Conversion of cholesterol to pregnenolone is the first rate-limiting step in steroid biosynthesis: 6 carbons are removed from cholesterol by mitochondrial membrane CYP450 enzyme (Fig. 18-2). Newly synthesized pregnenolone is then returned to the cytosol for subsequent zonal conversion by microsomal enzymes in each layer by F-layer enzymes and/or androgens by enzymes in the R-layer (Fig. 18-3). Because F-layer glucocorticoids powerfully suppress ACTH release, cortisol is the primary feedback regulator of ACTH-stimulated hormone production in the adrenal cortex. ACTH does not signifi-

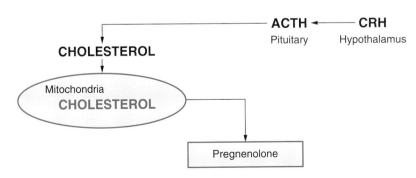

FIGURE 18-2. Conversion of cholesterol to pregnenolone.

cantly impact G-layer *aldosterone (Aldo)* synthesis, although certain glucocorticoids have mineralocorticoid actions.

Decreased activity of any enzymes required for biosynthesis can occur as an acquired or inherited (autosomal recessive) trait. Defects that decrease production of cortisol cause increases in ACTH and CRH secretion in an attempt to stimulate cortisol levels and lead to adrenal hyperplasia or overproduction of androgens, depending on the affected enzyme.

Evaluation of adrenal function requires measuring relevant adrenal hormones, metabolites, and regulatory secretagogues. Diagnosis is based on correlation of clinical and laboratory findings.[4]

Congenital Adrenal Hyperplasia

Congenital adrenal hyperplasia (CAH) is an inherited family of enzyme disorders causing decreased cortisol production. The clinical presentation depends on the affected enzyme as demonstrated in Figure 18-4. Laboratory findings reveal increased upstream substrates with overflow across open pathways and relatively decreased products downstream from the affected enzyme.[5] Partial defects can present after puberty. Ninety-five percent are a result of a 21-hydroxylase deficiency causing 17-OH progesterone and androgen buildup while cortisol decreases. Treatment with oral glucocorticoids replaces deficient cortisol and suppresses ACTH stimulated androgen excess.[6]

Only G-cells convert cholesterol to pregnenolone, the common steroid precursor, and then into aldosterone (15–20 mg/day) (Fig. 18-3). G-layer–specific Aldo synthesis occurs for several reasons. Low G-cell 17α-hydroxylase activity prevents substrate diversion into other pathways and low Aldo synthase activity in other zones assures the final oxidation of corticosterone to aldosterone is G-cell specific (Fig. 18-3).

Aldo secretion is regulated by the *renin-angiotensin system (RAS)*, which functions to maintain organ perfusion. Perceived volume depletion, low filtered salt, and sympathetic nerve stimulation is sensed as hypoperfusion by cells that stimulate renin production. Renin is a proteolytic enzyme secreted by renal cells in the juxtaglomerular apparatus. Renin initiates a sequence of cleavage steps of angiotensinogen or renin substrate to form angiotensin (A-I). *Angiotensin-converting enzyme (ACE)* converts A-I to A-II. A-II acts as a powerful vasoconstrictor to raise blood pressure and stimulate Aldo release. Chronic A-II stimulation or dietary salt restriction can cause Aldo hypersecretion and isolated G-layer hypertrophy.[7]

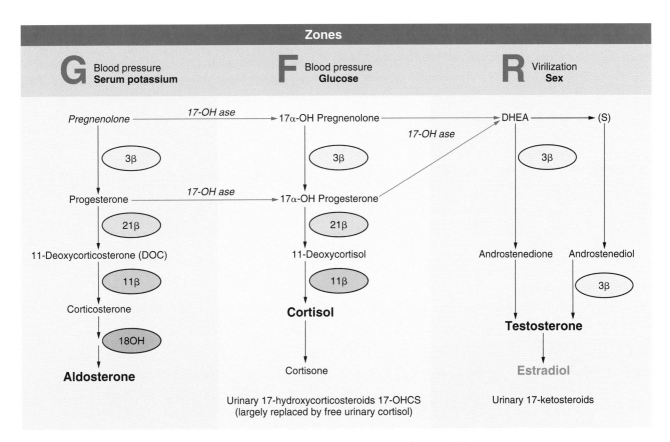

FIGURE 18-3. Conversion of cholesterol to pregnenolone and aldosterone.

Enzyme Defect	New Classification	HTN	Virilization	High Lab Value
3β-Hydroxysteroid dehydrogenase	3β-HSD II	N	Slight	DHEA
17α-Hydroxylase	CYP17	Y	No	Aldosterone
11β-Hydroxylase	CYP11B1GF	Y	Marked	11-DOC
21β-Hydroxylase	CYP21A2	N	Marked	17-OH-progesterone

FIGURE 18-4. Congenital adrenal hyperplasia syndromes.

Aldo acts on the kidney to increase blood pressure through volume expansion. This occurs by increasing sodium reabsorption; hence, water retention. Aldo also stimulates H^+ and K^+ excretion, causing metabolic alkalosis with volume expansion, *hypertension (HTN),* and hypokalemia. The phenomenon is enhanced with high sodium diets.

Angiotensin II, elevated serum potassium (K^+), progesterone, and dopamine stimulate aldosterone synthesis (Fig. 18-5). ANP, intracellular calcium, and certain drugs are Aldo suppressors, including ketoconazole, ACE inhibitors, *nonsteroidal anti-inflammatory drugs (NSAIDs),* and heparin.

Isolated Hypoaldosteronism

Insufficient Aldo secretion is seen with adrenal gland destruction, chronic heparin therapy following unilateral adrenalectomy (transient), and with G-layer enzyme deficiencies. Most often, it occurs in patients with mild renal insufficiency such as persons with diabetes who present with mild metabolic acidosis, high serum K^+, low urinary K^+ excretion (urine K^+ < urine Na+), and low reninemia. Pharmacologic treatment is with diet; bicarbonate; furosemide (K^+-wasting diuretic); or, occasionally, Florinef (synthetic mineralocorticoid), which enhances salt retention, K^+ and acid secretion.

Hyperaldosteronism

Patients with excess aldosterone production develop metabolic alkalosis, hypertension, and hypokalemia. They typically present with symptoms caused by low serum K^+, as outlined in Figure 18-6.

Causes of hypertension and unprovoked hypokalemia include:

- Primary aldosteronism (low renin)—autonomous oversecretion of Aldo.
- Secondary aldosteronism (elevated renin)—RAS-activated Aldo secretion.
- Pseudoaldosteronism (variable renin and Aldo levels)—renal tubular diseases causing urinary potassium loss by Aldo-independent mechanisms. In most cases, Aldo is low; however, two syndromes are associated with high Aldo levels: Bartter's syndrome (bumetanide-sensitive Cl^- channel mutation) and Gitelman's syndrome (thiazide-sensitive transporter mutation).

Documenting excess aldosterone excretion establishes the diagnosis of aldosteronism (urine measurements are superior to plasma measurements) but cannot discern between underlying etiologies. *Plasma renin activity (PRA)* measurements reflect the state of RAS activation and are helpful for that determination. Because PRA varies with volume status, upright position, and dietary sodium intake, an isolated PRA measurement has limited clinical value. PRA assessed relative to *plasma aldosterone (PA)* helps distinguish primary from other forms of aldosteronism.

Types of aldosteronism are diagrammed in Figure 18-7 according to their PA (*y*-axis) and PRA (*x*-axis) values in groups, according to those ratios).

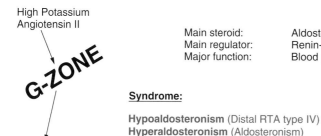

High Potassium
Angiotensin II

G-ZONE

Aldosterone

Main steroid: Aldosterone
Main regulator: Renin-angiotensin system (RAS)
Major function: Blood pressure and K^+ homeostasis

Syndrome:

Hypoaldosteronism (Distal RTA type IV)
Hyperaldosteronism (Aldosteronism)

Clinical Findings:

Hyperkalemia, renal salt wasting
HTN, hypokalemia, metabolic alkalosis

FIGURE 18-5. Cortex function and pathology by layer.

- Easy fatigability
- Muscle weakness (paralysis)
- Polyuria (loss of renal concentration ability and renal cysts)
- Palpitations (increased ventricular ectopy)
- Autonomic dysregulation (hypotension without reflex tachycardia)
- Impaired insulin secretion (decreased glucose tolerance)
- Aldosterone suppression

FIGURE 18-6. Signs and symptoms of hypokalemia.

DIAGNOSIS OF PRIMARY ALDOSTERONISM

Because 25% of HTN patients have low renin, the diagnosis of primary aldosteronism relies on three criteria[8]:

- HTN without edema.
- Low plasma renin that fails to increase with volume depletion.
- High aldosterone that fails to decrease with saline or angiotensin inhibition.

Diagnosis Algorithm

Urinary K^+ excretion measured in patients with HTN and unprovoked hypokalemia is a cost-effective screening test for aldosteronism. Urine $K^+ > 30$ mEq/day is inappropriate in hypokalemic patients and strongly suggests a hyperaldosteronemic state (spot urine $K^+ > Na^+$ is also suggestive). Urine $K^+ < 30$ mEq/day reflects renal K^+ retention, as seen with prior diuretic use or gastrointestinal loss.

Upright PA and RA ratio measured in a fluid-deprived patient (overnight dehydration increases RA) is defini-

tive in separating primary from other causes of aldosteronism, particularly when repeated following volume expansion (2 liters of normal saline over 4 hours), which normally suppresses aldosterone. A PA:PRA ratio >25 suggests primary aldosteronism. Most clinicians proceed to adrenal computed tomography (CT) or magnetic resonance imaging (MRI).

Captopril suppression is often confirmatory. Within three hours of taking 50 mg of Captopril (1 mg/kg), plasma Aldo remains high in primary *abnormal aldosterone production (Aldo-ism)* (PA:PRA ratio >25 ng/dL before and after test) but is suppressed in patients with other forms of HTN.

18-Hydroxycorticosterone levels can help define the causes of autonomous (nonsuppressible) aldosterone production. Levels >100 ng/dL suggest an *Aldo-producing adenoma (APA)*, whereas, idiopathic hyperaldosteronism (IHA) is more likely when levels are lower (<100 ng/dL). A correct diagnosis is critical for correct treatment. Surgery is curative for an autonomous functioning adenoma or unilateral hyperplasia; otherwise, drug therapy is used to antagonize (eg, spironolactone or amiloride with thiazide for IHA) or inhibit Aldo actions (eg, cortisone for glucocorticoid-responsive hyperaldosteronism).

Adrenal imaging (CT or MRI) is used to visualize adrenal gland anatomy. Structural abnormalities should compliment functional findings to establish a diagnosis. Pathology based on imaging studies alone can be misleading. Adrenal adenomas (nonsecreting) are routinely found in 10% of healthy patients; adrenal nodules can be

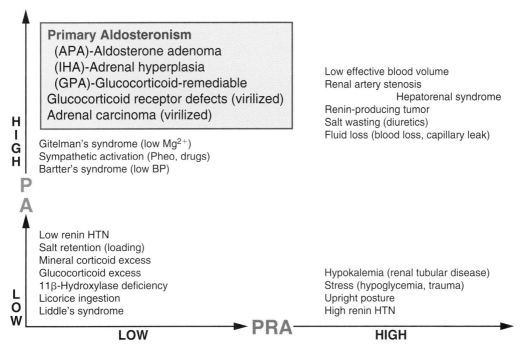

FIGURE 18-7. Types of aldosteronism according to PA:PRA ratio.

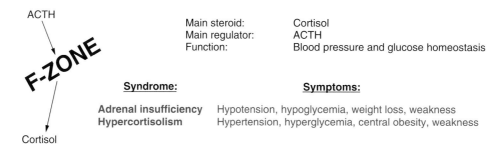

ACTH

F-ZONE

Cortisol

Main steroid: Cortisol
Main regulator: ACTH
Function: Blood pressure and glucose homeostasis

Syndrome: **Symptoms:**

Adrenal insufficiency   Hypotension, hypoglycemia, weight loss, weakness
Hypercortisolism   Hypertension, hyperglycemia, central obesity, weakness

FIGURE 18-8. F-zone disorders.

normal structural variants or result from abnormal gland stimulation. Occasionally, Aldo-secreting adenomas are missed because they are too small to resolve or hide within hyperplastic glands. If imaging is negative, the scan can be repeated in 6–12 months.

Scintigraphy or **adrenal vein sampling** is used for discordant results. In one study, 50% of patients diagnosed with APA by venous sampling had hyperplasia by CT.[8]

Cortisol synthesis (15–20 mg/day) is critical to hemodynamic and glucose homeostasis. F-zone disorders manifest with blood pressure and glucose abnormalities (Fig. 18-8). Glucocorticoids maintain blood glucose by inducing lipolysis and amino acid release from muscle breakdown for conversion into glucose (gluconeogenesis) and storage as liver glycogen.

Cortisol production is regulated by *adrenocorticotropic hormone (ACTH)*. ACTH is secreted in a pulsatile fashion by the pituitary gland. Diurnal variation causes ACTH and cortisol levels to be highest in the early morning (8:00 a.m.) and lowest at night (10:00 p.m. to 12:00 a.m.). ACTH pulse amplitude (not frequency) rises between 2:00 and 4:00 a.m. Additional peaks of ACTH follow protein-rich meals, *antidiuretic hormone (ADH)* stimulation, as well as CRH. Hypoglycemia indirectly stimulates ACTH by increasing CRH and ADH release. In addition, acute stress (physical and psychologic) directly stimulates ACTH secretion, causing cortisol levels to rise. Elevated glucocorticoids (endogenous and exogenous), in turn, suppress ACTH through feedback inhibition, decreasing proopiomelanocortin gene transcription in pituitary corticotroph cells and also by blocking the production, secretion, and stimulatory effects of CRH on ACTH synthesis and release in the pituitary.

ADRENAL INSUFFICIENCY (ADDISON'S DISEASE)

Adrenal insufficiency (low cortisol) results from a primary adrenal problem (destruction of 90% of the adrenal cortex) or is secondary to ACTH deficiency (abnormality at the hypothalamic–pituitary level).[9]

Symptoms of deficiency can be vague and misleading (Fig. 18-9). As cortisol is critical to normal glucose

homeostasis and maintenance of vascular tone, deficiency produces symptoms resembling failure to thrive, such as weakness, fatigue, anorexia, nausea, diarrhea, and abdominal pain accompanied by physical findings such as weight loss. Abnormal lab values depend on the underlying cause of low cortisol production and include hyponatremia, hyperkalemia, hypercalcemia, prerenal azotemia, and mild metabolic acidosis.

Autoimmune adrenalitis accounts for 70% of the cases of primary adrenal insufficiency; however, other conditions, including infectious diseases such as fungal (not candida), human immunodeficiency virus (HIV), and tuberculosis; bilateral adrenal hemorrhage; adrenoleukodystrophy; infiltrative processes; and metastasis, can also destroy the adrenal gland. Glucocorticoid therapy is the most common cause of secondary adrenal insufficiency; however, tumors, hemorrhage, infiltrative processes, developmental abnormalities, and malignancies also interfere with ACTH production by the pituitary gland.

Diagnosis of Adrenal Insufficiency

Low baseline levels (8:00 a.m., supine) are suggestive but not reliable for establishing a diagnosis of insufficiency. Random cortisol levels are only useful in excluding the diagnosis when elevated (>20 μg/dL). Cosyntropin is a synthetic stimulator of cortisol and aldosterone secretion, which tests the capacity of the adrenal gland to increase hormone production in response to stimulation. It is safe and offers reliable results regardless of food intake

Frequency	Symptoms	Signs
100%	Weakness Fatigue Anorexia	Weight loss
90%		Hyperpigmentation (primary adrenal insufficiency)
50%	Nausea Diarrhea	
10%	Pain	Adrenal calcification

FIGURE 18-9. Signs and symptoms of adrenal insufficiency.

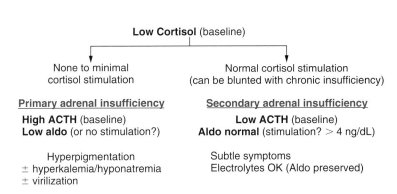

FIGURE 18-10. Differential diagnosis of low cortisol states.

or time of day. Hypoglycemia is also a potent stimulator of cortisol secretion but potentially dangerous. A stimulated free cortisol level <18 μg/dL indicates impaired adrenal function.

Following a blood draw for baseline cortisol, ACTH and aldosterone levels, cosyntropin (IV/IM) is given. Repeat samples are drawn at 30 and 60 minutes poststimulation. ACTH and aldosterone responses to cosyntropin aid in the differential diagnosis of low cortisol states as illustrated in Figure 18-10. Although good at identifying primary adrenal insufficiency, most causes of chronic secondary insufficiency (central) are associated with abnormal cortisol response to cosyntropin stimulation.

Metyrapone is used as an alternate diagnostic or confirmatory test for adrenal insufficiency. In normal adrenals, metyrapone blocks 11β-hydroxylase (Fig. 18-3), increasing *11-deoxycortisol (11-DOC)* (>7 μg/dL) while cortisol falls (<5 μg/dL). Secondary adrenal insufficiency is suggested in patients with a near-normal response to a 250 μg cosyntropin test, but with an abnormal response to metyrapone. Patients suspected of having central adrenal insufficiency should be screened with at least one head scan for pituitary disease unless they have a history of chronic exogenous glucocorticoid use.

The cause of primary adrenal gland destruction can often be distinguished by antibody titers and/or distinctive appearance with imaging. Autoimmune disease is suggested by findings such as small glands; infection, with large adrenal glands; and hemorrhage as shown by enlargement with characteristic intensity.

Treatment of Adrenal Insufficiency

In primary adrenal insufficiency, synthetic steroids from each cortex layer are replaced: G-Aldo (Florinef, 50–100 μg/day); F-cortisol (hydrocortisone, 20–25 mg/day; or prednisone, 5 mg/day); and R-DHEA (50–100 mg/day—*controversial*). In secondary insufficiency, steroidogenesis from the non-ACTH regulated layers remains intact, so only cortisol is replaced. Most clinicians double the dose of glucocorticoids during mild stress and give hydrocortisone 300 mg/day in divided doses for significant stresses.

HYPERCORTISOLISM

Unregulated release of CRH, ACTH, adrenal glucocorticoid secretion and exogenous intake causes hypercortisolism. Excess cortisol affects multiorgan systems, including immune (suppression, poor healing), dermatologic (thin, friable tissue, wide purple striae), vascular (vessel fragility, ecchymoses), adipose (increased fat with redistribution to upper back and central locations), muscle (wasting, proximal muscle weakness, heart failure), neurologic (peripheral neuropathy, autonomic dysregulation), bone (loss), renal (edema, HTN, calciuria), and metabolic (hyperglycemia and insulin resistance). Cortisol also has CNS actions, influencing pain perception and sense of well-being. Clinical presentation of hypercortisolism is variable, with no single feature common in all cases.

Multiple conditions are associated with high cortisol levels, with differing comorbidities and treatment options, as outlined in Figure 18-11. Determining the cause of hypercortisolism can be difficult, as laboratory values and clinical findings often overlap between syndromes.

CUSHING'S SYNDROME

Cushing's syndrome describes the complex of symptoms (Fig. 18-11) resulting from excess glucocorticoid production or prolonged exogenous steroid use. It is most commonly seen in three disorders: ACTH-secreting pituitary adenoma (68%); autonomous cortisol production from adrenal tumors or nodules (17%, ACTH is suppressed); and excess ectopic ACTH production (15%, usually malignant).[10,11]

Patients with Cushing's share striking similarity with patients with type 1 diabetes (insulin-resistant). They have a 4-fold increase in mortality even after successful therapy, primarily a result of *cardiovascular disease (CVD)*. Because mineralocorticoid receptors are equally responsive to glucocorticoids, excess cortisol can promote HTN in association with left ventricular hypertrophy. Electrocardiogram (ECG) abnormalities and loss of normal nocturnal fall in blood pressure is also seen. Untreated disease has a 50%, 5-year mortality.

Stress

Infection

Severe obesity (visceral)

Polycystic ovary syndrome (up to 40% have slightly elevated urine cortisol)

Chronic alcoholism (cortisol normalizes with abstinence)

Depression (up to 80% have abnormal cortisol levels, disappears with remission)

Iatrogenic Cushing's (<1% inhaled, topical, oral glucocorticoid use)

Cushing's Syndrome	Symptoms of Cushing's Syndrome	
	HTN	**(85–90%)**
	Central obesity	**(90%)**
	Glucose intolerance	**(80%)**
	Plethoric faces	**(80%)**
	Purple striae	**(65%)**
	Hirsuitism	**(65%)**
	Abnormal menses	**(60%)**
	Muscle weakness	**(60%)**

FIGURE 18-11. Conditions associated with hyper-cortisolism.

Iatrogenic Cushing's syndrome is rare (<1%) but may be difficult to discern from true disorders. All glucocorticoids, including synthetic, inhaled, and topical, can inhibit ACTH secretion; therefore, plasma ACTH, serum cortisol, and cortisol excretion may all be low (unless cortisol or cortisone is used). In contrast, urine contamination with topical hydrocortisone (vulvovaginal or perineal use) can falsely elevate urine cortisol values. Relatively greater urinary than serum cortisol and cortisone values suggest hydrocortisone addition in the urine. If suspected, synthetic glucocorticoids can be detected chromatographically.

Diagnosis of Cushing's Syndrome

Clinical symptoms are supported by laboratory findings of cortisol excess, loss of diurnal rhythm, and suppression resistance (once exogenous glucocorticoid administration is excluded because a universal diagnostic algorithm for Cushing's has not been established): (1) ACTH and cortisol are secreted in bursts and excess secretion may occur episodically; (2) each patient has unique metabolism, metabolites, and metabolic clearance rates; (3) stimulation and suppression thresholds often vary (nonsuppressible lesions can occasionally be suppressed, and normal patients can display suppression resistance); and (4) compliance and accuracy issues regarding sample collection and processing are common. Standard assessment tests for diagnosing Cushing's are listed below.[12]

Document Cortisol Excess
Urine free cortisol (and/or metabolites) (Fig. 18-3). Urine cortisol is a sensitive indicator of endogenous cortisolism. When serum cortisol exceeds the capacity of its carrier protein binding, free cortisol levels rise rapidly, increasing the free cortisol filtered into the urine. This value may be erroneous with high urine volume (>3 L) because patients who drink more than 5 L/day will have a 64% increase in urine cortisol. In contrast, urine *17-hydroxycorticosteroid (17-OHCS)* excretion occurs at a constant rate and is not effected by volume changes.

A 24-hour urine free cortisol is the most sensitive (95–100%) and specific (98%) screen for excess cortisol production. A revised method, collecting overnight (10:00 p.m. to 8:00 a.m.) urine samples for cortisol factored by urinary creatinine, appears equally valid (specificity and sensitivity of 97–100%). In one large study, 21–47% of Cushing's patients had at least one normal 24-hour urine cortisol; therefore, patients with intermediate values should be reevaluated 2–3 months later.[12]

Random plasma cortisol levels are of little value for the diagnosis of Cushing's. Levels in normal people vary widely during the day and overlap with levels found in patients with Cushing's.

Baseline a.m. cortisol concentrations have no diagnostic value unless they are clearly above the normal range.

Determine if Diurnal Rhythm Is Lost (Late-Night Values Remain High)
Plasma cortisol is highest between 6:00 and 8:00 a.m. and 50–80% lower between 10:00 p.m. and 12:00 a.m. Measuring late-night cortisol is justified by the fact that its normal evening nadir is lost in Cushing's syndrome and bilateral nodular hyperplasia, but preserved in obese and depressed patients.

Ideally, a blood sample (for cortisol and ACTH) is drawn between 11:00 p.m. and 12:00 a.m. Samples are stabilized, stored, and sent to the laboratory if the previously determined urine cortisol is elevated. Late-evening saliva or blood cortisol values may be more reliable than urine cortisol for diagnosis of Cushing's.

In two studies, a single midnight serum cortisol concentration (>7.5 μg/dL) was 90–96% sensitive and 100% specific for Cushing's.[12]

In another study of Cushing's patients (30 normal and 18 obese subjects), a single 11:00 p.m. salivary cortisol level, when combined with the 8:00 a.m. salivary cortisol concentration after a 1-mg overnight dexamethasone suppression test, had a sensitivity and specificity of 100%.[12]

Saliva cortisol is stable at room temperature for days and collection is noninvasive, can be performed at home, and has greater specificity (100%); however, it is less sensitive (92%) than serum or urine levels in detecting Cushing's. Midnight (12:00 a.m.) values <1.3 ng/mL by radioimmunoassay (RIA) or >1.5 ng/mL by competitive protein-binding assay helps exclude the diagnosis. Saliva measurements are useful in patients with suspected intermittent Cushing's who need to collect numerous samples over extended periods.

Determine Loss of Normal Cortisol Suppression by Dexamethasone

Dexamethasone acts as an exogenous cortisol substitute, suppressing ACTH if the pituitary gland is normal and cortisol secretion if the adrenal gland is normal.

An overnight dexamethasone suppression test is commonly used to screen patients for autonomous overproduction of cortisol. Dexamethasone (1 mg) given at about 11:00 p.m. acts to suppress the early morning ACTH stimulated rise in cortisol. Suppressed free cortisol <3.6 μg/dL measured between 8:00 and 9:00 a.m. is considered a negative test. Although it appears that repeated ingestion of dexamethasone minimizes individual differences in drug clearance, the low dose (1 mg) suppression test was 95% accurate and equally reliable as the standard 2-day, low-dose dexamethasone suppression (0.5 mg every 6 hours × 2 days, with normal urine free cortisol <10 μg on Day 2) per retrospective analysis of 426 Cushing's patients.

While the predictive value for a negative test nears 100%, false-positive results are common (up to 15%). Causes for this include testing errors, other cortisol suppression resistant states (eg, physical stress, anorexia nervosa, alcoholism, depression, acute illness, obesity, and renal insufficiency) and altered drug metabolism and drug interactions (eg, dilantin, barbiturates, carbamazepine, and rifampin).

Except in rare cases, a normal (overnight or 2-day) dexamethasone suppression test virtually excludes the possibility of Cushing's syndrome. Although not required for diagnosis, measured changes in saliva cortisol (normal, <2 ng/mL) and ACTH after dexamethasone suppression can be complimentary for a diagnosis.[13]

As in adrenal insufficiency, ACTH levels, both baseline and following low (1 mg) or high (8 mg) dexamethasone suppression can help determine an underlying etiology of cortisol excess states. One study demonstrated that high dose dexamethasone was only 57% specific for differentiating an ectopic from pituitary source of ACTH hypersecretion (Fig. 18-12).[12]

When Cushing's Is Confirmed, CRH Stimulation Tests Help Determine ACTH Dependency (Typically Not Necessary)

CRH stimulation is a newer and more helpful test for distinguishing types of Cushing's (central disease vs. primary adrenal syndrome). An 8:00 a.m., serum cortisol and ACTH level is drawn following CRH injection. In ACTH independent Cushing's syndrome, cortisol is high (>25 μg/dL) while ACTH is suppressed (<10 pg/mL), demonstrating ACTH production is not driving excess cortisol production. In this case, an adrenal etiology for excess cortisol is sought. In ACTH dependent Cushing's,

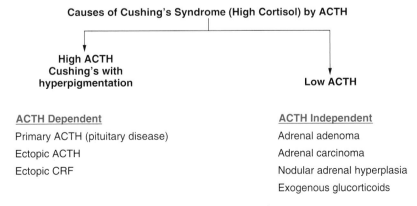

FIGURE 18-12. Differentiating source of ACTH secretion.

both cortisol (>25 μg/dL) and ACTH (>10 pg/mL) are elevated. Autonomous ACTH is from a pituitary or ectopic source.

To determine if ACTH excess results from a pituitary or ectopic source, a CRH stimulated bilateral, inferior, petrosal sampling (BIPSS) and peripheral vein sampling is performed. The results are expressed in a ratio. A petrosal sinus ACTH to peripheral vein ACTH ratio >3 is diagnostic for pituitary disease. A ratio <2.5 suggests an ectopic (nonpituitary) source of ACTH production. Remission rates for pituitary microadenoma approximate 85%; invasive adenomas <50% when resected. With additional treatment (pituitary x-irradiation), remission rates of invasive adenomas may slowly reach 85%.

For ectopic ACTH production, a neoplasm workup is performed; localization and surgical removal of autonomous ACTH producing lesions is attempted. Other treatment options include adrenalectomy and adrenal enzyme inhibitors.

Localization Procedures

- Adrenal Cushing's
  - Adrenal CT may discern tumor vs hyperplasia (R-layer DHEA(s) normal with F-layer adrenal adenomas).
  - Adrenal MRI T2-weighted image helps distinguish carcinoma. Cancer often involves other adrenal layers with the R-layer DHEA(s) being high in carcinoma; immunohistochemical markers, p53, and MIB-1 are also positive in carcinomas.
- Pituitary Cushing's
  - Pituitary MRI (detects 85% of microadenomas)
- Ectopic Cushing's
  - Chest CT (*eg,* ACTH bronchial adenoma, medullary thyroid carcinoma, and squamous cell carcinoma [SCC])

Algorithm for Cushing's Workup

Day 1:

8:00 a.m.: Completely empty bladder and start baseline urine collection.

11:00 p.m.: Collect saliva sample for cortisol level; ingest dexamethasone (1 mg); empty bladder; end baseline urine collection.

Optional extended workups: Begin overnight dexamethasone suppressed urine collection.

Day 2:

8:00 a.m.: Empty bladder (postsuppression urine cortisol complete); venous blood or saliva for cortisol; ACTH; dexamethasone (compliance); hold samples until needed.

See flowcharting interpretation of Cushing's workup (Fig. 18-13).

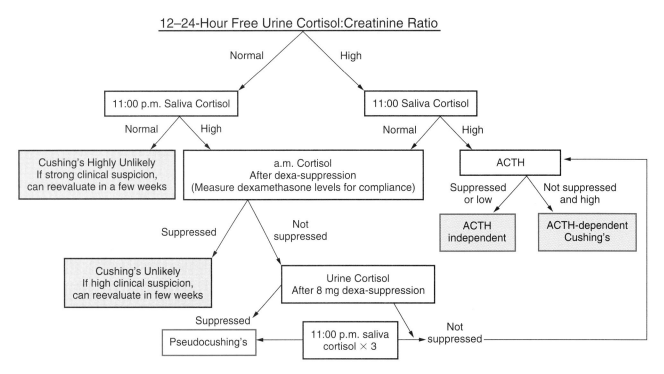

FIGURE 18-13. Cushing's syndrome workup. Note that dexamethasone serum levels (for standard test = 2 ng/mL; suppression test = 6.5 ng/mL) can be drawn at 8:00 a.m. (or 6 hours after the last dose) to help clarify or determine compliance. Normal dexamethasone saliva levels have not been determined.

Treatment

Options for primary (adrenal cortisol overproduction) and secondary (pituitary or ectopic ACTH overproduction) Cushing's are similar: surgery, radiation, and/or medications to suppress adrenal cortisol production or actions. Treatment strategies vary with clinical situations.

Lifelong replacement of glucocorticoids and mineralocorticoids (Florinef) is necessary in patients with bilateral adrenalectomy. Any patient undergoing bilateral adrenalectomy as a result of an ACTH-producing pituitary tumor should be routinely screened and closely followed for symptoms of increasing mass lesion of the pituitary gland (Nelson's syndrome). Finally, Cushing's can recur in adrenal rests; therefore, periodic, lifetime screening for adrenal overproduction is warranted in these patients.

Androgens are produced as by-products of cortisol synthesis that are regulated by ACTH. Although prolactin, pro-opiomelanocortin peptides, and T-lymphocytes are known stimulators of androgens, regulatory mechanisms of R-zone biosynthesis remains uncertain (Fig. 18-14). R-cells primarily produce DHEA and multiple 19-carbon steroids (androgens and estrogens) from 17α-hydroxylated pregnenolone and progesterone. DHEA is sulfated to DHEAS by sulfotransferase, an adrenal enzyme, and secreted daily (Fig. 18-1).

Both DHEA and DHEAS are precursors to more active androgens (*eg*, androstenedione, testosterone, and *5-dehydrotestosterone [5-DHT]*) and estrogens (*eg*, estradiol and estrone). Although DHEA and DHEAS have minimal androgenic activity, adverse effects are caused by conversion to active androgens in the adrenals and peripheral tissue, such as hair follicles, sebaceous glands, genitalia, adipose, and prostate tissue. Although men derive less than 5% of their testosterone from adrenal or peripheral sources, women rely on the adrenals for 40–65% of their daily testosterone production.[14]

Although observational data demonstrate adrenal androgen production increases in both genders in late childhood and correlates with the onset of pubic hair (adrenarche), it peaks in young adults and progressively declines with age.

ANDROGEN EXCESS

Androgen excess causes ambiguous genitalia in infants and precocious puberty in children of both sexes. Androgens stimulate organ development, linear growth, and epiphyseal fusion. Virilization in boys includes penile enlargement, androgen-dependent hair growth, and other secondary sexual characteristics. Girls develop hirsutism, acne, and clitorimegaly. Untimely overproduction can cause short stature by leading to early epiphyseal fusion.

In women, androgen overproduction can cause infertility, with masculinizing effects (*eg*, hirsutism, acne, male pattern baldness, menstrual irregularities, and virility).

In men, excess adrenal androgens can also cause infertility with feminizing effects by inhibiting pituitary gonadotropins, which effectively lowers testicular testosterone production. Despite overall androgen excess, males can experience hypogonadal symptoms, such as loss of muscle mass, decreased hair growth, decreased testes size, testicular testosterone production, and spermatogenesis, similar to hypercortisolism.

Diagnosis of Excess Androgen Production

Less than 10% of DHEA is produced by the gonads, therefore, high DHEA production strongly suggests adrenal hyperandrogenism, whereas elevated testosterone values are seen with either adrenal or gonadal hyperandrogenism.

Plasma DHEA or urine 17-ketosteroids can identify patients with adrenal causes of pathologic masculinization (females) and feminization (males).

Treatment for Adrenal Androgen Overproduction

Similar to the previously described disorders of overproduction, differentiation between ACTH dependent and independent secretion is assessed by dexamethasone suppression tests, then imaging studies are performed (CT, MRI). Adenomas and carcinomas are surgically removed. Glucocorticoid suppressible causes are treated accordingly. Exogenous contributors are discontinued and other nonadrenal conditions are treated. Drugs with

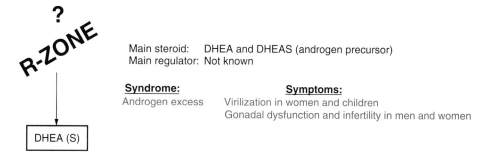

Main steroid: DHEA and DHEAS (androgen precursor)
Main regulator: Not known

Syndrome: **Symptoms:**
Androgen excess   Virilization in women and children
                     Gonadal dysfunction and infertility in men and women

FIGURE 18-14. R-zone biosynthesis. Manifestations of adrenal hyperandrogenism vary with age, onset, and gender.

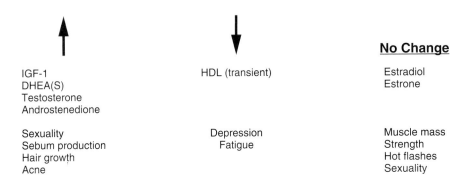

FIGURE 18-15. Effects of DHEA supplementation.

antiandrogenic properties (*eg*, minoxidil, spironolactone, birth control pills) are occasionally used.

Exogenous DHEA is a popular nutritional supplement with numerous purported properties (only a few studied), including vasodilatory, anti-inflammatory, antiaging, and antiatherosclerosis.

The clinical relevance of DHEA(S) interactions with nonandrogen/estrogen receptors remains unknown. DHEA (30–50 mg/day) is secreted as the major component of adrenal androgens. There is no evidence that this molecule is required for health or that it contributes to disease. No steroid receptor for DHEA has yet been identified. DHEA actions are attributed to its downstream products, testosterone and estrogen.

In normal and compromised patients (*eg,* adrenal insufficiency, glucocorticoid therapy, depression, older persons, and trained athletes), DHEA can increase the sense of well-being and raises or lowers a variety of serum markers (Fig. 18-15), although the changes are small. Supplementation (50–100 mg/day) in some androgen-deficient patients (*eg,* adrenal insufficiency, ACTH deficiency, and glucocorticoid therapy) may help ameliorate deficiency adverse effects and may inhibit glucocorticoid induced bone loss. However, DHEA can cause adverse androgenic effects in women, and the long-term consequences of supplementation remain unknown.

THE ADRENAL MEDULLA

The adrenal medulla is member of the amine precursor uptake and decarboxylation system. In response to stimulation, the medulla secretes catecholamines into the circulation in lieu of transmitting messages via efferent axons. It functions as an atypical sympathetic ganglion. Medullary catecholamine products serve as first responders to stress by acting within seconds (cortisol takes 20 minutes) to promote the fight-or-flight response, which increases cardiac output and blood pressure, diverts blood toward muscle and brain, and mobilizes fuel from storage.

Development

Sympathetic cells arise from primordial neural crest stem cells (sympathogonia), which migrate out of the CNS to a space behind the aorta where they differentiate into sympathoblasts (sympathetic ganglion cells) or pheochromoblasts (medulla chromaffin cells). Tumors that arise from either cell line share similar histologic and biochemical properties. Malignant neuroblastomas and benign ganglioneuromas arise from sympathoblasts, secrete homovanillic acid (HVA) and are rarely seen after adolescence. In contrast, tumors of chromaffin cells (*pheochromocytomas [Pheo]*) maintain the capacity to synthesize and store catecholamines (*norepinephrine [NE]* and *epinephrine [EPI]*) throughout life.[15]

Biosynthesis and Storage of Catecholamines

NE and EPI biosynthesis begins with the sequential conversion of phenylalanine substrates in a tightly regulated, compartmentalized manner. All reactions take place in the cytoplasm, except for the production of NE, which occurs within lipid vesicles or outer mitochondrial membranes, as illustrated in Figure 18-16.

In sympathetic neurons, cytoplasmic dopamine is sequestered into vesicles, converted into NE, and stored until nerve stimulation causes its release.

In medulla chromaffin cells, NE can passively diffuse into the cytosol. In the cytosol, NE is converted into EPI by a cortisol-dependent enzyme called PNMT. Any form of stress that increases cortisol levels stimulates EPI production. Free cytosolic EPI (like dopamine) is actively transported into secretory vesicles by *vesicle monoamine transporters (VMAT)* in pheochromocytes. The ratio of NE to EPI in the serum is normally 9:1 (98% from postganglionic neurons, 2% from the medulla). In adrenal insufficiency (low cortisol), that ratio increases to 45:1 in females and 24:1 in males.

Catecholamine Degradation

All catecholamines are rapidly eliminated from target cells and the circulation by three mechanisms:

1. reuptake into secretory vesicles.
2. uptake in nonneuronal cells (mostly liver).
3. degradation.

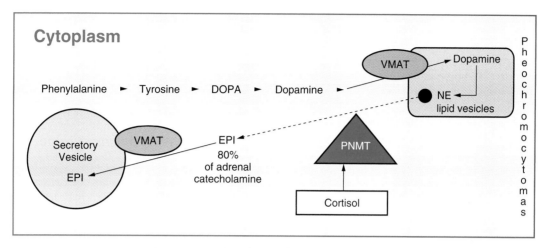

FIGURE 18-16. Biosynthesis and storage of catecholamines.

Degradation relies on two enzymes, *catechol methyltransferase (COMT)* (in nonneuronal tissues) and *monoamine oxidase (MAO)* (within neurons) to produce metabolites (metanephrines and VMA) from free catecholamines. Metabolites and free catecholamines are eliminated by direct filtration into the urine and excreted as free NE (5%); conjugated NE (8%); metanephrines (20%); and VMA (30%). Urine EPI (50%) is converted from NE by renal, not adrenal, *phenylethanolamine N-methyltransferase (PNMT)* before excretion (Fig. 18-17).

Urine and Plasma Catecholamine Measurements

Catecholamines are hydrophilic; circulate in low levels (50% albumin bound); have short half-lives (seconds to 2 minutes); and produce wide, rapidly fluctuating plasma levels that render accurate determination and interpretation technically challenging.

Urine catecholamines (free NE and EPI) are assayed using liquid chromatography or fluorometrics. Twenty-four hour urine catecholamine and metabolite levels are more reliable and are not altered by age or gender.

Most antihypertensive drugs and many other medications interfere with accurate catecholamine measurement. Substances causing autofluorescence (*eg,* tetracyclines, ephedrine, α-methlyldopa) can produce erroneous results when measured by fluorometric assays. Central α antagonists (clonidine) and thiazides are preferred agents to control hypertension during evaluation of conditions causing excessive sympathetic activation (high catecholamine states).

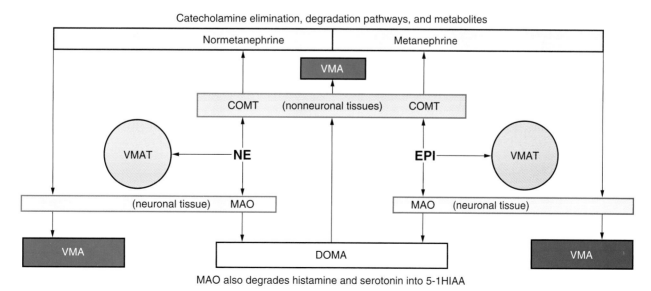

FIGURE 18-17. Catecholamine degradation. Free catecholamines (EPI and NE) are either sequentered into VMAT-containing vesicles or converted into metabolites, DOMA by neuronal MAOs and metanephrines by nonneuronal COMTs. These metabolites are ultimately degraded to VMA (DOMA by COMTs and metanephrines by MAOs) and excreted.

Causes of Sympathetic Hyperactivity

- Autonomic dysfunction
- Panic attack (emotions)
- Stress responses: hypoglycemia, injury, infarction, infection, psychosis, and seizures
- Drugs: decongestants, appetite suppressors, stimulants, bronchodilators, MAO inhibitors, thyroid hormone, cortisol, nicotine withdrawal, or short-acting sympathetic antagonists (clonidine or propranolol)
- Foods containing tyramine: imported beer, red wine, soy sauce, overripe/fermented foods, smoked or aged meats
- Pheochromocytoma (catecholamine producing tumor).

Pheochromocytomas are rare (<0.1% of hypertensive patients), catecholamine producing tumors arising from chromaffin tissue, which causes HTN in association with nonspecific clinical symptoms that mimic anxiety. Symptoms include palpitations, diaphoresis, and headaches. In a retrospective study, 40% of patients evaluated for pheochromocytoma met the criteria for panic disorder, compared with 5% of control patients with hypertension (Fig. 18-18).[16,17]

Patient presentation is highly variable, most have episodes of HTN (diastolic/orthostatic), palpitations, and diaphoresis, with nonspecific periods of symptoms initiated by various stimuli, including physical exertion, torso twisting, Valsalva, micturition, or coitus. Others have sustained HTN (some refractory to treatment) and many have no symptoms. Rarely, patients with Pheo present with episodic hypotension (exclusive EPI or dopamine secreting). Additional signs may include pallor, increased erythrocyte sedimentation rate, dilated cardiomyopathy, and erythrocytosis as a result of overproduction of erythropoietin. Pheo diagnosis is rarely confirmed.

Mechanisms of catecholamine secretion by persons with Pheo remain unclear (tumors are not innervated). Increased catecholamine synthesis, limited degradation capacity, and limited storage for excess NE and metabolites likely causes spillover into the blood, increasing circulating free NE and/or EPI along with other active peptides that causes symptoms. Because medullary catecholamines and adrenal cortical hormones serve similar functions producing similar effects, a rare patient with clinical and biochemical evidence of catecholamine hypersecretion may have an adrenocortical adenoma or carcinoma rather than a medullary tumor causing the symptoms. Pheo symptoms are related to the type of catecholamines secreted by the tumor and the receptors they activate.

Diagnosis of Pheochromocytoma

The best test for diagnosing Pheo is still uncertain. Although the majority of patients with pheochromocytoma have obvious diagnostic abnormalities on most tests, others can produce confounding results. When one test is equivocal, a different test should be performed if clinical suspicion remains high.[18,19]

Measuring both total plasma catecholamines (NE and EPI) and urine metanephrines is the most sensitive screening profile. Plasma catecholamines >2000 pg/mL in a rested, supine patient with an indwelling cannula is nearly diagnostic of pheochromocytoma. Of 287 patients with Pheo, 88% had elevated plasma NE and EPI, which increased to 100% during hypertensive episodes despite no correlation between blood pressure and basal catecholamine levels.[24] With borderline values (1000–2000 pg/mL), a clonidine suppression test can be helpful.

Plasma metanephrines, measured by HPLC or RIA, are touted as the most specific and sensitive diagnostic test. Yet, investigators at the Mayo Clinic found that plasma metanephrines lack specificity (15% false positive) and do not recommend it as a first line test but reserve it for high-risk patients or patients who cannot collect an accurate 24-hour urine specimen. Urine metanephrines (normal, >1.2 mg/day) may be the most sensitive urine test; it is less likely altered by drugs or certain foods. An overnight urine collection (8–12 hours) appears as accurate and more convenient than a 24-hour urine collection. Urine VMA by HPLC or fluorometric assay has the highest false-negative rate (up to 41%) of the urine catecholamine tests.[20]

Chromogranin A is co-stored and secreted in quantum with catecholamines. Eighty percent of pheochromocytoma patients have increased plasma chromogranin levels.

10%
Incidentally discovered (imaging, surgery, autopsy)
Multiple
Extra-adrenal (chest, neck abdomen, bladder)
Malignant (invasion, distant metastases)
Familial (Von Hippel-Lindau, MEN-II, parathyroid hyperplasia, medullary thyroid carcinoma, neurofibromatosis, paraganglioma)

90%
Intra-adrenal
Intra-abdominal (95%)
Single
Benign

FIGURE 18-18. Pheochromocytomas.

Serum chromogranin A is not routinely measured because it is less sensitive and specific for pheochromocytoma than direct catecholamine and metabolite measurements. In combination, serum chromogranin A and plasma catecholamines are specific (95%) but less sensitive (88%), likely because of high dependence on renal function. If the glomerular filtration rate is less than 80 mL/min, test sensitivity drops to 70%. Combined, resting plasma catecholamines >200 pg/mL and chromogranin A >20 pg/mL have a positive predictive value of 97% when GFR is normal.

If results of preceding tests are equivocal, pharmacologic tests are performed to separate patients with Pheo (low levels of biosynthetic activity) from those without Pheo who are experiencing similar symptoms secondary to increased sympathetic outflow (Clonidine, an antihypertensive agent, suppresses sympathetic outflow).

Clonidine suppression test (92% accurate) addresses the question, "is excess catecholamine production suppressible?" Because sympathetic activation is not responsible for pheochromocytoma catecholamine release, suppressing sympathetic activation via clonidine activation of central α_2 receptors will not lower NE levels in patients with pheochromocytoma despite improving the symptoms.

After stopping antihypertensive drugs for at least 12 hours, total plasma catecholamines are measured. Clonidine (0.3 mg) is administered and repeat levels are drawn 3 hours later. Patients without pheochromocytoma will have a fall in plasma total catecholamines to >500 pg/mL (this is inaccurate in patients with normal catecholamine levels).[21]

Biochemical confirmation of pheochromocytoma should be followed by radiologic localization. Although any site containing paraganglionic tissue may be involved, the most common extra-adrenal locations are the superior and inferior para-aortic areas (75%); bladder (10%); thorax (10%); and the head, neck, and pelvis (5%).

For localization of Pheo, either a CT (without dye) or MRI of the abdomen and adrenal glands is performed. On T2-weighted images, Pheos appear hyperintense, while other adrenal tumors look isointense compared with the liver. Either test detects most sporadic tumors (typically, ≥3 wide) with 98–100% sensitivity and 70% specificity. The lower specificity is due to relatively higher prevalence of adrenal *incidentalomas*. The ^{123}I-labeled MIBG (a NE analogue that concentrates in the adrenal and Pheos via VMAT) scintigraphy can be performed that is 100% specific for Pheo, but not sensitive enough for routine screening. PET-scanning with ^{18}F-fluorodeoxyglucose, 11C-hydroxyephedrine, or 6-[^{18}F]fluorodopamine may be helpful in identifying sites of metastatic disease.[22]

Treatment of Pheochromocytoma

Once pheochromocytoma is diagnosed, all patients are surgical candidates following appropriate medical preparation. Removal is a high-risk procedure. In the largest surgical series (147 pheochromocytoma patients) at one institution (1975–1997), overall perioperative mortality and morbidity rates were 2.4%.[18] Patients with severe preoperative hypertension, high-secretion tumors, or those undergoing repeat intervention were at highest risk for complications. Catecholamines fall to normal within one week of resection.

Although perioperative alpha blockade is widely recommended, fewer perioperative complications were observed in those not given α-blockers (study of 113 pheochromocytoma patients undergoing resection). A second regimen proposed by the Cleveland Clinic resulted in successful use of a calcium channel blocker for blood pressure control.

Outcome and Prognosis

Surgical removal of a pheochromocytoma is the primary therapy; nevertheless, excision does not necessarily lead to long-term cure of pheochromocytoma or HTN (even in patients with benign tumors). Patients with familial Pheos are more likely to have recurrence. In one series of 114 patients, pheochromocytoma recurred in 14% (48% of those were malignant). In patients without recurrence (86%), the hypertension-free survival was only 74% at 5 years and 45% at 10 years (family history of HTN and increasing age were risk factors). In 90 patients, the 20-year overall cause-specific survival rate was 80% regardless of pheochromocytoma location.[24] Long-term monitoring is indicated in all patients, even those who are apparently cured.

INCIDENTALOMA

Adrenal masses are often found incidentally at autopsy in asymptomatic patients. Approximately 10% of patients will have an adrenal tumor. With increasing use of routine CT and MRI scans, the number of adrenal adenomas discovered is expected to rise; most are nonfunctioning and benign. Of 61,054 abdominal CT scans done at the Mayo Clinic from 1985 to 1990, 3.4% had adrenal masses. Seventy-five percent were obvious metastatic cancer or known lesions, and 16.5% were incidentalomas (0.4% of scans). All adrenal masses are evaluated for malignancy and hypersecretion.[23]

If the incidental mass is greater than 3–6 cm, as seen on serial or functional scans, it is surgically removed.

Figure 18-19 illustrates a brief functional screen for adrenal masses, which assesses function of all adrenal layers and serves as a clinical summary.

CASE STUDY

Hypertension is common and most often presents as an independent medical condition. Occasionally, hypertension is a result of an underlying illness and requires different treatment. Because adrenal function is critical for (1) blood pressure, (2) potassium, and (3) glucose homeostasis, an adrenal etiology should be considered in all patients with blood pressure problems accompanied by electrolyte abnormalities, unexplained change in weight, failure to thrive, inappropriate virilization, and anxiety periods.

Eight different clinical scenarios are presented below. Each presentation is associated with a different diagnosis and treatment. A discussion of adrenal causes, diagnoses, and treatments for each are found within the chapter. Each Case Study completes the following opening statement: A 22-year-old woman (previously adopted, not currently taking medications, negative medical history) presents with . . .

CASE STUDY 18-1

. . . hypertension, with weakness and hypokalemia. The patient also has a high urine K^+ excretion without diuretics.

Question

1. What is the diagnosis?

CASE STUDY 18-2

. . . hypertension, with weakness and rapid onset of obesity. This patient also exhibits central fat pads, buffalo hump, plethora, thin skin, purple striae, easy bruising, osteoporosis, hyperglycemia/insulin resistance, and recurrent infections.

Question

1. What is the diagnosis?

CASE STUDY 18-3

. . . hypertension, with weakness, irregular menses, and hypokalemia. Her young age, borderline low cortisol, and low androgens also are significant.

Question

1. What is the diagnosis?

CASE STUDY 18-4

. . . hypertension, with periods of panic attacks and hot flashes. She also presents with headache, hyperglycemia, hyperthyroidism, and GI complaints.

Question

1. What is the diagnosis?

CASE STUDY 18-5

. . . hypertension, with virilization. This young woman presents with irregular menses diagnosed with polycystic ovary syndrome. She has a borderline low cortisol and elevated 17-OH progesterone.

Question

1. What is the diagnosis?

CASE STUDY 18-6

. . . hypertension and hyperkalemia. She has normal renal function (low urine K^+) and metabolic acidosis.

Question

1. What is the diagnosis?

CASE STUDY 18-7

. . . hypotension, failure to thrive, weight loss, and weakness. Her laboratory results reveal hyperkalemia, fasting hypoglycemia, and metabolic acidosis.

Question

1. What is the diagnosis?

CASE STUDY 18-8

. . . new virilization and hirsutism. Laboratory results show increased IGF-1 (insulin growth factor), DHEA(S), and testosterone levels. She is a health food enthusiast who experiments with nutritional supplements.

Question

1. What is the diagnosis?

Incidentaloma Function Evaluation

	Clinical Features	Screening Tests Negative Results
Pheochromocytoma	**HTN** (paroxysmal) with spells (sweating, HA, or palpitations)	24-hour urine metanephrines < 1 μg or 5.5 μmol/mg creatine
Cushing's syndrome	**HTN**, obesity (truncal) weakness	1 mg bedtime dexamethasone 8 a.m. cortisol < 3.6 μg/dL, or 24-hour urine free cortisol normal
Primary aldosteronism	**HTN**, hypokalemia, weakness	Serum potassium, *if low* urine K$^+$ excretion (<30 mEq)
Adrenocarcinoma	Virilization (+ above)	Plasma renin:aldosterone ratio < 30 Plasma DHEAS (< 9.2 μmol/L) Urine 17-ketosteroid < 20 mg

FIGURE 18-19. Brief functional screen for adrenal masses.

REVIEW QUESTIONS

1. When considering an endocrine cause for a patient's hypertension, which organ is the usual suspect? Does hypertension result from an overproduction or an underproduction state?

2. In general, what are some major warning signs of adrenal disease?

3. What is the common substrate from which all adrenal steroids are produced?

4. Outline each adrenal cortex end product by functional layer and list a specific regulator of each.

5. When produced, free catecholamines (NE and EPI) are short-lived. Outline their general fates and how they are measured.

6. Which adrenal steroid is responsible for epinephrine production?

REFERENCES

1. Kacsoh D. The adrenal gland. In: Dolan J, ed. Endocrine Physiology. New York: McGraw-Hill, 2000:360–448.
2. Orth D. Anatomy and development of the adrenal cortex. www.UpToDate.com, online 12.1, 12/03.
3. Miller W. The Adrenal Cortex. In: Felig P, ed. Endocrinology and Metabolism. New York: McGraw-Hill, 2001:387–493.
4. Lacroix A. The adrenal cortex: basic concepts and diagnostic procedures. In: Pinchera A, et al, eds. Endocrinology and Metabolism. London: McGraw-Hill, 2001:285–297.
5. Orth D. Adrenal steroid biosynthesis and congenital adrenal hyperplasia. www.UpToDate.com, online 12.1, 3/02.
6. Levine L. Congenital adrenal hyperplasia. In: Lavin M, ed. Manual of Endocrinology and Metabolism. Philadelphia: Lippincott Williams & Wilkins, 2002:147–163.
7. Stern N. The adrenal cortex and mineralocorticoid hypertension. In: Lavin M, ed. Manual of Endocrinology and Metabolism. Philadelphia: Lippincott Williams & Wilkins, 2002:115–139.

8. Kaplan N. Primary aldosteronism. In: Pine J, ed. Clinical Hypertension. Baltimore: Lippincott Williams & Wilkins, 1998:365–383.
9. Thomopoulos P. Adrenocortical insufficiency. In: Jeffers D, ed. Endocrinology and Metabolism. London: McGraw-Hill, 2001: 297–305.
10. Bertagna X. Cushing's syndrome. In: Pinchera A, et al, eds. Endocrinology and Metabolism. London: McGraw-Hill, 2001: 311–323.
11. Besser G. Cushing's syndrome. J Clin Endocrinol Metabol 1972;1:451.
12. Orth D. Establishing the diagnosis of Cushing's syndrome. www.UpToDate.com, online 12.1, 12/02.
13. Castro M, Quidute A, et al. Out-patient screening for Cushing's syndrome: sensitivity of the combination of circadian rhythm and overnight dexamethasone suppression salivary cortisol tests. J Clin Endocrinol Metabol 1999;84:878.

14. Chrovsos G. Dehydroepiandrosterone and its sulfate. www.UpToDate.com, online 12.1, 4/03.

15. Bravo E. The adrenal medulla: basic concepts. In: Pinchera A, et al, eds. Endocrinology and Metabolism. London: McGraw-Hill, 2001:337–341.

16. Kaplan N. Pheochromocytoma. In: Pine J, ed. Clinical Hypertension. Baltimore: Lippincott Williams & Wilkins, 1998:345–365.

17. Sowers K. Pheochromocytomas. In: Lavin M, ed. Manual of Endocrinology and Metabolism. Philadelphia: Lippincott Williams & Wilkins, 2002:139–145.

18. Bravo E. Diagnosis and Management of Pheochromocytoma. In: Pinchera A, et al, eds. Endocrinology and Metabolism. London: McGraw-Hill, 2001:341-349.

19. Fogarty J, Russo J, et al. Hypertension and pheochromocytoma testing: the association with anxiety disorders. Arch Fam Med 1994:3:55.

20. Sawka A. Fractionated plasma metanephrines are highly sensitive, but less specific than urinary total metanephrines and cate-cholamines in detection of pheochromocytoma. Program and Abstracts of The Endocrine Society's 83rd Annual Meeting, Denver, June 20–23, 2001, Abstract #P1-642. Denver, CO: The Endocrine Society, 2001:285.

21. Sjoberg R, Kidd G. The clonidine suppression test for pheochromocytoma: a review of its utility and pitfalls. Arch Int Med 1992:152:1193.

22. Pacak K, Eisenhofer G, Carrasquillo J, et al. 6-[^{18}F]fluoro-dopamine positron emission tomographic (PET) scanning for diagnostic localization of pheochromocytoma. Hypertension 2001:38:6–8.

23. Lutton J. The incidentally discovered adrenal mass. In: Pinchera A, et al, ed. Endocrinology and Metabolism. London: McGraw-Hill, 2001:323–329.

24. Young W, Kaplan N. Diagnosis and treatment of pheochromocytoma in adults. www.UpToDate.com, online 12.2, 1/04.

Gonadal Function

Dev Abraham, A. Wayne Meikle

OBJECTIVES

Upon completion of this chapter, the clinical laboratorian should be able to:

• Discuss the biosynthesis, secretion, transport, and action of the sex steroid and gonadotropins.
• Identify the location of the pituitary, ovaries, and testes.
• Describe the hypothalamic–pituitary–ovarian and hypothalamic–pituitary–testicular axes and how they regulate sex steroid and gonadotropin hormone production.

• Explain the principles of each diagnostic test for pituitary–gonadal axes dysfunction.
• Correlate laboratory information with regard to suspected gonadal disorders, given a patient's clinical data.
• Describe the appropriate laboratory testing protocol to effectively evaluate or monitor patients with suspected gonadal disease.

KEY TERMS

Amenorrhea	Gynecomastia	Leydig cell	Thecal cell
Androgen	Hirsutism	Luteal phase	Virilization
Corpus luteum	Hypogonadism	Ovulation	
Follicular phase	Inhibin	Sertoli cell	

THE OVARY

The ovaries are paired organs and, similar to the male gonads, perform dual functions: the production of the female gamete (the ovum) and the production of ovarian steroids.[1–3] Unlike in the male, the primordial reproductive cells in the female produce (in most cycles) a solitary gamete. Ovarian events are carefully orchestrated with menstrual events by a complex interplay of hormones among the ovaries, pituitary, and hypothalamus that prepares the uterus for implantation of the embryo. In the absence of such an event, the uterine lining is shed, resulting in menses.[4,5]

The length of the menstrual cycle is the time between any two consecutive cycles. The typical duration is about 28 days (± 3 days); mean menstrual flow is about 2–4 days.[4,5]

Functional Anatomy of the Ovary

The ovaries are ovoid structures (about 5 cm long) situated in the pelvic fossa. They are suspended by the broad ligament of the ovary and held in close relation to the position of the fimbrial end of the fallopian tubes, which are connected to the uterine cavity. The ovaries contain about 2–4 million primordial follicles.[2,6] With each cycle, a few primordial follicles are recruited for progressive maturation. Most follicles atrophy, with the exception of a single follicle (graafian follicle) that ultimately releases a mature ovum. The graafian follicle has an internal layer, the theca interna; an outer layer, the theca externa; and a central cavity that contains fluid derived from plasma. The secretory layer of the follicle is the granulosa layer.[2,5–7]

The developing ovum is attached to the inside of the graafian follicle cavity by granulosa cells called *cumulus cells*. In a precisely choreographed sequence of ovarian stimulation by follicle-stimulating hormones and leuteinizing hormones, the ovaries produce the principal steroid hormones, progesterone and estrogen. When the ovum is extruded, the graafian follicle undergoes a morphologic change to corpus luteum, with hypertrophy of the *theca cells* and granulosa cells. This process is called *luteinization*. The corpus luteum, rich in cholesterol, a substrate for continued production of progesterone and estrogen, maintains the endometrium for anticipated conception. If conception or implantation does not occur, the endometrium is shed and the corpus luteum atrophies to atretic follicle.

Hormonal Production by the Ovaries

As in the adrenal glands and the testes, the steroidogenic pathway and synthetic enzymes are present in the ovaries as well. Cholesterol is either synthesized from acetate source or actively transported from the low-density lipoprotein (LDL) particle in blood.[4,5,8,9]

Estrogen

Naturally synthesized estrogens are carbon-18 compounds. The principle estrogen produced in the ovary is estradiol. Estrone and estriol are mostly metabolites of intraovarian and extraglandular conversion. Estrogens promote development of secondary sexual characteristics in the female. Breast, uterine, and vaginal development are caused by estrogen effects; in particular, glandular and blood vessel development.[4,5,8,9] The lack of estrogen that naturally occurs with the onset of menopause leads to atrophic changes in these organs. The estrogens also affect the skin, vascular smooth muscles, bone cells, and the central nervous system (cognition). Estrogen is responsible for follicular phase changes in the uterus. Deficiency of estrogen results in irregular and incomplete development of the endometrium.[2,10]

Progesterone

Progesterone is a carbon-21 compound in the steroid family, which is produced by the corpus luteum. Progesterone induces secretory activity of the endometrial glands that have been primed by estrogen, which readies the endometrium for embryo implantation. Other effects include thickening of the cervical mucus, reduction of uterine contractions, and the thermogenic effect. Basal body temperature elevation that occurs after ovulation is a result of progesterone; this effect is used in clinical practice as a naturally occurring "luteinizing hormone kit" to signify the occurrence of ovulation. Progesterone is the dominant hormone responsible for the luteal phase of the cycle. Deficiency of progesterone results in failure of implantation of embryo.[2,4–6,8]

Androgens

Ovaries produce androgens that are all carbon-19 compounds—androstenedione, dehydroandrostenedione, testosterone, and dihydrotestosterone. Excess production of ovarian androgens in women leads to excess hair growth (hirsutism), loss of female characteristics (defeminization), and, in severe cases, frank male secondary sex features (masculinization, or *virilization*).[11–14] Unlike estrogen, which is not produced in the ovary after menopause, androgen synthesis continues well into advanced age.

Inhibins A and B, which are produced by the ovaries, are hormones that inhibit FSH production.[6,15] Activin is a hormone that enhances FSH secretion and induces steroidogenesis. Folliculostatin, relaxin, follicle regulatory protein, oocyte maturation factor, and meiosis-inducing substance are hormones that appear to have important, yet not clearly characterized functions.

The Menstrual Cycle

The menstrual cycle consists of two phases of parallel events that occur at the ovarian and endometrial sites. The first is the follicular (ovary) or proliferative (uterus) phase; the second is the luteal (ovary) or secretory (uterus) phase.[1,2,4–6,15,16]

The Follicular Phase

The estrogens secreted by the developing follicle increase the thickness of the endometrium by stimulation of the epithelial cells, growth of blood vessels, and development of endometrial glands. The intense secretory capacity of the uterine glands provides a secretion that aids the implantation of the embryo.

The Luteal Phase

The luteal phase follows the follicular phase, immediately after the extrusion of the ovum and the subsequent luteinization of the graafian follicle to form the corpus luteum. The corpus luteum maintains secretion of progesterone and aids in the implantation of the embryo. After about 14 days, the uterine endometrium is shed for the next cycle to begin. The typical duration of bleeding is 3–5 days, with blood loss of about 50 mL.

Hormonal Control of Ovulation

The central control of follicle-stimulating hormone (FSH) and luteinizing hormone (LH) secretion resides in the gonadotropin-releasing hormone (GnRH) pulse generator of the arcuate nuclei and medial preoptic nuclei of the hypothalamus.[1,2,4–6,15,16] Positive and negative feedback responses exist among estrogen, progesterone, and LH, FSH production. Because of the lack of estrogen after menopause, both FSH and LH levels rise.[1,15,16] The midcycle surge in LH production results in the culminating event of ovulation. FSH levels are elevated early in the follicular phase and diminish after ovulation. Any injury to the hypothalamus or stress (psychosocial or physical) leads to anovulation and amenorrhea.[10,17,18]

Pubertal Development in the Female

Tanner Staging

The staging system devised by Marshall and Tanner[9] is applied to monitor the growth stages of breast and pubic hair.

Staging of Breast Development

Stage 1: Papillary elevation.
Stage 2: Elevation of breast bud and papilla.
Stage 3: Elevation of breast tissue and papilla.
Stage 4: Elevation of papilla and areola form the breast; papilla is at or above the equator of the breast.
Stage 5: Areola is recessed into the breast and/or papilla is below the equator of the breast.

Staging of Pubic Hair Changes

Stage 1: Lanugo-type hair.
Stage 2: Dark terminal hair on labia majora.

Stage 3: Terminal hair covering labia majora and spreading to the mons pubis.
Stage 4: Terminal hair fully covering the labia majora and mons pubis.
Stage 5: Terminal hair covering the labia majora, mons pubis, and inner thighs.

Menstrual Cycle Abnormalities

The average menstrual cycle is 28 days long, with a range of 25–35 days considered normal. The average age when menopause occurs is between 45 and 55 years of age.[1,2,4–6,15,16]

Amenorrhea refers to absence of menses. When a woman has never menstruated, it is called *primary amenorrhea*.[7,17–20] When a women who has had at least one cycle of menstruation has a subsequent cessation for a minimum of 3–6 months, it is termed *secondary amenorrhea*.[10,17,18] Frequency of etiologic sites for amenorrhea are listed in Table 19-1. A diagnostic approach to secondary amenorrhea is outlined in Figure 19-1. *Oligomenorrhea* refers to infrequent or irregular menstrual bleeding, with cycle lengths in excess of 35–40 days. Uterine bleeding in excess of 7 days is dysfunctional and termed *menorrhagia*. In a patient with infertility, the diagnosis of inadequate luteal phase is made when the luteal phase is less than 10 days or when endometrial biopsy indicates the progression of endometrial changes is delayed in the preparation for implantation.

The principles underlying the evaluation of disorders of normal menstrual functions are the same for ovarian or pituitary dysfunction. The many causes of male and female infertility are shown in Table 19-2.

World Health Organization (WHO) Amenorrhea Classification[20,21]

Type 1. Hypothalamic hypogonadism (low or normal FSH and/or LH):
- Hypothalamic amenorrhea (anorexia nervosa, idiopathic, exercise induced).
- Kallmann's syndrome.
- Isolated gonadotropin deficiency.

TABLE 19-1. AMENORRHEA: ETIOLOGIC SITES OF ABNORMALITY

	PRIMARY	SECONDARY
Hypothalamus	27%	38%
Pituitary	2%	15%
PCOS	7%	30%
Ovary	43%	12%
Uterus/outflow	19%	7%

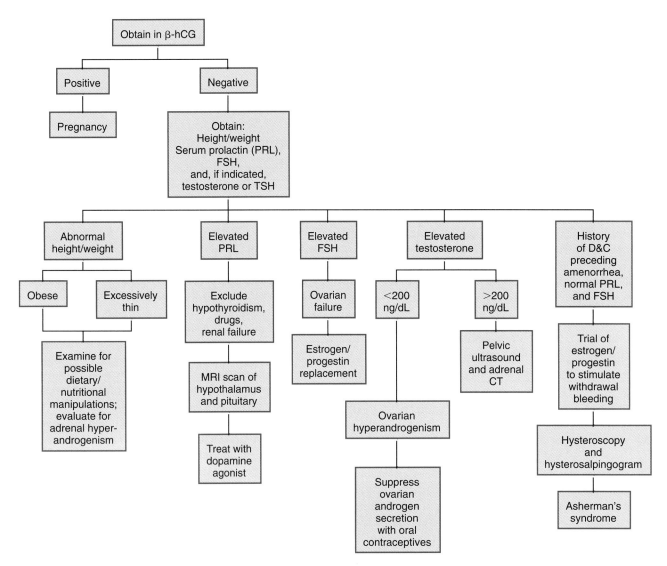

FIGURE 19-1. Diagnostic approach to secondary amenorrhea.

Type 2. Euestrogenic chronic anovulation (normal FSH and LH):
- Polycystic ovarian syndrome (LH > FSH in some patients 2:1 or above).
- Hyperthecosis.

Type 3. Hyperthalamic hypogonadism (FSH is commonly estimated to be elevated, but LH can also be elevated):
- Premature ovarian failure.
- Turner's syndrome.

Hypogonadotropic Hypogonadism

Many physiologic and pathologic causes induce secondary amenorrhea; most notably, weight loss either as a result of anorexia nervosa or secondary weight loss induced by various disease processes.[10,17,18,20–22] Intense physical exercise (commonly called *runner's amenorrhea*)

can also induce secondary amenorrhea. Pituitary tumors that disrupt secretion of FSH or LH can also induce hypogonadotropic hypogonadism. Prolactin production by prolactinomas can also have similar effects.[10,17] Any secondary cause of chronic hypogonadism can induce pathologic bone loss, resulting in osteopenia and, in severe cases, osteoporosis.

Primary Ovarian Failure

Primary ovarian failure can be a result of congenital chromosomal abnormality (Turner's syndrome) or premature menopause.[17,18,20,23] Patients with Turner's syndrome do not complain of the same hot flashes experienced by patients with secondary hypergonadotropic hypogonadism.[20] Elevation of FSH is a clue in the diagnosis of premature menopause. Premature ovarian failure can result along with other endocrine gland failure (hypoparathyroidism, hypothyroidism, hypoadrenalism, or mucocutaneous candidiasis).[6,17,18,20,22] Menopause is a

TABLE 19-2. ANDROGEN RESULTS IN HIRSUTISM AND VIRILIZATION

CONDITION	ANALYTE		
	TOTAL TESTOSTERONE	FREE TESTOSTERONE	DHEAS
Idiopathic hirsutism	↑	↑↑↑	↑
Polycystic ovary syndrome	↑	↑↑	↑
Congenital adrenal hyperplasia	↑↑	↑↑	↑↑↑
Virilizing tumors			
Ovarian	↑↑↑	↑↑↑	↑
Adrenal	↑↑	↑↑	↑↑↑

Modified from Demers LM. Hirsutism and Virilization, News and Views. Washington, D.C.: American Association for Clinical Chemistry, 1989.
DHEAS = dehydroepiandrosterone sulfate.

natural, inevitable event that results in elevation of FSH and LH levels, with low levels of estrogen.[1,6,16,24]

Polycystic Ovary Syndrome

This common disorder can present in many ways—infertility, hirsutism, chronic anovulation, glucose intolerance, hyperlipidemia or dyslipidemia, and hypertension.[11,13,14] The onset is often perimenarchial, chronic, and notable for slow progression. Investigations for this disorder involve estimation of free testosterone, sex hormone-binding globulin level, FSH and LH, fasting glucose, and insulin and lipid levels. Ovarian ultrasound reveals multiple cysts in most patients (about 30% of patients do not have ovarian cysts). Most patients with this disorder are overweight; however, patients with polycystic ovary syndrome (PCOS) of Eastern Asian or South American descent are of normal weight. Most symptoms and laboratory abnormalities are reversed with weight loss and increased physical activity. A

drug (Metformin), commonly used for the treatment of diabetes, is useful in this condition, even in the absence of diabetes.[13] It reportedly normalizes menstrual cycles and improves conception rates, although not FDA approved for this use.

Hirsutism

Hirsutism is abnormal, abundant, androgen-sensitive terminal hair growth in females, in areas where terminal hair follicles are sparse or not normally found. It is estimated that about 5–10% of women in the United States have hirsutism. Hirsutism is quantified by a practical measurement technique devised by Ferriman and Gallwey.[11,12,14,25] The most relevant areas of androgen-driven excess hair growth are in the midline of the body, resulting from an inherent preponderance of 5α-reductase activity, which converts testosterone to dehydrotestosterone (DHT). Hirsutism should only be considered in context to the ethnic origin of the women presenting for evaluation. Women of Italian, Eastern European, Eastern Indian, and Irish descent are endowed with more androgen-sensitive terminal hair than their northern European counterparts. Careful history elicitation of ethnic background in persons born in the United States is important before beginning a large-scale laboratory evaluation. Hormonal abnormalities associated with hirsutism are summarized in Table 19-3.

The Ferriman-Gallwey Scale

- Most commonly, nine areas are identified for assessment: lip, chin, neck, abdomen, upper and lower back, sideburn area, back, thigh, and middle of chest. A modified version of this scale uses additional areas.
- Points are scored on a scale of 1–4, based on thickness and pigmentation of the hair.
- A score of >8 indicates hirsutism.

Hirsutism Classification[11,12,14,25]

- Functional (normal androgen levels with excess hair growth) or true androgen excess (elevated androgens).
- Ovarian (LH-mediated) or adrenal (ACTH-mediated).

CASE STUDY 19-1

A 39-year-old woman presented with hot flashes and irregular menstrual cycles for 6 months. Clinical examination did not reveal abnormality. Laboratory evaluation reveals the following: CBC, normal; blood glucose, 89 mg/dL; TSH, 1.5 IU; FSH, 128 IU; and LH, 30 IU.

This clinical situation is consistent with one of the following:

1. PCOS

2. Prolactinoma

3. Pituitary tumor

4. Menopause

5. Hypothalamic hormone deficiency

TABLE 19-3. CAUSES OF INFERTILITY

TARGET	RESULT	CAUSE
Female		
Hypothalamus	Decreased GRH	Drugs Increased stress Diet
Pituitary	Decreased FSH, LH	Destructive tumor or vesicular lesion
Ovaries	Decreased estradiol or progesterone	Organ failure Organ dysgenesis Antiovarian antibodies Malnourishment, very low weight, metabolic disease
Fallopian tubes and uterus	Inadequate endometrium Tubal scarring and closure Decreased cervical mucus	Low progesterone output Pelvic inflammatory disease Cervical infections
Conception	Immobilization and destruction of sperm	Antisperm antibodies
Male		
Hypothalamus and pituitary	Azoospermia (no sperm) to oligospermia	Primary defects in hypothalamic or pituitary glands Exogenous androgens Testicular dysfunction, with decreased testicular production
Testes	Azoospermia (no sperm) to oligospermia Delayed or deficient sexual maturity; decreased testosterone	Orchitis; testicular infections, such as mumps; alcoholism and substance abuse Chromosomal defects
Prostate	Decreased seminal fluid	Infections of prostate or seminal vesicles
Urethrogenital tract	Retrograde or absent ejaculation	Physical abnormalities; chronic diabetes

- Peripheral conversion of androgens (obesity).
- Tumoral hyperandrogenism (ovarian, adrenal).
- Chorionic gonadotropin-mediated.

Causes of Hirsutism[11,12,14,25]
- Polycystic ovarian disease (PCOD), 35% of cases.
- Idiopathic, 60% of cases.
- Congenital adrenal hyperplasia, <1%; adrenal and ovarian neoplasms.
- Drugs.
  —Hirsutism: danazol, androgens, and androgenic progestins.
  —Hypertrichosis: streptomycin, penicillamine, diazoxide, and cyclosporine.
  —Minoxidil causes enlargement and pigmentation of vellus hair.

Estrogen Replacement Therapy

Estrogen replacement is still a contentious issue.[26-31] The Women's Health Initiative study enrolled 16,608 postmenopausal women who were placed on conventional replacement combinations. The outcome of the study was increased incidence of invasive breast cancer (hazards ratio, 1.26) and venous clot formation, no significant reduction of coronary artery disease, and reduction of bone loss and colon polyp formation. This therapy should be individualized to any given patient.

THE TESTES

The testes are paired, ovoidal organs that serve dual functions: (1) the production of sperm; and (2) the production of hormones that govern various processes in the human body that aid reproduction.[32] In the embryonic stage, the dominant male sex hormone, testosterone (T), aids in development and differentiation of the primordial gonads; after puberty and throughout adulthood and until late in older age, testosterone helps with sperm production and maintains secondary sexual characteristics.

Functional Anatomy of the Male Reproductive Tract

The testes are located outside the body, encased by a muscular sac. Blood flow is governed by an intricate plexus of arterial and venous blood flow that, together

CASE STUDY 19-2

A 49-year-old woman presented with increased hair growth for the past 6 months that started abruptly; she has male pattern hair loss, as well. On examination, she has temporal loss of hair and clitorimegaly. Laboratory evaluation reveals the following: Testosterone, 360 ng/dL; FSH, 12 IU; LH, 9 IU; and a normal prolactin level.

The next step in the evaluation is one of the following.

1. DHEA-S level

2. Repeat FSH and LH levels

3. Fasting blood sugar level

4. Fasting lipid level

5. Computed tomography of adrenal and ovaries

with contraction of the dartos muscle in the scrotal sac, regulates the temperature of the testicles at 2°C below core body temperature. This important function is vital to uninterrupted sperm production. Also encased in the muscular sheath is the spermatic cord, which has the ability to retract the testicles into the inguinal canal in case of threat of injury. Spermatogenesis occurs in the seminiferous tubules; the sperm move sequentially through the tubuli recti, rete testes, ductuli efferentes testes, the head, body, and tail of the epididymis, and, finally, into the vas deferens. Various secretory products of the seminal vesicles and prostate admix with sperm to form the final product (semen), which is deposited in the posterior vaginal wall during coitus. Seminal vesicle secretions are rich in vitamin C and fructose, important for the preservation of motility of the sperm.

Physiology of the Testicles

Spermatogenesis

Sperm are formed from stem cells called *spermatogonia*. The spermatogonia undergo mitosis and meiosis; finally, the haploid cells transform to form mature sperm.[33] The mature sperm has a head, body, and tail, with remarkable ability to swim to the only goal of forming a zygote with the haploid ovum. Certain spermatogonia stagger division so that sperm production is uninterrupted and continuous. The Sertoli cells are polyfunctional cells that aid in the development and maturation of sperm.

Hormonogenesis

Testosterone, the predominant hormone secreted by the testes, is controlled primarily by two pituitary hor-

mones: follicle-stimulating hormone (FSH) and luteinizing hormone (LH).[34,35] Because these hormones were first described in women, they are named in reference to the menstrual cycle. Both hormones are produced by a single group of cells in the pituitary called *gonadotrophs*. FSH acts primarily on germinal stem cells, and LH acts primarily on the Leydig cells that synthesize testosterone.

Hormonal Control of Testicular Function

The hypothalamus, located in the brain, generates a hormone called gonadotropin-releasing hormone (GnRH) in a pulsatile fashion. GnRH is released into the portal hypophysial system that, in turn, determines the production of LH and FSH from the pituitary gland. Impaired pulse generation of GnRH leads to inadequate production of LH and FSH, resulting in hypogonadism.[35,36] The first, and rate-limiting, step in the testicular steroidogenesis is conversion of cholesterol to pregnenolone. Cholesterol is either synthesized in the Leydig cells or the cholesterol in the blood is trapped by endocytosis. The LH binds to the glycoprotein receptor in the cell wall and induces intracellular cyclic AMP production that, in turn, activates protein kinase A, which catalyzes protein phosphorylation. This latter step induces testosterone synthesis. The testicular steroidogenesis pathway is similar to the pathway in the adrenal cortex and they share the same enzymatic systems. Testosterone is the principle androgen hormone in the blood. Testosterone is largely bound, with 2–3 % being free. About 50% of testosterone is bound to albumin and about 45% is bound to sex hormone-binding globulin (SHBG). The concentration of binding protein determines the level of total testosterone but not the free testosterone levels during laboratory estimation. Testosterone and *inhibin* are the two hormones secreted by the testes that provide feedback control to the hypothalamus and pituitary.

Testosterone concentration fluctuates in a circadian fashion, reflecting the parallel rhythms of LH and FSH levels. This fact should be considered when interpreting the blood level of testosterone. The highest level of testosterone is found at about 8 a.m. and the lowest level at about 8 p.m.

Cellular Mechanism of Testosterone Action

Testosterone enters the cell and converts to dihydrotestosterone (DHT). DHT complexes with an intracellular receptor protein; this complex binds to the nuclear receptor, effecting protein synthesis and cell growth.

Physiologic Actions of Testosterone

Prenatal development. Early in development, embryos have primordial components of the genital tracts of both sexes. The primitive gonads become distinguishable at about the 7th week of embryonic stage. Both chorionic gonadotropins and fetal LH stimulate production of testosterone by the fetal Leydig cells. Exposure of testosterone to the wolffian duct leads to differentiation of the various components of the male genital tract. *Sertoli cells* produce mullerian regression factor, which aids in regression of the female primordial genital tract. The scrotal skin is rich in a 5α-reductase, which converts testosterone to DHT. Fetal exposure to drugs that block this hormone leads to feminization of the male fetus.

Postnatal development. Testicular function is reactivated during puberty after a period of quiescence to produce testosterone that results in development of secondary sex hair (face, chest, axilla, and pubis); enhanced linear skeletal growth; development of internal and external genitalia; increased upper body musculature; and development of larynx and vocal cords, with deepening of voice.[37–39] Possible mood changes and aggressiveness are undesired effects that may occur during puberty. The linear growth effects of testosterone are finite, with epiphysial closure when genetically determined height is achieved. Hypogonadism during puberty leads to imprecise closure of growth plates, leading to tallness, long limbs, and disproportionate upper and lower body segments. Male secondary sexual characteristics can be staged by a system of development devised by Tanner.

Effect on spermatogenesis. Stimulation of Leydig cells induces production of testosterone. Testosterone, acting with FSH, has paracrine effects on the seminiferous and Sertoli cells inducing spermatogenesis. The intratesticular concentration of testosterone is 50- to 100-fold higher than that of peripheral blood. Maintenance of a high intratesticular level of testosterone is important for effective spermatogenesis. Exogenous overuse or abuse (athletes) of testosterone will reduce the high intratesticular concentration, leading to reduction of sperm production.

Effect on secondary sexual effects. Testosterone has growth-promoting effects on various target tissues. The secondary sex characteristics that develop during puberty are maintained into late adulthood by testosterone.[9] Exposure of scalp hair results in regression of the hair follicles (temporal recession). The prostate enlarges progressively during adulthood. Subsequent loss of secondary sexual characteristics should prompt evaluation for hypogonadism. Low testosterone levels lead to loss of bone mass and osteoporosis in males at any age.

Disorders of Sexual Development and Testicular Hypofunction

Pubertal development could be premature (precocious) or delayed, even if development is normal at birth.[41,42] Detailed descriptions of the sequence of hormonal pubertal abnormalities of hair, genitals, and breasts is be-

yond the scope of this text. The following are certain salient causes encountered in clinical practice:

Delayed puberty or hypogonadism, with increased gonadotropins (FSH and or LH)
  Klinefelter's syndrome
  Bilateral gonadal failure
    Primary testicular failure
    Anorchia
    Vanishing testicles
    Cancer cytotoxic agents
    Irradiation
    Trauma
    Infection (mumps orchitis)
Delayed puberty with normal or low FSH and/or LH levels
  Constitutional delayed puberty[43,44]
  Hypothalamic dysfunction
    Malnutrition
    Chronic systemic illness
    Severe obesity
    CNS tumors
  Hypopituitarism
    Panhypopituitarism
    Kallmann's syndrome (anosmia, cleft palate, and reduced FSH and LH levels)
    Isolated GH deficiency
  Hyperprolactinemia (prolactinoma or drug induced)
  Hypothyroidism
Miscellaneous[44]
  Prader-Willi syndrome
  Laurence-Moon syndrome
  LEOPARD syndrome
  Bloom syndrome
  Germ cell neoplasia
  Male pseudohermaphroditism
  Ataxia-telangiectasia
  Steroidogenic enzyme defects

The differential diagnosis of hypogonadism includes the above large and diverse group of disorders affecting the testicles and the hypothalamic-pituitary regulation of the testes. Certain important disorders are explained in the following section.

Hypergonadotropic Hypogonadism

The salient features of this subset of disorders include low testosterone along with elevated FSH or LH levels and impaired production of sperm.

Klinefelter's syndrome. This disorder occurs in about 1 of 400 men; it is caused by an extra chromosome. The most common karyotype is 47,XY.[45] Men with Klinefelter's syndrome have small (<2.5 cm), firm testicles. Gynecomastia (enlargement of the male breast) can also be present at the time of diagnosis. Due to reduced production of testosterone, FSH and LH levels are elevated.

CASE STUDY 19-3

A 24-year-old man presented with a history of hayfever, which had been treated with antihistamines. He relates diminished smell. He continues to grow slowly and pubertal development has been slow. The man denies erections or nocturnal emissions.

PE	Eunuchoidal man, appearing younger than age
Height	72 inches
Arm span	75 inches
Weight	180 lb
BP	130/82
Hair	Spare facial, axillary, and pubic
Genitalia	Penis, 3.1 cm (small)
Testes	Soft, 1 cm × 1.5 cm × 1.5 cm (normal, >4.5 × 3 cm × 3 cm)

Laboratory

Testosterone	157 ng/dL (normal, prepuberal <100; adult, 300–1000)
LH	<2 mU/mL (normal, prepubertal <5; adult, 3–18)
Prolactin	6 ng/mL (normal, 5–25)
TSH	1.2 mU/mL (normal, 0.3–5.0)

GnRH Stimulation

Time (Minutes)	LH	Normal
0, GnRH	<2 mU/mL	Pre-, <5
		Adult, 3–18
15	<2	Post-, 2.5 times
30	3	Baseline at
45	<2	some
60	3	point

After GnRH Priming

Time (Minutes)	LH	Normal
0	<2 mU/mL	Pre-, <5
		Adult, 3–18
15	10	LH rise
30	12	greater than
45	16	2.5 times
60	12	baseline

Management

Testosterone replacement therapy
Sexual maturity
Later desired fertility

GnRH pulsatile therapy produced a normal sperm count in 4 months and the man's wife became pregnant.

Questions

1. What is the level of the defect?

2. What is the significance of the body measurements?

3. What are the diagnostic considerations?

4. What test(s) might be obtained to make the diagnosis?

5. What constitutes normal fertility?

6. How will you counsel this man when he asks if he can have children?

These patients also have azoospermia and resultant sterility. Patients with mosaicism may produce some sperm and pregnancies have been reported in such patients. Elevated levels of FSH and LH induce increased aromatase activity, resulting in elevated estrogen levels. Men with Klinefelter's syndrome may have reduced bone density and breast cancer.

Testicular feminization syndrome. This is the most severe form of androgen-resistant syndrome, resulting in lack of testosterone action in the target tissue. As a result of the lack of testosterone effect, the physical development pursues the female phenotype, with fully developed breasts and female distribution of fat and hair. Most patients present for evaluation of primary amenorrhea; at which time, the lack of female internal genitalia becomes apparent. The testicles are often undescended and failure to promptly remove these organs results in malignant transformation. Biochemical evaluation reveals normal levels of testosterone with elevated FSH and LH levels. There is no utility or response to administration of exogenous testosterone.

5α-Reductase deficiency. The genotype is XY. A reduction of this enzyme results in reduction of testosterone level. Physical development is similar to the female phenotype until puberty when residual 5α-reductase activity sufficiently converts testosterone to dihydrotestosterone, resulting in development of male phenotype.

Myotonic dystrophy. Myotonic dystrophy is an autosomal dominantly inherited condition that presents with hypogonadism, muscle weakness, frontal balding, dia-

CASE STUDY 19-4

A 17-year-old man presented. A school physical examination showed less pubic and axillary hair than peers; penis and scrotum smaller; breast tissue since age 13; no erections or nocturnal emissions and no adolescent growth spurt. Sleeve and pant length increase every 4–6 months.

PMH, FH	NC
PE	
Height	73″
Arm span	74″
Weight	148 lb
BP	110/70
Pulse	69
Hair	Scant axillary and pubic
Breasts	Moderate gynecomastia, 3 cm
Genitalia	Penis, 4.5 cm
Testes	1.5 × 1 × 1 cm, bilaterally (normal, >4.5 × 2.5 × 2.5 cm)

Laboratory	
Testosterone, total	115 ng/dL (normal, 300–1000)
LH	42 mU/mL (normal, Adult, 3–18)
Karyotype	47,XXY

Questions

1. At what level is the defect in this case?

2. What diagnostic possibilities would explain the endocrine data?

3. What treatment(s) would be available to:
   a. treat his androgen deficiency?
   b. allow him to father children if he wanted fertility?

4. His appearance shows the defect occurred:
   a. prior to birth (during fetal life).
   b. after birth (postnatal).

betes, and muscle dystonia. Testicular failure presents in the fourth decade.

Testicular injury and infection. Mumps orchitis occurs in the postpubertal mumps infection. Viral orchitis may also occur in some patients. HIV infection is also described to destroy the testes. Radiation and chemotherapy for cancer can also damage the testes.

Sertoli-cell-only syndrome. This disorder is characterized by the lack of germ cells. Patients present with small testes, high FSH levels, azoospermia, and normal testosterone levels. Testicular biopsy is the only procedure to confirm this diagnosis.

Hypogonadotropic Hypogonadism

The hallmark of this group of disorders is the occurrence of low testosterone levels, together with low or inappropriately normal FSH and or LH levels.

Kallmann's syndrome. This syndrome is a result of an inherited, X-linked recessive trait that manifests as hypogonadism during puberty. The frequency of this syndrome is 1 of 10,000 males. The associated defects, such as anosmia (inability to smell) and midline defects (cleft palate and lip), should alert the clinician to suspect this disorder.[46,47] Certain patients also have red-green color blindness, congenital deafness, or cerebellar dysfunction.

Hyperprolactinemia. Prolactin elevation resulting from any cause (drug induced or prolactin producing tumors of the pituitary) can result in hypogonadotropic hypogonadism.[48,49]

Age. There is a gradual reduction of testosterone after age 30, with an average decline of about 110 ng/dL every decade. The Baltimore Longitudinal Study of Aging revealed reduced total testosterone levels of 19% at age 60, 28% at age 70, and 49% at age 80,[50,51] with free testosterone levels much lower in these patients. Age is also associated with elevation of SHBG by about 1% per year. Total testosterone levels may be normal in aging men but the free (unbound) levels of testosterone are more reliable indicators of biochemical reduction. The associated features of reduced secondary sex hair growth, loss of muscle bulk and strength, and loss of bone density are corroborative evidence indicative of the lack of tissue effects of testosterone. Testosterone deficiency is a constellation of clinical features of hypogonadism combined with low serum testosterone levels. The combination of biochemical and clinical evidence of testosterone should prompt consideration of testosterone replacement in older men.

Pituitary disease. Acquired hypogonadism can follow injury to the pituitary as a result of tumors, surgical trauma, vascular injury, autoimmune hypophysitis, or granulomatous or metastatic disease. Hemochromatosis is also a rare cause of pituitary dysfunction.

Diagnosis of Hypogonadism

Both clinical and biochemical features must be met (Fig. 19-2). Testosterone levels have a circadian rhythm and the time of sampling must be considered. Multiple estimations of free and bound testosterone levels should be done on different days before a diagnosis of hypogonadism is made.[52] The distinction between primary (disease or destruction of testes) versus secondary (disease or destruction of pituitary) is relatively easy to make. FSH and or LH levels are elevated in primary hypogonadism and are inappropriately normal or low with secondary etiology. Pituitary MRI should be done in secondary hypogonadism in young individuals. Older individuals often have secondary or tertiary (hypothala-

mic) dysfunction as a result of reduced hypothalamic pulse generator frequency, resulting in low or inappropriately normal FSH and or LH levels. Clinical signs and symptoms (eg, loss of secondary sex characteristics, osteoporosis) of hypogonadism should be corroborated with low testosterone levels, particularly when testosterone replacement therapy is contemplated.

Testosterone Replacement Therapy

The following modes of delivery are available for clinical use in the United States:

1. **Parenteral testosterone.** This is the most widely available and cost-effective (particularly if administered by spouse or partner) mode of administration. The cypionate and enanthate esters of testosterone are available for intramuscular injection. The peak level is achieved in 72 hours, and the effect lasts for a period of 1–2 weeks. When weekly administration provides a lesser peak or fluctuation in the level of testosterone between normal ranges, the usual dose is 50–100 mg

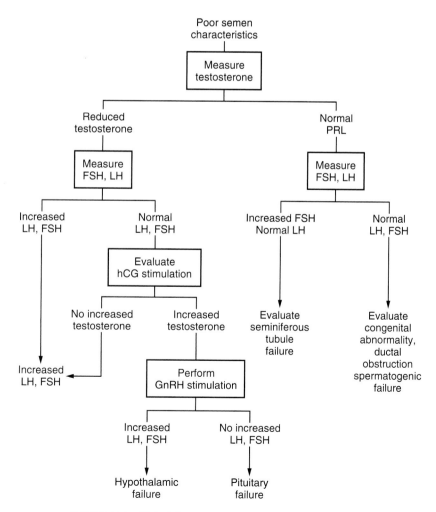

FIGURE 19-2. Clinical diagnostic evaluation of male hypogonadism.

every week or 200–250 mg once every 2 weeks. Testosterone dose should be based on lean body mass, not body weight. This is often achieved by administering a standard dose of testosterone, with minor dose escalations based on serum testosterone levels estimated midpoint between two injections; the goal is to maintain this level midpoint of the normal ranges of the assay being used.

2. **Transdermal testosterone therapy.** This mode of administration provides more physiologic levels of testosterone. The patch is permeability enhanced to aid in the absorption of testosterone through normal skin. Possible skin irritation often limits its use.

3. **Scrotal patch.** Scrotal skin is thin and easily absorbs testosterone. This mode of administration leads to higher dihydrotestosterone levels as a result of 5α-reductase-mediated conversion, in which the scrotal skin is rich. The scrotal skin must be shaved as needed to aid in adhesion of the patch, to which certain patients may disagree. Patients with Klinefelter's syndrome often have a poorly developed scrotal sac that is not large enough to accommodate the size of the patch.

4. **Testosterone gel.** This hydroalcoholic gel preparation is applied to nongenital skin once a day. The absorption is gradual and provides blood level of testosterone in the normal range for 24 hours. The main concern with this preparation is potential transmission to female partners or children on close skin contact.

5. **Oral preparations.** The use of this mode of delivery is currently discouraged due to potential hepatic complications. Hepatic function abnormalities, adenoma formation, and development of hemorrhagic cysts in the liver have been described. One particular preparation available in Europe, the undecenoate ester of testosterone, is absorbed into the lymphatic circulation, directly bypassing the hepatic portal circulation.

The complications of testosterone replacement are as follows:

- Polycythemia.
- Prostate enlargement.
- Possible growth promoting effect on preexisting, undiagnosed prostate cancer.
- Worsening of sleep apnea.
- Peripheral edema.

Monitoring Testosterone Replacement Therapy

Prostate-specific antigen (PSA), blood counts, and lipid levels should be monitored for 3–6 months after replacement of testosterone. Clinical evaluation for leg edema, worsening of sleep apnea, and prostate enlargement is also routinely recommended. Pharmacologic use of testosterone may also reduce sperm count by reducing the intratesticular testosterone concentration that is many fold higher than serum concentration. If PSA elevation is noted after testosterone replacement, prostate evaluation with possible biopsy is recommended. Active prostate cancer is a contraindication to testosterone replacement.

REVIEW QUESTIONS

1. If serum levels of estradiol do not increase after injection of human chorionic gonadotropin, the patient has:
   a. pituitary failure.
   b. primary ovarian failure.
   c. tertiary ovarian failure.
   d. secondary ovarian failure.

2. If a patient had a luteal phase defect, which hormone would most likely be deficient?
   a. Estrogen
   b. hCG
   c. FSH
   d. Prolactin
   e. Progesterone

3. Which of the following is the precursor for estradiol formation in the placenta?
   a. Maternal testosterone
   b. Maternal progesterone
   c. Placental hCG
   d. Fetal adrenal cholesterol
   e. Fetal adrenal DHEAS

4. Which of the following target tissues is incapable of producing steroidal hormones?
   a. Placenta
   b. Ovary
   c. Testis
   d. Adrenal cortex
   e. Adrenal medulla

5. The parent substance in the biosynthesis of androgens and estrogens is:
   a. cortisol.
   b. catecholamines.
   c. progesterone.
   d. cholesterol.

6. The biologically most active, naturally occurring androgen is:
   a. androstenedione.
   b. dehydroepiandrosterone.
   c. epiandrosterone.
   d. testosterone.

7. For the past 3 weeks, serum estriol levels in a pregnant woman have been steadily increasing. This is consistent with:
   a. a normal pregnancy.
   b. hemolytic disease of the newborn.
   c. fetal death.
   d. congenital cytomegalovirus infection.

8. Which of the following is secreted by the placenta and used for the early detection of pregnancy?
   a. Follicle-stimulating hormone (FSH)
   b. Human chorionic gonadotropin (hCG)
   c. Luteinizing hormone (LH)
   d. Progesterone

9. Chronic fetal metabolic distress is demonstrated by:
   a. decreased estrogen in maternal plasma and increased estriol amniotic fluid.
   b. increased estradiol in maternal plasma, with a corresponding increase of estriol in amniotic fluid.
   c. increased urinary estriol excretion and increased maternal serum estriol.
   d. decreased urinary estriol excretion and decreased maternal serum estriol.

10. Androgen secretion by the testes is stimulated by:
    a. luteinizing hormone (LH).
    b. follicle-stimulating hormone (FSH).
    c. testosterone.
    d. gonadotropins.

REFERENCES

1. Sherman BM, West JH, Korenman SG. The menopausal transition: analysis of LH, FSH, estradiol, and progesterone concentrations during menstrual cycles of older women. J Clin Endocrinol Metab 1976;42:629–636.
2. Gougeon A. Dynamics of follicular growth in the human: a model from preliminary results. Hum Reprod 1986;1:81–87.
3. Jost A, Vigier B, Prepin J, Perchellet JP. Studies on sex differentiation in mammals. Recent Prog Horm Res 1973;29:1–41.
4. Filicori M, Santoro N, Merriam GR, Crowley WF Jr. Characterization of the physiological pattern of episodic gonadotropin secretion throughout the human menstrual cycle. J Clin Endocrinol Metab 1986;62:1136–1144.
5. Taylor AE, Whitney H, Hall JE, Martin K, Crowley WF Jr. Midcycle levels of sex steroids are sufficient to recreate the follicle-stimulating hormone but not the luteinizing hormone midcycle surge: evidence for the contribution of other ovarian factors to the surge in normal women. J Clin Endocrinol Metab 1995;80:1541–1547.
6. Klein NA, Battaglia DE, Miller PB, Branigan EF, Giudice LC, Soules MR. Ovarian follicular development and the follicular fluid hormones and growth factors in normal women of advanced reproductive age. J Clin Endocrinol Metab 1996;81:1946–1951.
7. Peters H, Byskov AG, Grinsted J. Follicular growth in fetal and prepubertal ovaries of humans and other primates. Clin Endocrinol Metab 1978;7:469–485.
8. Apter D, Cacciatore B, Alfthan H, Stenman UH. Serum luteinizing hormone concentrations increase 100-fold in females from 7 years to adulthood, as measured by time-resolved immunofluorometric assay. J Clin Endocrinol Metab 1989;68:53–57.
9. Marshall WA, Tanner JM. Variations in pattern of pubertal changes in girls. Arch Dis Child 1969;44:291–303.
10. Santoro N, Filicori M, Crowley WF Jr. Hypogonadotropic disorders in men and women: diagnosis and therapy with pulsatile gonadotropin-releasing hormone. Endocr Rev 1986;7:11–23.
11. Hatch R, Rosenfield RL, Kim MH, Tredway D. Hirsutism: implications, etiology, and management. Am J Obstet Gynecol 1981;140: 815–830.
12. McKenna TJ. Screening for sinister causes of hirsutism. N Engl J Med 1994;331:1015–1016.
13. Nestler JE, Jakubowicz DJ. Decreases in ovarian cytochrome P450c17 alpha activity and serum free testosterone after reduction of insulin secretion in polycystic ovary syndrome. N Engl J Med 1996;335:617–623.
14. O'Driscoll JB, Mamtora H, Higginson J, Pollock A, Kane J, Anderson DC. A prospective study of the prevalence of clear-cut endocrine disorders and polycystic ovaries in 350 patients presenting with hirsutism or androgenic alopecia. Clin Endocrinol (Oxf) 1994;41:231–236.
15. Welt CK, McNicholl DJ, Taylor AE, Hall JE. Female reproductive aging is marked by decreased secretion of dimeric inhibin. J Clin Endocrinol Metab 1999;84:105–111.
16. Stanford JL, Hartge P, Brinton LA, Hoover RN, Brookmeyer R. Factors influencing the age at natural menopause. J Chronic Dis 1987;40:995–1002.
17. Groff TR, Shulkin BL, Utiger RD, Talbert LM. Amenorrhea-galactorrhea, hyperprolactinemia, and suprasellar pituitary enlargement as presenting features of primary hypothyroidism. Obstet Gynecol 1984;63:86S–89S.
18. Warren MP, Voussoughian F, Geer EB, Hyle EP, Adberg CL, Ramos RH. Functional hypothalamic amenorrhea: hypoleptinemia and disordered eating. J Clin Endocrinol Metab 1999;84:873–877.
19. Saenger P. Turner's syndrome. N Engl J Med 1996;335:1749–1754.
20. Timmreck LS, Reindollar RH. Contemporary issues in primary amenorrhea. Obstet Gynecol Clin North Am 2003;30:287–302.
21. Feichtinger W, Kemeter P, Salzer H, Friedrich F. Functional and hormonal differences between group I and group II amenorrhea (WHO classification) (author's transl). Wien Klin Wochenschr 1981;93:186–193.

22. Reindollar RH, Novak M, Tho SP, McDonough PG. Adult-onset amenorrhea: a study of 262 patients. Am J Obstet Gynecol 1986; 155:531–543.

23. Reindollar RH, Byrd JR, McDonough PG. Delayed sexual development: a study of 252 patients. Am J Obstet Gynecol 1981;140: 371–380.

24. Wise PM, Krajnak KM, Kashon ML. Menopause: the aging of multiple pacemakers. Science 1996;273:67–70.

25. Meldrum DR, Abraham GE. Peripheral and ovarian venous concentrations of various steroid hormones in virilizing ovarian tumors. Obstet Gynecol 1979;53:36–43.

26. Chlebowski RT, Hendrix SL, Langer RD, et al. Influence of estrogen plus progestin on breast cancer and mammography in healthy postmenopausal women: the Women's Health Initiative Randomized Trial. JAMA 2003;289:3243–3253.

27. Stjernquist M. After the early termination of the Women's Health Initiative study. New American recommendations for postmenopausal hormone therapy. Lakartidningen 2003;100:1790–1797.

28. Wassertheil-Smoller S, Hendrix SL, Limacher M, et al. Effect of estrogen plus progestin on stroke in postmenopausal women: the Women's Health Initiative: a randomized trial. JAMA 2003;289: 2673–2684.

29. Rapp SR, Espeland MA, Shumaker SA, et al. Effect of estrogen plus progestin on global cognitive function in postmenopausal women. The Women's Health Initiative Memory Study: a randomized controlled trial. JAMA 2003;289:2663–2672.

30. Shumaker SA, Legault C, Thal L, et al. Estrogen plus progestin and the incidence of dementia and mild cognitive impairment in postmenopausal women. The Women's Health Initiative Memory Study: a randomized controlled trial. JAMA 2003;289: 2651–2662.

31. Pines A. Lessons from the Women's Health Initiative (WHI) using hormone replacement therapy with regard to heart disease—the dream that has been broken? Harefuah 2003;142:163–165, 240.

32. Dewing P, Bernard P, Vilain E. Disorders of gonadal development. Semin Reprod Med 2002;20:189–198.

33. Sharpe RM, McKinnell C, Kivlin C, Fisher JS. Proliferation and functional maturation of Sertoli cells, and their relevance to disorders of testis function in adulthood. Reproduction 2003;125: 769–784.

34. Goncharova ND, Lapin BA, Khavinson V. Age-associated endocrine dysfunctions and approaches to their correction. Bull Exp Biol Med 2002;134:417–421.

35. Grumbach MM. The neuroendocrinology of human puberty revisited. Horm Res 57 2002;Suppl 2:2–14.

36. Tong S, Wallace EM, Burger HG. Inhibins and activins: clinical advances in reproductive medicine. Clin Endocrinol (Oxf) 2003; 58:115–127.

37. Labrie F. Extragonadal synthesis of sex steroids: intracrinology. Ann Endocrinol (Paris) 2003;64:95–107.

38. Hiort O, Holterhus PM. Androgen insensitivity and male infertility. Int J Androl 2003;26:16–20.

39. Lee DK, Chang C. Molecular communication between androgen receptor and general transcription machinery. J Steroid Biochem Mol Biol 2003;84:41–49.

40. Santoro N, Filicori M, Crowley WF Jr. Hypogonadotropic disorders in men and women: diagnosis and therapy with pulsatile gonadotropin-releasing hormone. Endocr Rev 1986;7:11–23.

41. Sultan C, Gobinet J, Terouanne B, et al. The androgen receptor: molecular pathology. J Soc Biol 2002;196:223–240.

42. Sultan C, Lumbroso S, Paris F, et al. Disorders of androgen action. Semin Reprod Med 2002;20:217–228.

43. Kelly BP, Paterson WF, Donaldson MD. Final height outcome and value of height prediction in boys with constitutional delay in growth and adolescence treated with intramuscular testosterone 125 mg per month for 3 months. Clin Endocrinol (Oxf) 2003;58: 267–272.

44. Zachmann M. Therapeutic indications for delayed puberty and hypogonadism in adolescent boys. Horm Res 1991;36:141–146.

45. Styne DM. Puberty and its disorders in boys. Endocrinol Metab Clin North Am 1991;20:43–69.

46. Seminara SB, Hayes FJ, Crowley WF Jr. Gonadotropin-releasing hormone deficiency in the human (idiopathic hypogonadotropic hypogonadism and Kallmann's syndrome): pathophysiological and genetic considerations. Endocr Rev 1998;19:521–539.

47. Labhart A. Male sex hormones and their derivatives. Pathophysiology and therapy. Fortschr Med 1978;96:2029–2034.

48. Heaton JP, Morales A. Endocrine causes of impotence (nondiabetes). Urol Clin North Am 2003;30:73–81.

49. Walsh JP, Pullan PT. Hyperprolactinaemia in males: a heterogeneous disorder. Aust N Z J Med 1997;27:385–390.

50. Harman SM, Metter EJ, Tobin JD, Pearson J, Blackman MR. Longitudinal effects of aging on serum total and free testosterone levels in healthy men. Baltimore Longitudinal Study of Aging. J Clin Endocrinol Metab 2001;86:724–731.

51. Morley JE. Androgens and aging. Maturitas 2001;38:61–71; discussion, 71–73.

52. Korenman SG, Morley JE, Mooradian AD, et al. Secondary hypogonadism in older men: its relation to impotence. J Clin Endocrinol Metab 1990;71:963–969.

SUGGESTED READINGS

Goldmann M. Basic Clinical Endocrinology.

Becker. Textbook in Endocrinology.

William's Textbook in Endocrinology.

Degroot's Textbook in Endocrinology.

Hypogonadism Guidelines. Endocr Prac 2002;8(6):455.

Harrison's Textbook of Medicine.

Meikle, AW. Androgen replacement therapy of male hypogonadism. In: Endocrine Replacement in Clinical Practice. Therapy. Ottawa, NJ: Humana Press, 333–368.

The Thyroid Gland

Daniel H. Knodel

OBJECTIVES

Upon completion of this chapter, the clinical laboratorian should be able to:
- Discuss the biosynthesis, secretion, transport, and action of the thyroid hormones.
- Know the location of the thyroid gland.
- Describe the hypothalamic–pituitary–thyroid axis and how it regulates thyroid hormone production.
- Explain the principles of each thyroid function test discussed.

- Correlate laboratory information with regard to suspected thyroid disorders, given a patient's clinical data.
- Describe the appropriate laboratory thyroid function testing protocol to use to effectively evaluate or monitor patients with suspected thyroid disease.

KEY TERMS

Follicular cells
Free T_4
Graves' disease
Hyperthyroidism
Hypothalamic–pituitary–
  thyroid axis
Hypothyroidism

Parathyroid glands
Subacute thyroiditis
Subclinical
  hyperthyroidism
Subclinical
  hypothyroidism
Thyroglobulin

Thyroidal peroxidase
  (TPO)
Thyrotoxicosis
Thyrotropin (TSH)
Thyrotropin-releasing
  hormone (TRH)
Thyroxine (T_4)

Thyroxine-binding
  globulin (TBG)
Thyroxine-binding
  prealbumin (TBPA)
Triiodothyronine (T_3)
TSH receptor antibodies

THE THYROID

The thyroid gland is responsible for the production of two hormones, thyroid hormone and calcitonin. Calcitonin is secreted by parafollicular C cells and is involved in calcium homeostasis. Thyroid hormone is critical in regulating body metabolism, neurologic development, and numerous other body functions. Clinically, conditions affecting thyroid hormone levels are much more common and are the major focus of this chapter.

Thyroid Anatomy and Development

The thyroid gland is positioned in the lower anterior neck and has a shape similar to a butterfly. It is divided into two lobes, one on either side of the trachea. A band of thyroid tissue, called the isthmus, bridges the lobes. Underneath the thyroid gland are the *parathyroid glands* (responsible for calcium balance) and the recurrent laryngeal nerves (innervation for the vocal cords). These later structures take on great significance during thyroid surgery when care must be exercised to avoid injury and resultant hypocalcemia or permanent hoarseness, respectively.

The fetal thyroid develops from an outpouching of the foregut at the base of the tongue and migrates to its normal location over the thyroid cartilage in the first 4–8 weeks of gestation. By week 11 of gestation, the thyroid gland begins to produce measurable amounts of thyroid hormone.[1] Thyroid hormone is critical to neurologic development of the fetus. Iodine is an essential component of thyroid hormone. In parts of the world where severe iodine deficiency exists, neither the mother nor the fetus can produce thyroid hormone and both develop hypothyroidism. The impact is most severe on the offspring because *hypothyroidism* leads to mental retardation and cretinism. Where iodine deficiency is not an issue, other problems can occur with thyroid development. For example, 1 of 4000 children is born with congenital hypothyroidism.[2] If the mother has normal thyroid function, the fetus will be protected during development by small amounts of maternal thyroid hormone crossing the placenta. Immediately postpartum, however, these newborns need to be started on appropriate doses of thyroid hormone or their neurologic development is significantly impaired. In the developed world, screening tests are preformed on all newborns to diagnose congenital hypothyroidism and prevent catastrophic complications by the timely institution of thyroid hormone therapy.

Thyroid Hormone Synthesis

Thyroid hormone is made mostly of the trace element iodine.[1] With this in mind, it is understandable that iodine metabolism plays a key role in thyroid function. Iodine is found in seafood, dairy products, breads that have been enriched with iodine, and vitamins. Of importance in health care, iodine is also present in high concentrations in contrast medium used to visualize arteries on heart catheterizations and computed tomography (CT) scans and in amiodarone, a medication used to treat certain heart problems. The recommended minimum intake of iodine is 150 µg/day, although most people in developed countries take in far more than this amount. If iodine intake drops below 50 µg/day, the thyroid gland will be unable to manufacture adequate amounts of thyroid hormone and thyroid hormone deficiency, *hypothyroidism*, will occur.[3]

Thyroid cells are organized into follicles. Follicles are spheres of thyroid cells surrounding a core of a viscous substance called *colloid*. The major component of colloid is *thyroglobulin*, a glycoprotein manufactured exclusively by thyroid *follicular cells*. Thyroglobulin is rich in the amino acid tyrosine. Some of these tyrosyl residues can be iodinated, producing the building blocks of thyroid hormone. On the outer side of the follicle, iodine is actively transported into the thyroid cell by the Na^+/I^- symporter located on the basement membrane. Inside the thyroid cell, iodide diffuses across the cell to the apical side of the follicle, which abuts the core of colloid. Here, catalyzed by a membrane-bound enzyme called *thyroidal peroxidase (TPO)*, concentrated iodide is oxidized and bound with tyrosyl residues on thyroglobulin. This results in production of monoiodothyronine (MIT) and diiodothyronine (DIT). This same enzyme also aids in the coupling of two tyrosyl residues to form *triiodothyronine (T_3)* (one MIT residue + one DIT residue) or *tetraiodothyronine (T_4)* (two DIT residues). These are the two active forms of thyroid hormone. This thyroglobulin matrix, with branches now holding T_4 and T_3, is stored in the core of the thyroid follicle. *Thyroid-stimulating hormone (TSH)* signals the follicular cell to ingest a microscopic droplet of colloid by endocytosis. Inside the follicular cell, these droplets are digested by intracellular lysosomes into T_4, T_3, and other products.[3] T_4 and T_3 are then secreted by the thyroid cell into the circulation (Fig. 20-1).

Activity of thyroid hormone is dependent on the location and number of iodine atoms. Approximately 80% of T_4 is metabolized into either T_3 (35%) or rT_3 (45%). Outer ring deiodination of T_4 (5'-deiodination) leads to production of 3,5,3'-triiodothyronine (T_3). T_3 is 3–8 times more metabolically active than T_4 and often considered to be the active form of thyroid hormone, while T_4 is the "pre" hormone (with thyroglobulin being the "prohormone"). However, inner ring deiodination of T_4 results in the production of metabolically inactive reverse T_3 (rT_3) (Fig. 20-2).

There are three forms of 5'-deiodinase. Type 1, 5'-deiodinase, the most abundant, is found mostly in the liver and kidney and is responsible for the largest contribution

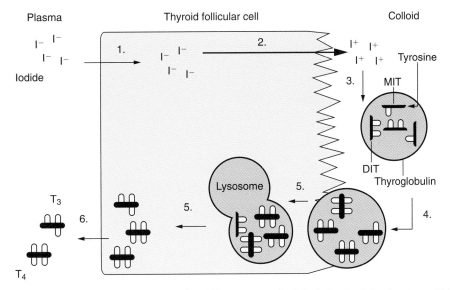

FIGURE 20-1. Biosynthesis of thyroid hormone. Thyroid hormone synthesis includes the following steps: (1) iodide (I-) trapping by thyroid follicular cells; (2) diffusion of iodide to the apex of the cell and transport into the colloid; (3) oxidation of inorganic iodide to iodine and incorporation of iodine into tyrosine residues within thyroglobulin molecules in the colloid; (4) combination of two diiodotyrosine (DIT) molecules to form tetraiodothyronine (thyroxine, T_4) or of monoiodotyrosine (MIT) with DIT to form triiodothyronine (T_3); (5) uptake of thyroglobulin from the colloid into the follicular cell by endocytosis, fusion of the thyroglobulin with a lysosome, and proteolysis and release of T_4 and T_3; and (6) release of T_4 and T_3 into the circulation.

to the circulating T_3 pool. Certain drugs (*eg,* propylthiouracil, glucocorticoids, and propranolol) can slow the activity of this deiodinase and are used in the treatment of severe hyperthyroidism. Type 2, 5'-deiodinase, is found in the brain and pituitary. Its function is to maintain constant levels of T_3 in the central nervous system. Its activity is decreased when levels of circulating T_4 are high and increased when levels are low. Activity of the deiodination enzymes gives another level of control on thyroid hormone activity other than hypothalamic–pituitary control through TRH and TSH (Fig. 20-2).[1]

Protein Binding of Thyroid Hormone

When released into the circulation, only 0.04% of T_4 and 0.4% of T_3 are unbound by proteins and available for hormonal activity. The three major binding proteins, in order of significance, are *thyroxine-binding globulin (TBG),*

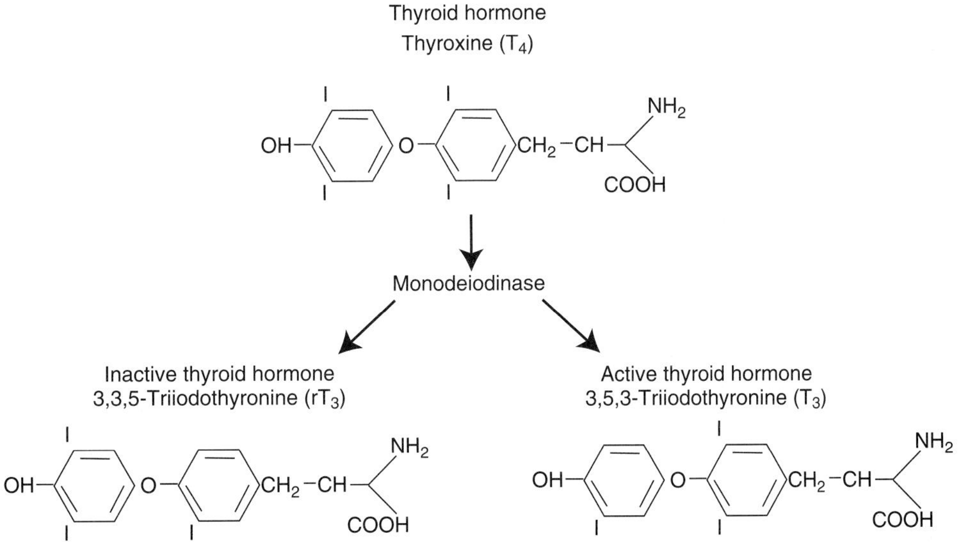

Thyroid hormone
Thyroxine (T_4)

$$OH\!\!-\!\!\bigcirc\!\!-\!\!O\!\!-\!\!\bigcirc\!\!-\!\!CH_2\!\!-\!\!CH\!\!-\!\!\overset{\displaystyle NH_2}{\underset{\displaystyle COOH}{|}}$$

Monodeiodinase

Inactive thyroid hormone
3,3,5-Triiodothyronine (rT₃)

Active thyroid hormone
3,5,3-Triiodothyronine (T₃)

FIGURE 20-2. Metabolism of thyroxine.

thyroxine-binding prealbumin (TBPA), and albumin. The quantity of T_4 and T_3 in the circulation can be significantly impacted by the amount of binding protein available for carrying these hormones. For example, high estrogen levels during pregnancy lead to increased thyroxine-binding protein production by the liver. High TBG levels bind more thyroid hormone, leading to high levels of total T_3 and total T_4. In the euthyroidal state, levels of the active free thyroid hormone remain in the normal range. Because measurement of free T_3 and free T_4 levels could potentially avoid confusion caused by abnormal levels of binding proteins, tests that attempt this feat are today's choice for measuring thyroid hormone levels.

Control of Thyroid Function

The key to correctly interpreting thyroid function testing is an understanding of the *hypothalamic–pituitary–thyroid axis.* This axis works to regular thyroid hormone production. *Thyrotropin-releasing hormone (TRH)* is synthesized by neurons in the supraoptic and supraventricular nuclei of the hypothalamus and stored in the median eminence of the hypothalamus. When secreted, this hormone stimulates cells in the anterior pituitary gland to manufacture and release *thyrotropin (TSH).* TSH, in turn, circulates to the thyroid gland and leads to increased production and release of thyroid hormone. When the hypothalamus and pituitary sense that there is an inadequate amount of thyroid hormone in circulation, TRH and TSH secretion increases and should lead to increased thyroid hormone production. If thyroid hormone levels are high, TRH and TSH release will be inhibited, leading to lower levels of thyroid hormone production. This feedback loop requires a normally functioning hypothalamus, pituitary, and thyroid gland, as well as, an absence of agents that mimic TSH action (Fig. 20-3).

Actions of Thyroid Hormone

Thyroid hormone circulates in the bloodstream. The free T_3 and *free T_4* are available to travel across the cell membrane. In the cytoplasm, T_4 is deiodinated into T_3, the active thyroid hormone. T_3 combines with its nuclear receptor on thyroid hormone-responsive genes, leading to production of messenger RNA and then, in turn, proteins that influence metabolism and development. Effects of thyroid hormone include tissue growth, brain maturation, increased heat production, increased oxygen consumption, and an increased number of β-adrenergic receptors. Clinically, patients who have excess thyroid hormone *(thyrotoxicosis)* will have symptoms of increased metabolism. Patients with hypothyroidism complain of symptoms of low metabolism.

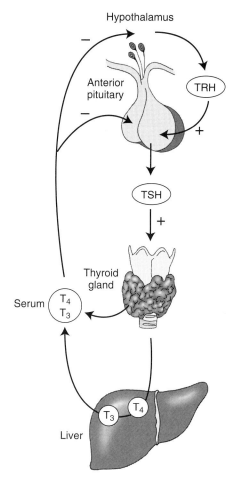

FIGURE 20-3. Hypothalamic–pituitary–thyroid axis. Thyrotropin-releasing hormone (TRH) stimulates the production and release of thyrotropin (TSH). TSH stimulates the thyroid gland to synthesize and secrete thyroid hormone. T_4 that is released by the thyroid gland is mostly converted to T_3 by the liver and kidney. T_3 and T_4 feedback inhibit TSH release directly through action at the pituitary and indirectly by decreasing TRH release from the hypothalamus. (Modified from Surks MI, Sievert R. Drugs and thyroid function. N Engl J Med 1995;333:1688.)

TESTS FOR THYROID EVALUATION

Blood Tests

TSH

The most useful test for assessing thyroid function is the TSH. Over the years, three generations of assays have been developed. All assays have been able to diagnose primary hypothyroidism (thyroid gland disease leading to low thyroid hormone production) with high levels of TSH. Second generation TSH immunometric assays, with detection limits of 0.1 mU/L, can effectively screen for hyperthyroidism, but third generation TSH chemiluminometric assays, with detection limits of 0.01, are less likely to give false-negative results and can more accurately distinguish between a patient with hyperthyroidism and euthyroidism. Second and third generation

TSH assays are routinely used to monitor and adjust thyroid hormone replacement therapy, as well as, screening for both hyperthyroidism and hypothyroidism.[4] Our confidence in these tests has given rise to new diagnoses for mild degrees of thyroid dysfunction, called *subclinical disease*. In *subclinical hypothyroidism*, the TSH is minimally increased, while free T_4 is normal. In *subclinical hyperthyroidism*, the TSH is suppressed, while free T_4 is normal. The value of the TSH assay is based on the fact that small changes in free T_4 levels (often within the normal range) induce a large reciprocal change in the TSH level.[5]

Serum T_4 and T_3

Serum total T_4 and T_3 levels are usually measured by radioimmunoassay (RIA), chemiluminometric assay, or similar immunometric technique. Because more than 99.9% of thyroid hormone is protein-bound, alterations in thyroid hormone-binding proteins, unrelated to thyroid disease, frequently lead to total T_3 and total T_4 levels outside of normal range. For this reason, efforts have been made to develop assays that measure free T_4 and free T_3, the biologically active forms of thyroid hormone.[6] Unfortunately, currently available kits have shortcomings in measuring free T_4 levels. That is, they have difficulty providing accurate free T_4 values through all known binding protein abnormalities.[7] Despite these shortcomings, free T_4 kits have replaced total T_4 determinations at the clinical level, secondary to ease of interpretation and lower processing cost. Kits that estimate free T_3 levels also have theoretic advantages, however, clinical utility is yet to be clearly defined.

Thyroglobulin

Thyroglobulin is synthesized and secreted exclusively by thyroid follicular cells. This prohormone in the circulation is proof of residual thyroid tissue, either benign or malignant. This fact makes thyroglobulin an ideal tumor marker for thyroid cancer patients. Patients with well-differentiated thyroid cancer, who have been treated successfully with surgery and radioactive iodine ablation, should have undetectable thyroglobulin levels.

Thyroglobulin is currently measured by double-antibody radioimmunoassay (RIA), enzyme-linked immunoassay (ELISA), immunoradiometric assay (IRMA), and immunochemiluminescent assay (ICMA) methods. The accuracy of the thyroglobulin assay is primarily dependent on the specificity of the antibody used and the absence of antithyroglobulin autoantibodies. Even with modern assays, antithyroglobulin autoantibodies lead to unreliable thyroglobulin results. For this reason, it is critically important to screen for autoantibodies whenever thyroglobulin is being measured. If antibodies are present, the value of the thyroglobulin assay is marginal. Approximately 25% of patients with well-differentiated thyroid cancer will have antithyroglobulin autoantibodies. This is approximately twice as high as in the general population. If a patient with well-differentiated thyroid cancer and antithyroglobulin autoantibodies has been successfully treated with surgery and radioactive iodine ablation, autoantibodies should disappear over time.[4]

Thyroid Autoimmunity

Many diseases of the thyroid gland are related to autoimmune processes. In autoimmune thyroid disease, antibodies are directed at thyroid tissue with variable responses. The most common cause of hyperthyroidism is an autoimmune disease called *Graves' disease*. The antibody in this condition is directed at the TSH receptor and stimulates the receptor, leading to growth of the thyroid gland and production of excessive amounts of thyroid hormone. This condition can be diagnosed with tests that detect antibodies to the TSH receptor. Thyroid-stimulating antibodies (TSAb, TSI) use a bioassay to determine presence of autoimmune hyperthyroidism. Tests for *TSH receptor antibodies* (TRAb, TSHR-Ab) can detect TSH receptor antibody whether they act to stimulate or block the TSH receptor. Both types of antibody assays will be positive in 70–100% of patients with Graves' disease. Chronic lymphocytic thyroiditis is at the other end of the autoimmune continuum. This is the most common cause of hypothyroidism in the developed world. In this condition, antibodies lead to decreased thyroid hormone production by the thyroid gland. The best test for this condition is the thyroid peroxidase antibody, which is present in 10–15% of the general population and 80–99% of patients with autoimmune hypothyroidism (Table 20-1).

OTHER TOOLS FOR THYROID EVALUATION

Nuclear Medicine Evaluation

Radioactive iodine is useful in assessing the metabolic activity of thyroid tissue and assisting in the evaluation and treatment of thyroid cancer. When radioactive iodine is given orally, a percentage of the dose is taken up by the thyroid gland. This percentage is called the radioactive

TABLE 20-1. PREVALENCE OF THYROID AUTOANTIBODIES

ANTIBODY	GENERAL POPULATION	GRAVES' DISEASE	AUTOIMMUNE HYPOTHYROIDISM
Antithyroglobulin	3%	12–30%	35–60%
Thyroid peroxidase (formerly, antimicrosomal)	10–15%	45–80%	80–99%
Anti-TSH receptor	1–2%	70–100%	6–60%

iodine uptake (RAIU). High uptake suggests that the gland is metabolically active and producing significant amounts of thyroid hormone. Low uptake suggests that the gland is metabolically inactive. Because TSH stimulates iodine uptake by the thyroid gland, it is important to interpret the scan in conjunction with this thyroid function test. An undetectable TSH should turn off the thyroid gland's uptake of iodine. If the uptake is high, with an undetectable TSH, the thyroid is acting autonomously (without regard for the usual feedback system) or through a TSH surrogate. In the case of Graves' disease, an immunoglobulin activates the TSH receptor on the thyroid gland, leading to high rates of thyroid hormone production and a high RAIU. The high level of thyroid hormone in the circulation feeds back on the pituitary and hypothalamus, turning off TSH. Unfortunately, this has no effect on the thyroid-stimulating immunoglobulin (TSH surrogate). If TSH is undetectable with low radioactive iodine uptake, the differential diagnosis includes excess oral thyroid hormone ingestion, high iodine intake, or a condition in which stored thyroid hormone is leaking from the thyroid gland (usually from one of several causes of *subacute thyroiditis*).

Radioactive iodine is also helpful in the evaluation of selected thyroid nodules. Thyroid nodules that take up significant amounts of radioactive iodine on thyroid scans (hot nodules) are unlikely to be thyroid cancer. Unfortunately, the converse does not hold true. Most thyroid nodules are cold or indeterminate on thyroid scan and yet the majority of these nodules are benign.

Thyroid Ultrasound

Thyroid ultrasounds are becoming more important in the assessments of thyroid anatomy and determination of the characteristics of any palpable thyroid abnormality. Thyroid ultrasounds can detect small, often clinically insignificant thyroid nodules. In up to 50% of clinically normal thyroid glands, small (<1 cm) thyroid nodules are seen.[8]

Fine-Needle Aspiration

Thyroid fine-needle aspiration biopsy (FNA) is often the first step and most accurate tool in the evaluation of thyroid nodules. The routine use of FNA biopsy allows prompt identification and treatment of thyroid malignancies and avoids unnecessary surgery in most patients with benign thyroid lesions. In this procedure, patients have small-gauge needles inserted into the nodules, and cells are aspirated for cytologic evaluation.

DISORDERS OF THE THYROID

Hypothyroidism

One of the most common diseases of the thyroid gland is hypothyroidism. This condition is diagnosed by a low free T_4 level (in primary or central hypothyroidism) and/or a high TSH (in primary hypothyroidism). Symptoms of hypothyroidism vary, depending on the degree of hypothyroidism and the rapidity of its development (Table 20-2). When thyroid hormone is significantly decreased, symptoms of cold intolerance, fatigue, dry skin, constipation, hoarseness, dyspnea on exertion, cognitive dysfunction, hair loss, and weight gain are reported. On physical examination, patients with severe hypothyroidism may have low body temperature, slow movements, bradycardia, delay in the relaxation phase of deep tendon reflexes, yellow discoloration of the skin (from hypercarotenemia), hair loss, diastolic hypertension, pleural and pericardial effusions, menstrual irregularities, and periorbital puffiness.

Hypothyroidism can lead to a variety of other abnormalities. Hypothyroidism, through inappropriate levels of antidiuretic hormone, can lead to hyponatremia.[9] Significant hypothyroidism can also lead to myopathy and high levels of creatine phosphokinase (CPK).[10] Anemia can also be seen in hypothyroidism.[11] The etiology of the anemia can be either a result of lower demand for oxygen carrying capacity or through associated autoimmune pernicious anemia. Hypothyroidism can also lead to hyperlipidemia,[12] especially when the TSH is greater than 10 mU/L. One study documented that 4.2% of patients with hyperlipidemia had hypothyroidism.[13] Another study documented that more than one half of patients with hy-

TABLE 20-2. SYMPTOMS AND SIGNS OF HYPOTHYROIDISM

SYMPTOMS	SIGNS
Cold intolerance	Slow movement and slow speech
Dyspnea on exertion	Delayed relaxation of tendon reflexes
Weight gain	Bradycardia
Cognitive dysfunction	Carotenemia
Mental retardation (infant)	Coarse skin
Constipation	Puffy face and loss of eyebrows
Growth failure	Periorbital edema
Dry skin	Enlargement of the tongue
Hoarseness	Diastolic hypertension
Edema	Pleural and pericardial effusions
Myalgia and paresthesia	Ascites
Depression	Galactorrhea
Menorrhagia	
Arthralgia	
Pubertal delay	

CASE STUDY 20-1

A 24-year-old woman presents 2 months postpartum with symptoms of hyperthyroidism. She does not have evidence of Graves' ophthalmopathy. Her TSH level is undetectable and free T_4 is two times the upper limits of normal.

Questions

1. What are possible causes for her thyrotoxicosis?

2. What tests would be useful to sort out the cause of thyrotoxicosis?

pothyroidism had hypercholesterolemia. In all of the conditions listed above (hyponatremia, unexplained high CPK levels, anemia, hyperlipidemia), it is prudent to evaluate for hypothyroidism as a secondary cause.

Hypothyroidism can be divided into primary, secondary, or tertiary disease, dependent on whether the defect is located in the thyroid gland, pituitary gland, or hypothalamus, respectively (Table 20-3). The most common cause of hypothyroidism in developed countries is chronic lymphocytic thyroiditis, or Hashimoto thyroiditis. This is an autoimmune disease of the thyroid gland, which is often associated with enlargement of the thyroid gland (goiter). TPO antibody testing will be positive in 80–99% of patients with chronic lymphocytic thyroiditis. Other common causes of hypothyroidism include iodine deficiency, thyroid surgery, and radioactive iodine treatment. Certain drugs can cause hypothyroidism (Table 20-3). Occasionally, patients will experience transient hypothyroidism associated with inflammation of the thyroid gland. Examples of transient hypothyroidism include recovery from nonthyroidal illness and the hypothyroid phase of one of several forms of subacute thyroiditis (painful thyroiditis, postpartum thyroiditis, and painless thyroiditis).

Hypothyroidism is common; 5–15% of women older than age 65 have this condition. For this reason, several organizations have recommended routine periodic assessment of thyroid function in women.[14,15]

Hypothyroidism is treated with thyroid hormone replacement therapy. Levothyroxine (T_4) is the treatment of choice. In primary hypothyroidism, the goal of therapy is to achieve a normal TSH. If hypothyroidism is of pituitary or hypothalamic origin (secondary or tertiary hypothyroidism), TSH levels will not be useful in managing the condition and a midnormal free T_4 level becomes the target of therapy. Levothyroxine has a half-life of approximately 7 days. When doses of thyroid hormone are changed, it is important to wait at least 5 half-lives before rechecking thyroid function tests to achieve a new steady state.

Thyrotoxicosis

Thyrotoxicosis is a complex of findings that result when peripheral tissue are presented with, and respond to, an excess of thyroid hormone. Thyrotoxicosis can be the result of excessive thyroid hormone ingestion, leakage of stored thyroid hormone from storage in the thyroid follicles, or excessive thyroid gland production of thyroid hormone. The latter form of thyrotoxicosis is called *hyperthyroidism*. The manifestations of thyrotoxicosis vary, depending upon the degree of thyroid hormone elevation and the status of the patient. Symptoms typically include anxiety; emotional lability; weakness; tremor; palpitations; heat intolerance; increased perspiration; and weight loss, despite a normal or increased appetite (Table 20-4).

Graves' Disease

Graves' disease is the most common cause of thyrotoxicosis. It is an autoimmune disease in which antibodies are produced that activate the TSH receptor. Features of

TABLE 20-3. ETIOLOGY OF HYPOTHYROIDISM

	CONDITION	COMMENTS
Primary	Chronic lymphocytic thyroiditis	TPOAb or TgAb are positive in 80–99% of patients
	Radioactive iodine thyroid for toxic goiter	History is key to diagnosis
	Subtotal thyroidectomy for toxic goiter	History and physical examination (neck scar) are key to diagnosis
	Excessive iodine intake	History and urinary iodine useful for diagnosis
	Subacute thyroiditis (painful, painless, or postpartum)	Hypothyroidism is usually transient
Secondary	Hypopituitarism	Caused by pituitary adenoma, pituitary radiation therapy, or pituitary destruction
Tertiary	Hypothalamic dysfunction	Rare

TABLE 20-4. SYMPTOMS AND SIGNS OF THYROTOXICOSIS

SYMPTOMS	SIGNS
Nervousness, irritability, restlessness, shortened attention span, behavior problems	Tachycardia
Tremor	Fine tremor
Palpitations	Warm, moist, flushed, smooth skin
Fatigue or weakness, decreased exercise tolerance	Lid lag, widened palpebral fissures
Weight loss with good appetite	Enlarged thyroid
Hyperdefecation	Brisk reflexes
Heat intolerance and perspiration	Muscular weakness, wasting
Menstrual change; usually oligomenorrhea	Dermopathy (Graves' disease)
Neck mass	Ophthalmopathy (Graves' disease)
Prominence of eyes	
Muscle weakness	

Graves' disease include thyrotoxicosis, goiter, ophthalmopathy (eye changes associated with inflammation and infiltration of periorbital tissue), and dermopathy (skin changes in the lower extremities that have an orange peel texture). There is a strong familial disposition to Graves' disease; 15% of patients will have a close relative with this condition. Females are 5 times as likely as males to develop this condition. Laboratory testing will usually document a high free T_4 and T_3 level, as well as undetectable TSH. TSI and TSH receptor antibodies are usually positive in this condition. RAIU will be elevated, and the thyroid scan will show diffuse uptake (Table 20-5).

Graves' ophthalmopathy can be particularly problematic.[16] Approximately 20–25% of patients with Graves'

CASE STUDY 20-2

A 67-year-old woman is referred for treatment of hyperlipidemia. Her cholesterol and triglycerides are high, despite treatment with lipid lowering medication. She is noted to have hair loss (wearing a wig) and hoarseness to her voice. She complains of cold intolerance and fatigue.

Questions

1. What testing would be helpful to screen for thyroid disease?

2. What treatment would you recommend?

3. What other laboratory abnormalities are commonly seen in hypothyroid patients other than hyperlipidemia and abnormal thyroid function tests?

hyperthyroidism have clinically obvious Graves' ophthalmopathy. With more sensitive testing, such as orbital computed tomography (CT) or magnetic resonance imaging (MRI) scans, most patients with Graves' hyperthyroidism have ophthalmopathy.[17] The findings in Graves' ophthalmopathy can include orbital soft tissue swelling, injection of the conjunctivae, proptosis (forward protrusion of the eye, secondary to infiltration of retroorbital muscles and fat), double vision (secondary to orbital muscle involvement and fibrosis), and corneal disease (often related to difficulty closing the eyelids). Treatment of Graves' ophthalmopathy is controversial. Occasionally, patients require surgical decompression of the orbits to prevent optic nerve injury and blindness.

Thyroid disease associated with Graves' disease is treated with medication, radioactive iodine, or surgery. Initially, most thyrotoxic patients are treated with β-blockers to control symptoms of adrenergic excess, such as tremor and tachycardia. Propylthiouracil (PTU) or methimazole (MMI) can be added to inhibit thyroid hormone biosynthesis and secretion.[18] These medications may also have immunomodulatory effects on the underlying autoimmune disease, helping promote remission of the condition after several months of therapy. Long-term remission rates vary but are generally run between 20% and 50% in the United States. Women seem to be more likely to achieve remission than men. Likewise, patients with small goiters and mild hyperthyroidism are more likely to achieve remissions. Low dietary iodine increases the chance of staying in long-term remission. Patients experiencing such a remission do not require therapy with thyroid hormone replacement.

When radioactive iodine or surgery is used, the goal is to destroy or remove enough thyroid tissue so that the patient becomes hypothyroid. Subsequent lifelong treatment with thyroid hormone replacement therapy is usu-

TABLE 20-5. DISORDERS ASSOCIATED WITH THYROTOXICOSIS

	CONDITION	PATHOGENIC MECHANISM	TSH LEVEL	RADIOACTIVE IODINE UPTAKE (RAIU)	OTHER TESTS IMPORTANT FOR DIAGNOSIS
Hyperthyroidism	Graves' disease	TSH receptor antibodies	Decreased	Increased	TRAb, TSI positive. Image on thyroid scan.
	Toxic adenoma	Benign tumor	Decreased	Increased	Image on thyroid scan.
	Toxic multinodular goiter	Foci of functional autonomy	Decreased	Increased	Image on thyroid scan.
	States of TSH excess	TSH-secreting pituitary tumor	Inappropriately high	Increased	MRI of pituitary
Nonhyper-thyroidism	Painful thyroiditis	Leakage of thyroid hormone.	Decreased	Decreased	Tg inappropriately high
	Postpartum thyroiditis	Leakage of thyroid hormone, autoimmune basis	Decreased	Decreased	TPO antibodies usually high
	Hormone ingestion	Hormone in food or medication	Decreased	Decreased	
	Ectopic thyroid tissue	Functioning metastasis of thyroid tumor; struma ovarii	Decreased	Decreased	Thyroid scan

ally required. Radioactive iodine therapy has been used for treatment of Graves' disease for longer than 50 years and is both generally safe and effective. Surgery is associated with risk of recurrent laryngeal nerve injury, leading to permanent hoarseness and/or injury to the parathyroid glands, causing hypocalcemia secondary to hypoparathyroidism. There are two situations in Graves' disease in which surgery is preferred to other forms of therapy. If there is concern that the patient may have thyroid cancer in addition to Graves' disease, surgery is the best way to insure removal of the potential cancer. In patients with severe ophthalmopathy, some experts in Graves' disease management prefer surgery because of concern that radioactive iodine treatment may cause an acute flaring of associated eye problems.

Toxic Adenomas and Multinodular Goiters

Toxic adenomas and multinodular goiters are two relatively common causes of hyperthyroidism. These conditions are caused by thyroid tissue that is autonomous in function. Neither TSH nor TSH receptor-stimulating immunoglobulin is required to stimulate thyroid hormone production. In some toxic nodules, mutations have been identified. These mutations have the same effect as chronic stimulation of the TSH receptor on thyroid hormone production. Clinically, toxic adenomas present in patients with hyperthyroidism and a palpable thyroid nod-

ule. On thyroid scan, the nodules are "hot," that is, they avidly take up radioactive iodine. The radioactive iodine uptake is also inappropriately high for the suppressed level of TSH. In toxic multinodular goiters, there are multiple areas within the thyroid gland that are autonomously producing thyroid hormone. Treatment for these two conditions involves surgery, radioactive iodine, or medication (MMI or PTU). Although the medications can block thyroid hormone production in these patients, they are not expected to lead to remission in these two conditions. Often, the toxic nodules produce so much thyroid hormone that the rest of the thyroid gland is suppressed and metabolically inactive. When radioactive iodine is given, it tends to destroy only the hyperactive (autonomous) portions of the thyroid gland, leaving normal (suppressed) thyroid tissue undamaged. The patient so treated, will often be left with normal thyroid function without the need for thyroid hormone replacement therapy.

DRUG-INDUCED THYROID DYSFUNCTION

Amiodarone-Induced Thyroid Disease

Several drugs other than PTU and methimazole can affect thyroid function. Amiodarone, used to treat cardiac arrhythmias, is one of these drugs.[19] It is fat-soluble and, therefore, has a long (50 days) half-life in the body. The fact that 37% of the molecular weight of amiodarone is iodine accounts for a significant part of the thyroid dysfunction seen. Iodine, when given in large doses, acutely leads to inhibition of thyroid hormone production. This is called the Wolff-Chaikoff effect. Amiodarone also blocks T_4 to T_3 conversion. The combination of these two actions leads to hypothyroidism in 8–20% of patients on chronic therapy. Amiodarone can also lead to hyperthyroidism in 3% of patients treated chronically with this medication. Certain patients develop hyperthyroidism as they escape the Wolff-Chaikoff effect and use the excess iodine for thyroid hormone production. Others develop hyperthyroidism if the medication leads to inflammation of the thyroid gland (subacute thyroiditis) and subsequent leakage of stored thyroid hormone into the circulation.

Subacute Thyroiditis

Several conditions occur that lead to transient changes in thyroid hormone levels.[20] These conditions are associated with inflammation of the thyroid gland, leakage of stored thyroid hormone, and then repair of the gland. Although nomenclature varies between authors, grouping together postpartum thyroiditis, painless thyroiditis, and painful thyroiditis as forms of subacute thyroiditis is one of the simplest classification schemes. These conditions are often associated with a thyrotoxic phase when thyroid hormone is leaking into the circulation, a hypothyroid phase when the thyroid gland is repairing itself, and a euthyroid phase when the gland is repaired. These phases can last for weeks to months.

Postpartum thyroiditis is the most common form of subacute thyroiditis. It occurs in 3–16% of women postpartum.[21] It is strongly associated with the TPO antibodies and chronic lymphocytic thyroiditis. Patients may experience thyrotoxicosis followed by hypothyroidism or simply hypothyroidism or hyperthyroidism. Thyroid hormone levels usually return to normal after several months, however, by 4 years postpartum, 25–50% of patients have persistent hypothyroidism, goiter, or both.[22] During the thyrotoxic phase, β-blockers can be used if treatment is necessary. During the hypothyroid phase, thyroid hormone replacement therapy can be given, usually for 3–6 months, unless permanent hypothyroidism evolves. The thyrotoxic phase of this condition, as well as other forms of subacute thyroiditis, can be distinguished from Graves' disease by a low RAIU and an absence of TSI- or TSH-receptor antibodies. Painless thyroiditis or subacute lymphocytic thyroiditis shares many characteristics of postpartum thyroiditis, except there is no associated pregnancy.

Painful thyroiditis, also called *subacute granulomatous, subacute nonsuppurative thyroiditis,* or *de Quervain's thyroiditis* is characterized by neck pain, low-grade fever, myalgia, a tender diffuse goiter, and swings in thyroid function tests (as discussed above). Viral infections are felt to trigger this condition. TPO antibodies are usually absent; erythrocyte sedimentation rate and thyroglobulin levels are often elevated.

NONTHYROIDAL ILLNESS

Hospitalized patients, especially critically ill patients, often have abnormalities in their thyroid function tests. Typically, the laboratory pattern is one of low T_4, FT_4 and (sometimes) TSH. Because illness decreases 5'-monodeiodinase activity, less T_4 is converted to active T_3. This leads to decreased levels of T_3 and higher levels of reverse T_3. There also seems to be an element of central hypothyroidism and thyroid hormone-binding changes associated with severe illness. It is believed that many of these changes are an appropriate adaptation to illness and thyroid hormone replacement therapy is not indicated.

THYROID NODULES

Thyroid nodules are common. Clinically apparent thyroid nodules are present in 6.4% of adult women and 1.5% of adult men, according to Framingham data.[23] Thyroid ultrasound finds unsuspected thyroid nodules in 20–45% of women and 17–25% of men.[24] The major concern with thyroid nodules is that they may represent a thyroid cancer. Fortunately, only 5–9% of thyroid nodules prove to be thyroid cancer. Fine-needle aspiration (FNA) of these nodules, with cytologic examination of the aspirate, has become a routine practice to help determine the nodules that require surgical removal from those that do not.[25]

SUMMARY

The thyroid gland is responsible for production of thyroid hormone. Two types of metabolically active thyroid hormones are produced—T_4 and T_3. Most T_4 released by the thyroid gland is converted in the periphery to metabolically active T_3. These hormones are critical in regulating body metabolism, neurologic development, and numerous other body functions. Thyroid hormone deficiency is common and usually diagnosed with an elevated TSH on lab testing. Patients with this condition often have symptoms related to slow metabolism. Thyrotoxicosis is the result of excess thyroid hormone. Clinically, patients with this condition have undetectable levels of TSH and elevated levels of T_3 and free T_4. Thyroid conditions tend to be very treatable. It is important to be familiar with the symptoms, diagnostic tests, and treatment algorithms of thyroid disease.

REVIEW QUESTIONS

1. All of the following statements about iodine are true EXCEPT:
   a. Iodine deficiency is one of the most common causes of hypothyroidism in the world.
   b. T_4 has 4 iodine molecules.
   c. Radioactive iodine treatment of Graves' disease is effective in less than 40% of patients treated with this agent.
   d. Radioactive iodine uptake is often useful in determining the cause of thyrotoxicosis.

2. The fetus:
   a. is dependent on thyroid hormone for normal neurologic development.
   b. does not develop a thyroid gland until the third trimester.
   c. is not susceptible to damage from radioactive iodine therapy given the mother.
   d. will be born with hypothyroidism in approximately 1 of 400 births in developed countries.

3. The thyroid gland:
   a. is an ineffective iodine trap.
   b. depends on thyroidal peroxidase (TPO) to permit iodination of the tyrosyl residues to make MIT and DIT.
   c. depends on thyroidal peroxidase (TPO) to permit the joining of two DIT residues to form T_3.
   d. usually functions independent of TSH levels.

4. The thyroid gland produces all of the following EXCEPT:
   a. TSH.
   b. thyroglobulin.
   c. T_3.
   d. T_4.

5. Hypothyroidism is generally associated with all of the following EXCEPT:
   a. weight gain.
   b. an elevation of TSH levels.
   c. TPO antibodies.
   d. TSH-receptor antibodies.

6. A 34-year-old woman presents with goiter, tachycardia, and weight loss of 2 months duration. TSH is undetectable and free T_4 is high. All of the following tests are useful in diagnosing the cause of the hyperthyroidism EXCEPT:
   a. TSH receptor antibodies.
   b. RAIU.
   c. fine-needle aspiration biopsy of the thyroid gland.
   d. TSH.

7. A 65-year-old woman presents with fatigue, hypothermia, pericardial effusions, and hair loss. Her thyroid function tests show a significantly elevated TSH and a low free T_4. All of the following laboratory test abnormalities may be associated with her underlying condition EXCEPT:
   a. an elevated cholesterol level.
   b. anemia.
   c. elevated CPK levels.
   d. elevated WBC.

8. A 26-year-old man presents with a 3-cm, right lobe, thyroid nodule and a normal TSH. What is the next test that should be performed?
   a. FNA of the nodule
   b. Free T_4 level
   c. Thyroid ultrasound
   d. Thyroid scan

9. The following are treatment options for hyperthyroidism associated with Graves' disease EXCEPT:
   a. PTU.
   b. β-blockers.
   c. radioactive iodine.
   d. thyroid hormone.

10. All of the following abnormalities might be expected in a severely ill patient EXCEPT:
    a. low T_4.
    b. low T_3.
    c. low TSH.
    d. low reverse T_3.

REFERENCES

1. Greenspan FS. The thyroid gland. In: Greenspan FS, Strewler GJ, eds. Basic & Clinical Endocrinology, 5th ed. New York: Appleton & Lange, 1997.
2. Lavin L. Manual of Endocrinology, 2nd ed. Boston: Little, Brown & Co., 1994:395.
3. Utiger TD. Thyroid hormone synthesis and physiology. www.UpToDate.com, online 11.1, 2002.
4. Ross DS. Laboratory assessment of thyroid function. www.UpToDate.com, online 11.1, 2002.
5. Spencer CA, LoPresiti JS, Patel A, et al. Applications of a new chemiluminometric thyrotropin assay to subnormal measurement. J Clin Endocrinol Metab 1990;70(2):453–460.
6. Ekins R. The free hormone hypothesis and measurement of free hormones (editorial). Clin Chem 1992;38(7):1289–1293.

7. Wong TK, Pekary AE, Hoo GS, et al. Comparison of methods for measuring free thyroxin in nonthyroidal illness. Clin Chem 1992; 38(5):720–724.

8. Tan GH, Gharib H. Thyroid incidentalomas: management approaches to nonpalpable nodules discovered incidentally on thyroid imaging. Ann Intern Med 1997;126:226.

9. Skowsky WR, Kikuchi TA. The role of vasopressin in the impaired water excretion of myxedema. Am J Med 1987;64(4): 613–621.

10. Khaleeli AA, Gohil K, McPhail G, et al. Muscle morphology and metabolism in hypothyroid myopathy: effects of treatment. J Clin Pathol 1983;36(5):519–526.

11. Green ST, Ng JP. Hypothyroidism and anaemia. Biomed Pharmacother 1986;40(9):326–331.

12. Diekman T, Lansberg PJ, Kastelein JJ, Wiersinga WM. Prevalence and correction of hypothyroidism in a large cohort of patients referred for dyslipidemia. Arch Intern Med 1995;155(14):1490–1495.

13. O'Brien T, Dinneen SF, O'Brien PC, Palumbo PJ. Hyperlipidemia in patients with primary and secondary hypothyroidism. Mayo Clin Proc 1993;68(9):860–866.

14. American College of Physicians. Clinical Guideline, Part 1. Screening for thyroid disease. Ann Intern Med 1998;129(2): 141–143.

15. Ladenson PW, Singer PA, Ain KB, et al. American Thyroid Association guidelines for detection of thyroid dysfunction. Arch Intern Med 2000;160(11):1573–1575.

16. Burch HB, Wartofsky L. Graves' ophthalmopathy: current concepts regarding pathogenesis and management. Endocr Rev 1993;14(6):747–793.

17. Villadolid MC, Yokoyama N, Izumi M, et al. Untreated Graves' disease patients without clinical ophthalmopathy demonstrate a high frequency of extraocular muscle (EOM) enlargement by magnetic resonance. J Clin Endocrinol Metab 1995;80(9):2830–2833.

18. Solomon BL, Evaul JE, Burman KD, Wartofsky L. Remission rates with antithyroid drug therapy: continuing influence of iodine intake? Ann Intern Med 1987;107(4):510–512.

19. Nademanee K, Singh BN, Callahan B, et al. Amiodarone, thyroid hormone indexes, and altered thyroid function: long-term serial effects in patients with cardiac arrhythmias. Am J Cardiol 1986; 58(10):981–986.

20. Burman KD. Overview of thyroiditis. www.UpToDate.com, online 11.1, 2002.

21. Gerstein HC. How common is postpartum thyroiditis? A methodologic overview of the literature. Arch Intern Med 1990;150(7): 1397–1400.

22. Othman S, Phillips DI, Parkes AB, et al. A long-term follow-up of postpartum thyroiditis. Clin Endocrinol (Oxf) 1990;32(5): 559–564.

23. Vander JB, Gaston EA, Dawber TG. The significance of nontoxic thyroid nodules. Ann Intern Med 1968;69:537.

24. Brander A, Viikinkoski P, Nickels J, et al. Thyroid gland: US screening in a random adult population. Radiology 1991;181:683.

25. Ezzat S, Sarti DA, et al. Thyroid incidentalomas: prevalence by palpation and ultrasonography. Arch Intern Med 1994;154:1838.

26. Gharif H. Changing concepts in the diagnosis and management of thyroid nodules. Endocrinol Metab Clin North Am 1997;26: 777.

Parathyroid Function and Control for Calcium Homeostasis

CHAPTER 21

Thomas P. Knecht, Lauren E. Knecht

CHAPTER OUTLINE

- **CALCIUM HOMEOSTASIS**
  Hormonal Control of Calcium Metabolism
- **ORGAN PHYSIOLOGY AND CALCIUM METABOLISM**
  Gastrointestinal
  Renal
  Bone
- **HYPERCALCEMIA**
  Signs and Symptoms of Hypercalcemia
  Causes of Hypercalcemia
- **HYPOCALCEMIA**
  Signs and Symptoms of Hypocalcemia
  Causes of Hypocalcemia
- **DRUGS THAT AFFECT CALCIUM METABOLISM**
- **METABOLIC BONE DISEASES**
  Rickets and Osteomalacia
  Osteoporosis
- **SUMMARY**
- **REVIEW QUESTIONS AND ANSWERS**
- **REFERENCES**

OBJECTIVES

Upon completion of this chapter, the clinical laboratorian should be able to:
- Describe the endocrine and organ physiology of calcium metabolism.
- Discuss the laboratory tools used to evaluate calcium metabolism.
- Apply the laboratory tools to clinical disease states of calcium metabolism.

KEY TERMS

1,25-Dihydroxy vitamin D (1,25(OH)$_2$D)
25-Hydroxy vitamin D
Bisphosphonates
Bone turnover
Calcium-sensing receptor
Cinacalcet
Cortical bone

Dual-energy x-ray absorptiometry (DEXA)
Hypercalcemia
Hypocalcemia
Lithium
Osteoblast
Osteoclast
Osteomalacia

Osteoporosis
Parathyroid hormone (PTH)
Parathyroid hormone-related protein (PTHrP)
Rickets
Teriparatide
Thiazide diuretics

Trabecular bone (also known as *cancellous bone*, although not used as commonly and not used in this chapter)
Vitamin D

CALCIUM HOMEOSTASIS

In classic physiologic fashion, under normal, healthy circumstances, with intact endocrine and organ physiology, calcium metabolism is in balance in the human and normal ranges are preserved. This chapter reviews the endocrine and organ physiology responsible for the control of blood calcium and how disorders of these systems can cause disease.[1] Any understanding of calcium metabolism requires a review of the organs involved in calcium homeostasis and the hormonal systems that affect the organ physiology (Fig. 21-1).

In understanding calcium homeostasis, it is essential to understand which parameter of "calcium" is the target of regulation. Blood calcium (serum calcium from an analyte standpoint) is teleologically what the endocrine/organ system network has evolved to maintain a "normal" range.[2,3] As hormones, glands, organs, and tissue are discussed, keep in mind that it is blood calcium that the body has an integrated network to maintain "within normal limits." The cellular and tissue effects of calcium, involving contractile machinery, structural roles, roles in enzymatic reactions, and so on, all depend on blood calcium being within normal limits.

The circulating (blood) pool of calcium is in constant flux. Calcium enters the blood pool, and calcium leaves the blood pool. Because blood calcium is the centric commodity in calcium homeostasis, it is useful to consider factors that put calcium into the blood (the "into blood" factors) and factors that remove calcium from the blood (the "out of blood" factors) (Fig. 21-1). The principal organs involved in this flux are the small intestine, the skeleton (bone), and the kidneys. All calcium that enters the body after birth arrives via gastrointestinal (GI) absorption. Dietary calcium, therefore, plays a crucial role in calcium homeostasis as the only "outside" source of calcium to the body. Bone, the chief reservoir of calcium in the body, can serve to remove calcium from the blood to be stored in bone and release calcium stored in bone to the blood. Other than inconsequential losses from the body via the GI tract, sweat, and saliva, the only real net loss of calcium from the body occurs via the kidneys in urine.

In reviewing calcium homeostasis, we will first review the hormones involved in the control of blood calcium, and then the organs that play the principal roles in calcium homeostasis. How hormonal regulation of organ/tissue function maintains blood calcium will be demonstrated and how various disease processes interfere with one or more steps in this regulatory network, and, in so doing, disrupt calcium homeostasis will be considered.

Hormonal Control of Calcium Metabolism

Two hormones play the dominant role in the endocrine regulation of calcium homeostasis: parathyroid hormone (PTH) and vitamin D. These hormones play vital roles in regulation of organ/tissue function to maintain blood calcium in the normal range.

Vitamin D

Before outlining *vitamin D* physiology, it should be noted that vitamin D is, in reality, a hormone. As is generally true of hormones, vitamin D is made at a site or sites different from the organs whose function it affects.[4] It is referred to as a vitamin based on historical terms, and the terminology has adhered. Vitamin D shares striking similarities in origin with steroid hormones; that is, vitamin D is a metabolic product of the cholesterol synthetic pathway. The tissues involved in vitamin D synthesis are the skin, liver, and kidneys (Fig. 21-2), and the tissue function affected is gut, bone, and parathyroids.[4]

De novo synthesis of vitamin D begins in the skin, where 7-dehydrocholesterol is transformed to vitamin D_3 by the action of ultraviolet light. Vitamin D_3 is biologically inert and must be further metabolized to the biologically active metabolite.

An enzyme in the liver, hepatic 25-hydroxylase, metabolizes vitamin D_3 to 25-hydroxy vitamin D. Hepatic 25-hydroxylase is not regulated by any component of the calcium homeostatic system and functions constitutively to hydroxylate vitamin D_3 at the 25-position of the sterol ring system. 25-hydroxy vitamin D is the blood test used to assess adequacy of vitamin D stores in the body. 25-hydroxy vitamin D levels are low in most forms of rickets and osteomalacia (vide infra).

An enzyme in the kidneys, renal 1α-hydroxylase, completes the metabolism of vitamin D to the active metabolite, *1,25-dihydroxy vitamin D (1,25(OH)$_2$D)*. Re-

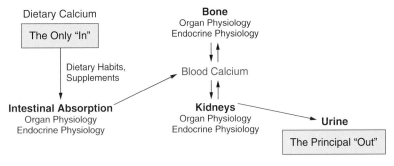

Dietary Calcium
The Only "In"

Dietary Habits, Supplements

Intestinal Absorption
Organ Physiology
Endocrine Physiology

Bone
Organ Physiology
Endocrine Physiology

Blood Calcium

Kidneys
Organ Physiology
Endocrine Physiology

▶ **Urine**

The Principal "Out"

FIGURE 21-1. Calcium homeostasis. Tissue and organs involved in calcium homeostasis (gut, skeleton, and kidneys) and how they relate to blood calcium. Also shown is the means of getting calcium de novo into the system (GI absorption) and elimination of calcium from the system (renal excretion) under normal physiologic conditions.

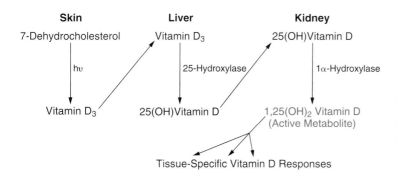

FIGURE 21-2. Vitamin D synthesis. Tissues involved in the synthesis of vitamin D and the steps that each tissue is responsible for. Also shown are enzymes responsible for the two enzymatically mediated steps (hepatic 25-hydroxylation and renal 1α-hydroxylation). The product of this pathway, 1,25(OH)$_2$ vitamin D, is responsible for the tissue-specific effects of vitamin D.

nal 1α-hydroxylase is an enzyme regulated by *parathyroid hormone (PTH);* PTH stimulates renal 1α-hydroxylase and, therefore, stimulates synthesis of the active metabolite of vitamin D, 1,25(OH)$_2$D.

Age, exposure to sunlight, and latitude can influence adequacy of vitamin D. Older individuals, those with little or no sunlight exposure, and those in more northern or southern latitudes are more likely to develop vitamin D deficiency (if not supplemented in the diet).

Vitamin D can also be obtained from dietary sources. Vitamin D is relatively rare in most typical foods consumed by North Americans, were it not for fortification. The only commonly encountered dietary sources of vitamin D are vitamins (especially multivitamins, or supplements specified to contain vitamin D), and vitamin D-fortified milk. Milk is fortified by ultraviolet irradiation, in a manner similar to ultraviolet light striking the skin and mediating the formation of vitamin D$_3$. Multivitamins generally supply 400 units of vitamin D$_3$, about the same amount obtained from a quart of vitamin D-fortified milk. Other than these more common sources, cod liver oil is also a source of vitamin D.

As referred to above, there are evolutionary similarities between vitamin D and steroid hormones. The cho-

lesterol biosynthetic pathway provides the precursors for vitamin D and steroid hormones. There is further evolutionary relationship, in that the vitamin D receptor is in the same supergene family as the receptors for steroid hormones, thyroid hormone, retinoid receptors, and several "orphan" receptors (these orphan receptors have no known ligand; some appear to function via regulation of phosphorylation status). As with all receptors in this supergene family, the vitamin D receptor is a nuclear receptor and carries out physiologic regulation by directing transcription of specific vitamin D responsive genes. 1,25(OH)$_2$D is the natural ligand for the vitamin D receptor.

The 1,25(OH)$_2$D–vitamin D receptor complex binds to the vitamin D response element upstream (5') of the transcription start site of vitamin D–influenced genes and influences gene transcription by interacting with other transcriptional elements and RNA polymerase to regulate transcription of the gene in question (Fig. 21-3).

The physiologic influence of vitamin D is carried out by only a few organ systems/tissues. In small intestinal epithelial (primarily duodenal) cells, 1,25(OH)$_2$D upregulates expression of numerous genes that stimulate transepithelial calcium transport from the intestinal lu-

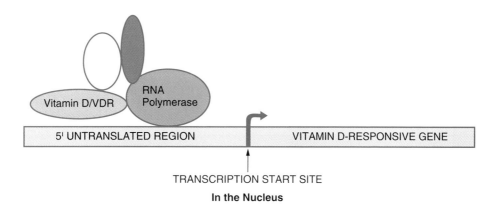

FIGURE 21-3. Vitamin D mechanism of action. DNA binding and interaction with other components of the transcriptional machinery of the vitamin D–vitamin D receptor complex are shown. Note the striking evolutionary similarity between this mechanism and that of other steroid and thyroid hormones. As prime examples, vitamin D inhibits transcription of the PTH gene in parathyroid tissue and stimulates transcription of the calcium transporter in the intestinal brush border epithelium.

men into the blood. The site of greatest absorption is the duodenum. $1,25(OH)_2D$ also stimulates absorption of phosphate.

In bone, $1,25(OH)_2D$ stimulates terminal differentiation of *osteoclast* precursors to osteoclasts. $1,25(OH)_2D$ also stimulates *osteoblasts* to influence osteoclasts to mobilize bone calcium. $1,25(OH)_2D$ does not directly affect *mature* osteoclast physiology. $1,25(OH)_2D$ plays an important role in bone mineralization; abnormal bone results when vitamin D is deficient or has defective metabolism.

As noted above, $1,25(OH)_2D$ increases blood calcium by augmenting intestinal absorption of luminal calcium. Blood calcium feeds back to parathyroid tissue and affects synthesis and secretion of PTH (further discussed below). However, $1,25(OH)_2D$ also has direct transcriptional control over PTH gene in the parathyroids. The $1,25(OH)_2D$–vitamin D receptor complex binds to the vitamin D response element upstream of the PTH gene and downregulates PTH gene transcription. This is a classic case of endocrine regulation of tissue function (Fig. 21-4): PTH stimulates production of $1,25(OH)_2D$, and $1,25(OH)_2D$, in turn, feeds back to decrease PTH secretion, all to maintain blood calcium in the normal range.

Parathyroid Hormone

Physiologically, PTH preserves blood calcium and phosphate in the normal range.[5] There are normally four parathyroid glands, usually found in the region of the thyroid gland (therefore, the name *parathyroid*). Sometimes, one or more parathyroid glands are found *within* the thyroid gland. Parathyroid glands may also be found outside their normal anatomic site, lying anywhere between the hyoid bone in the neck and the mediastinum.

To reemphasize, the name parathyroid refers only to anatomic proximity to the thyroid gland; there is no metabolic relationship between the thyroid gland and the parathyroids. When measuring PTH, the *intact* molecule (intact parathyroid hormone, intact PTH, PTH_i) should be the analyte assayed, not the older midmolecule assay or any other fragments of the intact molecule.[6]

PTH acts primarily to raise blood calcium; low blood calcium is the primary signal to the parathyroids to affect this response. PTH acts on bone (to cause bone resorption and increase blood calcium) and the kidneys (to increase fractional reabsorption of [glomerularly filtered] renal tubular calcium and, therefore, increase blood calcium). It also stimulates renal 1α-hydroxylation of 25-hydroxy vitamin D, to produce $1,25(OH)_2D$, the active metabolite of vitamin D; in so doing, PTH indirectly stimulates intestinal absorption of calcium, contributing to increasing blood calcium. PTH also lowers blood phosphate levels.

There is a *calcium-sensing receptor* in the parathyroid glands.[5] This receptor is in the seven-transmembrane spanning family of receptors. The calcium-sensing receptor senses ambient blood calcium and responds by contributing to regulation of PTH secretion. The PTH response to ambient calcium centers on a set point, with steeper PTH responses occurring near the middle of the normal range for blood calcium (Fig. 21-5). The calcium-sensing receptor senses if ambient calcium is too low and PTH secretion is increased. Increased circulating PTH increases bone resorption, causes renal retention of calcium (tubular reabsorption of calcium in glomerular filtrate), and stimulates intestinal absorption of calcium (via the effect of PTH on $1,25(OH)_2D$ production). In response to this concert, ambient calcium rises. Rising calcium, in turn, feeds back to the parathyroid glands. If blood calcium becomes too high, this is sensed by the calcium-sensing receptor and PTH secretion is suppressed, allowing more urinary loss of calcium and calcium to remain in bone and (by not stimulating production of $1,25(OH)_2D$) not stimulating intestinal absorption of calcium. The suppression of PTH by elevated calcium levels is used clinically to assess a cause of hypercalcemia (vide infra).

In summary, PTH regulates blood calcium concentration and vitamin D metabolism, which feed back to the parathyroids to regulate PTH secretion—yet another example of exquisite endocrine regulation of physiology.

As with all hormones, PTH mediates its effect by high affinity, saturable binding to a specific receptor.[5] The PTH receptor is a transmembrane protein receptor that mediates the PTH effect, at least in part, by activation of the enzyme adenylate cyclase and the second messenger pathway involving cyclic AMP (cAMP), with its effects on protein phosphorylation. An interesting example of molecular medicine is the disease *pseudohypoparathy-*

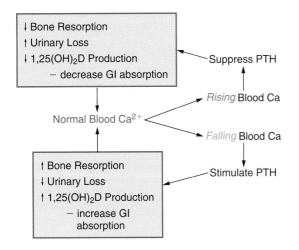

FIGURE 21-4. Calcium, PTH, and vitamin D feedforward and feedback loops. The endocrine response to shifts in blood calcium (rising or falling) is shown. A concerted hormone response, mediated at the organ level by the organs shown in Figure 21-1, helps restore blood calcium toward normal.

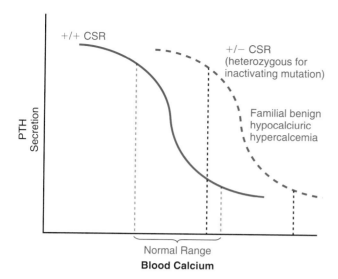

FIGURE 21-5. Calcium-sensing receptor: effect on PTH secretion. Shown is the response of parathyroid tissue (as demonstrated by PTH secretion) to blood calcium. The *set point* is determined by the parathyroid response mediated by the transmembrane calcium-sensing receptor. The *normal curve* is for heterozygosity for the "wild-type" calcium-sensing receptor (+/+). The *right-shifted curve* is shown for the case where there is heterozygosity for the receptor (familial benign hypocalciuric hypercalcemia): one wild-type copy of the gene and one inactivating mutation (+/–).

roidism, which will be discussed further in the section on hypocalcemia. This is a disease in which there is an inactivating mutation in the stimulatory G protein (Gs) that couples the PTH receptor to adenylate cyclase. Uncoupling the PTH receptor from adenylate cyclase makes the PTH target tissue unresponsive to PTH, although PTH is present and, in fact, elevated compared to normal (thus, *pseudo*hypoparathyroidism).[7]

ORGAN PHYSIOLOGY AND CALCIUM METABOLISM

As noted above, three organ systems dominate the organ system contribution to calcium metabolism: the GI tract, the kidneys, and bone.

Gastrointestinal

Normal intestinal function is required for calcium absorption.[8] Interruptions in intestinal function, such as may be seen with short bowel syndromes, genetic or physiologic defects, may affect calcium absorption. Normal vitamin D availability and metabolism is required for optimal calcium absorption. Adequate dietary calcium intake is required. Duodenal calcium can be roughly doubled by $1,25(OH)_2D$, from about 30% of that ingested to about 60–70% of that ingested. It should be noted that dietary phosphate can bind dietary calcium in the intestinal lumen, form the insoluble precipitate calcium phosphate, and prevent absorption of both calcium and phosphate. The insolubility of calcium phosphate is reflected in its solubility product constant, K_{sp}, which equals 1.2×10^{-29}. This is the basis for calcium carbonate use as a phosphate binder in patients with renal failure. For this reason, a diet high in phosphate (*eg,* a junk food diet or high consumption of dark soda pops) will tend to inhibit calcium absorption.

Renal

The kidneys play an essential role in calcium metabolism.[9] The role of the kidneys in vitamin D metabolism is crucial. This accounts for a major source of disordered calcium metabolism, renal failure (failure to make $1,25(OH)_2D$, suboptimal intestinal absorption of calcium, elevated

---

CASE STUDY 21-1

A 40-year-old woman presented to her physician complaining of terrible left flank pain that began the previous night. She reported the pain is worse than giving birth. She also reported blood in her urine earlier that day. She has felt fatigued, more forgetful, and as if her concentration has not been as good for about a year or so. She has no significant past medical history, is taking no medications, and family history is noncontributory. On physical exam, she looks to be in acute pain. There is marked tenderness on gentle percussion over the left costovertebral angle. Blood is drawn and notable for calcium, 11.2 mg/dL (normal, 8.5–10.2 mg/dL); albumin, 3.8 g/dL (normal, 3.5–4.8 g/dL), and intact PTH, 162 pg/mL (nor-

mal, 11–54 pg/mL). Renal function is normal (BUN, 25; creatinine, 0.9). Urine analysis is notable for blood, and >50 RBC per high power field. This prompts a 24-hour urine collection, which reveals calcium elevated at 483 mg/24 hours (normal, 100–250 mg/24 hours).

Questions

1. Which lab results are abnormal?

2. What is the presumptive diagnosis for this patient? The differential diagnosis?

3. What treatment is indicated for this disease?

PTH, inability of the failing kidneys to regulate calcium and phosphate excretion, ectopic calcium phosphate deposition in soft tissues, and poor bone health).

The kidneys respond to PTH in several key ways, preserving blood calcium and preventing hypocalcemia. The role of PTH in stimulating renal 1α-hydroxylation of 25(OH) vitamin D has been reviewed above. PTH also stimulates the tubular reabsorption of calcium from the glomerular filtrate, returning filtered calcium to the blood, preserving blood calcium, and preventing hypocalcemia.

In discussing renal physiology in relation to calcium homeostasis, it is important to differentiate between fractional reabsorption of calcium from the tubule and net excreted load of calcium. In hypercalcemia resulting from primary hyperparathyroidism and in the setting of hypercalcemia from most other causes, the filtered load of calcium is greatly increased. Although PTH stimulates tubular reabsorption of calcium, considering the greater filtered load, *net* calcium excretion is still increased compared with the normal (nonhyperparathyroid) state. Hypercalciuria results as a standard component of primary hyperparathyroidism. It should be noted that hypercalciuria from any cause poses an increased risk for calcium-containing kidney stones. This explains what may seem paradoxical increased fractional renal reabsorption of calcium and the increased risk of calcium stones in primary hyperparathyroidism. Indeed, hypercalcemia of almost any cause increases calcium stone risk.

Bone

A coupled process takes place throughout life in bone with bone formation and bone resorption, which is often referred to as *bone turnover*.[10] This process is normally tightly coupled, so that the one does not occur without the other. Bone formation is mediated by osteoblasts and bone resorption is mediated by osteoclasts (a cell in the monocyte/macrophage lineage). It is interesting that the osteoclasts required to mobilize skeletal calcium do not express receptors for either 1,25(OH)$_2$D or PTH, the principal hormones that stimulate bone resorption. Instead, these hormones act directly on the osteoblasts that, in turn, produce a complex array of cytokines, which then activate the osteoclasts and cause bone resorption and liberation of skeletal calcium. When the coupling of bone formation mediated by osteoblasts and bone resorption mediated by osteoclasts is uncoupled, so that the rate of resorption exceeds the rate of formation (favoring net resorption), the overall effect over time is to lose bone mass. Net bone resorption can affect skeletal health, leading to loss of bone mass and deteriorating skeletal microarchitecture, increasing fracture risk.

The two main types of bone in the skeleton are *trabecular bone* and *cortical bone*.[11] Cortical bone is the main type of bone in the long bones. Cortical bone is strong in the axial and cross-sectional dimensions and, therefore, well suited to the needs of the long bones. Trabecular bone consists of billions of crosshair connections, called *trabeculae*. Because of these interconnected trabeculae, trabecular bone is strong and the bone that gives compact bone, such as vertebral bodies in the spine, strength and integrity. Trabecular and cortical bone vary in their contribution to different skeletal sites. Long bones are essentially cortical and vertebral bodies in the spinal column are essentially trabecular. Other skeletal sites are a combination of cortical and trabecular bone, including the femoral neck, the distal radius, and the proximal humerus. It is primarily trabecular bone that is subject to bone loss due to hypogonadism (consider menopause) or pharmacologic doses of glucocorticoids (prednisone) that, in turn, are associated with increased fracture risk.

To summarize, calcium homeostasis is a complex balance between into blood and out of blood factors, which reflects integrated endocrine and organ physiology. It is this balance that achieves normal calcium metabolism; when disturbed, the result is alterations in calcium metabolism that can lead to various medical conditions that will be discussed below.

HYPERCALCEMIA

Hypercalcemia is the state of blood calcium levels above the normal range.[12] Ionized (free) calcium is the biologically active component of circulating calcium. About one half of circulating calcium is complexed (bound) with serum proteins, primarily albumin, with the remaining one half ionized (free). When total calcium is measured in a serum chemistry panel, remember that only about one half is ionized. Therefore, total calcium is of limited value unless its value is considered in the context of the patient's serum albumin. Patients with low serum albumin would be expected to have low total calcium and normal ionized calcium; vise versa for patients with high serum albumin. Ordering an ionized calcium level can eliminate this caveat. This is a direct measurement of free calcium and reflects calcium status, without the need to consider the fraction bound to serum proteins. Ionized calcium best correlates with biologic activity of calcium, as well as with symptoms of hypercalcemia or hypocalcemia when calcium is outside the normal range. Ionized calcium binding to proteins is a function of pH; more calcium binds at more alkaline pH and less at more acidic pH. Arterial blood, which should have a pH of 7.4, generally has more protein-bound calcium than venous blood, which should have a pH of about 7.2. Because of the arterial-venous difference in ionized calcium, it used to be measured in arterial blood. Now it is possible to measure ionized calcium in venous blood; the clinical lab calculates what the equivalent ionized calcium at pH 7.4 would be and reports that value.

Signs and Symptoms of Hypercalcemia

The signs and symptoms of hypercalcemia may be protean and depend on the degree of hypercalcemia. Clinically, the signs and symptoms vary among patients as to what levels of blood calcium incur (comorbid conditions may also influence the development of symptoms).[12] The signs and symptoms are generally described by organ system:

- Central nervous system (CNS): patients may have altered CNS function, including lethargy, decreased alertness, depression, confusion, forgetfulness, obtundation, and, in the extreme, coma.
- GI: patients may experience anorexia, constipation, and nausea and vomiting.
- Renal: calcium acts as a diuretic and impairs the ability of the kidneys to concentrate urine. This can lead to dehydration, which further worsens hypercalcemia. Hypercalciuria in the setting of most causes of hypercalcemia increases the risk of calcium-containing kidney stones.
- Skeletal: patients with most causes of hypercalcemia have increased bone resorption and, therefore, increased bone demineralization. This increases fracture risk.
- Cardiovascular: hypercalcemia may cause or exacerbate hypertension. The QT interval on the ECG may be shorted as a result of augmented calcium influx during myocardial depolarization.

Causes of Hypercalcemia

Endocrine Causes

As discussed above, endocrine causes of hypercalcemia relate to disorders affecting parathyroid and vitamin D function, as well as to other quasi-related phenomena. Drugs that can cause hypercalcemia are also discussed in this section.

Primary hyperparathyroidism[13] is the most common cause of hypercalcemia in the healthy outpatient setting. It is a condition resulting from adenoma, multiple adenomas, or hyperplasia of the parathyroids. The term *primary* refers to the fact that the physiologic defect lies with the parathyroid glands. These are usually benign (rarely malignant) and result in hypersecretion of PTH, independent of the normal feedback regulation by ambient calcium. In essence, this is usually a set point problem[5]: there appears to be a new set point recognized by the parathyroid cells in the abnormal parathyroid tissue; the abnormal tissue "thinks" normal ambient calcium is too low and brings it up to an abnormally high level by hypersecretion of PTH. In primary hyperparathyroidism (1° HPT), PTH is usually high, but may actually be in the high normal range. When you consider that high calcium should suppress normal parathyroid tissue (in an attempt to restore normal calcium levels—classic endocrine feedback reasoning), this helps you to see that a high normal PTH in the setting of hypercalcemia is abnormal; it is estimated that about 5–10% of patients with

---

CASE STUDY 21-2

A 58-year-old man has been a smoker for many years. Smoking three packs per day since he can remember, he insists his cigarettes "don't hurt me none, doc." He has been feeling ill lately, however, with loss of appetite, malaise, and weight loss. His mental status has been dulled recently, and he can't remember from "one minute to the next" what he is doing at his work. His baseline cough has been worse recently, and he has noticed blood streaking his sputum when he clears his sputum. He has no significant past medical history other than tobacco abuse. He takes no medications. His family history is only notable for his father dying of lung cancer at age 63 and his mother dying of emphysema at age 68.

On physical exam, he is a thin man who looks much older than his chronologic age. When he produces some sputum at the physician's request, it has a pink tinge and is streaked with blood. Chest exam reveals scattered wheezing and rales in the right upper lung region. He is diffusely weak on muscle strength testing. Labs are notable for: calcium, 16.8 mg/dL (normal, 8.5–10.2 mg/dL); albumin, 3.4 (normal, 3.5–4.8 g/dL); BUN, 27; and creatinine, 1.3. Chest x-ray reveals a 3-cm proximal right hilar mass with distal streaking. Further testing is prompted and reveals intact PTH undetectable at <1 pg/mL (normal, 11–54 pg/mL) and PTHrP elevated at 18.3 pmol/L (normal, 0.0–1.5 pmol/L).

Questions

1. Do you think this patient's smoking is related to his hypercalcemia?

2. What other lab results are abnormal?

3. What is this patient's diagnosis? His prognosis?

1° HPT may have PTH in the high normal range. The hypercalcemia of 1° HPT is generally not extreme unless compounded by additional factors, such as dehydration or renal insufficiency or failure. In 1° HPT, although the PTH increases fractional tubular reabsorption of calcium, the filtered load of calcium is much greater than normal, so that there is a net increase in calcium excretion in spite of the increased fractional reabsorption; hypercalciuria is an expected finding in 1° HPT. Classically, PTH also increases renal excretion of phosphate, and 1° HPT can lead to hypophosphatemia; however, this is diet dependent and, generally, serum phosphate is only helpful if measured in the fasting state (serum phosphate is not routinely measured in working up patients for 1° HPT). In 1° HPT, it is expected to find high blood calcium (ideally measured as ionized calcium), high (or high normal) PTH, and increased urinary calcium excretion (measured in a 24-hour urine collection); in the fasting state, hypophosphatemia may also be seen.

Primary hyperparathyroidism most often occurs sporadically, but may also occur in several genetic syndromes:

- Multiple endocrine neoplasia, type 1 (MEN 1) results in tumors of the parathyroids, pituitary, and pancreas. It results from loss of a tumor suppressor gene that maps to human chromosome 11[14]
- Multiple endocrine neoplasia, type 2A (MEN 2A) this results in tumors of the parathyroids, medullary thyroid hyperplasia or cancer, and pheochromocytoma. This results from an activating mutation in the *ret* protooncogene, which resides on human chromosome 10. The *ret* protooncogene can be routinely measured in the clinical lab. *Ret* should be measured whenever this condition is suspected, so that other family members, when appropriate, can be alerted and tested.[14]
- Familial hyperparathyroidism results in 1° HPT, without other associated tumors. The gene is unknown, but has been mapped to human chromosome 1[14]
- Familial benign hypocalciuric hypercalcemia (FBHH). This interesting syndrome is usually a result of mutations in the calcium-sensing receptor (vide supra). It is associated with mild hypercalcemia and hyperparathyroidism (Fig. 21-5), and *decreased* (or low normal) urinary calcium excretion.[15] The decreased urinary calcium excretion distinguishes FBHH from 1° HPT, making this test the one that distinguishes the two. As the name implies, the condition is benign and does not require treatment; it does not predispose to fractures or kidney stones. Recognition is critical, so that these patients don't get referred for parathyroidectomy!

Hypervitaminosis D is a condition resulting from intake of too much vitamin D, or by aberrant production of $1,25(OH)_2D$ as a result of extrarenal 1α-hydroxylation of 25-hydroxy vitamin D, usually associated with granulomatous conditions or abnormal lymphoid tissue.[16] It is difficult to get too much vitamin D in the diet, assuming all organ systems are functioning normally. The more commonly seen (although still fairly uncommon) cause of hypercalcemia with hypervitaminosis D is due to extrarenal 1α-hydroxylase activity in granulomas or lymphoid tissue. This is not the same 1α-hydroxylase enzyme found in the kidney whose activity is regulated by PTH and calcium; it is a different gene product and exhibits no feedback regulation by calcium. This 1α-hydroxylase activity functions constitutively to produce $1,25(OH)_2D$, which, in turn, can cause hypercalcemia by mechanisms previously discussed (*Endocrine Physiology* and *Organ Physiology*). Hypercalcemia resulting from excess vitamin D is predominately mediated by stimulation of GI absorption of calcium and by recruitment of osteoclasts, resulting in bone resorption.[16] $1,25(OH)_2D$ suppresses PTH gene transcription; therefore, the expected lab profile in a patient with hypervitaminosis D from ectopic 1α-hydroxylation of 25-hydroxy vitamin D is hypercalcemia, suppressed PTH, and elevated $1,25(OH)_2D$. The granulomatous conditions most frequently associated with this are sarcoidosis and tuberculosis.

Certain cancers may produce hormonally mediated hypercalcemia as a paraneoplastic syndrome. In some cases, these factors act more in a paracrine than a true endocrine fashion. In all of these cases, the factor(s) produced by the tumor are not subject to feedback regulation by calcium.

Multiple myeloma is a malignancy of B-lymphocytes that produce antibody (ie, plasma cells). These malignancies often produce hypercalcemia by secretion of cytokines that activate osteoclasts to resorb bone, and uncouple resorption from bone formation mediated by osteoblasts.[17] Because parathyroid tissue is not abnormal in these patients, PTH is appropriately suppressed in the hypercalcemia of multiple myeloma. The hypercalcemia may be extreme. The immunoglobulin light chains of the disease may also cause renal tubular necrosis and result in renal insufficiency, which worsens the hypercalcemia. Lytic bone lesions are seen on radiographs of affected bone.

Parathyroid hormone-related protein (PTHrP) is a common hormonal cause of the hypercalcemia associated with many malignancies[18,19]; it may also be produced by benign tumors and cause hypercalcemia.[20] PTHrP shares N-terminal sequence homology with PTH (thus, *PTH-related protein*). PTH and PTHrP both bind to the same receptor in kidney and bone; the receptor is also found in a variety of other tissue. The normal physiologic role of PTHrP is not clear. It probably plays a role in normal paracrine regulation of various tissue, including cartilage, skin, neurons in the CNS, and breast (calcium into breast milk). Cancers that are commonly associated with

PTHrP production (historically referred to as *humoral hypercalcemia of malignancy*) include squamous cell lung cancer, breast cancer, and renal cancer. Other tumors that may be associated with PTHrP-mediated hypercalcemia include pheochromocytoma, some islet cell tumors, and certain lymphomas. PTHrP secretion is not regulated in a feedback manner by blood calcium (Fig. 21-6). When PTHrP (which probably functions physiologically in a paracrine manner) is made by cancers, it is significantly overproduced to the extent that it circulates systemically, allowing it to act in an endocrine manner (from a clinical standpoint, primarily affecting bone and kidney,). It can be measured in blood when the humoral hypercalcemia of malignancy is suspected. PTHrP and PTH do not cross-react in immunoassays for each other, allowing each protein to be reliably measured in the clinical lab. PTHrP-mediated hypercalcemia is associated with a suppressed PTH. As with PTH-mediated hypercalcemia, PTHrP-mediated hypercalcemia is mainly a result of bone resorption and increased fractional renal tubular reabsorption of calcium. Cancers that make PTHrP and cause hypercalcemia are associated with a particularly poor prognosis. Symptoms associated with the syndrome include mental status changes, kidney stones, and fractures, as well as other cancer-related symptoms.

Organ System Causes

Milk-alkali syndrome is a rare cause of hypercalcemia, but is historically significant.[21] It was originally described in the 1920s in patients being treated for peptic ulcers with milk and/or cream and carbonate or bicarbonate salts. Consumption of high doses of calcium and absorbable antacids (*eg,* sodium bicarbonate; both agents are found together in calcium carbonate) may lead to hypercalcemia and metabolic alkalosis; milk-alkali syndrome is frequently associated with renal insufficiency. The actual mechanism of milk-alkali syndrome is some-

what unclear, but related, at least in part, to increased intestinal absorption and decreased renal clearance of calcium and bicarbonate. PTH is suppressed in the hypercalcemia of the milk-alkali syndrome.

Renal failure may cause various abnormalities in calcium metabolism, including hypercalcemia and hypocalcemia, depending on several factors.[21,22] It is not completely fair to say this is a nonhormonal cause of hypercalcemia because abnormal variations in PTH and vitamin D metabolism are usually encountered, as well. In renal failure, renal excretion of both calcium and phosphate is severely, if not totally, abolished. Calcium phosphate is insoluble and tends to precipitate in soft tissue. PTH is usually elevated in renal failure and, in balance with calcium phosphate precipitation and loss of urinary calcium excretion, may contribute to hypercalcemia. 1-Hydroxylation of 25-hydroxy vitamin D is abolished in renal failure, so that the active form of vitamin D is not produced. $1,25(OH)_2D$ is typically given to patients in renal failure and, therefore, can contribute to hypercalcemia.

Drugs That Cause Hypercalcemia

Various drugs can cause hypercalcemia.[21] These drugs will be discussed in greater detail (*Drugs That Affect Calcium Metabolism*).

Thiazide diuretics have a long history in the treatment of hypertension and can cause retention of glomerularly filtered calcium and cause or contribute to hypercalcemia. At routine doses used to treat hypertension, hypercalcemia is uncommon. Any other factors that could exacerbate the hypercalcemic effect of thiazides may increase the likelihood of thiazide-related hypercalcemia (*eg,* renal disease, primary hyperparathyroidism).

Lithium, at doses routinely used to treat bipolar affective disorder, may be associated with hypercalcemia. Lithium appears to shift the set point for calcium regulation of PTH secretion, favoring a higher level of blood calcium. It may also augment PTH signaling at PTH target tissue (particularly bone and kidney), increasing blood calcium.

High doses of vitamin A or the vitamin A analogs/metabolites in the retinoic acid family have been associated with hypercalcemia. In the hypercalcemia of vitamin A/retinoic acid, PTH and $1,25(OH)2D$ are suppressed, and PTHrP is not elevated. Vitamin A/retinoic acid appear to work via activation of osteoclasts and bone resorption.

HYPOCALCEMIA

Hypocalcemia is the state of blood calcium levels below the normal range.[23] This is probably best measured by ionized calcium; a total calcium is not diagnostic unless also accompanied by an albumin measurement.

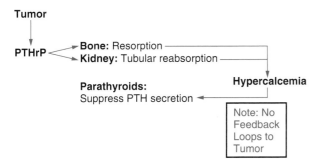

FIGURE 21-6. PTHrP endocrine pathophysiology. This demonstrates the effect of tumors that overproduce PTHrP. The pathophysiologic effect is via the same organ systems used by PTH to increase blood calcium. The difference between PTH and PTHrP is that PTH is subject to feedback regulation, whereas PTHrP is not subject to any feedback regulation by calcium (compare to Fig. 21-4).

Signs and Symptoms of Hypocalcemia

Signs and symptoms of hypocalcemia, regarding signs and symptoms associated with hypercalcemia, are protean and demonstrate individual variation at how low calcium must be for any particular signs or symptoms to appear.[23] The signs and symptoms of hypocalcemia are generally described by organ system:

- Neuromuscular: tetany (involuntary muscle contraction) affecting primarily the muscles in the hands, feet, legs, and back may be seen. Tapping on the 7th cranial nerve (facial nerve), just anterior to the ear may elicit twitching in the ipsilateral corner of the mouth (Chvostek's sign). Numbness and tingling in the face, hands, and feet may be seen. Inflation of a blood pressure cuff to 20 mm Hg above the patient's systolic blood pressure to induce a state of ischemia in the arm (metabolic acidosis), may cause spasm in the muscles of the wrist and hand (Trousseau's sign).
- CNS: irritability, seizures, personality changes, and impaired intellectual functioning may be seen.
- Cardiovascular: calcium not only plays a crucial role in the slow, inward calcium current of the QRS complex of ventricular depolarization, but also plays a crucial role in electromechanical coupling. In hypocalcemia, QT prolongation may be seen on the ECG. In the extreme, electromechanical dissociation (EMD) may be seen. Cardiac contractile dysfunction is rare but, in the extreme, can result in congestive heart failure. Cardiac dysfunction from hypocalcemia should be treated with emergent intravenous calcium.

Causes of Hypocalcemia

Endocrine Causes

PTH and vitamin D dominate the endocrine causes of hypocalcemia. It is important to start with discussing a key endocrine *response* to hypocalcemia (or the threat thereof). With the exception of hypocalcemia due to hypoparathyroidism, a key endocrine physiologic response to all (other) types of hypocalcemia is for the parathyroids to secrete more PTH to try to prevent or offset hypocalcemia. Elevated PTH in response to a threat of hypocalcemia is referred to as *secondary hyperparathyroidism,*[23] and, because of it, many patients with this response are found to have blood calcium within normal limits. Secondary hyperparathyroidism is distinguished from primary hyperparathyroidism in several important ways (Table 21-1). In primary hyperparathyroidism, PTH is elevated because of a disorder of parathyroid tissue (one or more parathyroid glands); in secondary hyperparathyroidism, the parathyroids are normal and healthy and PTH is elevated as a physiologic adaptation to the threat of hypocalcemia. In primary hyperparathyroidism, *hypercalcemia* is cured by removing the offending parathyroid(s). In secondary hyperparathyroidism, the hypocalcemia (or threat thereof) would get much worse and be more difficult to treat if the parathyroids were removed. Secondary hyperparathyroidism should be treated, when possible, by treating the underlying cause or threat of hypocalcemia and leaving the parathyroids alone.

Because the primary role of PTH is to prevent hypocalcemia, it is understandable that inadequate parathyroid function would cause, or cause a tendency

---

CASE STUDY 21-3

A 26-year-old man presented to his physician 3 weeks after having his thyroid surgically removed for thyroid cancer. His doctor swears she "got it all." However, since he went home from the hospital, he has noticed involuntary muscle cramping that is quite painful. He also feels numbness and tingling around his mouth and in his hands and feet. His girlfriend says he has been "crankier" for the last couple of weeks. His past medical history is only notable for the recent diagnosis of thyroid cancer and its resection 3 weeks prior to this visit. His only medication is L-thyroxine. Family history is noncontributory. On physical exam, he has a well-healing thyroidectomy scar. Tapping on the face, interior to the ears, causes twitching in the ipsilateral corner of the mouth (Chvostek's sign). There are no palpable masses in the thyroid bed. A blood pressure cuff inflated to

above the systolic pressure induces involuntary muscle contracture in the ipsilateral hand after 60 seconds (Trousseau's sign). Labs are notable for calcium, 5.6 mg/dL (normal, 8.5–10.2 mg/dL); albumin, 4.1 g/dL; BUN, 20; and creatinine, 1.0. Intact PTH is undetectable at <1 pg/mL.

Questions

1. Which lab results are abnormal?

2. What condition is he experiencing since his thyroidectomy?

3. What is the cause of this symptomatic condition?

4. What is the treatment for this patient, in addition to thyroxine medication?

TABLE 21-1. HYPERPARATHYROIDISM: PRIMARY (1°) VERSUS SECONDARY (2°)[a]

	1°HPT	2°HPT
Blood Calcium	High	Low or normal
PTH Level	High	High
Urinary Calcium	High	Usually low except
Abnormality/ Dysfunction	Parathyroidism	

[a]This table summarizes important distinctions between primary hyperparathyroidism (1° HPT) and secondary hyperparathyroidism (2° HPT) as judged by blood calcium and PTH, urinary calcium, and the location of the underlying defect.

toward, hypocalcemia.[24] The condition of inadequate (or loss of) parathyroid function, or hypoparathyroidism, can occur in several settings, the most common of which is postsurgical. Neck surgery may remove or irreparably damage the parathyroid glands. The most common setting is thyroid surgery, as a result of the anatomic proximity of the parathyroids to the thyroid gland. The importance of an experienced head and neck surgeon cannot be overemphasized to help minimize the possibility of unintentional parathyroid removal or damage. As with many endocrine glands, parathyroid tissue may be attacked by the immune system and result in autoimmune parathyroid destruction. Autoimmune hypoparathyroidism may cluster with other autoimmune diseases, including type 1 diabetes, autoimmune thyroid disease, and Addison's disease. Autoimmune hypoparathyroidism is somewhat rare compared with other more commonly seen autoimmune diseases. Treatment of hypoparathyroidism centers on maintaining normal blood calcium, without causing other adverse effects. PTH is not available clinically for replacement therapy (given the recent availability of human recombinant PTH_{1-34}, the use of PTH to treat hypoparathyroidism may occur soon). When the parathyroids are no longer present or functioning properly, the deficiency is treated with relatively high-dose vitamin D and calcium.[24] The vitamin D stimulates intestinal absorption of calcium. In the absence of PTH, however, the absorbed calcium may be excreted in the urine unimpeded, resulting in hypercalciuria that, in turn, may increase calcium-containing kidney stone risk. Therefore, there must be some balance of calcium and vitamin D intake to simultaneously prevent hypocalcemia and hypercalciuria. The goal is to generally maintain blood calcium toward the low end of normal to help achieve this balance.

Pseudohypoparathyroidism is a genetic disease that results in uncoupling the PTH receptor from adenylate cyclase, as a result of a mutant stimulatory G protein

(G_s).[7] In this disease, there is no physiologic effect of PTH; PTH binds its receptor but cannot activate the second messenger, cyclic AMP (cAMP). The patients have hypocalcemia and often hyperphosphatemia, similar to patients with hypoparathyroidism; however, when PTH is measured, it is high. Note that the high PTH is the physiologic response of normal, healthy parathyroid tissue to hypocalcemia because the defect lies in signaling via the PTH receptor and in not with the parathyroid glands. This is a classic example of a hormonal resistance syndrome. The patients with pseudohypoparathyroidism also have short stature and short 4th and 5th metacarpals. This is a rare condition, but an instructive case of molecular medicine and calcium metabolism. Treatment is with calcium and vitamin D, as described above for hypoparathyroidism.

Hypovitaminosis D broadly describes a collection of states which threaten the body with hypocalcemia, including low vitamin D availability,[25] defective metabolism of vitamin D,[26] or mutations in the vitamin D receptor[26]; these conditions cause insufficient vitamin D action (recall that the vitamin D effect is mediated by $1,25(OH)_2$ vitamin D binding to the vitamin D receptor, a member of the nuclear receptor supergene family, and regulating transcription of vitamin D-responsive genes). This causes the threat of hypocalcemia, met by developing secondary hyperparathyroidism, which will minimize or eliminate the hypocalcemia. Secondary hyperparathyroidism is an adaptive response to minimize the pathophysiology of defective vitamin D action and should never be treated with parathyroidectomy. Treatment depends on the underlying defect. Vitamin D insufficiency is treated by replacing vitamin D with dietary sources (vitamin D-fortified milk or vitamin supplements). Genetic defects in metabolizing vitamin D are treated by supplying the active metabolite, $1,25(OH)_2D$, bypassing the metabolic defect. Genetic defects in the vitamin D receptor can be more difficult to treat; generally, $1,25(OH)_2D$ is given in pharmacologic doses, and the response is variable.

The phenomenon of tertiary hyperparathyroidism should be briefly mentioned because it is frequently encountered in the literature. This condition (without implications as to the underlying pathophysiology) is usually encountered in patients with chronic renal insufficiency or failure. Renal insufficiency or failure is a common etiology for secondary hyperparathyroidism. There is some thought that prolonged stimulation of parathyroid function in secondary hyperparathyroidism may stimulate the development of a parathyroid adenoma or parathyroid hyperplasia, mimicking primary hyperparathyroidism in the setting of antecedent secondary hyperparathyroidism.[27] The authors question this supposed pathophysiology of tertiary hyperparathyroidism—it is as if chronic hypothyroidism may stimulate the development of pituitary thyrotroph adenomas or Addison's disease may stimulate the development of pituitary corticotroph adenomas or Grave's disease may stimulate the development of hyperfunctioning thyroid adenomas—this is not seen. Nevertheless, the literature is rife with reference to tertiary hyperparathyroidism. Unlike secondary hyperparathyroidism, tertiary hyperparathyroidism is almost invariably treated surgically.

Organ System Causes

Organ system causes of hypocalcemia relate back to the organ systems that play key roles in calcium homeostasis.

Intestinal problems, including short bowel syndromes, malabsorption syndromes, and dumping syndromes, can cause malabsorption of calcium and, therefore, the threat of hypocalcemia. Again, the threat of hypocalcemia is offset by the development of secondary hyperparathyroidism, which attempts to maintain blood calcium within normal limits by pulling calcium from bone and increasing renal tubular reabsorption of calcium. Treatment is generally with high-dose vitamin D and calcium.

Renal insufficiency or failure may cause hypocalcemia by hyperphosphatemia (recall the low-solubility product constant, K_{sp}, for calcium phosphate; $K_{sp} = 1.2 \times 10^{-29}$) and defective metabolism of vitamin D.[27] These patients also develop secondary hyperparathyroidism as an adaptive response. The serum calcium of patients treated with hemodialysis or peritoneal dialysis is easy to normalize (phosphate is not as easily managed by dialysis); transplantation usually corrects the defect. Treatment with calcitriol ($1,25(OH)_2D$) is often helpful but carries the attendant risk of developing *hyper*calcemia.

Another cause of hypocalcemia is a genetic defect in the renal tubule that causes an inability to normally recover filtered calcium out of tubular fluid. The filtered calcium is essentially lost in the urine. This also causes secondary hyperparathyroidism to prevent the hypocalcemia that would result from inappropriate wasting of calcium. The hyperparathyroidism augments GI absorption of calcium and bone resorption and ameliorates the tendency toward hypocalcemia but cannot increase tubular reabsorption of calcium because of the genetic defect. As expected, therefore, these patients have hypercalciuria and a tendency toward kidney stones. The treatment for this condition is hydrochlorothiazide (HCTZ) at doses higher than used to treat hypertension.[9] Treatment end points are normalization of urine calcium excretion and normalization of PTH.

DRUGS THAT AFFECT CALCIUM METABOLISM

Having discussed calcium homeostasis and hypercalcemia and hypocalcemia, certain important classes of drugs that affect calcium metabolism should be mentioned. These drugs can be related directly to the endocrine and organ physiology previously discussed.

Antiresorptive drugs inhibit osteoclast-mediated bone resorption.[28] Drugs in this broad category include drugs that have been available for several years to treat or prevent osteoporosis, including estrogen, *bisphosphonates*, selective estrogen receptor modulators (SERMS; the prototype is raloxifene), and calcitonin. These drugs act by various mechanisms on osteoclasts to prevent osteoclast-mediated bone resorption, therefore, the categorical name, *antiresorptive*. These drugs are used in various clinical settings to help prevent bone turnover and loss of skeletal mass and help lessen fracture risk. Notable clinical examples are postmenopausal osteoporosis, glucocorticoid-induced osteoporosis, and idiopathic osteoporosis. In some settings, several of these drugs may be used to treat hypercalcemia (vide supra). Specifically, several intravenously administered bisphosphonates are used to treat the hypercalcemia of malignancy. Subcutaneous calcitonin may also be used to treat dangerously

---

CASE STUDY 21-4

An 82-year-old woman living in a nursing home feels unsteady on her feet and doesn't go outside much anymore. Lactose intolerant, she has never been able to drink milk. She does not take any dietary supplements. She says, "I feel my age, doc," but otherwise has no specific complaints. On her annual lab assessment, calcium is found to be slightly low at 8.2 mg/dL (normal, 8.5–10.2 mg/dL), with albumin, 3.5 mg/dL (normal, 3.5–4.8 g/dL); BUN, 28; and creatinine, 1.1. This prompts further evaluation, which reveals intact PTH elevated at 181 pg/mL and 25(OH) vitamin D low at 6 ng/mL (normal, 20–50 ng/mL).

Questions

1. What diagnostic possibility is suggested from the initial lab results of her annual assessment?

2. This patient's differential diagnosis includes two diseases. What are they?

3. Is her renal function related to either of these two diseases?

4. How should this patient be treated?

high blood calcium, although tachyphylaxis rapidly develops and other means to lower calcium must be put into place at the time it is used.

There are also drugs that stimulate bone resorption, most commonly, glucocorticoids, such as prednisone and methylprednisolone. These drugs are widely used to treat inflammatory conditions, including asthma, rheumatoid arthritis, and lupus, as well as in the regimen of antirejection drugs used in patients with organ transplantations. Pharmacologic doses of glucocorticoids mimic the effect of high cortisol in endogenous Cushing's syndrome.[29] Prednisone (*eg*, glucocorticoid) affects calcium metabolism in various ways, one of which is to stimulate osteoclasts to resorb bone. This relatively uncouples bone formation and bone resorption, favoring bone resorption, and the result is a net loss of bone mass (and bone architecture). A major source of morbidity associated with pharmacologic doses of glucocorticoids is glucocorticoid-induced osteoporosis. Two bisphosphonates, alendronate and risedronate, are approved by the Food and Drug Administration (FDA) for treatment of glucocorticoid-induced bone loss. Other medications associated with accelerated bone resorption include anticonvulsants (particularly phenytoin), cyclosporin A, and various cytotoxic agents.

Lithium, a small monovalent cation in the alkaline earth family/first column of the periodic table, is used to treat bipolar affective disorder. At doses routinely used to treat bipolar affective disorder, lithium may be associated with hypercalcemia. Lithium appears to shift the set point for calcium regulation of PTH secretion, favoring a higher level of blood calcium. It may also augment PTH signaling at PTH target tissue (particularly bone and kidney), increasing blood calcium.

With a long history in hypertension treatment, thiazide diuretics can cause retention of glomerularly filtered calcium and cause or contribute to hypercalcemia. HCTZ is the commonly used agent in this class in the United States. At doses routinely used to treat hypertension, hypercalcemia is uncommon, although factors that could exacerbate the hypercalcemic effect of thiazides may increase the likelihood of thiazide-related hypercalcemia (*eg*, renal disease, primary hyperparathyroidism).[21] However, the cause of one problem may be the treatment of another. HCTZ is the treatment of choice for the genetic renal leak of calcium that causes hypercalciuria (and predisposition to calcium-containing kidney stones) and secondary hyperparathyroidism.

The FDA recently approved human recombinant PTH$_{1-34}$, or *teriparatide*, a drug that, for the first time, will can directly stimulate osteoblast-mediated bone formation.[30] Because it is a peptide hormone, it (like insulin) must be administered parenterally; it is injected subcutaneously in the same way as insulin. Although this seems paradoxical that PTH, the hormone described above to resorb bone, can also be used to build bone. This has to do with the pharmacokinetics of teriparatide. Recall that, in bone cells, only osteoblasts express PTH receptors. Teriparatide, administered once daily, has a short serum half-life of about 1–2 hours and is gone from the system in only a few hours. The once daily administration of teriparatide signals the osteoblasts to build bone; however, because of the duration of the signal, does not elicit the osteoblasts to send the cytokine signal to the osteoclasts (to which they would have responded by resorbing bone). Teriparatide stimulates the formation of cortical and trabecular bone without a coupled bone resorption response. It is only approved to treat severe osteoporosis; however, other uses, such as the treatment of hypoparathyroidism and to augment fracture healing, are being studied. Furthermore, it can be used in combination with an antiresorptive drug, which can further potentiate the effect of the drug on the skeleton.

An exciting new class of drugs, calcimimetics, is being developed to treat hyperparathyroidism. The congener in this class, *cinacalcet,* is an agonist at the calcium-sensing receptor.[31] By binding to the calcium-sensing receptor in parathyroid tissue, this agent signals to the parathyroid cell that there is adequate ambient calcium, downregulating PTH gene transcription and PTH secretion. This agent is undergoing clinical trials to assess its role in the nonsurgical treatment of primary hyperparathyroidism and as an adjunct for the treatment of parathyroid carcinoma and secondary hyperparathyroidism.

METABOLIC BONE DISEASES

Various disease states affect skeletal microarchitecture and macroarchitecture, strength, and integrity. The examples given here either make good teaching points or are commonly encountered in certain patient populations. These points will, in most cases, be related to the physiologic principles reviewed above.

Rickets and Osteomalacia

Rickets and *osteomalacia* are diseases of vitamin D metabolism.[25,26] Both diseases exhibit defects in skeletal mineralization (deposition of calcium and phosphate, or hydroxyapatite, in bone). One hallmark difference between these diseases is age of onset: Rickets is characterized by onset in childhood and osteomalacia by onset in adulthood. Various defects cause rickets and osteomalacia; because of time of onset, the skeletal manifestations differ. Rickets is associated with bony deformities because of bending of long bones under the influence of gravity. Because bones have formed by the time of the onset of osteomalacia, no such bony deformity is seen. Both conditions are generally associated with the development of secondary hyperparathyroidism. Fractures may result in either case because of poor bone structure; they are probably contributed to by secondary hyperparathyroidism. Hypocalcemia may be seen, but may also be masked by the effects of secondary hyperparathyroidism. Because of vitamin D-fortified milk and public awareness, both conditions have become less common than earlier in the 20th century. However, people of any age who do not get outside in the sunlight and who do not supplement their diet are at risk for vitamin D deficiency. Adequacy of vitamin D in the body is assessed by the blood level of 25-hydroxy vitamin D. Because secondary hyperparathyroidism is also expected in this setting, serum intact PTH and calcium and albumin or ionized calcium should be obtained for confirmation.

Rickets may also result from genetic defects in vitamin D metabolism or in vitamin D receptor.[26] Depending on the defect, the biochemical analysis for vitamin D adequacy (25(OH)vitamin D) may be normal. $1,25(OH)_2D$ may be low, normal, or high, depending on the genetic defect. Defects in vitamin D metabolism are best treated by supplying the metabolically active compound, $1,25(OH)_2D$ (calcitriol). Various vitamin D receptor defects have been described, including abnormal ligand binding, abnormal DNA binding, and abnormal transactivation of transcriptional machinery at the regulatory site of vitamin D responsive genes. The defect determines how well the patient will respond to pharmacologic doses of calcitriol.

Osteoporosis

Once considered an inevitable consequence of aging, *osteoporosis* is the most prevalent metabolic bone disease in adults. Osteoporosis is a silent disease until it causes a fracture, often at a degree of trauma that would not have caused a fracture in a nonosteoporotic skeleton (ie, the osteoporotic/fragility fracture). Osteoporosis is now recognized to be a specific disease with significant personal and public health consequences. With this recognition, significant advances have been made in diagnosis, prevention, and treatment of osteoporosis.

Osteoporosis affects an estimated 20–25 million Americans; (about 4:1 female:male predominance) and causes about $1\frac{1}{2}$, million fractures annually in the United States.[32] Most are vertebral compressions, with the next most frequent the hip, followed by distal forearm, ribs, and humerus. The most morbid osteoporotic fracture is the hip, with all hip fractures requiring surgery. Although about one half of vertebral compressions may be asymptomatic, the hip fracture carries a significant morbidity, as well as increased mortality. In fact, mortality from hip fracture is increased about 20% in the first year following the fracture, and it is estimated that deaths related to hip fracture are now equal with those from breast cancer.

There are several risk factors for reduced bone mass with attendant increased fracture risk,[32] but risk factor assessment alone is a poor predictor of osteoporosis. Accepted risk factors for decreased bone mass include hypogonadism (most often the postmenopausal state in women, but also hypogonadism in men), increasing age, family history of osteoporosis (although the gene(s) involved are not known), lean body habitus, Caucasian or Asian ethnicity, smoking, alcoholism, glucocorticoid excess (Cushing's syndrome or, more commonly, exogenous administration), hyperparathyroidism, disorders of

---

CASE STUDY 21-5

A 6-year-old girl is brought to a pediatrician by her parents who report that her height is not progressing as they think it should (or as it did for her 8-year-old sister) and her legs look bowed. The patient drinks milk and, other than her shorter stature and bowed legs, has the normal characteristics of her 6-year-old friends. She takes no medications. Family history is notable for cousins in the father's family with a similar problem. The pediatrician obtains labs that are notable for calcium, 7.2 mg/dL (normal, 8.5–10.2 mg/dL), with albumin, 4.1 g/dL (normal, 3.5–4.8 g/dL). Lower extremity x-rays show bowing of the long bones and generalized demineralization. This prompts the measurement of several other lab tests, which reveal intact PTH elevated at 866 pg/mL (normal, 11–54 pg/mL); 25(OH) vitamin D, normal at 35 ng/mL (normal, 20–57 ng/mL); and $1,25(OH)_2$ vita-

min D undetectable at <1 pg/mL (normal, 20–75 pg/mL).

Questions

1. What condition do the preliminary lab tests indicate?

2. What is the significance of 25(OH) vitamin D and $1,25(OH)_2$ vitamin D levels in the follow-up lab tests?

3. Describe the inborn error of metabolism with this patient.

4. What secondary condition will recur if vitamin D treatment is discontinued later in her life?

TABLE 21-2. LAB TESTS THAT MAY BE USEFUL IN EVALUATING PATIENTS FOR LOW BONE DENSITY OR FRACTURE[a]

BUN, creatinine
Bicarbonate
Calcium and albumin (or ionized calcium)
Globulin fraction (total protein–albumin)
Alkaline phosphatase, bone-specific alkaline phosphatase, osteocalcin
TSH, free T_4
Gonadotropins, estradiol or testosterone
Intact PTH
CBC, WBC differential
25-Hydroxy vitamin D
1,25-Dihydroxy vitamin D
24-hour urine calcium
Other lab tests depending on patient profile: PTHrP, urine free cortisol, serum protein electrophoresis, Bence Jones protein
Radiographs of skeletal site in question
Bone mineral densitometry (DEXA)
Other analyses depending on patient profile

[a]Listed are labs (not all-conclusive) that are useful in determining renal insufficiency, acidosis, hypercalcemia, increased globulin fraction, bone turnover, thyroid function, hyperparathyroidism, hypercalciuria, anemia, vitamin D adequacy, and others more specifically directed at any abnormalities found or considered.

vitamin D metabolism, endogenous hyperthyroidism (particularly in postmenopausal women), and some malignancies (including in the absence of bony metastases). Some of these factors have specific therapies, accentuating the importance of evaluating for and treating secondary causes of bone loss before simply initiating general therapy for osteoporosis. Several laboratory tests may be useful in diagnosing osteoporosis or other disease processes that may cause poor bone health (Table 21-2).

Osteoporosis can be diagnosed on the basis of a fracture that occurred at an inappropriate degree of trauma (*osteoporotic*, or *fragility* fracture). Such fractures do not include fractures that occur at an appropriate degree of trauma. The occurrence of a first fragility fracture predicts further fragility fractures. It is preferable to diagnose osteoporosis before the occurrence of a first fragility fracture. This is possible using dual-energy x-ray absorptiometry (DEXA) of the lumbar spine and the hip. This technique, commonly referred to as *bone mineral densitometry* (or bone mineral density or bone density), essentially measures bone mineralization. What DEXA really measures is grams of calcium per square centimeter of cross-sectional area of bone (g/cm^2) (ie, not a *density* (mass/volume, or g/cm^3) at all; however, the *density* terminology has remained. The minimal fracture risk in life is when bone density is at its greatest, generally about age 30 for both men and women, and is increased when bone mass is lost (Fig. 21-7). The diagnosis of osteoporosis based on bone densitometry is made by comparing the patient's bone density to the average race- and gender-matched peak bone density in life. This is reported as standard deviations above or below peak bone mass, as a T-score (+ = above the average peak in life; − = below the average peak in life). Normal bone density is above a T-score of −1.0. Osteoporosis is a T-score of −2.5 or below. An intermediate between normal and osteoporosis, osteopenia, is diagnosed as a T-score between −1.0 and −2.5.

Osteoporosis therapy is aimed at one goal: fracture prevention. Treatment should include modification of preventable risk factors, such as smoking, sedentary lifestyle, excessive alcohol, and adequate intake of calcium (generally, 1500 mg every day) and vitamin D (400 IU/day is the minimum recommended; optimal is probably closer to 800–1000 IU/day). Therapy may be include prevention of osteoporosis and treatment of established osteoporosis.

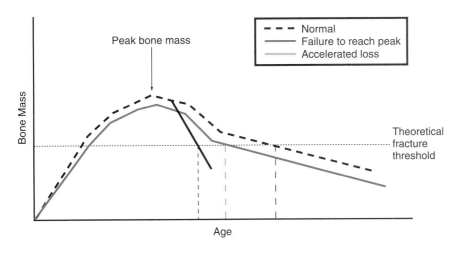

FIGURE 21-7. Bone mass as a function of age; perturbations that can affect bone mass. Shown is the accrual of bone mass with age to a peak that occurs in the mid-20s to early 30s (for both sexes) and the bone loss that occurs throughout life after the peak. Fracture risk increases as bone mass is lost. The "theoretical fracture threshold" is an artificial notion, but may be useful in demonstrating that at a given degree of trauma (varying from the simple act of weightbearing to increasing levels of impact), factors that are associated with low bone mass increase fracture risk and that the age that fracture risk is reached is relatively younger the earlier that lower bone mass is reached.

CASE STUDY 12-6

A 74-year-old woman slipped when mopping the kitchen floor and suffered a hip fracture, which was treated with open reduction and internal fixation (ORIF). After discharge from the hospital, she presented to her physician, asking if she has osteoporosis and, if so, what should be done. She takes no dietary supplements of calcium or vitamin D and only uses milk on her cereal. The woman has asthma, and has been treated with prednisone burst and tapers about 6 times in her life (as best she can recall). She went through menopause at age 49 and never took hormone replacement. Other than her hip, she reports no other fractures in adulthood but reports that she has lost about 2.5 inches in height. She thinks her mother had osteoporosis because she had a dowager's hump. The physician orders bone densi-

tometry, which shows PA spine T-score –3.8 and hip T-score (performed on the hip that was not broken!) –3.1. Labs revealed normal calcium and albumin, renal function, thyroid function, globulin fraction (total protein – albumin), and CBC. Alkaline phosphatase is slightly elevated, but she had a recent fracture.

Questions

1. What is this patient's diagnosis

2. Name 4–5 risk factors for this diagnosis

3. In addition to adequate calcium and vitamin D supplements, this patient would be a candidate for which new therapeutic drug?

The goal of osteoporosis prevention is to intervene before significant bone mass has been lost. The most commonly used pharmacologic therapies generally can be classified antiresorptive, in that they inhibit bone resorption mediated by osteoclasts.[28,29] These drugs include bisphosphonates (alendronate and risedronate), the selective estrogen receptor modulator (raloxifene), gonadal hormone replacement (estrogen ± progestin in women and testosterone in men), and calcitonin. Recently released, teriparatide (human recombinant PTH_{1-34}) is the first agent to become available for the treatment of osteoporosis that works by directly stimulating bone formation mediated by osteoblasts.[30] Experience with teriparatide is limited at this time. Contraindications to teriparatide include hypercalcemia; hyperparathyroidism; epiphyseal nonclosure (children); and osteosarcoma, a rare bone cancer.

Part osteoporosis treatment should include discussing fall prevention and recommending any measures that may

lessen the risk of falling, including walkers, handrails, night-lights, and hip pads.

SUMMARY

The key components of calcium homeostasis and metabolism have been reviewed and major organ systems and hormones involved in the regulation of blood calcium have been discussed. This chapter discussed the disease states of hypercalcemia and hypocalcemia and related them to the same organ systems and hormones, incorporating discussion of genetic and environmental factors affecting calcium homeostasis. Several disease states related to the organ systems and endocrine physiology and several drugs that can be used to treat these conditions have also been discussed. It is the hope of the authors that this brief treatise will help the reader to better relate to patient care regarding issues of calcium homeostasis.

REVIEW QUESTIONS

1. What principle hormones are involved in the normal physiologic regulation of calcium homeostasis?

2. What principle organs are involved in the maintenance of calcium homeostasis?

3. What tissue is involved in the production of the active metabolite of vitamin D?

4. What are the principle sources of vitamin D?

5. What is the best blood test for vitamin D adequacy?

6. What hormone is the most likely to be made by cancers and cause cancer-associated hypercalcemia? Is PTH elevated, normal, or suppressed in this condition?

7. What hormone is most likely to be produced by granulomatous diseases or lymphoid disorders and cause hypercalcemia? Is PTH elevated, normal, or suppressed in this condition?

8. Where does the defect lie in primary hyperparathyroidism? In secondary hyperparathyroidism?

9. What is the principle risk of hypercalciuria (increased urinary excretion of calcium)? How is hypercalciuria measured?

10. What is the most common cause of hypoparathyroidism?

11. What are the two types of bone? Which one is most rapidly lost in response to hypogonadism and glucocorticoid therapy.

12. Which cells in bone are responsible for bone resorption? For bone formation?

13. What is the most prevalent metabolic bone disease in the United States?

14. Name three drug categories that may inhibit bone resorption in osteoporotic patients.

15. Name the only drug currently approved for the treatment of severe osteoporosis that directly stimulates bone formation (*ie,* it is not an antiresorptive drug).

REFERENCES

1. Favus MJ, ed. Primer on the Metabolic Bone Diseases and Disorders of Mineral Metabolism, 4th ed. Philadelphia: Lippincott Williams & Wilkins, 1999:1–232.

2. Broadus AE. Mineral balance and homeostasis. In: Favus, MJ, ed. Primer on the Metabolic Bone Diseases and Disorders of Mineral Metabolism, 4th ed. Philadelphia: Lippincott Williams & Wilkins, 1999:74–80.

3. Portale AA. Blood calcium, phosphorus, and magnesium. In: Favus, MJ, ed. Primer on the Metabolic Bone Diseases and Disorders of Mineral Metabolism, 4th ed. Philadelphia: Lippincott Williams & Wilkins, 1999:15–18.

4. Holick MF. Vitamin D: photobiology, metabolism, mechanism of action, and clinical applications. In: Favus, MJ, ed. Primer on the Metabolic Bone Diseases and Disorders of Mineral Metabolism, 4th ed. Philadelphia: Lippincott Williams & Wilkins, 1999: 92–98.

5. Juppner H, Brown EM, Kronenberg HM. Parathyroid hormone. In: Favus, MJ, ed. Primer on the Metabolic Bone Diseases and Disorders of Mineral Metabolism, 4th ed. Philadelphia: Lippincott Williams & Wilkins, 1999:80–87.

6. Blind E, Gagel RF. Assay methods: parathyroid hormone, parathyroid hormone-related protein, and calcitonin. In: Favus, MJ, ed. Primer on the Metabolic Bone Diseases and Disorders of Mineral Metabolism, 4th ed. Philadelphia: Lippincott Williams & Wilkins, 1999:119–124.

7. Levine MA. Parathyroid hormone resistance syndromes. In: Favus, MJ, ed. Primer on the Metabolic Bone Diseases and Disorders of Mineral Metabolism, 4th ed. Philadelphia: Lippincott Williams & Wilkins, 1999:230–238.

8. Lemann J Jr, Favus MJ. The intestinal absorption of calcium, magnesium, and phosphate. In: Favus, MJ, ed. Primer on the Metabolic Bone Diseases and Disorders of Mineral Metabolism, 4th ed. Philadelphia: Lippincott Williams & Wilkins, 1999: 63–67.

9. Bushinsky DA. Calcium, magnesium, and phosphorus: renal handling and urinary excretion. In: Favus, MJ, ed. Primer on the Metabolic Bone Diseases and Disorders of Mineral Metabolism, 4th ed. Philadelphia: Lippincott Williams & Wilkins, 1999: 67–74.

10. Mundy GR. Bone remodeling. In: Favus, MJ, ed. Primer on the Metabolic Bone Diseases and Disorders of Mineral Metabolism, 4th ed. Philadelphia: Lippincott Williams & Wilkins, 1999: 30–38.

11. Baron R. Anatomy and ultrastructure of bone. In: Favus, MJ, ed. Primer on the Metabolic Bone Diseases and Disorders of Mineral Metabolism, 4th ed. Philadelphia: Lippincott Williams & Wilkins, 1999:3–10.

12. Shane, E. Hypercalcemia: pathogenesis, clinical manifestations, differential diagnosis, and management. In: Favus, MJ, ed. Primer on the Metabolic Bone Diseases and Disorders of Mineral Metabolism, 4th ed. Philadelphia: Lippincott Williams & Wilkins, 1999:183–187.

13. Bilezikian JP. Primary hyperparathyroidism. In: Favus, MJ, ed. Primer on the Metabolic Bone Diseases and Disorders of Mineral Metabolism, 4th ed. Philadelphia: Lippincott Williams & Wilkins, 1999:187–192.

14. Heath H III, Hobbs MR. Familial hyperparathyroid syndromes. In: Favus, MJ, ed. Primer on the Metabolic Bone Diseases and Disorders of Mineral Metabolism, 4th ed. Philadelphia: Lippincott Williams & Wilkins, 1999:192–195.

15. Marx SJ. Familial hypocalciuric hypercalcemia. In: Favus, MJ, ed. Primer on the Metabolic Bone Diseases and Disorders of Mineral Metabolism, 4th ed. Philadelphia: Lippincott Williams & Wilkins, 1999:195–198.

16. Adams JS. Hypercalcemia due to granuloma-forming disorders. In: Favus, MJ, ed. Primer on the Metabolic Bone Diseases and Disorders of Mineral Metabolism, 4th ed. Philadelphia: Lippincott Williams & Wilkins, 1999:212–214.

17. Mundy GR, Yoneda T, Guise TA. Hypercalcemia in hematologic malignancies and solid tumors associated with extensive localized bone destruction. In: Favus, MJ, ed. Primer on the Metabolic Bone Diseases and Disorders of Mineral Metabolism, 4th ed. Philadelphia: Lippincott Williams & Wilkins, 1999:208–212.

18. Strewler GJ, Nissenson RA. Parathyroid hormone-related protein. In: Favus, MJ, ed. Primer on the Metabolic Bone Diseases and Disorders of Mineral Metabolism, 4th ed. Philadelphia: Lippincott Williams & Wilkins, 1999:88–91.

19. Roberts MM, Stewart AF. Humoral hypercalcemia of malignancy. In: Favus, MJ, ed. Primer on the Metabolic Bone Diseases and Disorders of Mineral Metabolism, 4th ed. Philadelphia: Lippincott Williams & Wilkins, 1999:203–207.

20. Knecht TP, Behling CA, Burton DW, Glass CK, Deftos LJ. The humoral hypercalcemia of benignancy: a newly appreciated syndrome. Am J Clin Pathol 1996;105:487–492.

21. Stewart AF. Miscellaneous causes of hypercalcemia. In: Favus, MJ, ed. Primer on the Metabolic Bone Diseases and Disorders of Mineral Metabolism, 4th ed. Philadelphia: Lippincott Williams & Wilkins, 1999:215–219.

22. Goodman WG, Coburn JW, Slatopolsky E, Salusky IB. Renal osteodystrophy in adults and children. In: Favus, MJ, ed. Primer on the Metabolic Bone Diseases and Disorders of Mineral Metabolism, 4th ed. Philadelphia: Lippincott Williams & Wilkins, 1999:347–363.

23. Shane E. Hypocalcemia: pathogenesis, differential diagnosis, and management. In: Favus, MJ, ed. Primer on the Metabolic Bone

Diseases and Disorders of Mineral Metabolism, 4th ed. Philadelphia: Lippincott Williams & Wilkins, 1999:223–226.

24. Goltzman D, Cole DEC. Hypoparathyroidism. In: Favus, MJ, ed. Primer on the Metabolic Bone Diseases and Disorders of Mineral Metabolism, 4th ed. Philadelphia: Lippincott Williams &Wilkins, 1999:226–230.

25. Klein GL. Nutritional rickets and osteomalacia. In: Favus MJ, ed. Primer on the Metabolic Bone Diseases and Disorders of Mineral Metabolism, 4th ed. Philadelphia: Lippincott Williams & Wilkins, 1999:315–319.

26. Liberman UA, Marx SJ. Vitamin D-dependent rickets. In: Favus MJ, ed. Primer on the Metabolic Bone Diseases and Disorders of Mineral Metabolism, 4th ed. Philadelphia: Lippincott Williams & Wilkins, 1999:323–328.

27. Indridason OS, Quarles LD. Tertiary hyperparathyroidism and refractory secondary hyperparathyroidism. In: Favus MJ, ed. Primer on the Metabolic Bone Diseases and Disorders of Mineral Metabolism, 4th ed. Philadelphia: Lippincott Williams & Wilkins, 1999:198–202.

28. Watts NB. Pharmacology of agents to treat osteoporosis. In: Favus MJ, ed. Primer on the Metabolic Bone Diseases and Disorders of Mineral Metabolism, 4th ed. Philadelphia: Lippincott Williams & Wilkins, 1999:278–283.

29. Lukert BP. Glucocorticoid-induced osteoporosis. In: Favus MJ, ed. Primer on the Metabolic Bone Diseases and Disorders of Mineral Metabolism, 4th ed. Philadelphia: Lippincott Williams & Wilkins, 1999:292–296.

30. Neer RM, Arnaud CD, Zanchetta JR, et al. Effect of parathyroid hormone (1-34) on fractures and bone mineral density in postmenopausal women with osteoporosis. N Engl J Med 2001; 344:1434–1441.

31. Goodman WG. Calcimimetic agents and secondary hyperparathyroidism: treatment and prevention. Nephrol Dial Transplant 2002;17:204–207.

32. Wasnich RD. Epidemiology of osteoporosis. In: Favus MJ, ed. Primer on the Metabolic Bone Diseases and Disorders of Mineral Metabolism, 4th ed. Philadelphia: Lippincott Williams & Wilkins, 1999:257–259.

Liver Function

Edward P. Fody

O B J E C T I V E S

Upon completion of this chapter, the clinical laboratorian should be able to:

- Diagram the anatomy of the liver.
- Explain the physiologic functions of the liver to include bile secretion, synthetic activity, and detoxification.
- Discuss the basic disorders of the liver and which laboratory tests may be performed to diagnose them.
- Evaluate information to determine any disorder, given a patient's clinical data.

- Classify the three types of jaundice and discuss the causes.
- Explain the principles of the tests for bilirubin.
- Identify the enzymes most commonly used in the assessment of hepatobiliary disease.
- Differentiate the various types of hepatitis to include cause (*ie*, bacteria or virus), transmission, occurrence, alternate name, physiology, diagnosis, and treatment.

K E Y   T E R M S

Bile
Bilirubin
Cirrhosis
Conjugated bilirubin

Hepatitis
Hepatoma
Icterus

Kupffer cells
Lobule
Posthepatic

Prehepatic
Sinusoids
Urobilinogen

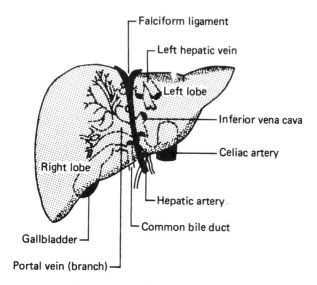

- Falciform ligament
- Left hepatic vein
- Left lobe
- Inferior vena cava
- Celiac artery
- Hepatic artery
- Common bile duct
- Right lobe
- Gallbladder
- Portal vein (branch)

FIGURE 22-1. Gross anatomy of the liver, showing major blood vessels and bile channels. (Adapted from Tietz NW. Fundamentals of Clinical Chemistry. Philadelphia: WB Saunders, 1976.)

In the past, the liver has been referred to as the center of courage, passion, temper, and love and even as the center of the soul. It was once believed to produce "yellow bile" necessary for good health. Today, we recognize the liver to be a complex organ responsible for many major metabolic functions in the body. More than 100 tests measuring these diverse functions have existed in the clinical laboratory at one time. However, many were abandoned in favor of those that have proven to be most clinically useful. This chapter discusses these more commonly used liver function tests, with particular emphasis on current methodology.

ANATOMY

The liver is the largest, most versatile organ in the body (Fig. 22-1). It consists of two main lobes that, together, weigh from 1400–1600 g in the normal adult. This reddish-brown organ is located under the diaphragm in the right upper quadrant of the abdomen. It has an abundant blood supply, receiving approximately 15 mL/minute from two major vessels: the hepatic artery and the portal vein. The hepatic artery, a branch of the aorta, contributes 20% of the blood supply and provides most of the oxygen requirement. The portal vein, which drains the gastrointestinal tract, transports the most recently absorbed material from the intestine to the liver. Within the connective tissue of the liver, these vessels give off numerous small branches that form a vascular network around so-called *lobules*.[1]

Structural Unit

The *lobule* (1–2 mm wide) forms the structural unit of the liver (Fig. 22-2). It comprises cords of liver cells (hepatocytes) radiating from a central vein. The boundary of

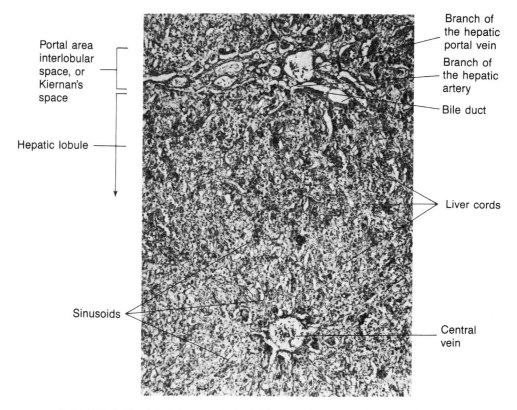

- Portal area interlobular space, or Kiernan's space
- Hepatic lobule
- Sinusoids
- Branch of the hepatic portal vein
- Branch of the hepatic artery
- Bile duct
- Liver cords
- Central vein

FIGURE 22-2. Liver lobule (panoramic view). (Photograph courtesy of James Furlong, MD.)

each lobule is formed by a portal tract made up of connective tissue that contains a branch of the hepatic artery, portal vein, and bile duct. Between the cords of liver cells are vascular spaces, called *sinusoids,* that are lined by endothelial cells and Kupffer cells. These spaces receive blood from the small branches of the hepatic artery and portal vein, which are located in the portal tracts. The *Kupffer cells* are phagocytic macrophages capable of ingesting bacteria or other foreign material from the blood that flows through the sinusoids. The blood from the sinusoids drains into the central veins (hepatic venule) and then to the hepatic veins and inferior vena cava. Primary bile canaliculi are conduits, 1–2 mm wide, located between the hepatocytes. The bile canaliculi interconnect extensively and increase in size until they connect with the larger bile ducts in the portal tracts.[2,3]

PHYSIOLOGY

The liver performs several hundred known functions each day, including numerous metabolic, secretory, and excretory functions. The total loss of the liver usually results in death from hypoglycemia within 24 hours. Although there are many liver functions, this chapter discusses those that have prime significance in liver disease.

Excretory and Secretory Function

One of the more important liver functions, and one that is disturbed in a large number of hepatic disorders, is the excretion of bile. *Bile* comprises bile acids or salts,[4] bile pigments (primarily bilirubin esters), cholesterol, and other substances extracted from the blood. Total bile production averages about 3 L per day, although only 1 L is excreted. The primary bile acids, cholic acid and chenodeoxycholic acid, are formed in the liver from cholesterol. The bile acids are conjugated with the amino acids glycine or taurine, forming bile salts. Bile salts (conjugated bile acids) are excreted into the bile canaliculi by means of a carrier-mediated active transport system. During fasting and between meals, a major portion of the bile acid pool is concentrated up to 10-fold in the gallbladder. Bile acids reach the intestine when the gallbladder contracts after each meal. Approximately 500–600 mL of bile enter the duodenum each day. Here, bile is intimately involved with digestion and absorption of lipids. When the conjugated bile acids (salts) come into contact with bacteria in the terminal ileum and colon, dehydration to secondary bile acids (deoxycholic and lithocolic) occurs, and these secondary bile acids are subsequently absorbed. The absorbed bile acids enter the portal circulation and return to the liver, where they are reconjugated and reexcreted. The enterohepatic circulation of bile occurs 2–5 times daily.[5–7]

Bilirubin, the principal pigment in bile, is derived from the breakdown of hemoglobin when aged red blood cells

are phagocytized by the reticuloendothelial system, primarily in the spleen, liver, and bone marrow. About 80% of the bilirubin formed daily comes from the degradation of hemoglobin. The remainder comes from destruction of heme-containing proteins (myoglobin, cytochromes, catalase) and catabolism of heme (Fig. 22-3).

When hemoglobin is destroyed, the protein portion—globin—is reused by the body. The iron enters the body's iron stores and is also reused. The porphyrin is broken down as a waste product and excreted. This action of split-

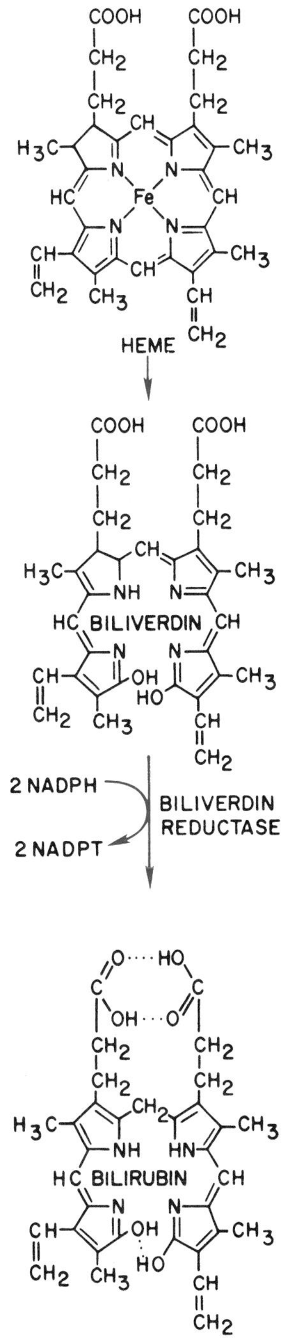

FIGURE 22-3. Catabolism of heme, leading to the formation of bilirubin.

ting the porphyrin ring and releasing the iron and globin forms biliverdin, which is easily reduced to bilirubin.

Bilirubin is transported to the liver in the bloodstream bound to proteins, chiefly albumin. It is then separated from the albumin and taken up by the hepatic cells. Two nonalbumin proteins, isolated from liver cell cytoplasm and designated Y and Z, account for the intracellular binding and transport of bilirubin. The conjugation (esterification) of bilirubin occurs in the endoplasmic reticulum of the hepatocyte. An enzyme, uridyldiphosphate glucuronyl transferase (UDPGT), transfers a glucuronic acid molecule to each of the two proprionic acid side chains in bilirubin, converting bilirubin into a diglucuronide ester. This product, bilirubin diglucuronide, is referred to as *conjugated bilirubin*. Conjugated bilirubin, which is water soluble, is secreted from the hepatic cell into the bile canaliculi and then passes along with the rest of the bile into larger bile ducts and eventually into the intestine. In the lower portion of the intestinal tract, especially the colon, the bile pigments are acted on by enzymes present in the intestinal bacteria. The first product of this reaction is mesobilirubin, which is reduced to form mesobilirubinogen and then urobilinogen, a colorless product. The oxidation of urobilinogen produces the red-brown pigment urobilin, which is excreted in the stool. A small portion of the urobilinogen is reabsorbed into the portal circulation and returned to the liver, where it is again excreted into the bile. There is, however, a small quantity that remains in the blood. This urobilinogen is ultimately filtered by the kidney and excreted in the urine (Fig. 22-4).

A total of 200–300 mg of bilirubin is produced daily in the healthy adult. A normally functioning liver is re-

quired to eliminate this amount of bilirubin from the body. This excretory function requires that bilirubin be in the conjugated form; that is, the water-soluble diglucuronide. Almost all the bilirubin formed is eliminated in the feces, and a small amount of the colorless product urobilinogen is excreted in the urine. Under normal circumstances, a low concentration of bilirubin (0.2–1.0 mg/dL) is found in the serum, the majority of which is in the unconjugated form. A small percentage (0.2 mg/dL) of this total bilirubin exists in normal serum as the conjugated form.[8]

When the bilirubin concentration in the blood rises, the pigment begins to be deposited in the sclera of the eyes and in the skin. This yellowish pigmentation in the skin or sclera is known as *jaundice,* or *icterus.*[9,10]

Jaundice may be caused by various pathophysiologic mechanisms. For example, there may be an increased bilirubin load on the liver cell or a disturbance in uptake and transport of bilirubin within the liver cell. In addition, there may be defects in conjugation or excretion of bilirubin into the bile. Further difficulties may be a result of obstruction of the large bile ducts before the bilirubin reaches the intestine. Several classifications of jaundice are found in the literature. One of the more frequently used classifications is based on the presumed site of physiologic or anatomic abnormality. In this classification, there are predominately three types of jaundice: prehepatic, hepatic, and posthepatic.[9]

Prehepatic jaundice results when an excessive amount of bilirubin is presented to the liver for metabolism, such as in hemolytic anemia. This type of jaundice is characterized by unconjugated hyperbilirubinemia. However, the serum bilirubin levels rarely exceed 5 mg/dL because the normal liver is capable of handling most of the overload. Unconjugated bilirubin is not water-soluble and is bound to albumin so that it is not filtered out of the blood by the kidney. Therefore, bilirubin will not appear in the urine in this type of jaundice.

The largest percentage of patients has hepatic jaundice. Hepatic jaundice may result from impaired cellular uptake, defective conjugation, or abnormal secretion of bilirubin by the liver cell.[10]

Gilbert syndrome is a relatively common disorder characterized by impaired cellular uptake of bilirubin. Affected individuals have no symptoms, but may have mild icterus. The elevated level of bilirubin is less than 3 mg/100 mL and unconjugated. Crigler-Najjar syndrome is a more serious disorder caused by a deficiency of the enzyme UDPGT. Two types have been described. Type I, in which there is a complete absence of the enzyme in the liver, is rare. No conjugated bilirubin is formed, and the bile is colorless. This type is uniformly fatal. In type II, Crigler-Najjar syndrome, there is a less severe deficiency of the enzyme and some conjugated bilirubin is formed. Dubin-Johnson syndrome and Rotor's syndrome are two

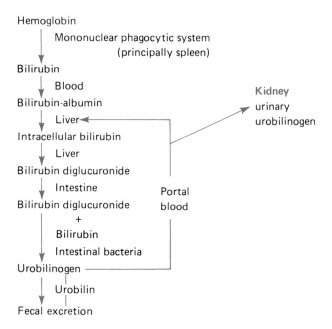

FIGURE 22-4. Metabolism of bilirubin.

hereditary disorders characterized by conjugated hyperbilirubinemia from defective excretion by the liver cell. Any cause of severe hepatocellular damage also may interfere with uptake, conjugation, or secretion of bilirubin. This will lead to unconjugated as well as conjugated hyperbilirubinemia.[11–16]

Posthepatic jaundice results from the impaired excretion of bilirubin caused by mechanical obstruction of the flow of bile into the intestine. This may be due to gallstones or a tumor. When bile ceases to flow into the intestine, there is a rise in the serum level of conjugated bilirubin and the stool loses its source of normal pigmentation and becomes clay-colored. Conjugated bilirubin appears in the urine, and urine urobilinogen levels decrease.[17] The various laboratory tests that assist in making the distinction between the different causes of jaundice are discussed later in this chapter.

Major Synthetic Activity

Among the many diverse metabolic functions carried out by the liver is the synthesis of many major biologic compounds, including proteins, carbohydrates, and lipids. The liver plays an important role in plasma protein production, synthesizing albumin and the majority of the α- and β-globulins. All the blood-clotting factors (except VIII) are synthesized in the liver. In addition, the deamination of glutamate in the liver is the primary source of ammonia, which is then converted to urea.

The synthesis and metabolism of carbohydrates is also centered in the liver. Glucose is converted to glycogen, a portion of which is stored in the liver and later reconverted to glucose as necessary. An additional important liver function is gluconeogenesis from amino acids.[18,19]

Fat is formed from carbohydrates in the liver when nutrition is adequate and the demand for glucose is being met from dietary sources. The liver also plays a key role in the metabolism of fat. It is the major site for the removal of chylomicron remnants and for the conversion of acetyl-CoA to fatty acids, triglycerides, and cholesterol. Further metabolism of cholesterol into bile acids also occurs in the liver. Very-low-density lipoproteins, which are responsible for transporting triglycerides into the tissues, are synthesized primarily in the liver. High-density lipoproteins are also made in the liver, as are phospholipids.[20]

The formation of ketone bodies occurs almost exclusively in the liver. When the demand for gluconeogenesis depletes oxaloacetate and acetyl-CoA cannot be converted rapidly enough to citrate, acetyl-CoA accumulates and a decyclase in the liver liberates ketone bodies into the blood.[21]

The liver is the storage site for all fat-soluble vitamins (A, D, E, and K) and several water-soluble vitamins, such as B_{12}. Another vitamin-related function is the conversion of carotene into vitamin A.

The liver is the source of somatomedin (an insulin-like factor that mediates the activity of growth hormone) and angiotensinogen, and is a major site of metabolic clearance of many other hormones. As the source of transferrin, ceruloplasmin, and metallothionein, the liver plays a key role in the transport, storage, and metabolism of iron, copper, and other metals.[22]

Many enzymes are synthesized by liver cells, but not all of them have been found useful in the diagnosis of hepatobiliary disorders. Those enzymes that have been used often include aspartate aminotransferase (AST, or serum glutamic-oxaloacetic transaminase [SGOT]) and alanine aminotransferase (ALT, or serum glutamic-

---

CASE STUDY 22-1

The following laboratory test results were obtained in a patient with severe jaundice, right upper quadrant abdominal pain, fever, and chills (Case Study Table 22-1.1).

Question

1. What is the most likely cause of jaundice in this patient?

CASE STUDY TABLE 22-1.1. LABORATORY RESULTS

Serum alkaline phosphatase	4 times normal
Serum cholesterol	Increased
AST (SGOT)	Normal or slightly increased
5'-Nucleotidase	Increased
Total serum bilirubin	25 mg/dL
Conjugated bilirubin	19 mg/dL
Prothrombin time	Prolonged but improves with a vitamin K injection

pyruvic transaminase [SGPT]), which escape into the plasma from damaged liver cells; alkaline phosphatase (ALP) and 5'-nucleotidase (5NT), which are induced or released when the canalicular membrane is damaged and biliary obstruction occurs; and γ-glutamyltransferase (GGT), which is increased in both hepatocellular and obstructive disorders.[23]

Detoxification and Drug Metabolism

Because the liver is interposed between the splanchnic circulation and the systemic blood, it serves to protect the body from potentially injurious substances absorbed from the intestinal tract and toxic by-products of metabolism. The most important mechanism in this detoxification activity is the microsomal drug-metabolizing system of the liver. This system is induced by many drugs (*eg,* phenobarbital) and other foreign compounds and is responsible for many detoxification mechanisms, including oxidation, reduction, hydrolysis, hydroxylation, carboxylation, and demethylation. These various mechanisms convert many noxious or comparatively insoluble compounds into other forms that are less toxic or more water-soluble and, therefore, excretable by the kidney. For example, ammonia, a toxic substance arising in the large intestine through bacterial action on amino acids, is carried to the liver by the portal vein and converted by hepatocytes into the innocuous compound urea.

Conjugation with moieties, such as glycine, glucuronic acid, sulfuric acid, glutamine, acetate, cysteine, and glutathione, occurs mainly in the cytosol or smooth endoplasmic reticulum. This mechanism is the mode of bilirubin and bile acid excretion.

DISORDERS OF THE LIVER

Jaundice

Jaundice, or *icterus,* refers to the yellowish discoloration of the skin and sclerae resulting from hyperbilirubinemia. Although the upper limit of normal for total serum bilirubin is 1 mg/dL, jaundice is not clinically apparent until the bilirubin level exceeds 2–3 mg/dL. In African American or Asian patients, yellowing of the sclerae may be the only clinical evidence of jaundice.[9] Jaundice is one of the oldest medical disorders known, having been described in ancient Greek, Roman, Chinese, and Hebrew texts. Hippocrates related jaundice to dysfunction of the liver.

Except in infants, hyperbilirubinemia is generally well tolerated and does not produce serious clinical adverse effects. However, in infants, hyperbilirubinemia (levels exceeding 15–20 mg/dL) may be associated with *kernicterus,* a serious disorder of the central nervous system resulting from increased bilirubin levels. This only occurs in infants because the immature central nervous system does not have a well-developed blood-brain barrier.[24–27]

Although all cases of jaundice result from hyperbilirubinemia, not all are caused by hepatic dysfunction. Although the majority of cases of jaundice are associated with liver disorders, hyperbilirubinemia may also result from erythrocyte destruction, or hemolysis, in patients with normal liver function. Distinction between hepatic and hemolytic disease in the patient presenting with jaundice is an important task for which the attending physician will rely heavily on laboratory results. This distinction is discussed in detail later in this chapter.[28,29]

Hypercarotenemia, a disorder caused by the excessive ingestion of vitamin A, may produce skin discoloration indistinguishable from that of hyperbilirubinemia. In hypercarotenemia, however, the sclerae are usually not discolored.

Cirrhosis

Cirrhosis is derived from the Greek word that means "yellow." However, in current usage, *cirrhosis* refers to the irreversible scarring process by which normal liver architecture is transformed into abnormal nodular architecture. One way to classify cirrhosis is by the appearance of the liver; that is, by the size of the nodules. These conditions are referred to as *macronodular* and *micronodular cirrhosis,* although mixed forms occur.[30]

Another way to classify cirrhosis is by etiology. In the United States, Canada, and Western Europe, the leading cause of cirrhosis is alcohol abuse, which leads to a micronodular type of cirrhosis.[31,32] Other causes of cirrhosis include hemochromatosis, postnecrotic cirrhosis (which occurs as a late consequence of hepatitis), and primary biliary cirrhosis (which is an autoimmune disorder). Other uncommon etiologies of cirrhosis exist. About 10–20% of cases cannot be classified as to etiology. Cirrhosis is a serious disorder and one of the ten leading causes of death in the United States. It causes many complications.

Portal hypertension results when blood flow through the portal vein is obstructed by the cirrhotic liver. This may result in splenomegaly, which may not be clinically significant, and esophageal varices, which may rupture and lead to fatal hemorrhage. The synthetic ability of the liver is reduced, causing hypoalbuminemia and deficiency of the clotting factors, which may lead to hemorrhage. Ascitic fluid may accumulate in the abdomen. Although some patients with cirrhosis are capable of prolonged survival, generally this diagnosis is an ominous one.[33,34]

Tumors

On a worldwide basis, primary malignant tumors of the liver, known as *hepatocellular carcinoma, hepatocarcinoma,* or *hepatoma,* are an important cause of cancer mortality. In the United States, these tumors are relatively uncommon. Most cases of hepatocellular carcinoma can be related to previous infection with a hepatitis virus. These tumors are especially common in parts of Africa and Asia and are infrequent in North America and Western Europe. However, the liver is frequently involved secondarily by tumors arising in other organs. Metastatic tumors to the liver from primary sites, such as the lung, pancreas, gastrointestinal tract, or ovary, are common. Benign tumors of the liver are relatively uncommon.[35,36]

Whether primary or secondary, any malignant tumor in the liver is a serious finding with a poor prognosis. Generally, the only hope for cure relies on surgical resection, which is usually impossible. Patients with malignancies of the liver usually have a survival measured in months.[37,38]

Reye's Syndrome

Reye's syndrome is a disorder of unknown cause, involving the liver and arising primarily in children, although cases have been reported in adults. It is a form of hepatic destruction that usually occurs following recovery from a viral infection, such as varicella (chickenpox) or influenza. It has been related to aspirin therapy. Shortly after the infection, the patient develops neurologic abnormalities, which may include seizures or coma. Liver functions are always abnormal, but the bilirubin level is not usually elevated. Without treatment, rapid clinical deterioration, leading to death, may occur.[39–42]

Drug- and Alcohol-Related Disorders

Many drugs and chemicals are toxic to the liver. This toxicity may take the form of overwhelming hepatic necrosis, leading to coma and death, or it may be subclinical and pass entirely unnoticed. Of all hepatic toxins, probably the most important is ethanol. In small amounts, alcohol may cause mild, inapparent injury. Heavier consumption leads to more serious damage, and prolonged,

heavy use may lead to cirrhosis. The exact amount of alcohol needed to cause cirrhosis is unknown, and only a minority of persons with alcoholism develop this condition. It is, however, a leading cause of morbidity and mortality in the United States.[32]

Certain drugs, including tranquilizers such as phenothiazines, certain antibiotics, antineoplastic agents, and anti-inflammatory drugs, may cause liver injury. Usually, this is mild and manifested only by elevation of liver function tests, which return to normal when the offending agent is discontinued. However, this occasionally may lead to massive hepatic failure or cirrhosis.[43–47]

One of the most common drugs associated with serious hepatic injury is acetaminophen. When taken in massive overdose, acetaminophen is virtually certain to produce fatal hepatic necrosis unless rapid treatment is initiated.[48,49]

ASSESSMENT OF LIVER FUNCTION

Analysis of Bilirubin

Brief Review of Classical Methodology

Because its yellow color is detectable by the human eye, concentrations of serum bilirubin have been estimated for centuries. In 1883, Ehrlich first described a reaction in urine samples of the formation of a red or blue pigment when bilirubin was coupled with a diazotized sulfanilic acid solution. In 1913, Van den Bergh applied the Ehrlich reaction to serum bilirubins. He also used alcohol as an accelerator for the coupling of bilirubin to diazotized sulfanilic acid. Malloy and Evelyn developed the first useful quantitative technique for bilirubin in 1937 by accelerating the reaction with a 50% methanol solution, a technique that avoided the precipitation of proteins that was a source of error in the Van den Bergh method. In 1938, Jendrassik and Grof used a procedure

---

CASE STUDY 22-2

The following laboratory test results were found in a patient with mild weight loss and nausea and vomiting, who later developed jaundice and an enlarged liver (Case Study Table 22-2.1).

Question

1. What disease process is most likely in this patient?

CASE STUDY TABLE 22-2.1. LABORATORY RESULTS

Total serum bilirubin	20 mg/dL
Conjugated bilirubin	10 mg/dL
Alkaline phosphatase	Mildly elevated
AST (SGOT)	Significantly elevated
ALT (SGPT)	Moderately elevated
Albumin	Decreased
γ-Globulin	Increased

containing caffeine-benzoate-acetate as an accelerator for the azo-coupling reaction.

Bilirubin also has been quantified by methods other than coupling to sulfanilic acid. These methods include a direct measurement of its natural color. This principle was successfully used in the development of the icterus index, which was introduced in 1919. The test involves diluting serum with saline until it visually matches the color of a .01% potassium dichromate solution. The number of times the serum must be diluted is called the *icterus index*. However, substances in the serum other than bilirubin, such as carotene, xanthophyll, and hemoglobin, also may contribute to the icterus index, limiting its clinical usefulness. This test is now obsolete. In recent years, bilirubin has been quantitated by dilution in a buffer, followed by direct measurement of the absorption, using a well-calibrated spectrophotometer. This method is used in the pediatric laboratory on newborns whose serum does not yet contain the interfering yellow lipochromes. The hemolysis that is so often a problem with pediatric specimens is "blanked out" by measuring a second wavelength. Noninvasive bilirubinometry is now possible.[50,51]

With several methods, it was determined that two types of bilirubin existed.[17] The fraction that produced a color in aqueous solution in the Van den Bergh method was described as *direct bilirubin*, whereas the fraction that produced a color only after alcohol was added was called *indirect bilirubin*. For many years, results of bilirubin determinations were reported as direct or indirect. This terminology is now outdated. Since 1956, it has been known that the direct reaction is given by the diglucuronide of bilirubin or conjugated bilirubin, which is water-soluble. The indirect reaction, however, is given by unconjugated bilirubin, which is water-insoluble but dissolves in alcohol to couple with the diazo reagent. Direct and indirect bilirubin should be reported as conjugated and unconjugated, respectively. Most commonly, conjugated and total bilirubin are reported.[52] Unconjugated bilirubin may be determined by subtracting conjugated bilirubin from total bilirubin.

Method Selection

Unfortunately, no single method for the determination of bilirubin will meet all the requirements of the clinical laboratory. For the evaluation of jaundice in newborns, the direct spectrophotometric method is satisfactory. The sources of error in this technique are turbidity, hemolysis, and yellow lipochrome pigments. Hemolysis and turbidity can be blanked out by measuring a second wavelength, but the yellow lipochromes cannot be blanked out. This method is, therefore, only valid for newborns whose serum does not contain lipochromes. In patients older than 1 month, a diazo-colorimetric procedure is necessary. Most investigators who have compared the dif-

ferent methods for the measurement of bilirubin agree that most techniques available today will give accurate results for total bilirubin, provided that good standards are available. The choice of method, then, should be based on whether one prefers a manual versus automated technique and whether direct bilirubin is to be determined. The choice of a direct bilirubin method poses the greatest problem because there is no reference method or adequate standardization available.

If a manual procedure is desired, then either the Evelyn-Malloy or Jendrassik-Grof method is suitable. The Jendrassik-Grof method is slightly more complex but has advantages over the Evelyn-Malloy method because it:

- is insensitive to sample pH changes.
- is insensitive to a 50-fold variation in protein concentration of the sample.
- has adequate optical sensitivity, even for low bilirubin concentrations.
- has minimal turbidity and a relatively constant serum blank.
- is not affected by hemoglobin up to 750 mg/dL.

Since the development of the original procedure by Jendrassik-Grof, a number of modifications have been made to speed the reaction, reduce interference, and so on. Several commercial bilirubin procedures now use a modified Jendrassik-Grof method. It seems to be a particularly popular technique for the discrete sampler analyzers currently on the market.

The recommended methods for total bilirubin determination using all automated machines will generally give equivalent results. The techniques for direct bilirubin are unfortunately not as reliable. The best method for measuring small amounts of conjugated serum bilirubin is a research method that uses high-performance liquid chromatography, but this method is too difficult for routine laboratory use. Most clinical laboratories use either the Evelyn-Malloy or the Jendrassik-Grof method. Because this chapter does not allow for a detailed description of all previously mentioned bilirubin test methodologies, it emphasizes only the most widely used principles for measuring adult and pediatric bilirubin.[52–55]

Jendrassik-Grof Method for Total and Conjugated Bilirubin Determination[56,57]

Principle. Serum or plasma is added to a solution of sodium acetate and caffeine–sodium benzoate, which is then added to diazotized sulfanilic acid to form purple azobilirubin. The sodium acetate buffers the pH of the diazotization reaction, whereas the caffeine–sodium benzoate accelerates the coupling of bilirubin with diazotized sulfanilic acid. This reaction is terminated by the addition of ascorbic acid, which destroys the excess diazo reagent. A strongly alkaline tartrate solution is then added to convert the purple azobilirubin to blue azobilirubin, and the intensity of the color is read at 600 nm.

Specimen Collection and Storage. A fasting serum specimen, which is neither hemolyzed nor lipemic in nature, is preferred. Before testing, serum should be stored in the dark and measured as soon as possible (within 2–3 hours) after collection. Serum may be stored in the dark in a refrigerator for up to 1 week and in the freezer for 3 months without appreciable change in the bilirubin concentration.

Comments and Sources of Error. Normal blood contains no conjugated bilirubin. Some conjugated bilirubin is reported as normal because current available methodology picks up some of the total bilirubin as a false positive. The best routine methods, however, keep this technical error to a minimum and report upper limits of normal of less than 0.2 mg/dL for conjugated serum bilirubin. This method compensates for lipochrome pigments, which are present in the serum of adults and children older than a few months of age. However, a hemolyzed specimen will cause a decrease in serum bilirubin by this method. In addition, because lipemia causes interference, fasting blood specimens are preferable. Serious loss of bilirubin occurs after exposure to fluorescent and indirect and direct sunlight. Therefore, it is imperative that exposure of samples and standards to light be kept to a minimum and that specimens and standards be refrigerated in the dark until the tests are performed.

Reference Range. Reference ranges for infants after 1 month and adults are shown in Table 22-1.

Direct Spectrophotometric Method for Determination of Total Bilirubin in Serum[52,57]

Principle. The absorbance of bilirubin in serum at 455 nm is proportional to its concentration. The serum of newborns does not contain lipochromes, such as carotene, that would increase the absorbance at 455 nm. The absorbance of hemoglobin at 455 nm is corrected by subtracting the absorbance at 575 nm.

Specimen. Serum is collected and stored with the same precautions as previously mentioned for adult specimens.

Comments and Sources of Error. Error will be introduced if the buffer is turbid. Because the method depends on the extinction coefficient of bilirubin, all volumes must be accurate and cuvets must be flat-surfaced,

with a path length of exactly 1 cm. A control should be used with a level near 20 mg/dL, which is a critical decision point for the clinician because exchange transfusion is necessary if this level is exceeded.

Precautions such as those mentioned in the previous method should also be followed for collection and storage of specimens. This method is relatively insensitive to hemolysis, which is often present in specimens obtained from infants, due to difficulty in skin puncture technique. However, it is significantly affected by the presence of lipochromes and, therefore, cannot be used in infants older than a few months of age.[52]

Reference Range. See Table 22-2.

Urobilinogen in Urine and Feces

Urobilinogen is a colorless end product of bilirubin metabolism that is oxidized by intestinal bacteria to the brown pigment urobilin. In the normal individual, part of the urobilinogen is excreted in the feces, and the remainder is reabsorbed into the portal blood and returned to the liver. A small portion that is not taken up by the hepatocytes is excreted by the kidney as urobilinogen. Increased levels of urinary urobilinogen are found in hemolytic disease and in defective liver-cell function, such as that seen in hepatitis. Absence of urobilinogen from the urine and stool is most often seen with complete biliary obstruction. Fecal urobilinogen is also decreased in biliary obstruction, as well as in hepatocellular disease.[6]

Most quantitative methods for urobilinogen are based on the reaction of this substance with *p*-dimethylaminobenzaldehyde to form a red color. This reaction was first described by Ehrlich in 1901. Many modifications of this procedure have been made over the years to improve specificity. Major improvements were made in 1925 by Terwen, who used alkaline ferrous hydroxide to reduce urobilin to urobilinogen and added sodium acetate to eliminate interference from such compounds as indole. The use of petroleum ether rather than diethyl ether for the extraction of urobilinogen was introduced in 1936 by Watson to help in the removal of other interfering substances. However, because studies indicate that the quantitative methods described do not completely recover urobilinogen from the urine, most laboratories use the less laborious, more rapid, semiquantitative method described next.[58–62]

TABLE 22-1. REFERENCE RANGES FOR BILIRUBIN

Conjugated	0–0.2 mg/dL (0–3 μmol/L)
Unconjugated	0.2–0.8 mg/dL (3–14 μmol/L)
Total	0.2–1.0 mg/dL (3–17 μmol/L)

TABLE 22-2. REFERENCE RANGES FOR INFANT TOTAL BILIRUBIN

INFANTS	PREMATURE, TOTAL	FULL TERM, TOTAL
24 hours	1–6 mg/dL	2–6 mg/dL
48 hours	6–8 mg/dL	6–7 mg/dL
3–5 days	10–12 mg/dL	4–6 mg/dL

Determination of Urine Urobilinogen (Semiquantitative)

Principle. Urobilinogen reacts with *p*-dimethyl amino-benzaldehyde (Ehrlich's reagent) to form a red color, which is then measured spectrophotometrically. Ascorbic acid is added as a reducing agent to maintain urobilinogen in the reduced state. The use of saturated sodium acetate stops the reaction and minimizes the combination of other chromogens with the Ehrlich's reagent.

Specimen. A *fresh* 2-hour urine is collected. This specimen should be kept cool and protected from light.

Comments and Sources of Error.

1. The results of this test are reported in Ehrlich units rather than in milligrams of urobilinogen because substances other than urobilinogen account for some of the final color development.
2. Compounds, other than urobilinogen, that may be present in the urine and react with Ehrlich's reagent include porphobilinogen, sulfonamides, procaine, and 5-hydroxyindoleacetic acid. Bilirubin will form a green color and, therefore, must be removed, as previously described.
3. Fresh urine is necessary, and the test must be performed without delay to prevent oxidation of urobilinogen to urobilin. Similarly, the spectrophotometric readings should be made within 5 minutes after color production because the urobilinogen-aldehyde color slowly decreases in intensity.

Reference Range. Urine urobilinogen, 0.1–1.0 Ehrlich units/2 hr or 0.54.0 Ehrlich units/day (0.86.8 mmol/day); 1 Ehrlich unit is equivalent to approximately 1 mg of urobilinogen.

Fecal Urobilinogen

Visual inspection of the feces usually suffices to detect decreased urobilinogen. However, the semiquantitative determination of fecal urobilinogen is available and involves the same principle described earlier for the urine.[11] It is carried out in an aqueous extract of fresh feces, and any urobilin present is reduced to urobilinogen by treatment with alkaline ferrous hydroxide before Ehrlich's reagent is added. A range of 75–275 Ehrlich units/100 g of fresh feces or 75–400 Ehrlich units per 24-hour specimen is considered a normal reference range.[62]

Measurement of Serum Bile Acids

Unfortunately, complex methods are required for the analysis of bile acids in serum. These involve extraction with organic solvents, partition chromatography, gas chromatography—mass spectroscopy, spectrophotometry, ultraviolet light absorption, fluorescence, radioimmunoassay, and enzyme immunoassay methods.[63–65] Although serum bile acid levels are elevated in liver disease, the total concentration is extremely variable and adds no diagnostic value to other tests of liver function. The variability of the type of bile acids present in serum, together with their existence in different conjugated forms, suggests that more relevant information of liver dysfunction may be gained by examining patterns of individual bile acids and their state of conjugation. For example, it has been suggested that the ratio of the trihydroxy to dihydroxy bile acids in serum will differentiate patients with obstructive jaundice from those with hepatocellular injury and that the diagnosis of primary biliary cirrhosis and extrahepatic cholestasis can be made on the basis of the ratio of the cholic to chenodeoxycholic acids. However, the high cost of these tests, the time required to do them, and the current controversy concerning their clinical usefulness render this approach unsatisfactory for routine use.

Enzyme Tests in Liver Disease

Any injury to the liver that results in cytolysis and necrosis causes the liberation of various enzymes. The measurement of these hepatic enzymes in the serum is used to assess the extent of liver damage and to differentiate hepatocellular (functional) from obstructive (mechanical) disease. The methods used to measure these enzymes, the normal reference ranges, and other general aspects of enzymology are considered in Chapter 10, *Enzymes*. Discussion in this chapter focuses on the characteristic changes in serum enzyme levels seen in various hepatic disorders.

The most common enzymes assayed in hepatobiliary disease include ALP and the aminotransferases. Used less often are γ-glutamyltransferase, lactate dehydrogenase (LD) and its isoenzymes, 5′-nucleotidase, ornithine carbamoyltransferase, and leucine aminopeptidase.[66–70]

Alkaline Phosphatase

ALP is found in a number of tissues but is used most often in the clinical diagnosis of bone and liver disease. Slight to moderate increases in ALP activity occur in many patients with hepatocellular disorders, such as hepatitis and cirrhosis, and transient increases may occur in all types of liver disease. The most striking elevations occur in extrahepatic biliary obstruction, such as a stone in the common bile duct, or in intrahepatic cholestasis, such as drug cholestasis or primary biliary cirrhosis. This enzyme is almost always increased in metastatic liver disease and may be the only abnormality on routine liver function tests. Because bone is a source of the enzyme, Paget disease, bony metastases, and other diseases associated with increased osteoblastic activity may produce high levels of ALP in the absence of liver disease. The enzyme is found in placenta, and pregnant women also have elevated levels.[71–74]

Aminotransferases (Transaminases)

AST (SGOT) and ALT (SGPT) are two enzymes widely used to assess hepatocellular damage. AST (SGOT) is found in all tissue, especially heart, liver, and skeletal muscle. ALT (SGPT) is primarily present in the liver and, to a lesser extent, in kidney and skeletal muscle, making it more "liver specific."

In the absence of acute necrosis or ischemia of other organs, elevated aminotransferase levels suggest hepatocellular damage. In severe viral hepatitis that causes extensive acute necrosis, significantly elevated serum aminotransferase levels may be found, whereas only moderate increases are found in less severe cases. Mild chronic or focal liver diseases, such as subclinical or anicteric viral hepatitis, alcoholic cirrhosis, granulomatous infiltration, and tumor invasion, may be associated with only mild abnormalities. Minimal elevations occur in biliary obstruction.

It is often helpful to conduct serial determinations of aminotransferases when following the course of a patient with acute or chronic hepatitis. However, one should exercise caution in interpreting these abnormal levels, because serum transaminases may actually decrease in some patients with severe acute hepatitis, owing to the exhaustive release of hepatocellular enzymes.[75–78]

5'-Nucleotidase. 5'-Nucleotidase is another phosphatase; it originates largely in the liver and is used clinically to determine whether an ALP elevation is caused by liver or bone disease. Levels of both 5'-nucleotidase and ALP are elevated in liver disease, whereas in primary bone disease, ALP level is elevated, but the 5'-nucleotidase level is usually normal or only slightly elevated. This enzyme is much more sensitive to metastatic liver disease than is ALP because, unlike ALP, its level is not significantly elevated in other conditions, such as pregnancy or childhood. In addition, some increase in enzyme activity may be noted after abdominal surgery.[79–81]

γ-Glutamyltransferase. γ-Glutamyltransferase (GGT) is found in high concentrations in the kidney and the liver and is elevated in the serum of almost all patients with hepatobiliary disorders. It is not specific for any type of liver disease but is frequently the first abnormal liver function test demonstrated in the serum of persons who consume large amounts of alcohol. The highest levels are seen in biliary obstruction. It is, therefore, a sensitive test for alcoholic liver disease. Measurement of this enzyme is also useful if jaundice is absent for the confirmation of hepatic neoplasms and is a useful test to confirm hepatic disease in patients with elevated alkaline phosphates.[82–86]

Leucine Aminopeptidase. Leucine aminopeptidase, widely distributed in human tissue, is found in the pancreas, gastric mucosa, liver, spleen, brain, large and small intestine, and kidney. Most investigators believe that the serum activity of leucine aminopeptidase cannot be used to differentiate hepatocellular from obstructive jaundice. Furthermore, the measurement of this enzyme does not provide any useful information that cannot be obtained by other tests, such as the determination of 5′-nucleotidase or γ-glutamyltransferase.[87]

Lactate Dehydrogenase. Measurement of total serum LD is usually not helpful diagnostically because LD is present in all organs and released into the serum from various tissue injuries. However, fractionation of LD into its five tissue-specific isoenzymes may give useful information about the site of origin of the LD elevation. LD-5 is mostly present in liver and skeletal muscle. An interpretation of isoenzyme patterns may be simple, with an elevated LD-5 in a patient with jaundice. However, the similarity of isoenzyme patterns between different tissue-damaging states may necessitate the use of additional laboratory tests for interpretation.

Moderate elevations of total serum LD levels are common in acute viral hepatitis and in cirrhosis, whereas biliary tract disease may produce only slight elevations. High serum levels may be found in metastatic carcinoma of the liver.[88]

Tests Measuring Hepatic Synthetic Ability

The measurement of the end products of hepatic synthetic activity can be used to assess liver disease. Although these tests are not sensitive to minimal liver damage, they are useful in quantitating the severity of hepatic dysfunction.

Most serum proteins are produced by the liver. A decreased serum albumin may be a result of decreased liver protein synthesis. The albumin level correlates well with the severity of functional impairment and is found more often in chronic rather than acute liver disease. The serum α-globulins also tend to decrease with chronic liver disease. However, a low or absent α-globulin suggests α-antitrypsin deficiency as the cause of the chronic liver disease. Serum γ-globulin levels are transiently increased in acute liver disease and remain elevated in chronic liver disease. The highest elevations are found in chronic active hepatitis and postnecrotic cirrhosis. In particular, IgG and IgM levels are more consistently elevated in chronic active hepatitis, IgM in primary biliary cirrhosis, and IgA in alcoholic cirrhosis.

Prothrombin time is commonly increased in liver disease because the liver is unable to manufacture adequate amounts of clotting factor or because the disruption of bile flow results in inadequate absorption of vitamin K from the intestine. Response of the prothrombin time to the administration of vitamin K is, therefore, of some value in differentiating intrahepatic disease with decreased synthesizing capacity from extrahepatic obstruction with decreased absorption of fat-soluble vitamins. A marked prolongation of the prothrombin time indicates severe diffuse liver disease and a poor prognosis.[89]

Tests Measuring Nitrogen Metabolism

The liver plays a major role in removing ammonia from the bloodstream and converting it to urea so that it can be removed by the kidneys. In liver failure, ammonia and other toxins increase in the bloodstream and may ultimately cause hepatic coma. In this condition, the patient becomes increasingly disoriented and gradually lapses into unconsciousness. The cause of hepatic coma is not fully defined, although ammonia is presumed to play a major role. However, the correlation between blood ammonia levels and the severity of the hepatic coma is poor. Therefore, the ammonia level is most useful when the patient serves as his own control and multiple measurements are made over time.[89–91]

The production of glutamine by an enzymatic intracellular reaction between ammonia and glutamic acid provides a mechanism for removal of ammonia from the central nervous system. Elevations of CSF glutamine have been described in hepatic encephalopathy and in some cases of Reye's syndrome. Glutamine levels can be measured by various methods, including acid hydrolysis and laser-induced fluorescence.[92]

Hepatitis

Hepatitis means "inflammation of the liver," which may be caused by viruses, bacteria, parasites, radiation, drugs, chemicals, autoimmune disease, or toxins. Among the viruses causing hepatitis are hepatitis types A, B, C, D (or delta), and E; cytomegalovirus; Epstein-Barr virus; and probably several others (Table 22-3).

Hepatitis A

Hepatitis A, also known as *infectious hepatitis* and *short-incubation hepatitis,* is usually transmitted by contaminated food or water. Epidemiologic data have suggested that a carrier state in hepatitis A is unlikely or is of a short duration. The hepatitis A virus (HAV) has been identified by electron microscopy as a spherical particle (27 nm wide) containing RNA. HAV has recently been cultured in vitro. However, this tissue-culture system is more a research tool than a diagnostic aid. The fecal shedding of the hepatitis A antigen is transient, and the antigen disappears from the stool after peak elevations of liver enzymes. The diagnosis of hepatitis A is made by

the serologic detection of hepatitis A antibody. The production of hepatitis A antibody (anti-HAV) represents a specific host response to HAV and is believed to confer immunity from reinfection. Use of immune electron microscopy of the stool and radioimmunoassays for the detection of this antibody suggests that different types of antibody (both IgM and IgG) may appear at different times during the course of the illness. The IgM⁻ specific antibody peaks in 1 week and disappears by 8 weeks, whereas the IgG antibody peaks within 1–2 months and persists for years.

The documentation of anti-HAV positivity indicates exposure to HAV, absence of infectivity, and presence of immunity to recurrent infection. Anti-HAV positivity neither implies previous clinically apparent hepatitis nor establishes an etiologic relationship between HAV and acute or chronic liver disease. The demonstration of seroconversion or fecal shedding of antigen during the acute phase of illness is the only reliable method of establishing an HAV etiology. Many people have anti-HAV antibodies without having had a clinically apparent infection.[93–98]

Hepatitis B

Hepatitis B is also known as *serum hepatitis* or *long-incubation hepatitis*. There are three major routes of transmission: parenteral, perinatal, and sexual. An additional fecal–oral route of transmission also exists, although this is not important from an epidemiologic basis. Infected patients manifest hepatitis B in virtually all body fluids, including blood, feces, urine, saliva, semen, tears, and breast milk.

The hepatitis B virus (HBV) consists of a 42-nm, double-shelved, spherical particle with a central core of deoxyribonucleic acid (DNA) surrounded by a protein coat. This particle, which is present in low concentrations in the serum of patients with active viral hepatitis, was originally called the *Dane particle*. Following an HBV infection, the core of the antigen is synthesized in the nuclei of hepatocytes and then passes into the cytoplasm of the liver cell, where it is surrounded by the protein coat. An antigen present in the core of the virus (HBcAg) and

TABLE 22-3. THE HEPATITIS VIRUSES

	NUCLEOTIDE	INCUBATION PERIOD	PRIMARY MODE OF TRANSMISSION	VACCINE	CHRONIC INFECTION	SEROLOGIC DIAGNOSIS AVAILABLE
Hepatitis A	RNA	2–6 weeks	Fecal–oral	Yes	No	Yes
Hepatitis B	DNA	8–26 weeks	Parenteral, sexual	Yes	Yes	Yes
Hepatitis C	RNA	2–15 weeks	Parenteral, ? sexual	No	Yes	Yes
Hepatitis D	RNA	—	Parenteral, sexual	Yes	Yes	Yes
Hepatitis E	RNA	3–6 weeks	Fecal–oral	No	?	Yes

a surface antigen present on the surface protein (HBsAg) have been identified by serologic studies. Another antigen, called the *e antigen (HbeAg)*, also has been identified.[29]

The clinical course of hepatitis B is extremely variable. Approximately two thirds of the cases may be asymptomatic or may produce only a mild flu-like illness. In the remaining one third of cases, a patient may develop a hepatitis-like syndrome of malaise, irregular fevers, right upper quadrant tenderness, jaundice, and dark urine.[98–101]

In approximately 1% of infected patients, the syndrome of fulminant hepatitis may develop. This is an overwhelming clinical illness with a high mortality.

Approximately 90% of patients infected with HBV recover within 6 months. This recovery is manifested by the development of antibody to hepatitis B surface antigen. Approximately 10% of the infected patients will develop chronic hepatitis, which is discussed later in the section, *Chronic Hepatitis B.*

Worldwide, HBV infection is fairly common and usually occurs at the time of birth. In some areas, such as parts of Africa, Asia, and the Pacific islands, up to 80% of the general population may show serologic evidence of past hepatitis infection. The chronic carrier rate is high. Such persons are at high risk for development of cirrhosis or hepatocellular carcinoma (hepatoma).[102]

In the United States, fewer than 10% of the population shows serologic evidence of past infection with the HBV. The chronic carrier rate is less than 1% of the general population. Persons at high risk for infection in this country include male homosexuals, intravenous drug abusers, children born to mothers who are hepatitis B surface antigen-positive at the time of delivery, immigrants from endemic areas, and sexual partners and household contacts of patients who have hepatitis B. Although transmission of hepatitis B by blood products still occurs, effective screening tests now make this rare. Health care workers, including laboratory personnel, may be at increased risk for developing hepatitis B, depending on their degree of exposure to blood and body fluids.[100]

An effective vaccine and also immunoglobulin exist for hepatitis B. The vaccine is highly effective in stimulating the production of hepatitis B surface antibody and, therefore, rendering the recipient immune. Following an acute exposure, such as a needlestick injury, the patient should receive both hepatitis vaccine and immunoglobulin. A similar treatment is highly effective in preventing the development of hepatitis in infants born to infected mothers.

It is especially important that all health care workers exposed to blood and body fluids take the hepatitis vaccine. Each year, thousands of cases of hepatitis B occur among health care workers, and several hundred die from its complications. This is entirely preventable. Everyone who works in the clinical laboratory should take the hepatitis vaccine.[97,101]

Hepatitis BsAg

Hepatitis BsAg (HBsAg), previously known as the *Australia antigen* and *hepatitis-associated antigen (HAA)*, is the antigen for which routine testing is performed on all donated units of blood. HBsAg is the first serologic marker to appear during the prodrome of acute hepatitis

---

CASE STUDY 22-3

The following laboratory results are obtained from a 19-year-old college student who consulted the Student Health Service because of fatigue and lack of appetite. She adds that she recently noted that her sclera appears somewhat yellowish and that her urine has become dark (Case Study Table 22-3.1).

Questions

1. What is the most likely diagnosis?

2. What additional factors in the patient's history should be sought?

3. What is the prognosis?

CASE STUDY TABLE 22-3.1. LABORATORY RESULTS

ALT (SGPT)	Elevated
AST (SGOT)	Elevated
Alkaline phosphatase	Minimally elevated
LD	Elevated
Serum bilirubin	5 mg/dL
Urine bilirubin	Increased
Hepatitis A antibody (IgG)	Negative
Hepatitis A antibody (IgM)	Positive
Hepatitis B surface antigen	Negative
Hepatitis B surface antibody	Negative
Hepatitis C antibody	Negative

B, and it identifies infected patients before the onset of clinical illness more reliably than any other. Although it has been shown that the isolated viral protein coat is not infectious, persons who chronically carry HBsAg in their serum must be considered potentially infectious because the presence of the intact virus cannot be excluded. Patients who recover from hepatitis B develop anti-HBs following the disappearance of the HBsAg at about the time of clinical recovery (Fig. 22-5). This antibody is common in the general population and is believed to confer immunity to future reinfection with HBV.[100]

Hepatitis BcAg

The core antigen, HBcAg, has not been demonstrated in the plasma of hepatitis victims or blood donors. This antigen is seen only in the nuclei of hepatocytes during an acute infection with hepatitis B. The antibody to the core antigen, anti-HBc, usually develops earlier in the course than the antibody to the surface antigen (Fig. 22-5). A recent serologic marker assay developed for general use is a test for IgM antibody to hepatitis B core antigen. In the proper clinical setting, this IgM assay has been shown to be specific for acute hepatitis B. Closely associated with the core antigen is a viral DN-dependent DNA polymerase. This viral enzyme is required for viral replication and is detectable in serum early in the course of viral hepatitis, during the phase of active viral replication.[98]

Hepatitis BeAg

Another marker of HBV infection is the e antigen. This antigen appears to be more closely associated with the core than the surface of the viral particle. The presence of the e antigen appears to correlate well with both the number of infectious virus particles and the degree of infectivity of HBsAg-positive sera. The presence of HBeAg in HBsAg carriers is an unfavorable prognostic sign and predicts a severe course and chronic liver disease. Conversely, the presence of anti-HBe antibody in carriers indicates a low infectivity of the serum (Fig. 22-6). The e antigen is detected in serum only when surface antigen is present (Fig. 22-7).

Hepatitis B Viral DNA Assay

It is possible to detect actual HBV DNA in the blood using nucleic acid hybridization or polymerase chain reactions. This provides a more sensitive measurement of infectivity and disease progression than serology. It may be used to monitor the effectiveness of antiviral therapy in patients with chronic HBV infection, but it supplements rather than replaces current HBV serologic assays.[103–105]

Hepatitis C

Until fairly recently, cases of viral hepatitis that could not be identified as type A or type B by serologic markers were logged in the general category of non-A or non-B hepatitis. Recently, the agent responsible for approximately 80% of these cases was identified as the ribonucleic acid (RNA) containing the *hepatitis C virus (HCV)*.

Tests for detecting those at risk for transmitting HCV are now available. They detect antibody to HCV and identify most infectious carriers.[106] Although much remains to be learned about hepatitis C, it appears most often to be transmitted parenterally. Sexual and fecal–oral routes also exist, and it may be transmitted by blood transfusion.[107–109]

Approximately 3% of blood donors in the United States are positive for HCV. Most of these patients are presumed to be infectious. The HCV antibody test will detect most infectious patients, although false-positive results do occur.[108]

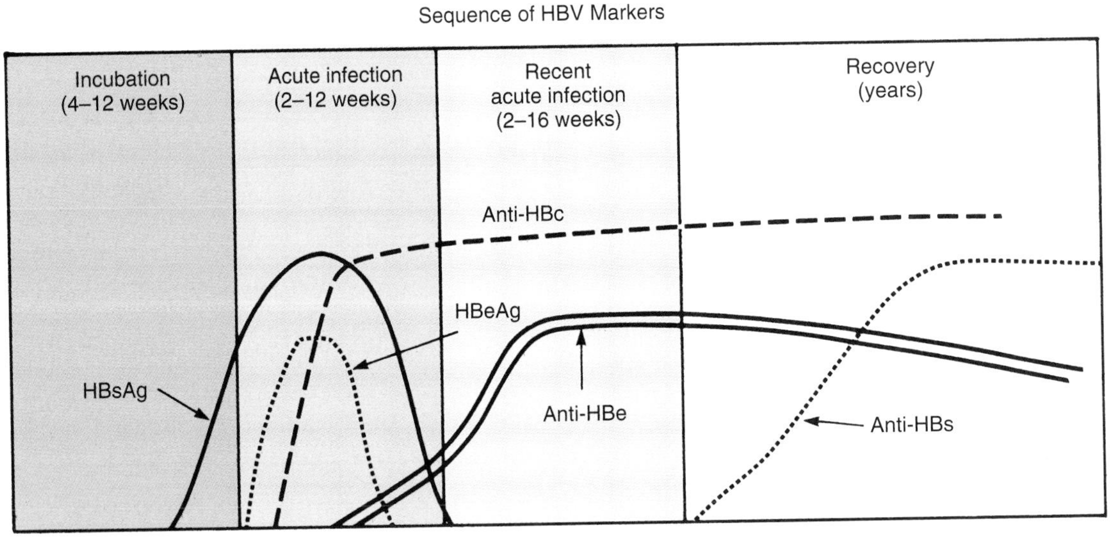

Sequence of HBV Markers

FIGURE 22-5. Serology of hepatitis B infection with recovery.

Sequence of HBV Surface Markers
Chronic Hepatitis

Incubation (4–12 weeks)	Acute illness (6 months)	Chronic hepatitis (years)

HBsAg

HBeAg

HBcAg

FIGURE 22-6. No antibody is formed against HBsAg. The persistence of HBeAg implies high infectivity and a generally poor prognosis. This patient would likely develop cirrhosis unless seroconversion occurs or treatment is given.

Clinically, acute hepatitis C is usually mild and may be entirely inapparent. However, infection has a high rate of progression to chronic hepatitis, cirrhosis, and carcinoma. Therefore, hepatitis C appears to be a major cause of chronic hepatitis in this country.[109,110]

Hepatitis C antibody is usually not detected in the first few months of infection but will almost always be present in the later stages. It is not protective and sometimes disappears several years following the resolution of the infection.

The serologic assay for HCV antibody is a screening test, and false-positives may occur. Therefore, positive results should be confirmed by a more specific method, such as the HCV recombinant immunoblast assay.[111]

Delta Hepatitis

Delta hepatitis, or hepatitis D (HDV), constitutes a unique example of satellite virus infection in human disease. HDV causes disease only in HBV-infected patients. It is incapable of causing any illness in patients who do not have hepatitis B.

HDV is an RNA virus with a high-degree of base-pair homology with HBV. When delta virus infection occurs in a patient who already has HBV infection, the delta virus uses HBV for replication. Then, both HBV and HDV are produced. Unlike the HBV, HDV appears directly toxic to human hepatocytes.

Two basic types of HDV infection exist, but both have the effect of worsening the prognosis of HBV. In coinfec-

Sequence of HBV Surface Markers
Chronic Hepatitis

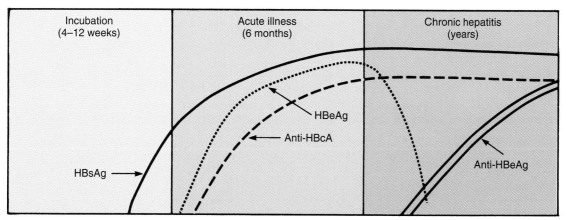

Incubation (4–12 weeks)	Acute illness (6 months)	Chronic hepatitis (years)

HBeAg

Anti-HBcA

Anti-HBeAg

HBsAg

FIGURE 22-7. Serology of chronic hepatitis with formation of antibody to HBeAg. This is a favorable sign and suggests that the chronic hepatitis may resolve. Complete recovery would be heralded by the disappearance of HBsAg and formation of its corresponding antibody.

CASE STUDY 22-4

The following results were obtained in the patient from Case Study 22-2 (Case Study Table 22-4.1).

Questions

1. What is the most likely diagnosis?

2. What is the prognosis?

3. What complications may develop?

CASE STUDY TABLE 22-4.1. LABORATORY RESULTS

Hepatitis A antibody (IgG)	Positive
Hepatitis A antibody (IgM)	Negative
Hepatitis B surface antigen	Positive
Hepatitis B surface antibody	Negative
Hepatitis Core antibody (IgM)	Positive
Hepatitis C antibody	Negative

---

tion, the patient acquires HBV and HDV simultaneously. A patient with this coinfection is more likely to develop serious complications and has a higher rate of progression to chronic hepatitis. However, the majority of the patients still recover.

The other possibility is superinfection, in which a patient who is a chronic HBV carrier is superinfected with the HDV. Fulminant hepatitis may develop or the progression to cirrhosis may be accelerated.

Epidemiologically, HDV infection appears concentrated in countries surrounding the Mediterranean, Black, and Red Seas. In the United States, between 10 and 20% of patients who are chronic HBV carriers will be serologically positive for HDV. The risk factors for HDV infection are generally the same as for HBV infection.[111–116]

Hepatitis E

The RNA-containing hepatitis E virus is transmitted primarily by the fecal–oral route. This illness is found mainly in underdeveloped countries, although sporadic cases have been reported, primarily among travelers, in the United States and Western Europe. The incubation period is short, generally between 21 and 42 days. The virus may be detected in feces and bile by about 7 days after infection.

Hepatitis E infection is generally mild, except in pregnant women, in whom it may be a devastating illness. Serologic tests are available for diagnosis.[113,117–124]

Worldwide, hepatitis E is an RNA-type virus associated with both acute and chronic hepatitis.

Chronic Hepatitis[102,104,125–129]

When evidence of hepatitis, such as elevated serum transaminase levels, is present for more than 6 months, *chronic hepatitis* is said to exist. Many different agents, including viruses, drugs, and alcohol, may cause chronic hepatitis. However, this discussion centers on viral causes.

Approximately 10% of HBV cases will progress to chronic hepatitis. The severity of the initial illness has nothing to do with the risk of developing chronicity.

CASE STUDY 22-5

A 36-year-old man consulted his family physician because of liver function abnormalities, which had been noted initially during a preinsurance physical examination 6 months ago. The following laboratory results are obtained, which are identical to those obtained 6 months previous (Case Study 22-5.1).

Questions

1. What is the most likely diagnosis?

2. What is the prognosis?

3. What complications may develop?

4. What additional tests should be done?

CASE STUDY TABLE 22-5.1. LABORATORY RESULTS

Hepatitis A antibody (IgG)	Positive
Hepatitis A antibody (IgM)	Negative
Hepatitis B surface antigen	Positive
Hepatitis B surface antibody	Negative
Hepatitis B core antibody (IgM)	Positive
Hepatitis C antibody	Negative

Therefore, many patients may develop chronic hepatitis without having been aware that they had hepatitis B infection. The serologic findings in patients with chronic hepatitis B are shown in Figure 22-7. These patients may be clinically sick or they may be apparently entirely healthy. However, as long as HBsAg is present, they are infectious and at risk for developing complications, including cirrhosis and hepatocellular carcinoma. Patients who manifest the e antigen are highly infectious and said to have the worst prognosis. The appearance of antibody to e antigen may herald recovery. Complete recovery occurs when hepatitis B surface antigen disappears and the corresponding antibody is detected. These patients are then immune to further infection. Although many patients with chronic hepatitis recover spontaneously, others may require aggressive treatment.

Worldwide, hepatitis B infection constitutes a major cause of morbidity and mortality. In underdeveloped countries, infection often occurs at the time of birth, and these children are at high risk for the development of cirrhosis or hepatocellular carcinoma.

Hepatitis C also has a high degree of chronicity. Although patients with chronic hepatitis C infection appear to be at high risk for cirrhosis, the role of hepatitis C in the development of hepatocellular carcinoma is much less clear. Interferon is currently used to treat chronic hepatitis. Hepatitis A is rarely, if ever, associated with chronic disease. Most patients with chronic hepatitis C have no signs or symptoms but manifest only mild elevations of liver function tests, especially transaminases. The degree of elevation has little predictive value in individual patients. About 80% of infected patients develop chronic hepatitis, although, in most cases, the disease does not progress. The percentage of patients progressing to cirrhosis varies widely in different studies but has been estimated to be as high as 40% after 40 years. Alcohol consumption increases the risk of cirrhosis. Liver biopsies are performed periodically in these patients, with the degree of inflammation and fibrosis correlating with the risk of cirrhosis.

Patients with chronic hepatitis C are usually treated with pegylated interferon and ribavirin. Therapy is monitored by estimating viral particles in plasma, using polymerase chain reaction (PCR).[121]

Other Forms of Hepatitis

Five forms of viral hepatitis (A, B, C, D, E) are well recognized. The role of G viruses is currently unclear. Hepatitis F is an enteric agent that may be transmitted to primates. Again, more needs to be learned about this agent and its role, if any, in human disease. Other forms of viral hepatitis, such as TT virus and SEN virus, may exist. The GB group of flavo-like viruses, GBV-A, GBV-B and GBV-C, are also associated with acute and chronic hepatitis. Little is known about these diseases. No diagnostic tests for them are commercially available at this time.[130–133]

SUMMARY

The liver is the largest and most versatile and complex organ in the body. It consists of two main lobes. The lobule, cords of liver cells or hepatocytes radiating from a central vein, forms the structural unit of the liver. There are several hundred known functions performed by the liver each day, including metabolic, secretory, and excretory functions. One of the most important functions of the liver is the excretion of bile. Bilirubin is the principal pigment in bile and is derived from the breakdown of hemoglobin when aged red blood cells are phagocytized by the reticuloendothelial system. There are two forms of bilirubin: conjugated and unconjugated. An increase in the concentration of bilirubin is known as jaundice. Jaundice may be caused by a variety of pathophysiologic mechanisms. There are three types of jaundice: prehepatic, hepatic, and posthepatic.

Among the many diverse metabolic functions of the liver is the synthesis of proteins, carbohydrates, and lipids. Many enzymes are synthesized by the liver, but not all have been found useful in the diagnosis of hepatobiliary disorders. Disorders of the liver include jaundice, cirrhosis, tumors, Reye's syndrome, and drug- and alcohol-related disorders. Analysis of bilirubin concentrations has been used for centuries to assess liver function. Two commonly used methodologies to assess bilirubin are Evelyn-Malloy and Jendrassik-Grof. Urobilinogen, a colorless end product of bilirubin metabolism, may also be measured to assess liver function. The measurement of hepatic enzymes in serum is used to assess the extent of liver damage and to differentiate hepatocellular (functional) from obstructive (mechanical) disease. The most common enzymes assayed in hepatobiliary disease include ALP and the aminotransferases (AST and ALT). Hepatitis, or inflammation of the liver, may be caused by viruses, bacteria, parasites, radiation, drugs, chemicals, or toxins. Among the viruses causing hepatitis are hepatitis types A, B, C, D (or delta), and E, cytomegalovirus, Epstein-Barr virus, and probably several others. Hepatitis A is usually transmitted by the fecal/oral root and causes a mild or inapparent infection with no tendency to chronic disease. Hepatitis B and C are primarily transmitted parenterally. Hepatitis B causes a serious illness in a minority of patients; however, in many patients, the infection is mild or even inapparent. Acute infection with hepatitis C is usually mild to inapparent. Hepatitis B has a slight tendency to chronic disease, while most patients with hepatitis C infection develop chronic infection.

Delta hepatitis is a unique satellite virus that causes a superinfection in patients already infected with hepatitis B. Hepatitis E is primarily transmitted by the fecal/oral root and causes serious disease only in pregnant women.

Chronic hepatitis is a major cause of morbidity and mortality worldwide. Chronic hepatitis is a major risk factor for the development of hepatocellular carcinoma.

REVIEW QUESTIONS

1. Hyperbilirubinemia in newborns usually:
   a. results in permanent brain damage.
   b. is caused by hemolysis.
   c. is caused by biliary atresia.
   d. produces no serious consequences.
   e. must be treated if serum bilirubin levels exceed 5 mg/dL.

2. Cirrhosis is derived from the Greek word meaning:
   a. yellow.
   b. hard.
   c. large.
   d. tumor.
   e. liver.

3. All of the following statements concerning urobilinogen are correct EXCEPT:
   a. colorless.
   b. produced by oxidative actions of intestinal bacteria.
   c. undergoes significant enterohepatic circulation.
   d. urinary levels increased in biliary obstruction.
   e. fecal levels decreased in biliary obstruction.

4. Elevated levels of CSF glutamine are found in patients with:
   a. hepatic encephalopathy.
   b. brain tumors.
   c. strokes.
   d. schizophrenia.
   e. renal failure.

5. Which form of hepatitis is caused by a DNA virus?
   a. Hepatitis A
   b. Hepatitis B
   c. Hepatitis C
   d. Hepatitis D
   e. Hepatitis E

6. In patients with hepatitis B, hepatitis e antigen is found in serum only when which of the following is also present?
   a. Surface antigen
   b. Antibody to surface antigen
   c. Antibody to hepatitis E
   d. Hepatitis C antibody (IgG)
   e. Hepatitis C antibody (IgM)

7. Which of the following enzymes is most useful in establishing the hepatic origin of an elevated serum alkaline phosphatase?
   a. Alanine aminotransferase
   b. Aspartate aminotransferase
   c. Ornithine carbamoyltransferase
   d. γ-Glutamyltranspeptidase
   e. Lactate dehydrogenase

8. Hepatitis E infection is likely to produce serious consequences in:
   a. children.
   b. pregnant women.
   c. travelers in third world countries.
   d. older people.
   e. patients who take aspirin.

9. Worldwide, most primary malignant tumors of the liver are related to:
   a. alcoholism.
   b. gallstones.
   c. previous infection with a hepatitis virus.
   d. Reye's syndrome.
   e. malaria.

10. Ehrlich reagent is used in the measurement of:
    a. bilirubin.
    b. urobilinogen.
    c. ammonia.
    d. bile acids.

REFERENCES

1. Barnard SE, Becker YT, Blair KT, et al. The effect of low dose epinephrine infusion on hepatic hemodynamics. Transplant Proc 1998;30(5):2306–2308.
2. Emond JC, Renz JF. Surgical anatomy of the liver and its application to hepatobiliary surgery transplantation. Semin Liver Dis 1994;14(2):158–168.
3. Barwick K, Rosai, J. Ackerman's Surgical Pathology, 8th ed. St Louis: CV Mosby, 1996:857–942.
4. De Wit LT, Douma DJ, Groen AK, et al. Hepatic bile versus gallbladder bile: a comparison of protein and lipid concentration and composition in cholesterol gallstone patients. Hepatology 1998;28(1):11–16.
5. Balistreri WF. Fetal and neonatal bile acid synthesis and clinical implications. J Inherited Metab Dis 1991;14:459–477.
6. Hofmann AF. Bile acid secretion, bile flow and biliary lipid secretion in humans. Hepatology 1990;12(3, Pt 2):17S–22S, discussion, 22S–25S.
7. Fuchs M. Bile acid regulation of hepatic physiology: III. Regulation of bile acid synthesis: past progress and future challenges. Am J Physiol Gastrointest Liver Physiol 2003;284(4):G551–G557.
8. Ahlfors CE. Measurement of plasma unbound unconjugated bilirubin. Anal Biochem 2000;15;279(2):130–135.
9. Lyche KD, Brenner DA. A logical approach to the patient with jaundice. Contemp Intern Med 1992;4(5):43–58.

10. Beckingham IJ, Ryder SD. ABC of diseases of liver, pancreas, and biliary system. Investigation of liver and biliary diseases. BMJ 2001;322(7277):33–36.

11. Doumas BT, Wu TW. The measurement of bilirubin fractions in serum. Crit Rev Clin Lab Sci 1991;28:415–446.

12. Mathew P. The genetic basis of Gilbert's syndrome. N Engl J Med 1996;334(12):802–803.

13. Adachi Y, Koiwai O, Sato H. The genetic basis of Gilbert's syndrome. Lancet 1996;347(9001):557–558.

14. Emi Y, Ikushiro S, Iyanagi T. Biochemical and molecular aspects of genetic disorders of bilirubin metabolism. Biochim Biophys Acta 1998;1407(3):173–184.

15. Gollan JL, Green RM. Crigler-Najjar disease type I: therapeutic approaches to genetic liver diseases into the next century. Gastroenterology 1997;112(2):649–651.

16. Berg CL. The physiology of jaundice: molecular and functional characterization of the Crigler-Najjar syndromes. Hepatology 1995;22(4, Pt 1):1338–1340.

17. Westwood A. The analysis of bilirubin in serum. Ann Clin Biochem 1991;28(Pt 2):119–130.

18. Cherrington AD, Connolly CC, Moore MC. Autoregulation of hepatic glucose production. Eur J Endocrinol 1998;138(3):240–248.

19. Kjaer M. Hepatic glucose production during exercise. Adv Exp Med Biol 1998;441:117–127.

20. Ascher N, Carithers RL Jr, Hoofnagle JH, et al. Fulminant hepatic failure: summary of a workshop. Hepatology 1995;21(1):240–252.

21. Gorski J, Oscai LB, Palmer WK. Hepatic lipid metabolism in exercise and training. Med Sci Sports Exerc 1990;22(2):213–221.

22. Bonkovsky HL. Iron and the liver. Am J Med Sci 1991;301(1):32–43.

23. Rochling FA. Evaluation of abnormal liver tests. Clin Cornerstone 2001;3(6):1–12.

24. Arai N, Hayashi M, Kumada S, et al. Neuropathology of the dentate nucleus in developmental disorders. Acta Neuropathol (Berl) 1997;94(1):36–41.

25. Burns D, Perlman JM, Rogers BB. Kernicteric findings at autopsy in two sick near term infants. Pediatrics 1997;99(4):612–615.

26. Gourley, GR. Bilirubin metabolism and kernicterus. Adv Pediatr 1997;44:173–229.

27. Ostrow JD, Tiribelli C. New concepts in bilirubin and jaundice: report of the Third International Bilirubin Workshop, April 6–8, 1995, Trieste, Italy. Hepatology 1996;24(5):1296–1311.

28. Black ER. Diagnostic strategies and test algorithms in liver disease. Clin Chem 1997;43(8, Pt 2):1555–1560.

29. Neuschwander-Tetri BA. Common blood tests for liver disease. Which ones are most useful? Postgrad Med 1995;98(1):49–56, 59, 63.

30. Popper H. General pathology of the liver. Light microscopic aspects serving diagnosis and interpretation. Semin Liver Dis 1986;6:175–184.

31. Menon KV, Gores GJ, Shah VH. Pathogenesis, diagnosis, and treatment of alcoholic liver disease. Mayo Clin Proc 2001;76(10):1021–1029.

32. Lieber CS. Alcohol and the liver: 1994 update. Gastroenterology 1994;106(4):1085–1105.

33. Bosch J. Medical treatment of portal hypertension. Digestion 1998;59(5):547–555.

34. Barnes DS, Geisinger MA, Henderson JM. Portal hypertension. Curr Probl Surg 1998;35(5):379–452.

35. Del Olmo JA, Escudero A, Gilabert S, et al. Incidence and risk factors for hepatocellular carcinoma in 967 patients with cirrhosis. J Cancer Res Clin Oncol 1998;124(10):560–564.

36. Carriaga MT, Henson DE. Liver, gallbladder, extrahepatic bile ducts, and pancreas. Cancer 1995;75:171–190.

37. Blair T, Blanke C, Chappam WC, et al. Hepatocellular carcinoma outcomes based on indicated treatment strategy. Am Surg 1998;64(12):1128–1134; discussion 1134–1135.

38. Fan ST, Lau H, Ng IO, et al. Long term prognosis after hepatectomy for hepatocellular carcinoma: a survival analysis of 204 consecutive patients. Cancer 1998;83(11):2302–2311.

39. Bruce JC, Glasgow JF, Hall SM, et al. The changing clinical pattern of Reye's syndrome 1982–1990. Arch Dis Child 1996;74(5):400–405.

40. Salmona M, Tacconi MT, Visentin M. Reye's and Reye-like syndromes, drug-related diseases? (Causative agents, etiology, pathogenesis, and therapeutic approaches). Drug Metab Rev 1995;27(3):517–539.

41. Smith TC. Reye syndrome and the use of aspirin. Scott Med J 1996;41(1):4–9.

42. Stumpf DA. Reye syndrome: an international perspective. Brain Dev 1995;17(Suppl):77–78.

43. Amacher DE. Serum transaminase elevations as indicators of hepatic injury following the administration of drugs. Regul Toxicol Pharmacol 1998;27(2):119–130.

44. Garcia Rodriguez LA, Jick H, Ruigomez A. A review of epidemiologic research on drug-induced acute liver injury using the general practice research database in the United Kingdom. Pharmacotherapy 1997;17(4):721–728.

45. Arner P, Large V. Regulation of lipolysis in humans. Pathophysiological modulation in obesity, diabetes, and hyperlipidaemia. Diabetes Metab 1998;24(5):409–418.

46. Dossing M, Sonne J. Drug-induced hepatic disorders. Incidence, management and avoidance. Drug Saf 1993;9(6):441–449.

47. Goodman ZD. Drug hepatotoxicity. Clin Liver Dis 2002;6(2):381–397.

48. Anker AL, Smilkstein MJ. Acetaminophen. Concepts and controversies. Emerg Med Clin North Am 1994;12(2):335–349.

49. Lee WM. Review article: drug-induced hepatotoxicity. Aliment Pharmacol Ther 1993;7(5):477–485.

50. Hansen TW. Mechanisms of bilirubin toxicity: clinical implications. Clin Perinatol 2002;29(4):765–778, viii.

51. Bertini G, Rubaltelli FF. Non-invasive bilirubinometry in neonatal jaundice. Semin Neonatol 2002;7(2):129–33.

52. Doumas BT, Lott JA. Direct and total bilirubin tests: contemporary problems. Clin Chem 1993;39(4):641–647.

53. Slaughter, MR. Sensitivity of conventional methods for bilirubin measurements. J Lab Clin Med 1996;127(2):233.

54. Ryder KW, et al. Erroneous laboratory results from hemolyzed, icteric, and lipemic specimens. Clin Chem 1993;39(1):175–176.

55. Ross JW, et al. The accuracy of laboratory measurements in clinical chemistry: a study of 11 routine chemistry analytes in the College of American Pathologists chemistry survey with fresh frozen serum, definitive methods, and reference methods. Arch Pathol Lab Med 1998;122(7):587–608.

56. Schlebusch H, et al. Comparison of five routine methods with the candidate reference method for the determination of bilirubin in neonatal serum. J Clin Chem Clin Biochem 1990;28(4):203–210.

57. Harrison SP, et al. Three direct spectrophotometric methods for determination of total bilirubin in neonatal and adult serum, adapted to the Technicon RA-1000 Analyzer. Clin Chem 1989;35(9):1980–1986.

58. Misdraji J, Nguyen PL. Urinalysis. When-and when not-to order. Postgrad Med 1996;100(1):173–6,181–2,185–8.

59. Rumley A. Urine dipstick testing: comparison of results obtained by visual reading and with the Bayer CLINITEK 50. Ann Clin Biochem 2000;37(Pt 2):220–221.

60. Binder L, Glass B, Haynes J, et al. Failure of prediction of liver function test abnormalities with the urine urobilinogen and urine bilirubin assays. Arch Pathol Lab Med 1989;113(1):73–76.

61. Fevery J, Kotal P. Quantitation of urobilinogen in feces, urine, bile and serum by direct spectrophotometry of zinc complex. Clin Chim Acta 1991;14:202(1–2):1–9.

62. Binder L, Glas B, Haynes J, et al. Abnormalities of urine urobilinogen and urine bilirubin assays and their relation to abnormal results of serum liver function tests. South Med J 1988; 81(10):1229–1232.

63. Lee BL, New AL, Ong CN. Comparative analysis of conjugated bile acids in human serum using high-performance liquid chromatography and capillary electrophoresis. J Chromatogr B Biomet Sci Appl 1997;704(1–1):35–42.

64. Polkowska G, Polkowska W, Kudlicka A, Wallner G, Chrzasteck-Spurch H. Range of serum bile acid concentrations in neonates, infants, older children, and in adults. Med Sci Monit 2001;7 Suppl 1:268–270.

65. Azer SA, Klaassen CD, Stacey NH. Biochemical assay of serum bile acids: methods and applications. Br J Biomed Sci 1997; 54(2):118–132.

66. Burke MD. Liver function: test selection and interpretation of results. Clin Lab Med 2002;22 (2):377–390.

67. Aliberti G, Corvisieri P, de Michele LV, et al. Lactate dehydrogenase and its isoenzymes in the marrow and peripheral blood from haematologically normal subjects. Physiol Res 1997;46(6):435–438.

68. Aranda-Michel J, et al. Tests of the liver: use and misuse. Gastroenterologist 1998;6(1):34–43.

69. Collier J, Bassendine M. How to response to abnormal liver function tests. Clin Med 2002;2(5):406–409.

70. Pratt DS, Kaplan MM. Evaluation of abnormal liver-enzyme results in asymptomatic patients. N Engl J Med 2000;342(17): 1266–1271.

71. Moss DW. Diagnostic aspects of alkaline phosphatase and its isoenzymes. Clin Biochem 1987;20(4):225–230.

72. Mercer DW. Serum isoenzymes in cancer diagnosis and management. Immunol Ser 1990;53:613–629.

73. Artiss JD, Epstein E, Kiechle FL, et al. The clinical use of alkaline phosphatase enzymes. Clin Lab Med 1986;6(3):491–505.

74. Raymond FD, Moss DW, Fisher D. Separation of alkaline phosphatase isoforms with and without intact glycan-phosphatidylinositol anchors in aqueous polymer phase systems. Clin Chim Acta 1994;227(1–2):111–120.

75. Sherman KE. Alanine aminotransferase in clinical practice. A review. Arch Intern Med 1991;151(2):260–265.

76. Mandell BF. Alanine aminotransferase: a nonspecific marker of liver disease. Arch Intern Med 1992;152(1):209–213.

77. Rej R. Aminotransferases in disease. Clin Lab Med 1989;9(4): 667–687.

78. Panteghini M, et al. Clinical and diagnostic significance of aspartate aminotransferase isoenzymes in sera of patients with liver diseases. J Clin Chem Clin Biochem 1984;22(2):153–158.

79. Bacq Y, et al. Liver function tests in normal pregnancy: a prospective study of 103 pregnant women and 103 matched controls. Hepatology 1996;23(5):1030–1034.

80. Panteghini M. Electrophoretic fractionation of 5'-nucleotidase. Clin Chem 1994;40(2):190–196.

81. Sunderman FW Jr. The clinical biochemistry of 5'-nucleotidase. Ann Clin Lab Sci 1990;20(2):123–139.

82. Stewart SH. Racial and ethnic differences in alcohol-associated aspartate aminotransferase and gamma-glutamyltransferase evaluation. Arch Intern Med 2002;162(19):2236–2239.

83. Harasymiw J. The early detection of heavy alcohol consumption using routine clinical laboratory test results. Am Clin Lab 2002; 21(6):22–24.

84. Whitfield JB. Gamma glutamyltransferase. Crit Rev Clin Lab Sci 2001;38(4):263–355.

85. Cabrera-Abreu JC, Green A. Gamma-glutamyltransferase: value of its measurement in paediatrics. Ann Clin Biochem 2002;39(Pt 1):22–25.

86. Conigrave KM, Degenhardt LJ, Whitfield JB, et al. WHO/ISBRA study group. CDT, GGT, and AST as markers of alcohol use: the WHO/ISBRA collaborative project. Alcohol Clin Exp Res 2002; 25(3):332–339.

87. Alhava E, Partanen K, Pasanen P, et al. Value of serum alkaline phosphatase, aminotransferases, gamma-glutamyltransferase, leucine aminopeptidase, and bilirubin in the distinction between benign and malignant diseases causing jaundice and cholestasis: results from a prospective study. Scand J Clin Lab Invest 1993; 53(1):35–39.

88. Schwartz MK. Lactic dehydrogenase. an old enzyme reborn as a cancer marker? Am J Clin Pathol 1991;96(4):441–443.

89. Anand AC, Neuberger JM, Nightingale P. Early indicators of prognosis in fulminant hepatic failure: an assessment of the King's criteria. J Hepatol 1997;26(1):62–68.

90. Green A. When and how should we measure plasma ammonia? Ann Clin Biochem 1988;25:(Pt 3):199–209.

91. da Fonseca-Wollheim F. The influence of pH and various anions on the distribution of $NH4+$ in human blood. Eur J Clin Chem Biochem 1995;33(5):289–294.

92. Tucci S, et al. Measurement of glutamine and glutamate by capillary electrophoresis and laser induced fluorescence detection in cerebrospinal fluid of meningitis sick children. Clin Biochem 1998;31(3):143–150.

93. Koff RS. Hepatitis A. Lancet 1998;351(9116):1643–1649.

94. Alter MJ, Bell BP, Fleenor M, et al. The diverse patterns of hepatitis A epidemiology in the United States—implications for vaccination strategies. J Infect Dis 1998;178(6):1579–1584.

95. Lemon SM. Type A viral hepatitis: epidemiology, diagnosis, and prevention. Clin Chem 1997;43(8, Pt 2):1494–1499.

96. Macedo G, Ribeiro T. Hepatitis A: insights into new trends in epidemiology. Eur J Gastroenterol Hepatol 1998;10(2):175.

97. Dolan SA. Vaccines for hepatitis A and B. The latest recommendations on safe and extended protection. Postgrad Med 1997; 102(6):74–80.

98. Kurstak C, Kurstak E, Hossain A. Progress in diagnosis of viral hepatitis A, B, C, D and E. Acta Virol 1996;40(2):107–115.

99. Gregorio GV, Mieli-Vergani G, Mowat AP. Viral hepatitis. Arch Dis Child 1994;70(4):343–348.

100. Davis GL. Hepatitis B: diagnosis and treatment. South Med J 1997;90(9):866–870; quiz 871.

101. Gitlin N. Hepatitis B: diagnosis, prevention, and treatment. Clin Chem 1997;43(8, Pt 2):1500–1506.

102. Colantoni A, De Maria N, Idilman R, et al. Pathogenesis of hepatitis B and C-induced hepatocellular carcinoma. J Viral Hepat 1998;5(5):285–299.

103. Bengtstrom M, Jalava T, Kallio A, et al. A rapid and quantitative solution hybridization method for detection of HBV DNA in serum. J Virol Methods 1992;36(2):171–180.

104. Campelo C, Cisterna R, Gorrino MT, et al. Detection of hepatitis B virus DNA in chronic carriers by the polymerase chain reaction. Eur J Clin Microbiol Infect Dis 1992;11(8):740–744.

105. Aspinall S, Mphahlele MJ, Peenze I, et al. Detection and quantitation of hepatitis B virus DNA: comparison of two commercial hybridization assays with polymerase chain reaction. J Viral Hepat 1995;2(2):107–111.

106. McHutchison JG, Person JL, et al. Improved detection of hepatitis C virus antibodies in high risk populations. Hepatology 1992;15:19–25.

107. Alter MJ, Krzysztof K, Margolis HS, et al. The natural history of community-acquired hepatitis C in the United States. N Engl J Med 1992;327:1899–1905.

108. Yen T, Keeffe EB, Ahmed A. The epidemiology of hepatitis C virus infections. J Clin Gastroenterol 2003;36(1):47–53.

109. Cardoso M, Dengler T, Kerowgan M, et al. Estimated risk of transmission of hepatitis C virus by blood transfusion. Vox Sang 1998;74(4):213–216.

110. Holland PV. Post-transfusion hepatitis: current risks and causes. Vox Sang 1998;74(Suppl 2):135–141.

111. Vyas GN, Yang G. Immunodiagnosis of viral hepatitides A to E and non-A to -E. Clin Diagn Lab Immunol 1996;3(3):247–256.

112. Bernardez-Hermida I, Perez-Gracia MT. Serological markers for diagnosis of acute delta hepatitis infection. Eur J Clin Microbiol Infect Dis 1993;12(8):650–651.

113. Herrera JL. Serologic diagnosis of viral hepatitis. South Med J 1994;87(7):677–684.

114. Casey JL. Hepatitis delta virus. Genetics and pathogenesis. Clin Lab Med 1996;16(2):451–464.

115. Negro F, Rizzetto M. Diagnosis of hepatitis delta virus infection. J Hepatol 1995;22(1 Suppl):136–139.

116. Linares A, Navascues CA, Rodrigo L, et al. Epidemiology of hepatitis D virus infection: changes in the last 14 years. Am J Gastroenterol 1995;90(11):1981–1984.

117. Emerson SU, Ghabrah TM, Purcell RH, et al. Comparison of tests for antibody to hepatitis E virus. J Med Virol 1998;55(2):134–137.

118. Alter MJ, Holland PV, Mast EE, et al. Evaluation of assays for antibody to hepatitis E virus by a serum panel. Hepatitis E Virus Antibody Serum Panel Evaluation Group. Hepatology 1998;27(3):857–861.

119. McPherson RA. Laboratory diagnosis of human hepatitis viruses. J Clin Lab Anal 1994;8(6):369–377.

120. Renz M, Seelig HP, Seelir R. PCR in the diagnosis of viral hepatitis. Ann Med 1992;24(3):225–230.

121. Burkholder BT, Favorov MO, Holland PV, et al. Prevalence of and risk factors for antibody to hepatitis E virus seroreactivity among blood donors in Northern California. J Infect Dis 1997;176(1):34–40.

122. Balayan MS. Epidemiology of hepatitis E virus infection. J Viral Hepat 1997;4(3):155–165.

123. Bradley DW. Hepatitis E virus: a brief review of the biology, molecular virology, and immunology of a novel virus. J Hepatol 1995;22(1 Suppl):140–145.

124. Dawson GJ, De Guzman IJ, Holzer TJ, et al. Diagnosis of acute hepatitis E infection utilizing enzyme immunoassay. Dig Dis Sci 1994;39(8):1691–1693.

125. Maddrey WC. Safety of combination interferon alfa-2b/ribavirin therapy in chronic hepatitis C: relapsed and treatment-naïve patients. Semin Liver Dis 1999;19:67–75.

126. Corrao G, Arico S. Independent and combined action of hepatitis C virus infection and alcohol consumption on the risk of symptomatic liver cirrhosis. Hepatology 1994;20:1115–1120.

127. Seeff LB. The natural history of chronic hepatitis C virus infection. Clin Liver Dis 1997;1:587–602.

128. Poynard R, Ratziu V, Charlotte R, et al. Rates and risk factors of liver fibrosis progression in patients with chronic hepatitis C. J Hepatol 2001;34:730–739.

129. Forns X, Ampurdanes S, Sanchez-Tapias JM, et al. Long-term follow-up of chronic hepatitis C in patients diagnosed at a tertiary-care center. J Hepatol 2001;35:265–271.

130. Castano G, Dawson GJ, Flichman D, et al. Detection of hepatitis G virus RNA in patients with acute non-A-E hepatitis. J Viral Hepat 1998;5(3):161–164.

131. Loya F. Does the hepatitis G virus cause hepatitis? Tex Med 1996;92(12):68–73.

132. Doo EC, Lian TJ, Shiffs ER, Sorrell MF, Maddrey WC. The hepatitis viruses. In: Schiff ER, Sorrell MF, Maddrey WC, eds. Schiff's Diseases of the Liver. Philadelphia: Lippincott Williams & Wilkins, 2003:917–940.

133. Alter HJ, Umemura T, Tanaka Y. Putative new hepatitis virus. In: Schiff ER, Sorrell MF, Maddrey WC, eds. Schiff's Diseases of the Liver. Philadelphia: Lippincott Williams & Wilkins, 2003:891–905.

Cardiac Function

Lynn R. Ingram

OBJECTIVES

Upon completion of this chapter, the clinical laboratorian should be able to:
- Explain the origin of six general symptoms of cardiac disease.
- Discuss the etiology and physiologic effects of the following cardiac conditions:
  - Congenital heart disease
  - Hypertensive heart disease
  - Infectious heart diseases
  - Coronary heart disease
  - Congestive heart failure
- Identify nine risk factors for coronary heart disease.
- List six features of an ideal cardiac marker.

- Compare and contrast the specificity and sensitivity of the most commonly used serum cardiac markers.
- Assess the clinical utility of the various cardiac markers to assess myocardial infarction.
- Analyze the role of the clinical laboratory in the assessment of a patient with cardiac disease.
- Assess the usefulness of point-of-care cardiac markers and the role of the clinical laboratory in the use of these methods.
- Name and define the purpose of the most common types of drugs used to treat cardiac disease.

KEY TERMS

Acute coronary
  syndrome
β-Adrenergic blocking
  drugs
Angina pectoris
Antiplatelet therapy
Arrhythmias
Atherosclerosis
Atrial septal defects
  (ASD)
B-naturiuretic peptide
Carbonic anhydrase
  isoenzyme III

Cardiac catheterization
Cardiac glycosides
Cardiac markers
Cardiomyopathy
CK isoforms
CK-MB
Coarctation of the aorta
Congestive heart failure
Creatine kinase (CK)
D-Dimer
Diuretics
Essential hypertension
Fibrinogen

Glycogen phosphorylase
  isoenzyme BB
Heart fatty acid–binding
  protein
Homocysteine
Hs-CRP
Infectious endocarditis
Ischemia-modified
  albumin
Myocardial infarction
Myocarditis
Myoglobin

Myosin light chains
  (MLC)
Pericarditis
Persistent ductus
Rheumatic heart disease
Secondary hypertension
Tetralogy of Fallot
Thrombolytic agents
Troponin I (TnI)
Troponin T (TnT)
Vasodilators
Ventricular septal defect
  (VSD)

HEART DISEASE

Heart disease is a common and debilitating condition that affects millions of patients each year; however, obtaining an accurate and timely diagnosis remains difficult. The patient's medical history and radiologic and laboratory test results often do not provide enough information to ensure the most beneficial medical care, especially for patients presenting with chest pain. An early and accurate diagnosis of these patients would improve prognosis and quality of life, as well as reduce risks for development of further cardiac and constitutional problems.

The issues of reimbursement and managed care have stimulated interest in the development of new diagnostic markers for cardiac disease that will differentiate patients who need further procedures, such as coronary artery bypass grafting, angioplasty, or thrombolytic therapy, from those patients who can safely be managed medically. Therefore, selection of appropriate *cardiac markers* that provide the most cost-effective and clinically useful indicators of myocardial function is critical.

This chapter reviews common cardiac diseases, diagnostic tests by the clinical laboratory, and routine treatments for heart disease.

Symptoms of Heart Disease

Patients with cardiac disease are often asymptomatic until a relatively late stage in their condition. The most frequent symptoms manifested in heart disease are dyspnea, chest pain, palpitations, syncope, fatigue, and edema (Table 23-1).

Dyspnea is an awareness of or difficulty in breathing. It can be a result of cardiac or respiratory disease and is a normal response during exercise in healthy individuals. Dyspnea as a result of cardiac disease may occur only on exercise or can be present at rest in advanced disease. Left ventricular heart failure causes pulmonary edema, reducing lung elasticity, increasing the amount of effort necessary to breathe, and increasing the respiratory rate due to stimulation of pulmonary receptors. Orthopnea, breathlessness when a patient lies flat, occurs when blood is redistributed in the supine position, increasing the pressure of abdominal contents against the diaphragm. Paroxysmal nocturnal dyspnea is an accumulation of fluid in the lungs at night, often waking the patient from sleep, fighting for breath. Wheezing as a result of bronchial edema and a productive, blood-tinged cough are also common.[1]

Cyanosis, a bluish discoloration of the skin, is the obvious result of dyspnea and is caused by an increased amount of nonoxygenated hemoglobin in the blood. Central cyanosis is a result of right-to-left shunting of blood or impaired pulmonary function; peripheral cyanosis is caused by shunting or local vasoconstriction. Cyanosis becomes apparent when 5 g/dL, or more, of reduced hemoglobin is present.[2]

Angina pectoris is the most common symptom associated with ischemic heart disease. It is a gripping or crushing, central chest pain that may be felt around or deep within the chest. The pain may radiate to the neck or jaw or, less commonly, to the back or abdomen, and is

TABLE 23-1. SYMPTOMS OF HEART DISEASE

COMMON SYMPTOMS	UNUSUAL SYMPTOMS
Dyspnea	Cough
Syncope	Abdominal pain
Cyanosis	Hemoptysis
Pain	Headache
Palpitations	Sweating
Fatigue	Vision and speech disturbances
Edema	Weakness of extremities Weight loss Nausea/vomiting Fever

associated with heaviness, paresthesia, or pain in one (usually the left) or both arms. It is typically worsened by exercise and relieved by rest. The pain is most often caused by a lack of oxygen to the myocardium as a result of inadequate coronary blood flow.[1]

A palpitation may be an increased awareness of a normal heartbeat or the sensation of a slow, rapid, or irregular heart rate. The most common arrhythmia felt as palpitations are premature ectopic beats.[1] Premature beats are usually felt as missed beats because the early beat is followed by a pause before the next normal beat, which is rather forceful because of the longer diastolic filling period.

The most common syncopal attacks are vasovagal in nature (simple faints) and not a result of serious disease. They can be caused by venous pooling or provoked by fright or shock and are often accompanied by dizziness, nausea, sweating, ringing in the ears, a sinking feeling, and yawning. Cardiovascular syncope is usually sudden and brief, and the classic variety is a result of a disturbance of cardiac rhythm, such as a slowed heart rate. Without warning, the patient falls to the ground with a slow or absent pulse and, after a few seconds, the patient recovers consciousness. Often, there are no sequelae.[1]

Fatigue is a common, but nonspecific, cardiac symptom. Lethargy is associated with heart failure, persistent cardiac arrhythmia, and cyanotic heart disease. It may be a result of both poor cerebral and peripheral perfusion and poor oxygenation of blood.[1]

Retained fluid accumulates in the feet and ankles of ambulant patients and over the sacrum of bed-bound patients. The edema associated with heart disease is often absent in the morning because the fluid is reabsorbed when lying down, but becomes progressively worse during the day. When severe, the calf and thigh may become edematous and ascites or a pleural effusion may develop.[1]

A cough may be the primary complaint in some patients with pulmonary congestion. A nonproductive cough differentiates these patients from those with infectious pulmonary conditions. Hemoptysis occurs in congestive heart failure and is especially common in patients with mitral stenosis.[3]

Nocturia is also common in patients with congestive heart failure. Anorexia, abdominal fullness, right upper quadrant tenderness, and weight loss are seen in patients with advanced heart failure but are rare in mild or early heart disease.

CONGENITAL HEART DISEASE

Congenital heart defects are the cause of approximately 2% of all cardiac disease[4] and occur in about 8% of live births.[5] There is an overall male predominance, although some specific lesions occur more frequently in females, and it is a common cause of death in the first year of life. Congenital heart disease includes valvular defects that interfere with the normal flow of blood, septal defects

that allow mixing of oxygenated blood from the pulmonary circulation with unoxygenated blood from the systemic circulation, shunts, abnormalities in position or shape of the aorta or pulmonary arteries, or a combination of these conditions.[6] Many variations and degrees of severity are possible.

The etiology of congenital cardiac disease is often unknown; however, most defects appear to be multifactorial and reflect a combination of both genetic and environmental influences. Because the heart develops early in embryonic life and is completely formed and functioning by week 10 of gestation, all congenital heart defects develop before week 10 of pregnancy. Factors that are closely associated with the development of congenital heart disease include maternal rubella infections, maternal alcohol abuse, drug treatment and radiation, and certain genetic and chromosomal abnormalities.

The rubella virus, the causative agent of German measles, has been known to be a cause of congenital heart defects for a long time. Infection of the mother during the first 3 months of pregnancy is associated with a high incidence of congenital heart disease in the baby. Apparently, the virus crosses the placenta, enters the fetal circulation, and damages the developing heart.[4]

Fetal alcohol syndrome is often associated with heart defects, as well. Alcohol affects the fetal heart by directly interfering with its development. Although the exact teratogenic mechanism of fetal alcohol syndrome remains unknown,[4] it has been proposed that alcohol is toxic to fetal heart cells and destroys them. Many therapeutic and illegal drugs ingested by the mother can cross the placenta to harm the fetal heart.

Chromosomal abnormalities are associated with several developmental syndromes, many of which include heart disease. The best-known example is Down's syndrome—or trisomy 21 syndrome—which is often associated with atrial septum defects.[4]

The symptoms of congenital heart disease may be evident at birth or during early infancy, or they may not become evident until later in life. Signs and symptoms common to many congenital heart diseases include cyanosis, pulmonary hypertension, clubbing of fingers, embolism or thrombus formation, reduced growth, or syncope.[1] The most common congenital cardiac lesions are ventricular and atrial septal defects, persistent ductus arteriosus, coarctation of the aorta, valvular defects, and tetralogy of Fallot.[1]

Ventricular septal defect (VSD), commonly known as *a hole in the heart,* is the most common congenital cardiac malformation. In this condition, blood flows through the septal defect from the left ventricle to the right ventricle, causing less blood to be pumped from the left ventricle and reducing output to the systemic circulation. More blood enters the pulmonary circulation, which overloads and irreversibly damages the pulmonary vessels, causing pulmonary hypertension. Some small VSDs will close spontaneously, but moderate or large VSDs should be surgically repaired before the development of severe pulmonary hypertension.[1]

Atrial septal defects (ASD) are often first diagnosed in adulthood. This abnormality causes left-to-right shunting of blood between the atria. Pulmonary hypertension and atrial arrhythmia are common when the patient is older than age 30 years, but most children with this condition are asymptomatic. A significant ASD should be surgically repaired as soon as possible after diagnosis.[1]

The ductus arteriosus connects the pulmonary artery to the descending aorta. In fetal life, the ductus turns blood away from the pulmonary circulation into the systemic circulation, where blood is reoxygenated as it passes through the placenta. At birth, the high oxygen content in the blood triggers closure of the duct. If the duct is malformed or does not contain sufficient elastic tissue, it will not close. A persistent duct produces continuous aorta-to-pulmonary artery shunting, resulting in severe left heart failure *(persistent ductus)*. Many times, there are no symptoms until later in life when heart failure or infective endocarditis develops. Premature babies are often born with persistent ductus arteriosus that are

anatomically normal but are immature in that they lack the mechanism to close. These babies may be treated with indomethacin, which stimulates prostaglandin production and closure of the duct or the duct can be corrected surgically with little risk.[1]

Coarctation of the aorta is a narrowing of the aorta at the insertion of the ductus arteriosus. In most cases, this condition is associated with a bicuspid, rather than tricuspid, aortic valve.[7] This condition may remain asymptomatic for many years and treatment is surgical excision of the coarctation.

Congenital valve problems may be classified as stenosis (narrowing of a valve that restricts the forward flow of blood) or valvular incompetence (a valve that fails to close completely, allowing blood to leak backward). Mitral valve prolapse, abnormally enlarged and floppy valve leaflets that balloon backward with pressure, is common.[6] *Tetralogy of Fallot* is the most common cyanotic congenital heart abnormality in children who survive beyond the neonatal period. It is a combination of four defects: VSD, right ventricular outflow obstruction, abnormal positioning of the aorta above the VSD, and right ventricular hypertrophy (Fig. 23-1).[1]

Tetralogy of Fallot

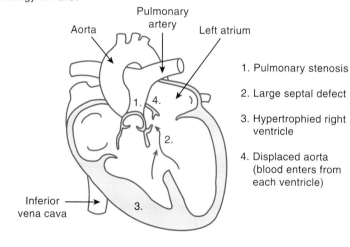

1. Pulmonary stenosis

2. Large septal defect

3. Hypertrophied right ventricle

4. Displaced aorta (blood enters from each ventricle)

FIGURE 23-1. Tetralogy of Fallot compared with normal cardiac anatomy. (Reprinted with permission from Mulvihill ML. Human Diseases: A Systemic Approach, 3rd ed. Norwalk, CT: Appleton & Lange, 1991.)

Normal anatomy of heart

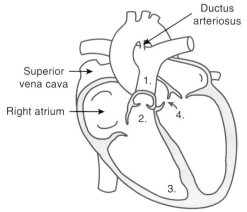

1. Pulmonary artery open

2. Complete septum

3. Right ventricle wall narrower than left

4. Blood enters aorta from left ventricle only

CASE STUDY 23-1

A 15-month-old girl with a heart murmur since birth was evaluated for repeated pulmonary infections, failure to grow, cyanosis, and mild clubbing of fingers and toes. She had been on digitalis therapy by the referring physician. The x-ray showed a moderately enlarged heart and an enlarged pulmonary artery. Pertinent laboratory data were obtained.

Total protein (6.0–8.3 g/dL)	5.4
Albumin (3.5–5.2 g/dL)	3.0
Hemoglobin (14–18 g/dL)	19.2
Hematocrit (40–54%)	59
Erythrocyte count (4.3–5.7 × 10^6/mm^3)	6.4

A cardiac catheterization was performed, and a large ventricular septal defect was found.

Questions

1. How does this congenital defect affect the body's circulation?

2. Why are the red cell measurements increased in this patient?

3. What treatment will be suggested for this patient?

4. What is this patient's prognosis?

This combination of lesions leads to increased right ventricular pressure and right-to-left shunting of blood through the VSD. The pulmonary circulation receives a small amount of unoxygenated blood from the right ventricle, and the systemic circulation receives a larger amount of blood, consisting of mixed oxygen and unoxygenated blood.[6] Children with this condition may present with dyspnea, fatigue, and hypoxic episodes on exertion. Complete surgical correction is possible, even in infancy.[1]

CONGESTIVE HEART FAILURE

Congestive heart failure results when the heart is unable to pump blood effectively. It is characterized by fluid accumulation, initially in the lungs and subsequently throughout the body. It is estimated that 4.6 million persons are being treated for heart failure and more than 550,000 persons are diagnosed annually with congestive heart failure.[8]

When the heart is unable to pump efficiently, cardiac output decreases. When the left side of the heart fails, excess fluid accumulates in the lungs, resulting in pulmonary edema and reduced output of blood to the systemic circulation. The kidneys respond to this decreased blood flow with excessive fluid retention, making the heart failure worse. When the right side of the heart fails, excess fluid accumulates in the systemic venous circulatory system and generalized edema results. There is also diminished blood flow to the lungs and to the left side of the heart, resulting in decreased cardiac output to the systemic arterial circulation.

Congestive heart failure may occur if the heart muscle is weak or if the heart is stressed beyond its ability to react. The most common causes of congestive heart failure

are coronary artery disease, cardiomyopathies, myocarditis, valvular disease, and cardiac arrhythmias (Table 23-2).

Coronary artery disease is the most common cause of heart failure in the United States. Management and prognosis for congestive heart failure caused by coronary artery disease is poor, with a 5-year mortality of about 50%.[9] Atherosclerosis of coronary arteries leads to ischemia, a process that replaces active cardiac muscle with fibrous tissue that does not function as cardiac muscle. Occlusion of the cardiac vessels reduces blood flow

TABLE 23-2. CAUSES OF CONGESTIVE HEART FAILURE

Coronary Artery Disease

Cardiomyopathies
  Dilated cardiomyopathy
    Autoimmune response
    Small blood vessel disease
    Alcohol-induced
  Restrictive cardiomyopathy
    Abnormality of the myocardium
    Infiltration of myocardium with abnormal protein
    Endomyocardial disease
    Thrombus or tumor
  Hypertrophic cardiomyopathy
    Autosomal dominant inheritable condition

Inflammatory Heart Disease
  Cardiac infections
  Immunologic injury to myocardium
  Valvular incompetence

Cardiac Conduction Dysfunctions/Arrhythmias

Congenital Heart Disease

and forces the heart muscle into anaerobic metabolism, producing waste products that can also damage the tissue cells. Decreasing cardiac muscle mass increases the load carried by the remaining tissue, resulting in increased cardiac stress and damage. The combination of these factors underscores the seriousness of congestive heart failure in ischemia.

Cardiomyopathies result from an abnormality of the heart muscle. If the heart is unable to contract efficiently, the heart dilates disproportionately and results in an enlarged heart with relatively thin cardiac walls. They are grouped as dilated cardiomyopathies, restrictive cardiomyopathies, or hypertrophic cardiomyopathies.

Dilated cardiomyopathy may be the result of an autoimmune response; small blood vessel disease; or direct myocardial toxicity, such as seen in alcohol-induced cardiomyopathy and anthracycline cardiotoxicity. Presenting symptoms of dilated cardiomyopathy are dyspnea on exertion, orthopnea, paroxysmal nocturnal dyspnea, and chest discomfort similar to angina.

Patients with restrictive cardiomyopathy have increased diastolic pressure, resulting in inefficient filling of the ventricles and less blood being distributed to the body. This condition can be caused by amyloidosis, endometrial fibrosis, glycogen storage, fibroelastosis, neoplastic infiltration and collagen-vascular diseases.[9] Hemochromatosis, an infiltration of iron into tissue, can also affect heart muscle and lead to loss of contractility and muscle function.

Hypertrophic cardiomyopathy is characterized by enlargement of the ventricular septum that is out of proportion to the other ventricular walls and often is called *asymmetric septal hypertrophy.* This condition appears to be inherited as an autosomal dominant trait in most cases. It may be a result of myocarditis caused by infections, immunologic injury to the tissue, or it may be idiopathic. It can also develop in patients with valvular heart disease. Valvular malfunctions alter the blood volume that the heart must regulate. Such patients will progress to cardiac failure as blood volume changes alter the blood load for ventricles and atria.

Arrhythmia, or malfunction of the cardiac conduction system, may also result in congestive heart failure. Arrhythmia may be caused by ischemia, infarction, infiltrates, electrolyte imbalances, or chemical toxins.

Clinical indications of congestive heart failure range from mild symptoms that appear only on exertion to the most advanced conditions in which the heart is unable to function without external support. Congestive heart failure is readily detectable if it involves a patient with myocardial infarction, angina, pulmonary problems, or arrhythmia, but congestive heart failure is most commonly investigated because of dyspnea, edema, cough, or angina. Other symptoms, such as exercise intolerance, fatigue, and weakness, are common (Table 23-3).

TABLE 23-3. CONDITIONS CONTRIBUTING TO CONGESTIVE HEART FAILURE

Hypertension
Connective tissue diseases
Anemia/polycythemia
Endocrine disorders
Malnutrition
Drug/alcohol toxicity
Obesity
Pulmonary disease

ACUTE CORONARY SYNDROME

Ischemic heart disease involves a progression of pathologic conditions that includes erosion and rupture of coronary artery plaques, activation of platelets, and thrombi. This progression is termed *acute coronary syndrome* and ranges from unstable angina to extensive tissue necrosis in acute myocardial infarction. The clinical laboratory is critical in the diagnosis of these conditions, assessment of reperfusion after thrombolytic therapy, infarct sizing, identification of reinfarctions, and risk stratification.[10]

Coronary heart disease is caused by a lack of nutrients and oxygen reaching the heart muscle and resulting in myocardial ischemia. Ischemia is a reduced blood supply to one area of the heart and is often a result of atherosclerosis, thrombosis, spasms, or embolisms but may also be a result of anemia, carboxyhemoglobinemia, or hypotension, which causes reduced blood flow to the heart. Increased demand for oxygen and nutrients as a result of extreme exercise or thyrotoxicosis may also cause ischemia.

Most frequently, ischemia is the result of abnormal coronary arteries, usually caused by an obstruction in one or more of these arteries. *Atherosclerosis* is a thickening and hardening of the artery walls caused by deposits of cholesterol-lipid-calcium plaque in the lining of the arteries.[11] The following nine risk factors predispose individuals to develop these arterial plaques:

1. **Age.** Atherosclerosis may develop in early life but becomes a more significant risk factor with increasing age. It is a more common finding after age 40 years and is found almost universally in older persons in the Western world.[1]
2. **Sex.** Men tend to be more affected by atherosclerosis than premenopausal women of comparable age. After menopause, the difference tends to disappear. Women are thought to be protected by higher levels of high-density lipoprotein (HDL) cholesterol until estrogen levels drop at menopause.[4]

3. **Family history.** Atherosclerosis is often found in members of the same family but a direct inheritance pattern has yet to be shown. Family lifestyles play a role in this process, and it is difficult to distinguish genetic from lifestyle factors in predicting coronary artery disease. Some conditions are directly inherited, such as familial hypercholesterolemia and familial combined hyperlipidemia.[1]

4. **Hyperlipidemia.** An increased serum cholesterol concentration has been shown to have a strong association with atherosclerosis. Lowering the serum cholesterol, especially the low-density lipoprotein (LDL) cholesterol fraction, has been shown to decrease the incidence of coronary artery disease and slow the progression of coronary atherosclerosis.[9] The relationship between plaque formation and triglyceride levels is not as well defined.

5. **Smoking.** There is a direct relationship between number of cigarettes smoked and the risk of coronary artery disease in men that is related to the decrease in HDL-cholesterol levels, increased LDL-cholesterol levels, increased platelet adhesion, vasoconstriction, and increased *fibrinogen* and clot formation caused by smoking.[9] This relationship is not as well defined in women or in those who smoke pipes or cigars.

6. **Hypertension.** Both systolic and diastolic hypertension is associated with increased risk for atherosclerosis for both men and women.[9]

7. **Sedentary lifestyle.** Regular exercise has shown some protection against the development of heart disease and, conversely, a sedentary lifestyle is a strong factor in the development of coronary heart disease.

8. **Diabetes mellitus.** Because of the strong relationship between diabetes and vascular disease, there is also an increased risk for coronary artery disease in patients with diabetes, especially in those whose diabetes is poorly controlled.

9. **Response to stress.** Aggressive, ambitious, compulsive persons have almost twice the risk for coronary disease as persons who do not express these characteristics.

Regardless of the etiology of the ischemia, there are three general results of cardiac ischemia: congestive heart failure, angina pectoris, and myocardial infarction (Fig. 23-2). Congestive heart failure results when there is reduced oxygen supply to the cardiac muscle, causing it to fail to pump the blood efficiently.

Angina pectoris is a symptom of inadequate perfusion of the heart muscle, resulting in chest pain. Typical angina pectoris occurs with increased physical exertion or stress and usually rapidly resolves with rest. In patients with coronary artery disease, the narrowed cardiac vessels do not allow for increased blood flow into the cardiac muscle at times of additional physical or emotional stress, causing the pain. Other types of angina include variant angina, nocturnal angina, and unstable angina. Variant angina is not related to exertion or any increase in stress but is caused by spasm of a coronary artery. It is often longer in duration than normal angina and the pain is more severe. Nocturnal angina generally occurs in patients with severe coronary disease and wakes patients from sleep with severe chest pain. Unstable angina is the most severe form and pain is often present at rest. The pain is often provoked by mild increases in exercise or stress and can even be initiated by ingesting a large meal. The pain is long lasting and severe and does not respond as well or as quickly to standard treatments. Many patients with unstable angina will rapidly progress to myocardial infarction. Although angina is not easily differentiated from myocardial infarction in some cases, there are no classic electrocardiogram (ECG) changes or enzyme elevations in angina and cardiac damage does not usually occur unless it is prolonged or severe.

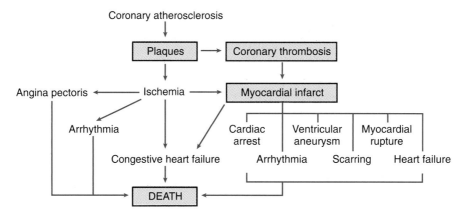

FIGURE 23-2. Presentation of coronary heart disease. Coronary heart disease may present as angina pectoris, congestive heart failure, or myocardial infarct. (Reprinted with permission from Damjanov I. Pathology for the Health Related Professions. Philadelphia: WB Saunders, 1996.)

Myocardial infarction, or heart attack, occurs when blood flow to an area of the cardiac muscle is suddenly blocked, leading to ischemia and death of myocardial tissue. The heart tissue becomes inflamed and necrotic at the point of obstruction and is followed by the release of cellular enzymes and proteins into the blood. The damaged area of the heart quickly loses its ability to contract and conduct electrical impulses and oxygen supplies are depleted. This type of damage is irreversible and the area of necrosis is eventually replaced by fibrous scar tissue.

The severity of damage from a myocardial infarction varies greatly and is primarily related to the size and location of the infarct. If the left anterior descending coronary artery is blocked, the anterior and lateral walls of the heart, ventricular septum, and anterolateral papillary muscle are affected. If the dominant right coronary artery is affected, damage to the inferoposterior wall, posteromedial papillary muscle, and inferior septum results. If any collateral circulation has developed because of chronic reduced blood flow in that particular area of the heart, the resulting damage will be less significant than if no collateralization has occurred.

Most infarctions involve all three layers of the heart. Patients usually present with varying degrees of chest pain severity of several hours duration and other symptoms such as left arm pain, shortness of breath, hypotension, sweating, nausea, and vomiting. Certain patients, especially patients with diabetes or hypertension and patients who are older, will have no chest pain and few symptoms. Although many patients would indicate that there were no warning signs of an impending cardiac event, most will admit to a recent history of dyspnea, unstable angina, and a vague sense of ill health. Complications of a myocardial infarction are common and include sudden death due to ventricular arrhythmias and fibrillation, heart block if conduction fibers are located in the area of the infarct, and other conduction irregularities, resulting in arrhythmia, congestive heart failure, and thromboembolism.[6]

HYPERTENSIVE HEART DISEASE

Hypertension is defined by the World Health Organization as systolic pressure greater than 160 mm Hg and diastolic pressure greater than 95 mm Hg. It is one of the most common cardiovascular diseases, and it is estimated that approximately 50% of middle-aged persons have hypertension. The prevalence of hypertension increases with age, from 4% in persons aged 20–29 years to 65% in persons older than age 80 years.[12] It is more common in the Black population than in White or Hispanic groups. Hypertension may affect all organs, but especially the kidneys, brain, and heart.

The most important factor that determines blood pressure is peripheral resistance, and it is this increased peripheral resistance that results in heart disease. It increases the workload of the left ventricle, eventually resulting in hypertrophy and dilation. The increase in size of the left ventricle causes the mitral valve to allow regurgitation of blood into the left atrium that, over time, results in dilatation and increased pressure in the left atrium, as well. This increased pressure is transferred to

---

CASE STUDY 23-2

A 59-year-old woman came to the emergency department of a local hospital complaining of pain and a feeling of heaviness in her abdomen for several days. She reported no weakness, chest pain, or left arm pain. She has no chronic health problems except of seasonal allergies and a slightly elevated total cholesterol. Her ECG showed characteristic changes indicative of AMI.

CARDIAC ENZYMES	8:30 P.M.; APRIL 11	6:30 A.M.; APRIL 12
Total CK (54–186 U/L)	170	106
CK-MB (0–5 ng/mL)	6.3	3.8
% CK-MB (<6%)	3.7%	3.6%
Myoglobin (<70 µg/L)	52	41
Troponin T (0–0.1 µg/L)	0.8	2.3

Questions

1. Do the symptoms and personal history of this patient suggest AMI?

2. Based on the preceding laboratory data, would this diagnosis be AMI?

3. Why or why not?

the pulmonary circulation and, thus, affects the right side of the heart. Another complicating factor in this process is that hypertension is also associated with an increased prevalence of atherosclerosis, further increasing risk for heart disease.

There are often no symptoms associated with increased blood pressure, but dizziness, headaches, palpitations, restlessness, nervousness, and tinnitus may be present. There is a strong association between hypertension and obesity, heavy alcohol consumption, smoking, and sedentary lifestyles.

Ninety to ninety-five percent of patients with hypertension have no known cause for the condition which is known as primary, or essential, hypertension.[13] Primary hypertension is multifactorial in nature, with both cardiac and peripheral vasculature factors influencing the blood pressure. The interplay among these many factors is poorly defined, and genetics, racial, gender, and environmental factors also complicate the picture. Persons that have an identified source of their hypertension are classified as having *secondary hypertension.* Renal disease, the most common cause of secondary hypertension, is associated with sodium retention. Malignant hypertension is a serious condition seen when severe renal disease causes renal cell inflammation and destruction and is associated with high mortality unless vigorously treated. Primary aldosteronism will result in sodium retention and, therefore, in hypertension, as a result of abnormal control of the renal excretion of the major electrolytes. Pheochromocytoma is an uncommon cause of striking increases in blood pressure resulting from increased excretion of catecholamines from a chromaffin tumor.

INFECTIVE HEART DISEASE

Infectious agents continue to be implicated in a variety of heart diseases (Table 23-4). The most common infectious diseases involving the heart are rheumatic heart disease, infectious endocarditis, and pericarditis; however, there is increasing interest in determining if an infectious factor may be associated with cardiac conditions such as coronary heart disease.[14]

Rheumatic fever is an inflammatory disease of children and young adults that occurs as a result of complications from infection with group A streptococci. A decline in the incidence of rheumatic fever since the early 1900s results from a reduced number of all streptococcal infections and the effective use of antibiotics against these infections. Although restricted to pharyngeal involvement in most persons, in certain individuals, this organism progresses to affect the heart, joints, skin, and central nervous system. Rheumatic fever is not caused by a direct infection of the heart with the streptococcus organism nor is it a result of a cardiac toxin produced by the microorganism, but is related to an autoimmune reaction stimulated by group A

TABLE 23-4. INFECTIOUS AGENTS ASSOCIATED WITH HEART DISEASE

Pericarditis/Myocarditis

Mycoplasma pneumoniae	*Chlamydia trachomatis*
Mycobacterium tuberculosis	*Streptococcus pneumoniae*
Staphylococcus aureus	Enterobacteriaceae
Coxsackievirus A and B	Echovirus
Adenovirus	Influenza
Coccidioides immitis	*Aspergillus* species
Candida species	*Cryptococcus neoformans*
Histoplasma capsulatum	*Trypanosoma cruzi*

Infective Endocarditis

Tococcus viridans	*Streptococcus faecalis*
Staphylococcus aureus	*Staphylococcus epidermidis*
Histoplasma species	*Brucella* species
Candida species	*Aspergillus* species
Coxiella burnetii	

Rheumatic Heart Disease

Group A β-hemolytic streptococcus

Coronary Heart Disease

Chlamydia pneumoniae	*Helicobacter pylori*
Cytomegalovirus	Herpes simplex virus type 2

streptococci.[1] It is thought that antibodies against the streptococcal antigens cross-react with similar antigens found in the heart and initiate a cell-mediated immune response involving macrophages and lymphocytes.[4]

Rheumatic heart disease affects all layers of the heart. Inflammation of the inner surface of the heart (endocarditis), especially the valves of the left heart, leads to ulceration and growth of vegetations on the heart lining and eventually to irreversible valve damage. *Myocarditis* caused by rheumatic heart disease may result in cardiac conduction problems or arrhythmia because of necrotic aggregates of lymphocytes and macrophages found in the myocardium.

Diagnosis of rheumatic heart disease is based on finding at least two of the following major symptoms: polyarthritis, carditis, chorea (involuntary movements caused by brain lesions), subcutaneous rheumatoid nodules, or erythema marginatum (a connective tissue and skin disease).[4] Other symptoms may include joint pain, fever, elevated erythrocyte sedimentation rate, immunologic evidence of a recent streptococcal infection, and characteristic electrocardiogram (ECG) changes. Treatment options are few and surgical repair of valvular damage is often required.

Infectious endocarditis is an inflammation of the inner lining of the heart chambers and valves and may be caused by several microorganisms. Streptococci and staphylococci are common causes, as are gram-negative bacteria and some fungi.[4] These organisms attach to the endocardium, invade the valves, and form vegetations of fibrin, platelets, blood cells, and microorganisms. These vegetations interfere with the function of the valves and may dislodge, forming emboli that can cause widespread infection or infarction of other organs. Two types of infective endocarditis are subacute and acute. Symptoms of subacute endocarditis are vague and insidious in many cases. Low-grade fevers, fatigue, anorexia, and spleno-megaly are common early in the condition, and heart murmurs and congestive heart failure may develop in advanced infections. Acute endocarditis has a sudden onset of spiking fevers, chills, and drowsiness. Both types of infectious endocarditis respond to appropriate antibiotic therapy if treated early.

Pericarditis is usually secondary to another condition, often other cardiac conditions. It may be caused by bacteria, viruses, or fungi and is associated with several autoimmune disorders, such as systemic lupus erythematosus. Accumulation of fluid in the pericardial sac is the defining aspect of this condition and the various types of fluid within the sac will differentiate the type of pericarditis. Purulent exudates indicate bacterial infections, clear serous fluids are caused by viral infections, and a serofibrinous exudate is associated with severe damage as in rheumatic heart disease.

Symptoms of pericarditis vary with the underlying cause but tachycardia, chest pain, shortness of breath, and cough are common. Large amounts of fluid can lead to distended neck veins, faint heart sounds, and ECG changes.[6]

Infectious agents have recently become the objects of interest in the continued search for additional causes of and effective treatments and preventive strategies for coronary artery disease. Viruses, such as herpes viruses and coxsackie B virus, and the bacteria *Chlamydia pneumoniae* and *Helicobacter pylori* have been widely studied. Chronic infection has been found to be significantly associated with development of atherosclerosis and the clinical complications of unstable angina, myocardial infarction, and stroke. For the most part, these are still just associations and specific causative relationships have not been established.[15]

DIAGNOSIS OF HEART DISEASE

Because of its dire consequences, great efforts have been made to determine the best tools for the early and accurate diagnosis of acute myocardial infarction (AMI). The World Health Organization has established three criteria for the diagnosis of AMI:

1. **History:** The history is typical if acute, severe, and prolonged chest pain is present.
2. **ECG:** Unequivocal changes are the development of abnormal, persistent Q waves, or equivalents, in at least two contiguous leads of the standard ECG, and evolving injury current lasting longer than 1 day.
3. **Serum cardiac markers:** Unequivocal change consisting of serial enzyme/protein changes, with an initial rise and subsequent fall of serum concentrations.[16]

Because a single, diagnostic laboratory test that will quickly and accurately assess cardiac function does not exist, a combination of cardiac markers is required. The search for a cardiac marker that would be useful in evaluating many types of heart conditions continues; the following features would be required for an ideal marker:

- The marker should be absolutely heart specific to allow reliable diagnosis of myocardial damage in the presence of skeletal muscle injury.
- The marker should be highly sensitive to detect even minor heart damage.
- The marker should be able to differentiate reversible from irreversible damage.
- In acute myocardial infarction, the marker should allow monitoring of reperfusion therapy and estimation of infarct size and prognosis.
- The marker should be stable and the measurement rapid, easy to perform, quantitative, and cost effective.
- The marker should not be detectable in patients who do not have myocardial damage.[17]

Most efforts to date have been placed on the development of such an ideal cardiac marker for the early and accurate diagnosis of AMI. Many factors must be considered in the selection of the most clinically diagnostic, effective, and cost-efficient laboratory tests for patients with chest pain. The time that has elapsed after onset of chest pain; any concomitant diseases; the possibility of skeletal muscle injury; the ease of measurement and turnaround time for results; and assay specificity, sensitivity, and interferences are only a few considerations in these decisions.[18]

The National Academy of Clinical Biochemistry recommends that two biochemical markers be used for routine diagnosis of AMI: an early marker that is reliably increased within 6 hours after onset of symptoms and a definitive marker that remains increased after 6–9 hours but has high sensitivity and specificity for myocardial injury and remains abnormal for several days.[16]

Laboratory Diagnosis of Acute Myocardial Infarction

Enzymes

Although the angiotensin sensitivity test (AST) was the first marker used for laboratory diagnosis of AMI, it lacks cardiac specificity and presently has no clinical significance for AMI diagnosis. Lactate dehydrogenase (LD) was also used to indicate AMI. It is a cytoplasmic enzyme found in most cells of the body, including the heart, and, therefore, is not specific for the diagnosis of cardiac disease. Although LD isoenzyme determinations increase specificity for cardiac tissue, with the LD1 and LD2 subfractions being most indicative of cardiac involvement, the National Academy of Clinical Biochemistry recommends that LD and LD isoenzymes no longer have a role in diagnosis of cardiac diseases.[16]

Creatine kinase (CK) is a cytosolic enzyme involved in the transfer of energy in muscle metabolism. It is a dimer comprised of two subunits (the B, or brain form, and the M, or muscle form), resulting in three CK isoenzymes. The CK-BB (CK1) isoenzyme is of brain origin and only found in the blood if the blood-brain barrier has been breached. CK-MM (CK3) isoenzyme accounts for most of the CK activity in skeletal muscle, whereas CK-MB (CK2) has the most specificity for cardiac muscle, even though it accounts for only 3–20% of total CK activity in the heart.[17] As a marker of early AMI, total CK shows sensitivity of only about 40% and specificity of only 80%.[18]

CK-MB is a valuable tool for the diagnosis of AMI because of its relatively high specificity for cardiac injury. Extensive experience with CK-MB has established it as the benchmark and gold standard for other cardiac markers. However, it takes at least 4–6 hours from onset of chest pain before CK-MB activities increase to significant levels in the blood. Peak levels occur at 12–24 hours, and serum activities usually return to baseline levels with 2–3 days (Fig. 23-3). Although the specificity of CK-MB

for heart tissue is greater than 85%,[18] it is also found in skeletal muscle and false-positive results may be caused by analytic interferences and clinical conditions such as muscle disease and acute or chronic muscle injuries.

During recent years, CK-MB activity assays have been increasingly replaced by CK-MB mass assays that measure the protein concentration of CK-MB rather than its catalytic activity. These laboratory procedures are based on immunoassay techniques using monoclonal antibodies and have fewer interferences and higher analytic sensitivity than activity-based assays. Mass assays can detect an increased concentration of serum CK-MB about 1 hour earlier than activity-based methods, and persistently normal CK-MB mass concentrations over a period of 6–8 hours have a negative predictive value of 97%.[19]

To increase specificity of CK-MB for cardiac tissue, it has been proposed that that a ratio (relative index) of CK-MB mass/CK activity be calculated. If this ratio exceeds 3, it is indicative of AMI rather than skeletal muscle damage.

CK isoforms are present in all sera and are produced as a part of the normal clearance mechanism for CK isoenzymes. There is only one CK-MB (MB$_2$) and one CK-MM (MM$_3$) isoform in myocardium. There are inherent problems with using CK isoforms as a cardiac marker, such as the lack of heart-specificity for CK-MB, the small content of CK-MB in normal myocardium tissue, and detectable levels of CK-MB in normal individuals. However, CK isoforms may be effectively used as indicators of reperfusion after thrombolytic therapy in patients with confirmed AMI.[17]

Cardiac Proteins

Several proteins may be monitored in suspected cases of AMI to give significant diagnostic information. *Myoglobin*, an oxygen-binding heme protein that accounts for 5–10% of all cytoplasmic proteins, is rapidly released from striated muscles (both skeletal and cardiac muscle) when damaged. However, because of its small size, myoglobin is rapidly cleared by the kidneys, making it an unreliable long-term marker of cardiac damage. Because of the abundance of myoglobin in cardiac and skeletal muscle tissue, the upper reference limit of serum myoglobin directly reflects the patient's muscle mass and, therefore, varies with gender, age, and physical activity.[20] Although there is some evidence that there are several forms of myoglobin, a cardiac-specific myoglobin has not been identified. The usefulness of myoglobin as a cardiac marker was established in the mid-1970s when a radioimmunoassay technique was developed for its determination, but it was only when rapid, quantitative, and automated assays became available that myoglobin gained acceptance as a routinely used diagnostic assay for AMI.[21]

Myoglobin is significantly more sensitive than CK and CK-MB activities during the first hours after chest pain

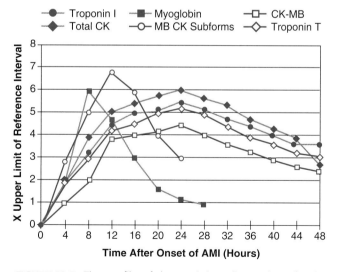

FIGURE 23-3. Time profiles of characteristic cardiac markers after AMI. Illustrated here is the plasma temporal profiles of commonly used cardiac diagnostic markers, namely, CK-MB, total CK, troponin I, troponin T, myoglobin, and CK-MB subforms. Early diagnosis of infarction (≤6 hours) is only potentially possible with two of the markers, namely, CK-MB subforms and myoglobin. (Reprinted with permission from Roberts R. Rapid MBCK subform assay and the early diagnosis of myocardial infarction. Clin Lab Med 1997;17(4):669–683.)

onset. It starts to rise within 1–4 hours and is detectable in essentially all AMI patients between 6 and 9 hours from chest pain onset, returning to baseline levels within 18–24 hours[18] (Fig. 23-3). If myoglobin concentration remains within the reference range 8 hours after onset of chest pain, AMI can essentially be ruled out. Although the early sensitivities of CK-MB mass, CK isoforms, and myoglobin are comparable, CK-MB determinations are preferable over myoglobin in patients who are admitted later than 10–12 hours after chest pain onset because the myoglobin concentration may have already returned to reference ranges within that time frame.[18] Myoglobin should not be used for early diagnosis of AMI in patients with renal disease, especially those persons in renal failure, because myoglobin will be consistently increased as a result of decreased clearance by the diseased kidneys. The rapid disappearance of myoglobin from serum allows it to be used as an indicator of reinfarction. A persistently normal myoglobin concentration will rule out reinfarction in patients with recurrent chest pain after AMI.

Muscle fibers convert the chemical energy of adenosine triphosphate (ATP) into mechanical work. As this occurs, enzymes, electrolytes, and proteins are activated or converted into materials that stimulate muscle fiber contraction. Actomyosin ATPase, calcium, actin, myosin, and a complex of three proteins known as the *troponin complex* are major players in this conversion. The three polypeptides of the troponin complex are troponin T, troponin I, and troponin C. Troponin C is not heart specific. Unlike CK-MB, the serum troponins are not found in the serum of healthy individuals. Although traditional enzymes are thought to be released from tissue only after irreversible myocardial damage has occurred, the cardiac troponins may be released in reversible ischemia as well as irreversible myocardial necrosis.

Troponin T (TnT) allows for both early and late diagnosis of AMI. Serum concentrations of TnT begin to rise within a few hours of chest pain onset and peak by day 2. A plateau lasting from 2 to 5 days usually follows, and the serum TnT concentration remains elevated beyond 7 days before returning to reference values (Fig. 23-3). The early appearance of TnT gives no better diagnostic information than CK-MB or myoglobin concentrations within the first 4 hours after chest pain onset, but the sensitivity of TnT for detecting myocardial infarct is 100% from 12 hours to 5 days after chest pain onset.[18] Also, the degree of elevation of TnT after AMI is significant, often up to a 200-fold increase over the upper limit of reference intervals.[20]

TnT concentrations are particularly useful for diagnosing myocardial infarction in patients who do not seek medical attention within the usual 2- to 3-day window during which total CK and CK-MB are elevated.[17] It is also useful in the differential diagnosis of myocardial damage in patients with cardiac symptoms as well as skeletal muscle injury because the TnT result will clearly

and specifically indicate the extent of the cardiac damage as opposed to muscle damage.[22] Cardiac TnT also has value in monitoring patients after reperfusion of an infarct-related coronary artery. In AMI patients with early reperfusion, TnT appears and peaks in serum significantly earlier than in those patients with delayed or incomplete reperfusion. A significant increase in TnT after the start of thrombolytic therapy indicates acceptable reperfusion of the infarct-related coronary artery.[23] The degree of elevation of TnT on days 3–4 after AMI can also be used as a practical and cost-effective estimate of myocardial infarct size.[24]

Troponin I (TnI) is only found in the myocardium in adults, making it extremely specific for cardiac disease. It is also found in much higher concentrations than CK-MB in cardiac muscle, making it a sensitive indicator of cardiac injury. TnI is not found in detectable amounts in the serum of patients with multiple injuries or athletes after strenuous exercise, in patients with acute or chronic skeletal muscle disease, in patients with renal failure, or in patients with elevated CK-MB, unless myocardial injuries are also present.[18] TnI is a good biochemical assessment of cardiac injury in critically ill patients, those with multiple organ failure, and situations in which CK/CK-MB elevations may be difficult to interpret.

After an AMI, the TnI increases above the reference range between 4 and 6 hours after chest pain onset, peaks at 12–18 hours, and returns to within reference limits in about 6 days, depending on AMI size[18] (Fig. 23-3). TnT tends to remain elevated longer and maintain higher sensitivity after day 7 after infarct than TnI.[18]

An ultrasensitive TnI assay has been developed which improves early sensitivity in assessing myocardial damage. The immunoluminometric (ILMA) assay improves the accuracy of TnI for monitoring myocardial damage during certain types of chemotherapy and congestive heart failure.[22]

Cardiac myosin light chains (MLC) are also involved with muscle contractions. They were first thought to be unique myocardial proteins, but recent research has determined that MLC is no more specific for cardiac injury than CK-MB determinations. Like the troponins, MLC is released from reversibly ischemic tissue. Although rapid testing of MLC is available, MLC determination does not offer any advantage over cardiac troponin assays. Therefore, MLC remains of limited clinical significance as a routine cardiac marker.[18]

Markers of Inflammation and Coagulation Disorders

Because the classic risk factors for acute coronary syndromes, such as gender, age, family history, and hyperlipidemia, are found in only 50% of all AMI patients, the ability to predict an individual's risk of AMI is currently

CASE STUDY 23-3

An 83-year-old man with known severe coronary artery disease, diffuse small vessel disease, and significant stenosis distal to a vein graft from previous CABG surgery, was admitted when his physician referred him to the hospital after a routine office visit. His symptoms included 3+ pedal edema, jugular vein distention, and heart sound abnormalities. Significant laboratory data obtained upon admission were as follows:

Urea nitrogen (6–24 mg/dL)	53
Creatinine (0.5–1.4 mg/dL)	2.2
Total protein (6.0–8.3 g/dL)	5.8
Albumin (3.5–5.3 g/dL)	3.2
Glucose (60–110 mg/dL)	312
Calcium (4.3–5.3 mEq/L)	4.1
Phosphorus (2.5–4.5 mg/dL)	2.4
Total CK (54–186 U/L)	134
CK-MB (0–5 ng/L)	4
% CK-MB (<6%)	3%
Myoglobin (<70 μg/L)	62
Troponin T (0–0.1 μg/L)	0.2

Questions

1. Do the symptoms of this patient suggest AMI?

2. Based on the preceding laboratory data, would this diagnosis be AMI? Why or why not?

3. Based on the preceding laboratory data, are there other organ system abnormalities present?

4. What are the indicators of these organ system abnormalities?

5. Is there a specific laboratory test that might indicate congestive heart failure in this patient?

poor. The search continues for additional tools to aid in predicting risk and preventing an event. There is accumulating data that the inflammatory response plays a critical role in the pathogenesis of ischemic heart disease. Patients with unstable angina show atherosclerotic plaques, with a significant infiltration of inflammatory cells and elevated systemic levels of acute-phase reactants.[25] Substances related to the activation of coagulation and fibrinolytic functions may also be of clinical value in monitoring acute coronary ischemia.

Hs-CRP

Studies have evaluated several acute-phase proteins as potential markers for cardiovascular risk assessment, and there is evidence that C-reactive protein (CRP) is a reliable predictor of acute coronary syndrome risk. CRP is an acute-phase reactant produced primarily by the liver. It is stimulated by interleukin-6 and increases rapidly with inflammation. The plasma concentration of CRP is determined mainly by its synthesis rate and, provided normal liver function exists, is a sensitive marker for ongoing chronic inflammation that is not affected by ischemic injury.[26] It rises significantly in response to injury, infection, or other inflammatory conditions and is not present in appreciable amounts in healthy individuals.

Although it is a nonspecific response to inflammation, its presence indicates an inflammatory process within the body. The increases in CRP have been proven to be minimal in acute coronary syndromes, often remaining within the established reference range. Reliable, automated high sensitivity assays for CRP (hs-CRP) have been developed that allow detection of the small increases of CRP often seen in cardiac disease.

Epidemiologic data document a positive association between hs-CRP and the prevalence of coronary artery disease. Elevated baseline levels of hs-CRP are correlated with higher risk of future cardiovascular morbidity and mortality among those with and without clinical evidence of vascular disease. In patients with established vascular disease, each standard deviation increase in baseline hs-CRP is associated with a 45% increase in relative risk of nonfatal myocardial infarction or sudden cardiac death over 2 years of follow-up.[27]

hs-CRP also demonstrates prognostic capacity in those who do not yet have a diagnosis of vascular disease. A mild elevation of baseline levels of hs-CRP among apparently healthy individuals is associated with higher long-term risk for future cardiovascular events. This predictive capacity offers patients the ability to receive treatment to reduce inflammation and, thus, their risk.[27]

CASE STUDY 23-4

A 68-year-old man presented to the emergency department with sudden onset of chest pain, left arm pain, dyspnea, and weakness while away from home on a business trip. His prior medical history is not available, but he admits to being a 2-pack/day smoker for longer than 20 years.

Cardiac markers were performed at admission and 8 hours postadmission with the following results:

CARDIAC MARKERS	7:30 A.M.; SEPTEMBER 26	4:00 P.M.; SEPTEMBER 26
CK-MB (0–5 ng/L)	5.3	9.2
Myoglobin (<70 µg/L)	76	124
Troponin T (0–0.1 µg/L)	<0.1	1.3

Questions

1. Do these results indicate a specific diagnosis?

2. If so, what is the diagnosis?

3. What myoglobin, CK-MB, and troponin T results would be expected if assayed at 4 p.m. on September 27?

4. Can any assumptions be made about the patient's lifestyle/habits/health that would increase his risk for this condition?

5. Are there any assays that might indicate his risk for further events of this type?

Fibrinogen

Fibrinogen is a soluble glycoprotein produced in the liver and involved in platelet aggregation and coagulation. It is also an acute-phase protein produced in response to inflammation. A relationship has been established between elevated levels of fibrinogen and risk of cardiovascular disease and may serve as a marker of long-term prognosis. Prospective studies in healthy men show that a single fibrinogen measurement may predict increased risk of cardiovascular events as much as 16 years later.[28] Including measurement of fibrinogen in screening for cardiovascular risk may be valuable in identifying persons who may benefit from aggressive preventive strategies.

D-Dimer

D-Dimer is the end product of the ongoing process of thrombus formation and dissolution that occurs at the site of active plaques in acute coronary syndromes. Because this process precedes myocardial cell damage and release of protein contents, it can be used for early detection. It remains elevated for days so it may be an easily detectable physiologic marker of an unstable plaque even when the troponins or CK-MB are not increased, potentially identifying high-risk patients who otherwise might be missed.[29] D-Dimer lacks specificity for cardiac damage as it is increased in other conditions that cause thrombosis. Elevations of D-Dimer have been shown to be useful in predicting risk for future cardiac events.[30]

Markers of Congestive Heart Failure

BNP

Brain-type, or B natriuretic peptide (BNP), is a peptide hormone secreted primarily by the cardiac ventricles. It acts on the renal glomerulus to stimulate urinary excretion of sodium and to increase urine flow without affecting the glomerular filtration rate, blood pressure, or renal blood flow.

Plasma concentrations of BNP are increased in diseases characterized by an expanded fluid volume (renal failure, hepatic cirrhosis with ascites, primary aldosteronism, and congestive heart failure), reduced renal clearance of peptides (renal failure), or stimulation of peptide production (ventricular hypertrophy or strain, ectopic production from tumors, thyroid disease, excessive circulating glucocorticoid, or hypoxia).[31]

Diagnosis of congestive heart failure (CHF) is difficult because of its nonspecific symptoms, as well as the lack of a specific biochemical marker for CHF. Studies show that plasma concentrations of BNP are elevated in patients with heart failure, especially in those patients with severe symptoms.[32] Evidence suggests that patients with a BNP concentration below approximately 20 pmol/L are unlikely to have CHF and those with results above this concentration have a high probability of CHF.[31] BNP results should be able to differentiate those patients who should undergo further diagnostic assessments from those who are unlikely to have cardiac failure. BNP may also be clinically relevant in determining the prognosis of patients, especially those with a diagnosis of CHF or those who have experienced a recent AMI. The recent development of a reliable and rapid assay for BNP makes it likely that it will become a commonplace biochemical marker used in the diagnosis of CHF.

Other Markers

The search for the "perfect" cardiac marker continues with the development of several assays to aid in the diagnosis of myocardial injury. This perfect marker will be more rapidly detectable than currently available assays, be completely specific for cardiac muscle damage, and be easily performed (see Table 23-6).

Glycogen Phosphorylase Isoenzyme BB (GPBB)

GPBB is a glycolytic enzyme that plays an essential role in the regulation of carbohydrate metabolism by mobilizing glycogen. It is not specific for cardiac tissue, but it is significantly more sensitive than CK, CK-MB mass, myoglobin, and TnT in patients with AMI during the first 3–4 hours after the onset of chest pain. In most AMI patients, GPBB increases between 1 and 4 hours from chest pain onset and returns to within the reference level within 1–2 days.

Heart Fatty Acid–Binding Protein

Heart fatty acid–binding protein (H-FABP) is a low-molecular-weight protein found in large quantities in the cytoplasm of myocardial and muscle cells that is involved in fatty acid metabolism and lipid homeostasis. Although H-FABP is not cardiac-specific, the H-FABP content of skeletal muscle is only 10–30% of that found in cardiac muscle, whereas the skeletal muscle content of myoglobin is approximately twice that of cardiac tissue. Thus, H-FABP is expected to be a more sensitive and specific marker than myoglobin for use in the early detection of myocardial injury.[33] It increases rapidly upon cellular damage, usually within 2–4 hours, peaks within 5–10 hours, and returns to normal within 24–36 hours after onset of chest pain. The magnitude of the increase in plasma H-FABP has also demonstrated a good correlation with the size of the infarction.[34]

Carbonic Anhydrase (CA) Isoenzyme III

CA is a soluble enzyme that catalyzes the hydration of carbon dioxide to bicarbonate and a proton and is involved in pH regulation, transport of ions, water and electrolyte balance, and metabolism of carbohydrates, urea, and lipids.[35] There are seven CA isoenzymes with a wide range of tissue distribution but a major site of CA activity is skeletal muscle. CAIII is not found in cardiac muscle and, therefore, can be used to differentiate between skeletal muscle and cardiac muscle damage when performed in conjunction with a more heart-specific analyte such as myoglobin. In the patient with actual or possible coexisting skeletal muscle injury, TnT or TnI would still be the markers of choice for confirming or excluding myocardial damage.[18]

Ischemia-Modified Albumin

A recently identified biochemical marker for ischemia, *ischemia-modified albumin* (IMA), is in the final stages of investigation. IMA is produced when albumin comes into contact with ischemic tissue, altering it and making it more resistant to binding metals. The mechanism for production of IMA is distinct from other early markers, such as CK-MB and troponins, which are products of myocardial tissue necrosis. IMA is produced continually during ischemia and rises within 2–3 hours of an ischemic event. One study shows that a negative IMA test at presentation to the emergency department had a 96% negative predictive value for a negative troponin result 6 hours later.[36] Future data is needed to determine whether IMA is specific for cardiac ischemia or if it is related to all tissue ischemia.

Homocysteine

Homocysteine is a naturally occurring amino acid found in blood, which is associated with vitamin B_{12}, B_6, and folic acid. An elevated homocysteine level is a potential risk factor for coronary heart disease, cerebral vascular disease, carotid artery disease, and peripheral vascular disease by promoting plaque formation. It is known that vitamin supplementation with folic acid, B_{12} and B_6 reduces homocysteine concentrations but the benefit of such treatment remains uncertain.[37]

Patient-Focused Cardiac Tests

It is widely accepted that early diagnosis of patients with AMI will result in less cardiac tissue damage, fewer complications, reduced hospital length of stay, and faster recovery. Also, treatment options, such as thrombolytic therapy or angioplasty, that can prevent further damage to the heart must be administered in a timely fashion. Typically, 90% of patients admitted to the hospital require biochemical testing to confirm or exclude AMI.[38] The American College of Cardiology and the American Heart Association recommend that the initial patient evaluation be performed within 20 minutes of arrival to the emergency department (ED) and that the optimum turnaround time (TAT) from patient arrival to the availability of test results for cardiac markers should be less than 30 minutes.[39] The National Academy of Clinical Biochemistry Standards of Laboratory Practice recommends that cardiac marker results should be available within 1 hour of sampling.[16] The pressure to comply with these standards is great, as well as difficult to achieve, in large institutions with busy EDs. Point-of-care (POC) testing for cardiac markers is one strategy to reduce turnaround time and the recent development of devices for performing whole blood cardiac assays at the patient's bedside has made it feasible to meet these strict guidelines.

Several medical and technical issues must be addressed when POC cardiac testing is considered. There are both qualitative and quantitative test systems available and systems that produce a panel of cardiac marker results, as well as discrete, single analyte results. Laboratorians and clinicians must collaborate to determine which cardiac markers are offered at their institution. Determining diagnostic cut-off values for AMI on POC results and correlating those results with those that may be performed in the clinical laboratory at a later time are also concerns.

Under the Clinical Laboratory Improvement Amendments Act (CLIA), POC cardiac marker testing is classified as moderately complex testing, not as a waived test. This classification requires more stringent regulatory guidelines and is more difficult to implement and maintain in POC settings. Issues such as maintaining ongoing proficiency testing, quality control, and operator competency will require greater oversight by the laboratory.[39]

The Role of the Laboratory in Monitoring Heart Disease

The laboratory's role in monitoring heart function primarily involves measuring the effects of the heart on other organs, such as the lungs, liver, and kidney. Arterial blood gases measure the patient's acid-base and oxygen status and are used to determine the respiratory acidosis and elevated carbon dioxide levels that are often seen in patients with heart disease. The patient with edema will develop electrolyte and osmolality changes as a result of fluid retention and ionic redistribution. Decreased cardiac output results in sodium retention by the kidneys, but also causes increased fluid retention; therefore, the serum sodium generally stays within the reference ranges or may be slightly decreased. Serum electrolyte determinations, including sodium, potassium, chloride, and calcium, are important to monitor diuretic and drug therapy in patients with heart disease.[4]

Elevations of aspartate aminotransferase (AST), alanine aminotransferase (ALT), and alkaline phosphatase (ALP) are often seen in patients with chronic right ventricular failure[4] and the γ-glutamyltransferase (GGT) value may be twice the value of the upper limit of the normal range in congestive heart failure, suggesting liver congestion and damage.

Lipid evaluation will assess risk for coronary artery disease. Maintenance of near-normal HDL-cholesterol, LDL-cholesterol, and triglyceride levels is highly recommended for cardiac patients. Determination of a lipoprotein similar to LDL, called lipoprotein (a), may also be indicated as it is an independent risk factor associated with development of premature coronary artery and vascular disease.

The patient who has secondary heart failure due to thyroid dysfunction can be identified by a highly sensitive thyroid-stimulating hormone assay. The laboratory is also invaluable for monitoring therapeutic drugs following the diagnosis of heart disease.

The routine complete blood count is important for detecting anemia and infection. Hemolysis may indicate additional testing for hemoglobinuria and myoglobinuria, indicators of cardiovascular damage and myocardial disease. An increase in white blood cells may indicate peri-carditis, endocarditis, or valvular infections. If kidney dysfunction has occurred as a result of the heart disease, anemia due to decreased production of renal erythropoietin may develop.

An infection associated with pericarditis, endocarditis, and valvular problems would be identified by blood cultures. Cultures of specimens from the pericardium and endocardium might also be performed if a pericardial infection is suspected.

The laboratory's role during the treatment of heart disease may also extend to providing blood components when surgical intervention is needed. Bypass grafts, correcting valvular defects, and other surgical procedures to correct heart failure may involve the use of blood components during the surgery and the patient's recovery.

TREATMENT

When cardiac disease is diagnosed, certain lifestyle changes are recommended to improve both quality of life and longevity. Exercise is effective in reducing the risk for further cardiac disease and for rehabilitation after myocardial infarction and other chronic cardiac disorders. Smoking cessation is an important step in reducing risks of complications and worsening of cardiac conditions. Dietary considerations are a necessary component of controlling the symptoms of cardiac disease. Weight reduction will reduce the workload of the heart and dietary restriction of sodium and fats are recommended. The use of drug therapy to reduce LDL-cholesterol concentrations may be necessary if reduced ingestion of animal and saturated fats does not lower concentrations to an acceptable level. Stress management is also encouraged, both to minimize anxiety associated with heart conditions and to control reactions to stressful life situations.

The strong correlation between hypertension and heart disease requires strict control of hypertension. Treatment for *essential hypertension* is aimed at reducing risk factors, such as weight reduction, salt and alcohol restriction, and increased exercise.

In the past 20 years, more than 30 studies have been performed comparing cardiovascular disease in postmenopausal women on estrogen replacement therapy with nonestrogen users that indicate the incidence of coronary artery disease among estrogen users is approximately one half of nonusers. It has been long recognized that these results may be a result of the fact that the population of estrogen users is inherently healthier than those who do not use estrogen replacement therapy. Yet, recent studies have shown no benefit of estrogen therapy versus placebo in reducing the risk of cardiovascular disease. At present, the conclusion is that coronary artery disease is not prevented by estrogen among older women with established heart disease.[40]

CASE STUDY 23-5

A 48-year-old woman was seen by her primary physician for a routine physical. Her father and his brother died before the age of 55 with AMI and another uncle had CABG surgery at age 52. Because of this family history, she requested any testing that might indicate a predisposition or increased risk factors for early cardiac disease. She does not smoke, does not have hypertension, is approximately 20 pounds overweight, and exercises moderately. The following test results were obtained.

Total cholesterol (<200 mg/dL)	187 mg/dL
HDL cholesterol (30–75 mg/dL)	52 mg/dL
LDL cholesterol (60–130 mg/dL)	95 mg/dL
Lipoprotein (a) (<30 mg/dL)	34 mg/dL
Triglycerides (60–160 mg/dL)	203 mg/dL
Glucose (60–110 mg/dL)	83 mg/dL
Total CK (15–130 IU/L)	65 IU/L
CK-MB (<8 IU/L)	1.9 IU/L
% CK-MB (0–6%)	3%
Homocysteine (<15 μmol/L)	18 μmol/L
Fibrinogen (2–4.5 mg/dL)	4.3 mg/dL
D-Dimer (0–250 μg/mL)	160 μg/mL
hs-CRP (0.016–0.76 mg/dL)	0.91 mg/dL

Questions

1. Do any of the results obtained indicate a high risk for development of cardiac disease? If so, which results?

2. Does this patient have risk factors for early cardiac disease that can be modified by diet or lifestyle modifications? If so, what changes can be made?

3. Is there any specific treatment that can be instituted to reduce this patient's risk?

4. How should this patient be monitored?

Drug Treatment

Multidrug treatment is routine to control the many and varied problems associated with cardiac disease. It usually consists of a combination of vasodilators, diuretics, β blockers, calcium channel antagonists, cardiac glycosides, and anticoagulants (Table 23-5).

Nitrates are coronary artery dilators that increase the blood supply to the heart and decrease blood pressure. Sublingual nitroglycerine is frequently used for relief of angina and is a part of the routine treatment of congestive heart failure and myocardial infarction. Topical ointments and skin patches may also be used to supply a consistent dosage of nitroglycerine to treat unstable angina and limit cardiac damage due to ischemia.

The most commonly used *vasodilators* are the angiotensin-converting enzyme (ACE) inhibitors, such as hydralazine or captopril. These drugs dilate the peripheral arteries and veins, decreasing the amount of effort that the heart expends to pump blood and are often an integral part of the treatment of cardiac conditions such as congestive heart failure and myocardial infarction.

β-Adrenergic blocking drugs reduce heart rate or the force of contractions, reducing oxygen demand for the heart by blocking the β receptors in the sinus mode and the myocardium. This group of drugs is used to treat tachycardia, ectopic beats, and arrhythmias, as well as angina pain and hypertension. Propranolol is a typical β blocker.

Calcium channel antagonists will decrease smooth muscle contractions and result in vasodilation. These drugs bind to the calcium channel subunits to limit the ability of calcium to cross the cell membrane. They are most often used to treat hypertension, angina, and supraventricular tachycardia.[41]

Cardiac glycosides, particularly digoxin, are used to increase heart contractility and slow the conduction impulses. Digoxin is the most commonly prescribed cardiac glycoside because of its convenient pharmacokinetics, alternative routes of administration, and widespread availability of serum drug level measurements.[42] Most patients with congestive heart failure, atrial fibrillation or tachycardia, hypertension, or cardiac ischemia will receive a drug of this type to control symptoms.

TABLE 23-5. DRUG TREATMENT OF CARDIAC DISEASE

CLASSIFICATION OF DRUG	ACTION OF DRUG	EXAMPLE
Vasodilator	Increase blood supply to heart muscle; decrease blood pressure	Nitroglycerine; angiotensin-converting enzyme inhibitors, such as hydralazine or captopril
Diuretic	Reduce blood volume and edema	Furosemide; thiazides
β Blocker	Reduce heart rate and the force of cardiac contractions	Propranolol
Calcium channel antagonist	Decrease smooth muscle contractions	Nifedipine
Cardiac glycoside	Increase contractility of the heart and slow conduction impulses	Digoxin
Anticoagulant	Reduce formation of prothrombin and prevent thrombosis andthromboembolism	Heparin; warfarin
Antiplatelet therapy	Reduce platelet activation and aggregation	Aspirin

Diuretics are given to help the kidneys clear excess water and sodium to reduce blood volume and, thereby, reduce the workload placed on the heart. Diuretics provide relief of symptoms in both pulmonary edema and congestive heart failure. It is important to monitor electrolyte balance and hydration to prevent too aggressive diuresis.

Numerous trials have demonstrated that early thrombolysis-induced reperfusion reduces infarct size and mortality. *Thrombolytic agents,* such as streptokinase, urokinase, or tissue plasminogen activator, may be indicated to lyse blood clots in AMI, acute pulmonary embolism, acute deep vein thrombosis, or arterial thrombosis or embolism.[41] The use of thrombolytic agents in patients with AMI, as compared with standard medical therapy, re-

duces overall mortality by 18%.[43] The greatest benefit occurs when these agents are administered within 3 hours after onset of symptoms.[44]

Antiplatelet therapy, often aspirin, is effective in reducing the risk for progression of atherosclerosis to myocardial infarction. It reduces platelet activation and aggregation, a significant factor in thrombotic processes and, as a result, reduces risk for ischemic heart disease.[41]

The use of heparin, warfarin, or other anticoagulants reduces the formation of prothrombin or inhibits the action of thrombin. Anticoagulant therapy is recommended to prevent venous thrombosis and thromboembolism and extension and recurrence of an infarct and to reduce mortality associated with these conditions.[45]

TABLE 23-6. ADDITIONAL MARKERS OF HEART DISEASE

MARKER	SIGNIFICANCE
hs-CRP	Inflammation Predictor of risk of future ACS
Fibrinogen	Inflammation Predictor of risk and prognosis of cardiac disease
D-Dimer	Indicator of plaque instability Identifies high-risk patients when other markers are not present
B-natriuretic peptide	Diagnostic for congestive heart failure
Glycogen phosphorylase isoenzyme BB	Sensitive indicator of AMI within 1-4 hours of onset of pain
Heart fatty acid–binding protein	Sensitive and specific indicator of cardiac injury
Degree of elevation reflects size of infarct in AMI	Degree of elevation reflects size of infarct in AMI
Carbonic anhydrase III	Differentiates cardiac damage vs. skeletal muscle damage
Ischemia-modified albumin	Indicator of ischemia Negative result "rules out" AMI
Homocysteine	Risk factor of coronary heart disease and vascular disease

Surgical Treatment

Coronary artery bypass graft surgery (CABG) was introduced in the late 1960s and has become a standard treatment for ischemic heart disease since that time. This surgical technique relieves symptoms and decreases mortality associated with ischemic heart disease by replacing the occluded coronary arteries with unaffected artery grafts. Patients with stable and unstable angina pectoris, AMI, "silent" ischemia, survivors of sudden cardiac death, congenital coronary anomalies, and congestive heart failure are frequently candidates for this surgery.[46]

Percutaneous transluminal coronary angioplasty (PTCA) is a surgical procedure in which an angioplasty balloon is inserted into a coronary artery and expanded. This opens the lumen of the obstructed vessel and restores blood flow to the affected area. There is some disagreement as to the long-term benefits of PTCA as compared with those of CABG, but in single coronary vessel disease, PTCA may be the treatment of choice.

Transmyocardial laser revascularization is a promising investigational technique in which a laser creates channels in the left ventricle to provide a blood supply to the adjacent myocardium. This revascularization has been shown to decrease the size of ischemic regions in patients who were not candidates for more conventional therapies.

Orthotopic heart transplantation is an option for treatment of advanced heart disease when medical and surgical treatments have failed or when patients have significant contraindications for these procedures. Currently, the 1-year survival rate after cardiac transplantation is 82% and the 3-year survival rate is 74%.[47] The limited availability of sufficient donor hearts is currently the limiting factor for this treatment option.

SUMMARY

The goal of an accurate and timely diagnosis for heart conditions is currently not achieved in all patients, especially those with acute chest pain. A thorough knowledge of the anatomy and function of the heart and the causes and effects of heart disease continues to be a most valuable tool in identifying and treating heart disease. The judicious use of laboratory and other diagnostic data is critical to the identification of patients who need further care and those who may safely be discharged. In patients who are exhibiting chest pain, recognizing the time-related patterns of increasing cardiac markers used today is an important factor in indicating the appropriate treatment for each individual patient. However, the symptoms and the risk factors identified often may not correlate with the laboratory and radiologic data obtained.

Advances in surgical and pharmacologic treatments for heart conditions will increase the life expectancy, as well as the quality of life, in patients with advanced heart disease. The future will bring development of more sensitive assays that have absolute specificity for cardiac disease, which will result in an accurate diagnosis in all patients.

REVIEW QUESTIONS

1. A serum troponin T concentration is of most value to the patient with a myocardial infarction when:
   a. the onset of symptoms is within 3–6 hours of the sample being drawn.
   b. the CK-MB has already peaked and returned to normal concentrations.
   c. the myoglobin concentration is extremely elevated.
   d. the troponin I concentration has returned to normal concentrations.

2. A normal myoglobin concentration 8 hours after onset of symptoms of a suspected myocardial infarction will:
   a. essentially rule out an acute myocardial infarction.
   b. provide a definitive diagnosis of acute myocardial infarction.
   c. be interpreted with careful consideration of the troponin T concentration.
   d. give the same information as a total CK-MB.

3. Which of the following analytes has the highest specificity for cardiac injury?
   a. Troponin I
   b. CK-MB mass assays
   c. Total CK-MB
   d. AST

4. Which of the following is NOT a consideration when investigating point-of-care (POC) testing for cardiac markers?
   a. Ease and costs of testing
   b. Time required to obtain results
   c. Maintaining regulatory requirements because it is considered a waived test
   d. Correlation of results obtained by POC methods to those obtained in the main laboratory

5. Which of the following tests do not monitor inflammation levels or coagulation factors that may contribute to acute coronary syndromes?
   a. hs-CRP
   b. Ischemia-modified albumin
   c. D-Dimer
   d. Fibrinogen

6. Rheumatic heart disease is a result of infection with which of the following organisms?
   a. *Staphylococcus aureus*
   b. Group A streptococci
   c. *Pseudomonas aeruginosa*
   d. *Chlamydia pneumoniae*

7. Angina, a common symptom of congestive heart failure, is often relieved by the administration of:
   a. diuretics.
   b. β-adrenergic blocking drugs.
   c. cardiac glycosides.
   d. nitrates.

8. Which of the following cardiac markers is the most useful indicator of congestive heart failure?
   a. Fibrinogen
   b. D-Dimer
   c. Glycogen phosphorylase isoenzyme BB
   d. B-natriuretic peptide

9. Which of the following cardiac markers is the best indicator of the size of the infarction in AMI?
   a. Fibrinogen
   b. B-natriuretic peptide
   c. Heart fatty acid–binding protein
   d. Troponin I

10. Which of the following is NOT a feature of an ideal cardiac marker?
    a. Absolute specificity
    b. High sensitivity
    c. Close estimation of the magnitude of cardiac damage
    d. Ability to predict future occurrence of cardiac disease

REFERENCES

1. Camm AJ. Cardiovascular disease. In: Kumar PJ, Clark ML, eds. Clinical Medicine, 2nd ed. London: Bailliere Tindall, 1990:511.
2. Braunwald E. The clinical examination. In: Goldman L, Braunwald E, eds. Primary Cardiology. Philadelphia: WB Saunders, 1998:30.
3. Carabello BA. Recognition and management of patients with valvular heart disease. In: Goldman L, Braunwald E, eds. Primary Cardiology. Philadelphia: WB Saunders, 1998:375.
4. Damjanov I. Pathology for the Health-Related Professions. Philadelphia: WB Saunders, 1996.
5. Marelli AJ, Moodie DS. Adult congenital heart disease. In: Topol, EJ, ed. Textbook of Cardiovascular Medicine, 2nd ed. Philadelphia: Lippincott Williams & Wilkins, 2002:711.
6. Gould BE. Pathophysiology for the Health-Related Professions. Philadelphia: WB Saunders, 1997.
7. Therrien J, Webb GD. Congenital heart disease in adults. In: Braunwald E, Zipes DP, Libby P, eds. Heart Disease: A Textbook of Cardiovascular Medicine, 6th ed. Philadelphia: WB Saunders, 2001:1599.
8. Givertz MM, Colucci WS, Braunwald E. Clinical aspects of heart failure: high-output heart failure; pulmonary edema. In: Braunwald E, ed. Heart Disease: A Textbook of Cardiac Medicine, Vol 1, 6th ed. Philadelphia: WB Saunders, 2001:535.
9. Gazes PC. Clinical Cardiology: A Cost-effective Approach. New York: Chapman & Hall, 1997.
10. Christenson RH, Duh SH. Evidence-based approach to practice guides and decision thresholds for cardiac markers. Scand J Clin Lab Invest 1999;59(Suppl 230):90–102.
11. Thomas CL, ed. Taber's Cyclopedic Medical Dictionary, 18th ed. Philadelphia: FA Davis, 1997;168.
12. Wilson PWF. An epidemiologic perspective of systemic hypertension, ischemic heart disease and heart failure. Am J Cardiol 1997; 80(9B):3J–7J.
13. Black HR. Approach to the patient with hypertension. In: Goldman L, Braunwald E. Primary Cardiology. Philadelphia: WB Saunders, 1998;134.
14. Ellis RW. Infection and coronary heart disease. J Med Microbiol 1997;46:535–539.
15. Muhlestein JB. Chronic infection and coronary artery disease. Med Clin N Am 2000;84(1):123–148.
16. Wu AHB, Apple FS, Gibler WB, et al. National Academy of Clinical Biochemistry Standards of Laboratory Practice: recommendations for the use of cardiac markers in coronary artery disease. Clin Chem 1999;45(7):1104–1121.
17. Mair J. Progress in myocardial damage detection: new biochemical markers for clinicians. Crit Rev Clin Lab Sci 1997;34:1–66.
18. Karras DJ, Kane DL. Serum markers in the emergency department: diagnosis of acute myocardial infarction. Emerg Med Clin N Am 2001;19(2):321–337.
19. Zimmerman J, Fromm R, Meyer D, et al. Diagnostic marker cooperative study for the diagnosis of myocardial infarction. Circulation 1999;99:1671–1677.
20. O'Neil BJ, Ross, MA. Cardiac markers protocols in a chest pain observation unit. Emerg Med Clin N Am 2001;19(1):67–86.
21. Delanghe JR, Chapelle JP, Vanderschueren SC. Quantitative nephelometric assay for determining myoglobin evaluated. Clin Chem 1990;36(9):1675–1678.
22. Puschendorf B. Strategies for cardiac marker measurement. Clin Chem Lab Med 1999;37(11/12):997-999.
23. Antman EM, Braunwald E. Acute myocardial infarction. In: Braunwald E, Zipes DP, Libby P, eds. Heart Disease: A Textbook of Cardiovascular Medicine, 6th ed. Philadelphia: WB Saunders, 2001:1134.
24. Remppis A, Ehlermann P, Giannitsis E. et al. Cardiac troponin T levels at 96 hours reflect myocardial infarct size: a pathoanatomical study. Cardiology 2000;93:249–253.
25. Liuzzo G, Rizzello V. C-reactive protein and primary prevention of ischemic heart disease. Clin Chim Acta 2001;311:45–48.
26. Speidl WS, Graf S, Hornykewycz S, et al. High-sensitivity C-reaction protein in the prediction of coronary events in patients with premature coronary artery disease. Am Heart J 2002;144(3):449–455.

27. Morrow DA, Ridker PM. C-reactive protein, inflammation, and coronary risk. Med Clin N Am 2000;84(1):149–161.

28. Sehnal E, Slany J. Fibrinogen-the key to familiar CHD or just another shadow in Plato's allegory? Eur Heart J 2002;23(16):1231–1233.

29. Newby LK. Cardiac marker testing: where should we focus? Am Heart J 2000;140(3):351–353.

30. Ridker PM. Inflammation, aspirin, and the risk of cardiovascular disease in apparently healthy men. N Engl J Med1997;336(14):973–979.

31. Cowie MR, Mendez GF. BNP and congestive heart failure. Prog Cardiovascular Dis 2002;44(4):293–332.

32. Wei C-M, Heublein DM, Perella MA. Natriuretic peptide system in human heart failure. Circulation 1993;88:1004–1009.

33. Ishii J, Wang J, Naruse H, et al. Serum concentrations of myoglobin vs. human heart-type cytoplasmic fatty acid-binding protein in early detection of acute myocardial infarction. Clin Chem 1997;43:1372–1378.

34. Ghani F, Wu AHB, Graff L, et al. Role of heart-type fatty acid-binding protein in early detection of acute myocardial infarction. Clin Chem 2000;46:718–719.

35. Sly WS, Peiyi YH. Human carbonic anhydrases and carbonic anhydrase deficiencies. Ann Rev Biochem 1995;64:375–401.

36. Check W. Getting a jump on cardiovascular disease. CAP Today 2002;16(3):1.

37. Tribouilloy CM, Peltier M, Peltier MCI, et al. Plasma homocysteine and severity of thoracic aortic atherosclerosis. Chest 2000;118(6):1685–1689.

38. Collinson PO. Testing for cardiac markers at the point of care. Clin Lab Med 2001;21(2):351–362.

39. Lewandrowski K. Cardiac markers: the next opportunity of point-of-care testing. Clin Lab News 2003;29(1):10–11.

40. Knopp RH, Aikawa K. Estrogen, female gender, and heart disease. In: Topol EJ, ed. Textbook of Cardiovascular Medicine, 2nd ed. Philadelphia: Lippincott Williams & Wilkins, 2002:179.

41. Opie LH. Pharmocologic options for treatment of ischemic disease. In: Smith TW, ed. Cardiovascular Therapeutics: A Companion to Braunwald's Heart Disease. Philadelphia: WB Saunders, 1996:22.

42. Kelly RA, Smith TW. The pharmacology of heart failure drugs. In: Smith TW, ed. Cardiovascular Therapeutics: A Companion to Braunwald's Heart Disease. Philadelphia: WB Saunders, 1996:176.

43. Topol EJ, Van de Werf, FJ. Acute myocardial infarction. In: Topol EJ, ed. Textbook of Cardiovascular Medicine, 2nd ed. Philadelphia: Lippincott Williams & Wilkins, 2002:394.

44. Ryan TJ. Management of acute myocardial infarction: synopsis of ACC and AHA practice guidelines. Postgrad Med 1997;102(5):84–96.

45. Schafer AJ, Ali NM, Levine GN. Hemostasis, thrombosis, fibrinolysis, and cardiovascular disease. In: Braunwald E, Zipes DP, Libby P, eds. Heart Disease: A Textbook of Cardiovascular Medicine, 6th ed. Philadelphia: WB Saunders, 2001:2118.

46. Solomon AJ, Gersh BJ. Ischemic heart disease: surgical options. In: Smith TW, ed. Cardiovascular Therapeutics: A Companion to Braunwald's Heart Disease. Philadelphia: WB Saunders, 1996:65.

47. Miniati DN, Robbins RC, Reitz BA. Heart and heart-lung transplantation. In: Braunwald E, Zipes DP, Libby P, eds. Heart Disease: A Textbook of Cardiovascular Medicine, 6th ed. Philadelphia: WB Saunders, 2001:629.

Renal Function

Carol J. Skarzynski

Alan H. B. Wu

OBJECTIVES

Upon completion of this chapter, the clinical laboratorian should be able to:

- Diagram the anatomy of the nephron.
- Describe the physiologic role of each of part of the nephron: glomerulus, proximal tubule, loop of Henle, distal tubule, and collecting duct.
- Describe the mechanisms by which the kidney maintains fluid and electrolyte balance in conjunction with hormones.
- Discuss the significance and calculation of glomerular filtration rate and estimated glomerular filtration rate.

- Relate the clinical significance of total urine proteins, urine albumin microalbuminuria, myoglobin clearance, serum β$_2$-microglobulin, and cystatin C.
- List the tests in a urinalysis and microscopy profile and understand the clinical significance of each.
- Describe diseases of the glomerulus and tubules and how laboratory tests are used in these disorders.
- Distinguish between acute and chronic renal failure.
- Discuss the therapy of chronic renal failure with regard to renal dialysis and transplantation.

KEY TERMS

Acute renal failure
Aldosterone
Antidiuretic hormone (ADH)
Chronic kidney disease
Countercurrent multiplier system
Creatinine clearance

Cystatin C
Diabetes mellitus
Erythropoietin
Estimated glomerular filtration rate (EGFR)
Glomerular filtration rate (GFR)
Glomerulonephritis

Glomerulus
Hemodialysis
Hemofiltration
Loop of Henle
Microalbumin
β$_2$-Microglobulin (β$_2$-M)
Myoglobin
Nephrotic syndrome

Prostaglandin
Renal threshold
Renin
Rhabdomyolysis
Tubular reabsorption
Tubular secretion
Tubule
Vitamin D

TABLE 24-1. KIDNEY FUNCTIONS

Urine formation
Fluid and electrolyte balance
Regulation of acid-base balance
Excretion of the waste products of protein metabolism
Excretion of drugs and toxins
Secretion of hormones
Renin
Erythropoietin
1,25-Dihydroxy vitamin D_3
Prostaglandins

The kidneys are vital organs that perform a variety of important functions (Table 24-1). The most prominent functions are removal of unwanted substances from plasma (both waste and surplus), homeostasis (maintenance of equilibrium) of the body's water, electrolyte and acid-base status, and participation in hormonal regulation. In the clinical laboratory, kidney function tests are used in assessment of renal disease, water balance, and acid-base disorders and in situations of trauma, head injury, surgery, and infectious disease. This chapter focuses on renal anatomy and physiology and the analytic procedures available to diagnose, monitor, and treat kidney dysfunction.

RENAL ANATOMY

The kidneys are paired, bean-shaped organs located retroperitoneally on either side of the spinal column. Macroscopically, a fibrous capsule of connective tissue encloses each kidney. When dissected longitudinally, two regions can be clearly discerned—an outer region called the cortex and an inner region called the medulla (Fig. 24-1A). The pelvis can also be seen. It is a basin-like cavity at the upper end of the ureter into which newly formed urine passes. The bilateral ureters are thick-walled canals, connecting the kidneys to the urinary bladder. Urine is temporarily stored in the bladder until voided from the body by way of the urethra. Figure 24-1B shows the arrangement of nephrons in the kidney, functional units of the kidney that can only be seen microscopically. Each kidney contains approximately 1 million nephrons. Each nephron is a complex apparatus comprised of five basic parts expressed diagrammatically in Figure 24-2.

- The *glomerulus*—a capillary tuft surrounded by the expanded end of a renal *tubule* known as *Bowman's capsule.* Each glomerulus is supplied by an afferent arteriole carrying the blood in and an efferent arteriole carrying the blood out. The efferent arteriole branches into peritubular capillaries that supply the tubule.
- The *proximal convoluted tubule*—located in the cortex.
- The long *loop of Henle*—comprised of the thin *descending limb,* which spans the medulla, and the *ascending limb,* which is located in both the medulla and the cortex, comprised of a region that is thin and then thick.
- The *distal convoluted tubule*—located in the cortex.
- The *collecting duct*—formed by two or more distal convoluted tubules as they pass back down through the cortex and the medulla to collect the urine that drains from each nephron. Collecting ducts eventually merge and empty their contents into the renal pelvis.

The following section describes how each part of the nephron normally functions.

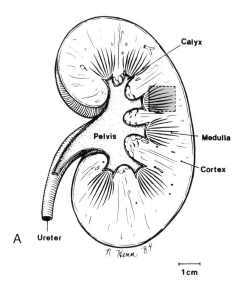

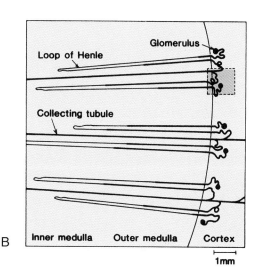

FIGURE 24-1. Anatomy of the kidney.

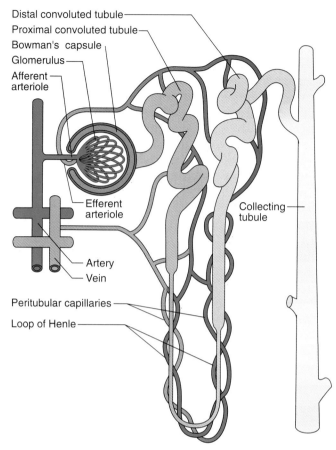

Distal convoluted tubule
Proximal convoluted tubule
Bowman's capsule
Glomerulus
Afferent arteriole
Efferent arteriole
Collecting tubule
Artery
Vein
Peritubular capillaries
Loop of Henle

FIGURE 24-2. Representation of a nephron and its blood supply.

RENAL PHYSIOLOGY

There are three basic renal processes:

1. glomerular filtration
2. tubular reabsorption
3. tubular secretion.

Figure 24-3 illustrates how three different substances are variably processed by the nephron. Substance A is *filtered* and *secreted*, but not reabsorbed; substance B is *filtered* and a *portion reabsorbed*; and substance C is *filtered* and *completely reabsorbed*.[1] The following is a description

of how specific substances are regulated in this manner to maintain homeostasis.

Glomerular Filtration

The glomerulus is the first part of the nephron and functions to filter incoming blood. Several factors facilitate filtration. One factor is the unusually high pressure in the glomerular capillaries, which is a result of their position between two arterioles. This sets up a steep pressure difference across the walls. Another factor is the semipermeable glomerular basement membrane, which has a molecular size cutoff value of approximately 66,000 daltons, about the molecular size of albumin. This means that water, electrolytes, and small dissolved solutes, such as glucose, amino acids, low-molecular-weight proteins, urea, and creatinine, pass freely through the basement membrane and enter the proximal convoluted tubule. Other blood constituents, such as albumin; many plasma proteins; cellular element; and protein-bound substances, such as lipids and bilirubin, are too large to be filtered. In addition, because the basement membrane is negatively charged, negatively charged molecules, such as proteins, are repelled. Of the 1200–1500 mL of blood that the kidneys receive each minute (approximately one quarter of the total cardiac output), the glomerulus filters out 125–130 mL of an essentially protein-free, cell-free fluid, called *glomerular filtrate*. The volume of blood filtered per minute is the *glomerular filtration rate (GFR)*, and its determination is essential in evaluating renal function, as discussed in the section on *Analytic Procedures*.

Tubular Function

Proximal Convoluted Tubule

The proximal tubule is the next part of the nephron to receive the now cell-free and, essentially protein-free, blood. This filtrate contains waste products, which are toxic to the body above a certain concentration, and substances that are valuable to the body. One function of the proximal tubule is to return the bulk of each valuable substance back to the blood circulation. Thus, 75% of the

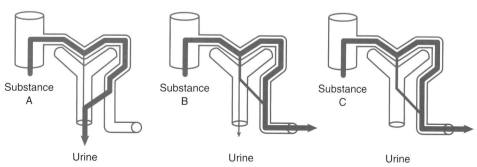

Substance A   Substance B   Substance C

Urine   Urine   Urine

FIGURE 24-3. Renal processes of filtration, reabsorption, and secretion.

water, sodium, and chloride; 100% of the glucose (up to the renal threshold); almost all of the amino acids, vitamins, and proteins; and varying amounts of urea, uric acid, and ions, such as magnesium, calcium, potassium, and bicarbonate, are *reabsorbed*. Almost all (98–100%) of uric acid, a waste product, is actively reabsorbed, only to be secreted at the distal end of the proximal tubule.

When the substances move from the tubular lumen to the peritubular capillary plasma, the process is called *tubular reabsorption*. With the exception of water and chloride ions, the process is active; that is, the tubular epithelial cells use energy to bind and transport the substances across the plasma membrane to the blood. The transport processes that are involved normally have sufficient reserve for efficient reabsorption, but they are saturable. When the concentration of the filtered substance exceeds the capacity of the transport system, the substance is then excreted in the urine. The plasma concentration above which the substance appears in urine is known as the *renal threshold,* and its determination is useful in assessing both tubular function and nonrenal disease states. A renal threshold does not exist for water because it is always transported passively through diffusion down a concentration gradient. Chloride ions in this instance diffuse in the wake of sodium.

A second function of the proximal tubule is to *secrete* products of kidney tubular cell metabolism, such as hydrogen ions, and drugs, such as penicillin. The term *tubular secretion* is used in two ways: (1) Tubular secretion describes the movement of substances from peritubular capillary plasma to the tubular lumen, and (2) tubular secretion also describes when tubule cells secrete products of their own cellular metabolism into the filtrate in the tubular lumen. Transport across the membrane of the cell is again either active or passive.

Loop of Henle

Countercurrent Multiplier System. The osmolality in the medulla in this portion of the nephron increases steadily from the corticomedullary junction inward and facilitates the reabsorption of water, sodium, and chloride. The hyperosmolality that develops in the medulla is continuously maintained by the loop of Henle, a hairpin-like loop between the proximal tubule and the distal convoluted tubule. The opposing flows in the loop, the downward flow in the descending limb, and the upward flow in the ascending limb, is termed a *countercurrent flow*. To understand how the hyperosmolality is maintained in the medulla, it is best to look first at what happens in the ascending limb. Sodium and chloride are actively and passively reabsorbed into the medulla interstitial fluid along the entire length of the ascending limb. Because the ascending limb is relatively impermeable to water, little water follows and the medulla inter-

stitial fluid becomes hyperosmotic compared with the fluid in the ascending limb. The fluid in the ascending limb becomes hypotonic or dilute as sodium and chloride ions are reabsorbed without the loss of water, so the ascending limb is often called the *diluting segment*. The descending limb, in contrast to the ascending limb, is highly permeable to water and does not reabsorb sodium and chloride. The high osmolality of the surrounding interstitial medulla fluid is the physical force that accelerates the reabsorption of water from the filtrate in the descending limb. Interstitial hyperosmolality is maintained because the ascending limb continues to pump sodium and chloride ions into it. This interaction of water leaving the descending loop and sodium and chloride leaving the ascending loop to maintain a high osmolality within the kidney medulla produces hypoosmolal urine as it leaves the loop. This process is called the *countercurrent multiplier system*.[2]

Distal Convoluted Tubule

The distal convoluted tubule is much shorter than the proximal tubule, with two or three coils that connect to a collecting duct. The filtrate entering this section of the nephron is close to its final composition. About 95% of the sodium and chloride ions and 90% of water have already been reabsorbed from the original glomerular filtrate. The function of the distal tubule is to effect small adjustments to achieve electrolyte and acid-base homeostasis. These adjustments occur under the hormonal control of both *antidiuretic hormone (ADH)* and *aldosterone*. Figure 24-4 describes the action of these hormones.

ADH. ADH is a peptide hormone secreted by the posterior pituitary, mainly in response to increased blood osmolality; ADH is also released when blood volume decreases by more than 5–10%. Large decreases of blood volume will stimulate ADH secretion even when plasma osmolality is decreased.[3] ADH stimulates water reabsorption. The walls of the distal collecting tubules are normally impermeable to water (like the ascending loop of Henle), but they become permeable to water in ADH. Water diffuses passively from the lumen of the tubules, resulting in more concentrated urine and decreased plasma osmolality.

Aldosterone. This hormone is produced by the adrenal cortex under the influence of the renin–angiotensin mechanism. Its secretion is triggered by decreased blood flow or blood pressure in the afferent renal arteriole and by decreased plasma sodium. Aldosterone stimulates sodium reabsorption in the distal tubules and potassium and hydrogen ion secretion. Hydrogen ion secretion is linked to bicarbonate regeneration and ammonia secretion, which also occur here. In addition to these ions, small amounts of chloride ions are reabsorbed.

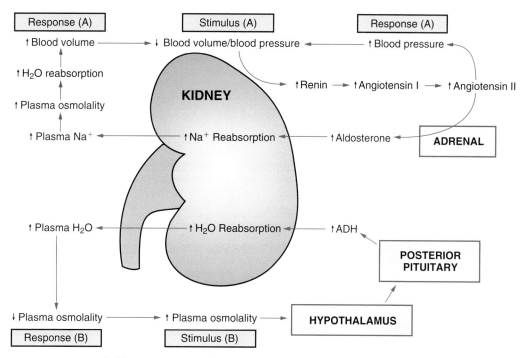

FIGURE 24-4. ADH and aldosterone control of the renal reabsorption of water and Na$^+$. (Reprinted with permission from Kaplan A, et al. The kidney and tests of renal function. In: Kaplan A, Jack R, Opheim KE, Toivola B, Lyon AW, eds. Clinical Chemistry: Interpretation and Techniques, 4th ed. Baltimore: Williams & Wilkins, 1995:158, Fig. 6.2.)

Collecting Duct

The collecting ducts are the final site for either concentrating or diluting urine. The hormones *ADH* and *aldosterone* act on this segment of the nephron to control reabsorption of water and sodium. Chloride and urea are also reabsorbed here. Urea plays an important role in maintaining the hyperosmolality of the renal medulla. Because the collecting ducts in the medulla are highly permeable to urea, urea diffuses down its concentration gradient out of the tubule and into the medulla interstitium, increasing its osmolality.[4]

Elimination of Nonprotein Nitrogen Compounds

Nonprotein nitrogen compounds (NPN) are waste products formed in the body as a result of the degradative metabolism of nucleic acids, amino acids, and proteins. Excretion of these compounds is an important function of the kidneys. The three principal compounds are urea, creatinine, and uric acid.[5,6] For a more detailed treatment of their biochemistry and disease correlations, see Chapter 9, *Nonprotein Nitrogen Compounds*.

Urea

Urea makes up the majority (>75%) of the NPN waste excreted daily as a result of the oxidative catabolism of protein. Urea synthesis occurs in the liver. Proteins are broken down to amino acids, which are then deaminated to form ammonia. Ammonia is readily converted to urea, avoiding toxicity. The kidney is the only significant route of excretion for urea. It has a molecular weight of 60 and, therefore, is readily filtered by the glomerulus. In the collecting ducts, 40–60% of urea is reabsorbed. The reabsorbed urea contributes to the high osmolality in the medulla, which is one of the processes of urinary concentration mentioned earlier (see *Loop of Henle*).

Creatinine

Muscle contains creatine phosphate, a high-energy compound for the rapid formation of adenosine triphosphate (ATP). This reaction is catalyzed by creatine kinase (CK) and is the first source of metabolic fuel used in muscle contraction. Creatinine is formed from creatine as shown below.

$$\text{Creatine phosphate} + \text{ADP} + \text{H}^+ \xrightleftharpoons{\text{CK}}$$

$$\text{creatine} + \text{ATP} \xrightarrow{\text{nonenzymatic}} \text{creatinine} \qquad \textbf{(Eq. 24–1)}$$

Every day, up to 20% of total muscle creatine (and its phosphate) spontaneously dehydrates and cycles to form the waste product creatinine. Therefore, creatinine levels are a function of muscle mass and remain approximately the same in an individual from day-to-day unless muscle mass or renal function changes. Creatinine has a molecular weight of 113 and is, therefore, readily filtered by the glomerulus. Unlike urea, creatinine is not reabsorbed by the tubules. However, a small amount of creatinine is secreted by the kidney tubules at high serum concentrations.

Uric Acid

Uric acid is the primary waste product of purine metabolism. The purines, adenine and guanine, are precursors of nucleic acids ATP and guanosine triphosphate (GTP), respectively. Uric acid has a molecular weight of 168. Like creatinine, it is readily filtered by the glomerulus, but it then undergoes a complex cycle of reabsorption and secretion as it courses through the nephron. Only 6–12% of the original filtered uric acid is finally excreted. Uric acid exists in its ionized and more soluble form, usually sodium urate, at urinary pH >5.75 (the first pK_a of uric acid). At pH <5.75, it is undissociated. This fact has clinical significance in the development of urolithiasis (formation of calculi) and gout.

Water, Electrolyte, and Acid-Base Homeostasis

Water Balance

The kidney's contribution to water balance in the body is through water loss or water conservation, which is regulated by the hormone ADH. ADH responds primarily to changes in osmolality and intravascular volume. Increased plasma osmolality or decreased intravascular volume stimulates secretion of ADH from the posterior pituitary. ADH then increases the permeability of the distal convoluted tubules and collecting ducts to water, resulting in increased water reabsorption and excretion of more concentrated urine. In contrast, the major system regulating water intake is thirst, which appears to be triggered by the same stimuli that trigger ADH secretion.

In states of dehydration, the renal tubules reabsorb water at their maximal rate, resulting in production of a small amount of maximally concentrated urine (high urine osmolality, 1200 mOsmol/L).[7] In states of water excess, the tubules reabsorb water at only a minimal rate, resulting in excretion of a large volume of extremely dilute urine (low urine osmolality, down to 50 mOsmol/L).[8–10] The continuous fine-tuning possible between these two extreme states results in the precise control of fluid balance in the body (Fig. 24-5).

Electrolyte Balance

The following is a brief overview of the notable ions involved in maintenance of electrolyte balance within the body. For a more comprehensive treatment of this subject, refer to Chapter 13, *Electrolytes.*

Sodium. Sodium is the primary extracellular cation in the human body and is excreted principally through the kidneys. Sodium balance in the body is controlled only through excretion. The *renin-angiotensin-aldosterone* hormonal system is the major mechanism for control of sodium balance.

Potassium. Potassium is the main intracellular cation in the body. The precise regulation of its concentration is

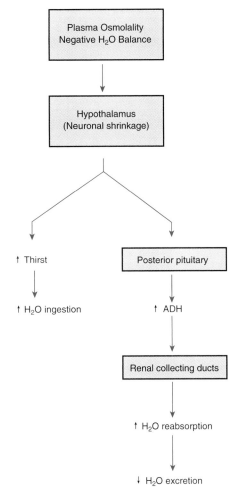

FIGURE 24-5. ADH control of thirst mechanism.

of extreme importance to cellular metabolism and is controlled chiefly by renal means. Like sodium, it is freely filtered by the glomerulus and then actively reabsorbed throughout the entire nephron (except for the descending limb of the loop of Henle). Both the distal convoluted tubule and the collecting ducts can reabsorb and excrete potassium, and this excretion is controlled by aldosterone. Potassium ions can compete with hydrogen ions in their exchange with sodium (in the proximal convoluted tubule); this process is used by the body to conserve hydrogen ions and, thereby, compensate in states of metabolic alkalosis.

Chloride. Chloride is the principal extracellular anion and is involved in the maintenance of extracellular fluid balance. It is readily filtered by the glomerulus and is passively reabsorbed as a counter ion when sodium is reabsorbed in the proximal convoluted tubule. In the ascending limb of the loop of Henle, potassium is actively reabsorbed by a distinct chloride "pump," which also reabsorbs sodium. This pump can be inhibited by loop diuretics, such as furosemide. As expected, the regulation of chloride is controlled by the same forces that regulate sodium.[7,10]

Phosphate, Calcium, and Magnesium. The phosphate ion occurs in higher concentrations in the intracellular than the extracellular fluid environments. It exists as either a protein-bound or a non–protein-bound form; homeostatic balance is chiefly determined by proximal tubular reabsorption under the control of parathyroid hormone (PTH). Calcium, the second-most predominant intracellular cation, is the most important inorganic messenger in the cell. It also exists in protein-bound and non–protein-bound states. Calcium in the non–protein-bound form is either ionized and physiologically active or nonionized and complexed to small, diffusible ions, such as phosphate and bicarbonate. The ionized form is freely filtered by the glomerulus and reabsorbed in the tubules under the control of PTH. However, renal control of calcium concentration is not the major means of regulation. PTH- and calcitonin-controlled regulation of calcium absorption from the gut and bone stores is more important than renal secretion or reabsorption. Magnesium, a major intracellular cation, is important as an enzymatic cofactor. Like phosphate and calcium, it exists in both protein-bound and ionized states. The ionized fraction is easily filtered by the glomerulus and reabsorbed in the tubules under the influence of PTH. See Chapter 21, *Parathyroid Function and Control for Calcium Homeostasis,* for more detailed information.

Acid-Base Balance

Many nonvolatile acidic waste products are formed by normal body metabolism each day. Carbonic acid, lactic acid, ketoacids, and others must be continually transported in the plasma and excreted from the body, causing only minor alterations in physiologic pH. The renal system constitutes one of three means by which constant control of overall body pH is accomplished. The other two strategies involved in this regulation are the respiratory system and the acid-base buffering system.[11]

The kidneys manage their share of the responsibility for controlling body pH by dual means: conserving bicarbonate ions and removing metabolic acids. For a more in-depth examination of these processes, refer to Chapter 14, *Blood Gases, pH, and Buffer Systems.*

Regeneration of Bicarbonate Ions. In a complicated process, bicarbonate ions are first filtered out of the plasma by the glomerulus. In the lumen of the renal tubules, this bicarbonate combines with hydrogen ions to form carbonic acid, which subsequently degrades to carbon dioxide (CO_2) and water. This CO_2 then diffuses into the brush border of the proximal tubular cells, where it is reconverted by carbonic anhydrase to carbonic acid and then degrades back to hydrogen ions and regenerated bicarbonate ions. This reaction is detailed as follows:

$$H_2O + CO_2 \xrightarrow{CA} H_2CO_3 \longleftrightarrow H^+ + HCO_3^- \quad \textbf{(Eq. 24–2)}$$

This regenerated bicarbonate is transported into the blood to replace what was depleted by metabolism; the accompanying hydrogen ions are secreted back into the tubular lumen and from there enter the urine. Filtered bicarbonate is "reabsorbed" into the circulation, helping to return blood pH to its optimal level and effectively functioning as another buffering system.

Excretion of Metabolic Acids. Hydrogen ions are manufactured in the renal tubules as part of the regeneration mechanism for bicarbonate. These hydrogen ions, as well as others that are dissociated from nonvolatile organic acids, are disposed of by several different reactions with buffer bases.

Reaction With Ammonia (NH_3). The glomerulus does not filter NH_3. However, this substance is formed in the renal tubules when the amino acid glutamine is deaminated by glutaminase. This NH_3 then reacts with secreted hydrogen ions to form ammonium ions (NH_4^+) which are unable to readily diffuse out of the tubular lumen and, therefore, are excreted into the urine.

$$\text{Glutamine} \xrightarrow{\text{Glutaminase}} \text{glutamic acid} + NH_3$$

$$NH_3 + H^+ + NaCl \rightarrow NH_4Cl + Na^+ \quad \textbf{(Eq. 24–3)}$$

This mode of acid excretion is the primary means by which the kidneys compensate for states of metabolic acidosis.

Reaction With Monohydrogen Phosphate (HPO_4^{2-}). Phosphate ions filtered by the glomerulus can exist in the tubular fluid as disodium hydrogen phosphate (Na_2HPO_4) (dibasic). This compound can react with hydrogen ions to yield dihydrogen phosphate (monobasic), which is then excreted. The released sodium then combines with bicarbonate to yield sodium bicarbonate and is reabsorbed.

$$Na_2HPO_4 + H^+ \longleftrightarrow NaH_2PO_4 + Na^+ \quad \textbf{(Eq. 24–4)}$$

These mechanisms can excrete increasing amounts of metabolic acid until a maximum urine pH of approximately 4.4 is reached. After this, renal compensation is unable to adjust to any further decreases in blood pH and metabolic acidosis ensues. Few free hydrogen ions are excreted directly in the urine.

Endocrine Function

In addition to numerous excretory and regulatory functions, the kidney has endocrine functions as well. It is both a primary endocrine site, as the producer of its own hormones, and a secondary site, as the target locus for hormones manufactured by other endocrine organs. The kidneys synthesize renin, erythropoietin, 1,25-dihydroxy vitamin D_3, and the prostaglandins.

Renin. *Renin* is the initial component of the *renin-angiotensin-aldosterone* system. Renin is produced by the juxtaglomerular cells of the renal medulla when extracellular fluid volume or blood pressure decreases. It catalyzes the synthesis of angiotensin by cleavage of the circulating plasma precursor angiotensinogen. Angiotensin is converted to angiotensin II by angiotensin-converting enzyme (ACE). Angiotensin II is a powerful vasoconstrictor that increases blood pressure and stimulates release of aldosterone from the adrenal cortex. Aldosterone, in turn, promotes sodium reabsorption and water conservation.[8,10] For a more detailed look at the complexities of this feedback loop, see Chapter 18, *Adrenal Function.*

Erythropoietin. *Erythropoietin* is a single-chain polypeptide produced by cells close to the proximal tubules, and its production is regulated by blood oxygen levels. Hypoxia produces increased serum concentrations within 2 hours. Erythropoietin acts on the erythroid progenitor cells in the bone marrow, increasing the number of red blood cells. In chronic renal insufficiency, erythropoietin production is significantly reduced. Recently, recombinant human erythropoietin has been developed and is now in routine use in chronic renal failure patients. Before this therapy, anemia was a clinical reality in these patients.[5,8] Erythropoietin concentrations in blood can be measured by immunoassays.

1,25-Dihydroxy Vitamin D₃

The kidneys are the sites of formation of the active form of *vitamin D;* 1,25 $(OH)_2$ vitamin D_3.[3,5] This form of vitamin D is one of three major hormones that determine phosphate and calcium balance and bone calcification in the human body. Chronic renal insufficiency is, therefore, often associated with *osteomalacia* (inadequate bone calcification, the adult form of rickets), owing to the continual distortion of normal vitamin D metabolism.

Prostaglandins. The *prostaglandins* are a group of potent cyclic fatty acids formed from essential (dietary) fatty acids, primarily arachidonic acid. They are formed in almost all tissue and their actions are diverse. The prostaglandins produced by the kidneys increase renal blood flow, sodium and water excretion, and renin release. They act to oppose renal vasoconstriction due to angiotensin and norepinephrine.

ANALYTIC PROCEDURES

Several tests are available that assess the various aspects of nephron function, including glomerular filtration and proximal and distal tubular secretion and reabsorption.

Clearance Measurements

All laboratory methods used for evaluation of renal function rely on the measurement of waste products in blood, usually urea and creatinine, which accumulate when the kidneys begin to fail. Renal failure must be advanced, with only about 20–30% of the nephrons still functioning, before the concentration of either substance begins to increase in the blood. The rate at which creatinine and urea are removed or cleared from the blood into the urine is termed *clearance*. Clearance is defined as that volume of plasma from which a measured amount of substance can be completely eliminated into the urine per unit of time expressed in mL/minute.[5] Measurement of clearance is used to estimate the rate of glomerular filtration.

Creatinine

Creatinine is a nearly ideal substance for the measurement of clearance. It is an endogenous metabolic product synthesized at a constant rate for a given individual and cleared essentially only by glomerular filtration (it is not reabsorbed and is only slightly secreted by the proximal tubule). Analysis of creatinine is simple and inexpensive using colorimetric assays.

Creatinine Clearance and GFR

Calculation of *creatinine clearance* has become the standard laboratory method to determine *glomerular filtration rate (GFR)*. This value is derived by mathematically relating the serum creatinine concentration to the urine creatinine concentration excreted during a period of time, usually 24 hours. Specimen collection, therefore, must include both a 24-hour urine specimen and a serum creatinine value, ideally collected at the midpoint of the 24-hour urine collection. The urine container (clean, dry, and free of contaminants or preservatives) must be kept refrigerated throughout the duration of both the collection procedure and the subsequent storage period until laboratory analysis can be performed. The concentration of creatinine in both serum and urine is measured by the applicable methods discussed in Chapter 9, *Nonprotein Nitrogen Compounds*. The total volume of urine is carefully measured, and the *creatinine clearance* is calculated using the following formula:

$$C_{Cr} \text{ (mL/minute)} = \frac{U_{Cr} \text{ (mg/dL)} \times V_{Ur} \text{ (mL/24 hours)}}{P_{Cr} \text{ (mg/dL)} \times 1440 \text{ minutes/24 hours}} \times \frac{1.73}{A}$$

(Eq. 24–5)

where C_{Cr} = creatinine clearance
  U_{Cr} = urine creatinine concentration
  V_{Ur} = urine volume excreted in 24 hours
  P_{Cr} = serum creatinine concentration
  1.73/A = normalization factor for body surface area

1.73 is the generally accepted average body surface in square meters

A is the actual body surface area of the individual determined from height and weight.

If the patient's body surface area varies greatly from the average (eg, obese or pediatric patients), this correction for body mass must be included in the formula.

Nomograms for the more exact determination of body surface area from weight and height values can be found in Appendix G, *Nomogram for the Determination of Body Surface Area.*

- Reference ranges for creatinine clearance are:
- Male: 97 mL/minute per 1.73 m² to 137 mL/minute per 1.73 m²
- Female: 88 mL/minute per 1.73 m² to 128 mL/minute per 1.73 m²
- Creatinine clearance normally decreases with age, with a decrease of about 6.5 mL/minute per 1.73m² for each decade of life.

Estimated Glomerular Filtration Rate
The National Kidney Foundation recommends that *estimated* GFR (*EGFR*) be calculated each time a serum creatinine is reported. (Additional information is available at the National Kidney Foundation Web site: The equation is used to predict GFR and is based on serum creatinine, age, body size, gender, and race, without the need of a urine creatinine. Because the calculation does not require a timed urine collection, it should be used more often than the traditional creatinine clearance and result in earlier detection of chronic kidney disease. See *Chronic Kidney Disease* below for interpretation of GFR (usually by EGFR).[12]

$$\text{GFR (mL/minute)} = \frac{(140 - \text{Age}) \times \text{Weight (kg)}}{72 \times S_{Cr} \text{ (mg/dL)}} \times$$

$$(0.85 \text{ if female})* \qquad \textbf{(Eq. 24–6)}$$

Urea
Urea clearance was one of the first clearance tests performed. Urea is freely filtered at the glomerulus and approximately 40% reabsorbed by the tubules. For this reason, it does not provide a full clearance assessment and is no longer widely used.

Older clearance tests used administration of inulin, sodium [¹²⁵I] iothalamate, or *p*-aminohippurate to assess glomerular filtration or tubular secretion. These tests are time-consuming, expensive, and difficult to administer and, for the most part, have been discontinued.

Urine Electrophoresis

Owing to the efficiency of renal glomerular filtration and tubular reabsorption, normal urinary protein excretion is only about 50–150 mg/24 hours. Proteinuria may develop when there are defects in renal reabsorption or glomerular capillary permeability or when there is a significant increase in serum immunoglobulins. As a result, urine electrophoresis is used primarily to distinguish between acute glomerular nephropathy and tubular proteinuria. It is also used to screen for abnormal mono-

clonal or polyclonal globulins. Positive identification and subtyping of the urinary paraproteins can be performed by immunofixation electrophoresis.

β₂-Microglobulin

β₂-Microglobulin (β₂-M) is a small, nonglycosylated peptide (molecular weight, 11,800 daltons) found on the surface of most nucleated cells. The plasma membrane sheds β₂-M as a relatively intact molecule into the surrounding extracellular fluid. Because this process is fairly constant in adults; levels of β₂-M remain stable in normal patients. Elevated levels in serum indicate increased cellular turnover as seen in myeloproliferative and lymphoproliferative disorders, inflammation, and renal failure. As a small, endogenous peptide, β₂-M is easily filtered by the glomerulus. About 99.9% is then reabsorbed by the proximal tubules and catabolized. Measurement of serum β₂-M is used clinically to assess renal tubular function in renal transplant patients, with elevated levels indicating organ rejection. β₂-M has been found in some studies to be a more efficient marker of renal transplant rejection than serum creatinine values because it does not depend on lean muscle mass or daily variation in excretion.[13,14]

Myoglobin

Myoglobin is a low-molecular-weight protein (16,900 daltons) associated with acute skeletal and cardiac muscle injury. Myoglobin functions to bind and transport oxygen from the plasma membrane to the mitochondria in muscle cells. In *rhabdomyolysis*, myoglobin release from skeletal muscle is sufficient to overload the proximal tubules and cause acute renal failure. Early diagnosis and aggressive treatment of elevated myoglobin may prevent or lessen the severity of renal failure. Recently, myoglobin clearance has been proposed as an effective early indicator of myoglobin-induced acute renal failure. A high clearance or a low clearance and low serum concentration indicates low risk and a low clearance and high serum concentration indicates high risk.[15] Serum and urine myoglobin can be measured easily and rapidly by immunoassays. Urine myoglobin can also be measured by dipstick methods after removing hemoglobin, but this method has a lack of sensitivity and specificity.

Microalbumin

The term *microalbuminuria* describes small amounts of albumin in urine. Urine *microalbumin* measurement is important in the management of patients with diabetes mellitus, who are at serious risk of developing nephropathy over their lifetimes. Type 1 has a 30–45% risk, and Type 2 has a 30% risk. In the early stages of nephropathy, there is renal hypertrophy, hyperfunction, and increased

*From Cockcroft-Gault (Nephron 1976; 16:31)

thickness of the glomerular and tubular basement membranes. In this early stage, there are no overt signs of renal dysfunction. In the next 7–10 years, there is progression to glomerulosclerosis, with increased glomerular capillary permeability. This permeability allows small (micro) amounts of albumin to pass into the urine. If detected in this early phase, rigid glucose control, along with treatment to prevent hypertension, can be instituted and progression to end-stage renal disease (ESRD) prevented.[16] The American Diabetes Association's criteria for the frequency of testing of all persons with diabetes for urinary albumin, recommends testing at initial patient evaluation and yearly thereafter for all postpubertal patients who have had diabetes for at least 5 years.[17]

Quantitative albumin-specific immunoassays, usually using nephelometry or immunoturbidimetry, are widely used. Urinary albumin concentrations of 50–200 mg/24 hour are predictive of diabetic nephropathy.[18] A 24-hour urine collection is preferred, but a random urine sample that uses a ratio of albumin to creatinine can be also be used. An albumin/creatinine ratio of 20–30 mg/g is indicative of microalbuminuria.[19] Although many urine dipstick methods are not sensitive enough to detect these low levels of albumin, newer dipstick methods are now available for specific detection of albumin and the albumin/creatinine ratio.

Cystatin C

Cystatin C is a low-molecular-weight protein produced by nucleated cells. It is freely filtered by the glomerulus and reabsorbed and catabolized by the proximal tubule. Produced at a constant rate, levels remain stable if kidney function is normal. Recent studies have shown measurement of cystatin C to be at least as useful as serum creatinine and creatinine clearance in detecting early changes in kidney function. Cystatin C can be measured by immunoassay methods.[20]

Urinalysis

Urinalysis (UA) permits a detailed, in-depth assessment of renal status with an easily obtained specimen. UA also serves as a quick indicator of an individual's glucose status and hepatic-biliary function. Routine UA includes assessment of physical characteristics, chemical analyses, and a microscopic examination of the sediment from a (random) urine specimen.

Physical Characteristics

Specimen Collection. The importance of a properly collected and stored specimen for UA cannot be overemphasized. Initial morning specimens are preferred, particularly for protein analyses, because they are more concentrated from overnight retention in the bladder. The specimen should be obtained by a clean midstream catch or catheterization. The urine should be freshly collected into a clean, dry container with a tight-fitting cover. It must be analyzed within 1 hour of collection if held at room temperature or else refrigerated at 2°–8°C for not more than 8 hours before analysis. If not assayed within these time limits, several changes will occur. Bacterial multiplication will cause false-positive nitrite tests, and urease-producing organisms will degrade urea to ammonia and alkalinize the pH. Loss of CO_2 by diffusion into the air adds to this pH elevation, which, in turn, causes cast degeneration and red-cell lysis.

The urine container must be sterile if the urine is to be cultured. Specimens for routine UA are usually random, or spot, collections.

Visual Appearance. Color intensity of urine correlates with concentration: the darker the color, the more concentrated the specimen. The various colors observed in urine are a result of different excreted pigments. Yellow and amber are generally due to urochromes (derivatives of urobilin, the end product of bilirubin degradation), whereas a yellowish-brown to green color is a result of bile pigment oxidation. Red and brown after standing are due to porphyrins, whereas reddish-brown in fresh specimens comes from hemoglobin or red cells. Brownish-black after standing is seen in *alkaptonuria* (a result of excreted homogentisic acid) and in malignant melanoma (in which the precursor melanogen oxidizes in the air to melanin). Drugs and some foods, such as beets, also may alter urine color.

Odor. Odor ordinarily has little diagnostic significance. The characteristic pungent odor of fresh urine is due to volatile aromatic acids, in contrast to the typical ammonia odor of urine that has been allowed to stand. Urinary tract infections impart a noxious, fecal smell to urine, whereas the urine of diabetics often smells fruity as a result of ketones.

Turbidity. The cloudiness of a urine specimen depends on pH and dissolved solids composition. Turbidity generally may be due to gross bacteriuria, whereas a smoky appearance is seen in hematuria. Thread-like cloudiness is observed when the specimen is full of mucus. In alkaline urine, suspended precipitates of amorphous phosphates and carbonates may be responsible for turbidity, whereas in acidic urine, amorphous urates may be the cause.[13]

Volume. The volume of urine excreted indicates the balance between fluid ingestion and water lost from the lungs, sweat, and intestine. Most adults produce from 750–2000 mL/24 hours, averaging about 1.5 L per person. (For a routine UA, a 10-mL to 12-mL aliquot from a well-mixed sample is optimal for accurate analysis of sedimentary constituents.) Polyuria is observed in diabetes mellitus and insipidus (in insipidus, as a result of lack of ADH), as well as in chronic renal disease, *acromegaly* (overproduction of the growth hormone somatostatin), and *myxedema* (hypothyroid edema). Anuria or *oliguria* (<200 mL/day) is found in nephritis, ESRD, urinary tract obstruction, and acute renal failure.

Specific Gravity. The specific gravity (SG) of urine is the weight of 1 mL of urine in grams divided by the weight of 1 mL of water. SG gives an indication of the density of a fluid that depends on the concentration of dissolved total solids. SG varies with the solute load to be excreted (consisting primarily of NaCl and urea), as well as with the urine volume. It is used to assess the state of hydration/dehydration of an individual or as an indicator of the concentrating ability of the kidneys.

Laboratory Methods. The most commonly encountered analytic method consists of a refractometer, or total solids meter. This operates on the principle that the refractive index of a urine specimen will vary directly with the total amount of dissolved solids in the sample. This instrument measures the refractive index of the urine as compared with water on a scale that is calibrated directly into the ocular and viewed while held up to a light source. Correct calibration is vital for accuracy. Most recently, an indirect colorimetric reagent strip method for assaying SG has been added to most dipstick screens. Unlike the refractometer, dipsticks measure only ionic solutes and do not take into account glucose or protein.

Disease Correlation. Normal range for urinary SG is 1.005–1.030. Dilute specimens are classified in the range of 1.000–1.010, whereas concentrated samples fall between 1.025 and 1.030. SG can vary in pathologic states. Low SG can occur in diabetes insipidus, in which it may never exceed the range of 1.001–1.003, and in pyelonephritis and glomerulonephritis, in which the renal concentrating ability has become dysfunctional. High SG can be seen in diabetes mellitus, congestive heart failure, dehydration, adrenal insufficiency, liver disease, and nephrosis. SG will increase about 0.004 units for every 1% change in glucose concentration and about 0.003 units for every 1% change in protein. Fixed SG (*isosthenuria*) around 1.010 is observed in severe renal damage, in which the kidney excretes urine that is iso-osmotic with the plasma. This generally occurs after an initial period of anuria because the damaged tubules are unable to concentrate or dilute the glomerular filtrate.[9,13]

pH. Determinations of urinary pH *must* be performed on fresh specimens because of the significant tendency of urine to alkalinize on standing. Normal urine pH falls within the range of 4.5–8.0. Acidity in urine (pH, <7.0) is primarily caused by phosphates, which are excreted as salts conjugated to Na^+, K^+, Ca^{2+}, and NH_4^+. Acidity also reflects the excretion of the nonvolatile metabolic acids pyruvate, lactate, and citrate. Owing to the Na^+/H^+ exchange pump mechanism of the renal tubules, pH (H^+ ion concentration) increases as sodium is retained. Pathologic states, in which increased acidity is observed, include systemic acidosis, as seen in diabetes mellitus, and renal tubular acidosis. In renal tubular acidosis, the tubules are unable to excrete excess H^+ even though the body is in metabolic acidosis, and urinary pH remains around 6.

Alkaline urine (pH, >7.0) is observed postprandially as a normal reaction to the acidity of gastric HCl dumped into the duodenum and then into the circulation. Urinary tract infections and bacterial contamination also will alkalinize pH. Medications such as potassium citrate and sodium bicarbonate will reduce urine pH. Alkaline urine is also found in *Fanconi's syndrome*, a congenital generalized aminoaciduria resulting from defective proximal tubular function.

Chemical Analyses

Routine urine chemical analysis is rapid and easily performed with commercially available reagent strips or dipsticks. These strips are plastic coated with different reagent bands directed toward different analytes. When dipped into urine, a color change signals a deviation from normality. Colors on the dipstick bands are matched against a color chart provided with the reagents. Automated and semiautomated instruments that detect by reflectance photometry provide an alternative to the color chart and offer better precision and standardization. Abnormal results are followed-up by specific quantitative or confirmatory urine assays. The analytes routinely tested are glucose, protein, ketones, nitrite, leukocyte esterase, bilirubin/urobilinogen, and hemoglobin/blood.

Glucose and Ketones. These constituents are normally absent in urine. The clinical significance of these analytes and their testing methods are discussed in Chapter 11, *Carbohydrates.*

Protein. Reagent strips for UA are used as a general qualitative screen for proteinuria. They are primarily specific for albumin, but they may give false-positive results in specimens that are alkaline and highly buffered. Positive dipstick results should be confirmed by more specific chemical assays, as described in Chapter 8, *Amino Acids and Proteins,* or more commonly by microscopic evaluation to detect casts.

Nitrite. This assay semiquantitates the amount of urinary reduction of nitrate (on the reagent strip pad) to nitrite by the enzymes of gram-negative bacteria. This scheme is shown in the following reaction:

$$\text{Nitrite} + p\text{-arsanilic acid} \longleftrightarrow \text{diazonium compound}$$
$$+ \ N\text{-1-naphthylethylenediamine} \longleftrightarrow \text{pink color}$$

(Eq. 24–7)

A negative result does not mean that no bacteriuria is present. A gram-positive pathogen, such as *Staphylococcus, Enterococcus,* or *Streptococcus,* may not produce nitrate-reducing enzymes; alternatively, a spot urine sample may not have been retained in the bladder long enough to pick up a sufficient number of organisms to register on the reagent strip.[13]

Leukocyte Esterase. White blood cells, especially phagocytes, contain esterases. A positive dipstick for esterases indicates possible white blood cells in urine.

Bilirubin/Urobilinogen. Hemoglobin degradation ultimately results in the formation of the waste product bilirubin, which is then converted to urobilinogen in the gut through bacterial action. Although most of this urobilinogen is excreted as urobilin in the feces, some is excreted in urine as a colorless waste product. This amount is normally too small to be detected as a positive dipstick reaction. In conditions of prehepatic, hepatic, and posthepatic jaundice, however, urine dipstick tests for urobilinogen and bilirubin may be positive or negative, depending on the nature of the patient's jaundice. A more in-depth view of bilirubin metabolism and assay methods is given in Chapter 22, *Liver Function*. Reagent strip tests for bilirubin involve diazotization and formation of a color change. Dipstick methods for urobilinogen differ, but most rely on a modification of the Ehrlich reaction with *p*-dimethylaminobenzaldehyde.[13]

Hemoglobin/Blood. Intact or lysed red blood cells produce a positive dipstick result. The dipstick will be positive in cases of renal trauma/injury, infection, or obstruction that result from calculi or neoplasms.

Sediment Examination

Centrifuged, decanted urine aliquot leaves behind a sediment of formed elements that is used for microscopic examination.

Cells. For cellular elements, evaluation is best accomplished by counting and then taking the average of at least ten microscopic fields.

Red Blood Cells. Erythrocytes greater in number than 0–2/high-powered field (hpf) are considered abnormal. Such hematuria may result simply from severe exercise or menstrual blood contamination. However, it also may be indicative of trauma, particularly vascular injury, renal/urinary calculi obstruction, pyelonephritis, or cystitis. Hematuria in conjunction with leukocytes is diagnostic of infection.

White Blood Cells. Leukocytes greater in number than 0–1/hpf are considered abnormal. These cells are usually polymorphonuclear phagocytes, commonly known as *segmented neutrophils*. They are observed when there is acute glomerulonephritis, urinary tract infection, or inflammation of any type. In hypotonic urine (low osmotic concentration), white blood cells can become enlarged, exhibiting a sparkling effect in their cytoplasmic granules. These cells possess a noticeable Brownian motion and are called *glitter cells*, but they have no pathologic significance.

Epithelial Cells. Several types of epithelial cells are frequently encountered in normal urine because they are continuously sloughed off the lining of the nephrons and urinary tract. Large, flat, squamous vaginal epithelia are often seen in urine specimens from female patients; and samples heavily contaminated with vaginal discharge may show clumps or sheets of these cells. Renal epithelial cells are round, uninucleate cells; and, if present in numbers greater than 2/hpf, indicate clinically significant active tubular injury or degeneration. Transitional bladder epithelial cells (urothelial cells) may be flat, cuboidal, or columnar and also can be observed in urine on occasion. Large numbers will be seen only in cases of urinary catheterization, bladder inflammation, or neoplasm.

Miscellaneous Elements. Spermatozoa are often seen in the urine of both males and females. They are usually not reported because they are of no pathologic significance. In males, however, their presence may indicate prostate abnormalities. Yeast cells are also frequently found in urine specimens. Because they are extremely refractile and of a similar size to red blood cells, they can easily be mistaken under low magnification. Higher power examination for budding or mycelial forms differentiates these fungal elements from erythrocytes. Parasites found in urine are generally contaminants from fecal or vaginal material. In fecal contaminant category, the most commonly encountered organism is *Enterobius vermicularis* (pinworm) infestation in children. In the vaginal contaminant category, the most common is the intensely motile flagellate, *Trichomonas vaginalis*. A true urinary parasite, sometimes seen in patients from endemic areas of the world, is the ova of the trematode *Schistosoma haematobium*. This condition will usually occur in conjunction with a significant hematuria.[13]

Bacteria. Normal urine is sterile and contains no bacteria. Small numbers of organisms seen in a fresh urine specimen usually represent skin or air contamination. In fresh specimens, however, large numbers of organisms, or small numbers accompanied by white blood cells and the symptoms of urinary tract infection, are highly diagnostic for true infection. Clinically significant bacteriuria is considered more than 20 organisms/hpf or, alternatively, 10^5 or greater registered on a microbiologic colony count. Most pathogens seen in urine are gram-negative coliforms (microscopic "rods") such as *Escherichia coli* and *Proteus* species. Asymptomatic bacteriuria, in which there are significant numbers of bacteria without appreciable clinical symptoms, occurs somewhat commonly in young girls, pregnant women, and patients with diabetes. This condition must be taken seriously because, if left untreated, it may result in pyelonephritis and, subsequently, permanent renal damage.

Casts. Casts are precipitated, cylindrical impressions of the nephrons. They comprise Tamm-Horsfall mucoprotein (*uromucoid*) from the tubular epithelia in the ascending limb of the loop of Henle. Casts form whenever there is sufficient renal stasis, increased urine salt or protein concentration, and decreased urine pH. In patients with severe renal disease, truly accurate classification of casts may require use of "cytospin" centrifugation and Papanicolaou test for adequate differentiation. Unlike cells, casts should be examined under low power and are most often located around the edges of the coverslip.

Hyaline. The matrix of these casts is clear and gelatinous, without embedded cellular or particulate matter. They may be difficult to visualize unless a high-intensity lamp is used. Their presence indicates glomerular leakage of protein. This leakage may be temporary (as a result of fever, upright posture, dehydration, or emotional stress) or may be permanent. Their occasional presence is not considered pathologic.

Granular. These casts are descriptively classified as either coarse or finely granular. The type of embedded particulate matter is simply a matter of the amount of degeneration that the epithelial-cell inclusions have undergone. Their occasional presence is not pathologic; however, large numbers may be found in chronic lead toxicity and pyelonephritis.

Cellular. Several different types of casts are included in this category. *Red blood cell* or *erythrocytic casts* are always considered pathologic because they are diagnostic for glomerular inflammation that results in renal hematuria. They are seen in subacute bacterial endocarditis, kidney infarcts, collagen diseases, and acute glomerulonephritis. *White blood cell* or *leukocytic casts* are also always considered pathologic because they are diagnostic for inflammation of the nephrons. They are observed in pyelonephritis, nephrotic syndrome, and acute glomerulonephritis. In asymptomatic pyelonephritis, these casts may be the only clue to detection. Epithelial-cell casts are sometimes formed by fusion of renal tubular epithelia after desquamation; occasional presence is normal. Many, however, are observed in severe desquamative processes and renal stases that occur in heavy metal poisoning, renal toxicity, eclampsia, nephrotic syndrome, and amyloidosis. *Waxy casts* are uniformly yellowish, refractile, and brittle appearing, with sharply defined, often broken edges. They are almost always pathologic because they indicate tubular inflammation or deterioration. They are formed by renal stasis in the collecting ducts and are, therefore, found in chronic renal diseases. *Fatty casts* are abnormal, coarse, granular casts with lipid inclusions that appear as refractile globules of different sizes. *Broad (renal failure) casts* may be up to 2–6 times wider than "regular" casts and may be cellular, waxy, or granular in composition. Like waxy casts, they are derived from the collecting ducts in severe renal stasis.

Crystals

Acid Environment. Crystals seen in urines with pH values of less than 7 include calcium oxalate, which are normal colorless octahedrons or "envelopes"; they may have an almost star-like appearance. Also seen are amorphous urates, normal yellow-red masses with a grain of sand appearance. Uric acid crystals found in this environment are normal yellow to red-brown crystals that appear in extremely irregular shapes, such as rosettes, prisms, or rhomboids. Cholesterol crystals in acid urine are clear, flat, rectangular plates with notched corners. They may be seen in nephrotic syndrome and in conditions producing chyluria and are always considered abnormal. Cystine crystals are also sometimes observed in acid urine; they are highly pathologic and appear as colorless, refractile, nearly flat hexagons, somewhat similar to uric acid. These are observed in *cystinuria* (an inherited aminoaciduria resulting in mental retardation) and *homocystinuria* (a rare defect of cystine reabsorption resulting in renal calculi).

Alkaline Environment. Crystals seen in urines with pH values greater than 7 include amorphous phosphates, which are normal crystals that appear as fine, colorless masses, resembling sand. Also seen are calcium carbonate crystals, which are normal forms that appear as small, colorless dumbbells or spheres. Triple phosphate crystals are also observed in alkaline urines; they are colorless prisms of 3–6 sides, resembling "coffin lids." Ammonium biurate crystals are normal forms occasionally found in this environment, appearing as spiny, yellow-brown spheres, or "thorn apples."

Other. Sulfonamide crystals are abnormal precipitates shaped like yellow-brown sheaves, clusters, or needles, formed in patients undergoing antimicrobial therapy with sulfa drugs. These drugs are seldom used today. Tyrosine/leucine crystals are abnormal types shaped like clusters of smooth, yellow needles or spheres. These are sometimes seen in patients with severe liver disease.[13]

PATHOPHYSIOLOGY

Glomerular Diseases

Disorders or diseases that directly damage the renal glomeruli may, at least initially, exhibit normal tubular function. With time, however, disease progression involves the renal tubules, as well. The following syndromes have discrete symptoms that are recognizable by their patterns of clinical laboratory findings.[5,8]

Acute Glomerulonephritis

Pathologic lesions in acute *glomerulonephritis* primarily involve the glomerulus. Histologic examination shows large, inflamed glomeruli with a decreased capillary lumen. Abnormal laboratory findings usually include rapid onset of hematuria and proteinuria (usually albumin, and generally <3 g/day). The rapid development of a decreased GFR, anemia, elevated blood urea nitrogen (BUN) and serum creatinine, oliguria, sodium and water retention (with consequent hypertension and some localized edema), and, sometimes, congestive heart failure are typical. Numerous hyaline and granular casts are generally seen on UA. The actual red blood cell casts are regarded as highly suggestive of this syndrome.

Acute glomerulonephritis is often related to recent infection by group A β-hemolytic streptococci. It is theorized that circulating immune complexes trigger a strong inflammatory response in the glomerular basement membrane, resulting in a direct injury to the glomerulus itself. Other possible causes include drug-related exposures, acute kidney infections due to other bacterial (and, possibly, viral) agents, and other systemic immune complex diseases, such as systemic lupus erythematosus (SLE) and subacute bacterial endocarditis (SBE).

Chronic Glomerulonephritis

Lengthy glomerular inflammation may lead to glomerular scarring and the eventual loss of functioning nephrons. This process often goes undetected for lengthy periods because only minor decreases in renal function occur at first and only slight proteinuria and hematuria are observed. Gradual development of uremia (or *azotemia,* excess nitrogen compounds in the blood) may be the first sign of this process.

Nephrotic Syndrome

Nephrotic syndrome (Fig. 24-6) can be caused by a several different diseases that result in injury and increased permeability of the glomerular basement membrane. This defect almost always yields several abnormal findings, such as extremely massive proteinuria (>3.5 g/day) and resultant hypoalbuminemia. The subsequent decreased plasma oncotic pressure causes a generalized edema as a result of the movement of body fluids out of vascular and into interstitial spaces. Other hallmarks of this syndrome are hyperlipidemia and lipiduria. Lipiduria takes the form of oval fat bodies in the urine. These bodies are de-

generated renal tubular cells containing reabsorbed lipoproteins. Primary causes are associated directly with glomerular disease states.

Tubular Diseases

Tubular defects occur to a certain extent in the progression of all renal diseases as the GFR falls. In some instances, however, this aspect of the overall dysfunction becomes predominant. The result is decreased excretion/reabsorption of certain substances or reduced urinary concentrating capability. Clinically, the most important defect is renal tubular acidosis (RTA), the primary tubular disorder affecting acid-base balance. This disease can be classified into two types, depending on the nature of the tubular defect:

- *distal RTA,* in which the renal tubules are unable to keep up the vital pH gradient between the blood and tubular fluid
- *proximal RTA,* in which there is decreased bicarbonate reabsorption, resulting in hyperchloremic acidosis. In general, reduced reabsorption in the proximal tubule is manifested by findings of abnormally low serum values for phosphorus and uric acid and by glucose and amino acids in the urine. In addition, there may be some proteinuria (usually <2 g/day).

Acute inflammation of the tubules and surrounding interstitium also may occur as a result of analgesic drug or radiation toxicity, methicillin hypersensitivity reactions, renal transplant rejection, and viral-fungal-bacterial infections. Characteristic clinical findings in these cases are decreases in GFR, urinary concentrating ability, and metabolic acid excretion; leukocyte casts in the urine; and inappropriate control of sodium balance.[5,8]

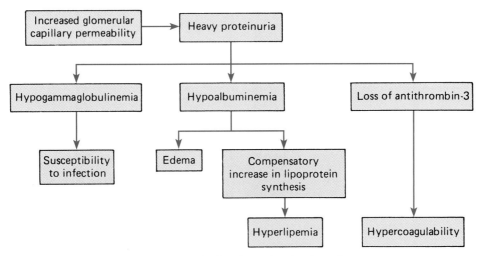

FIGURE 24-6. Pathophysiology of nephrotic syndrome.

Urinary Tract Infection/Obstruction

Infection

The site of infection may be either in the kidneys (*pyelonephritis*) or in the urinary bladder (*cystitis*). In general, a microbiologic colony count of more than 10^5 colonies/mL is considered diagnostic for infection in either locale. *Bacteriuria* (as evidenced by positive nitrite dipstick findings for some organisms), hematuria, and *pyuria* (leukocytes in the urine, as shown by positive leukocyte esterase dipstick) are all frequently encountered abnormal laboratory results in these cases. In particular, white blood cell (leukocyte) casts in the urine is considered diagnostic for pyelonephritis.[5,8,13]

Obstruction

Renal obstructions can cause disease in one of two ways. They may either gradually raise the intratubular pressure until nephrons necrose and chronic renal failure ensues, or they may predispose the urinary tract to repeated infections.

Obstructions may be located in the upper or lower urinary tract. Blockages in the upper tract are characterized by a constricting lesion below a dilated collecting duct. Obstructions of the lower tract are evidenced by the residual urine in the bladder after cessation of *micturition* (urination); symptoms include slowness of voiding, both initially and throughout urination. Causes of obstructions can include neoplasms (such as prostate/bladder carcinoma or lymph node tumors constricting ureters), acquired diseases (such as urethral strictures or renal calculi); and congenital deformities of the lower urinary tract. The clinical symptoms of advancing obstructive disease include decreased urinary concentrating capability, diminished metabolic acid excretion, decreased GFR, and reduced renal blood flow. Laboratory tests useful in determining the nature of the blockage are urinalysis, urine culture, BUN, serum creatinine, and CBC. Final diagnosis is usually made by radiologic imaging techniques.[3,6,10]

Renal Calculi

Renal calculi, or kidney stones, are formed by the combination of various crystallized substances, which are listed in Table 24-2. Of these, calcium oxalate stones are by far the most commonly encountered, particularly in the tropics and subtropics.

It is currently believed that recurrence of calculi in susceptible individuals is a result of several causes, but mainly a reduced urine flow rate (related to a decreased fluid intake) and saturation of the urine with large amounts of essentially insoluble substances. Chemical analysis of stones is important in determining the cause of the condition. Specialized x-ray diffraction and infrared spectroscopy techniques are widely used for this purpose. Clinical symptoms are, of course, similar to those encountered in other obstructive processes: hematuria, urinary tract infections, and characteristic abdominal pain.[5,8,13]

Renal Failure

Acute Renal Failure

Acute renal failure is a sudden, sharp decline in renal function as a result of an acute toxic or hypoxic insult to the kidneys, defined as occurring when the GFR is reduced to less than 10 mL/minute. This syndrome is subdivided into three types, depending on the location of the precipitating defect.

- *Prerenal failure*: the defect lies in the blood supply before it reaches the kidney. Causes can include cardiovascular system failure and consequent hypovolemia.
- *Primary renal failure*: the defect involves the kidney. The most common cause is acute tubular necrosis; other causes include vascular obstructions/inflammations and glomerulonephritis.
- *Postrenal failure*: the defect lies in the urinary tract after it exits the kidney. Generally, acute renal failure occurs as a consequence of lower urinary tract obstruction or rupture of the urinary bladder.

Toxic insults to the kidney that are severe enough to initiate acute renal failure include hemolytic transfusion reactions, myoglobinuria due to rhabdomyolysis, heavy metal/solvent poisonings, antifreeze ingestion, and analgesic and aminoglycoside toxicities. These conditions directly damage the renal tubules. Hypoxic insults include conditions that severely compromise renal blood flow, such as septic/hemorrhagic shock, burns, and cardiac failure.

TABLE 24-2. TYPES OF KIDNEY STONES

STONE COMPOSITION	CAUSE OF STONE FORMATION
Calcium oxalate	Hyperparathyroidism
	High urine calcium
	Vitamin D toxicity
	Sarcoidosis
	Osteoporosis
Magnesium ammonium phosphate	Infectious processes
Calcium phosphate	Excess alkali consumption
	Infection with urease-producing organisms
Uric acid	Gout
	High levels of uric acid in blood and urine
Cystine	Inherited cystinuria

A 52-year-old man with a history of AIDS, hypertension, diabetes mellitus, and alcohol abuse was found unconscious in his home by his roommate. In the emergency department, he was hypotensive (103/60), febrile (T = 101°), and unresponsive. CT scan of the abdomen showed cholecystitis and gallstones. Laboratory data is listed below. (Case developed by Cynthia Batangan Santos, MD, Pathology Resident, Hartford Hospital Department of Pathology and Laboratory Medicine, Hartford, CT. Modified and printed with permission.)

The patient was diagnosed with acute renal failure. He was given IV fluids; BUN fell to 68 mg/dL and creatinine to 2.2 mg/dL. The patient's blood culture report was positive for *E. coli*. He was treated with tobramycin and cefepime. The patient contin

ued to deteriorate and died 5 days after admission. Cause of death was multiorgan failure secondary to AIDS, sepsis, and alcoholic cirrhosis.

Questions

1. What is the significance of the patient's elevated CK? Explain why the doctor ordered a CKMB and troponin level. What can you conclude about the patient's cardiac status?

2. What is the cause of his acute renal failure?

3. What is the significance of the patient's large urine hemoglobin?

4. How would you interpret this patient's liver function tests considering his clinical history?

Drugs of Abuse: Serum Ethanol	Negative: 84 mg/dL	Urinalysis: Hemoglobin WBC RBC	Large: 4 hpf (0–4) 2 hpf (0–4)
CK	3308 U/L (24–204)	BUN	71 mg/dL (8–21)
CKMB	15 ng/mL (0–7.5)	Creatinine	4.1 mg/dL (0.9–1.5)
CKMB rel. index	0.5 (0–4)	ALP	443 U/L (45–122)
Troponin T	<0.01 ng/mL (0–0.4)	AST	305 U/L (9–45)
pH	7.50	ALT	78 U/L (8–63)
PCO_2	27 mm Hg	GGT	724 U/L (11–50)
Total CO_2	15 mmol/L	Total bilirubin	2.7 mg/dL (0.2–1.0)
		Direct bilirubin	2.4 mg/dL (0–0.2)

The most commonly observed symptoms of acute renal failure are oliguria and anuria (<400 mL/day). The diminished ability to excrete electrolytes and water results in a significant increase in extracellular fluid volume, leading to peripheral edema, hypertension, and congestive heart failure. Most prominent, however, is the onset of the *uremic syndrome* or ESRD, in which increased BUN and serum creatinine values are observed along with the preceding symptoms. The outcome of this disease is either recovery or, in the case of irreversible renal damage, progression to chronic renal failure.[5,8]

Chronic Renal Failure (Chronic Kidney Disease)
Chronic kidney disease (the preferred terminology) is a clinical syndrome that occurs when there is a gradual decline in renal function over time (Fig. 24-7) Early detection and treatment are needed to prevent progression to ESRD and complications such as coronary vascular disease. The National Kidney Foundation has formulated guidelines for earlier diagnosis, treatment, and prevention of further disease progression. See Table 24-3 for the five stages of chronic kidney disease. GFR and evidence of kidney damage based on measurement of proteinuria or other markers form the basis of the classifications.[21]

The conditions that can precipitate acute renal failure also may lead to chronic renal failure.[5,14] Several other causes for this syndrome are listed in Table 24-4.

Diabetes Mellitus
Diabetes mellitus can have profound effects on the renal system. Patients with type 1 diabetes suffer from an insulin deficit. Approximately 45% of patients with type 1 will develop progressive deterioration of kidney function (*diabetic nephropathy*) within 15–20 years after diagnosis. A smaller percentage of persons with type 2 diabetes will also develop this condition. The effects are primarily glomerular, but they may affect all kidney structures as well and are theorized to be caused by the abnormally hyperglycemic environment that constantly bathes the vascular system.[5,8]

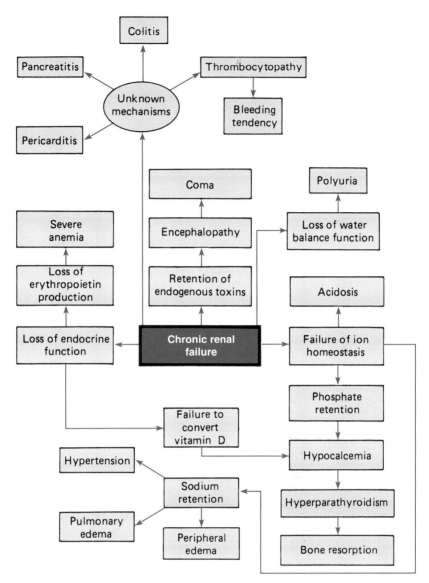

FIGURE 24-7. Pathophysiology of chronic kidney disease.

TABLE 24-3. SYSTEMATIC CLASSIFICATION OF CKD STAGES

STAGE	DESCRIPTION	GFR (mL/minute per 1.73 m²)
	At increased risk[a]	≥90 (with risk factors)
1	Kidney damage with normal or ↑ GFR	>90
2	Kidney damage with normal or ↓ GFR	60–89
3	Moderate ↓ GFR	30–59
4	Severe ↓ GFR	15–29
5	Kidney failure	<15

[a]At-risk patients should be screened. Stages 1–5 illustrate the progression of CKD. (Source: National Kidney Foundation. K/DOQI Clinical Practice Guidelines for Chronic Kidney Disease: Executive Summary. New York, 2002:16.)

TABLE 24-4. ETIOLOGY OF CHRONIC RENAL FAILURE

ETIOLOGY	EXAMPLES
Renal circulatory diseases	Renal vein thrombosis, malignant hypertension
Primary glomerular diseases	SLE, chronic glomerulonephritis
Renal sequelae to metabolic disease	Gout, diabetes mellitus, amyloidosis
Inflammatory diseases	Tuberculosis, chronic pyelonephritis
Renal obstructions	Prostatic enlargement, calculi
Congenital renal deformity	Polycystic kidneys, renal hypoplasia
Miscellaneous conditions	Radiation nephritis

A 45-year-old man presented to the hospital with alcohol withdrawal. After drinking a pint of brandy daily for the past 5–6 years, he decided to stop drinking 4 days ago. He experienced tremors and then visual and auditory hallucinations. On arrival at the hospital, he was diaphoretic and tachycardic, with a pulse rate of 102. His chemistry results are shown below.

Na^+	130 mmol/L	Total protein	7.1 g/dL
K^+	3.7 mmol/L	Albumin	3.7 g/dL
Cl^-	90 mmol/L	ALP	63 U/L
CO_2	20 mmol/L	AST	42 U/L
BUN	81 mg/dL	ALT	16 U/L
Creatinine	4.0 mg/dL	GGT	131 U/L
Magnesium	1.4 mg/dL	CK	591 U/L
Alcohol	Negative	Total bilirubin	0.5 mg/dL

Medical history included arthritis, hypertension, depression, and alcoholism. He had been taking an anti-inflammatory medication for arthritis and an antidepressant. Overnight, he became agitated and required increasing doses of a benzodiazepine, together with physical restraints for behavior control. The next morning, he was transferred to the ICU where he was evaluated for acute renal failure. The patient was rehydrated and his arthritis and antidepressant medications were withheld. Lab test results are listed below:

Na^+	139 mmol/L	Creatinine	1.4 mg/dL
K^+	3.5 mmol/L	CK	1626 U/L
Cl^-	107 mmol/L	CKMB	3.4 ng/mL
CO_2	23 mmol/L	Relative index	0.2
BUN	16 mg/dL		

Questions

1. Is the patient still in acute renal failure?

2. What was the cause of his acute renal failure?

3. Why has the patient's electrolyte status improved?

4. Why is his CK highly elevated?

Typically, diabetes affects the kidneys by causing them to become glucosuric, polyuric, and nocturic. These states are caused by the heavy demands made on the kidneys to diurese hyperosmotic urine. In addition, a mild proteinuria (*microalbuminuria*) often develops between 10 and 15 years after the original diagnosis (see *Microalbumin* above). Hypertension often manifests next, further exacerbating the renal damage. Eventually, chronic renal insufficiency or nephrotic syndrome may evolve, and each may be identified by their characteristic symptoms and laboratory findings. Early treatment of diabetes that focuses on tight control of blood glucose and prevention of high blood pressure may prolong the onset of chronic renal failure.

Renal Hypertension

Renal disease-induced hypertension can be caused by either decreased perfusion to all or part of the kidney (ischemia). Lack of perfusion may be caused by trauma damage or narrowing of an artery or intrarenal arterioles. Chronic ischemia of any kind results in nephron dysfunction and eventual necrosis. The resulting changes in blood and body fluid volumes within the kidney trigger the activation of the renin-angiotensin-aldosterone system, setting off vasoconstriction that is manifested as persistent hypertension.

Renal hypertension can be evaluated by monitoring serum aldosterone, Na^+, and renin levels. As a result of the effect of aldosterone, there will be increased serum Na^+, decreased serum K^+, and increased urine K^+.

Therapy of Acute Renal Failure

Dialysis. In patients with acute renal failure, uremic symptoms, uncontrolled hyperkalemia, and acidosis have traditionally been indications that the kidneys are unable to excrete the body's waste products and a substitute method in the form of dialysis was necessary. Dialysis is often instituted before this stage, however. Several forms of dialysis are available; however, they all use a semipermeable membrane surrounded by a dialysate bath.

In traditional *hemodialysis* (removal of waste from blood), the membrane is synthetic and outside the body. Arterial blood and dialysate are pumped at high rates (150–250 mL/minute and 500 mL/minute, respectively) in opposite directions. The blood is returned to the venous circulation and the dialysate discarded. The diffusion of low-molecular-weight solutes (<500 daltons) into the dialysate is favored by this process, but mid-molecular-weight solutes (500–2000 daltons) are inadequately cleared. Creatinine clearance is about 150–160 mL/minute.

In peritoneal dialysis, the peritoneal wall acts as the dialysate membrane and gravity is used to introduce and remove the dialysate. Two variations of this form are available, continuous ambulatory peritoneal dialysis (CAPD) and continuous cycling peritoneal dialysis; however, the process is continuous in both, being performed 24-hours a day, 7-days a week. This method is not as rigorous as the traditional method. Small solutes (eg, potassium) have significantly lower clearance rates compared with the traditional method, but more large solutes are cleared and steady-state levels of blood analytes are maintained.

Continuous arteriovenous *hemofiltration* (ultrafiltration of blood), continuous venovenous hemofiltration, continuous arteriovenous hemodialysis, and continuous venovenous hemodialysis together make up the slow continuous renal replacement therapies developed to treat acute renal failure in critically ill patients in intensive care settings. In these methods, the semipermeable membrane is again outside the body. Solutes up to 5000 daltons (the pore size of the membranes) and water are slowly (10 mL/minute) and continuously filtered from the blood in the first two methods, causing minimal changes in plasma osmolality. Volume loss can be replaced in the form of parenteral nutrition and intravenous medications. The final two methods are similar to the filtration methods, but a continuous trickle of dialysis fluid is pumped past the dialysis membrane, resulting in continuous diffusion and a doubling of the urea clearance.

Therapy of End-Stage Renal Disease (ESRD)

For patients with irreversible renal failure, dialysis and transplantation are the only two therapeutic options. Initiation of either treatment occurs when the GFR falls to 5 mL/minute (10–15 mL/minute in patients with diabetic nephropathy).

Dialysis. Traditional hemodialysis or its more recent, high-efficiency form, as well as peritoneal dialysis are the available methods. The clinical laboratory used in conjunction with a hemodialysis facility must be able to adequately monitor procedural efficiency in a wide variety of areas. Renal dialysis has basic goals, and specific laboratory tests should be performed to evaluate the achievement of each goal.

Transplantation. The most efficient hemodialysis techniques provide only 10–12% of the small solute removal of two normal kidneys and considerably less removal of larger solutes. Even patients who are well dialyzed have physical disabilities and decreased quality of life. Kidney transplantation offers the greatest chance for full return to a healthy, productive life. However, this option is limited by the significant shortage of donor organs. For ESRD patients, waiting for an organ donation can vary from several months to several years.

CASE STUDY 24-3

A 78-year-old woman with a history of hypertension, aortic thoracic graft, and esophageal reflux disease complained of fever (100()) and weakness. She had been treated 3 weeks before at the hospital for a urinary tract infection. She was admitted to the hospital for a diagnostic workup and transfusion. Her laboratory results are listed below:

Na$^+$	129 mmol/L	Hct	25.6%
K$^+$	3.7 mmol/L	Hgb	8.5 g/dL
Cl$^-$	97 mmol/L	WBC	9,700
CO$_2$	19 mmol/L		
BUN	52 mg/dL		
Creatinine	3.2 mg/dL		

Urine culture was positive for *Citrobacter*. Urinalysis results are listed below:

Color	Hazy/yellow
Specific gravity	1.015
pH	5
Blood	Large
Protein	2+
Glucose	Negative
Ketones	Negative
Nitrates	Negative
RBC	>25
WBC	1–4
Casts	Granular, 1–4

The patient's renal function continued to decline, and she was put on hemodialysis. A renal biopsy was performed that showed end-stage crescent glomerulonephritis. Two days later, the patient suffered a perforated duodenal ulcer that required surgery and blood transfusion. Subsequently, she developed coagulopathy and liver failure. Her condition continued to deteriorate in the next few days, and she died following removal of life support.

Questions

1. Looking at the urinalysis, what is the significance of the 2+ protein and >25 RBCs?

2. What is the most likely cause of glomerulonephritis?

3. Why was the patient put on hemodialysis?

Renal transplantation is from a compatible donor to a recipient suffering from irreversible renal failure. The organ can be from a cadaver or a live individual (80% and 20%, respectively, of all kidney transplants in the United States). For this procedure to be successful, the body's immune response to the transplanted organ must be suppressed. Therefore, the donor and recipient are carefully screened for ABO blood group, human leukocyte antigen (HLA) compatibility, and preformed HLA antibodies. The HLA system is the major inhibitor to transplantation.

Although kidney transplants have the capacity to function for decades, the mean half-life of a cadaveric transplant is approximately 7 years. The mortality rate is not significantly different from hemodialysis. Three-year graft survival figures vary from 65% to 85%, with live grafts doing better. It has been reported that there is no difference in patient survival among hemodialysis, CAPD, and cadaveric kidney transplantation. Live related-donor transplantation is associated with a better patient survival than other ESRD therapeutic options.

SUMMARY

The kidney plays a vital role in the maintenance of water and electrolyte balance, homeostasis, and removal of waste products. The kidney produces several important hormones (eg, renin and 1,25-dihydroxy vitamin D) needed to perform these tasks. Other renal hormones (eg, erythropoietin) are important for other physiologic functions.

Renal function tests focus largely on glomerular clearances, as assessed by creatinine and urea measurements, and tubular functions, as assessed by protein measurements (eg, urine electrophoresis). The analysis of urine for analytes, such as pH, glucose, ketones, and bilirubin, continue to be important screening tests for many nonrenal diseases, such as diabetes mellitus, ketoacidosis (and other acid-base imbalances), hemolysis, and liver disease. Newer protein assays, such as urine microalbumin, serum β_2-M, cystatin C, and serum and urine myoglobin, can provide important prognostic information useful for patient management. Microalbuminuria is useful for early detection of diabetic nephropathy, β_2-M is useful for early renal transplant rejection, and myoglobin clearance rates are helpful in predicting rhabdomyolysis-induced acute renal failure.

Common renal diseases include infectious and inflammatory processes to the glomerulus, tubules, and urinary tract, obstructions to normal kidney function, and acute and chronic renal failure. In situations of chronic renal failure, aggressive therapeutic approaches based on dialysis and transplantation have enabled prolonged survival of what was once a terminal condition. Variations in dialysis techniques have made this process more available and convenient and, with the implementation of powerful immunosuppressive drugs, widespread renal transplantation is now limited only by the availability of appropriate donor organs.

REVIEW QUESTIONS

1. Calculate creatinine clearance, given the following information: serum creatinine, 1.2 mg/dL; urine creatinine, 120 mg/dL; urine volume, 1750 mL/24 hr; body surface area, 1.80 m².

2. Predict GFR in a 50-year-old woman who weighs 60 kg. Her serum creatinine level is 2.5 mg/dL.

3. The measurement of serum cystatin C, a small protein produced by nucleated cells, is useful for:
   a. calculating creatinine clearance.
   b. diagnosing end-stage renal disease.
   c. monitoring dialysis patients.
   d. detecting an early decrease in kidney function.

4. Acute renal failure can be classified into three types. List each type and give an example of each.
   a. _____
   b. _____
   c. _____

5. The proximal tubule functions to:
   a. concentrate salts.
   b. reabsorb 75% of salt and water.

   c. form the renal threshold.
   d. reabsorb urea.

6. The normal glomerular filtration rate is approximately:
   a. 2 mL/minute.
   b. 125 mL/minute.
   c. 800 mL/minute.
   d. 1200 mL/minute.

7. Renal clearance is the:
   a. volume of urine produced per day.
   b. amount of creatinine in urine.
   c. volume of plasma from which a substance is removed per unit of time.
   d. urine concentration of a substance divided by the urine volume per unit of time.

8. Renin release by the kidney is stimulated by:
   a. increased plasma sodium concentration.
   b. a decrease in extracellular fluid volume or pressure.
   c. increased dietary sodium.
   d. renal tubular reabsorption.

9. The set of results that most accurately reflects severe renal disease is:

	serum creatinine	creatinine clearance	BUN
a.	1.0 mg/dL	110 mL/minute	17 mg/dL
b.	2.0 mg/dL	120 mL/minute	14 mg/dL
c.	1.0 mg/dL	95 mL/minute	43 mg/dL
d.	3.7 mg/dL	44 mL/minute	88 mg/dL

10. Creatinine clearance results are corrected using a patient's body surface area to account for differences in:
    a. age.
    b. dietary intake.
    c. sex.
    d. muscle mass.

REFERENCES

1. Vander A, et al. Human Physiology: The Mechanisms of Body Function, 7th ed. New York: McGraw-Hill, 1998:503, 508, 519.

2. Kaplan A, et al. Clinical Chemistry: Interpretation and Techniques, 4th ed. Baltimore: Williams & Wilkins, 1995:156–157.

3. DuFour DR. Professional Practice in Clinical Chemistry: A Companion Text, Water and Electrolyte Balance. Washington, D.C.: AACC, 1999.

4. Davies A, Blakely A, Kidd C. Human Physiology. London: Harcourt Publishers, 2001:747.

5. Rock RC, Walker WG, Jennings CD. Nitrogen metabolites and renal function. In: Tietz NW, ed. Fundamentals of Clinical Chemistry, 3rd ed. Philadelphia: WB Saunders, 1987:669.

6. Russell PT, Sherwin JE, Obernolte R, et al. Nonprotein nitrogenous compounds. In: Kaplan LA, Pesce AJ, eds. Clinical Chemistry: Theory, Analysis, and Correlation, 2nd ed. St. Louis: CV Mosby, 1989:1005.

7. Fraser D, Jones G, Kooh SW, et al. Calcium and phosphate metabolism. In: Tietz NW, ed. Fundamentals of Clinical Chemistry, 3rd ed. Philadelphia: WB Saunders, 1987:705.

8. First MR. Renal function. In: Kaplan LA, Pesce AJ, eds. Clinical Chemistry: Theory, Analysis, and Correlation, 3rd ed. St. Louis: CV Mosby, 1996:484.

9. Kaplan LA. Measurement of colligative properties. In: Kaplan LA, Pesce AJ, eds. Clinical Chemistry: Theory, Analysis, and Correlation, 2nd ed. St. Louis: CV Mosby, 1989:207.

10. Kleinman LI, Lorenz JM. Physiology and pathophysiology of body water and electrolytes. In: Kaplan LA, Pesce AJ, eds. Clinical Chemistry: Theory, Analysis, and Correlation, 2nd ed. St. Louis: CV Mosby, 1989:313.

11. Sherwin JE, Bruegger BB. Acid-base control and acid-base disorders. In: Kaplan LA, Pesce AJ, eds. Clinical Chemistry: Theory, Analysis, and Correlation, 2nd ed. St. Louis: CV Mosby, 1989:332.

12. Lab Tests Online: GFR and EGFR at a glance. Available at: http://www.labtestsonline.org.

13. Schumann GB, Schweitzer SC. Examination of urine. In: Kaplan LA, Pesce AJ, eds. Clinical Chemistry: Theory, Analysis, and Correlation, 2nd ed. St. Louis: CV Mosby, 1989:820.

14. Frauenhoffer E, Demers LM. Beta$_2$-microglobulin. ASCP Check Sample Continuing Education Program, Clinical Chemistry, No. CC 865 (CC173). Chicago, IL, 1986.

15. Wu AHB, Laios I, Green S, et al. Immunoassays for serum and urine myoglobin: myoglobin clearance assessed as a risk factor for acute renal failure. Clin Chem 1994;40:796.

16. Skogen W. Urinary albumin and diabetic nephropathy. Clin Lab News 1995;21(3):6–7.

17. American Diabetes Association. Position statement: standards of medical care for patients with diabetes mellitus. Diabetes Care 1994;17:616–623.

18. Bennett PH, et al. Screening and management of microalbuminuria in patients with diabetes mellitus: recommendations to the Scientific Advisory Board of the National Kidney Foundation from an Ad Hoc Committee of the Council on Diabetes Mellitus of the National Kidney Foundation. Am J Kidney Disease 1995;25:107.

19. Emancipator K. Laboratory diagnosis and monitoring of diabetes mellitus. Am J Clin Pathol 1999;112:665.

20. Lab Tests Online: Cystatin C at a glance. Available at: http://www.labtestsonline.org/understanding/analytes/cystatin_c/glance.

21. Mitchum C. Implementing the new kidney disease testing guidelines. Clin Lab News 2002; September:14.

CHAPTER 25

Pancreatic Function

Edward P. Fody

CHAPTER OUTLINE

- **PHYSIOLOGY OF PANCREATIC FUNCTION**
- **DISEASES OF THE PANCREAS**
- **TESTS OF PANCREATIC FUNCTION**
  Secretin/CCK Test
  Fecal Fat Analysis
  Sweat Electrolyte Determinations
  Serum Enzymes
  Other Tests of Pancreatic Function

- **SUMMARY**
- **REVIEW QUESTIONS**
- **REFERENCES**
- **SUGGESTED READINGS**

OBJECTIVES

Upon completion of this chapter, the clinical laboratorian should be able to:
- Discuss the physiologic role of the pancreas in the digestive process.
- List the hormones excreted by the pancreas, together with their physiologic roles.

- Describe the following pancreatic disorders and list the associated laboratory tests that would aid in diagnosis: acute pancreatitis, chronic pancreatitis, pancreatic carcinoma, cystic fibrosis, and pancreatic malabsorption.

KEY TERMS

Cholecystokinin (CCK)   Pancreatitis   Secretin   Steatorrhea
Islets of Langerhans

The pancreas is a large gland that is involved in the digestive process, but located outside of the gastrointestinal (GI) system. It is composed of both endocrine and exocrine tissue. The endocrine functions of the pancreas include production of insulin and glucagon; both hormones are involved in carbohydrate metabolism. Exocrine function involves the production of many enzymes used in the digestive process. This chapter discusses the physiology of pancreatic function, diseases of the pancreas, and tests of pancreatic function.

PHYSIOLOGY OF PANCREATIC FUNCTION

As a digestive gland, the pancreas is only second in size to the liver, weighing about 70–105 g. It is located behind the peritoneal cavity across the upper abdomen at about the level of the first and second lumbar vertebrae, about 1–2 inches above the umbilicus. It is located in the curve made by the duodenum (Fig. 25-1). The pancreas is composed of two morphologically and functionally different tissues: endocrine tissue and exocrine tissue.

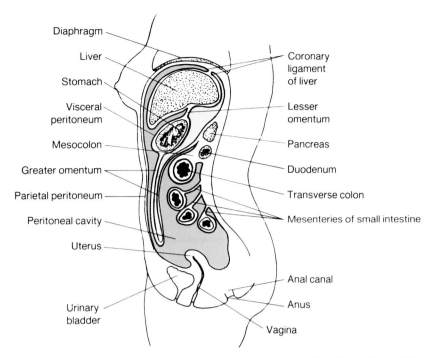

FIGURE 25-1. Peritoneum and mesenteries. The parietal peritoneum lines the abdominal cavity, and the visceral peritoneum covers abdominal organs. Retroperitoneal organs are covered by the parietal peritoneum. The mesenteries are membranes that connect abdominal organs to each other and to the body wall. (Reprinted with permission from Thompson JS, Akesson EJ, eds. Thompson's Core Textbook of Anatomy, 2nd ed. Philadelphia: JB Lippincott, 1990:115.)

The *endocrine* (hormone-releasing) component is by far the smaller of the two and consists of the *islets of Langerhans*, which are well-delineated, spherical or ovoid clusters composed of at least four different cell types. The islet cells secrete at least four hormones into the blood: insulin, glucagon, gastrin, and somatostatin. The larger, *exocrine* pancreatic component (enzyme-secreting) secretes about 1.5–2 L/day of fluid, which is rich in digestive enzymes, into ducts that ultimately empty into the duodenum.

This digestive fluid is produced by pancreatic acinar cells (grape-like clusters), which line the pancreas and are connected by small ducts. These small ducts empty into progressively larger ducts, eventually forming one major pancreatic duct and a smaller accessory duct. The major pancreatic duct and the common bile duct open into the duodenum at the major duodenal papilla (Fig. 25-2). Normal, protein-rich, pancreatic fluid is clear, colorless, and watery, with an alkaline pH that can reach up to 8.3. This alkalinity is caused by the high concentration of sodium bicarbonate present in pancreatic fluid, which is used eventually to neutralize the hydrochloric acid in gastric fluid from the stomach as it enters the duodenum. The bicarbonate and chloride concentrations vary reciprocally so that they total about 150 mmol/L.

Pancreatic fluid has about the same concentrations of potassium and sodium as serum. The digestive enzymes, or their proenzymes secreted by the pancreas, are capable

of digesting the three major classes of food substances (proteins, carbohydrates, and fats) and include: (1) the proteolytic enzymes trypsin, chymotrypsin, elastase, collagenase, leucine aminopeptidase, and some carboxypeptidases; (2) lipid-digesting enzymes, primarily lipase and lecithinase; (3) carbohydrate-splitting pancreatic amylase; and (4) several nucleases (ribonuclease), which separate the nitrogen-containing bases from their sugarphosphate strands.

Pancreatic activity is under both nervous and endocrine control. Branches of the vagus nerve can cause a

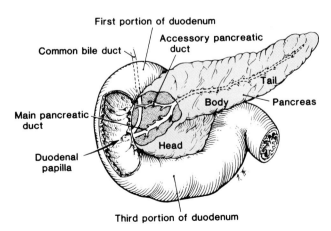

FIGURE 25-2. Diagram of the pancreas and its relationship to the duodenum.

small amount of pancreatic fluid secretion when food is smelled or seen, and these secretions may increase as the bolus of food reaches the stomach. Most of the pancreatic action, however, is under the hormonal control of *secretin* and *cholecystokinin* (CCK; formerly called *pancreozymin*). Secretin is responsible for the production of bicarbonate-rich and, therefore, alkaline pancreatic fluid, which protects the lining of the intestine from damage. Secretin is synthesized in response to the acidic contents of the stomach reaching the duodenum. It can also affect gastrin activity in the stomach. This pancreatic fluid contains few digestive enzymes. CCK, in the presence of fats or amino acids in the duodenum, is produced by the cells of the intestinal mucosa and is responsible for release of enzymes from the acinar cells by the pancreas into the pancreatic fluid.

DISEASES OF THE PANCREAS

Other than trauma, only three diseases cause more than 95% of the medical attention devoted to the pancreas. If they affect the endocrine function of the pancreas, these diseases can result in altered digestion and nutrient metabolism. The role of the pancreas in diabetes mellitus is discussed in Chapter 11, *Carbohydrates*.

1. *Cystic fibrosis* (known by various other terms, such as *fibrocystic disease of the pancreas* and *mucoviscidosis*) is an inherited autosomal recessive disorder, characterized by dysfunction of mucous and exocrine glands throughout the body. The disease is relatively common and occurs in about 1 of 1600 live births. It has various manifestations and can initially present in such widely varying ways as intestinal obstruction of the newborn, excessive pulmonary infections in childhood, or, uncommonly, as pancreatogenous malabsorption in adults. The disease causes the small and large ducts and the acini to dilate and convert into small cysts filled with mucus, eventually resulting in the prevention of pancreatic secretions reaching the duodenum or, depending on the age of the patient, a plug that blocks the lumen of the bowel, leading to obstruction. As the disease progresses, there is increased destruction and fibrous scarring of the pancreas and a corresponding decrease in function. Cystic fibrosis is transmitted as an autosomal recessive disorder with a high degree of penetrance. It occurs primarily in persons of Northern European descent. The cystic fibrosis gene known as CFTR occurs on chromosome 7, and more than 900 mutations causing this disorder have been identified; however, some occur more commonly than others. In areas of high frequency, such as Brittany in Western France, more than 10% of the population may carry a cystic fibrosis mutation, and 1 in 3,000 infants may be affected, making it the most common genetic disorder in these populations. Genetic screening is now widely carried out.[1–3]

2. *Pancreatic carcinoma* is the fifth most frequent form of fatal cancer and causes about 27,000 deaths each year in the United States, which represents about 5% of all deaths from malignant neoplasms. The 5-year survival rate is less than 2%; more than 90% of patients die within 1 year of diagnosis. Most pancreatic tumors arise as adenocarcinomas of the ductal epithelium. Because the pancreas has a rich supply of nerves, pain is a prominent feature of the disease. If the tumor arises in the body or tail of the pancreas, detection does not often occur until an advanced stage of the disease because of its central location and the associated vague symptoms. Cancer of the head of the pancreas is usually detected earlier because of its proximity to the common bile duct. Signs of these tumors are jaundice, weight loss, anorexia, and nausea. Jaundice is associated with signs of posthepatic hyperbilirubinemia (intrahepatic cholestasis) and low levels of fecal bilirubin, resulting in clay-colored stools. However, findings are not specific for pancreatic tumors, and other causes of obstruction must be ruled out.

Islet cell tumors of the pancreas affect the endocrine capability of the pancreas. If the tumor occurs in beta cells, hyperinsulinism is often seen, resulting in low blood glucose levels, sometimes followed by hypoglycemic shock. Pancreatic α-cell tumors, which overproduce gastrin, are called *gastrinomas;* they cause *Zollinger-Ellison syndrome* and can be duodenal in origin. These tumors are associated with watery diarrhea, recurring peptic ulcer, and significant gastric hypersecretion and hyperacidity. Pancreatic α-cell glucagon-secreting tumors are rare; the hypersecretion of glucagon is associated with diabetes mellitus.

3. *Pancreatitis*, or inflammation of the pancreas, is ultimately caused by autodigestion of the pancreas as a result of reflux of bile or duodenal contents into the pancreatic duct. Pathologic changes can include acute edema, with large amounts of fluid accumulating in the retroperitoneal space and an associated decrease in effective circulating blood volume; cellular infiltration, leading to necrosis of the acinar cells, with hemorrhage as a possible result of necrotic blood vessels; and intrahepatic and extrahepatic pancreatic fat necrosis. Pancreatitis is generally classified as acute (no permanent damage to the pancreas), chronic (irreversible injury), or relapsing/recurrent, which can also be acute or chronic. It commonly occurs in midlife. Painful episodes can occur intermittently, usually reaching a maximum within minutes or hours, lasting for several days or weeks, and frequently accompanied by nausea and vomiting. Pancreatitis is often associated with alcohol abuse or biliary tract disease, but patients with hyperlipoproteinemia and those with hyperparathyroidism are also at a significantly increased risk for this disease.

Other etiologic factors associated with acute pancreatitis include mumps, obstruction caused by biliary tract

CASE STUDY 25-1

A 38-year-old man entered the emergency department with the complaint of severe, boring, midabdominal pain of 6 hours' duration. A friend, who had driven him to the hospital, stated that the patient fainted 3 times as he was being helped into the automobile. The patient had a 15-year history of alcoholism and drank 1–2 pints of whiskey every day. He had last been hospitalized for acute alcoholism 3 months ago, at which time he had relatively minor abnormalities of liver function. On this admission, his blood pressure was 80/40 mm Hg; pulse, 110 beats/minute and thready; and respirations, 24 breaths/minute and shallow. Clinical laboratory test results are shown in Case Study Table 25-1.1.

Questions

1. What is the probable disease?

2. What is the cause for the low serum calcium?

3. What is the cause for the increased blood urea nitrogen?

CASE STUDY TABLE 25-1.1. LABORATORY RESULTS

Serum amylase	640 units (3.5–260)
Serum sodium	133 mEq/L (135–145)
Potassium	3.4 mEq/L (3.8–5.5)
Calcium	4.0 mEq/L (4.5–5.5)
Blood urea nitrogen	32 mg/dL (8–25)
White blood cell count	16,500
Hemoglobin	12 g/dL

disease, gallstones, pancreatic tumors, tissue injury, atherosclerotic disease, shock, pregnancy, hypercalcemia, hereditary pancreatitis, immunologic factors associated with postrenal transplantation, and hypersensitivity. Symptoms of acute pancreatitis include severe abdominal pain that is generalized or in the upper quadrants and often radiates toward the back or down the right or left flank. The etiology of chronic pancreatitis is similar to that of acute pancreatitis, but chronic excessive alcohol consumption appears to be the most common predisposing factor.

Laboratory findings include increased amylase, lipase, triglycerides, and hypercalcemia, which is often associated with underlying hyperparathyroidism. Hypocalcemia may be found and has been attributed to the sudden removal of large amounts of calcium from the extracellular fluid because of impaired mobilization or as a result of calcium fixation by fatty acids liberated by increased lipase action on triglycerides. Hypoproteinemia is attributable mainly to the notable loss of plasma into the retroperitoneal space. A shift of arterial blood flow from the inflamed pancreatic cells to less affected or normal cells causes oxygen deprivation and tissue hypoxia in the area of damage, including the surrounding organs and tissue.

All three conditions can result in severely diminished pancreatic exocrine function, which can significantly compromise digestion and absorption of ingested nutrients. This is the essence of the general malabsorption syndrome, which embodies abdominal bloating and discomfort; the frequent passage of bulky, malodorous feces; and weight loss. Failure to digest or absorb fats, known as *steatorrhea*, renders a greasy appearance to feces (more than 5 g of fecal fat per 24 hours). The malabsorption syndrome typically involves abnormal digestion or absorption of proteins, polysaccharides, carbohydrates, and other complex molecules, as well as lipids. Severely deranged absorption and metabolism of electrolytes, water, vitamins (particularly fat-soluble vitamins A, D, E, and K), and minerals can also occur. Malabsorption can involve a single substance, such as vitamin B_{12}, which results in a megaloblastic anemia (pernicious anemia), or lactose caused by a lactase deficiency. In addition to pancreatic exocrine deficiency, the malabsorption syndrome can be caused by biliary obstruction, which deprives the small intestine of the emulsifying effect of bile, and various diseases of the small intestine, which inhibit absorption of digested products.

TESTS OF PANCREATIC FUNCTION[1,2]

Depending on etiology and clinical picture, pancreatic function may be suspect when there is evidence of increased amylase and lipase. The reader is referred to Chapter 10, *Enzymes*, for an in-depth discussion of these enzymes. Other laboratory tests of pancreatic function

A 56-year-old man who is an alcoholic presents with a 2-week history of midabdominal pain. He also describes clay-colored stools, mild icterus, nausea, vomiting, and a 10-pound weight loss. Laboratory findings are shown in Case Study Table 25-2.1.

Questions

1. What organ system is primarily involved?

2. What are the major diagnostic considerations?

3. What do the laboratory results mean? What additional laboratory tests would be useful in establishing a diagnosis?

4. What other studies or procedures might be required?

CASE STUDY TABLE 25-2.1. LABORATORY RESULTS

TEST	RESULT	REFERENCE RANGE
Serum bilirubin	4.2 mg/dL	0.3–1.0 mg/dL
Serum lactate dehydrogenase	625 IU/L	0–200 IU/L
Serum alanine aminotransferase	76 IU/L	0–46 IU/L
Serum alkaline phosphatase	462 IU/L	0–80 IU/L
Serum amylase	80 IU/L	0–85 IU/L
Urine bilirubin	3+	Negative

include those used for detection of malabsorption (eg, examination of stool for excess fat, D-xylose test, and fecal fat analysis), tests measuring other exocrine function (eg, secretin, CCK, fecal fat, trypsin, and chymotrypsin), tests assessing changes associated with extrahepatic obstruction (eg, bilirubin), and endocrine-related tests (eg, gastrin, insulin, and glucose) that reflect changes in the endocrine cells of the pancreas.

Direct evaluation of pancreatic fluid may include measurement of the total volume of pancreatic fluid and the amount or concentration of bicarbonate and enzymes, which requires pancreatic stimulation. Stimulation may be accomplished using a predescribed meal or administration of secretin, which allows for volume and bicarbonate evaluation, or secretin stimulation followed by CCK stimulation, which adds enzymes to the pancreatic fluid evaluation. The advantage of these tests, both of which require intubation of the patient, is that the chemical and cytologic examinations are performed on actual pancreatic secretions. Cytologic examination of the fluid can often establish the presence, or at least the suspicion, of malignant neoplasms, although the precise localization of the primary organ of involvement (ie, pancreas, biliary system, ampulla of Vater, or duodenum) is not possible by duodenal aspiration.

Because of advances in imaging techniques, these stimulation tests are used less often; none have proved especially useful in diagnosis of mild or acute pancreatic disease in which the acute phase has subsided. Most of the tests have found clinical utility in excluding the pancreas from diagnosis. The sweat test, used for screening cystic fibrosis, is not specific for assessing pancreatic involvement but, when used along with the clinical picture at the time of testing, can provide important diagnostic information. The following pancreatic function tests are reviewed briefly: secretin/CCK test, fecal fat analysis, sweat chloride determinations, and amylase and lipase interpretation.

Secretin/CCK Test

The secretin/CCK test is a direct determination of the exocrine secretory capacity of the pancreas. The test involves intubation of the duodenum without contamination by gastric fluid, which would neutralize any bicarbonate. The test is performed after a 6-hour or overnight fast. Pancreatic secretion is stimulated by intravenously administered secretin in a dose varying from 2–3 U/kg of body weight, followed by CCK administration. If a simple secretin test is desired, the higher dose of secretin is given alone.

No one protocol has been uniformly established for the test. Pancreatic secretions are collected variously for 30, 60, or 80 minutes after administration of the stimulants, either as 10-minute specimens or as a single, pooled collection. The pH, secretory rate, enzyme activities (eg, trypsin, amylase, or lipase), and amount of bicarbonate are determined. The average amount of bicarbonate excreted per hour is about 15 mM for men and 12 mM for women, with an average flow of 2 mL/kg. Assessment of enzymes must be taken in view of total volume output. Decreased pancreatic flow is associated with pancreatic obstruction and increase in enzyme concentrations. Low concentrations of bicarbonate and enzymes are associated with cystic fibrosis, chronic pancreatitis, pancreatic cysts, calcification, and edema of the pancreas.[1]

Fecal Fat Analysis

Fecal lipids are derived from four sources: unabsorbed ingested lipids, lipids excreted into the intestine (predominantly in the bile), cells shed into the intestine, and metabolism of intestinal bacteria. Patients on a lipid-free diet still excrete 1–4 g of lipid in the feces in a 24-hour period. Even with a lipid-rich diet, the fecal fat does not normally exceed about 7 g in a 24-hour period. Normal fecal lipid is composed of about 60% fatty acids; 30% sterols, higher alcohols, and carotenoids; 10% triglycerides; and small amounts of cholesterol and phospholipids. Although significantly increased fecal fat can be caused by biliary obstruction, severe steatorrhea is usually associated with exocrine pancreatic insufficiency or disease of the small intestine.

Qualitative Screening Test for Fecal Fat

Various screening tests have been devised for detecting steatorrhea. These tests commonly use fat-soluble stains (*eg*, Sudan III, Sudan IV, Oil Red 0, or Nile blue sulfate), which dissolve in and color lipid droplets. Of greater importance than the particular technical procedure is the level of experience and dependability of the clinical laboratorian performing the test.

Sudan Staining for Fecal Fat[3,4]

Neutral fats (triglycerides) and many other lipids stain yellow-orange to red with Sudan III because the dye is much more soluble in lipid than in water or ethanol. Free fatty acids do not stain appreciably unless the specimen is heated in the presence of the stain with 36% acetic acid. The slide may be examined warm or cool and the number of fat droplets assessed. As the slide cools, the fatty acids crystallize out in long, colorless, needle-like sheaves. Detection of meat fiber is accomplished by a third aliquot of fecal sample mixed on the slide with 10% alcohol and a solution of eosin stained for 3 minutes. The meat fiber should stain as rectangular cross-striated fibers. Splitting the sample and detecting neutral fats, fatty acids, and undigested meat fibers can provide diagnostic information. Increases in fats and undigested meat fibers are indicative of patients with steatorrhea of pancreatic origin. A representative fecal specimen is used for analysis.

Normal feces can have up to 40 or 50 small (1–5 mm), neutral lipid droplets per high-powered microscope field. Steatorrhea is characterized by an increase in the number and size of stainable droplets, often with some fat globules in the 50- to 100-mm range. Fatty acid assessment greater than 100 stained small droplets, along with the presence of meat fiber, is expected in patients with steatorrhea.

Quantitative Fecal Fat Analysis[3,4]

The definitive test for steatorrhea is the quantitative fecal fat determination, usually on a 72-hour stool collection, although the collection period may be increased to up to 5 days. There are two basic methods for the quantitation of fecal lipids. In the gravimetric method, fatty acid soaps (predominantly calcium and magnesium salts of fatty acids) are converted to free fatty acids, followed by extraction of most of the lipids into an organic solvent, which is then evaporated so that the lipid residue can be weighed. In titrimetric methods, lipids are saponified with hydroxide, and the fatty acid salts are converted to free fatty acids using acid. The free fatty acids, along with various unsaponified lipids, are then extracted with an organic solvent, and the fatty acids are titrated with hydroxide after evaporation of the solvent and redissolving of the residue in ethanol. The titration methods obviously measure only saponifiable fatty acids and, consequently, render results about 20% lower than those from gravimetric methods. A further objection is that titrimetric methods use an assumed average molecular weight for fatty acids to convert moles of fatty acids to grams of lipid.

At one time, it was common to measure the amount of free fatty acids as a percentage of total lipids on the presumption that a high percentage of free fatty acids indicates adequate pancreatic lipase activity. This method is no longer considered reliable because of spurious results, particularly caused by lipase produced by intestinal bacteria.

It is essential that patients be placed on a lipid-rich diet for at least 2 days before instituting the fecal collection. The diet must contain at least 50 g, and preferably 100 g, of lipid each day. Fecal collections should extend for three or more successive days.

There are various ways to express fecal lipid excretion. Expressing lipid excretion as a percentage of wet or dry fecal weight is open to serious challenge because of wide variations in both fecal water content and dry residue as a result of dietary intake. The most widely accepted approach is to report the grams of fecal fat excreted in a 24-hour period.

Gravimetric Method of Sobel[5] for Fecal Fat Determination (Modified)[6]

The entire fecal specimen is emulsified with water. An aliquot is acidified to convert all fatty acid soaps to free fatty acids, which are then extracted with other soluble lipids into petroleum ether and ethanol. After evaporation of the organic solvents, the lipid residue is weighed. All feces for a 3-day period are collected in tared containers. The containers *must not* have a wax coating. The specimen must be kept refrigerated.

Total lipid does not change significantly during 5 days' storage of the specimen at refrigerator temperatures. Patients must not ingest castor oil, mineral oil, or other oily laxatives and must not use rectal suppositories containing oil or lipid for 2 days before the test and during the test.

The reference range for fecal lipids in adults is 1–7 g/24 hours.

Sweat Electrolyte Determinations[6–9]

Measurement of the sodium and chloride concentration in sweat is the most useful test for the diagnosis of cystic fibrosis. Significantly elevated concentrations of both ions occur in more than 99% of affected patients. The twofold to fivefold increases of sweat sodium and chloride are diagnostic of cystic fibrosis in children. Even in adults, no other condition causes increases in sweat chloride and sodium above 80 mEq/L. Sweat potassium is also increased, but less significantly so, and is not generally relied on for diagnosis. Contrary to some assertions, sweat electrolyte determinations do not distinguish heterozygote carriers of cystic fibrosis from normal homozygotes.

Older methods for acquiring sweat specimens required skilled technologists who frequently performed the test. Induction of sweat included applying plastic bags or wrapping the patient in blankets, which was fraught with serious risks of dehydration, electrolyte disturbances, and hyperpyrexia. In 1959, pilocarpine administration by iontophoresis was reported as an efficient method for sweat collection and stimulation.[10,11] Iontophoresis employs an electric current that causes pilocarpine to migrate into a limited skin area, usually the inside of the forearm, toward the negative electrode from a moistened pad on the positive electrode. A collection vessel is then applied to the skin. The sweat is then analyzed for chloride. For confirmation, the test should be repeated. Commercially available surface electrodes that analyze the sweat chloride are readily available. For details, the reader is referred to Chapter 27, *Body Fluid Analysis*.

It is widely accepted that sweat chloride concentrations greater than 60 mmol/L are diagnostic of cystic fibrosis in children.[12] Sweat sodium and chloride concentrations in female patients undergo fluctuation with the menstrual cycle and reach a peak 5–10 days before the onset of menstruation but do not overlap with the ranges associated with cystic fibrosis.

Serum Enzymes[11]

Amylase is the serum enzyme most commonly relied on for detecting pancreatic disease. It is not, however, a function test. Amylase is particularly useful in the diagnosis of acute pancreatitis, in which significant increases in serum concentrations occur in about 75% of patients. Typically, amylase in serum increases within a few hours of the onset of the disease, reaches a peak in about 24 hours, and because of its clearance by the kidneys, returns to normal within 3–5 days, often making urine amylase a more sensitive indicator of acute pancreatitis. The magnitude of the enzyme elevation cannot be correlated with the severity of the disease.

Determination of the renal clearance of amylase is useful in detecting minor or intermittent increases in the serum concentration of this enzyme. To correct for diminished glomerular function, the most useful expression is the ratio of amylase clearance to creatinine clearance, as follows:

$$\frac{\text{\% Amylase clearance}}{\text{Creatinine}} = 100 \times \frac{\text{UA}}{\text{SA}} \times \frac{\text{SC}}{\text{UC}} \quad \text{(Eq. 25–1)}$$

where UA = urine amylase
SA = serum amylase
SC = serum creatinine
UC = urine creatinine

Normal values are less than 3.1%. Significantly increased values, averaging about 8% or 9%, occur in acute pancreatitis but also may occur in other conditions, such as burns, sepsis, and diabetic ketoacidosis.

The use of serum lipase in the clinical detection of pancreatic disease has been compromised in the past by technical problems inherent in the various analytic methods. Improved analytic methods appear to indicate that

CASE STUDY 25-3

Parents brought their 7-year-old son to the pediatrician with the complaint of frequent fevers and failure to grow. The child had three bouts of pneumonia during the past 2 years and was bothered by chronic bronchitis, which caused him to cough up copious amounts of thick, yellow, mucoid sputum. Despite a big appetite, he had gained only 1–2 pounds in the past 2 years and was of short, frail stature. He especially liked salty foods. He usually had 3 or 4 bulky, foul-smelling bowel movements daily. A 9-year-old sister was in excellent health.

Questions

1. What is the most likely disease?

2. What clinical laboratory test would be most informative, and what results would be expected?

3. What other clinical laboratory tests would likely be abnormal?

lipase increases in serum about as soon as amylase in acute pancreatitis and that increased levels persist somewhat longer than those of amylase. Consequently, some physicians consider lipase more sensitive than amylase as an indicator of acute pancreatitis or other causes of pancreatic necrosis.

Both amylase and lipase may be significantly increased in serum in many other conditions (*eg,* opiate administration, pancreatic carcinoma, intestinal infarction, obstruction or perforation, and pancreatic trauma). Amylase levels are also frequently increased in mumps, cholecystitis, hepatitis, cirrhosis, ruptured ectopic pregnancy, and macroamylasemia. Electrophoresis of total amylase, if available, would reveal an increased p-type isoenzyme that, along with the lipase, remains elevated longer than the total amylase in acute pancreatitis. Lipase levels are often significantly increased in bone fractures and in association with fat embolism.

Other Tests of Pancreatic Function

Case Study Table 25-2.1 summarizes several laboratory tests that might be helpful in diagnosis of pancreatic disorders. Other tests, which differentiate pancreatic from enteric malabsorption, must be performed and are discussed in detail in Chapter 26, *Gastrointestinal Function.* One such test is the D-xylose absorption test. D-Xylose is a pentose sugar that does not require pancreatic enzymes for absorption. In a patient with a suspected malabsorption syndrome, a normal D-xylose points toward pancreatic insufficiency.

The starch tolerance test was devised to differentiate pancreatogenous from intestinal malabsorption. In theory, a patient with inadequate delivery of pancreatic amylase into the small intestine would have a much lower increase in blood glucose levels after ingestion of a purified starch preparation than a person with normal amounts of amylase. The results are compared with those of a standard glucose tolerance test. Unfortunately, this reference approach is confused by the fact that the glucose tolerance test is frequently abnormally flat in patients with intestinal malabsorption, as well as in more than half of patients with pancreatic insufficiency. Another problem is that gelation of the starch, on cooling, interferes with digestion and absorption. Also, starch digestion is initiated

by salivary secretion, which continues in the intestine of patients with gastric anacidity. Consequently, this test is rarely used.

Determining proteolytic enzyme activity in feces was formerly a common procedure for evaluating pancreatic exocrine function, particularly in the diagnosis of cystic fibrosis. One such procedure determines fecal proteolytic activity by its ability to digest gelatin on an x-ray film to produce clearing of the film. Unfortunately, the results are of limited reliability because many intestinal bacteria produce proteolytic enzymes, and bacteria also destroy pancreatic enzymes. More specific assays have been devised, but these have received limited acceptance.

Radiographic tests, including chest and abdominal x-rays, ultrasound, duodenography, computerized tomography, endoscopy, angiography, and pancreatic biopsy, are essential tools for proper diagnosis of pancreatic disorders.[13]

SUMMARY

The pancreas is a digestive gland that weighs 70–105 g. It is composed of two morphologically and functionally different tissues: endocrine tissue and exocrine tissue. The endocrine component consists of the islets of Langerhans, which secrete at least four hormones into the blood: insulin, glucagon, gastrin, and somatostatin. The larger exocrine pancreatic component secretes digestive enzymes into ducts that ultimately empty into the duodenum. Pancreatic activity is under both nervous and endocrine control. Other than trauma, only three diseases cause more than 95% of the medical attention devoted to the pancreas: cystic fibrosis, pancreatic carcinoma, and pancreatitis. The role of the pancreas in diabetes mellitus is discussed in Chapter 11, *Carbohydrates.* Depending on the etiology and clinical picture, pancreatic function may be suspected when there is evidence of increased amylase and lipase. Tests of pancreatic function include those used for detection of malabsorption (*eg,* D-xylose, excess fat, meat fiber, and fecal fat), tests for measuring other exocrine function (*eg,* secretin, CCK, trypsin, and chymotrypsin), tests assessing changes associated with extrahepatic obstruction (*eg,* bilirubin), and endocrine-related tests that reflect changes in the endocrine cells of the pancreas (*eg,* gastrin, insulin, glucose, and cortisol).

REVIEW QUESTIONS

1. Laboratory findings in pancreatitis include all of the following EXCEPT:
   a. increased amylase.
   b. increased lipase.
   c. increased triglycerides.
   d. increased cortisol.

2. Which of the following tests is a direct determination of the exocrine secretory capacity of the pancreas?
   a. Amylase
   b. Quantitative fecal fat analysis
   c. Secretin/CCK test
   d. None of the above.

3. Which of the following statements concerning cystic fibrosis is NOT correct?
   a. Occurs predominantly in populations of Northern European extraction
   b. Frequently diagnosed by measurement of sweat chloride
   c. Affects males and females about equally
   d. Caused by a variety of mutations on chromosome 7
   e. Genetic screening is usually unsuccessful

4. Cystic fibrosis is *least likely* to produce which of the following conditions?
   a. Intestinal obstruction in the newborn
   b. Pulmonary infections
   c. Scarring of the pancreas
   d. Hepatic cirrhosis
   e. Intestinal malabsorption

5. The proper time period for the collection of a fecal fat specimen is:
   a. 24 hours.
   b. 36 hours.
   c. 48 hours.
   d. 72 hours.
   e. 96 hours.

6. The main pancreatic duct drains into the:
   a. duodenum.
   b. stomach.
   c. gallbladder.
   d. colon.
   e. liver.

REFERENCES

1. Scotet V, Gillet D, Dugueperoux I, et al. Spatial and temporal distribution of cystic fibrosis and of its mutations in Brittany, France: a retrospective study from 1960. Hum Genet 2002; 111(3):247–254.
2. Corbetta C, Seia M, Bassotti A, et al. Screening for cystic fibrosis in newborn infants: results of a pilot programme based on a two tier protocol (IRT/DNA/IRT) in the Italian population. J Med Screen 2002;9(2):60–63.
3. Gregg AR, Simpson JL. Genetic screening for cystic fibrosis. Obstet Gynecol Clin North Am 2002;29(2):329–340.
4. Boyd EJ, Wormsley KG. Laboratory tests in the diagnosis of the chronic pancreatic diseases. Part 1. Secretagogues used in tests of pancreatic secretion. Int J Pancreatol 1987;2(3):137–148.
5. Chesner I, Lawson N. Tests of exocrine pancreatic function. Ann Clin Biochem 1994;31(Pt 4):305–314.
6. Simko V. Sudan stain and quantitative fecal fat. Gastroenterology 1990;98(6):1725–1723.
7. Huang G, Khouri MR, Shiau YF. Sudan stain of fecal fat: new insight into an old test. Gastroenterology 1989;96(2 Pt 1):421–427.
8. Boyd EJ, Rinderknecht H, Wormsley KG. Laboratory tests in the diagnosis of the chronic pancreatic diseases. Part 3. Tests on pure pancreatic juice. Int J Pancreatol 1987;2(5–6):291–304.
9. Farrell PM, Gregg RG, Koscik R, et al. Newborn screening for cystic fibrosis in Wisconsin: comparison of biochemical and molecular methods. Pediatrics 1997;99(6):819–824.
10. James TJ, Taylor RP. Enzymatic measurement of sweat sodium and chloride. Ann Clin Biochem 1997;34(Pt 2):211.
11. Stern RC. The diagnosis of cystic fibrosis. N Engl J Med 1997;336 (7):487–491.
12. Burnett RW, LeGrys VA. Current status of sweat testing in North America: results of the College of American Pathologists Needs Assessment Survey. Arch Pathol Lab Med 1994;118(9):865–867.
13. Boyd EJ, Wormsley KG. Laboratory tests in the diagnosis of the chronic pancreatic diseases. Part 2. Tests of pancreatic secretion. Int J Pancreatol 1987;2(4):211–251.
14. Boyd EJ, Rinderknecht H, Wormsley KG. Laboratory tests in the diagnosis of the chronic pancreatic diseases. Part 4. Tests involving the measurement of pancreatic enzymes in body fluid. Int J Pancreatol 1988;3(1):1–16.
15. Boyd EJ, Wormsley KG. Laboratory tests in the diagnosis of the chronic pancreatic diseases. Part 5. Stool enzyme measurements. Int J Pancreatol 1988;3(2–3):101–103.
16. Boyd EJ, Rinderknecht H, Wormsley KG. Laboratory tests in the diagnosis of the chronic pancreatic diseases. Part 6. Differentiation between chronic pancreatitis and pancreatic cancer. Int J Pancreatol 1988;3(4):259–240.

SUGGESTED READINGS

DiMagno EP, Layer P. Human exocrine pancreatic enzyme secretion. In: Go VLW, DiMagno EP, Gardner JD, et al, eds. The Pancreas: Biology, Pathobiology and Disease, 2nd ed. New York: Raven Press, 1993:275–300.

Owyang C, Williams JA. Pancreatic secretion. In: Yamada T, Alpers DH, Laine L, et al, eds. Textbook of Gastroenterology. Philadelphia: Lippincott Williams & Wilkins, 1999:355–379.

Pandol SJ. Pancreatic physiology and secretory testing. In: Feldman M, Friedman LS, Sleisenger MH, eds. Sleisenger & Fordtran's Gastrointestinal and Liver Diseases: Pathophysiology, Diagnosis, Management, 7th ed. Philadelphia: WB Saunders, 2002:871–880.

Gastrointestinal Function

Edward P. Fody

OBJECTIVES

Upon completion of this chapter, the clinical laboratorian should be able to:
- Describe the physiology and biochemistry of gastric secretion.

- List the tests used to assess gastric and intestinal function.
- Explain the clinical aspects of gastric analysis.
- Evaluate a patient's condition, given clinical data.

KEY TERMS

Gastrin	Lactose tolerance test	Secretagogues	Zollinger-Ellison
Intrinsic factor	Pepsin	D-Xylose absorption test	syndrome

The gastrointestinal (GI) system is composed of the mouth, esophagus, stomach, small intestine, and large intestine. Digestion, which is primarily a function of the small intestine, is the process by which starches, proteins, lipids, nucleic acids, and other complex molecules are degraded to simple constituents (molecules) for absorption and use in the body. This chapter discusses the physiology and biochemistry of gastric secretion, intestinal physiology, pathologic aspects of intestinal function, and tests of gastric and intestinal function.

PHYSIOLOGY AND BIOCHEMISTRY OF GASTRIC SECRETION[1]

Gastric secretion occurs in response to various stimuli:

- Neurogenic impulses from the brain transmitted by means of the vagal nerves (eg, responses to the sight, smell, or anticipation of food).
- Distention of the stomach with food or fluid.
- Contact of protein breakdown products, termed *secretagogues*, with the gastric mucosa.

- The hormone *gastrin* is the most potent stimulus to gastric secretion; it is secreted by specialized G cells in the gastric mucosa and the duodenum in response to vagal stimulation and contact with secretagogues.

Inhibitory influences include high gastric acidity, which decreases the release of gastrin by the gastric G cells. Gastric inhibitory polypeptide is secreted by K cells in the middle and distal duodenum and proximal jejunum in response to food products such as fats, glucose, and amino acids. Vasoactive intestinal polypeptide, produced by H cells in the intestinal mucosa, directly inhibits gastric secretion, gastrin release, and gastric motility.

Gastric fluid has a high content of hydrochloric acid, pepsin, and mucus. Hydrochloric acid is secreted against a hydrogen ion gradient as great as 1 million times the concentration in plasma (*ie,* gastric fluid can reach a pH of 1.2–1.3 under conditions of augmented or maximal stimulation). *Pepsin* refers to a group of relatively weak proteolytic enzymes, with pH optima from about 1.6 to 3.6, that catalyze all native proteins except mucus. The most important component of gastric secretion in terms of body physiology is *intrinsic factor,* which greatly facilitates the absorption of vitamin B_{12} in the ileum.

CLINICAL ASPECTS OF GASTRIC ANALYSIS[2–5]

Gastric analysis is used in clinical medicine mainly for the following purposes:

- Gastric analysis was widely used in clinical medicine, but has now been largely replaced by fiber optic endoscopy and improved radiologic procedures.
- Gastric analysis is used clinically mainly to detect hypersecretion characteristic of the *Zollinger-Ellison syndrome.* This syndrome involves a gastrin-secreting neoplasm, usually located in the pancreatic islets, and exceptionally high plasma gastrin concentrations. Basal 1-hour secretion usually exceeds 10 mEq, and the ratio of basal 1-hour to maximal secretion usually exceeds 60% (*ie,* the stomach is not really in the basal state but rather is pathologically stimulated by the high plasma gastrin level).

Gastric analysis is also used occasionally to evaluate pernicious anemia in adults. Gastric atrophy is present in this condition, and the stomach fails to secrete intrinsic factor, which binds to vitamin B_{12} to prevent its degradation by gastric acid. The pH of gastric fluid in this condition typically does not fall below 6, even with maximum stimulation. Rarely, gastric analysis may aid in determining the type of surgical procedure required for ulcer treatment.

Previously, various substances were used to stimulate gastric secretion (*eg,* caffeine, alcohol, and test meals), but these are submaximal stimuli and obsolete. From 1953 until the late 1970s, histamine acid phosphate was used as a maximal stimulus to gastric secretion. Because of adverse effects, some of them severe, histamine has now been replaced by pentagastrin, which is a synthetic pentapeptide composed of the four C-terminal amino acids of gastrin linked to a substituted alanine derivative.

Normal gastric fluid is translucent, pale gray, and slightly viscous and often has a faintly acrid odor. Residual volume should not exceed 75 mL. Residual specimens occasionally contain flecks of blood or are green, brown, or yellow from reflux of bile during the intubation procedure. The presence of food particles is abnormal and indicates obstruction.

TESTS OF GASTRIC FUNCTION

Measuring Gastric Acid in Basal and Maximal Secretory Tests[2–5]

After an overnight fast, gastric analysis is usually performed as a 1-hour basal test, followed by a 1-hour stimulated test subsequent to pentagastrin administration (6 μg/kg subcutaneously). Test results reveal wide overlap among healthy subjects and diseased patients, except for anacidity (*eg,* in pernicious anemia) and the extreme hypersecretion found in Zollinger-Ellison syndrome. Gastric peptic ulcer is usually associated with normal secretory volume and acid output. Duodenal peptic ulcer is usually associated with increased secretory volume in both the basal and maximal secretory tests; considerable overlap occurs, nevertheless, with the normal range.

Measuring Gastric Acid[2]

In stimulated-secretion specimens, the ability of the stomach to secrete against a hydrogen ion gradient is determined by measuring the pH. The total acid output in a timed interval is determined from the titratable acidities and volumes of the component specimens. After intubation, the residual secretion is aspirated and retained. Secretion for the subsequent 10–30 minutes is discarded to allow for adjustment of the patient to the intubation procedure. Specimens are ordinarily obtained as 15-minute collections for a period of 1 hour.

The gastrin response to intravenous secretin stimulation may be used to investigate patients with mildly elevated serum gastrin levels. In this test, pure porcine secretin is injected intravenously, and gastrin levels are collected at 5-minute intervals for the next 30 minutes. In patients with Zollinger-Ellison syndrome, the gastrin level increases at least 100 pg/mL over the basal level. Patients with ordinary peptic ulceration, achlorhydria, or other conditions show a slight decrease in gastrin concentration.[6]

The volume, pH, and titratable acidity and the calculated acid output of each specimen are reported, as is the total volume and acid output for each test period (sum of the component specimens). There is considerable variation in gastric acid output among healthy subjects in both the basal and maximal secretory tests. Nevertheless, in the basal test, most healthy subjects secrete 0–6 mEq of acid in a total volume of 10–100 mL. In the maximal 1-hour test, using histamine or pentagastrin as the stimulus, most men secrete 1–40 mEq of acid in a total volume of 40–350 mL. Women and older persons usually secrete somewhat less acid than young men.

Plasma Gastrin[6–9]

Measurement of plasma gastrin levels is invaluable in diagnosing Zollinger-Ellison syndrome, in which fasting levels typically exceed 1000 pg/mL and can reach 400,000 pg/mL, compared with the normal range of 50–150 pg/mL. Gastrin is usually not increased in simple peptic ulcer disease. Increased plasma gastrin levels do occur in most pernicious anemia patients but decrease toward normal when hydrochloric acid is artificially instilled into the stomach.

INTESTINAL PHYSIOLOGY

Digestion, predominantly a function of the small intestine, is the process in which starches, proteins, lipids, nucleic acids, and other complex molecules are degraded to monosaccharides, amino acids and oligopeptides, fatty acids, purines, pyrimidines, and other simple constituents. For most large molecules, digestion is necessary for absorption to occur. Each day, the duodenum receives about 7–10 L of ingested water and food and secretion from the salivary glands, stomach, pancreas, and biliary tract. The materials then enter the jejunum and ileum, where another 1–1.5 L of secretion is added. Ultimately, however, only about 1.5 L of fluid material reaches the *cecum,* which is the first portion of the colon or large intestines. This considerable absorptive capability is possible because the small intestine (about 20 feet long) has numerous mucosal folds, minute projections from the luminal surface called *villi,* and microscopic projections on the mucosal cells called *microvilli,* all of which greatly increase the secretory and absorptive surface to an estimated 200 m². Absorption takes place by passive diffusion for some substances and by active transport for others. In addition, the small intestine actively secrete electrolytes and other metabolic products. The large intestine (about 5 feet long) has two major functions: water resorption, in which the 1.5 L of fluid received by the cecum is reduced to about 100–300 mL of feces, and storage of feces before defecation. The abdominal structures that constitute the alimentary tract are shown diagrammatically in Figure 26-1.

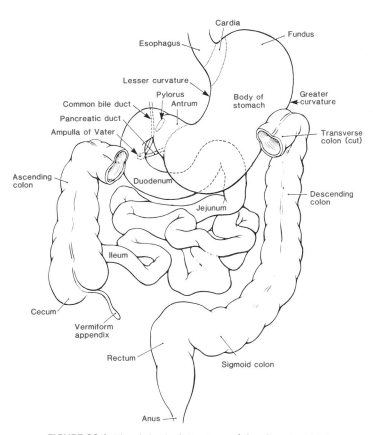

FIGURE 26-1. The abdominal structures of the alimentary tract.

CASE STUDY 26-1

A 34-year-old man was admitted for diagnostic evaluation with the complaint of epigastric pain of 2 years' duration, which was variously described as gnawing or burning. He had been diagnosed with a duodenal peptic ulcer 18 months ago; at that time, therapy of antacids and dietary revision provided considerable alleviation of symptoms. More recently, the pain had become more persistent and awakened the patient 4–6 times each night. Radiologic studies revealed a 2.5-cm ulcer crater in the first portion of the duodenum and a 0.5-cm ulcer in the antrum of the stomach. Serum electrolytes were normal. Hemoglobin was 8.3 g/dL with normal red blood cell indices. White blood count was 13,100. Gastric analy-

sis revealed 640 mL of secretion in the basal hour, with an acid output of 38 mEq, and 780 mL of secretion in the 1-hour pentagastrin stimulation test, with an acid output of 48 mEq.

Questions

1. What is the probable disease?

2. In view of existing data, what other test would be virtually diagnostic for this disease?

3. What is the explanation for decreased hemoglobin and increased white blood cell count?

CLINICOPATHOLOGIC ASPECTS OF INTESTINAL FUNCTION

Clinical chemistry testing of intestinal function focuses almost entirely on the evaluation of absorption and its derangements in various disease states. As discussed in Chapter 25, *Pancreatic Function*, diseases of the exocrine pancreas and biliary tract may also cause malabsorption. Intestinal diseases that may cause the malabsorption syndrome are highly varied in their etiology, pathogenesis, and severity. These intestinal diseases and disorders include tropical and nontropical or celiac sprue, Whipple's disease, Crohn's disease, primary intestinal lymphoma, small intestinal resection, intestinal lymphangiectasia, ischemia, amyloidosis, and giardiasis. In addition to the malabsorption syndrome, which ordinarily causes impaired absorption of fats, proteins, carbohydrates, and other substances, specific malabsorption states also occur (eg, acquired deficiency of lactase, which prevents normal absorption of lactose, and Hartnup syndrome, a genetic disorder that involves deficient intestinal transport of phenylalanine and leucine).

TESTS OF INTESTINAL FUNCTION

Lactose Tolerance Test[10]

The disaccharidases, lactase (which cleaves lactose into glucose and galactose) and sucrase (which cleaves sucrose into glucose and fructose), are produced by the mucosal cells of the small intestine. Congenital deficiencies of these enzymes are rare, but acquired deficiencies of lactase are commonly found in adults. Affected patients experience abdominal discomfort, cramps, and diarrhea after ingesting milk or milk products. About 10–20% of American Caucasians and 75% of African Americans are affected.

Lactose tolerance testing was used to establish this diagnosis, but the test is subject to many false-positive and false-negative results. This test has largely been replaced by hydrogen breath testing.

D-Xylose Absorption Test[11,12]

D-Xylose is a pentose sugar that is ordinarily not present in the blood in any significant amount. As with other monosaccharides, pentose sugars are absorbed unaltered in the proximal small intestine and do not require the intervention of pancreatic lytic enzymes. Therefore, the ability to absorb D-xylose is of value in differentiating malabsorption of intestinal etiology from that of exocrine pancreatic insufficiency. Because only about one half of orally administered D-xylose is metabolized or lost by action of intestinal bacteria, significant amounts are excreted unchanged in the urine. Some protocols have used the measurement of only the D-xylose excreted in the urine during the 5 hours following ingestion of a 25-g dose by a fasting adult (0.5 g/kg in a child). Even with normal renal function, false-positive and false-negative results frequently occur. Blood levels measured one or more times after ingestion of D-xylose (eg, at 30 minutes, 1 hour, 2 hours) significantly improve the diagnostic reliability of the test. Some protocols use smaller doses of D-xylose to avoid abdominal cramps, intestinal hypermotility, and osmotic diarrhea that frequently accompany the 25-g dose.

D-Xylose Test

After ingestion of a specified solution of D-xylose, blood specimens are obtained and urine is collected for a 5-hour period to determine the extent of D-xylose absorption. The concentration of D-xylose is determined by heating protein-free supernates of urine and plasma to convert xylose to furfural, which is then reacted with *p*-bromoaniline to form a pink product, the absorbance of which is measured at 520 nm. Thiourea is added as an antioxidant to prevent the formation of interfering chromogens. After an overnight fast, the patient voids and drinks a D-xylose solution: 25 g of D-xylose in 250 mL of water for adults and 0.5 g/kg for children, or other dose as established. The patient drinks an equivalent amount of water during the next hour. No additional food or fluids are to be taken until the test is completed. Urine is collected for 5 hours after the D-xylose ingestion. A blood specimen is collected in potassium oxalate at 2 hours (commonly, 1 hour is chosen for children).

Normal blood concentrations of D-xylose in association with decreased urine excretion suggest impairment of renal function or incomplete urine collection. Aspirin therapy diminishes renal excretion of D-xylose, whereas indomethacin decreases intestinal absorption. After ingestion of a 25-g dose of D-xylose, healthy adults should excrete at least 4 g in the 5-hour period. For infants and children, the excretion following a dose of 0.5 g/kg for various ages expressed as percentages of ingested dose are shown in Table 26-1. Blood levels for healthy adults vary widely, but a blood concentration of less than 25 mg/dL at 2 hours should be considered abnormal after the 25-g dose. With the 0.5 g/kg dose, infants younger than 6 months should have a blood concentration of at least 15 mg/dL at 1 hour, infants older than 6 months and children should achieve levels of at least 30 mg/dL.[5,11]

Serum Carotenoids

Carotenoids are various yellow to orange or purple pigments that are widely distributed in animal tissue; they are synthesized by many plants and impart a yellow color to some vegetables and fruits. The major carotenoids in human serum are lycopene; xanthophyll; and beta-carotene, the chief precursor of vitamin A in humans. Being fat soluble, carotenoids are absorbed in the small intestine in association with lipids. Malabsorption of lipids typically results in a serum concentration of carotenoids lower than the reference range of 50–250 mg/dL. Starvation, dietary idiosyncrasies, and fever also cause diminished serum concentrations. The test does not distinguish among the various etiologies of malabsorption.

Fecal Fat Analysis

As discussed in Chapter 25, *Pancreatic Function,* increased fecal fat loss, or steatorrhea, is an integral manifestation of the general malabsorption syndrome. However, neither the presence of steatorrhea nor the documentation of its severity is of benefit in distinguishing among the various etiologies of malabsorption, with the exception that severe steatorrhea is rarely caused by biliary obstruction.

Other Tests of Intestinal Malabsorption

Deficiencies of numerous analytes can occur in association with intestinal malabsorption. Measurement of these analytes is usually of value, not so much in confirming the diagnosis of malabsorption as in determining the extent of nutritional deficiency and, thus, the need for replacement therapy. Diminished appetite and dietary intake are usually more severe in patients who have malabsorption with an intestinal etiology. Body wasting or cachexia may be severe. Frequently, because loss of albumin into the intestinal lumen and diminished dietary intake of protein accompany the diminished absorption of oligopeptides and amino acids, a negative nitrogen balance occurs together with decreased serum total proteins and albumin. A serum albumin of less than 2.5 g/dL is much more characteristic of intestinal disease than of pancreatic disease. In association with severe disease of the small intestine, deficiencies of fat-soluble vitamins A, D, E, and K occur. Vitamin K deficiency, in turn, causes deficiencies of vitamin K–dependent coagulation factors II (prothrombin), VII (proconvertin), IX (plasma thromboplastin component), and X (Stuart-Prower factor), which are reflected in abnormal prothrombin time and partial thromboplastin time tests.

In severe small intestinal disease, such as tropical or celiac sprue, malabsorption of folate and vitamin B_{12} can occur, and megaloblastic anemia is rather common and is of some benefit in distinguishing intestinal from pancreatic disease. Absorption of iron is usually diminished, and the tendency toward low serum iron levels may be aggravated by intestinal blood loss. Intestinal absorption of calcium is often diminished as a result of calcium binding by unabsorbed fatty acids and accompanying vitamin D deficiency and decreased serum magnesium. Because sodium, potassium, water absorption and metabolism may also be seriously deranged, serum sodium and potassium levels are decreased and dehydration occurs. Impaired absorption of carbohydrates in intestinal diseases, such as sprue, results in decreased to flat blood concentration curves in glucose, lactose, and sucrose tolerance tests.

TABLE 26-1. D-Xylose Results for Pediatric Patients[2,4]

AGE	REFERENCE RANGE
Younger than 6 months	11–33%
6–12 months	20–32%
1–3 years	20–42%
3–10 years	25–45%
Older than 10 years	25–50%

CASE STUDY 26-2

A 26-year-old woman appeared in the outpatient clinic with the complaint of abdominal discomfort; diarrhea; and an 18-pound, unintentional weight loss during the past 2–3 years. She related a similar period of 5 or 6 years of abdominal distress and diarrhea in childhood, but this essentially disappeared when she was about 12–13 years old. She was now having 3–5 bowel movements daily, which were described as bulky, malodorous, and floating. She weighed 106 pounds and was 67 inches tall. She never had surgical procedures. Physical examination revealed poor skin turgor, general pallor, and a protuberant abdomen. Abnormal clinical laboratory values included those in Case Study Table 26-2.1.

Fecal examination revealed no ova or parasites, and bacteriologic culture revealed no pathogens.

Questions

1. What is the disease process?

2. What is the probable etiology in this case?

3. What is the cause of the abnormal coagulation tests?

4. What is the probable major cause for the anemia, and what are other possible contributing causes?

CASE STUDY TABLE 26-2.1. LABORATORY RESULTS

ANALYTE	RESULT
Hemoglobin	8.1 g/dL
Hematocrit	30%
RBC count	$4.1 \times 10^6/\mu L$
Serum sodium	134 mEq/L
Potassium	3.4 mEq/L
Serum carotenoids	14 µg/dL
Fecal fat	22 g/24 hours
D-Xylose absorption test (25-g dose)	5-hour excretion of 1.3 g and blood level at 2 hours of 8 mg/dL
Prothrombin time	15.8 seconds (12–14 seconds)
Activated partial thromboplastin time	56 seconds (30–45 seconds)

SUMMARY

Gastric secretion occurs in response to various stimuli. Gastric analysis is performed to detect the hypersecretion characteristic of Zollinger-Ellison syndrome. Measurement of plasma gastrin levels is also used in the diagnosis of Zollinger-Ellison syndrome. Digestion is predominantly a function of the small intestine. Clinical chemistry testing of intestinal function focuses almost entirely on the evaluation of absorption and its derangements in various disease states. Intestinal diseases and disorders include Whipple's disease, Crohn's disease, sprue, amyloidosis, and giardiasis. Several malabsorption syndromes or states also exist (eg, acquired deficiency of lactase and Hartnup syndrome). Tests of intestinal function include the D-xylose test, serum carotenoids, and fecal fat analysis.

REVIEW QUESTIONS

1. Which of the following tests is only of the absorptive ability of the intestine?
    a. Lactose tolerance test
    b. D-Xylose test
    c. Fecal fat (72-hour collection)
    d. Serum carotenoids
    e. Serum albumin

2. The smallest amount of D-xylose is normally absorbed by patients:
    a. younger than 1 year of age.
    b. between 1 and 3 years of age.
    c. between 3 and 5 years of age.
    d. between 5 and 10 years of age.
    e. who are adults.

3. In a gastric acidity test, a patient produces 50 mL of gastric fluid. A 5-mL aliquot of this fluid requires 10 mL of 0.1 N NaOH to titrate to pH 7.0. Calculate the acid output in milliequivalents (mEq).
   a. 2
   b. 4
   c. 6
   d. 8
   e. 10

4. The results in the previous question could be found in all of the following conditions EXCEPT:
   a. Zollinger-Ellison syndrome.
   b. peptic ulcer.
   c. previous pentagastrin stimulation.
   d. pernicious anemia.
   e. a healthy person.

5. In which of the following would gastrin levels be increased?
   a. Peptic ulceration
   b. Zollinger-Ellison syndrome
   c. Achlorhydria
   d. Amyloidosis

6. Normal blood concentrations of D-xylose, with decreased urine D-xylose excretion, suggests:
   a. incomplete urine collection.
   b. impaired renal function.
   c. lactose intolerance.
   d. a and b.

7. A serum albumin of less than 2.5 g/dL would be most indicative of:
   a. intestinal disease.
   b. pancreatitis.
   c. peptic ulcer.
   d. pancreatic carcinoma.

8. Regarding gastric acid basal and maximal secretory tests, peptic ulcer is usually associated with:
   a. increased secretory volume for both the basal and maximal tests.
   b. normal secretory volume and acid output.
   c. decreased secretory volume for both the basal and maximal tests.
   d. none of the above.

REFERENCES

1. Schubert ML, Shamburek RD. Control of acid secretion. Gastroenterol Clin North Am 1990;19(1):1–25.
2. Hung PD, Schubert ML, Mihas AA. Zollinger-Ellison syndrome. Curr Treat Options Gastroenterol 2003;6(2):163–170.
3. Metz DC, Starr JA. A retrospective study of the usefulness of acid secretory testing. Aliment Pharmacol Ther 2000;14(1):103–111.
4. Hirschowitz BI, Simmons J, Mohnen J. Long-term lansoprazole control of gastric acid and pepsin secretion in ZE and non-ZE hypersecretors: a prospective 10-year study. Aliment Pharmacol Ther 2001;15(11):1795–1806.
5. Rosenfeld L. Gastric tubes, meals, acid, and analysis: rise and decline. Clin Chem 1997;43(5):837–842.
6. Berger AC, Gibril F, Venzon DJ, et al. Prognostic value of initial fasting serum gastrin levels in patients with Zollinger-Ellison syndrome. J Clin Oncol 2001;19(12):3051–3057.
7. Cadiot G, Mignon M. Diagnostic and therapeutic criteria in patients with Zollinger-Ellison syndrome and multiple endocrine neoplasia type 1. J Intern Med 1998;243(6):489–494.
8. Hung PD, Schubert ML, Mihas AA. Zollinger-Ellison syndrome. Curr Treat Options Gastroenterol 2003;6(2):163–170.
9. Metz DC, Buchanan M, Purich E, Fein S. A randomized controlled crossover study comparing synthetic porcine and human secretins with biologically derived porcine secretin to diagnose Zollinger-Ellison syndrome. Aliment Pharmacol Ther 2001:15(5):669–676.
10. Korpela R, Peuhkuri K, Poussa T. Comparison of a portable breath hydrogen analyser (Micro H2) with a Quintron MicroLyzer in measuring lactose maldigestion, and the evaluation of a Micro H2 for diagnosing hypolactasia. Scand J Clin Lab Invest 1998;58(3):217–224.
11. Kuno C, Watanabe J, Yuasa H. Comparative assessment of D-xylose absorption between small intestine and large intestine. J Pharm Pharmacol 1997;49(1): 26–29.
12. Hamanaka Y, Oka M, Suzuki T, et al. Oral absorption tests: absorption site of each substrate. Nutrition 1998;14(1):7–10.

SUGGESTED READINGS

Chey WD, Chey WY. Tests of gastric and exocrine pancreatic function and absorption. In: Yamada T, Alpers DH, Laine L, et al, eds. Textbook of Gastroenterology. Philadelphia: Lippincott Williams & Wilkins, 1999:2924–2937.

Feldman M. Gastric secretion. In: Feldman M. Friedman LS, Sleisenger MH, eds. Sleisenger & Fordtran's Gastrointestinal and Liver Diseases: Pathophysiology, Diagnosis, Management, 7th ed. Philadelphia: WB Saunders, 2002:715–731.

Body Fluid Analysis

Frank A. Sedor

OBJECTIVES

Upon completion of this chapter, the clinical laboratorian should be able to:

- Identify the source of amniotic fluid, cerebrospinal fluid, sweat, synovial fluid, pleural fluid, pericardial fluid, and peritoneal fluid.
- Describe the physiologic purpose of amniotic fluid, cerebrospinal fluid, sweat, synovial fluid, pleural fluid, pericardial fluid, and peritoneal fluid.

- Discuss the clinical utility of testing amniotic fluid, cerebrospinal fluid, sweat, synovial fluid, pleural fluid, pericardial fluid, and peritoneal fluid.
- Interpret the patient's status, given the results of a foam stability index, L/S ratio, and sweat test.
- Differentiate between a transudate and an exudate.

KEY TERMS

Amniocentesis
Amniotic fluid
Ascites
Effusion
Exudate

Hypoglycorrhachia
L/S ratio
Otorrhea
Pericardial fluid
Peritoneal fluid

Pleural fluid
Respiratory distress
  syndrome
Rhinorrhea

Serous fluid
Synovial fluid
Thoracentesis
Transudate

This chapter attempts to acquaint the reader with several fluids that are often analyzed in the clinical chemistry laboratory. In general, the source, physiologic purpose, and clinical utility of laboratory measurements for each of these body fluids is emphasized.

AMNIOTIC FLUID

The amniotic sac provides an enclosed environment for fetal development. This sac is bilayered as the result of a fusion of the amnionic (inner) and chorionic (outer) membranes at an early stage of fetal development. The fetus is suspended in *amniotic fluid* (AF) within the sac. The AF provides a cushioning medium for the fetus and serves as a matrix for influx and efflux of constituents.

Obviously, the mother must be the ultimate physiologic source for AF. Depending on the interval of the gestational period, the fluid may be derived from different sources. At initiation of pregnancy, some maternal secretion across the amnion contributes to the volume. Shortly after formation of the placenta, embryo, and fusion of membranes, AF is largely derived by transudation across the fetal skin. In the last half of pregnancy, the skin becomes substantially less permeable, and fetal micturition, or urination, becomes the major volume source. The fate of the fluid also varies with period of gestation. A bidirectional exchange is presumed to occur across the membranes and at the placenta. Similarly, during early pregnancy, the fetal skin is involved. In the last half of pregnancy, the mechanism of fetal swallowing is the major fate of AF. There is a dynamic balance established between production and clearance; fetal urination and swallowing maintain this balance. The continual swallowing maintains intimate contact of the AF with the fetal gastrointestinal tract, buccal cavity, and bronchotracheal tree. This contact is evidenced by the sloughed material from the fetus that provides us with the "window" to fetal developmental and functional stages.

Cells found in the fluid originate with the fetus, and the chemical content reflects the continual swallowing and clearance of fluid. A sample of fluid is obtained by transabdominal *amniocentesis* (amniotic sac puncture), which is performed under aseptic conditions. Before an attempt is made to obtain fluid, the positions of the placenta, fetus, and fluid pockets are visualized using ultrasonography. Aspiration of anything except fluid could lead to erroneous conclusions, as well as possible harm to the fetus.

Amniocentesis and subsequent AF analysis is performed to test for: (1) congenital diseases, (2) neural tube defects, (3) hemolytic disease, (4) gestational age, and (5) fetal pulmonary development. The first, diagnosis of genetic abnormality, is accomplished by cell culture. Fluid obtained between 14 and 20 weeks of pregnancy is harvested for cells of fetal origin. The cells are cultured, collected for chromosomal analysis, and are lysed so that enzyme contents may be determined to evaluate for metabolic defects. This procedure has been largely supplanted by the use of chorionic villus sampling (CVS) and cytogenetic analysis. CVS may pose a risk to the fetus, and first-trimester amniocentesis may provide a sample with less interfering substances.

Screening for neural tube defects (NTDs) is initially performed using maternal serum. The presence of elevated levels of α-fetoprotein (AFP) was originally thought to indicate NTDs such as spina bifida and anencephaly. Elevated maternal serum AFP can also be closely correlated with abdominal hernias into the umbilical cord, cystic hygroma, and poor pregnancy outcome. Low maternal serum AFP is associated with an increased incidence of Down's syndrome and other aneuploidies. The protocol for AFP testing is generally considered to include: (1) maternal serum AFP, usually with the assay of hCG, unconjugated estriol, and inhibin; (2) repeat, if positive; (3) diagnostic ultrasound; and (4) amniocentesis for confirmation. Interpretation of maternal serum AFP testing is complex, being a function of age, race, weight, gestational age, and level of nutrition.

Testing of amniotic fluid AFP (AFAFP) is the confirmatory procedure. AFP is a product of first the fetal yolk sac and then the fetal liver. It is released into the fetal circulation and presumably enters the AF by transudation. Entry into the maternal circulation could be by placenta crossover or from the AF. If there were an open defect (*eg*, spina bifida) that caused an increase in AFAFP, there would be a concomitant increase in maternal serum AFP. Under normal conditions, AFAFP would be cleared by fetal swallowing and metabolism. An increased presence overloads this mechanism, causing AFAFP elevation. Assay of the protein is normally done by immunologic means. The lack of treatment of a positive presence and the lack of 100% specificity increase the need for extreme care in analysis. Societal and clinical concerns mandate that the highest levels of quality control be practiced.

This concern generated the need for a second test to affirm NTDs and abdominal wall defects. The method used is the assay for a central nervous system (CNS)-specific acetylcholinesterase (AChE). The NTD allows direct or, at least less difficult, passage of AChE into the AF. Analysis for CNS-specific AChE in the AF then offers a degree of confirmation for AFAFP. The methods used for CNS AChE include enzymatic, immunologic, and electrophoretic with inhibition. The latter includes the use of acetylthiocholine as substrate and BW284C51, a specific CNS inhibitor, to differentiate the serum pseudocholinesterase from the CNS-specific AChE.

Analysis of AF to screen for hemolytic disease of the newborn (erythroblastosis fetalis) was the first recognized laboratory procedure performed on AF. Hemolytic disease of the newborn is a syndrome of the fetus resulting from ABO incompatibility of the maternal and fetal blood. Maternal antibodies to fetal erythrocytes cause a hemolytic reaction that can vary in severity. The resultant hemoglobin breakdown products, predominantly bilirubin, appear in the AF and provide a measure of the severity of the incompatibility reaction.

The most commonly employed method is a direct spectrophotometric scan of undiluted AF and subsequent calculation of the relative bilirubin amount. Classically, absorbance due to bilirubin is reported instead of a concentration of bilirubin. The method consisted of scanning AF from 700 nm to 350 nm against a water

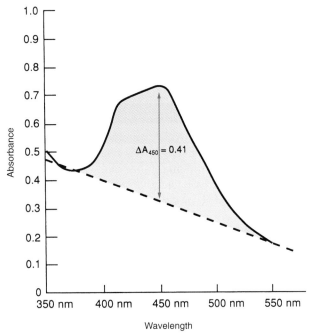

FIGURE 27-2. ΔA_{450nm} from AF bilirubin scan.

blank. The resultant absorbances can be used differently to derive the necessary information. The common method, the method of Liley,[1] requires the plotting of the observations at 5-nm intervals against wavelength, using semilogarithmic paper. A baseline is constructed from 550 nm to 350 nm; the change at 450 nm is a result of bilirubin.

Care must be used in the interpretation of the spectra. A decision for treatment can be made based on the degree of hemolysis and gestational age. The rather limited treatment options are immediate delivery, intrauterine transfusion, or observation. The transfusion can be accomplished by means of the umbilical artery and titrated to desired hematocrit. Several algorithms have been proposed to aid in decision making (Fig. 27-1). An example of an uncomplicated bilirubin scan is shown in Figure 27-2. The most commonly encountered interferences are maternal urine (from bladder interdiction), fetal or maternal blood, and meconium (fetal fecal material). Although light does not interfere per se, safeguards against exposure to light, especially sunlight, must be maintained before analysis. Light may degrade the bilirubin present, causing an underestimation of hemolytic disease severity.

Examples of interferences, compared with a normal specimen, are given in Figure 27-3. Each laboratory should compile its own catalog of real examples for spectrophotometric analysis. The presence of blood is identified by Soret absorbances of hemoglobin at 410–415 nm; the presence of urine is identified by the broad curve and confirmed by creatinine, urea, and protein analyses; and

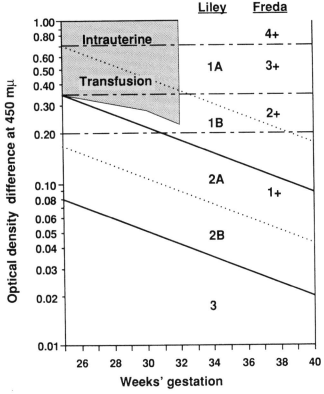

FIGURE 27-1. Assessment of fetal prognosis. Liley method: *1A, above broken line,* condition desperate, immediate delivery or transfusion; *1B, between broken and continuous lines,* hemoglobin >8 g/100 mL, delivery or transfusion *(stippled area)* urgent; *2A, between continuous and broken lines,* hemoglobin 8–10 g/100 mL, delivery 36–37 weeks; *2B, between broken and continuous lines,* hemoglobin 11–13.9 g/100 mL, delivery 37–39 weeks; *3, below continuous line,* not anemic, delivery at term.

Freda method: *4+, above upper horizontal line,* fetal death imminent, immediate delivery or transfusion; *3+, between upper and middle horizontal lines,* fetus in jeopardy, death within 3 weeks, delivery or transfusion as soon as possible; *2+, between middle and lower horizontal lines,* fetal survival for at least 7–10 days, repeat test, possible indication for transfusion; *1+, below lower horizontal line,* fetus in no immediate danger of death. (Modified from Robertson JG. Evaluation of the reported methods of interpreting spectrophotometric tracings of amniotic fluid in rhesus isoimmunization. Am J Obstet Gynecol 1966;95:120.)

the presence of meconium is identified by the distinctly greenish color and flat absorbance curve.

In management of pregnancy, it is important to know gestational age. Laboratory results are often used in age evaluation. The elucidation of an analyte to reflect gestational age has resulted in the cataloging of as many constituents as are known in serum. Four parameters have been used with some degree of frequency: creatinine, urea, uric acid, and osmolality. Creatinine is thought to reflect fetal muscle mass; urea, protein; uric acid, nucleoproteins; and osmolality, a combination of all these. The problem in the use of these parameters is the wide range of concentration for given gestational ages. The ranges are so wide that significant overlap occurs, leading to inability to make accurate predictions. In practice, creatinine is the parameter used. A fluid with a level of 2 g/dL is assumed mature. Note that this is not effective in AF volume aberrations (*eg*, oligohydramnios or small AF volume). Ultrasonography has become the better tool to estimate fetal size and gestational age.

The primary reason for AF testing is the need to assess fetal pulmonary maturity. All the organ systems are at jeopardy from prematurity, but the state of the fetal lungs is a priority from the clinical perspective. The availability of laboratory tests that give an indication of maturity has also fostered this emphasis. Consequently, the laboratory is asked whether sufficient specific phospholipids are reflected in the AF to prevent atelectasis (alveolar collapse)

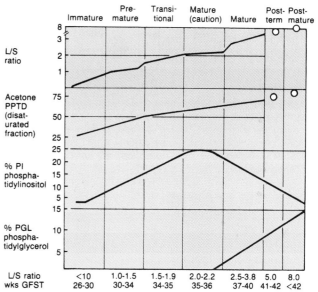

FIGURE 27-4. The form used to report the lung profile. The four determinations are plotted on the *ordinate* and the weeks of gestation on the *abscissa* (as well as the *L/S ratio* as an "internal standard"). When plotted, these fall with a high frequency into a given grid that then identifies the stage of development of the lung as shown in the upper part of the form. The designation "mature (caution)" refers to patients other than those with diabetes who can be delivered *if necessary* at this time; if the patient has diabetes, she can be delivered with safety when the values fall in the "mature" grid. (Reprinted with permission from Kulovich MV, Hallman MB, Gluck L. The lung profile I. Normal pregnancy. Am J Obstet Gynecol 1979;135:57. Copyright © 1977 by the Regents of the University of California.)

if the fetus were to be delivered. This question is important when preterm delivery is contemplated because of other risk factors in pregnancy, such as preeclampsia or premature rupture of membranes. Risk factors to fetus or mother can be weighed against interventions, such as delay of delivery, or against at-risk postdelivery therapies, such as exogenous surfactant therapy, high-frequency ventilation, or extracorporeal membrane oxygenation.

Alveolar collapse in the neonatal lung may occur on the changeover to air as an oxygen source at birth if the proper quantity and type of phospholipid (surfactant) is not present. The ensuing condition, which may vary in degree of severity, is called *respiratory distress syndrome*. It also has been referred to as *hyaline membrane disease* because of the hyaline membrane found in affected lungs. Lung maturation is a function of differentiation, beginning near the 24th week of pregnancy, of alveolar epithelial cells into type I and type II cells. The type I cells become equipped for gas exchange, and the type II cells become the producers of surfactant. As the lungs mature, increases occur in phospholipid concentration, particularly the compounds phosphatidylglycerol and lecithin, especially dipalmitoylphosphatidylcholine[2] (Fig. 27-4). These two compounds, present in 10% and 70%, respec-

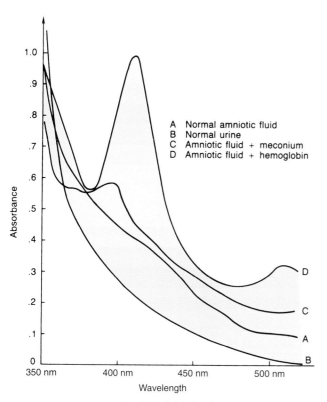

FIGURE 27-3. Amniotic fluid absorbance scans.

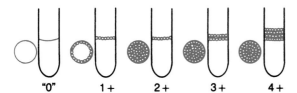

FIGURE 27-5. Grading system used in evaluating the FS-50 test. (Reprinted with permission from Statland, et al. Evaluation of a modified foam stability [FS-50] test. An assay performed on amniotic fluid to predict fetal pulmonary maturity. Am J Clin Pathol 1978;69:51. Reprinted with permission from the *American Journal of Clinical Pathology*.)

tively, of total phospholipid concentration, are most important as surfactants. Their presence in high enough levels acts in concert to allow contraction and reexpansion of the neonatal alveoli. To conceptualize their importance, remember the difficulty in blowing up a new toy balloon relative to a balloon that has been partially inflated. For the newborn, the normal amount of proper surfactant allows contraction of the alveoli without collapse. The next inspiration is the difference between a partially inflated versus a flattened new balloon. Insufficient surfactant allows alveoli to collapse, requiring a great deal of energy to reexpand the alveoli upon inspiration. This not only creates an extreme energy demand on a newborn but probably also causes physical damage to the alveoli with each collapse. The damage may lead to "hyaline" deposition, or the newborn may not have the strength to continue inspiration at the energy cost. The end result of either can be fatal.

The approaches to assessing fetal pulmonary status may be divided into functional assays and biochemical assays. Functional assays provide a direct physical measure of AF in an attempt to assess surfactant ability to decrease surface tension. Examples of this group are surface tension, fluorescence polarization, and foam stability index. These tests reflect the gross concentration of surfactants rather than specific phospholipid levels. Belonging to the latter group are assays that quantitate dipalmitoylphosphatidylcholine (the major lecithin), phosphatidylglycerols, all or most of the phospholipids, and the classic ratio of lecithins to sphingomyelins (*L/S ratio*). Each group of tests has its advocacy and extensive citations in the literature. All attempt to indicate the major changes in phospholipid concentrations that occur at about 36 weeks' gestation and indicate fetal pulmonary maturation (Fig. 27-5). With all tests, centrifugation of the AF to remove debris is necessary.

Excessive force (anything greater than that needed to remove debris) can change the lipid profile by causing the lipids present to fractionate as a result of centrifugal force. The difference in ratios observed at 1000 versus 3000 g can radically alter clinical interpretation. Before

adoption of any method for AF analysis, a protocol for centrifugal separation to include relative force (*not* revolutions per minute) and duration of centrifugation must be adopted and rigorously followed.

The foam stability index (FSI),[3] a variant of Clements' original "bubble test,"[4] appears acceptable as a rapid, inexpensive, informative assay. This qualitative, technique-dependent test requires only common equipment. The assay is based on the ability of surfactant to generate a surface tension lower than that of a 0.47-mole fraction ethanol-water solution. If sufficient surfactant is present, a stable ring of foam bubbles remains at the air–liquid interface. As surfactant increases (fetal lung maturity probability increases), a larger mole fraction of ethanol is required to overcome the surfactant-controlled surface tension. The highest mole fraction used while still maintaining a stable ring of bubbles at the air–liquid interface is reported as the FSI (Table 27-1). The test is dependent on technique and can also be skewed by contamination of any kind in the AF (*eg*, blood or meconium contamination). Interpretation of the FSI bubble patterns is difficult and technique dependent. Results can vary among clinical laboratorians. Most laboratories have found a FSI of 0.47 or 0.48 to represent a borderline maturity status. It is imperative that laboratory-specific reference intervals be determined. Values greater than borderline indicate increasing probability of maturity.

The quantitative tests were given emphasis primarily by the work of Gluck.[5] The phospholipids of importance are phosphatidylglycerol (PG), phosphatidylcholine (PC, lecithin), and sphingomyelin (SP). Relative amounts of PG and PC increase dramatically with pulmonary maturity, whereas SP concentration is relatively constant. Increases in PG and PC correspond to larger amounts of surfactant being produced by the alveolar type II cells as fetal lungs mature.

The classic technique for separation and evaluation of the lipids involves thin-layer chromatography (TLC) of an extract of the AF. The extraction procedure removes most interfering substances and results in a concentrated lipid solution. Current practices use either one- or two-dimensional TLC for identification. Laboratory needs determine if a one-dimensional or a two-dimensional method is performed. An example of the phospholipids separation by one-dimensional TLC is shown in Figure 27-6.[6]

TABLE 27-1. FSI DETERMINATION

	TUBE 1	TUBE 2	TUBE 3
Vol AF	0.50	0.50	0.50
Vol 95% EtOH	0.51	0.53	0.55
FSI	0.47	0.48	0.49

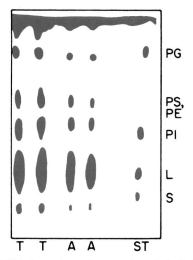

FIGURE 27-6. Thin-layer chromatogram of amniotic fluid phospholipids. Standard phospholipids (*ST*), total extract (*T*), and acetone-precipitable compounds (*A*) in amniotic fluid are shown. The phospholipid standards contained, per liter, 2 g each of lecithin and P1, 1 g each of PG and sphingomyelin, and 0.3 g each of PS and PE. 10 mL of the standard was spotted. (Reprinted with permission from Tsai MY, Marshall JG. Phosphatidylglycerol in 261 samples of amniotic fluid. Clin Chem 25[5]:683. Copyright 1979 American Association for Clinical Chemistry.)

The classic breakpoint for judgment of maturity has been a L/S ratio of 2. The presence of PG is an additional marker. PG was initially presumed to indicate maturity, but later reports have modified this. An initial PG level of at least 3% is usually needed. This may also be method dependent. There are always exceptions and outliers, however. It is important to remember that the classic L/S ratio measures total lecithin versus sphingomyelin. Some methods include selective oxidation and removal of the nonsaturated phospholipids, so that a direct measurement of dipalmitoylphosphatidylcholine can be measured. It is difficult to compare these assays empirically.

There are still conflicting reports about decision levels for the phospholipid measurements when applied to certain pathologies, particularly diabetes. Earlier reports suggested that diabetes caused certain stresses that required a L/S ratio of greater than 2 and PG greater than 6% to be comparable with a nondiabetic situation. Whether the reports were reflecting the difficulty in management of diabetes or a real effect on fetal maturity is unknown. The most recent reports appear to agree that, in diabetes, the L/S ratio interpretation is unchanged, but the lecithin fraction may have a lesser proportion of the dipalmitoyl species than is usual.

CASE STUDY 27-1

A 26-year-old woman, pregnant for the first time, presented at the emergency department in possible labor. Her blood pressure was 180/110 mm Hg, and her temperature was 99.6°F. Her history revealed an anxious woman, with pregnancy of unknown duration, who had never seen a physician. She admitted to rapid weight gain over the past 2 weeks but said that she had been feeling well until then. Recently, she felt faint and experienced episodes of vertigo. Urinalysis was significant for 3+ glucose and protein. Hematology revealed a low hemoglobin level and a moderately low platelet count, but leukocyte levels were normal. A chemistry panel revealed Na, 132 mmol/L; K, 3.0 mmol/L; Cl, 100 mmol/L; CO_2, 29 mmol/L; BUN, 7 mg/dL; creatinine, 0.5 mg/dL; and glucose, 351 mg/dL. A decision was made to admit her and perform several more tests. The following laboratory results (upper limit of reference interval given) were obtained:

L/S ratio	=	1.8 with PG = 2%
AF creatinine	=	1.5
FSI	=	0.47
AST	=	40 (35)
ALT	=	40 (35)
ALP	=	250 (100)
Mg^{2+}	=	1.6 (2.2)
Ca^{2+}	=	9.0 (10.5)
PO_4	=	4.0 (4.3)
Alb	=	3.2 (5.0)

After 24 hours of bed rest, the patient's BP fell to 140/90, and the contractions subsided.

Questions

1. Do the laboratory results indicate a normal pregnancy?

2. Comment on the maturity of the fetus.

Because the analysis of AF for a L/S ratio is so terribly technique dependent, it is absolutely mandatory for the laboratory to thoroughly evaluate the methodology used. It is more important to relate that methodology to the particular clinical setting in developing interpretative intervals. It is not unusual to see a nominal L/S ratio maturity level of 2.0 ± 0.3 at one hospital, compared with 2.2 ± 0.2 at another center using the same method. Close cooperation with the medical staff is necessary in defining the ranges to be employed.

Application of fluorescence polarization technique to AF provides another type of measurement. This procedure, as used on a commercially available polarimeter with complete reagent system (Abbott Laboratories), offers a rapidly performed test (less than 1 hour) on a versatile analyzer that is relatively technique-free. Its use has become so widespread that it has been suggested as the initial test to be used in a testing cascade.[7] The method used is based on the partition of a synthetic lecithin-like fluorescent dye between phospholipid aggregates and albumin. Dye associated with the phospholipid aggregates decreases polarization; with albumin, polarization increases. Total polarization is compared with a set of lipid:albumin standards to yield a unitless value. As the fetal lung matures, the amount of surfactant (phospholipid) increases, and, therefore, the polarization is affected. The use of this system is widespread, in part, based on the accessibility to all laboratories, straightforward analytic procedure, and consistency in result interpretation. Recently, a protocol for interpretation based on gestational age has been reported.[8]

The predictive value is compromised by blood or meconium (lipids) or fetal pathologies, causing altered albumin levels such as urinary tract anomalies. Additionally, if the AF is centrifuged, not filtered, lipid level is altered, and, therefore, polarization is decreased.

Another recently advanced functional measurement has been the quantitation of lamellar bodies. These packets of surfactant, released by the type 2 cells, are about the size of platelets and, therefore, should be quantifiable using the platelet channel of a hematology analyzer. Tentative breakpoints for an uncontaminated AF at 30,000–50,000 "platelet equivalents" have been suggested. Research is continuing to validate the assay. A standardized protocol has been developed in an effort to make the assay transferable between laboratories.[9]

Reference intervals, or cut-points, are set for "normal" pregnancies. All of the tests perform reasonably well in ruling out immaturity. However, all tests have failings with false-negative rates; specifically, when associated with deliveries that did not develop respiratory distress syndrome, although predicted to do so based on an immature result. Two excellent reviews are recommended for discussions regarding lung maturity tests and when they should be used and the effects of conditions such as pregnancy-induced hypertension.[10,11]

CEREBROSPINAL FLUID

Cerebrospinal fluid (CSF) is the liquid that occupies the spaces of the CNS. As such, it surrounds all facets of the brain and spinal cord. These spaces are continuous and, therefore, reflect all aspects of the CNS. CSF performs at least four major functions: (1) physical support and protection, (2) method for excretion, (3) provision of a controlled chemical environment, and (4) intracerebral and extracerebral transport (Fig. 27-7).

The major and most obvious function of CSF is as a buoyant cushion for the brain. The denser brain floats in the less dense fluid, allowing movement within the skull. The significance is demonstrated by the result of a blow to the head. The initial shock is transferred to the entire brain, instead of inflicting damage to one area. It may be bruised at the side opposite the blow, depending on the force imparted.

The second major function of CSF is the maintenance of a constant gross chemical matrix for the CNS. Serum

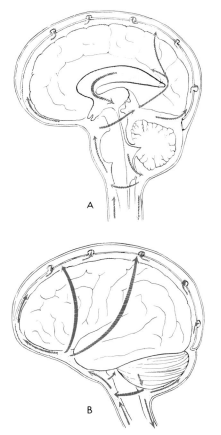

FIGURE 27-7. Major pathways of CSF. (**A**) Sagittal view; (**B**) lateral view. (Reprinted with permission from Milhorat TH. Hydrocephalus and the Cerebrospinal Fluid. Baltimore: Williams & Wilkins, 1972:25.)

components may vary greatly, but constituent levels of CSF are maintained within narrow limits.

The excretory function is not well defined, but it is presumed to be effective, especially in pathologic states. Because there is no lymphatic system in the brain, only two paths are available for elimination of wastes: capillary exchange and excretion by means of CSF. The transport function is described as a neuroendocrine role. The CSF is involved in the distribution of hypophyseal hormones within the brain and the clearance of hormones from the brain to the blood.

The total CSF volume is about 150 mL, or about 8% of the total CNS cavity volume. The fluid is formed predominantly at the choroid plexus deep within the brain and by the ependymal cells lining the ventricles.

CSF is formed at an average rate of about 0.4 mL/minute, or 500 mL/day. Formation is a result of selective ultrafiltration of plasma and active secretion by the epithelial membranes. Absorption of CSF occurs at outpouchings in the dura called *arachnoid villi,* and CSF drains into the venous sinuses of the dura. The villi also function to clear particulate matter, such as cellular debris. Reabsorption, like formation, is selective and specific. Obviously, if a constant volume is maintained at a formation rate of 500 mL/day, resorption is constant.

Specimens of CSF are obtained by lumbar puncture, usually at the interspace of vertebrae L3–L4 or lower, using aseptic technique. The fluid obtained is usually separated into three aliquots: (1) for chemistry and serology, (2) for bacteriology, and (3) for microscopy. It is paramount to remember that this matrix is of limited volume and should be analyzed immediately. Any remaining sample should be preserved because of its limited availability. The order of the tubes reflects the presumed order for minimalization of interference from less than optimal collection technique, with tube 3 presumably least contaminated by cells of intervening tissue.

Laboratory investigation of CSF is indicated for cases of suspected CNS infection, demyelinating disease, malignancy, and hemorrhage in the CNS. Historically, it is usually performed before radiologic procedures such as myelography, but the diagnostic utility in these cases is extremely small. As with all patient samples entering the laboratory, visual examination of the specimen is the first and often the most important observation made. The CSF, if normal, is clear, colorless, free of clots, and free of blood. Differences from these standards indicate a probable pathology and merit further examination. Cloudy fluids usually require microscopic examination, whereas a yellow to brown or red color may indicate blood.

The two most common reasons for blood and hemoglobin pigments to be found in CSF are traumatic tap and subarachnoid hemorrhage. Traumatic tap is the artifactual presence of blood or derivatives due to interdiction of blood vessels during the lumbar puncture. Hemorrhage results from a breakdown of the barrier of the CNS and circulatory system from trauma, for example. Obviously, the latter is serious. The two can be differentiated by observation and, possibly, testing. Bright red color and erythrocytes in decreasing number as the fluid is sampled indicate a traumatic tap. Xanthochromia or hemoglobin breakdown pigments indicate that erythrocyte lysis and metabolism have previously occurred, at least 2 hours earlier. Excluding a prior traumatic tap or hyperbilirubinemia (>20 mg/dL), xanthochromia would indicate hemorrhage.

Biochemical (chemical) analysis of CSF has led to compilations of the scope of possible constituents. In clinical practice, however, the number of useful indicators becomes small. The tests of interest are glucose, protein (total and specific), lactate, lactate dehydrogenase, glutamine, and the acid-base parameters. Most often used are glucose and proteins. Before any analysis, the fluid should be centrifuged to avoid contamination by cellular elements. The enzyme lactate dehydrogenase has been suggested as a tumor marker, but it is relatively nonspecific. It is also elevated in bacterial infection, although other parameters are more specific. The level of glutamine should reflect the level of CNS ammonia removed by glutamine formation from glutamate. This would be elevated in the hepatic encephalopathy of Reye's syndrome. The test has largely been supplanted by the relative ease and simplicity of reliable plasma ammonia determinations. Determination of the specific acid-base parameters obtained using a blood-gas instrument is relevant because of the vital environment of the CSF and the effect on control of respiration. The lack of buffering capacity of the CSF and the stringent requirements for sample integrity in the procedures for collection and analysis render routine usage of this series of tests impractical.

The tests that have been most reliable diagnostically and accessible analytically are those for CSF glucose, total protein, and specific proteins. Glucose enters the spinal fluid predominantly by a facilitative transport as compared with a passive (diffusional) or active (energy-dependent) transport. It is carried across the epithelial membrane by a stereospecific carrier species. The carrier mechanism is responsible for transport of lipid-insoluble materials across the membrane into the CSF. Generally, this is a "downhill" process consistent with a concentration gradient. The CSF glucose concentration is about two thirds that of plasma.

Because an isolated CSF glucose concentration may be misleading, it is recommended that a plasma sample be obtained at the same time, so that plasma and CSF glucose levels can be evaluated as a set. Normal CSF glucose is considered greater than 45 mg/dL (2.5 mmol/L). Increased glucose levels are not clinically informative, usually providing only confirmation of hyperglycemia. This generality must be tempered by two factors: (1) equilibration after glucose loading usually takes 3–4 hours; and (2) with increasing blood glucose levels, the CSF glucose increases, but not proportionally. The first is important in cases of meals taken close to the time of sampling. The second is significant because it implies that the plasma/CSF glucose ratio decreases as gross hyperglycemia occurs.

The decreasing CSF/plasma glucose ratio as plasma glucose increases is consistent with a saturable carrier process. It would not be unusual for the ratio to be 0.4:0.6 with massive plasma glucose levels (more than 600 mg/dL), but a CSF glucose level of 80 mg/dL, with plasma level of 300 mg/dL, is clinically significant and would merit concern.

Decreased CSF glucose levels (*hypoglycorrhachia*) can be the result of: (1) disorder in carrier-mediated transport of glucose into CSF, (2) active metabolism of glucose by cells or organisms, or (3) increased metabolism by the CNS. The mechanism of transport decrease is still under intense discussion, but it is speculated to be the cause in tuberculous meningitis and sarcoidosis. Acute purulent, amebic, fungal, and trichinotic meningitis are examples of consumption by organisms, whereas diffuse meningeal neoplasia and brain tumor are examples of consumption by CNS tissue. Consumption of glucose is usually accompanied by an increased lactate level because of anaerobic glycolysis by organisms or cerebral tissue. An increased lactate level with a normal to decreased glucose level has been suggested as a readily accessible indicator for bacterial versus viral meningitis.[12] Analysis of glucose and lactate in CSF is easily accomplished by techniques used for plasma and serum. It is important that provision for analysis of glucose or lactate in CSF be immediate or that the specimen be preserved with an antiglycolytic, such as fluoride ion.

Protein levels in CSF reflect both the selective ultrafiltration of the CSF epithelial barrier and their secretory ability. All protein usually found in plasma is found in CSF, except at much decreased levels. Total protein is about 0.5%, or $1/200$ that of plasma. The specific protein concentrations in CSF are not proportional to the plasma levels because of the specificity of the ultrafiltration process. Correlation is best accomplished using hydrodynamic ratios of the protein species rather than molecular weight. Because of the relationship of CSF proteins to serum, serum analysis should accompany specific CSF protein analysis. A decreased level of CSF total protein can arise from: (1) decreased dialysis from plasma; (2) increased protein loss (*eg*, removal of excessive volumes of CSF); or (3) leakage of CSF from a tear in the dura, otorrhea, or rhinorrhea. The last reason is most common. A dural tear can occur as a result of a previous lumbar puncture or

from severe trauma. *Otorrhea* and *rhinorrhea* refer to leakage of CSF from the ear or into the nose, respectively. Identification of the source of the leak is best done by an analysis for τ-transferrin, a protein unique to the CSF.

An increased level of CSF total protein is a useful nonspecific indicator of pathologic states. Increases may be caused by: (1) lysis of contaminant blood from traumatic tap, (2) increased permeability of the epithelial membrane, (3) increased production by CNS tissue, (4) obstruction, or (5) decrease in rate of removal. Contamination from blood is significant because of the 200:1 concentration ratio. The presence of any amount of blood can elevate CSF protein levels. The epithelial membrane becomes more permeable from bacterial or fungal infection or cerebral hemorrhage, whereas an increase in CNS production occurs in subacute sclerosing panencephalitis (SSPE) or multiple sclerosis (MS). There may also be combinations of permeability and production, such as the collagen-vascular diseases. An obstructive process, such as tumor or abscess, would also cause increased protein. The last mentioned cause of increased levels of CSF total protein, decreased absorption, is theoretically possible but has not been demonstrated.

Diagnostically more sensitive information can be obtained by analysis of the protein fractions present. A comparison to the serum pattern is necessary for accurate conclusions. Under normal conditions, prealbumin and a unique form of transferrin (τ protein) are present in CSF in higher concentration than in serum. Although the respective proteins can be determined in both serum and CSF, the proteins of greatest interest are albumin and immunoglobulin G (IgG). Because albumin is produced solely in the liver, its presence in CSF must occur by means of membrane transport. IgG, however, can arise by local synthesis from plasma cells within the CSF. The measurement of albumin in both serum and CSF is then used to normalize the IgG values from each matrix to determine the source of the IgG. This IgG–albumin index is primarily used to aid the diagnosis of demyelinating diseases, such as multiple sclerosis and SSPE. MS is the most common inflammatory demyelinating disease of the CNS.

$$\frac{\text{CSF IgG/serum IgG}}{\text{CSF albumin/serum albumin}} = \text{CSF index}$$

$$\text{Normal} = 0.5 \qquad \text{(Eq. 27-1)}$$

Increases in serum protein cause increases in the CSF levels because of permeability. However, increased CSF IgG, without concomitant CSF albumin increase, suggests local production (multiple sclerosis or SSPE). Increases in permeability and production are found with bacterial meningitis. Methods to analyze IgG and albumin CSF levels are the same as for serum but are optimized for the lower levels found.

A 32-year-old man was in good health until about 1 year ago, when he entered an accelerated computer programming training program. Within the last year, he began to notice episodic blurring of vision, mild vertigo, and headache. He attributed his complaints of sensory loss in his hands and a feeling of weakness after physical exertion to being "out of shape." He decided to see his physician after an attack of blurred vision accompanied by a feeling of paralysis, which was followed by pins and needles in his left leg. An optic examination was negative. Neurologic examination led to a spinal tap being performed for laboratory findings and myelography. The latter was negative. The laboratory results were as follows:

CSF	=	Clear, colorless fluid, apparently free of debris; culture yields no growth
WBC	=	Normal
Glucose	=	60 mg/dL (plasma = 80 mg/dL)
IgG/Alb ratio	=	1.7
IgG		Oligoclonal banding present

Questions

1. What is the significance of the normal CSF protein and variant IgG/Alb ratio?

2. What pathology is consistent with these results?

Increased CSF protein levels or clinical suspicion usually indicates the need for electrophoretic separation of the respective proteins. At times, this separation demonstrates multiple banding of the IgG band. This observation is referred to as *oligoclonal proteins* (a small number of clones of IgG from the same cell type with nearly identical electrophoretic properties). This occurrence is usually associated with inflammatory diseases and multiple sclerosis or SSPE. These types of disorders would stimulate the immunocompetent cells. The recognition of an oligoclonal pattern supersedes the report of normal protein levels and is cause for concern if the corresponding serum separation does not demonstrate identical banding.

Another protein thought to be specific for multiple sclerosis is myelin basic protein (MBP). Initial reports suggested high specificity, but MBP also has been found in nondemyelinating disorders and does not always occur in demyelinating disorders. MBP levels are used by some to monitor therapy of multiple sclerosis. Current international guidelines for the diagnosis of MS recognize both an elevated IgG Index and the presence of CSF oligoclonal bands different from serum as supporting evidence.

SWEAT

The common eccrine sweat glands function in the regulation of body temperature. They are innervated by cholinergic nerve fibers and are a type of exocrine gland. Sweat has been analyzed for its multiple inorganic and organic contents but, with one notable exception, has not proved a clinically useful model. That exception is the analysis of sweat for chloride and sodium levels in the diagnosis of cystic fibrosis (CF). The sweat test is the single most accepted common diagnostic tool for the clinical identification of this disease. Normally, the coiled lower part of the sweat gland secretes a "presweat" upon cholinergic stimulation. As the presweat traverses the ductal part of the gland going through the dermis, various constituents are resorbed. In CF, the electrolytes, most notably chloride and sodium ions, are improperly resorbed owing to a mutation in the cystic fibrosis transmembrane conductance regulator (CFTR) gene, which controls a cyclic AMP-regulated chloride channel.

CF (mucoviscidosis) is an autosomal recessive inherited disease that affects the exocrine glands and causes electrolyte and mucous secretion abnormalities. This exocrinopathy is present only in the homozygous state. The frequency of the carrier (heterozygous) state is estimated at 1 of 20 in the United States. The disease predominantly affects Caucasians. The observed rate of expression ranks CF as the most common lethal hereditary disease in the United States, with death usually occurring by the third decade. The primary cause of death is pneumonia, secondary to the heavy, abnormally viscous secretion in the lungs. These heavy secretions cause obstruction of the microairways, predisposing the CF patient to repeated episodes of pneumonia. The third part of the diagnostic triad is pancreatic insufficiency. Again, abnormally viscous secretions obstruct pancreatic ducts. This obstruction ostensibly causes pooling and autoactivation of the pancreatic enzymes. The enzymes then cause destruction of the exocrine pancreatic tissue.

Diagnostic algorithms for CF continue to rely on abnormal sweat electrolytes, pancreatic or bronchial abnormalities, and family history. The use of blood immunoreactive trypsin, a pancreatic product, has been proposed as both a method for newborn screening and a diagnostic adjunct. The rapidly developing area of molecular genetics provides the definitive methodology. The gene defect causing CF has been localized on chromosome 7, and the most common mutations causing CF have been DNA "fingerprinted." It is anticipated that within the next decade, direct DNA analysis will catalog all mutations and provide definitive screening and diagnosis. Although it has been reported that a form of CF with normal sweat chloride exists, the sweat chloride test remains the most accessible laboratory tool for CF discovery.[13]

The sweat glands, although affected in their secretion, remain structurally unaffected by CF. Analysis of sweat for both sodium and chloride is valid but, historically, chloride was and is the major element, leading to use of the sweat chloride test. Because of its importance, a standard method has been suggested by the Cystic Fibrosis Foundation. It is based on the pilocarpine nitrate iontophoresis method of Gibson and Cooke.[14] Pilocarpine is a cholinergic-like drug used to stimulate the sweat glands. The sweat is absorbed on a gauze pad during the procedure. Other tests (*eg*, osmolality or conductivity) that reflect the sodium and chloride concentrations have been proposed, but the sweat chloride test remains the reference method.

After collecting sweat by iontophoresis, chloride and sodium analysis is performed. Many methods have been suggested, and all are dependent on laboratory requirements. Generally, the sweat is leached into a known volume of distilled water and analyzed for chloride (chloridometer) and sodium (flame photometry). In general, values greater than 60 mmol/L are considered positive for both ions.

Although a value of 60 mmol/L is generally recognized for the quantitative pilocarpine iontophoretic test, it is important to consider several factors in interpretation. Not only will there be analytic variation around the cutoff, an epidemiologic borderline area will also occur. Considering this, the range of 45–65 mmol/L for chloride would be more appropriate in determining the need for repetition. Other variables must be considered. Age generally increases the limit—so much so that it is increasingly difficult to classify adults. Obviously, the patient's state of hydration also affects sweat levels. Because the complete procedure is technically demanding, expertise should be developed before the test is clinically available. A complete description of sweat collection and analysis, including procedural justifications, is available for review.[15]

SYNOVIAL FLUID

Joints are classified movable or immovable. The movable joint contains a cavity that is enclosed by a capsule; the inner lining of the capsule is synovial membrane. This cavity contains *synovial fluid,* which is formed by ultrafiltration of plasma across the synovial membrane. The membrane also secretes a mucoprotein rich in hyaluronic

acid into the dialysate, which causes the synovial fluid to be viscous. The membrane is composed of three different cell types: type A cells are rich in vacuoles and lysosomes and function as phagocytes; type B cells are rich in rough endoplasmic reticulum and presumed to be secretory in function; and type C cells appear to be hybrids of types A and B in appearance and function. Synovial fluid is assumed to function as a lubricant for the joints and as a transport medium for delivery of nutrients and removal of cell wastes. The volume of fluid found in a large joint, such as the knee, rarely exceeds 3 mL. Normal fluid is clear, colorless to pale yellow, viscous, and nonclotting. Variations are indicative of pathologic conditions.

Collection of a sample is accomplished by arthrocentesis of the joint under aseptic conditions. The sample should be preserved immediately with heparin for culture, with ethylenediaminetetraacetic acid (EDTA) for microscopic analysis, or with fluoride for glucose analysis. Microscopic examination is the most rewarding in diagnostic significance. Although many analytes have been chemically determined, the ratio of synovial fluid to plasma glucose (normally, 0.9:1) remains the most useful. Decreased ratios are found in inflammatory (*eg*, gout, rheumatoid arthritis, systemic lupus erythematosus) and purulent (bacterial, viral arthritis) conditions. Standard methods for glucose analysis are applicable.

SEROUS FLUIDS

The lungs, heart, and abdominal cavity are surrounded by single-celled, membranous, bilayered sacs permeable to serum constituents. When *serum* dialyzes across these membranes, the fluid formed is called *serous fluid;* specifically, pleural (lung), pericardial (heart), and peritoneal (abdominal) fluid.

Picture the sacs as a balloon containing a small amount of water. Push a football into the balloon, and the balloon expels the residual air until only water remains (Fig. 27-8). The water spreads to fill the resultant

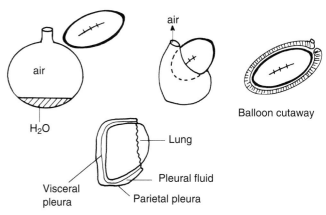

FIGURE 27-8. Example of serous fluid formation.

"balloon bilayer potential space." The serous membranes are analogous to the balloon; the internal organs, to the football. The pleural (lung) sac is continuous at the hilus of the bronchial tree; the pericardium, at the major vessels; and the peritoneum, around each organ. All are expandable and present "potential spaces" for fluid or gases to collect. The formation of serous fluid is a continuous process driven by the hydrostatic pressure of the systemic circulation and maintenance of oncotic pressure due to protein. The potential space is usually filled; that is, no gases are present. The fluid reduces or eliminates friction caused by expansion and contraction of the encased organs. A disturbance of the dynamic equilibrium that causes an increase in fluid is an abnormal state. An increase in fluid volume is called *effusion*.

Pleural Fluid

The outer layer of the pleural sac, the parietal layer, is served by the systemic circulation; the inner, visceral layer, by the bronchial circulation. Pleural fluid is essentially interstitial fluid of the systemic circulation. With normal conditions, there is 3–20 mL of pleural fluid in the pleural space. The fluid exits by drainage into the lymphatics of the visceral pleura and the visceral circulation. Any alteration in the rate of formation or removal of the pleural fluid affects the volume, causing an effusion. It is then necessary to classify the nature of the effusion by analysis of the pleural fluid. The fluid is removed from the pleural space by needle and syringe after visualization by radiology. This procedure is called *thoracentesis*; the fluid is called *thoracentesis fluid*, or *pleural fluid*. Specifically preserved aliquots of the fluid are used for future testing as follows: (1) heparinized for culture, (2) EDTA for microscopy, (3) sodium fluorescein (NaF) for glucose and lactate, and (4) untreated for further biochemical testing.

The classification of the fluid as transudate or exudate is crucial. *Transudates* are secondary to remote (nonpleural) pathology and indicate that treatment should begin elsewhere. An *exudate* indicates primary involvement of the pleura and lung, such as infection, and demands immediate attention. For example, any mechanical disturbance in the formation of fluid (*eg,* hypoproteinemia causing decreased oncotic pressure) would increase pleural fluid volume. This would be a transudative process. An exudative process would be the obstruction of the lymphatic drainage as a result of malignancy, such as lymphoma (Table 27-2). Further testing, including chemical, microscopy, and culture, is then required to identify the etiology.

The assignment of fluid to either the transudate or exudate category had previously been based on the protein concentration of the fluid. This criterion has been re-

TABLE 27-2. CAUSES OF PLEURAL EFFUSIONS

TRANSUDATIVE	EXUDATIVE
Congestive heart failure[a]	Bacterial pneumonia[a]
Nephrotic syndrome	Tuberculosis
Hypoproteinemia	Pulmonary abscess
Hepatic cirrhosis	Malignancy (lymphatic obstruction)
Chronic renal failure	Viral/fungal infection
	Pulmonary infarction
	Pleurisy
	Pulmonary malignancy
	Lymphoma
	Pleural mesothelioma

[a]Most common cause.

placed by the use of a series of fluid/plasma (F/P) ratios known as Light's criteria. Specifically, if the F/P for total protein is greater than 0.5, the ratio for lactate dehydrogenase (LD) is greater than 0.6, or if the pleural fluid LD/upper limit serum LD ratio reference interval is greater than 0.67, the fluid is an exudate. A serum albumin–pleural fluid albumin ratio (albumin gradient of ≥1.2) usually indicates transudates. However, this criteria misidentifies about 10% of cases, particularly congestive heart failure. Further characterization of the exudate by the chemistry laboratory may involve analysis for glucose, lactate, amylase, triglyceride, or pH. A decrease in glucose (increase in lactate) would suggest infection or inflammation. An increase in amylase compared with that of serum suggests pancreatitis. Grossly elevated triglyceride levels (2–10 × serum) could indicate chylothorax. The use of pH measurements, performed as one would a blood-gas level determination, has gained favor. Succinctly, pH less than 7.2 suggests infection, and pH greater than 7.4 suggests malignancy. The methodologies for these analyses are the same as those employed for the serum and blood constituents and, therefore, are feasible in the clinical laboratory.

Pericardial Fluid

The relationship of the pericardium, *pericardial fluid,* and the heart is similar to that with the lungs. Mechanisms of formation and drainage are the same; however, pericardial sampling and laboratory analysis is rare.

Peritoneal Fluid

The clinical questions to be answered are usually as follows: (1) What is causing ascites? (2) Is infection present? (3) Is there risk for infection?[16]

Excess fluid (>50 mL) in the peritoneal cavity indicates disease. The excess fluid is called *ascites,* and the fluid is called *ascitic fluid.* The process of obtaining samples of this fluid by needle aspiration is *paracentesis.* Usually, the fluid is visualized by ultrasound to confirm its presence and volume before paracentesis is attempted.

Theoretically, the same mechanisms that cause serous effusions in other potential spaces are operative for the peritoneal cavity. Specifically, a disturbance in the rate of dialysis secondary to a primary, remote pathology is a transudate, as compared with a primary pathology of the peritoneal membrane (exudate). The multiple factors that apply to this large space, including renal function, tend to cloud the distinction. The most common cause of ascites with a normal peritoneum is portal hypertension. Obstructions to hepatic flow, such as cirrhosis, congestive heart failure, and hypoalbuminemia for any reason, demonstrate the highest incidence.

The exudative causes of ascites are predominantly metastatic ovarian cancer and infective peritonitis. The differentiation of the two is analogous to the measures of protein and LD described for pleural fluid. The ability to differentiate, however, has been challenged. The serum-ascites albumin gradient (SAAG, or serum albumin–fluid albumin) of 1.1 g/dL or more used to indicate portal hypertension is the most accepted measurement. A neutrophil count greater than 0.5×10^9/liter indicates peritonitis.

SUMMARY

In addition to serum and plasma, the clinical chemistry laboratory often analyzes other body fluids, such as AF, CSF, sweat, synovial fluid, and serous fluids. AF provides a cushioning medium for fetal development.

Amniocentesis and subsequent AF analysis are performed to test for congenital disease, neural tube defects, hemolytic disease, gestational age, and fetal pulmonary development. CSF is a liquid that occupies the spaces of the CNS, which includes the brain and spinal cord. Functions of the CSF include physical support and protection, method of excretion, provision of a controlled chemical environment, and intracerebral and extracerebral transport. The total volume of CSF is about 150 mL.

Specimens of CSF are obtained by lumbar puncture. Laboratory investigation of CSF is indicated for cases of suspected CNS infection, demyelinating disease, malignancy, and hemorrhage in the CNS. The tests most reliable diagnostically and accessible analytically are those for CSF glucose, total protein, and specific proteins. Sweat is a product of the common eccrine sweat glands, which function in the regulation of body temperature. The sweat test is the most accepted diagnostic tool for CF. Within the movable joint, is a cavity filled with synovial fluid, which is formed by ultrafiltration of plasma across the synovial membrane. Normal fluid is clear, colorless to pale yellow, viscous, and nonclotting. Any variations are indicative of pathologic conditions. Collection of this fluid is accomplished by arthrocentesis. The lungs, heart, and abdominal cavity are surrounded by a single-celled, membranous, bilayered sac, which is permeable to serum constituents.

The fluid formed when serum dialyzes across these membranes is serous fluid; specifically, pleural (lung), pericardial (heart), and peritoneal (abdominal) fluids. Formation of serous fluid is a continuous process and driven by the hydrostatic pressure of the systemic circulation and maintenance of oncotic pressure due to protein. Under normal conditions, there is 3–20 mL of pleural fluid in the pleural space. Removal of the fluid is called thoracentesis. The relationship of the pericardium and pericardial fluid with the heart is similar to that with the lungs; pericardial sampling in the laboratory is rare. An excess of fluid in the peritoneal cavity indicates disease. This is called ascites. The fluid is ascitic fluid and is obtained by a procedure called paracentesis.

REVIEW QUESTIONS

1. Laboratory testing for assessment of fetal lung maturity is based on:
   a. differentiation products of type I pneumocytes.
   b. production of acetylcholinesterase.
   c. production of AFP.
   d. products of type II pneumocytes.
   e. presence of meconium.

2. Amniotic fluid:
   a. provides a cushion for the fetus.
   b. is a mixture of maternal and fetal fluids.
   c. is assessed by umbilical catheterization.
   d. a and b.
   e. a, b, and c.

3. Lamellar body counts reflect:
   a. platelet count of the fetus.
   b. platelet count of the mother.
   c. meconium count of the fetus.
   d. surfactant phospholipid packets.
   e. all of the above.

4. Blood in CSF is commonly observed after:
   a. administration of indocyanine green.
   b. traumatic tap.
   c. hemolytic anemia.
   d. lumbar puncture.
   e. low pH.

5. CSF glucose is measured to access:
    a. transport efficiency.
    b. diabetes.
    c. traumatic tap.
    d. hemochromatosis.
    e. infection.

6. Increased CSF protein is pathognomonic for:
    a. multiple sclerosis.
    b. collagen vascular disease.
    c. fungal infection.
    d. all of the above.
    e. none of the above.

7. CF is characterized by:
    a. elevated sweat chloride levels.
    b. homozygous expression of an autosomal recessive trait.
    c. pancreatic insufficiency.
    d. all of the above.
    e. a and c only.

8. Synovial fluid:
    a. is formed by plasma ultrafiltration.
    b. lubricates the pneumocytes.
    c. is rich in hyaluronic acid.
    d. all of the above.
    e. a and c only.

9. Serous fluids:
    a. are derived from serum.
    b. provide lubrication and protection.
    c. fill the potential space.
    d. all of the above.
    e. a and b only.

10. Pleural fluid transudate:
    a. reflects primary involvement of the pleura.
    b. is characterized by an increased LD F/P ratio.
    c. is characterized by an increased glucose F/P ratio.
    d. is characterized by a total protein F/P ratio of 0.5.
    e. all of the above.

11. Analysis of paracentesis fluid is performed to:
    a. determine cause of fluid presence.
    b. assess infection risk.
    c. determine lung involvement.
    d. all of the above.
    e. a and b.

12. The most common cause of ascites is:
    a. portal hypertension.
    b. venous return.
    c. parietal cell differentiation.
    d. eccrine infection.
    e. type A cell leakage.

REFERENCES

1. Liley AW. Liquor amnil analysis in the management of the pregnancy complicated by rhesus sensitization. Am J Obstet Gynecol 1961;82:1359.
2. Kulovich MV, Hallman MB, Gluck L. The lung profile. I. Normal pregnancy. Am J Obstet Gynecol 1979;135:57.
3. Statland BE, Freer DE. Evaluation of two assays of functional surfactant in amniotic fluid: surface-tension lowering ability and the foam stability index test. Clin Chem 1979;25:1770.
4. Clements JA, Plataker ACG, Tierney DF, et al. Assessment of the risk of the respiratory distress syndrome by a rapid test for surfactant in amniotic fluid. N Engl J Med 1972;286:1077.
5. Gluck L, Kulovich MV, Borer RC Jr, et al. Diagnosis of the respiratory distress syndrome by amniocentesis. Am J Obstet Gynecol 1971;109:440.
6. Tsai MY, Marshall JG. Phosphatidylglycerol in 261 samples of amniotic fluid from normal and diabetic pregnancies, as measured by one-dimensional thin layer chromatography. Clin Chem 1979;25:682.
7. Herbert WNP, Chapman JF, Schnoor MM. Role of the TDX FLM assay in fetal lung maturity. Am J Obstet Gynecol 1993;168:808.
8. Kaplan LA, Chapman JT et al. Prediction of respiratory distress syndrome using the Abbot FLM II amniotic fluid assay. Clin Chem Acta 2002;326:61–68.
9. Neerhof ME, Dohnal JC, Ashwood ER, et al. Lamellar body counts: a consensus on protocol. Obstet Gynecol 2001;97(2):318–320.
10. Assessment of Fetal Lung Maturity. ACOG Educational Bulletin, No. 230, November 1996.
11. Field NT, Gilbert WM. Current status of amniotic fluid tests of fetal lung maturity. Clin Obstet Gynecol 1977;40(2):366–386.
12. Bailey EM, Domenico P, Cunha BA. Bacterial or viral meningitis. Postgrad Med 1990;88:217.
13. Highsmith WE, Burch L, Zhou Z, et al. A novel mutation in the cystic fibrosis gene in patients with pulmonary disease but normal sweat chloride concentrations. N Engl J Med 1994;331:974.
14. Gibson LE, Cooke RE. A test for concentration of electrolytes in cystic fibrosis of the pancreas utilizing pilocarpine by iontophoresis. Pediatrics 1959;23:545.
15. NCCLS. Sweat testing: Sample collection and quantitative analysis approved guidelines. NCCLS Document C34-A2. Villanova, PA: National Committee for Clinical Laboratory Standards, 2000.
14. Habeeb, KS, Herrera, JL. Management of ascites: paracentesis as a guide. Postgrad Med 1997;101(1):191–2, 195–200.

SUGGESTED READINGS

American Society of Human Genetics. Policy statement for maternal serum alpha-fetoprotein screening programs and quality control for laboratories performing maternal serum and amniotic fluid alpha-fetoprotein assays. Am J Hum Genet 1987;40:75.

Brown LM, Duck-Chong CG. Methods of evaluating fetal lung maturity. Crit Rev Clin Lab Sci 1982;17(1):85.

Committee for a Study of Evaluation of Testing for Cystic Fibrosis. Report. J Pediatr 1976;88(4):711.

Daveson H. Physiology of the Cerebrospinal Fluid. London: Churchill, 1967.

Fairweather DVI, Eskes TKAB, eds. Amniotic Fluid Research and Clinical Application, 2nd ed. New York: Excerpta Medica, 1978.

Freeman JA, Beeler MF, eds. Laboratory Medicine/Urinalysis and Medical Microscopy, 2nd ed. Philadelphia: Lea & Febiger, 1983.

Freer DE, Statland BE. Measurement of amniotic fluid surfactant. Clin Chem 1981;27:1629.

Guyton AC. Textbook of Medical Physiology, 5th ed. Philadelphia: WB Saunders, 1976.

Halsted JA, Halsted CH, eds. The Laboratory in Clinical Medicine, 2nd ed. Philadelphia: WB Saunders, 1981.

Health and Public Policy Committee, American College of Physicians. Diagnostic thoracentesis and pleural biopsy in pleural effusions. Ann Intern Med 1985;103:799.

Platt PN. Examination of synovial fluid in the role of the laboratory in rheumatology. Clin Rheum Dis 1983;9(1):51.

Queenan JT, ed. Modern Management of the Rh Problem, 2nd ed. Hagerstown, MD: Harper & Row, 1977.

Rocco VK, Ware AJ. Cirrhotic ascites. Ann Intern Med 1986;105:573.

Rodriguez EM, van Wimersma Greidanus TB. Cerebrospinal fluid and peptide hormones. In: Frontiers of Hormone Research. New York: S Karger, 1982:9.

Russell JC, Cooper CC, Ketchum CH, et al. Multicenter evaluation of TDX test for assessing fetal lung maturity. Clin Chem 1989;35:1005.

Teloh HA. Clinical pathology of synovial fluid. Ann Clin Lab Sci 1975;5(4):282.

Webster HL. Laboratory diagnosis of cystic fibrosis. Crit Rev Clin Lab Sci 1983;18(4):313.

Wiswell TE, Mediola J Jr. Respiratory distress syndrome in the newborn: innovative therapies. Am Fam Physician 1993;47:407.

Wood JH, ed. Neurobiology of the Cerebrospinal Fluid, Vol 2. New York: Plenum Press, 1983.

Specialty Areas of Clinical Chemistry

CHAPTER 28

Therapeutic Drug Monitoring

David P. Thorne

OBJECTIVES

Upon completion of this chapter, the clinical laboratorian should be able to:

- Discuss the characteristics of a drug that make therapeutic drug monitoring essential.
- Identify the factors that influence the absorption of an orally administered drug.
- Relate the factors that influence the rate of drug elimination.
- Define drug distribution and the factors that influence it.

- Calculate volume of distribution, elimination constant, and drug half-life.
- Relate the concentration of a circulating drug to pharmacokinetic parameters.
- Name the therapeutic category of each drug presented in this chapter.
- Describe the major toxicities of the drugs presented in this chapter.
- Identify the features of each drug presented in this chapter that may influence their serum drug concentration.

KEY TERMS

Drug absorption
Drug distribution
Drug elimination

Peak drug level
Pharmacokinetics

Therapeutic drug
  monitoring

Therapeutic range
Trough drug levels

Therapeutic drug monitoring (TDM) involves the analysis, assessment, and evaluation of circulating concentrations of drugs in serum, plasma, or whole blood. The purpose of these actions is to ensure that a given drug dosage produces maximal therapeutic benefit and minimal toxic adverse effects.[1,2] For most drug therapies, dosage regimens have been established that are safe and effective in most of the population, therefore, TDM is unneeded. With certain drugs, however, the correlation between dosage and therapeutic effects or toxic outcomes is weak and it is difficult to predict what dose should be used. In these situations, trial and error, in conjunction with direct observation, may work. For example, if a standard drug dose does not display therapeutic benefit and increasing the dose does provide benefit without toxic effects, an appropriate dosage adjustment has been made. Unfortunately, this system may be inappropriate in all situations. If overdosing or underdosing results in severe consequences to the patient, trial and error is not justified. If this is the case, TDM based on strong correlations between circulating concentrations of drug and therapeutic benefit or toxic adverse effects assists in the determination of an appropriate dosage regimen. The standard dosage is statistically derived from observations in a healthy population.[2] Disease states may produce altered physiologic conditions in which the standard dose does not produce the predicted concentration in circulation.[3] In these cases, individualizing a dosage regimen is warranted.[4] Again, TDM provides a basis for establishing a rational dosage regimen to fit individual situations.[5]

The following are the common indications for TDM:

- The consequences of overdosing and underdosing are serious.
- There is a small difference between a therapeutic and toxic dose.
- There is a poor relationship between the dose of drug and circulating concentrations but a good correlation between circulating concentrations and therapeutic or toxic effects.
- There is a change in the patient's physiologic state that may unpredictably affect circulating drug concentrations.
- A drug interaction is or may be occurring.
- TDM helps in monitoring patient compliance.

A common feature of all aspects of TDM is the quantitative evaluation of circulating concentrations of drugs. When taken together with clinical context, this provides a basis for rational problem solving and optimizing patient outcomes.[6] This process requires that several key factors be taken into consideration, such as the route of administration, rate of absorption, distribution of drug within the body, and rate of elimination (Fig. 28-1). This chapter begins by focusing on these factors and how they influence the circulating concentration of a drug. The re-

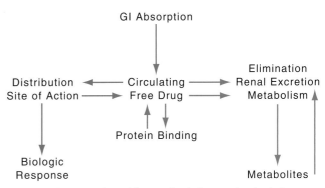

FIGURE 28-1. Overview of factors that influence the circulating concentration of an orally administered drug. *GI,* gastrointestinal.

mainder of the chapter surveys selected drugs commonly subject to TDM.

ROUTES OF ADMINISTRATION

For a drug to express a therapeutic benefit, it must be at the appropriate concentration at its site of action. Measuring drug concentration at the site of action would be ideal. Unfortunately, for most drugs, this can't be done. The circulatory system offers a convenient route that can effectively deliver most drugs to its site of action. The goal of most therapeutic regimens is to acquire a blood, plasma, or serum concentration that has been correlated with an effective concentration at the site of action. Drugs can be administered by several routes. Each presents with different characteristics that influence circulating concentrations. Drugs can be injected directly into the circulation (intravenous, IV), into muscles (intramuscular, IM), or just under the skin (subcutaneous, SC). They can also be inhaled or absorbed through the skin (transcutaneous). Rectal delivery (suppository) is commonly used in infants and in situations in which oral delivery is unavailable. Oral administration is the most common route of delivery. The focus of the current discussion is on oral and IV administration.

ABSORPTION

For orally administered drugs, the efficiency of *absorption* from the gastrointestinal tract is dependent on many factors. The formulation of the drug is a key issue. Tablets and capsules require dissolution before being absorbed. Liquid solutions have a tendency to be more rapidly absorbed. Some drugs are subject to uptake by transport mechanisms intended for dietary constituents; however, most are absorbed by passive diffusion. This process requires that the drug be in a hydrophobic (nonionized) state. Because of gastric acidity, weak acids are efficiently absorbed in the stomach. Weak bases are preferentially absorbed in the intestine, where the pH is more neutral. For most drugs, absorption from the gastrointestinal tract occurs in a predictable manner in healthy people. However, changes in intestinal motility, pH, inflammation, as well as food or other drugs may dramatically change absorption characteristics.[7] In these cases, the use of TDM may assist in establishing an effective dosage regime.

All substances, including drugs, absorbed from the intestine (except the rectum) enter the hepatic portal system. In this system, all the blood from the gastrointestinal tract is routed through the liver before it enters into general circulation. Certain drugs are subject to significant hepatic uptake and metabolism during this passage through the liver. This process is known as *first-pass metabolism.*[8]

For certain drugs, there may be a wide degree of variance in these processes, even within a normal population. In addition, many of the absorptive characteristics of a drug may change with age, pregnancy, or pathologic conditions. In these instances, predicting the final circulating concentration from a standard oral dose can be difficult. With the use of TDM, however, effective oral dosage regimens can be determined.

FREE VERSUS BOUND DRUGS

Most drugs in circulation are subject to binding with serum constituents. Although many potential species may be formed, most are drug–protein complexes. An important aspect needed to understand drug dynamics is that only the free fraction can interact with its site of action and result in a biologic response. It is the free fraction that best correlates with both the therapeutic and toxic effects of a drug. For many drugs, the percentage free is dependent on physiologic and biochemical parameters. At a standard dose, total plasma content may be within the *therapeutic range,* but the patient experiences toxic adverse effects (high free fraction) or does not realize a therapeutic benefit (low free fraction). This may occur secondary to changes in serum protein content. Changes in serum-binding proteins may occur during inflammation, malignancies, pregnancy, hepatic disease, nephrotic syndrome, and malnutrition. The percentage free may also be influenced by the concentration of substances that compete for binding sites, which may be other drugs or endogenous substances, such as urea, bilirubin, or hormones. Free drug measurements should be considered for drugs that are highly protein bound and for which clinical signs are inconsistent with total drug concentrations.

DRUG DISTRIBUTION

The free fraction of circulating drugs is subject to diffusion out of the vasculature into interstitial and intracellular spaces. The ability to leave circulation is largely dependent on the lipid solubility of the drug. Drugs that are highly hydrophobic can easily traverse cellular membranes and partition into lipid compartments, such as adipose and nerve cells. Drugs that are polar but not ionized also cross cell membranes but do not sequester into lipid compartments. Ionized species diffuse out of the vasculature but at a slow rate. The volume of distribution (V_d) index is used to describe the distribution characteristics of a drug. It is expressed mathematically as follows:

$$V_d = D/C_t \qquad \text{(Eq. 28–1)}$$

where: V_d = volume of distribution (in liters),
$\quad$ D = an injected dose (milligrams [mg] or grams [g]),
$\quad$ C = concentration in plasma (mg/L or g/L)

Drugs that are hydrophobic can have a large V_d. Substances that are ionized or are primarily bound in plasma have small V_d values.

DRUG ELIMINATION

Drugs can be cleared from the body by various mechanisms. Independent of the clearance mechanism, decreases in the serum concentration of drugs most often occur as a first-order process (exponential rate of loss). This implies that the rate of change of drug concentration over time varies continuously in relation to the concentration of the drug. First-order elimination follows the following general equation:

$$\Delta C/\Delta T = -kC \qquad \text{(Eq. 28–2)}$$

This equation defines how the change in concentration per unit time ($\Delta C/\Delta T$) is directly related to the concentration of drug (C) and the constant (k). The k value is a simple proportionality factor that describes the percentage change (negative because it is decreasing) per unit time; it is commonly referred to as the *elimination constant* or the *rate of elimination.* The graphic solution to this equation is an exponential function that declines in the predicted curvilinear manner, asymptotically approaching zero (Fig. 28-2). The graph shown in Figure 28-2 illustrates a rapid rate of change at high drug concentrations and slow rates of change at low drug concentrations. Plotting it in semilogarithmic dimensions (Fig. 28-3) can linearize this function.

Hepatic metabolism or renal filtration, or a combination of the two, eliminates most drugs. For certain drugs, elimination by these routes is highly variable. In addition, functional changes in these organs may result in changes in the rate of elimination. In these situations, information regarding elimination rate and estimating the circulating concentration of a drug after a given time period are important factors in establishing an effective and safe dosage regimen. Equation 28-2 and Figures 28-2 and 28-3 are useful in determining the rate of elimination and the concentration of a drug after the time period. The following equation illustrates how the equation is used.

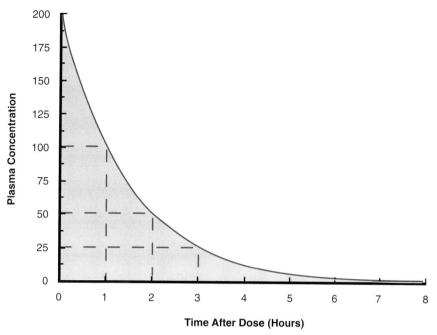

FIGURE 28-2. First-order drug elimination. This graph demonstrates exponential rate of loss on a linear scale. *Hash-marked lines* are representative of half-life.

Integration of Equation 28-2 yields the following:

$$C_T = C_0 e^{-kT} \qquad \textbf{(Eq. 28–3)}$$

where: C_0 = the initial concentration of drug,
$\quad$ C_T = the concentration of drug after the time period (T),
$\quad$ k = the elimination constant, and
$\quad$ T = the time period evaluated.

This is the most useful form of the elimination equation. From it, we can calculate the elimination constant or, if k is known, we can determine the amount of drug that will be present after a certain time period.

Example:

The concentration of gentamicin is 10 μg/mL at 12:00. At 16:00, the gentamicin concentration is 6 μg/mL. What is the elimination constant (k) for gentamicin in this patient?

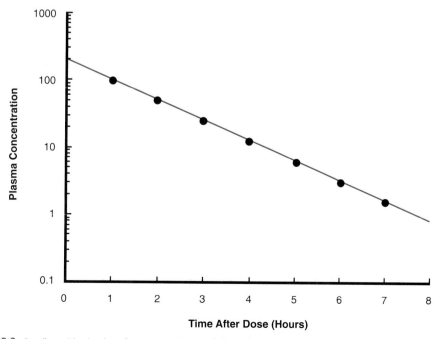

FIGURE 28-3. Semilogarithmic plot of exponential rate of drug elimination. The slope of this plot is equal to the rate of elimination (k).

Using Equation 28-3:

$C_0 = 10$

$C_T = 6$

$T = 4$ hours

Substituting these values into the equation produces:

$6 = 10\,e^{-k\,(4\text{ hours})}$

Dividing both sides by 10 produces:

$0.6 = e^{-k\,(4\text{ hours})}$

To eliminate the exponential sign, we would take the natural logarithm of both sides:

$\ln 0.6 = -k\,(4\text{ hours})$

Solving the natural log:

$-0.51 = -k\,(4\text{ hours})$

Multiplying through by -1:

$0.51 = k\,(4\text{ hours})$

Dividing both sides by 4 hours:

$0.13/h = k$

This calculated value for k indicates the patient is eliminating 13% of serum gentamicin per hour.

In this same patient on the same day, what would be the predicted serum concentration of gentamicin at midnight (24:00)?

For C_0, we can use either the 12:00 or 16:00 value as long as the correct corresponding time value is used. In this example, we will use the 16:00 value of 6 μg/mL.

$C_0 = 6$ μg/mL

$T = 8$ hours

$k = 0.13/h$

Substituting into Equation 28-3:

$C_T = 6\,e^{-0.13/\text{hour}\,(8\text{ hours})}$

Solving for the exponent:

$C_t = 6\,e^{-1.04}$

Note that the time unit (hours) has canceled. Solving for the exponent:

$C_T = 6\,(0.35)$

$C_t = 2.1$ μg/mL

Note that the concentration units have carried through.

Although the elimination constant (k) is a useful value, it is not common nomenclature in the clinical setting. Instead, the term *half-life* is used. This represents the time needed for the serum concentration to decrease by one half. It can be determined graphically (Fig. 28-2) or by conversion of the elimination constant (k) to half-life ($T_{1/2}$) using the formula given in Equation 28-4. Of these two methods, the calculation provides an easy and accurate way to determine half-life.

$$T_{1/2} = 0.693/k \qquad \textbf{(Eq. 28–4)}$$

Metabolic Clearance

Xenobiotics are substances not normally found within human systems, yet capable of entering biochemical pathways intended for endogenous substances. Most drugs are xenobiotics. There are many potential biochemical pathways in which drugs can be acted on. The biochemical pathway responsible for a large portion of drug metabolism is the hepatic mixed function oxidase (MFO) system. The basic function of this system involves taking hydrophobic substances and, through a series of enzymatic reactions, converting them into water-soluble substances. These products are then either pumped into the bile or released into the general circulation, where they are eliminated by renal filtration.

There are many enzymes involved in the MFO system. They are commonly divided into two functional groups or phases. Phase I reactions produce reactive intermediates. Phase II reactions conjugate functional groups to these reactive sites, the products of which are water soluble. The reactive intermediates can be conjugated with various functional groups; glutathione, glycine, phosphate, and sulfate are common. The MFO system is a nonspecific system that allows many different endogenous and exogenous substances to go through this series of reactions. Although there are many potential substrates for this pathway, the products formed from an individual substance are specific. For example, acetaminophen is a substrate for MFO and always forms a glutathione conjugate. In addition, if the conjugating group for a given drug becomes depleted, the phase I products continue to be produced. In this situation, accumulation of phase I products may result in toxic adverse effects.

It is also noteworthy that the MFO system is inducible. This is seen as an increase in the synthesis and activity of the rate-limiting enzymes within this pathway. The most common inducers are xenobiotics that are substrates for this pathway. Certain drugs may stimulate their own rate of elimination. Due to biologic variability in the degree of induction, TDM could again assist in establishing an appropriate dosage regime.

Because many potential substrates can enter the MFO system, many drug–drug interactions occur within this pathway.[9] Competitive and noncompetitive interactions may occur. This results in altered rates of elimination of the involved drugs.[10] In most instances, the degree of alteration in unpredictable. Again the value of TDM is apparent.

Implied in this discussion are that changes in hepatic status can result in changes in the concentration of circulating drugs eliminated by this pathway.[11] Induction of the MFO system typically results in accelerated clearance and a corresponding shorter half-life. In the opposite manner, hepatic disease states characterized by a loss of functional tissue may result in slow rates of clearance and corresponding longer half-lives.[8] In these situations, TDM aids in dosage adjustment.

For some drugs, there is considerable variance in the rate of hepatic and nonhepatic drug metabolism within a normal population. This results in a highly variable rate of clearance, even in the absence of disease. Establishing dosage regimens for these drugs is, in many instances, aided by the use of TDM. With the use of molecular genetics, it is now possible to identify common genetic variants of some drug-metabolizing pathways.[12] Identification of these individuals may assist in establishing an individualized dosage regimen.

Renal Clearance

The plasma free fraction of parent drugs or their metabolites is subject to glomerular filtration, renal secretion, or both.[13] For those drugs not secreted or subject to reabsorption, the elimination rate of free drug directly relates to the creatinine clearance rate. Decreases in glomerular filtration rate directly results in increased serum half-life and concentration. The aminoglycoside antibiotics and cyclosporine are examples of drugs with this behavior.

PHARMACOKINETICS

Pharmacokinetics is the mathematic modeling of drug concentration in circulation. This process assists in establishing or modifying a dosage regimen. It takes into consideration all factors that determine the concentration of a serum drug and its rate of change. Many factors previously discussed in this chapter would be included in this field of study. Figure 28-3 is an idealized plot of elimination after an IV bolus. It assumes there is no distribution of this drug. A drug that does distribute outside of vascular space would produce an elimination graph such as in Figure 28-4. The rapid rate of change seen immediately after the initial IV bolus is a result of distribution and elimination. The rate of elimination (k) can only be determined after distribution is complete. Figure

28-5 is a plot of serum concentration as it would appear after oral administration of a drug. As absorbed drug enters the circulation, it is subject to simultaneous distribution and elimination. Serum concentrations rise when the rate of absorption exceeds distribution and elimination. The concentration declines as the rate of elimination and distribution exceeds absorption. The rate of elimination can only be determined after absorption and distribution are complete.

Most drugs are not administered as a single bolus but are delivered on a scheduled basis (*eg,* once every 8 hours). With this type of administration, serum drug concentration oscillates between a maximum (*peak drug level*) and a minimum (*trough drug level*). The goal of a multiple dosage regimen is to achieve a trough that is in the therapeutic range and a peak that is not in the toxic range. Evaluation of this oscillating function cannot be done immediately after initiation of a scheduled dosage regimen. About seven doses are required before a steady state oscillation is acquired. The basis of this number (seven doses) is demonstrated in Figure 28-6.

After the first oral dose, absorption and distribution occur, followed only by elimination. Before the concentration of drug drops significantly, the second dose is given. The peak of the second dose is additive to what remained from the first dose. Because elimination is first order, the higher concentration produces an increased rate of elimination. The third through seventh scheduled doses all have the same effect, increasing serum concen-

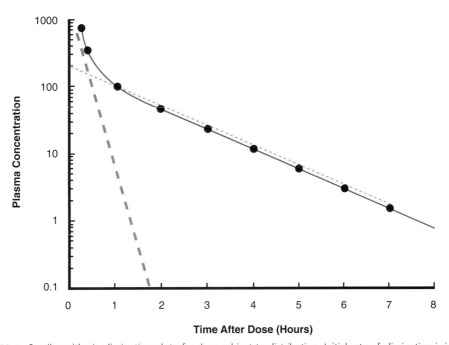

FIGURE 28-4. Semilogarithmic elimination plot of a drug subject to distribution. Initial rate of elimination is influenced by distribution *(dashed line)* and terminal elimination rate *(dotted line)*. After distribution is complete (1.5 hours), elimination is first order.

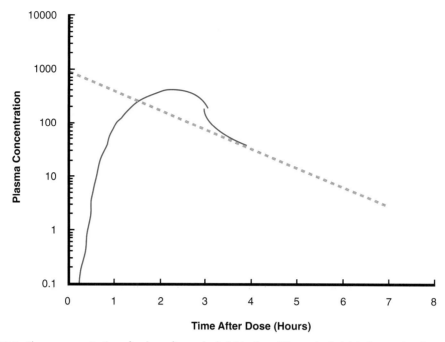

FIGURE 28-5. Plasma concentration of a drug after oral administration. After oral administration at time 0, serum concentration increases *(solid line)* after a brief lag period. Plasma concentrations peak when rate of elimination and distribution exceed rate of absorption. First-order elimination *(dotted line)* occurs when absorption and distribution are complete.

tration and the rate of elimination. By the end of the seventh dose, the amount of drug administered in a single dose is equal to the amount eliminated during the dosage period. At this point, steady state is established and peak and trough concentrations can be evaluated.

SAMPLE COLLECTION

Timing of specimen collection is the single most important factor in TDM. In general, trough concentrations for most drugs are drawn right before the next dose; peak

concentrations are drawn 1 hour after an orally administered dose. This rule of thumb must always be used within the clinical context of the situation. A commonly used drug that is an exception to this rule is digoxin. Drugs that are absorbed slowly may require several hours before peak drug levels can be evaluated. In all situations, determination of serum concentrations should be done only after steady state has been achieved.

Serum or plasma is the specimen of choice for the determination of circulating concentrations of most drugs. Care must be taken that the appropriate container is used

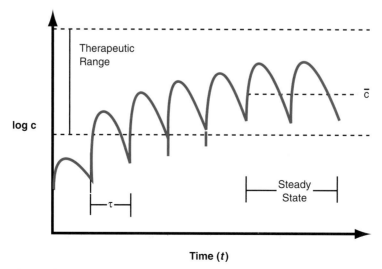

FIGURE 28-6. Steady-state kinetics in a multiple-dosage regimen. The character τ indicates the dosage interval. Equal doses at this interval reach steady state after 6 or 7 dosage intervals. $\bar{c}$, mean drug concentration.

when collecting these specimens. Certain drugs have a tendency to be absorbed into the gel of certain serum separator collection tubes. It is necessary to follow vendor recommendations when this effect is possible. Failure to do so may result in falsely low values. Heparinized plasma is suitable for most drug analysis. The calcium-binding anticoagulants add a variety of anions and cations that may interfere with analysis or cause a drug to distribute differently between cells and plasma. As a result, ethylenediaminetetraacetic acid (EDTA), citrated and oxalated plasma are not usually acceptable specimens.

CARDIOACTIVE DRUGS

Many cardiac conditions are treated with drugs. Of these drugs, only a few require TDM.[14] The cardiac glycosides and the antiarrhythmics are two classes of drugs for which assessment of serum concentration aids in decisions regarding their dosage regimen.[15]

Digoxin

Digoxin is a cardiac glycoside used in the treatment of congestive heart failure.[16] It functions by inhibiting membrane Na^+-K^+-ATPase. This causes a decrease in intracellular potassium, resulting in increased intracellular calcium in cardiac myocytes. The increased calcium im-

proves cardiac contractility (inotropic effect). This effect is seen in the serum concentration range of 0.8–2 ng/mL. Higher serum concentrations (3 ng/mL) decrease the rate of ventricular depolarization. Although this level can be used to control ventricular tachycardia, it is done infrequently because of toxic adverse effects that become apparent at serum concentrations of greater than 2 ng/mL. Digoxin toxicity affects many organ and cell types. Nausea, vomiting, and visual disturbances are common. Cardiac effects, such as premature ventricular contractions (PVCs) and atrioventricular node blockage, are also common.

Absorption of orally administered digoxin is variable. It is influenced by dietary factors, gastrointestinal motility, and the formulation of the drug. In circulation, about 25% is protein bound. The nonbound (free) form of serum digoxin is sequestered into muscle cells. At equilibrium, the tissue concentration is 15–30 times greater then plasma. Elimination of digoxin occurs primarily by renal filtration of the plasma free form. The remainder is metabolized to several products by the liver. The half-life of plasma digoxin is 38 hours in an average adult. The major contributing factor to the half-life is the slow release of tissue digoxin back into circulation.

Because of variable gastrointestinal absorption of digoxin, establishing a dosage regimen usually requires

---

CASE STUDY 28-1

A patient with congestive heart failure has been successfully treated with digoxin for several years. Laboratory records indicate semiannual peak digoxin levels have all been in the therapeutic range. This patient recently developed renal failure, and admission testing was performed. Selected serum or blood laboratory results from this specimen are shown in Case Study Table 28-1.1. Although digoxin is high, the physician indicates the patient is not exhibiting signs or symptoms of toxicity.

Questions

1. If these results were derived from a random specimen, how may the time since the last dose effect the interpretation of the digoxin results?

2. Other than time, what additional factors should be taken into consideration when interpreting the digoxin results?

3. What additional laboratory test would aid in the interpretation of this case?

CASE STUDY TABLE 28-1.1. LABORATORY RESULTS

TEST	RESULT	REFERENCE RANGE
Sodium	129	135–145 mEq/L
Potassium	5.5	3.5–5 mEq/L
Chloride	113	97–107 mEq/L
Blood pH	7.25	7.35–7.45
TCO_2	16	21–31 mmol/L
Urea Nitrogen	180	5–20 mg/dL
Creatinine	4.5	0.6–1 mg/dL
Osmolality	275	282–300 mOsm/kg
Digoxin	2.5	0.9–2 ng/mL

assessment of serum concentrations after initial dosing to ensure that effective and nontoxic serum concentrations are achieved.[17] In addition, changes in glomerular filtration rate can have a dramatic effect on serum concentration; frequent dosage adjustments, in conjunction with serum levels, need to be done in patients with renal disease. The therapeutic actions and toxicities of digoxin can be influenced by the concentration of serum electrolytes. Low serum potassium and magnesium potentiate digoxin actions. In these conditions, adjustment of serum concentrations below the therapeutic range may be necessary to avoid toxicity. Thyroid status may also influence digoxin actions. Hyperthyroid patients display a resistance to digoxin actions; hypothyroid patients are more sensitive.

The timing for evaluation of peak digoxin levels is crucial. In an average adult, serum levels peak between 2 and 3 hours after an oral dose. However, uptake into tissue is a relatively slow process. As a result, peak serum concentrations do not correlate with tissue concentrations. It has been established that the serum concentration 8 hours after an orally administered dose correlates with tissue concentration, therefore, peak levels are usually evaluated at this time. Peak levels collected before this time are misleading and not valid.

Immunoassay is used to measure total digoxin concentration in serum. With most commercial assays, cross-reactivity with hepatic metabolites is minimal; however, newborns, pregnant women, and patients with uremia or late-stage liver disease produce an endogenous substance that cross-reacts with the antibodies used to measure serum digoxin.[18] In patients with these digoxin-like immunoreactive substances, falsely elevated concentrations are common.

Lidocaine

Lidocaine is used to correct ventricular arrhythmia and to prevent ventricular fibrillation. This is particularly important in patients with acute myocardial infarction. Lidocaine cannot be administered orally due to almost complete hepatic removal of the absorbed drug (first-pass metabolism). Lidocaine is commonly delivered by continuous intravenous infusion after a loading dose; therefore, plasma levels remain relatively constant during administration. The primary reasons for monitoring plasma lidocaine concentration are to ensure it is in the therapeutic range of 1.5–4 μg/mL and to avoid toxicity, which exists just above the therapeutic range. Plasma lidocaine in the range of 4–8 μg/mL is associated with central nervous system depression. Plasma concentrations greater then 8 μg/mL are associated with seizures and severe decreases in blood pressure and cardiac output. Lidocaine is primary eliminated by hepatic metabolism. The concentration of plasma lidocaine is dependent on the rate of administration and the rate of hepatic clearance. Changes in renal function have little effect on plasma lidocaine. The primary product of hepatic metabolism of lidocaine is monoethylglycinexylidide (MEGX). Although this substance has little therapeutic activity, its toxicity is additive to the parent drug. The sum of lidocaine and MEGX must be taken into consideration when evaluating possible toxic reactions. Lidocaine and MEGX can be assayed by chromatography or immunoassay. Many lidocaine assays also measure MEGX. Consult the method description in the package insert or operator's manual.

Quinidine

Quinidine is a naturally occurring drug that can be used to treat various cardiac arrhythmic situations.[19] The two most common formulations are quinidine sulfate and quinidine gluconate. Oral administration is the most common route of delivery. Gastrointestinal absorption is complete and rapid for the sulfate. Peak serum concentrations are reached about 2 hours after an oral dose of the sulfate. The gluconate is a slow-release formulation. Peak serum concentration is reached 4–5 hours after an oral dose. The most predominant toxic adverse effects of quinidine are nausea, vomiting, and abdominal discomfort. Cardiovascular toxicity, such as PVCs, may be seen at twice the upper limit of the therapeutic range. In most instances, monitoring of quinidine involves only determination of the trough level to ensure it is within the therapeutic range. Peak assessment is performed only when symptoms of toxicity are present. Because of its slow rate of absorption, trough levels of the gluconate are usually drawn 1 hour after the last dose.

Absorbed quinidine is about 70% bound to serum proteins. Most is eliminated by hepatic metabolism. Induction of this system, such as by barbiturates, increases the clearance rate. Impairment of this system, as seen in late-stage liver disease, may extend the half-life of this drug. Plasma quinidine concentration can be determined by chromatography or immunoassay.

Procainamide

Like quinidine, procainamide is used to treat cardiac arrhythmia. Oral administration is the most common. Gastrointestinal absorption is rapid and complete. Peak plasma concentrations occur at about 1 hour. Absorbed procainamide is about 20% bound to plasma proteins. It is eliminated by a combination of renal filtration and hepatic metabolism. N-acetyl procainamide (NAPA) is an hepatic metabolite of the parent drug, with antiarrhythmic activity similar to procainamide. The total antiarrhythmic potential of this drug must take into consideration the parent drug and this metabolite. Alteration in either renal or hepatic function may lead to increased

A patient is receiving procainamide for treatment of cardiac arrhythmia. An intravenous loading dose resulted in a serum concentration of 6.0 μg/mL. The therapeutic range for procainamide is 4–8 μg/mL, and its half-life is 4 hours. Four hours after the initial loading dose, another equivalent dose was given as an intravenous bolus. This resulted in a serum concentration of 7.5 μg/mL.

Questions

1. Does the serum concentration after the second dose seem appropriate? If not, what would be the predicted serum concentration at this time?

2. What factors would influence the rate of elimination of this drug?

serum concentration of the parent drug and its metabolites. Increased concentration results in myocardial depression and arrhythmia.[20] Both procainamide and its active metabolite can be measured by immunoassay.

Disopyramide

Disopyramide is another drug used to treat cardiac arrhythmias. It is commonly used as a quinidine substitute when quinidine adverse effects are excessive. It is most commonly administered as an oral preparation. Gastrointestinal absorption is complete and rapid. It binds to several plasma proteins. Binding is highly variable within individuals and is concentration dependent: as serum concentration increases, so does the percentage free. As a result, it is difficult to correlate total serum concentration with therapeutic benefit and toxicity. In most patients, total serum concentrations in the range of 3–5 μg/mL have been determined to be effective and nontoxic; however, interpretation of disopyramide results should take the clinical perspective into consideration. The primary toxicities of disopyramide are dose dependent. Anticholinergic effects, such as dry mouth and constipation, may be seen at serum concentrations greater than 4.5 μg/mL. Cardiac effects, such as bradycardia and atrioventricular node blockage, are usually seen at serum concentrations greater than 10 μg/mL. Disopyramide is primarily eliminated by renal filtration and, to a lesser extent, by hepatic metabolism. In conditions with low glomerular filtration rate, the half-life is prolonged and serum concentrations rise. Plasma disopyramide concentration can be determined by chromatography or immunoassay.

ANTIBIOTICS[21]

Aminoglycosides

Aminoglycosides are a group of chemically related antibiotics used for the treatment of infections with gram-negative bacteria that are resistant to less toxic antibiotics. There are many individual agents within this classification. The most commonly encountered in a clinical setting are gentamicin, tobramycin, amikacin, and

kanamycin.[22] All share a common mechanism of action but vary in effectiveness against different strains of bacteria. All share a common nephrotoxicity and ototoxicity. The ototoxic effect involves disruption of inner ear cochlear and vestibular membranes, which results in hearing and balance impairment.[23] These effects are irreversible. Cumulative effects may be seen with repeated high-level exposure. Nephrotoxicity is also of major concern. Aminoglycosides impair the function of proximal tubules of the kidney, which may result in electrolyte imbalance and possibly proteinuria. These effects are usually reversible; however, extended high-level exposure may result in necrosis of these cells and subsequent renal failure. Toxic concentrations are usually considered any concentration above the therapeutic range.

Because aminoglycosides are not well absorbed from the gastrointestinal tract, administration is limited to the IV or IM route, therefore, these drugs are not used in an outpatient setting. Aminoglycosides are eliminated by renal filtration. In patients with compromised renal function, appropriate adjustments must be made based on serum concentrations. Chromatography and immunoassay are the primary methods used for aminoglycoside determinations.

Vancomycin

Vancomycin is a glycopeptide antibiotic that is effective against gram-positive cocci and bacilli. Because of poor oral absorption, vancomycin is administered by IV infusion. Unlike other drugs, a clear relationship between serum concentration and toxic adverse effects has not been firmly established. Indeed, many of the toxic effects occur in the therapeutic range (5–10 μg/mL). The major toxicities of vancomycin are red-man syndrome, nephrotoxicity, and ototoxicity. Red-man syndrome is characterized by an erythemic flushing of the extremities. The renal and hearing effects are similar to those of the aminoglycosides. It appears that the nephrotoxic effects occur more frequently at trough concentrations that are greater than 10 μg/mL. The ototoxic effect occurs more frequently when peak serum concentrations exceed

40 µg/mL. Because vancomycin has a long distribution phase, in most instances, only trough levels are monitored to ensure the serum drug concentration is within the therapeutic range.[24] Vancomycin is primarily eliminated by renal filtration and excretion. It is assayed by immunoassay and chromatographic methods.

ANTIEPILEPTIC DRUGS

Epilepsy, convulsions, and seizures are prevalent neurologic disorders. Because these drugs are used as prophylactics, therapeutic ranges are considered guidelines. Effective concentrations are determined as the concentration that works with no or acceptable adverse effects.[25] Most antiepileptic drugs are analyzed by immunoassay or chromatography.

Phenobarbital

Phenobarbital is a slow-acting barbiturate that effectively controls several types of seizures. Absorption of oral phenobarbital is slow but complete. For most patients, peak serum concentration is reached about 10 hours after an oral dose. Circulating phenobarbital is 50% bound. It is eliminated primarily by hepatic metabolism. However, renal filtration is also significant. With compromised renal or hepatic function, the rate of elimination is decreased. The half-life of serum phenobarbital is 70–100 hours. Because of the slow absorption and long half-life, serum concentrations do not change dramatically within a dosing interval. Therefore, only trough levels are usually evaluated unless toxicity is suspected. Toxic adverse effects of phenobarbital include drowsiness, fatigue, depression, and reduced mental capacity.

Phenobarbital clearance occurs by the hepatic MFO system. It is noteworthy that it is also a potent inducer of this system. After initiation of therapy, dose adjustment is usually required after the induction period is complete. For most individuals, this is 10–15 days after the first dose

Primidone is an inactive proform of phenobarbital. After absorption of an oral dose, this drug is rapidly converted to its active form, phenobarbital. Primidone is used in preference of phenobarbital when steady state kinetics need to be established quickly. Primidone is rapidly absorbed and converted to the active drug. Both primidone and phenobarbital need to be measured to assess the total potential amount of phenobarbital in circulation.

Phenytoin

Phenytoin (Dilantin) is used to treat seizure disorders. It is also used as a short-term prophylactic agent in brain injury to prevent loss of functional tissue. Phenytoin is primarily administered as an oral preparation. Gastrointestinal absorption is variable and sometimes incomplete. Circulating phenytoin has a high but variable degree of protein binding (87–97%). Like most drugs, the unbound (free) fraction is the biologically active portion of total serum concentration. Reduced protein binding may occur with anemia, with hypoalbuminemia, and with other drugs. Toxicity may be observed when the total serum drug concentration is within the therapeutic range. The major toxicity of phenytoin is initiation of seizures. Seizures in a patient being treated with phenytoin may be a result of subtherapeutic or toxic levels. Additional adverse effects of phenytoin include hirsutism, gingival hyperplasia, vitamin D, and folate deficiency. Phenytoin is eliminated by hepatic metabolism in a unique manner. At therapeutic concentrations, this elimination pathway may become saturated (zero-order kinetics). Therefore, relatively small changes in dosage or elimination may have dramatic effects on plasma concentration.

CASE STUDY 28-3

A child, who has been successfully treated for seizure disorders with oral phenytoin for several years, has had severe diarrhea for the past 2 weeks. Subsequent to this, the patient had a seizure. Evaluation of serum phenytoin at the time of the seizure revealed a low value. The dose was increased until serum concentrations were within the therapeutic range. The diarrhea was resolved. Several days after this, the patient had another seizure.

Questions

1. What is the most probable cause of the initial low serum phenytoin?

2. Would determination of free serum phenytoin aid in resolving the cause of the initial seizure?

3. What assays other than the determination of serum phenytoin would aid in this situation?

4. What is the most probable cause of the seizure after the diarrhea has been resolved?

For most patients, total serum concentrations of 10–20 g/mL are effective. In many situations, however, the effective range of total serum concentration must be individualized to suit the clinical situation. The therapeutic range for free serum phenytoin is 1–2 μg/mL. This has been well correlated with the pharmacologic actions of this drug. In patients with altered serum protein binding, determination of the free fraction aids in dosage adjustment.

Fosphenytoin is an injectable proform of phenytoin that is rapidly metabolized in serum, releasing the parent drug.[26] It takes about 75 minutes for this conversion to take place. Most immunoassays for phenytoin do not detect this proform. Thus, peak levels should be evaluated only after the conversion to the active drug is complete.

Valproic Acid

Valproic acid is used for the treatment of petit mal and absence seizures.[27] It is administered as an oral preparation. Gastrointestinal absorption is rapid and complete. Circulating valproic acid is highly protein bound (93%). The percentage bound decreases in renal failure, in late liver disease, and with other drugs that may compete for its binding site. It is eliminated by hepatic metabolism. The therapeutic range for valproic acid is relatively wide (50–120 μg/mL). Determination of serum concentration is primarily done to ensure that toxic levels (more than 120 μg/mL) are not present. Nausea, lethargy, and weight gain are the most common adverse effects. Pancreatitis, hyperammonemia, and hallucinations have been associated with high serum levels (more than 200 μg/mL). Hepatic dysfunction occasionally occurs in some patients even at therapeutic serum concentrations, therefore, hepatic indicators should be checked frequently for the first 6 months after initiation of therapy. Many factors may influence the nonbound (free) fraction of total serum valproic acid. Therefore, determination of the free fraction provides a more reliable index of therapeutic and toxic concentrations.

Carbamazepine

Carbamazepine is an effective treatment in various seizure disorders. Because of its serious toxic adverse effects, it is less frequently used, except when patients do not respond to other drugs. Orally administered carbamazepine is absorbed with a high degree of variability. Circulating carbamazepine is 70–80% protein bound. It is eliminated primarily by hepatic metabolism. Many forms of liver dysfunction may result in serum accumulation. Carbamazepine is an inducer of its own metabolism. Thus, frequent plasma levels must be analyzed on initiation of therapy until the induction period has come to completion.

Carbamazepine toxicity is diverse and variable. Certain effects occur in a dose-dependent manner; others do not. There are several idiosyncratic effects of carbamazepine, which effect a portion of the population at therapeutic concentrations, including rashes, leukopenia, nausea, vertigo, and febrile reactions. Of these, leukopenia is the most serious. Leukocyte counts are commonly done during the first 2 weeks of therapy to detect this possible toxic effect. Liver function testing is also done during this period. Mild, transient liver dysfunction is commonly seen during this period. Large and persistent increases in liver indices or a significant leukopenia commonly result in discontinuation of the drug. The therapeutic range for carbamazepine is 4–12 μg/mL.[28] Plasma concentrations greater than 15 μg/mL are associated with hematologic dyscrasias and possible aplastic anemia.

Ethosuximide

Ethosuximide is used for control of petit mal seizure. It is administered as an oral preparation. The therapeutic range is 40–100 μg/mL. The toxicities associated with high plasma concentrations are rare, tolerable, and self-limiting. TDM of ethosuximide is done to ensure that serum concentrations are in the therapeutic range.

PSYCHOACTIVE DRUGS

Lithium

Lithium is an orally administered drug used to treat manic-depression (bipolar disorder). Absorption is complete and rapid. Lithium is a cationic metal that does not bind to proteins. Distribution is uniform throughout the total body water. It is eliminated predominately by renal filtration and is subject to reabsorption. Compromises in renal function usually result in accumulation. Correlations between serum concentration and therapeutic response have not been well established. However, serum concentrations in the range of 0.8–1.2 mmol/L are effective in a large portion of the patient population. The purpose of TDM for lithium is to avoid serum concentrations associated with toxic effects.[29] Serum concentrations in the range of 1.2–2 mmol/L may cause apathy, lethargy, speech difficulties, and muscle weakness. Serum concentrations greater then 2 mmol/L are associated with muscle rigidity, seizures, and possible coma. Determination of serum lithium is commonly done by ion-selective electrode. Flame emission photometry and atomic absorption are also viable methods.

Tricyclic Antidepressants

Tricyclic antidepressants (TCAs) are a class of drugs used to treat depression, insomnia, extreme apathy, and loss of libido. From a clinical laboratory perspective, imipramine, amitriptyline, and doxepin are the most relevant.[24] Desipramine and nortriptyline are active metabolic products of imipramine and amitriptyline, respectively, and must also be included. The TCAs are orally administered drugs with a variable degree of absorption. In many patients, they slow gastric emptying and intestinal motility, which significantly slows their rate of absorption. As a result, peak serum concentrations are reached in the range of 2–12 hours.

The TCAs are highly protein bound (85–95%). For most TCAs, the therapeutic effects are not seen for the first 2–4 weeks after initiation of therapy. The correlations between serum concentration and therapeutic effects of most TCAs are moderate to weak. They are eliminated by hepatic metabolism. Many of the metabolic products formed have therapeutic actions. The rate of metabolism of these agents is variable and influenced by a wide variety of factors. As a result, the half-life of TCAs varies considerably among patients. The rate of elimination can also be influenced by the coadministration of other drugs that are eliminated by hepatic metabolism. The toxicity of TCAs are dose dependent. At serum concentrations about twice the upper limit of the therapeutic range, drowsiness, constipation, blurred vision, and memory loss are common adverse effects. Higher levels may cause seizure, cardiac arrhythmia, and unconsciousness.

Because of the high variability in half-life and absorption, plasma concentrations of the TCAs should not be evaluated until a steady state has been achieved. At this point, therapeutic efficacy is determined from clinical evaluation of the patient, and potential toxicity is determined by serum concentration. Many of the immunoassays for TCAs use polyclonal antibodies, which cross-react among the different TCAs and their metabolites. In this analytic system, the results are reported out as "total tricyclics." Other immunoassays use an extraction step to separate parent drugs from the metabolites. Interpretation of these results after extraction requires an in-depth understanding of the assay. Chromatographic methods provide simultaneous evaluation of both the parent drugs and metabolites, which provides a basis for unambiguous interpretation of results.[30]

BRONCHODILATORS

Theophylline

Theophylline is used in the treatment of asthma and other chronic obstructive pulmonary diseases. It is effective in both acute situations and prophylactically. In acute asthma attacks, theophylline therapy is usually initiated intravenously and then changed to oral administration. Oral theophylline is absorbed completely but at a variable rate, which is dependent on the formulation of the drug and dietary factors. Absorbed theophylline is

50% protein bound in plasma. It is eliminated by a combination of renal filtration and hepatic metabolism. Small changes in serum protein content and glomerular filtration rate have little influence on plasma concentrations. The primary reason for monitoring serum theophylline is to ensure that concentrations are not in the toxic range. The therapeutic range for theophylline is 10–20 μg/mL. Toxic effects are noted at serum concentrations greater the 20 μg/mL. Symptoms of toxicity include nausea, vomiting, and diarrhea. Serum concentrations greater than 30 μg/mL are associated with cardiac arrhythmia, seizures, and a poor prognosis.

IMMUNOSUPPRESSIVE DRUGS

Transplantation medicine is a rapidly emerging discipline within clinical medicine. The clinical laboratory plays many important roles that determine the success of any transplantation program.[31] Among these responsibilities, monitoring of the immunosuppressive drugs used to prevent rejection is of key concern. Most of these drugs require establishment of individual dosage regimens to optimize therapeutic outcomes and minimize toxicity.[32]

Cyclosporine

Cyclosporine is a cyclic polypeptide that has potent immunosuppressive activity. Its primary clinical use is suppression of host-versus-graft rejection of heterotopic transplanted organs. It is administered as an oral preparation. Absorption of cyclosporine is in the range of 5–50%. Because of this high variability, the relationship between oral dose and blood concentration is poor, therefore, TDM is an important part of establishing an initial dosage regime. Circulating cyclosporine sequesters in cells, including erythrocytes. Erythrocyte content is highly temperature dependent; therefore, evaluation of plasma concentration requires rigorous control of specimen temperature. To avoid this preanalytic variable, whole blood is the specimen of choice. Correlations have been established between whole blood concentration and therapeutic and toxic effects. Cyclosporine is eliminated by hepatic metabolism to inactive products.

Immunosuppression requirements differ depending on the organ transplanted. Cardiac, liver, and pancreas transplants have the highest requirement (300 ng/mL). Whole blood concentrations in the range of 350–400 ng/mL have been associated with toxic effects. The toxic effects of cyclosporine are primarily renal tubular and glomerular dysfunction, which may result in hypertension. Several immunoassays are available for determination of whole blood cyclosporine concentration. Many cross-react with inactive metabolites. Chromatographic methods are available; they provide separation and quantitation of the parent drug from metabolites.

Tacrolimus

Tacrolimus (FK-506) is an orally administered immuno-suppressive drug that is 100 times more potent than cyclosporine; therefore, the dosage is far less than that of cyclosporine.[33] Early use of tacrolimus suggested a low degree of toxicity compared with cyclosporine at therapeutic concentrations. However, after extensive use in clinical practice it has been demonstrated that both have comparable degrees of nephrotoxicity at therapeutic concentrations. At concentrations above therapeutic, tacrolimus has been associated with thrombus formation.

Many aspects of tacrolimus pharmacokinetics are similar to cyclosporine. Gastrointestinal uptake is highly variable. Whole blood concentrations correlate well with therapeutic and toxic effects. Tacrolimus is eliminated almost exclusively by hepatic metabolism. Metabolic products are primarily secreted into the bile. Increases in immunoreactive tacrolimus may be seen in cholestasis as a result of cross-reactivity with several of these products. Because of the high potency of tacrolimus, circulating therapeutic concentrations are low. This limits the methodologies capable of measuring whole blood concentrations. The most original method is HPLC/MS; however, several immunoassays are also available.[34]

ANTINEOPLASTICS

Assessment of therapeutic benefit and toxicity of most antineoplastic drugs is not aided by TDM because correlations between plasma concentration and therapeutic benefit are hard to establish.[35] Many of these agents are rapidly metabolized or incorporated into cellular macromolecular structures within seconds to minutes of their administration. In addition, the therapeutic range for many of these drugs includes concentrations associated with toxic effects. Considering that most antineoplastic agents are administered IV as a single bolus, the actual delivered dose is more important than circulating concentrations.

Methotrexate

Methotrexate is one of the few antineoplastic drugs in which TDM offers benefits to a therapeutic regimen.[36] High-dose methotrexate followed by leucovorin rescue has been shown to be an effective therapy for various neoplastic conditions. The basis of this therapy involves the relative rate of mitosis of normal versus neoplastic cells. In general, neoplastic cells divide more rapidly than normal cells. Methotrexate inhibits DNA synthesis in all cells. Neoplastic cells, as a result of their rapid rate of division, have a higher requirement for DNA and are susceptible to depravation of this essential constituent before normal cells. The efficacy of methotrexate therapy is dependent on a controlled period of inhibition, one

that is selectively detrimental to neoplastic cells. This is accomplished by administration of leucovorin, which reverses the actions of methotrexate at a specific time after methotrexate infusion. This is referred to as *leucovorin rescue*. Failure to stop methotrexate actions results in cytotoxic effects to most cells. Evaluation of serum methotrexate concentration, after the inhibitory time period has passed, is used to determine how much leucovorin is needed to counteract many of the toxic effects of methotrexate.

SUMMARY

TDM is a process used to generate indices that are used as the basis for establishing a rational, individualized drug regimen to ensure optimal patient outcomes.[37] For most drugs, this process is unneeded. Standardized dosage regimes, which are statistically derived from a healthy population, provide therapeutic benefit without toxicity the majority of the time. However, the standardized dose does not work in all situations; the following are a few examples:

- Drugs that produce severe adverse effects at dosages close to those which result in therapeutic benefit. In these instances, trial and error may be an inappropriate method to establish a safe and effective dosage regimen. This is especially true if the drug is administered orally and if the rate of drug absorption is highly variable.
- Standard drug dosages predict circulating concentrations in healthy, average people. For individuals who vary from these characteristics, adsorption, distribution and elimination may be unpredictable. Monitoring serum concentrations of these drugs when establishing a dosage regimen is an important component of therapy with these agents.
- Many drugs are subject to biotransformation (metabolism). For most drugs, the products of these reactions are neither toxic nor pharmacologically active. However, if metabolic products are active or toxic, these must be taken into consideration.

Although only several prescribed drugs are commonly subject to TDM, the scope of this field is expanding as toxic effects become better defined and therapeutic ranges are further refined. An additional advantage of TDM is it allows for the safe use of drugs that would otherwise be unusable. This expands the drugs available to treat disease and, in many instances, improves patient care.[38]

The basic principles of TDM, which address absorption, distribution, and elimination, can also be applied to nontherapeutic substances that have entered the body.[39] Indeed, the use of these concepts is central to the study of poisons.

REVIEW QUESTIONS

1. Drug X has a half-life ($T_{1/2}$) of 2 days. The concentration at noon today is 10 μg/mL. What would be the expected concentration of drug X at noon tomorrow?
   a. 7.5 μg/mL
   b. 7 μg/mL
   c. 5 μg/mL
   d. 3.5 μg/mL

2. Salicylic acid is a common component of many over-the-counter drugs. In a patient suffering from gastric achlorhydria, what would be the predicted serum concentration of this drug after a standard dose?
   a. Greater then expected
   b. Less then expected
   c. No change

3. Which of the following drugs would be correctly classified as an antiepileptic?
   a. Digoxin
   b. Disopyramide
   c. Chloramphenicol
   d. Phenytoin
   e. Tacrolimus

4. Of the following, what would be the most appropriate time for evaluation of a peak digoxin level after oral administration?
   a. Immediately before the next dose
   b. Immediately after a dose
   c. 8 hours after a dose
   d. 3 days after a dose

5. Of the following statements concerning lidocaine, which is/are TRUE?
   a. Lidocaine is only administered as an oral preparation.
   b. Phenobarbital is one of the products of lidocaine metabolism.
   c. The toxicity of lidocaine is related to the concentration of the parent drug and one of its metabolites—MEGX.
   d. All of the above are true.
   e. Only a and c are true.

6. Of the following statements concerning procainamide, which is/are TRUE?
   a. Procainamide is an antibiotic.
   b. N-Acetylprocainamide is an active product of procainamide metabolism.
   c. The primary toxicity of procainamide is bone marrow suppression.
   d. All of the above are true.
   e. Only a and c are true.

7. Of the following statements concerning lithium, which is/are TRUE?
   a. Lithium is an element.
   b. Lithium is used as a drug to treat depression and mania.
   c. Lithium concentration in serum is most commonly evaluated by ion-specific electrode.
   d. All of the above are true.
   e. Only a and c are true.

8. What is the purpose for the determination of serum concentrations of the antineoplastic drug methotrexate?
   a. To ensure that serum concentrations are in the therapeutic range
   b. To ensure that serum concentrations are not in the toxic range
   c. To determine the amount of leucovorin needed to halt methotrexate action
   d. All of the above
   e. Only a and c

9. I am an immunosuppressive drug used to control host-versus-graft rejection of transplanted organs. Renal toxicity is my primary problem. I am commonly assayed by chromatographic techniques using whole blood as the specimen. What am I?
   a. Cyclosporine
   b. Carbamazepine
   c. Tacrolimus
   d. Any of the above
   e. Either a or c

10. A patient, who has been successfully receiving gentamicin for the past 2 weeks, has suddenly developed a renal condition in which glomerular filtration rate has significantly decreased. What would be the expected adjustment in dosage in response to this?
    a. The dosage should be increased.
    b. The time interval between dosages should be increased.
    c. Phenobarbital should be coadministered to stimulate hepatic metabolism.
    d. No dosage adjustment is required.
    e. The drug should be discontinued.

11. Salicylate and bilirubin compete for the same binding site on serum albumin. What effect would prehepatic jaundice have on salicylate?
    a. An increase in the rate of clearance of salicylate
    b. A decrease in the pharmacologic response to salicylate
    c. An increase in the free concentration of salicylate
    d. All of the above
    e. Only a and c

12. A drug with a small volume of distribution:
    a. is confined to the vasculature.
    b. diffuses out of the vasculature into interstitial space.
    c. diffuses out of the vasculature into intracellular space.
    d. selectively partitions into the fatty compartment.
    e. is rapidly eliminated in exhaled breath

13. Twenty milligrams of a drug is injected intravenously. One hour after injection, blood is drawn and assayed for the drug. The concentration in this specimen was 0.4 mg/L. What is the volume of distribution for this drug?
    a. 0.8 L
    b. 8 L
    c. 20 L
    d. 50 L
    e. Unable to determine with the data provided

14. A new orally administered drug has been introduced in your institution. It is unclear whether TDM is needed for this drug. What factors should be taken into consideration when addressing this question?
    a. Consequences of a subtherapeutic concentration in circulation
    b. Severity of toxic adverse effects
    c. Predictability of serum concentrations after a standard oral dose
    d. Proximity of toxic range to therapeutic range
    e. All of the above should be taken into consideration

REFERENCES

1. Gentry CA, Rodvold KA. How important is TDM in the prediction and avoidance of adverse reactions? Drug Saf 1995;12:359–363.
2. Jelliffe R. Goal-oriented, model-based drug regimens: setting individualized goals for each patient. Ther Drug Monit 2000;22:325–329.
3. Walson PD. Therapeutic drug monitoring in special populations. Clin Chem 1998;44:415–419.
4. Marshall A. Laying the foundations for personalized medicines. Nat Biotechnol 1997;15:954–957.
5. Schumacher GE, Barr JT. Total testing process applied to therapeutic drug monitoring: impact on patient outcomes and economics. Clin Chem 1998;44:370–374.
6. Tonkin AL, Bocher F. Therapeutic drug and patient outcomes: a review of the issues. Clin Pharmacokinet 1994;27:169–174.
7. Feldman EB. How grapefruit juice potentiates drug bioavailability. Nutr Rev 1997;55:398–400.
8. Kwan KC. Oral bioavailability and the first-pass effect. Drug Metab Dispos 1997;25:1329–1336.
9. Fraser AG. Pharmacokinetic interactions between alcohol and other drugs. Clin Pharmacokinet 1997;33:79–90.
10. Tucker GT, Advances in understanding drug metabolism and its contribution to variability in patient response. Ther Drug Monit 2000;22:110–113.
11. Huet PM, Villeneuve JP, Fenyves D. Drug elimination in chronic liver disease. J Hepatol 1997;26(Suppl 2):63–72.
12. Kalow W. Pharmacogenetics. Pharmacol Rev 1997;49:369–379.
13. Ibrahim S, Honig P, Huang SM, Gillespie W, et al. Clinical Pharmacology studies in patients with renal impairment: past experiences and regulatory perspective. J Clin Pharmacol 2000;40:7–10.
14. Valdes R, Jortani SA, Gheorhiade M. Standards of laboratory practice: cardiac drug monitoring. National Academy of Clinical Biochemistry. Clin Chem 1998;44:1096–1109.
15. Keyler DE, VanDeVoort JT, Howard JE, et al. Monitoring blood levels of selected drugs: remember to factor in many confounding variables. Postgrad Med 1998;103:209–212, 215–219.
16. Cohn JN. Overview of the treatment of heart failure. Am J Cardiol 1997;80:2L–6L.
17. Caufield JS, Gums JG, Grauer K. The serum digoxin concentration: ten questions to ask. Am Fam Physicians 1997;56:495–503.
18. Jortani SA, Valdes R. Digoxin and its related endogenous factors. Crit Rev Clin Lab Sci 1997;34:225–274.
19. Grace AA, Camm AJ. Quinidine. N Engl J Med 1998;338:35–45.
20. Kolecki PF, Curry SC. Poisoning by sodium channel blocking agents. Crit Care Clin 1997;13:829–848.
21. Hammett CA, Johns T. Laboratory guidelines for monitoring antimicrobial drugs. National Academy of Clinical Biochemistry. Clin Chem 1998;44:1129–1140.
22. Beggs EJ, Barclay ML. Aminoglycosides: 50 years on. Br J Clin Pharmacol 1995;39:597–603.
23. Priuska EM, Schacht J. Mechanism and prevention of aminoglycocide ototoxicity. Ear Nose Throat J 1997;76:164–171.
24. Andres I, Lopex R, Pou L, et al. Vancomycin monitoring: one or two serum levels? Ther Drug Monit 1997;19:614–619.
25. Schwabe SK, Challenges in the clinical development of new antiepileptic drugs. Ther Drug Monit 2002;24(1):81–84.
26. Luer MS. Fosphenytoin. Neurol Res 1998;20:178–182.
27. Sundqvist A, Tomson T, Lundkvist B. Valproate as monotherapy for juvenile myoclonic epilepsy: dose effect study. Ther Drug Monit 1998;20:149–157.
28. Bialer M, Levy RH, Perucca E. Does carbamazepine have a narrow therapeutic plasma concentration range? Ther Drug Monit 1998;20:56–59.
29. Linder MW, Keck PE. Standards of laboratory practice: antidepressant drug monitoring. National Academy of Clinical Biochemistry. Clin Chem 1998;44:1073–1084.
30. Schatzberg AF, Pharmacological principles of antidepressant efficacy. Human Psychopharmacol 2002;(Suppl 2):17–22.
31. Cronin DC, Faust TW, Brady, L et al. Modern immunosuppression. Clin Liver Dis 2000;4:619–655.
32. Shaw LM, Kaplan B, Kaufman D. Toxic effects of immunosuppressive drugs: mechanisms and strategies for controlling them. Clin Chem 1996;42(8 Pt 2):1316–1321.
33. Jusko WJ, Thomson AW, Fung J, et al. Consensus document: therapeutic monitoring of tacrolimus (FK-506). Ther Drug Monit 1995;17:606–614.

34. Cogill JL, Taylor PJ, Westly IS, et al. Evaluation of the tacrolimus II microparticle enzyme assay in liver and kidney transplant recipients. Clin Chem 1998;44:1942–1946.

35. McLeod HL. Therapeutic drug monitoring opportunities in cancer therapy. Pharmacol Ther 1997;74:39–54.

36. Lovell DJ. Ten years experience with methotrexate. Rev Rheum Engl Ed 1997;64(Suppl 10):186S–188S.

37. Schumacher GE, Barr JT. Bayesian and threshold probabilities in therapeutic drug monitoring: when can serum drug concentration alter clinical decisions. Am J Hosp Pharm 1994;51:321–327.

38. Moyer TP, Oliver LK. Supporting pharmaceutical studies from FDA submissions: diversifying the drug monitoring laboratory. Clin Chem 1998;44:433–436.

39. Dixit R, Riviere J, Anderson ME. Toxicokinetics and physiologic based toxicokinetics in toxicology and risk assessment. J Toxicol Environ Health B Crit Rev 2003;6:1–40.

SUGGESTED READINGS

Hardman JG, Limbird LE, Gillman AG, eds. Goodman & Gilman's The Pharmacological Basis of Therapeutics, 10th ed. New York: Pergamon Press. 2002.

Birkett DJ. Pharmacokinetics Made Easy. New York: McGraw-Hill, 2003.

Winter ME. Basic Clinical Pharmacokinetics, 3rd ed (reissued). Philadelphia: Lippincott Williams & Wilkins, 1994, ISBN 0-915486-22-9.

Toxicology

David P. Thorne

OBJECTIVES

Upon completion of this chapter, the clinical laboratorian should be able to:
- Define the term toxicology.
- List the major toxicants.
- Define the pathologic mechanisms of the toxicants discussed in the chapter.
- Discuss the laboratory methods used to evaluate toxicity.

- Explain the difference between quantitative and qualitative tests in toxicology.
- Critically evaluate clinical laboratory data in poisoning cases and provide recommendations for further testing.
- Define the role of the clinical laboratory in the evaluation of exposure to poisons.

KEY TERMS

Dose-response relationship

Drugs of abuse
Poison

TD_{50}

Toxicology

Toxicology is the study of poisons. The scope of this field is very broad. There are four major disciplines within toxicology: mechanistic, descriptive, forensic, and clinical toxicology. Mechanistic toxicology elucidates the cellular and biochemical effects of toxins. These studies provide a basis for rational therapy design and the development of tests to assess the degree of exposure of poisoned individuals. Descriptive toxicology uses the results from animal experiments to predict what level of exposure will cause harm in humans. This process is known as *risk assessment*. Regulatory toxicologists are responsible for interpreting the data from mechanistic and descriptive studies to establish standards that define the level of exposure that will not pose a risk to public health or safety. Typically, these toxicologists work for, or in conjunction with, government agencies. Forensic toxicology is primarily concerned with the medicolegal consequences of toxin exposure. A major focus of this area is establishing and validating the analytic performance of the methods used to generate evidence in legal situations, including the cause of death. Clinical toxicology is the study of interrelationships between toxin exposure and disease states. This area emphasizes not only diagnostic testing but also therapeutic intervention.

Within the organizational scheme of a typical medical laboratory, toxicology is usually considered part of chemistry, mainly because the methods used to evaluate toxins qualitatively and quantitatively are best suited to this area. However, appropriate diagnosis and management of poisoning victims, in many instances, requires an integrated approach from all sections of the clinical laboratory.[1]

EXPOSURE TO TOXINS

Exposure to toxic agents can occur for various reasons. From a clinical standpoint, about 50% of poisoning cases are intentional suicide attempts. Accidental exposure accounts for about 30% of cases. The remainder of cases are a result of homicide or occupational exposure. Of these, suicide has the highest mortality rate. Accidental exposure occurs most frequently in children; however, an accidental drug overdose of either therapeutic or illicit drugs is relatively common in adults. Occupational exposure primarily occurs in industrial and agricultural settings.

ROUTES OF EXPOSURE

Toxins can enter the body by several routes. Ingestion, inhalation, and transdermal absorption are the most common. Of these, ingestion is the most often seen in a clinical setting. For most toxins to exert a systemic effect, they must be absorbed into circulation. Absorption of toxins from the gastrointestinal tract occurs by several mechanisms. Some are taken up by processes intended for dietary nutrients. However, most are absorbed by pas-

sive diffusion. This process requires that the substance cross cellular barriers. Hydrophobic substances have the ability to diffuse across cell membranes and, therefore, can be absorbed anywhere along the gastrointestinal tract. Ionized substances cannot passively diffuse across membranes. Weak acids can become protonated in gastric acid. The result is a nonionized species, which can be absorbed in the stomach. In a similar manner, weak bases favor absorption in the intestine, where the pH is largely neutral or slightly alkaline. Other factors can influence absorbance of toxins from the gastrointestinal tract, including rate of dissolution, gastrointestinal motility, resistance to degradation in the gastrointestinal tract, and interaction with other substances. Toxins that are not absorbed from the gastrointestinal tract do not produce systemic effects but may produce local effects, such as diarrhea, bleeding, or malabsorption of nutrients, which may cause systemic effects secondary to toxin exposure.

DOSE-RESPONSE RELATIONSHIP

A *poison* can be defined as any substance that causes a harmful effect upon exposure. Although this basic definition is useful, other factors must be taken into consideration. Among these, dose is a key issue. The concept that any substance has the potential to cause harm if given at the correct dosage (even water) is a central theme in toxicology. There is a need to establish an index of the relative toxicity of substances to allow assessment of their potential to cause pathologic effects. Several systems are available. Most correlate the dose of a toxin that will result in a harmful response. One such system correlates a single acute oral dose range with the probability of a lethal outcome in an average 70-kg man (Table 29-1). This is a useful system to compare the relative toxicities of substances. The predicted response in this system is death, which is valid. However, most toxins can express pathologic effects other than death at lower degrees of exposure; therefore, other indices have been developed.

A more in-depth characterization can be acquired by evaluating data from a cumulative frequency histogram

TABLE 29-1. TOXICITY RATING SYSTEM

TOXICITY RATING	LETHAL ORAL DOSE IN AVERAGE ADULT
Super toxic	<5 mg/kg
Extremely toxic	5–50 mg/kg
Very toxic	50–500 mg/kg
Moderately toxic	0.5–5 g/kg
Slightly toxic	5–15 g/kg
Practically nontoxic	>15 g/kg

Adapted from Klaassen CD. Principles of toxicology. In: Klaassen CD, Amdur MO, Doull J, eds. Toxicology: The Basic Science of Poisons, 3rd ed. New York: Macmillan, 1986:13.

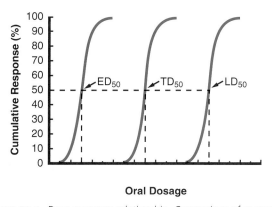

FIGURE 29-1. Dose-response relationship. Comparison of responses of a therapeutic drug over a range of doses. The ED_{50} is the dose of drug in which 50% of treated individuals will experience benefit. The TD_{50} is the dose of drug in which 50% of individuals will experience toxic adverse effects. The LD_{50} is the dose of drug in which 50% of individuals will result in morbidity.

of toxic responses over a range of doses. This experimental approach is typically used to evaluate several responses over a wide range of concentrations. One response monitored is the toxic response. This is the response that has been associated with an early pathologic effect at lower than lethal doses. This response has been determined to be an indicator of the toxic effects specific for that toxin. For a substance that exerts early toxic effects by damaging liver cells, the response monitored may be increases in serum alanine aminotransferase (ALT) or γ-glutamyltransferase (GGT) activity. The dose-response relationship implies that there will be an increase in the toxic response as the dose is increased. It should be noted that not all individuals display a toxic response at the same dose. The population variance can be seen in a cumulative frequency histogram of the percentage of people producing a toxic response over a range of concentrations (Fig. 29-1). The TD_{50} is the dose that would be predicted to produce a toxic response in 50% of the population. If the monitored response is death, the LD_{50} is the dose that would predict death in 50% of the population. Similar experiments can be used to evaluate the doses of therapeutic drugs. The ED_{50} is the dose that would be predicted to be effective or have a therapeutic benefit in 50% of the population. The therapeutic index is the ratio of the TD_{50} to the ED_{50}. Drugs with a large therapeutic index have few toxic adverse effects when the dose of drug is in the therapeutic range.

Acute and Chronic Toxicity

Acute toxicity and *chronic toxicity* are terms used to relate the duration and frequency of exposure to observed toxic effects. Acute toxicity is usually associated with a single, short-term exposure to a substance, the dose of which is sufficient to cause immediate toxic effects. Chronic toxicity is usually associated with repeated frequent exposure for extended periods, at doses that are insufficient to cause an immediate acute response. In many instances, chronic exposure is related to an accumulation of the toxicant or the toxic effects. Chronic toxicity may affect different systems then those associated with acute toxicity. Dose-response relationships have been established for many toxic substances in both acute and chronic situations.

ANALYSIS OF TOXIC AGENTS

In most instances, analysis of toxic agents in a clinical setting is a two-step procedure.[2] The first step is a screening test, which is a rapid, simple, qualitative procedure intended to detect specific substances or classes of toxicants. In general, these procedures have good analytic sensitivity but lack specificity. A negative result can rule out a drug or toxicant; however, a positive result should be considered a presumptive positive until confirmed by a second, more specific method.

A variety of analytic methods can be used for screening and confirmatory testing. Immunoassays are commonly used to screen for drugs. In some instances, these assays are specific for a single drug (*eg*, tetrahydrocannabinol [THC]). In most cases, however, drugs within general classes are detected (*eg*, barbiturates, opiates). Thin-layer chromatography is a relatively simple, inexpensive method of detecting various drugs and other organic compounds. Gas chromatography is a widely used, well-established technique for the qualitative and quantitative determination of many volatile substances. The reference method for the qualitative identification of most organic compounds is gas chromatography, using a mass spectrometer as the detector.

TOXICOLOGY OF SPECIFIC AGENTS

Many chemical agents encountered on a regular basis have potential adverse effects. The focus of this section is to survey the commonly encountered nondrug toxins seen in a clinical setting, as well as those that present as medical emergencies with acute exposure.

Alcohol

The toxic effects of alcohol are both general and specific. Exposure to alcohol, like exposure to most volatile organic solvents, initially causes disorientation, confusion, and euphoria, which can progress to unconsciousness, paralysis, and, with high-level exposure, even death. Most alcohols display these effects at about equivalent molar concentrations. This similarity suggests a common depressant effect on the central nervous system (CNS) that appears to be mediated by changes in membrane properties. In most cases, recovery from CNS effects is rapid and complete after cessation of exposure.

Distinct from the general CNS effects are the specific toxicities of each type of alcohol, which are usually mediated by biotransformation of alcohols to toxic products. There are several pathways by which short-chain aliphatic alcohols can be metabolized. Of these, hepatic conversion to an aldehyde, by alcohol dehydrogenase (ADH), and further conversion to an acid, by hepatic aldehyde dehydrogenase (ALDH), is the most significant.

$$\text{Alcohol} \xrightarrow{\text{ADH}} \text{Aldehyde} \xrightarrow{\text{ALDH}} \text{Acid} \qquad \textbf{(Eq. 29–1)}$$

Ethanol exposure is common.[3] Excessive ethanol consumption, with its associated consequences, is a leading cause of economic, social, and medical problems throughout the world. The economic impact is estimated to exceed $100 billion per year in terms of lost wages and productivity. Many social and family problems are associated with excessive ethanol consumption. The burden to the health care system is significant. Ethanol-related disorders are consistently one of the top-10 leading causes of hospital admissions. About 20% of all hospital admissions have some degree of alcohol-related problems. It is estimated that 80,000 Americans die each year, either directly or indirectly, as a result of abusive alcohol consumption. This correlates to about a fivefold increase in premature mortality. In addition, consumption of ethanol during pregnancy may lead to fetal alcohol syndrome or fetal alcohol effects, both of which are associated with delayed motor and mental development in children.

Correlations have been made between blood-alcohol concentration and the clinical signs and symptoms of acute intoxication. A blood-alcohol level in the range of 80–100 mg/dL has been established as the statutory limit for operation of a motor vehicle in most states. This is associated with a diminution of judgment and motor performance. The determination of blood ethanol concentration by the laboratory in cases of drunk driving requires an appropriate chain of custody, documentation of quality control, and proficiency testing records.[4] About one half of the 40,000–50,000 annual automobile related fatalities in the use involve alcohol as a factor.

Besides the short-term effects of ethanol, most pathophysiologic consequences of ethanol abuse are associated with chronic consumption over a long period. In an average adult, this correlates to the consumption of about 50 grams of ethanol per day for about 10 years. Consumption to this degree has been associated with compromised function in various organ, tissue, and cell types. However, the liver is the most sensitive organ. The pathologic sequence starts with the accumulation of lipids in hepatocytes. With continued consumption, this may progress to alcoholic hepatitis. About 20% of individuals with long-term, high-level intake develop this form of toxic hepatitis. Of those who do, progression to cirrhosis is common. Cirrhosis can be characterized as

an irreversible fibrosis leading to a loss of functional hepatic mass. Progress through this sequence is associated with changes in many laboratory tests related to hepatic function.

Several laboratory indicators of excessive ethanol consumption have sufficient diagnostic sensitivity and specificity to identify excessive ethanol consumption as the cause of a disease state.[5] Most are related to the progression of ethanol-induced liver disease. Table 29-2 lists common laboratory indicators of prolonged hazardous consumption.

Several mechanisms have been proposed to mediate the pathologic effects of long-term ethanol consumption. Of these, adduct formation with acetaldehyde appears to play a key role. Hepatic metabolism of ethanol is a two-step enzymatic reaction. The final product is acetic acid. Acetaldehyde is a reactive intermediate in this pathway. Most ethanol is converted to acetic acid in this pathway; however, a significant portion of the intermediate is released in the free state.

$$\text{Ethanol} \longrightarrow \text{Acetaldehyde} \longrightarrow \text{Acetate} \qquad \textbf{(Eq. 29–2)}$$
$$\searrow \text{Acetaldehyde adducts}$$

Extracellular acetaldehyde is a transient species as a result of rapid adduct formation with amine groups of proteins. Formation of acetaldehyde adducts has been shown to change the structure and function of various proteins. Many of the pathologic effects of ethanol have been correlated with the formation of these adducts.

TABLE 29-2. COMMON INDICATORS OF ETHANOL ABUSE

TEST	COMMENTS
GGT	Increases can be seen before the onset of pathologic consequences.
	Increases in serum activity can occur in many non–ethanol-related conditions.
AST	Increases in serum activity can occur in many non–ethanol-related conditions.
AST/ALT ratio	A ratio of greater than 2.0 is highly specific for ethanol-related liver disease.
HDL	High serum HDL is specific for ethanol consumption.
MCV	Increased erythrocyte MCV is commonly seen with excessive ethanol consumption.
	Increases are not related to folate or vitamin B_{12} deficiency.

CASE STUDY 29-1

A patient with a provisional diagnosis of depression was sent to the laboratory for a routine workup. The complete blood cell count was unremarkable except for an elevated erythrocyte mean cell volume (MCV). Results of urinalysis were unremarkable. The serum chemistry testing revealed slightly increased aspartate amino transferase (AST), total bilirubin, and high-density lipoprotein (HDL) levels. All other chemistry results, including glucose, urea, creatinine, cholesterol, pH, PCO$_2$, alanine aminotransferase (ALT), sodium, and potassium, were within the normal reference range. The physician suspects ethanol abuse; however, the patient claims to be a noncon-

sumer. Subsequent testing revealed a serum GGT 3 times the upper limit of normal. No ethanol was detected in serum. Screening tests for infectious forms of hepatitis were negative.

Questions

1. Are the above results consistent with a patient who is consuming hazardous quantities of ethanol?

2. Is further testing needed to rule in or out ethanol abuse? If so, what tests would you recommend?

Methanol is a common solvent. It may be ingested accidentally as a component of many commercial products or as a contaminant of homemade liquors. Methanol is initially metabolized by hepatic ADH to the intermediate formaldehyde. Formaldehyde is rapidly converted to formic acid by hepatic ALDH. The formation of formic acid causes severe acidosis, which may lead to death. Formic acid is also responsible for an optic neuropathy that may lead to blindness.

Isopropanol, also known as rubbing alcohol, is commonly available. It is metabolized by hepatic ADH to acetone, which is its primary metabolic end product. Both isopropanol and acetone have CNS depressant effects similar to ethanol. However, acetone has a long half-life. Intoxication with isopropanol, therefore, may result in severe acute-phase ethanol-like symptoms that may persist for an extended period.

Ethylene glycol (1,2-ethanediol) is a common component of hydraulic fluid and antifreeze. Ingestion by children is relatively common because of its sweet taste. The immediate effects of ethylene glycol ingestion are similar to those of ethanol. However, metabolism by hepatic ADH and ALDH results in the formation of several toxic species, including oxalic acid and glycolic acid, which results in severe metabolic acidosis. This is complicated by the rapid formation and deposition of calcium oxalate crystals in renal tubules. With high levels of consumption, calcium oxalate crystal formation may result in renal tubular damage.

Determination of Alcohols

From a medicolegal perspective, determination of blood ethanol concentration must be accurate and precise.[6] Serum, plasma, and whole blood are acceptable specimens. Correlations have been established between ethanol concentration in these specimens and impairment of psychomotor function. Because ethanol uni-

formly distributes in total body water, serum, which has a greater water content than whole blood, has a higher concentration per unit volume. Most states have standardized the acceptable specimen types admissible as evidence.

When acquiring a specimen for ethanol determination, the venipuncture site should be cleaned with an alcohol-free disinfectant. Because of the volatile nature of short-chain aliphatic alcohols, specimens must be capped at all times to avoid evaporation. Sealed specimens can be refrigerated or stored at room temperature for up to 14 days without loss of ethanol. Nonsterile specimens or those intended to be stored for long periods of time should be preserved with sodium fluoride to avoid increases in ethanol content that result from contaminating bacterial fermentation.

Several analytic methods can be used for the determination of ethanol in serum. Among these, the enzymatic, gas chromatography, and osmometry methods are the most commonly used. When osmolarity is measured by freezing point depression, increases in serum osmolarity correlate well with increases in serum ethanol concentration. The degree of increase in osmolality due to ethanol is expressed as the difference between the measured and the calculated osmolality; the difference is called the *osmolar gap*. Serum osmolality increases by about 10 mOsm/kg for each 60 mg/dL increase in serum ethanol.

$$\text{Osmolar gap} = \text{measured osmolarity} - \text{calculated osmolarity} \quad \text{(Eq. 29–3)}$$

This relationship is not specific for ethanol. Increases in the osmolar gap can also occur with certain metabolic imbalances; therefore, use of the osmolar gap for the determination of serum or blood ethanol concentration lacks analytic specificity. However, it is a useful screening test.

Gas chromatography is the reference method for ethanol determination. This method can simultaneously quantitate other alcohols, such as methanol and isopropanol. This analysis starts with dilution of the serum or blood sample with a saturated solution of sodium chloride in a closed container. Volatiles within the liquid specimen partition into the air space (head space) of the closed container. Sampling of this head space provides clean specimens with little or no matrix effect. Quantitation of peaks can be done by constructing a standard curve or by ratio to an internal standard (n-propanol) as shown in Figure 29-2.

Enzymatic methods for the determination of ethanol are common. The enzyme used in this assay is a nonhuman form of ADH. This enzyme oxidizes ethanol to acetaldehyde with reduction of NAD^+ to NADH.

$$\text{Ethanol} + NAD^+ \xrightarrow{\text{ADH}} \text{acetaldehyde} + \text{NADH} \quad \textbf{(Eq. 29–4)}$$

The NADH produced can be monitored directly by absorbance at 340 nm or can be coupled to an indicator reaction. This form of ADH is relatively specific for ethanol (Table 29-1). Intoxication with methanol or isopropanol produces a negative or low result; therefore, a negative result by this method does not rule out ingestion of other alcohols. There is good agreement between the enzymatic reactions of ethanol and gas chromatography. The enzymatic reactions can be fully automated and do not require specialized instrumentation.

Carbon Monoxide

Carbon monoxide is produced by incomplete combustion of carbon-containing substances. The primary environmental sources of carbon monoxide include gasoline

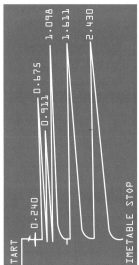

Retention Time (min)	Analyte
0.675	Methanol
0.911	Acetone
1.098	Ethanol
1.611	Isopropanol
2.430	n-Propanol

FIGURE 29-2. Headspace gas chromatography of alcohol. The concentration of each alcohol can be determined by comparison to the response from the internal standard n-propanol.

TABLE 29-3. SYMPTOMS OF CARBOXYHEMOGLOBINEMIA

COHb (%)	SYMPTOMS AND COMMENTS
0.5	Typical in nonsmokers
5–15	Range of values seen in smokers
10	Shortness of breath with vigorous exercise
20	Shortness of breath with moderate exercise
30	Severe headaches, fatigue, impairment of judgment
40–50	Confusion, fainting on exertion
60–70	Unconsciousness, respiratory failure, death with continuous exposure
80	Immediately fatal

engines, improperly ventilated furnaces, and wood or plastic fires. Carbon monoxide is a colorless, odorless, and tasteless gas that is rapidly absorbed into blood from inspired air. Carbon monoxide expresses its toxic effects by high-affinity binding to divalent iron within heme proteins, such as cytochromes, myoglobin, and hemoglobin.[7] Of these, binding to hemoglobin produces the most significant toxic outcome.

When carbon monoxide binds to hemoglobin, it is called *carboxyhemoglobin (COHb)*. The affinity of carbon monoxide for hemoglobin is 245 times greater than for oxygen. Air is about 20% oxygen by volume. If inspired air contained 0.1% carbon monoxide by volume, this would result in a 50% carboxyhemoglobinemia at equilibrium. For this reason, carbon monoxide is considered a very toxic substance. Because both carbon monoxide and oxygen compete for the same binding site, exposure to carbon monoxide results in a decrease in the concentration of oxyhemoglobin. Furthermore, binding of carbon monoxide to hemoglobin increases the affinity of oxygen to hemoglobin, a shift to the left on the hemoglobin–oxygen dissociation curve. The net effect of carbon monoxide exposure is a decrease in the amount of oxygen delivered to tissue, producing hypoxia. The major toxic effects of carbon monoxide exposure are seen in organs with high oxygen demand, such as the brain and heart.[8] The concentration of carboxyhemoglobin (expressed as the percentage of COHb present to the capacity of the specimen to form COHb) and corresponding symptoms are detailed in Table 29-3.

Several methods are available for the evaluation carbon monoxide poisoning. Carboxyhemoglobin has a cherry-red appearance. This is the basis of a spot test for excessive carbon monoxide exposure; 5 mL of 40% NaOH is added to 5 mL of a 1/20 aqueous dilution of whole blood. Persistence of a pink solution is consistent with a carboxyhemoglobin level of 20% or greater. There are two primary quantitative assays for carboxyhemoglobin: differential spectrophotometry and gas chromatography. The only treatment for carbon monoxide poisoning is 100% oxygen therapy. In severe cases, hyperbaric oxygen may be used.

Gas chromatography is accurate and precise and the reference method for the determination of carboxyhemoglobin. Carbon monoxide is released from hemoglobin after treatment with potassium ferricyanide. After analytic separation, carbon monoxide is detected by changes in thermal conductivity. Spectrophotometric methods work on the principle that different forms of hemoglobin present with different spectral absorbency curves. By measuring absorbance at four to six different wavelengths, the concentration of the different species of hemoglobin (including carboxyhemoglobin) can be determined by calculation. This is the most common method used and is the basis for several automated systems.

Caustic Agents

Caustic agents are found in many household products and occupational settings. Even though any exposure to a strong acid or alkaline substance is associated with injury, aspiration and ingestion present the greatest hazard. Aspiration is usually associated with pulmonary edema and shock, which can rapidly progress to death. Ingestion produces lesions in the esophagus and gastrointestinal tract, which may produce perforations. This results in hematemesis, abdominal pain, and possibly shock. Onset of metabolic acidosis or alkalosis occurs rapidly after ingestion. Corrective therapy for ingestion is usually by dilution.

Cyanide

Cyanide is classified as a supertoxic substance[9] that can exist as a gas or solid or in solution. Exposure can occur by inhalation, ingestion, or transdermal absorption. Cyanide is used in many industrial processes.[10] It is also a component of some insecticides and rodenticides. Cyanide is also produced as a pyrolysis product from the burning of some plastics, including urea foams used as insulation in homes. Thus, carbon monoxide and cyanide exposure may account for a significant portion of the toxicities associated with smoke inhalation. Ingestion of cyanide is a common suicide agent.

Cyanide expresses toxicity by binding to heme iron. Binding to mitochondrial cytochrome oxidase causes an uncoupling of oxidative phosphorylation. This results in rapid depletion of cellular adenosine triphosphate as a result of the inability of oxygen to accept electrons. Increases in cellular oxygen tension and venous PO_2 occur as a result of lack of oxygen utilization. At low levels of exposure, patients experience headaches, dizziness, and respiratory depression, which can rapidly progress to seizure, coma, and death at slightly greater doses. Cya-

nide clearance is primary mediated by rapid enzymatic conversion to thiocyanate, a nontoxic product rapidly cleared by renal filtration. Cyanide toxicity is associated with acute exposure at concentrations sufficient to exceed the rate of clearance by this enzymatic process.

Evaluation of cyanide exposure requires a rapid turnaround time. There are several methods available. Ion-specific electrode methods and photometric analysis following two-well microdiffusion separation are the most common. Chronic low-level exposure can be evaluated by determination of urinary thiocyanate concentration.

Metals

Arsenic

Arsenic may exist bound to or as a primary constituent of many different organic and inorganic compounds. It exists in both naturally occurring and manmade substances; therefore, exposure to arsenic may occur in various settings. Environmental exposure through air and water is prevalent in many industrialized areas.[11] Occupational exposure occurs in agriculture and the smelting industries. It is also a common homicide and suicide agent.

Absorption of arsenic depends on the form of the compound. Organic arsenic-containing compounds are rapidly absorbed by passive diffusion. Other forms are absorbed at a slower rate. Clearance of arsenic is primarily by renal filtration of the free, ionized state. Arsenic expresses toxic effects by high-affinity binding to the thiol groups in proteins; therefore, the portion available for filtration in serum is low. This results in a long half-life in the body; the whole body content of arsenic may be cumulative with chronic exposure.

Arsenic binding to proteins often results in a change in structure and function. Because many proteins are capable of binding arsenic, the toxic symptoms of arsenic poisoning are nonspecific. Many cellular and organ systems are effected. Fever, anorexia, and gastrointestinal distress are seen with chronic or acute ingestion at low levels. Peripheral and central damage to the nervous system, renal effects, hemopoietic effects, and vascular disease leading to death are associated with high levels of exposure.

Analysis of arsenic is most commonly done by atomic absorption spectrophotometry. Blood and urine are acceptable specimens to evaluate short-term exposure. Hair and fingernail content have been found useful in the assessment of long-term exposure.

Cadmium

Cadmium is a metal found in many industrial processes, with its main use in electroplating and galvanizing. It is commonly encountered during the mining and processing of many metals. Cadmium is a pigment found in paints and plastics and is the cathodal material of nickel-cadmium batteries. It is a significant environmental pollutant.[12]

Excessive exposure occurs most frequently by inhalation of cadmium particulates in industry and by ingestion of contaminated food. Cadmium expresses its toxicity primarily by binding to proteins; however, it can also bind to other cellular constituents. Cadmium distributes throughout the body but has a tendency to accumulate in the kidney, where most of its toxic effects are expressed.[13] An early finding of cadmium toxicity is manifested by renal tubular dysfunction. Tubular proteinuria, glucosuria, and aminoaciduria are typically seen. Evaluation of excessive cadmium is most commonly accomplished by determination of whole blood or urinary content using atomic absorption spectrophotometry.

Lead

Lead is a common environmental contaminant.[14] It was a common constituent of household paints before 1972 and is still found in commercial and art paints. Gasoline was leaded until 1978. Residuals from automobile exhaust can still be found in high concentrations on highways. Plumbing constructed of lead pipes or joined with leaded connectors can significantly contribute to the lead concentration of water. Lead is a by-product or component of many industrial processes. The lead content of foods is highly variable. In the United States, the average daily intake for an adult is between 75–120 μg/day. This level of intake is not associated with overt toxicity.[15] Because lead is present in all biologic systems and because no physiologic or biochemical function has been found, the key issue is what dose causes a toxic effect. Susceptibility to lead toxicity is dependent primarily on age. Adults are largely tolerant to the effects of lead compared with children.[16]

Exposure to lead can occur by any route; however, ingestion of contaminated dietary constituents accounts for most exposures. Gastrointestinal absorption of lead is influenced by various factors. Adults absorb 5–15% of ingested lead. Children have a greater degree of absorption. Infants absorb 30–40%. Factors controlling rate of absorption are unclear.[17] Absorbed lead binds with high affinity to many macromolecular structures. It distributes throughout the body. Lead distributes into two theoretical compartments. One is the skeleton, which is the largest pool. Lead combines with the matrix of bone and can persist in this compartment for a long period. The half-life of lead in bone is longer than 20 years. The other theoretical compartment is soft tissue. The half-life of lead in this compartment is somewhat variable; the average half-life in soft tissue is 120 days.

Elimination of lead occurs primarily by renal filtration. Because only a small fraction of total body lead presents in circulation, the elimination rate is slow. Considering the relatively constant rate of exposure and the slow elimination rate, total body lead accumulates over a lifetime. The largest accumulation occurs in bone. Significant ac-

cumulation also occurs in kidney, bone marrow, circulating erythrocytes, and peripheral and central nerves.

Lead toxicity is multifaceted and occurs in a dose-dependent manner (Fig. 29-3). Most toxic effects are a result of binding to proteins, which results in a change in structure and function. The neurologic effects of lead are of particular importance. Lead exposure causes encephalopathy characterized by a cerebral edema and ischemia. Severe lead poisoning can result in stupor, convulsions, and coma. Lower levels of exposure may not present with these symptoms. However, low-level exposure may result in subclinical effects typified by behavioral changes, hyperactivity, attention deficit disorder, and a decrease in intelligence quotient scores. Children appear particularly sensitive to these effects[9] and are now evaluated for lead poisoning before entry into school. Higher levels of exposure have been associated with demyelinization of peripheral nerves, which results in a decrease in nerve conduction velocity.

Lead is a potent inhibitor of many enzymes; this inhibition mediates many toxic effects. Noteworthy are the effects on vitamin D metabolism and the heme synthetic pathway. This results in changes in bone and calcium metabolism and in anemia. Decreased serum concentrations of both 25-hydroxy and 1,25-dihydroxy vitamin D are seen in excessive lead exposure. The anemia is primarily caused by an inhibition of the heme synthetic pathway, which results in increases in the concentration of several intermediates in this pathway, including aminolevulinic acid and protoporphyrin. Increases in protoporphyrin result in high concentrations of zinc protoporphyrin in circulating erythrocytes. Zinc protoporphyrin is a highly fluorescent compound. Measurement of this fluorescence has been used to screen for lead toxicity. Increased urinary aminolevulinic acid is a highly sensitive and specific indicator of lead toxicity that correlates well with blood levels. Another hematologic finding is the presence of basophilic stippling in erythrocytes as a result of inhibition of erythrocytic pyrimidine nucleotidase. This enzyme is responsible for removal of residual DNA after extrusion of the nucleus. Basophilic stippling is a sensitive indicator of lead exposure.

Excessive lead exposure has also been associated with hypertension, carcinogenesis, birth defects, and compromised immunity. Lead causes several toxic renal effects.[18] Early stages are associated with tubular dysfunction, resulting in glycosuria, aminoaciduria, and hyperphosphaturia. Late stages are associated with tubular atrophy and glomerular fibrosis. The fibrosis may result in a decreased glomerular filtration rate.

Treatment of lead poisoning involves removal from exposure and treatment with therapeutic chelators, such as ethylenediaminetetraacetic acid (EDTA) and dimercaptosuccinic acid (DMSA). These substances are capable of removing lead from soft tissue and bone by form-

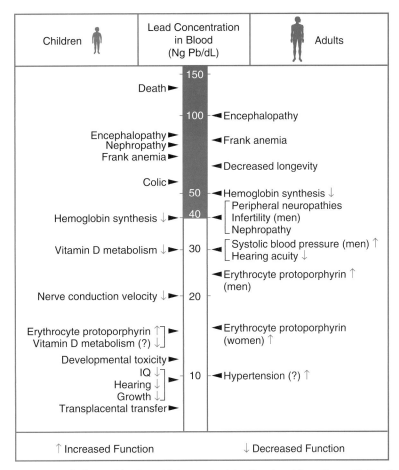

FIGURE 29-3. Comparison of effects of lead on children and adults. (Reprinted from Royce SE, Needleman HL, eds. Case Studies in Environmental Medicine: Lead Toxicity. Washington, D.C.: U.S. Public Health Service, ATSDR, 1990.)

ing low-molecular-weight, high-affinity complexes that can be cleared by renal filtration. The efficacy of this therapy is determined by monitoring the urinary concentration of lead.

The assessment of total body burden of lead poisoning is best evaluated by the quantitative determination of lead concentration in whole blood. The use of urine is also valid but correlates closer to the level of recent exposure. Care must be taken during specimen collection to ensure that the specimen does not become contaminated from exogenous sources. Lead-free containers are recommended for this purpose.

Several methods can be used to measure lead concentration. Chromogenic reactions and anodic stripping voltametry methods have been used, but they lack clinical utility because they lack analytic sensitivity. At present, graphite furnace atomic absorption spectrophotometry (AAS) is the most common method used.

Mercury

Mercury is a metal that exists in three forms: elemental (liquid at room temperature), inorganic salts, or a component of organic compounds. Exposure occurs prima-

rily by inhalation and ingestion. Consumption of contaminated foods is the major source of exposure in the general population. Inhalation and accidental ingestion of inorganic and organic forms in industrial settings is the most common reason for toxic levels.[19] Each form of mercury has different toxicologic characteristics. Elemental mercury (Hg^0) can be ingested without significant effects. Inhalation of elemental mercury is insignificant because of its low vapor pressure. Cationic mercury (Hg^{2+}) is moderately toxic. Organic mercury, such as methyl mercury (CH_3Hg^+), is very toxic.[20] Considering that the most common route of exposure to mercury is by ingestion, the primary factor that determines toxicity is gastrointestinal absorbance.

Elemental mercury is largely not absorbed because of its viscous liquid nature. Inorganic mercury is only partially absorbed. Although not significantly absorbed, inorganic mercury still has significant local toxicity in the gastrointestinal tract. The portion that is absorbed distributes uniformly throughout the body. The organic forms of mercury are rapidly and efficiently absorbed by passive diffusion. Systemic organic mercury partitions into hydrophobic compartments. This results in high concentrations in brain and peripheral nerves. In these lipophilic compartments, organic mercury is biotransformed to the divalent state, allowing it to bind to neuronal proteins.[21] Elimination of systemic mercury occurs primarily by renal filtration of bound low-molecular-weight species or the free (ionized) state. Considering that most mercury is bound to protein, the elimination rate is slow. Therefore, chronic exposure exerts a cumulative effect.

Mercury toxicity is a result of protein binding, which results in a change of structure and function. The most significant result of this interaction is the inhibition of many enzymes. Binding to intestinal proteins after ingestion of inorganic mercury results in acute gastrointestinal disturbances. Ingestion of moderate amounts may result in severe bloody diarrhea because of ulceration and necrosis of the gastrointestinal tract. In severe cases, this may lead to shock and death. The absorbed portion of ingested inorganic mercury affects many organs. Clinical findings include tachycardia, tremors, thyroiditis, and, most significantly, a disruption of renal function. The renal effect is associated with glomerular proteinuria and loss of tubular function. Organic mercury may also have a renal effect at high levels of exposure. However, neurologic symptoms are the primary toxic effects of this hydrophobic form. Low levels of exposure cause tremors, behavioral changes, mumbling speech, and loss of balance. Higher levels of exposure result in hyporeflexia, hypotension, bradycardia, renal dysfunction, and death. Analysis of mercury is by atomic absorption, using whole blood or an aliquot of a 24-hour urine specimen or anodal stripping voltametry. Analysis of mercury by atomic absorption requires special techniques as a result of the volatility of elemental mercury.

Pesticides

Pesticides are substances that have been intentionally added to the environment to kill or harm an undesirable life form. Pesticides can be classified into several categories, such as insecticides and herbicides. These agents have been applied to the control of vector-borne disease and urban pests and to improve agricultural productivity. Pesticides can be found in occupational settings and in the home; therefore, there are frequent opportunities for exposure. Contamination of food is the major route of exposure for the general population. Inhalation, transdermal absorption, and ingestion as a result of hand-to-mouth contact are common occupational and accidental routes of exposure.[22]

Ideally, the actions of pesticides would be target specific. Unfortunately, most are nonselective and result in toxic effects to many nontarget species, including humans. Pesticides come in many different forms with a wide range of potential toxic effects.[23] The health effects of short-term, low-level exposure to most of these agents have yet to be well elucidated. Extended low-level exposure to low levels may result in chronic disease states. Of primary concern is high-level exposure, which may result in acute disease states or death. The most common victims of acute poisoning are people who are applying pesticides and do not take appropriate precautions to avoid exposure. Ingestion by children at home is also common. Pesticide ingestion is also a common suicide vehicle.

There is a wide variation in the chemical configuration of pesticides, ranging from simple salts of heavy metals to complex high-molecular-weight organic compounds. Insecticides are the most prevalent of pesticides. Based on chemical configuration, the organophosphates, carbamates, and halogenated hydrocarbons are the most common insecticides. Organophosphates are the most abundant pesticides and are responsible for about one third of all pesticide poisonings.

Organophosphates and carbamates function by inhibition of acetylcholinesterase, an enzyme present in both insects and mammals. In mammals, acetylcholine is a neurotransmitter found in both central and peripheral nerve. It is also responsible for stimulation of muscle cells and several endocrine/exocrine glands. The actions of acetylcholine are terminated by the actions of membrane-bound, postsynaptic acetylcholinesterase. Inhibition of this enzyme by these agents results in the prolonged presence of acetylcholine on its receptor, which produces a wide range of systemic effects. Low levels of exposure are associated with salivation, lacrimation, and involuntary urination and defecation. Higher levels of exposure result in bradycardia, muscular twitching, cramps, apathy, slurred speech, and behavioral changes. Death due to respiratory failure may also occur.

Absorbed organophosphates bind with high affinity to several proteins, including acetylcholinesterase. Protein-binding prevents direct analysis of organophosphates. Thus, exposure is evaluated indirectly by measurement of acetylcholinesterase inhibition. Inhibition of this enzyme has been found to be a sensitive and specific indicator of organophosphate exposure. Because acetylcholinesterase is a membrane-bound enzyme, serum activity is low. To increase the analytic sensitivity of this assay, erythrocytes that have high surface activity are commonly used. Evaluation of erythrocytic acetylcholinesterase activity for detection of organophosphate exposure, however, is not commonly available because of low demand and the lack of an automated method.

An alternative test that has become commonly available is measurement of serum pseudocholinesterase (SChE) activity. This enzyme is inhibited by organophosphates in a similar manner to the erythrocytic enzyme. Unlike the erythrocytic enzyme, however, changes in the serum activity of SChE lack sensitivity and specificity for organophosphate exposure. Pseudocholinesterase is found in liver, pancreas, brain, and serum. The biologic function of this enzyme is not well defined. Decreased levels of SChE can occur in acute infection, pulmonary embolism, hepatitis, and cirrhosis. There are also several variants of this enzyme that demonstrate diminished activity. Thus, decreases in SChE are not specific for organophosphate poisoning. The normal reference range for SChE is between 4,000 and 12,000 U/L. The intraindividual variation (the degree of variance within an average individual) is about 700 U/L. Symptoms associated with organophosphate toxicity occur at about a 40% reduction in activity. An individual whose normal SChE exists on the high side of the normal reference range and who has been exposed to toxic levels of organophosphates may still have SChE activity in the normal reference range. Because of these factors, determination of SChE activity lacks sensitivity in the diagnosis of organophosphate poisoning. Therefore, SChE is considered a screening test, and clinical context must be taken into consideration when interpreting the results. Immediate antidotal therapy can be initiated in cases of suspected organophosphate poisoning with decreased activity of SChE. However, continuation of therapy and documentation of such poisoning should be confirmed by testing of the erythrocytic enzyme.

TOXICOLOGY OF THERAPEUTIC DRUGS

Many overdose situations are the result of accidental or intentional excessive dosage of pharmaceutical drugs. All drugs are capable of toxic effects at the right dosage. This discussion focuses on the therapeutic drugs most commonly seen in clinical overdose situations.

Salicylates

Aspirin (acetylsalicylic acid) is a commonly used analgesic, antipyretic, and anti-inflammatory drug. It functions by decreasing thromboxane and prostaglandin formation through inhibition of cyclooxygenase. At recommended doses, there are several noteworthy adverse effects, including interference with platelet aggregation and gastrointestinal function. There is also an epidemiologic relationship between aspirin, childhood viral infections (*eg*, varicella and influenza), and the onset of Reye's syndrome.

Acute ingestion of high doses of aspirin is associated with various toxic effects through several different mechanisms.[24] Because it is an acid, excessive salicylate ingestion is associated with a metabolic acidosis. Salicylate is also a direct stimulator of the respiratory center. The hyperventilation produces a respiratory alkalosis. In many instances, the net result is immediate mixed acid-base disturbance. Salicylates also inhibit the Krebs cycle, resulting in excess conversion of pyruvate to lactate. In addition, at high levels of exposure, salicylates stimulate mobilization and use of free fatty acid, resulting in excess ketone body formation. All these factors contribute to a metabolic acidosis that may lead to death. Treatment for overdose involves neutralizing and eliminating the excess acid and maintaining electrolyte balance.

Correlations have been established between serum concentrations of salicylates and toxic outcomes. Several methods are available for the quantitative determination of salicylate in serum. Gas or liquid chromatography methods provide the highest analytic sensitivity and specificity but have not found clinical utility because of equipment expense and technical difficulty. Several immunoassay methods are available; the most common is a chromogenic assay known as the *Trinder reaction,* which reacts salicylate with ferric nitrate to form a colored complex that is then evaluated spectrophotometrically.

Acetaminophen

Acetaminophen, either solely or in combination with other compounds, is a commonly used analgesic drug. In healthy subjects, therapeutic dosages have few adverse effects. Overdose of acetaminophen, however, is associated with a severe hepatotoxicity (Fig. 29-4).

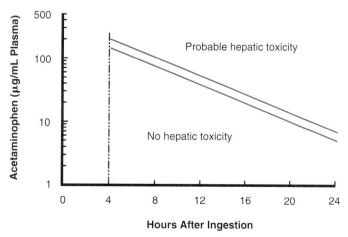

FIGURE 29-4. Rumack-Matthew nomogram. Prediction of acetaminophen-induced hepatic damage based on serum concentration. (Reprinted with permission from Rumack BH, Matthew H. Acetaminophen poisoning and toxicity. Pediatrics 1975;55:871.)

Absorbed acetaminophen is bound with high affinity to various proteins, resulting in a low free fraction. Thus, renal filtration of the parent drug is minimal. Most is eliminated by hepatic uptake, biotransformation, conjugation, and excretion. Acetaminophen can follow several different pathways through this process; each forming a different product. The pathway of major concern is the hepatic mixed-function oxidase system. In this system, acetaminophen is first transformed to reactive intermediates, which are then conjugated with reduced glutathione. In overdose situations, glutathione can become depleted, yet reactive intermediates continue to be produced. This results in an accumulation of reactive intermediates inside the cell. Because some intermediates are free radicals, this results in a toxic effect to the cell that leads to necrosis of the liver, the organ in which these reactions are occurring.[25]

The time frame for the onset of hepatocyte damage is relatively long. In an average adult, serum indicators of hepatic damage do not become abnormal until 3–5 days after ingestion of a toxic dose. The initial symptoms of acetaminophen toxicity are vague, nonspecific, and not predictive of hepatic necrosis. The serum concentration of acetaminophen that results in depletion of glutathione has been determined for an average adult. Unfortunately, acetaminophen is rapidly cleared from serum and determination of serum acetaminophen is often made many hours after ingestion. In these situations, it is unknown whether toxic concentrations of acetaminophen were present at some previous time. To aide in this situation, nomograms are available that predict hepatotoxicity based on serum concentrations of acetaminophen at a known time after ingestion. It is also noteworthy that chronic, heavy consumers of ethanol metabolize acetaminophen at a more rapid rate than average, resulting in a more rapid formation of reactive intermediates and an increased possibility of depleting glutathione at a lower dose than normal. Therefore, alcoholic patients are more susceptible to acetaminophen toxicity, and using the nomogram for interpretation in these patients is inappropriate.[26]

The reference method for the quantitation of acetaminophen in serum is high-performance liquid chromatography. This method, however, is not widely used in clinical settings because of expense and technical difficulty. Immunoassay is currently the most common analytic method used for serum acetaminophen determination. Competitive enzyme or fluorescence polarization immunoassay systems are most frequently used.

TOXICOLOGY OF DRUGS OF ABUSE

Assessment of drug abuse is of medical interest for many reasons. In drug overdose, it is essential to identify the responsible agent to ensure appropriate treatment. In a similar manner, identification of drug abuse in nonoverdose situations provides a rationale for treatment for addiction. For these reasons, testing for *drugs of abuse* is commonly done. This typically involves screening of a single urine specimen for many substances by qualitative screening procedures. In most instances, this procedure only detects recent drug use, therefore, with abstinence of relatively short duration, many abusing patients may not be identified. In addition, a positive drug screen cannot discriminate between a single casual use and chronic abuse. Identification of chronic abuse usually involves several positive test results in conjunction with clinical evaluation. In a similar manner, a positive drug screen does not determine the time frame or dose of the drug taken.

Drug abuse or overdose can occur with prescription, over-the-counter, or illicit drugs. The focus of this discussion is on substances with addictive potential.

The use of drugs for recreational or performance enhancement purposes is relatively common. The National Institute on Drug Abuse reports that about 30% of the population older than high school-age have used an illicit drug. Testing for drug abuse has become commonplace in professional, industrial, and athletic settings. The potential punitive measures associated with this testing may involve or result in civil or criminal litigation. Therefore, the laboratory must ensure that data are legally admissible and defendable. This requires the use of analytic methods that have been validated as accurate and precise. It also requires documentation of specimen security. Protocols and procedures must be established that prevent and detect specimen adulteration and that may prevent drug detection. Measurement of urinary temperature, pH, specific gravity, and creatinine is commonly done to ensure that these specimens have not been diluted or treated with substances that may interfere with testing. Specimen collection should be monitored and a chain-of-custody established to guard against specimen exchange.

Testing for drugs of abuse can be done by several methods. A two-tiered approach of screening and confirmation is usually employed.[27] Screening procedures should be simple, rapid, inexpensive, and capable of being automated. They are often referred to as *spot tests*. In general, screening procedures have good analytic sensitivity with marginal specificity; a negative result can rule out an analyte with a reasonable degree of certainty. These methods usually detect classes of drugs based on similarities in chemical configuration. This allows detection of parent compounds and congeners, which have similar effects. Considering that many designer drugs are modified forms of established drugs of abuse, these methods increase the scope of the screening process. A drawback to this type of analysis is that it may also detect chemically related substances that have no or low abuse

TABLE 29-4. PREVALENCE OF COMMON DRUGS OF ABUSE

SUBSTANCE	PREVALENCE (%)[a]
Alcohol	75–80
Marijuana	20–26
Cocaine	5–13
Benzodiazepines	1–5
Barbiturates	0.5–5
Opiates	0.1–2
Phencyclidine	0.1–2
Amphetamines	0.1–1
Other stimulants	0.8–2
Other sedative hypnotics	0.6–2

[a]This table provides approximate frequencies of relevant drugs of abuse encountered in the clinical laboratory. The percentage values estimate the prevalence of use in college-age individuals, the most common users, who by survey claim to have used drugs within the last 30 days, and individuals who tested positive in the same age-group. (Adapted from NIDA Capsules and InfoFacts Web sites: URL http://www.nida.nih.gov; accessed 4/12/04.)

potential; therefore, interpretation of positive test results requires integration of clinical context and further testing. Confirmation testing uses methods that have high sensitivity and specificity; many of these tests provide quantitative as well as qualitative information. Confirmatory testing requires the use of a method different from that used in the screening procedure.

There are several general analytic procedures commonly used for analysis of drugs of abuse. Chromogenic reactions, the generation of a colored product usually by a chemical reaction, are occasionally used as screening procedures. Immunoassay-based procedures are widely used both as screening and confirmatory assays. In general, immunoassays offer a high degree of sensitivity and are easily automated. A wide variety of chromatography techniques are used for the qualitative identification and quantitation of drugs. Thin-layer chromatography is an inexpensive method for the screening of many drugs and has the advantage that no instrumentation is required. Liquid and gas chromatography allow complex mixtures of drugs to be separated and quantitated. These methods are generally labor intensive and not well suited to screening.

Many drugs have the potential for abuse.[28] Trends in drug abuse vary geographically and between different socioeconomic groups. For a clinical laboratory to provide an effective toxicology service requires knowledge of the drug or drug groups likely to be found within the patient population it serves. Fortunately, the process of selecting which drugs to test for has been aided by national studies that have identified the drugs of abuse most commonly seen in the population (Table 29-4). This provides the basis for test selection in most situations. The following discussion focuses on select drugs with a high potential for abuse.

Amphetamines

Amphetamine and methamphetamine are therapeutic drugs used for narcolepsy and attentional deficit disorder. These drugs are stimulants with a high abuse potential.[29] They produce an initial sense of increased mental and physical capacity along with a perception of well-being. These initial effects are followed by restlessness, irritability, and possibly psychosis. Abatement of these late effects is often countered with repeated use. Tolerance and psychological dependence develop with chronic use. Overdose, although rare in experienced users, results in hypertension, cardiac arrhythmias, convulsions, and possibly death. Various compounds chemically related to amphetamines are components of over-the-counter medications, including ephedrine, pseudoephedrine, and phenylpropanolamine. These amphetamine-like compounds are common in allergy and cold medications.

CASE STUDY 29-2

An emergency department case with a provisional diagnosis of overdose with an over-the-counter cold medicine undergoes a drug screen. Test results from immunoassay screening were negative for opiates, barbiturates, benzodiazepines, THC, and cocaine, but positive for amphetamines. The salicylate level was 15 times the upper limit of the therapeutic range. Results for acetaminophen and ethanol were negative.

Questions

1. What would be the expected results of arterial blood gas analysis?

2. What would be the expected results of a routine urinalysis?

3. What are some of the possible reasons the amphetamine screen is positive?

Identification of amphetamine abuse involves analysis of urine for the parent drugs. Immunoassay systems are commonly used as the screening procedure. Because of variable cross-reactivity with over-the-counter medications that contain amphetamine-like compounds, a positive result by immunoassay is considered presumptive. Confirmation of immunoassay-positive tests are most commonly done by liquid or gas chromatography.

Anabolic Steroids

Anabolic steroids are a group of compounds related chemically to the male sex hormone testosterone. These artificial substances were developed in the 1930s as therapy for male hypogonadism. It was soon discovered that use of these compounds in healthy subjects increases muscle mass. In many instances, this results in an improvement in athletic performance. Recent studies have reported that 6.5% of adolescent boys and 1.9% of girls reported the use of steroids without a prescription.[30]

Most illicit steroids are obtained through the black market from underground laboratories and foreign sources. The quality and purity of these drugs is highly variable. In most instances, the acute toxic effects of these drugs are related to inconsistent formulation, which may result in high dosages and impurities. A variety of both physical and psychological effects have been associated with steroid abuse. Chronic use of steroids has been associated with a toxic hepatitis. Chronic use has also been associated with accelerated atherosclerosis and abnormal aggregation of platelets, both of which predispose to stroke and myocardial infarction. In addition, steroid abuse causes an enlargement of the heart. In this condition, heart muscle cells develop faster than the associated vasculature. This may lead to ischemia of heart muscle cells, which predisposes cardiac arrhythmias and possible sudden death. In males, chronic steroid use is associated with testicular atrophy, sterility, and impotence. In females, it causes development of masculine traits, breast reduction, and sterility.

Identification of steroid abusers by laboratory testing is limited to chromatographic methods. Both gas and liquid systems have been used.[31] Gas chromatography with mass spectrometry is the most commonly used method.

Cannabinoids

Cannabinoids are a group of psychoactive compounds found in marijuana.[32] Of these, tetrahydrocannabinol (THC) is the most potent and abundant. Marijuana, or its processed product hashish, can be smoked or ingested. A sense of well-being and euphoria is the subjective effect of exposure. It is also associated with impair-

ment of short-term memory and intellectual function. Effects of chronic use have not been well established. Overdose has not been associated with specific physiologic toxic outcomes. Tolerance and a mild dependence may develop with chronic use. THC is a lipophilic substance, which is rapidly removed from circulation by passive distribution into hydrophobic compartments, such as brain and fat. This results in slow elimination as a result of redistribution back into circulation and subsequent hepatic metabolism.

The half-life of THC in circulation is 1 day after a single use and 3–5 days in chronic, heavy consumers. Hepatic metabolism of THC produces several products that are primarily eliminated in urine. The major urinary metabolite is 11-nor-Δ-tetrahydrocannabinol-9-carboxylic acid (THC-COOH). This metabolite can be detected in urine for 3–5 days after a single use or for up to 4 weeks in a chronic, heavy consumer after abstinence. Immunoassay for THC-COOH is the basis of the screening test for marijuana consumption. Gas chromatography with mass spectrometry is used for confirmation. Both methods are sensitive and specific. Because of the low limit of detection of these methods, it is possible to find THC-COOH in urine as a result of passive inhalation. Urinary concentration standards have been established that can discriminate between passive and direct inhalation.

Cocaine

Cocaine is an effective local anesthetic with few adverse effects at therapeutic concentrations. At higher circulating concentrations, it is a potent CNS stimulator that elicits a sense of excitement and euphoria.[33] Cocaine is an alkaloid salt that can be administered directly (eg, by insufflation or intravenous injection) or inhaled as a vapor when smoked in the free-base form (crack). It has high abuse potential. The half-life of the circulating cocaine is brief: 0.5–1 hour. Acute cocaine toxicity is associated with hypertension, arrhythmia, seizure, and myocardial infarction. Both subjective and toxic effects are expressed when circulating concentrations are rising. Because of its short half-life, maintaining the subjective effects over a single extended period requires repeated dosages of increasing quantity, therefore, correlations between serum concentration and the subjective or toxic effects cannot be established. Because rate of change is more important than serum concentration, a primary factor that determines the toxicity of cocaine is the dose and route of administration. Intravenous administration presents with the greatest hazard, closely followed by smoking.

Cocaine's short half-life is a result of rapid hepatic hydrolysis to inactive metabolites. This is the major route of elimination. Only a small portion of the parent drug can be found in urine after an administered dose. The primary product of hepatic metabolism is benzoylecgonine, which is primarily eliminated in urine. The half-life of benzoylecgonine is 4–7 hours. The presence of this metabolite in urine is a sensitive and specific indicator of cocaine use. It can be detected in urine for up to 3 days after a single use. In chronic heavy abusers, it can be detected in urine for up to 20 days after the last dose. The primary screening procedure for identification of cocaine use is detection of benzoylecgonine in urine by immunoassay. Confirmation testing is done by gas chromatography with mass spectrometry.

Opiates

Opiates are a class of substances capable of analgesia, sedation, and anesthesia.[34] All are derived from or chemically related to substances derived from the opium poppy. The naturally occurring substances include opium, morphine, and codeine. Heroin, hydromorphone (Dilaudid), and oxycodone (Percodan) are chemically modified forms of the naturally occurring opiates. Meperidine (Demerol), methadone (Dolophine), propoxyphene (Darvon), pentazocine (Talwin), and fentanyl (Sublimaze) are the common synthetic opiates. Opiates have a high abuse potential. Chronic use leads to tolerance with physical and psychological dependence. Acute overdose presents with respiratory acidosis due to depression of respiratory centers, myoglobinuria, and possibly an increase in serum indicators of cardiac damage (CKMB, troponin). High-level opiate overdose may lead to death caused by cardiopulmonary failure. Treatment of overdose includes the use of the opiate antagonist naloxone.

Laboratory testing for opiates usually involves initial detection (screening) by immunoassay. Most immunoassays are primarily designed to detect morphine and codeine. However, cross-reactivity as a result of similarities in chemical structure allows detection of many of the opiates: naturally occurring, chemically modified, and synthetic. Gas chromatography with mass spectrometry is the confirmatory method of choice.

Phencyclidine

Phencyclidine (PCP) is an illicit drug with stimulant, depressant, anesthetic, and hallucinogenic properties. It has high abuse potential. Adverse effects are commonly noted at doses that produce the desired subjective effects, such as agitation, hostility, and paranoia. Overdose is associated with stupor and coma. PCP can be ingested or inhaled by smoking PCP-laced tobacco or marijuana. It is a lipophilic drug that rapidly distributes into fat and brain. Elimination is slow as a result of redistribution into circulation and hepatic metabolism. About 10–15%

of an administered dose is eliminated unchanged in urine. Hepatic metabolism forms various products. Identification of PCP abuse is by detection of the parent drug in urine. In chronic heavy users, PCP can be detected 7–30 days after abstinence. Immunoassay is used as the screening procedure. Gas chromatography with mass spectrometry is the confirmatory method.

Sedative Hypnotics

Many therapeutic drugs can be classified as sedative hypnotics or tranquilizers. All members of this class are CNS depressants. They have a wide range of therapeutic roles and are commonly used. Most of these drugs have abuse potential, ranging from high to low. These drugs become available for illegal use through diversion from approved sources. Barbiturates and benzodiazepines are the most common type of sedative hypnotics abused. Although barbiturates have a higher abuse potential, benzodiazepines are more commonly found in abuse and overdose situations. This appears to be a result of availability. There are many individual drugs within the barbiturate and benzodiazepine classification. Secobarbital, pentobarbital, and phenobarbital are the more commonly abused barbiturates. Diazepam (Valium), chlordiazepoxide (Librium), and lorazepam (Ativan) are commonly abused benzodiazepines. Overdose with sedative hypnotics initially presents with lethargy and slurred speech, which can rapidly progress to coma. Respiratory depression is the most serious toxic effect of most of these agents. Hypotension can occur with barbiturates. The toxicity of many of these agents is potentiated by ethanol.

Immunoassay is the most common screening procedure for both barbiturates and benzodiazepines. Broad cross-reactivity within members of each group allows for detection of many individual drugs. Liquid or gas chromatography can be used for confirmatory testing.

SUMMARY

Poisoning cases account for a significant number of hospital admissions and visits to physician offices.[35] The clinical laboratorian serves multiple roles that affect patient outcome in these cases. Identification and quantitation of the toxin is a primary responsibility. In addition, the laboratorian should be ready to suggest testing regimens that may further define the diagnosis and provide a basis for monitoring the efficacy of therapy. Providing an effective clinical toxicology service requires an understanding of the patient population served and a basic understanding of the toxic mechanisms of the poisons commonly encountered.[36]

1. Compound A is reported to have an oral LD_{50} of 5 mg/kg body weight. Compound B is reported to have an LD_{50} of 50 mg/kg body weight. Of the following statements regarding the relative toxicity of these two compounds, which is TRUE?
   a. Ingestion of low amounts of compound A would be predicted to cause more deaths then an equal dose of compound B.
   b. Ingestion of compound B would be expected to produce no toxic effects at a dose of greater than 100 mg/kg body weight.
   c. Neither compound A nor compound B is toxic at any level of oral exposure.
   d. Compound A is more rapidly adsorbed from the gastrointestinal tract than compound B.
   e. Compound B would be predicted to be more toxic than compound A if the exposure route were transdermal.

2. Which of the following statements best describes the TD_{50} of a compound?
   a. The dosage of a substance that is lethal to 50% of the population
   b. The dosage of a substance that would produce therapeutic benefit in 50% of the population
   c. The dosage of a substance that would be predicted to cause a toxic effect in 50% of the population
   d. The percentage of individuals who would experience a toxic response at 50% of the lethal dose
   e. The percentage of the population who would experience a toxic response after an oral dosage of 50 mg

3. Of the following analytic methods, which is most commonly used as the confirmatory method for identification of drugs of abuse?
   a. Scanning differential colorimetry
   b. Ion-specific electrode
   c. Gas chromatography with mass spectrometry
   d. Immunoassay
   e. Nephelometry

4. A weakly acidic toxin (pK = 4.0) that is ingested will:
   a. not be absorbed because it is ionized.
   b. not be absorbed unless a specific transporter is present.
   c. be passively absorbed in the colon (pH = 7.5).
   d. be passively absorbed in the stomach (pH = 3.0).
   e. be absorbed only if a weak base is ingested at the same time.

5. What is the primary product of methanol metabolism by the alcohol-aldehyde dehydrogenase system?
   a. Acetone
   b. Acetaldehyde
   c. Oxalic acid
   d. Formaldehyde
   e. Formic acid

6. Which of the following statements concerning cyanide toxicity is/are TRUE?
   a. Inhalation of smoke from burning plastic is a common cause of cyanide exposure.
   b. Cyanide is a relatively nontoxic compound that requires chronic exposure to produce a toxic effect.
   c. Cyanide expresses its toxicity by inhibition of oxidative phosphorylation.
   d. All of the above are true.
   e. Only a and c are true.

7. Which of the following laboratory results would be consistent with acute high-level oral exposure to an inorganic form of mercury (Hg^{2+})?
   a. High concentrations of mercury in whole blood and urine
   b. Proteinuria
   c. Positive occult blood in stool
   d. All of the above are true
   e. All of the above are false

8. A child presents with microcytic, hypochromia anemia. The physician suspects iron-deficiency anemia. Further laboratory testing reveals a normal total serum iron and iron-binding capacity; however, the zinc protoporphyrin level was very high. A urinary screen for porphyrins was positive. Erythrocytic basophilic stippling was noted on the peripheral smear. Which of the following laboratory tests would be best applied to this case?
   a. Urinary thiocyanate
   b. Carboxyhemoglobin
   c. Whole blood lead
   d. Urinary anabolic steroids
   e. Urinary benzoylecgonine

9. A patient with suspected organophosphate poisoning presents with a low SChE level. However, the confirmatory test, erythrocyte acetylcholinesterase, presents with a normal result. Excluding analytic error, which of the following may explain these conflicting results?
   a. The patient has late-stage hepatic cirrhosis.
   b. The patient was exposed to low levels of organophosphates.

c. The patient has a variant of SChE that displays low activity.

d. All of the above are correct.

e. Only a and c are correct.

10. A patient enters the emergency department in a coma. The physician suspects a drug overdose. Immunoassay screening tests for opiates, barbiturates, benzodiazepines, THC, amphetamines, and PCP were all negative. No ethanol was detected in serum. Can the physician rule out drug overdose as the cause of this coma with these results?

a. Yes

b. No

c. Maybe

REFERENCES

1. Kirk M, Pace S. Pearls, pitfalls and updates in toxicology. Emerg Med Clin North Am 1997;15:427.

2. Brettell TA, Saferstein R. Forensic science. Anal Chem 1997;69:123R.

3. McKenna M, Chick J, Buxton M, et al. The SECCAT survey: the cost and consequences of alcoholism. Alcohol 1996;31:565.

4. Urry FM, Wong Y. Current issues in alcohol testing. Lab Med 1995;26:194.

5. Thorne D, Kaplan K. Laboratory indicators of ethanol consumption. Clin Lab Sci 1999;12:351.

6. Church AS, Witting MD. Laboratory testing in ethanol, methanol, ethylene glycol and isopropanol toxicities. J Emerg Med 1997;15:687.

7. Jaffe FA. Pathogenicity of carbon monoxide. Am J Forensic Med Pathol 1997;18:406.

8. Balzan MV, Agius G, Galea A. Carbon monoxide poisoning: easy to treat but difficult to recognize. Postgrad Med J 1996;72:470.

9. Satarug S, Baker J, Urbenjapol S, et al. A global perspective on cadmium pollution and toxicity in non-occupationally exposed populations Toxicol Lett 2003;137:65.

10. Herber RF, Christensen JM, Sabbioni E. Critical evaluation of cadmium concentration in blood for use in occupational health. Int Arch Occup Environ Health 1997;69:372.

11. Vahter M. Mechanisms of arsenic biotransformation. Toxicology 2002;181:211.

12. Cabrera C, Ortega E, Lorenzo ML, et al. Cadmium contamination of vegetable crops, farmlands, and irrigation waters. Rev Environ Contam Toxicol 1998;154:55.

13. Lauwerys RR, Bernard AM, Roels HA, et al. Cadmium: exposure markers as predictive indicators of nephrotoxic effects. Clin Chem 1994;40:1391.

14. Silbergeld EK. Preventing lead poisoning in children. Annu Rev Public Health 1997;18:187.

15. De Gennaro L. Lead and the developing nervous system. Growth Dev Aging 2002;66:43.

16. Piomeli S. Childhood lead poisoning. Pediatr Clin North Am 2002;49:1285.

17. Diamond GL, Goodrum PE, Felter SP, et al. Gastrointestinal absorption of metals. Drug Chem Toxicol 1997;20:345.

18. Loghman M. Renal effects of environmental and occupational lead exposure. Environ Health Perspect 1997;105:928.

19. Ratcliffe HE, Swanson GM, Fischer LJ. Human exposure to mercury: a critical assessment of the evidence of adverse health effects. J Toxicol Environ Health 1996;49:221.

20. Watanabe C, Satoh H. Evolution of our understanding of methyl mercury as a health threat. Environ Health Perspect 1996;104(Suppl 2):367.

21. Mottet NK, Vahter ME, Charleston JS, et al. Metabolism of methyl mercury in the brain and its toxic significance. Met Ions Biol Syst 1997;34:371.

22. Blondell J. Epidemiology of pesticide poisoning in the United States, with special reference to occupational cases. Occup Med 1997;12:209.

23. Cabrera C, Ortega E, Lorenzo ML. Monitoring for pesticide exposure. AAOHN J 1996;44:599.

24. Temple AR. Acute and chronic effects of aspirin toxicity and their treatment. Arch Intern Med 1981;141:P364.

25. Diener H, Limmroth V. Analgesics. Curr Med Res Opin 2001;17:13.

26. Johnson SC, Pelletier LL. Enhanced hepatotoxicity of acetaminophen in the alcoholic patient. Medicine 1997;76:185.

27. Eshridge KD, Gutherie SK. Clinical issues associated with urine testing of substances of abuse. Pharmacotherapy 1997;17:497.

28. Repetto MR, Repetto M. Habitual, toxic and lethal concentrations of 103 drugs of abuse in humans. J Toxicol Clin Toxicol 1997;37:1.

29. Cho AK, Segal DS, eds. Amphetamine and Its Analogs: Psychopharmacology, Toxicology and Abuse. New York: Academic Press, 1994.

30. Brower K. Anabolic steroid abuse and dependence. Curr Psychiatry Rep 2002;5:377.

31. Bowers LD. Analytic advances in detection of performance-enhancing compounds. Clin Chem 1997;43:1299.

32. Brown T, Dobs A. Endocrine effects of marijuana. J Clin Pharmacol, 2002;42:90S.

33. Boghdadi MS, Henning RJ. Cocaine: pathophysiology and clinical toxicology. Heart Lung 1997;26:484.

34. Kalant H. Opium revisited: a brief review of its nature, composition nonmedical use and the relative risks. Addiction 1997;92:267.

35. Vernon DD, Gleich MC. Poisoning and drug overdose. Crit Care Clin 1997;13:647.

36. Mokhlesi B, Leikin J, Murray P, Corbridge T. Adult toxicology in critical care. Chest 2003;123:897

SUGGESTED READINGS

Casarett LJ, Klaassen CD, Doull J, eds. Casarett and Doull's Toxicology: The Basic Science of Poisons, 6th ed. New York: McGraw-Hill, 2001.

Pradyot P. A Comprehensive Guide to the Hazardous Properties of Chemical Substances, 2nd ed. New York: John Wiley & Sons, 1999.

Sipes IG, McQueen CA, Gandolfi AJ. Comprehensive Toxicology. New York: Pergamon, 1997.

Circulating Tumor Markers: Basic Concepts and Clinical Applications

James T. Wu

CHAPTER OUTLINE

OBJECTIVES

Upon completion of this chapter, the clinical laboratorian should be able to
- Discuss the incidence of cancer in the United States.
- Explain the role of tumor markers in cancer management.
- Identify the characteristics or properties of an ideal tumor marker.
- State the major clinical value of tumor markers.
- Name the major tumors and their associated markers.
- Describe the major properties, methods of analysis, and clinical use of CEA, AFP, CA125, CA19–9, PSA, β-hCG, and PALP.
- Explain the use of enzymes and hormones as tumor markers.

KEY TERMS

Cancer
DNA index (DI)
Neoplasm

Oncofetal antigen
Oncogene
Protooncogene

Staging
Tumor-associated antigen

Tumor marker
Tumor-specific antigen

BASIC CONCEPTS

Growth Regulation

There are two major processes involved in cell growth: proliferation and differentiation. *Cancer* is a disease of abnormal growth. When the growth and development of a normal cell loses control, tumor cells begin to emerge, which is called *tumorigenesis.*

Neoplasia and Hyperplasia

Neoplasia and hyperplasia are two similar biologic processes. The major difference between them is how growth is controlled. Hyperplasia involves the multiplication of cells in an organ or tissue, which may consequently have increased in volume. Neoplasia, however, involves the possibility of normal cells undergoing cancerous proliferation as hyperplasia taking place under less controlled conditions; it is, therefore, a form of pathologic hyperplasia. Therefore, hyperplasia serves a useful purpose and is controlled by stimuli, whereas neoplasia is unregulated and serves no purpose. In other words, the elevation of tumor markers in the case of hyperplasia is transient, whereas neoplasia will be a long lasting phenomenon if not treated.

Differences Between Normal and Cancer Cells

When either differentiation or proliferation becomes unregulated, there is a risk for normal cells to be converted to tumor cells. This process is usually associated with changes of the genetic components of the cell that account for the different behaviors and functions observed in cancer. Conceivably, the major modifications that distinguish normal cells from cancer cells could be entirely accounted for by various phenomena related to the genetic blue prints of the cell, such as the mutation of cellular oncogenes and abnormal regulation of their expression or a rearrangement of oncogenic DNA sequences.

Benign and Malignant Tumors

Most tumor cells undergo a benign stage, gradually progress to malignancy, and eventually become metastasized if not treated.[1] The genetic instability associated with tumor cells can make tumor cells more susceptible to additional mutations, which may lead ultimately to malignant disease. During the benign stage, tumors remain at the primary site and present a smaller risk to the host. At this early stage, the patient stands a good chance of being successfully treated, such as by the complete removal of the tumor. Therefore, the early detection of a benign tumor is critical to cancer prevention in general and to high-risk families in particular. All benign tumors are well differentiated and composed of cells resembling the mature normal cells from the tissue of origin of the neoplasm.

Metastasis

Most cancer deaths are associated with metastatic disease. Multiple genetic changes are the main reasons for growth regulation imbalances, leading to uncontrolled proliferation. Metastasis is, therefore, a multistep processes involving numerous tumor cell–host cell and cell–matrix interactions. For tumor cells to metastasize,[2] the tumor cells at the primary site have to first penetrate their adjacent surroundings, including the epithelial basement membrane and the interstitial stroma. They then invade blood or lymphatic vessels and are carried to distant sites, until they are finally arrested in the venous/capillary beds or solid tissue of a distant organ. In this new environment, these tumor cells must again penetrate the vascular walls to proliferate at the new distant site. In general, the larger, more aggressive, or rapidly growing the primary neoplasm, the greater the likelihood that the tumor cells will metastasize. It should also be noted that metastasis is a highly selective process. Cells isolated from individual tumors may differ in many ways, with respect to capacity for invasion and metastasis, growth rate, cell surface receptors, immunogenicity, and response to cytotoxic drugs.[2]

Signal Transduction Pathway

The pathway of signal transduction controls both cell cycle and apoptosis (Fig. 30-1). The pathway is an orderly and specific transmission of growth-regulatory messages from outside the cell to the machinery controlling replication inside the cell nucleus.[3]

In this pathway, extracellular stimuli bind to and activate their corresponding receptors with inducible protein-tyrosine kinase activity at the cell surface. These stimuli include hormones, such as insulin and adrenal medullary hormones, cytokines, transforming growth factor β, epidermal growth factor, c-erbB-2, nerve growth factor, and even antigens. A signal from the receptor is then relayed, amplified, and integrated, resulting in the expression of target genes in the nucleus and subsequent biologic responses instructing the cell to proliferate or cease proliferation.

Until recently, the linear path from growth factor and membrane receptor all the way to DNA replication is nearly complete. On binding of the stimulus to the receptor, the transmission of signal is carried out by protein phosphorylation. A wave of protein activation takes place, involving activation of the enzymatic function of many protein kinases. For example, a large number of extracellular signals initially react with signaling pathways and use G proteins (ras) to lead to diverse biologic consequences.

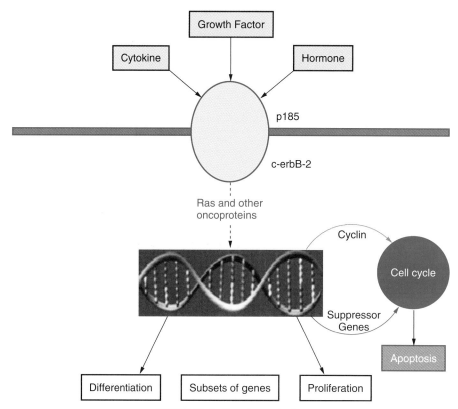

FIGURE 30-1. Signal transduction.

Cell Cycle

The cell cycle is one of the most important determining factors controlling cell proliferation. The cell cycle involves the passage of a cell through a complete round of replication. In most mammalian cells, the cell cycle is composed of four phases: an interphase section, composed of the G_1, S, and G_2 phases, and a fourth phase, M, or mitosis (Fig. 30-2). The G_1 phase is defined as the interval between the conclusion of mitosis and the start of DNA replication, and the S phase is the interval during which the nuclear genome is replicated. The G_2 phase is the interval between completion of nuclear DNA replication and the onset of mitosis. In most replicating cell populations, there is a pool of nonreplicating cells that maintains the ability to reenter replication. These reversibly quiescent cells occupy a special metabolic compartment or fifth phase, known as G_o. Completion of the cell cycle requires the coordination of various macromolecular syntheses, assemblies, and movements. Coordination of these complex processes is achieved by a series of changes in cyclin-dependent kinases (CDKs).[4] The active forms of the CDKs are a complex of at least two proteins, a kinase and a cyclin. These components of the cell cycle are encoded by a separate category of genes that, when mutated, will not only increase genetic instability but also acceler-

ate cellular evolution and the progression to malignancy. Tumors, in short, result from the absence of certain cell cycle controls.[5] Defects in the cell cycle machinery may, therefore, help cause cancer. Mutations in the cyclin gene have been found in a variety of cancers.

Apoptosis

The balance between cell proliferation and cell death is, in effect, by apoptosis. Apoptosis, a programmed cell or physiologic death, is a natural self-destruct system present in all cells.[6] Failure of cells to undergo apoptotic cell death may lead to cancer. It is the natural process the body employs for the replacement of cells and the deletion of damaged cells inherent in the normal functioning of multicellular organisms. Apoptosis is a control mechanism for tissue remodeling during growth and development. Therefore, apoptosis provides a way for the body to eliminate cells that have been produced in excess, that have developed improperly, or that have sustained genetic damage.

Currently, several markers related to apoptosis include p53 protein, Bcl 2, and Fas/Fas ligand. They can be both inducers and inhibitors of cell-death. These markers would have tremendous potential for diagnosis, prognosis, and therapeutic application.

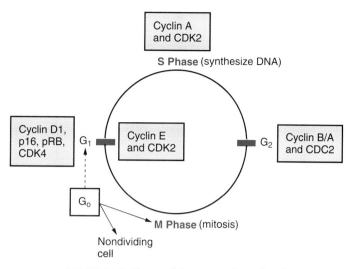

FIGURE 30-2. Phases of the mammalian cell cycle.

Angiogenesis

Angiogenesis is a fundamental process by which new blood vessels are formed.[6,7] Tumor growth and metastasis are angiogenesis-dependent. Angiogenesis is critical, not only for the growth of solid tumors, but also for the shedding of cells from the primary tumor and the development of metastases at distant sites.[8] The new blood vessels embedded in a tumor provide a gateway for tumor cells to enter the circulation and to metastasize to distant sites. The degree of angiogenesis in an initial primary tumor correlates with metastatic spread and survival rates in patients. A tumor must continuously stimulate the growth of new capillary blood vessels for the tumor to grow.

Assessment of tumor angiogenesis may, therefore, prove valuable in selecting patients with early breast carcinoma for aggressive therapy. The most well-known angiogenic factors are vascular endothelial growth factor (VEGF), acidic and basic fibroblast growth factor (aFGF and bFGF), and transforming growth factor α (TGF-α), all of which transform normal cells into transformed phenotypes.

Adhesion

Adhesion molecules are a specific class of transmembrane glycoprotein involved wherever cells are moving and interacting, as in wound healing, inflammation, and cancer metastasis. They regulate the migration of leukocytes to sites of inflammation or into lymphatic tissue. Increasing evidence has shown that the appearance of certain membrane molecules is related to metastatic potential or a sign of the conversion of normal to malignant cells. Many studies have confirmed that the expression of these adhesion molecules on the cell membrane has impacted the behavior of the tumor cell.

Three classes of adhesion molecules are known: selectins, integrins, and the immunoglobulin superfamily. Each class possesses unique structural elements and characteristics. Soluble adhesion molecules can be found in blood and tissue fluids.

CASE STUDY 30-1

A 72-year-old woman complained of intermittent diarrhea and constipation for the last 2 weeks and a weight loss of 22 pounds over the last 6 months. Physical examination was unremarkable except for a guaiac-positive stool. A colonoscopy was performed, which identified a circumferential mass in the sigmoid colon. A biopsy was performed, which identified the mass as an adenocarcinoma. A carcinoembryonic antigen (CEA) level was obtained as part of her initial surgical workup.

Questions

1. Is the CEA test useful as a screening test for colon carcinoma?

2. What other conditions can result in elevated CEA levels?

3. How is CEA used to monitor patients after surgery for colon cancer?

4. What other laboratory tests should be considered in the initial surgical workup of this patient?

SPECIFICITY AND SENSITIVITY

It is essential that both the meaning of test sensitivity and tumor marker specificity be understood before discussing their applications. In fact, the clinical utility of a tumor marker becomes almost totally dependent on the specificity and sensitivity of the tumor marker. When a tumor marker assay is said to be 100% sensitive, the assay will detect all patients with a particular type of cancer, whereas an assay that is 100% specific will identify only the patients with the specific type of tumor and not those with benign or nonmalignant diseases. It is unfortunate that none of the tumor markers discovered so far can approach the 100% specificity and sensitivity of an ideal tumor marker.

CLINICAL UTILITIES OF TUMOR MARKERS

Screening

Up to the present time, none of the tumor markers discovered had sufficient specificity and sensitivity for screening in the general population. Screening is not recommended for most tumor markers, especially in an asymptomatic population. In addition to the lack of desired specificity and sensitivity of tumor markers, the low prevalence of cancer in general would also discourage screenings for cancer. It was also feared that the nonspecific nature of most tumor marker tests could cause unnecessary alarm or anxiety in the general population.

Nevertheless, there are exceptions in which successful cancer screening has been carried out by measuring tumor markers in carefully defined populations.

α-Fetoprotein (AFP)

The screening for primary hepatoma in Asian countries is based on the measurement of serum AFP. It is thought to be a good example of such an exception as a result of the high incidence of liver cancer in that area of the world. Additional information and study is required to confirm this.

Prostate-Specific Antigen (PSA) and Free PSA

Because of tissue specificity, PSA became the first tumor marker recommended for screening for prostate cancer in men older than age 50.[9] The purpose was to detect prostate cancer at early curable stages, when the tumor is still confined inside the organ. So-called PSA is actually present in the blood circulation in two major forms: free PSA and a PSA–α_1-antichymotrypsin (PSA–ACT) complex. Measuring the free PSA percentage (free PSA/total PSA $\times$ 100) or free PSA to PSA–ACT ratio may help differentiate benign prostate hyperplasia (BPH) from prostate cancer.[10]

Susceptibility Genes

Several familial cancers are associated with germline mutations in various genes. The most prominent of these are the genes for susceptibility to breast and ovarian cancer, such as BRCA1 and BRCA2. In the colon, the adenomatous polyposis coli (APC) gene can be inherited and predispose to cancer. Screening tests for BRCA1 and BRCA2 are now available to screen these families for the identification of carriers.

Monitoring Treatment

One of the two most useful applications of tumor markers involves their use in monitoring the course during treatment of the cancer patient. The measurement of serum tumor markers during treatment gives an indication of the effectiveness of the antitumor drug used and provides a guide for the selection of the most effective drug for each individual case (ie, it supplies a means to determine therapeutic efficacy).

CASE STUDY 30-2

A 69-year-old Caucasian man presented to the medical clinic with complaints of increased and difficult urination. Further questioning revealed the need to urinate several times a night. Although he has had the problem for some time, it has recently become worse. A serum prostate-specific antigen (PSA) was obtained and a digital rectal examination was performed. The PSA level was elevated at 15 ng/mL (reference range, <4 ng/ml) and the digital exam revealed an enlarged prostate without palpable nodules.

Questions

1. Can serum PSA be used alone as a screening test for prostate cancer?

2. What are some causes for an elevated serum PSA level?

3. If this patient's cancer is limited to the prostate, should PSA levels be monitored after radical prostatectomy and/or radiation therapy?

4. What other laboratory tests should be performed in this patient's initial workup?

Detection of Recurrence

Monitoring tumor markers for the detection of recurrence following the surgical removal of the tumor is the second most useful application of tumor markers. Because patients being monitored have already had their cancer identified, the specificity of the tumor marker is less important than sensitivity. It is desirable to monitor the patient using a highly sensitive tumor marker test to detect recurrence as early as possible. It should be noted that the appearance of most circulating tumor markers have a lead time of several months (3–6 months) prior to the stage at which many of the physical procedures can be used for the detection of the cancer.

Prognosis

For cancer patients, determination of prognosis is based on the assessment of tumor aggressiveness, which, in turn, determines how a patient should be treated. Prognostic factors measured in the clinical laboratory also indicate risk and predict the length of a relapse-free, as well as overall, survival period at the time of primary therapy. This practice has gained in popularity in recent years. For example, prognostic factors (or risk factors) are routinely measured in the breast tumor cytosol to help determine the proper endocrine or chemotherapy for patients following tumor removal.

Because the serum concentration of tumor markers increases with tumor progression and usually reaches the highest levels when tumors become metastasized, the serum levels of tumor markers at diagnosis are likely to reflect the aggressiveness of the tumor and help predict the outcome for the patients. High levels of serum tumor marker measured during diagnosis would indicate the presence of a malignant or metastatic tumor associated with a poor prognosis.

Early Detection

Detecting phenotypes in the blood circulation corresponding to early mutations of a cancer allows the detection of early neoplasm at the curable stage.[11] It should be noted that several risk factors may lead to tumorigenesis, which can be identified and eliminated with diet adjustment and lifestyle change. Most risk factors are related to inflammation and oxidative stress. Measurement of all mutant phenotypes and risk factors in the circulation would help identify individuals at risk for cancer or detect early tumors in benign state.

Target Therapy

Previously, drugs used in chemotherapy were predominantly DNA-active drugs that were considerably toxic and had limited efficacy. Recently, monoclonal antibodies and enzyme inhibitors interacting with signal transduction pathway molecules, cell cycle apoptosis, angiogenesis, and adhesion have entered clinical trials. Conceivably, interrupting the permanent, or constitutive signals that drive tumor cell growth will be a more effective antitumor therapy. Inhibition of tumor cell proliferation may also be effective by introducing agents (or genes) that turn off the signaling pathway or pathways that specifically drive proliferation within a given tumor or tumor type. The prevailing new rationale is aimed at the development of target-selective "smart" drugs on the basis of characterized mechanisms of action. The specific defect of the tumor identified by these new tumor markers should, therefore, lead to the design of more specific drugs, including antibodies and small molecules, which inhibit growth factor receptors and receptor tyrosine kinases.

TYPES OF TUMOR MARKERS

The most noticeable phenotypic expression associated with cancer cells is related to cell growth regulation. Any molecule that can be identified with malignant transformation, proliferation, de-differentiation, and metastases of tumor cells can be used as a tumor marker. The clinical value of any given tumor marker depends on its intended clinical use, as well as its specificity and sensitivity.

Enzymes, Serum Proteins, and Hormones

Warburg was the first to note that malignant tumors usually exhibit a high rate of glycolytic activity in the presence of oxygen. Since then, glycolytic enzymes have been monitored during the management of certain cancer patients.[12] Even in recent years, several enzymes and isoenzymes were still being used extensively as tumor markers (Tables 30-1 and 30-2). Although it was realized that these ubiquitous serum enzymes were not specific for cancer, their levels often reflected tumor progression and paralleled the clinical status of the patient. Therefore, they are clinically useful for monitoring the success of therapy. Methods for measuring these tumor markers in the early days were limited to enzymatic activity and electrophoresis, both tests of relatively low sensitivity. An increasing number of immunoassays have been developed for enzymes and isoenzymes, more recently using specific monoclonal antibodies for the purpose of further improving test sensitivity and specificity.

More than one mechanism accounts for the elevation of enzymes in cancer. In most instances, the elevation is related to the higher proliferation rate of tumor cells. However, the elevation of certain enzymes may be a result of oncofetal expression and others may be related to gene mutation. Isoenzymes with different tissue specificities (*eg*, lactate dehydrogenase [LD], creatine kinase [CK], and alkaline phosphatase [ALP]) can also be identified with many malignant diseases.[13] Studies have shown re-

TABLE 30-1. ENZYMES AS TUMOR MARKERS

ENZYME	ASSOCIATED MALIGNANT DISEASE
Prostatic acid phosphatase	Prostate carcinoma, late stage
Lysozyme	Colon cancer; monocytic and myelomonocytic leukemia
Lactate dehydrogenase	Acute leukemia; malignant lymphoma; germ cell tumors; metastatic colon, breast, and lung cancers
5'-Nucleotide phosphodiesterase	Lung cancer; liver metastases
Sialyltransferase	Nonspecific
Fucosyltransferase	Multiple malignant tumors
Thymidine kinase	Hodgkin's lymphoma; certain leukemias; small cell carcinoma of the lung
Terminal deoxynucleotidyl transferase	Lymphoblastic cancer

peatedly that the elevation of certain specific isoenzymes is responsible for the observed increases of overall enzyme activities in many malignant diseases. Conceivably, measuring specific isoenzymes instead of the overall enzymatic activity would improve the specificity of the test.

Carcinoembryonic Proteins

Under normal conditions, the expression of all proteins is subjected to genetic regulation. At a certain stage of cell development, the initiation of cellular differentiation will selectively turn off the expression of certain phenotypes (suppression) and allow only a few to continue. This well regulated process, however, will be lost to varying degrees when the normal cell is transformed into a tumor cell, depending on the stage of the tumor. In other words, the expression of some proteins, slated to be turned-off during normal developmental processes, may be reactivated in tumor cells. The detection of almost equal amounts of oncodevelopmental gene products during both fetal development and carcinogenesis lead us to believe that there is a common, gene-related, basic

TABLE 30-2. SERUM ISOENZYMES AS TUMOR MARKERS

ISOENZYME	ASSOCIATED MALIGNANT DISEASES
CK-BB	Adenocarcinoma of the prostate, lung and stomach; not specific
Type 2 macro-CK (oligomeric mitochondrial CK)[a]	Metastatic liver cancer and various carcinomas
Type I macro-CK (complex between CK-BB and IgG)	Various neoplastic diseases
Mitochondrial CK-IgA complex	Detected in various carcinomas. Appears to be a prognosticator for patients with advanced tumors.
Galactosyltransferase II[b]	Ovarian, liver, and esophageal cancers
Placental ALP (PALP)[c]	Advanced colorectal cancer; not specific.
Placental-like ALP (Regan isoenzyme)	Highest frequency was found in germ cell tumors (eg, seminomas) and ovarian cancers; not specific.
Liver ALP	Liver metastases. Also elevated in seminomas and ovarian cancers
Bone ALP	Osteosarcoma; bone metastases
LD-1	Testicular germ cell tumors (seminomas, yolk sac tumor)
LD-4 and LD-5 isoenzymes	Elevated in most cancers at advanced stage

[a]Data are from Kanemitsu F. Clinical significance and characteristics of creatine kinase-immunoglobulin complexes in sera from patients with malignant tumors. Clin Chim Acta 1986;160:19–26.

[b]Data are from Uemura M, Yamasaki M, Yoshida S, et al. An enzyme immunoassay for galactosyltransferase isoenzyme II, and its clinical application to cancer diagnosis. Clin Chem 1990;36:598–601.

[c]The placental-like isozyme has different biochemical and immunochemical properties compared to the placental ALP. However, there is 98% homology in amino acid sequence between these two enzymes.

CASE STUDY 30-3

A 25-year-old man was found to have an elevated lactate dehydrogenase (LD) of 350 IU/L (reference range, 93–139 IU/L) that was confirmed with a second sample. LD electrophoresis was performed and revealed an elevation in the LD-1 isoenzyme above the normal range. Electrocardiogram (ECG) studies were negative for acute myocardial infarct. Creatine kinase (CK) electrophoresis showed only a CK-MM band. On physical examination, the man was found to have a tumor mass in the left scrotum. Serum α-fetoprotein (AFP) and β-human chorionic gonadotropin (β-hCG) tests were ordered.

Questions

1. What is the most likely primary diagnosis for this patient?

2. What kind of benign diseases should be considered in the differential diagnosis? Why?

3. Can the type of testicular tumor be determined based on the serum AFP and β-hCG results?

4. Can a final diagnosis be made based only on the tumor marker findings? If not, why not?

---

process in development, as well as in carcinogenesis. For the same reason, malignant transformation may be treated as a special phase of development.

Many of these carcinoembryonic proteins, such as carcinoembryonic antigen (CEA) and AFP, do not have clearly defined physiologic functions. Most of these molecules are present in nanogram and picogram concentrations in the blood circulation. Quantification of their concentrations circulating in the blood for both diagnosis and patient management requires the sensitivity of radioimmunoassays (RIAs) or enzyme immunoassays (EIAs).[14] However, the specificity and sensitivity of these carcinoembryonic proteins are not 100%; they are, nevertheless, much higher than that of enzymes, serum proteins, and hormones when used as tumor markers. The serum concentration of these carcinoembryonic proteins not only correlates well with tumor activity but also has the potential for predicting prognosis.

Monoclonal Defined Tumor Markers

Several epitopes that appear on the tumor marker can be identified by monoclonal antibodies. They were developed originally in an attempt to replace CEA for the

TABLE 30.3. MONOCLONAL TUMOR MARKER IMMUNOASSAYS

MONOCLONAL KIT	ASSOCIATED MAJOR MALIGNANT DISEASE
CA 125	Ovarian carcinoma
Hybri-BREScan (CA 549) or CA 15-3[a]	Breast carcinoma
Hybri-CMark (CA 195) or CA 19-9[a]	Pancreatic carcinoma
CA 72-4	Gastric carcinoma
Free PSA	Differentiate between BPH and prostatic carcinoma

[a]Hybritech (San Diego, CA).

management of patients with various carcinomas. These monoclonal antibodies have indeed provided a greater degree of specificity and sensitivity than the CEA assay in the management of patients with breast, ovarian, and pancreatic carcinomas (Table 30-3).

It should be noted that more then one type of molecule expresses the same epitope; in fact, many tumor-associated epitopes are also shared by various tumor markers derived from different tumors. Consequently, monoclonal assays may react with different molecules as long as they both express the same epitope.

Nonspecific Tumor Markers

Certain tumor markers are detectable nonspecifically in many cancers, much less specific than most tumor markers used routinely for cancer patient management; their concentrations are nevertheless sensitive to changes of the tumor activity. Many of these nonspecific tumor markers are inexpensive and simple to measure, and are, therefore, useful for monitoring therapy and detecting recurrence for patients with known diagnosis. For example, lipid-associated sialic acid in the plasma (LASA-P) can be quantified with a simple, rapid, and inexpensive calorimetric procedure and its serum concentration is closely parallel to the serum concentrations of many tumor markers of higher specificity.

Cell-Specific Tumor Markers

Most tumor markers described above are tumor markers related to carcinomas, which are derived from epithelial cells. However, both neuroendocrine and squamous cells can be found in various tumors and can progress to malignancy. For example, squamous cell antigen (SCCA) is the marker for squamous cell carcinoma (SCC), and chromogranin A (CgA) and neuron-specific enolase (NSE) are markers of neuroendocrine cell carcinoma.

RECOMMENDATIONS FOR TEST ORDERING

It is important to know how to order a tumor marker test for the management of cancer patients. Several factors need to be considered during test ordering.

Ordering Serial Tests

Because most tumor markers are nonspecific, it is difficult to differentiate between malignant diseases and benign diseases based solely on elevated results of a single test.

Using the Same Kit

It has been found that patients may be mistreated due to the inconsistent laboratory results obtained from different laboratories using different commercial kits.

Half-Life of the Tumor Marker

Tumor marker serum levels are routinely measured to determine the success of surgical tumor removal. To make certain that the determined concentration is not affected by the residual concentration of the tumor marker circulating in the blood prior to surgery, the preexisting tumor marker needs sufficient time to clear from circulation before obtaining a blood specimen from the patient for measurement. To determine the proper interlude after surgery and before testing, the half-life of the tumor marker in the blood circulation needs to be taken into consideration. It is conceivable that, in addition to the half-life of the tumor marker, the preexisting concentration and the upper normal limit of the tumor marker may also play a role in determining the length of time before a specimen is obtained from the patient after surgery for testing.

Hook Effect

One drawback of the popular sandwich-type solid phase immunoassay is its association with the hook effect. The hook effect tends to give a falsely low value when the serum concentration of the tumor marker rises above a certain elevated level. The consequence of a hook effect can be serious, especially when levels fall within the normal range and are misinterpreted as normal when, in fact, the patient has a malignant disease. For example, it is not unusual to find specimens that measure over 100,000 U/mL of CA 19-9 in patients with pancreatic carcinoma. In those patients, falsely low CA 19-9, as a result of the hook effect, may be reported. It is important, therefore, to determine at what level of tumor marker the hook effect will start to occur for the kit that is being used for measurements. The measurement of tumor markers at two different dilutions, with at least a 10-fold difference, will ordinarily avoid the hook effect. It should be noted that there is no hook effect in immunoassays based on a competitive binding format.

FREQUENTLY ORDERED TUMOR MARKERS

Individual Tumor Markers

α-Fetoprotein (AFP)

AFP is a major fetal serum protein, as well as one of the major carcinoembryonic proteins. Elevated AFP can be found in patients with primary hepatoma carcinoma cell (HCC) and yolk sac-derived germ cell tumors. AFP is the most useful serum marker for diagnosis and management of HCC. However, AFP is also transiently elevated during pregnancy and in many benign liver diseases, such as hepatitis and liver cirrhosis. Because of the high prevalence of liver cancer in China and other countries in Southeast Asia, AFP testing has been used successfully to screen for hepatoma in that region of the world. The upper normal for serum AFP is approximately 15 ng/mL for adults. Newborns and young infants have much higher serum AFP values. At about 8 months, the value of serum AFP approaches adult levels.[15]

β₂-Microglobulin (β2M)

β2M is a low-molecular-weight protein (11,800 D) and the constant light chain of the human histocompatibility locus antigen (HLA) expressed on the surface of most nucleated cells. The surfaces of lymphocytes and monocytes are particularly rich in β2M. β2M is a nonspecific tumor marker because it is elevated, not only in solid tumors but also in lymphoproliferative diseases and a variety of inflammatory disorders, including rheumatoid arthritis, systemic lupus erythematosus, Sjögren's syndrome, and Crohn's disease. β2M is stable in serum but degrades rapidly in the urine at pH <6.0. A more sensitive assay is required for measuring β2M in urine. The normal serum β2M concentration is approximately 0.9–2.5 mg/L.

Cancer Antigen 125 (CA 125)

CA 125 was first defined by a murine monoclonal antibody OC 125 raised against a serous ovarian carcinoma cell line. This epitope is associated with a high-molecular-weight (>200 kD) mucin-like glycoprotein expressed in coelomic epithelium during embryonic development and human ovarian carcinoma cells. CA 125 is a glycoprotein antigen in which a carbohydrate moiety is also part of the antigenic determinant. Elevated serum CA 125 is found in greater than 80% of nonmucinous epithelial ovarian carcinomas, such as the serous cystadenocarcinoma of the ovary. CA 125 is not specific for ovarian carcinoma; however, the appearance of elevated CA 125 has been found to precede clinical diagnoses of recurrent diseases from 1 to 4 months.

CA 125 may be useful for detecting ovarian tumors at an early stage and for monitoring treatments without surgical restaging. Upper normal limit for serum CA 125 is 35 U/mL.

Cancer Antigen 15-3 (CA 15-3)

CA 15-3 represents distinct epitopes on a high-molecular-weight (300–450 kD) mucin glycoprotein (polymorphic epithelial mucin) expressed by various adenocarcinomas, especially those associated with the breast. Elevated serum CA 15-3 levels (>25 U/mL) are observed in 70–80% of patients with metastatic breast cancer. However, CA 15-3 levels can also be elevated in chronic hepatitis, liver cirrhosis, sarcoidosis, tuberculosis, and systemic lupus erythematosus. CA 15-3 is currently used to monitor the clinical course of patients with breast cancer. CA 15-3 is a more sensitive and specific marker for monitoring the clinical course of patients with metastatic breast cancer and is a more sensitive marker for metastasized breast cancer than CEA.

Cancer Antigen 19-9 (CA 19-9)

The molecule carrying the CA 19-9 epitope appears as a mucin in the sera of cancer patients but as a ganglioside in tumor cells. CA 19-9 is related to Lewis blood group substances, and only serum antigen from cancer patients belonging to the $Le(a^-b^+)$ or $Le(a^+b^-)$ blood group will be CA19-9 positive. There, the assay for CA 19-9 measures a carbohydrate antigenic determinant expressed on a high-molecular-weight mucin.[16] CA 19-9, like other mucin antigens, is not organ specific and is elevated in various adenocarcinomas, including pancreatic, lung, colorectal, and gastric carcinomas. The highest sensitivity of CA 19-9 was found in pancreatic and gastric cancers. Serum CA 19-9 concentrations are not only highly and frequently elevated in both gastric and pancreatic carcinomas, but are also useful for monitoring the success of therapy and detecting recurrence in these cancer patients. The upper normal limit for serum CA 19-9 is 37 U/mL.

Carcinoembryonic Antigen (CEA)

CEA is a glycoprotein with a molecular weight of approximately 200 kD. CEA is the first of the so-called carcinoembryonic proteins discovered by Gold and Freedman.[17,18] CEA is still the most widely used tumor marker for gastrointestinal (GI) cancer today; however, most CEA assays using polyclonal antibodies have been replaced by assay using monoclonal anti-CEA antibodies. CEA was originally thought to be a specific marker for colorectal cancer; however, after further studies, it turned out to be a nonspecific marker. High levels of CEA (>10 ng/mL) are frequently associated with malignancy. Liver damage can impair CEA clearance and lead to increased levels in the blood circulation. Increased CEA concentrations have been observed in persons who are heavy smokers and in certain patients following radiation treatment and chemotherapy. Upper normal range for serum CEA is 2.5–5 ng/mL, depending on the kit used.

Chromogranin A

Chromogranin A is a major soluble protein of the chromaffin granule, a catecholamine-storage vesicle. Chromogranin A can be released from the adrenal medulla, together with catecholamines, on stimulation of the splanchnic nerve. It has been a useful index of sympathoadrenal catecholamine release in laboratory animals. However, chromogranin A is not confined to chromaffin cells of the adrenal medulla and sympathetic neurons; it is also present in various neuroendocrine tissue. Chromogranin A is a useful marker of exocytotic sympathoadrenal activity in patients with pheochromocytoma. Plasma chromogranin A is also elevated in patients with peptide-producing tumors. Elevated serum levels of chromogranin A have also been found in endocrine pancreatic tumor, carcinoid tumors, and small cell lung cancer.

Estrogen Receptor (ER)

ER is a protein (70 kD) that is localized in the nuclei of mammary and uterine tissue. Both ER and PgR (progesterone receptor) are also transcription factors that, on binding to DNA, activate DNA and modulate specific gene expressions. Measurement of ER and PR in the breast tumor cytosol is used to identify those patients most likely to benefit from endocrine therapy. Approximately 55–60% and 80% of patients whose primary tumors demonstrated ER and both ER and PgR, respectively, will respond to hormone therapy. Patients whose primary tumors are ER/PgR-rich also experienced longer disease-free intervals after mastectomy and longer overall survival than those with receptor-poor cancer.

Human Chorionic Gonadotropin (hCG)

hCG, a sialoglycoprotein (45 kD) consisting of noncovalently linked α and β dissimilar subunits, is secreted by trophoblast cells of the normal placenta. Both malignant and nonmalignant trophoblast cells synthesize and secret, not only the biologic active dimer but also the free α and β subunits. hCG is elevated in the urine and serum during pregnancy, but present only in trace amounts (<0.3 IU/2) in normal sera. However, elevated hCG can be found in trophoblastic tumors, choriocarcinoma, and germ cell tumors of the ovary and testis. More than 60–70% of patients with nonseminomas and occasionally those with seminomas have elevated free β-hCG. Ectopic β-hCG is also occasionally elevated in ovarian cancer and some lung cancers. It is free β-hCG, not free α-hCG or total hCG, that is sensitive and specific for aggressive neoplasms. Free β-hCG is not detectable (<100 ng/L) in the serum of healthy subjects.

Homovanillic Acid (HVA)

In adults, HVA and vanillylmandelic acid (VMA) are excreted in larger than normal amounts in patients with tumors originating from the neural crest. Measurement of urinary VMA and HVA is considered useful for detection and monitoring of patients with pheochromocytoma. Their measurement is also useful for the diagnosis of neuroblastoma in children.

Lipid-Associated Sialic Acid in Plasma (LASA-P)

Sialic acids (N-acetylneuraminic acids) are the acylated derivatives of neuraminic acid and the terminal residues at the nonreducing end of the carbohydrate chains in many glycoproteins, glycolipids, and proteoglycans. Sialoglycoproteins on the tumor cell surface have a long history of association with invasiveness and metastases. LASA-P is found elevated in various malignant diseases, such as in the breast, GI, or lungs. It is also altered in leukemia, lymphoma, Hodgkin's disease, and melanoma, as well as in nonmalignant inflammatory diseases. Apparently, LASA-P is not specific to any specific type of tumor and is used in conjunction with other tumor markers for increased levels of sensitivity and specificity.

Neuron-Specific Enolase (NSE)

NSE is the γ subunit of an enolase isoenzyme in the glycolytic pathway, which is found predominantly in neurons and neuroendocrine cells. NSE is also detected in several cells, including those that make up the amine precursor uptake and decarboxylation (APUD) systems and cells of the diffuse neuroendocrine system.

Elevated levels of NSE can be found in tumors originating from the neuroendocrine cell system, including glucagonomas and insulinomas. The highest levels were found in oat cell, small cell, and lung carcinoma. Elevated serum NSE can also be found in children with neuroblastoma; more than one half of those children had NSE levels greater than 100 ng/mL. A few patients with other lung cancers could also have elevated serum NSE levels; however, no elevations were found in patients with benign lung diseases.

Progesterone Receptor (PgR)

PgR is a member of a superfamily of ligand-activated nuclear transcription factors and is composed of specific domains involved in DNA, hormone-binding, and transactivation. PgR is detected in the human as two distinct proteins of different molecular weights of approximately 94 and 120 kD, respectively. Because synthesis of PgR in breast tumors is ER dependent, PgR is an even more sensitive indicator than ER of potential responsiveness to endocrine therapy. When patients were positive for both ER and PgR, almost 80% responded to various hormonal therapies, whereas the response rate was only about 60% in patients positive for ER only.

Prostate-Specific Antigen (PSA)

Free PSA is a single-chain glycoprotein (about 33–34 kD) that is functionally a kallikrein-like serine protease produced exclusively by the epithelial cells lining the acini and ducts of the prostate gland; it is a major protein in seminal plasma. Because free PSA is a serine protease, free PSA complexes with various protease inhibitors and forms complexes in the serum. The major PSA complex detected in the serum is PSA–ACT complex. All current commercial kits for serum PSA are actually measuring both free PSA and PSA–ACT, so-called total PSA (tPSA). tPSA is perhaps the best tumor marker discovered so far. The tissue specificity of tPSA makes it the most useful tumor marker available for the diagnosis and management of prostate cancer. Lack of cancer specificity is the only drawback with tPSA. Benign conditions, such as benign prostate hyperplasia (BPH), prostatitis, and infarction, can also give rise to elevated serum tPSA levels. Because of its tissue specificity, the tPSA assay is particularly useful for monitoring the success of surgical prostatectomy and for detecting recurrence. Complete removal of the prostate should result in an undetectable tPSA level; any measurable tPSA after radical prostatectomy would indicate residual prostatic tissue or metastasis. In those patients, increasing tPSA concentrations after a successful surgery strongly indicates a recurrent disease. The use of serum tPSA in combination with digital rectal examination (DRE) has been recommended as a screening tool for detecting clinically significant prostate cancer. Screening permits the treatment of organ confined, potentially curable prostate cancer discovered in men with a life expectancy of longer than 10 years. Measuring free PSA (fPSA) and calculation of % fPSA ([fPSA/tPSA] × 100) is useful to differentiate between BPH and prostate tumor.

Squamous Cell Carcinoma Antigen (SCCA)

SCC antigen is a near neutral subfraction of the TA-4 tumor antigen, which can be purified from squamous cell carcinoma tissue of the uterine cervix. The SCCA is useful for monitoring squamous cell carcinomas of the head and neck, lung, esophagus, and anal canal. Serum concentrations of SCCA are highest in patients with metastases. As many as 50% of patients with renal failure could have increased SCCA serum concentrations.[19] More than 70% of patients with advanced cervical cancer have elevated SCCA. Serial serum SCCA assays correlate with progression and regression of cervical cancer during chemotherapy. In one study, more than 90% of patients with recurrent disease showed elevated SCCA levels. However, SCCA is also elevated in some nonmalignant conditions, including extensive liver disease.

Vanillylmandelic Acid (VMA)

Both VMA and HVA are acidic metabolites of catecholamines. They are excreted in elevated concentrations by patients with neuroblastoma and pheochromocytoma and, therefore, can be used as tumor markers for diagnosis and for monitoring patients during treatment. The determination of urinary VMA is a useful diagnostic test in patients with neuroblastoma and pheochromocytoma.

REVIEW QUESTIONS

1. Cancer accounts for what percentage of deaths in the United States annually?
   a. 5%
   b. 13%
   c. 20%
   d. 23%

2. Tumor marker tests are used to:
   a. aid in staging of cancer.
   b. monitor response to therapy.
   c. detect recurrent disease.
   d. all of the above.

3. Tumor markers may be defined as:
   a. analytic tests (*eg*, flow cytometry) used to mark cancer cells.
   b. radioactive substances and chemicals used to help the physician identify cancer cells.
   c. biologic substances synthesized and released by cancer cells or substances produced by the host in response to cancer cells.
   d. none of the above.

4. Which of the following is an oncofetal antigen?
   a. α-Fetoprotein
   b. LD
   c. PAP
   d. Neuron-specific enolase

5. Which of the following tumor markers is found in both carcinoma and embryonic tissue and is useful as a prognostic indicator in colorectal carcinoma?
   a. AFP
   b. CEA
   c. PAP
   d. CA 120

6. The major clinical use for CA 125 is monitoring treatment response of:
   a. ovarian carcinoma.
   b. colorectal cancer.
   c. prostatic cancer.
   d. breast cancer.

7. Which of the following tumor markers is used in the management of patients with prostatic cancer?
   a. Prostatic acid phosphatase
   b. Prostate-specific antigen
   c. CA 549
   d. Tissue polypeptide antigen

8. Which of the following enzymes is commonly used as a tumor marker?
   a. Lipase
   b. LD
   c. Aldolase
   d. Catalase

9. A tumor marker used in the assessment of choriocarcinoma or hydatidiform mole is:
   a. β-hCG.
   b. CEA.
   c. AFP.
   d. IgG.

10. DNA analysis (measuring nuclear DNA content) may be used to:
    a. diagnose cancer.
    b. mark cancer cells for removal by surgery.
    c. discriminate between benign and malignant disease.
    d. detect alterations in genes.

REFERENCES

1. Vogelstein B, Fearon ER, Hamilton SE, et al. Genetic alterations during colorectal-tumor development. N Engl J Med 1988;319:525–532.
2. Fidler IJ, Hart IR. Biological diversity in metastatic neoplasms: origins and implications. Science 1982;217:998–1003.
3. Druker MI, Carpenter G. Role of growth factors and their receptors in the control of normal cell proliferation and cancer. Clin Physiol Biochem 1987;5:130–139.
4. Dutta A, Chandra R, Leiter LM, et al. Cyclins as markers of tumor proliferation: immunocytochemical studies in breast cancer. Proc Natl Acad Sci USA 1995;92:5386–5390.
5. Hartwell LH, Kastan MB. Cell cycle control and cancer. Science 1994;266:1821–1828.
6. Folkman J, Shing Y. Angiogenesis. J Biol Chem 1992;267:10931–10934.
7. Folkman J. Angiogenesis in cancer, vascular, rheumatoid and other disease. Nature Med 1995a;1:27–33.
8. Weider N, Semple JP, Welch WR, et al. Tumor angiogenesis and metastasis-correlation in invasive breast carcinoma. N Engl J Med 1991;324:1–8.
9. Catalona W, Smith D, Ratliff T, et al. Measurement of prostate-specific antigen in serum as a screening test for prostate cancer. N Engl J Med 1991;324:1156–1162.
10. Catalona WJ, Smith DS, Wolfert RL, et al. Evaluation of percentage of free serum prostate-specific antigen to improve specificity of prostate cancer screening. JAMA 1995;274:1214–1220.
11. Berlin NI. Early diagnosis of cancer. Prev Med 1974;3:185–196.
12. Coombes RC, Powles TJ, Gazet JC, et al. Biochemical markers in human breast cancer. Lancet 1977;1:132–137.
13. Fishman WH, Inglis NI, Stolbach LL, et al. A serum alkaline phosphatase isoenzyme of human neoplastic cell origin. Cancer Res 1968;28:150–154.
14. Thomson DMP, Krupey J, Freedman SO, et al. The radioimmunoaasy of circulating carcinoembryonic antigen of the human digestive system. Proc Natl Acad Sci USA 1969;64:161–167.

15. Wu JT, Roan Y, Knight JA. Serum AFP levels in normal infants: their clinical and physiological significance. Symposium XIV. In: Mizejewski GJ, Porter IH, eds. AFP and Congenital Disorders. Birth Defect Institute. New York: Academic Press, 1985:111.

16. Feller WF, Henslee HE, Kinders RJ, et al. Mucin glycoproteins as tumor markers. In: Herberman RB, Mercer DW, eds. Immunodiagnosis of Cancer, 2nd ed. New York: Marcel Dekker, 1990: 631–672.

17. Gold P, Freedman SO. Demonstration of tumour specific antigens in human colonic carcinomata by immunological tolerance and absorption techniques. J Exp Med 1963;121:439–461.

18. Gold P, Freedman SO. Specific carcinoembryonic antigens of the human digestive system. J Exp Med 1965;122:467–481.

19. Molina R, Fillella X, Torres MD, et al. SCC antigen measured in malignant and nonmalignant diseases. Clin Chem 1990;36: 251–254.

SUGGESTED READINGS

Wu JT, Nakamura R, eds. Human Circulating Tumor Markers: Current Concepts and Clinical Applications. Chicago: ASCP Press, 1997.

Wu JT, ed. Circulating Tumor Markers of the New Millennium: Target Therapy, Early Detection, and Prognosis. Washington, D.C.: AACC Press, 2002.

Vitamins, Essential Fats, and Macronutrients

Larry H. Bernstein

CHAPTER

31

CHAPTER OUTLINE

- ■ ENERGY REQUIREMENTS
- ■ ENERGY OF FUELS
- ■ VITAMINS
  Fat-Soluble Vitamins
  Water-Soluble Vitamins
  Recommended Dietary Allowance
  Vitamin Metabolism
  Special Diets
- ■ ESSENTIAL FATTY ACIDS
- ■ THE MALNUTRITION RISK
  Those at Risk for Malnutrition
  Systemic Inflammatory Response and the
  Nutritionally Dependent Adaptive Dichotomy

Stress Hypermetabolism
- ■ NUTRITIONAL ASSESSMENT
  Malnutrition Risk Prevention Program
  Creatine/Height Index
  Immunologic Testing
  Body Composition
  Functional Tests
  Protein Markers in Nutritional Assessment
  Total Parenteral Nutrition
- ■ SUMMARY
- ■ REVIEW QUESTIONS
- ■ REFERENCES

OBJECTIVES

Upon completion of this chapter, the clinical laboratorian should be able to:

- Discuss the contribution of individual nutrient classes to human metabolism.
- Discuss therapeutic nutrition support by enteral and parenteral routes.
- List biochemical parameters used to monitor nutritional status.
- Describe the biochemical roles of vitamins.
- Correlate alterations in vitamin status with circumstances of increased metabolic requirements, age-related physiologic changes, or pathologic conditions.

- Describe drug–nutrient interactions that influence vitamin status.
- Delineate laboratory procedures used in the assessment of vitamin status.
- Discuss the role of the laboratory in nutritional assessment and monitoring.
- List the populations at risk for malnutrition.
- Identify the plasma protein changes as a result of stress.
- Describe some of the electrolyte and mineral abnormalities associated with TPN.

KEY TERMS

Anabolism
Basal metabolic rate
  (BMR)
Body mass index (BMI)
Catabolism
Enteral feeding

Essential nutrients
Hypervitaminosis
Hypovitaminosis
kcal (kilocalorie)
Kwashiorkor
Malnutrition

Marasmus
Nitrogen balance
Nutrient
Osteomalacia
Pellagra
Recommended dietary
  allowance (RDA)

Rickets
Scurvy
Total parenteral nutrition
  (TPN)
Vitamin

The current emphasis on nutrition and health has resulted in the increasing importance of *nutritional assessment.* Clinicians and the public alike are now more aware of how nutrition can affect both health and healing. Nutritional components of the diet include both macronutrients and micronutrients. Macronutrients used for energy include carbohydrates, proteins, and fats. Micronutrients, required by the body in only minute concentrations of milligrams or less, are vitamins, minerals, and trace elements. The first part of this chapter discusses the micronutrients, including biochemistry, deficiency, toxicity, and methods of analysis. Various minerals (*ie,* inorganic elements or compounds) and trace elements (*eg,* iron, zinc, copper) are discussed in Chapter 15, *Trace Elements.* The second part of this chapter discusses assessment of the macronutrients.

The risk of *malnutrition* is associated with unexpected complications, such as pneumonia, urinary infection, sepsis, and systemic inflammatory response syndrome (SIRS). Although severe malnutrition may be recognized merely by extreme or significant weight loss, loss of strength, and loss of function, a moderate degree of malnutrition is often unnoticed at time of admission. Therefore, reliance on anthropometric measurements, once considered to be standard indicators of serious malnutrition, has been replaced by a combination of subjective global assessment and biochemical parameters. Biochemical measurements make a greater contribution to monitoring the patient's response to nutritional supplementation.

ENERGY REQUIREMENTS

The World Health Organization (WHO) defines the energy requirement of an individual as: "The level of energy intake that will balance energy expenditure when the individual has a body size and composition, and a level of physical activity, consistent with long-term good health."[1] The body is in energy balance when the energy intake is in equilibrium with energy expenditure. Excess calories are stored as depot fat and reflected in an increase in the *body mass index (BMI)*. There is a strong association between excess BMI, hypertension, and insulin-resistance. Starvation leads to a marasmic state, with loss of fat and somatic protein, decreasing the BMI. Trauma, stress, and sepsis increase energy expenditure.[2–4] Energy expenditure can be determined by direct calorimetry (heat-generated), indirect calorimetry (from measurement of oxygen consumption and carbon dioxide production), and isotope-dilution methods, using double-labeled water.

Indirect calorimetry measures substrate oxidation and energy expenditure by CO_2 production from measurement of respiratory gas exchange rates. The method assumes the CO_2 expired is proportional to the rate of respiration. The assumption depends on O_2 disappearing from the inspired air being used exclusively for biologic

oxidations so that all expired CO_2 is derived from combustion of substrates. It is also assumed that all nonprotein nitrogen excreted into the urine is derived only from the oxidation of free amino acids, which is 16% of the nitrogen content. Indirect calorimetry measures the net loss of substrate by oxidation, regardless of cycling that may occur along the way. Indirect calorimetry and the Fick principle both measure oxygen consumption (VO_2) and carbon dioxide production (VCO_2). Indirect calorimetry measures oxygen consumption (VO_2) and transpulmonary O_2 gradient from respiratory gas exchange. Fick proposed to measure the VO_2 and VCO_2 from gas exchange and the transpulmonary O_2 and CO_2 gradient by heart catheterization. In this idealized model, O_2 input and CO_2 output is measured, and the cardiac output (CO) provides the flow rate.

ENERGY OF FUELS

Respiratory quotient (RQ), defined as VCO_2/VO_2, is the measure of efficiency of respiration. The calorimetric RQ is between 0.69 and 1.00. The energy expenditure being measured by the VO_2, a value of less than 1.0, is incomplete combustion. RQ is important for calculating the nutritional requirements in providing assisted nutritional support. The RQ for fat is 0.7, whereas the RQ for carbohydrate is 1.0. We have to weigh the advantage of the administration of fat versus carbohydrate energy sources. Fat has an advantage over carbohydrate because it is a dense calorie source and efficiently oxidized, based on low RQ. The effect of excessive carbohydrate calories is excessive CO_2 production, which drives a hyperpnea, detrimental to the pulmonary compromised patient. Lipid has a rate of administration that is rate-limited by its clearance. Excessive fat administration is immunosuppressive.

VITAMINS

Vitamins have a wide range of functions in biologic tissue, serving as cofactors in many enzymatic reactions, so that these enzymes have low catalytic activity in cellular reactions if vitamins are not present. These compounds and their biologically inactive precursors must be partially obtained from food sources and, in some instances, from bacterial synthesis. When vitamin cellular and activity levels from diet or intestinal absorption are inadequate, it is termed *vitamin deficiency.* The term *vitamin* has an historical basis in deficiency states that were relieved by specific food intake. The most notable examples are: *scurvy* (vitamin C), sailors and lime consumption (limeys); *rickets,* vitamin D in the early industrial age; beriberi, alcoholics and thiamine; *pellagra,* niacin; night blindness, vitamin A; megaloblastic anemia, folic acid; spina bifida; and pernicious anemia (with neuropathy), vitamin B_{12}. Abnormal increases of metabolism requiring high supplies of one of these cofactors may be termed *vi-*

tamin insufficiency or *vitamin dependency*, depending on the level of supply demanded for physiologic function.[5,6]

Variabilities in clinical expression of vitamin abnormalities result from differences in specific cause, degree, and duration of vitamin inadequacy; the simultaneous presence of nutritional insufficiencies; and increased metabolic demands imposed by conditions such as pregnancy, infection, and cancer. The clinical symptoms of vitamin deficiencies are usually nonspecific in early stages and in mild, chronic deficiency states. A combination of dietary history, physical examination, and laboratory measurements is often required to diagnose vitamin deficiency. Vitamin metabolism is complex, and vitamin supplementation of foods is common. It is not unusual to find vitamin toxicities from inappropriate use of vitamin supplementation.

For simplicity, vitamins of diverse chemical structure are classified as either water soluble or fat soluble. Fat-soluble vitamins include A, D, E, and K. Those vitamins soluble in water include the B complex of vitamins—thiamine, riboflavin, niacin, vitamins B_6 and B_{12}, biotin, folate, and vitamin C. Water-soluble vitamins are readily excreted in the urine and less likely than fat-soluble vitamins to accumulate to toxic levels in the body. Vitamins, classified as fat or water soluble, and the symptoms usually seen in deficiency states are shown in Table 31-1.[7]

Investigating the dietary deficiency of vitamins (*hypovitaminosis*) is sustained primarily from knowledge of dietary sources and dietary practices that produce inadequate intake or absorption. Recommended dietary allowances are defined by the Food and Nutrition Board as levels of intake of *essential nutrients* based on available scientific knowledge to be sufficient to meet the nutritional needs of healthy individuals.[5,6]

Information on the dietary intake requirements needed to avoid deficiency symptoms and to maintain specific functions define the dietary allowances of these vitamins. The recommended dietary allowances are established to meet the needs of 97.5% of the population; however, in certain instances, they are higher if the *nutrient* is poorly absorbed or insufficiently used.[7]

Chemical determination of human vitamin states has been approached in the following ways:

- Measurement of active cofactors or precursors in biologic fluids or blood cells.
- Measurement of urinary metabolites of the vitamin.
- Measurement of a biochemical function requiring the vitamin (*eg*, enzymatic activity), with and without in vitro addition of the cofactor form.
- Measurement of urinary excretion of vitamin or metabolites after a test load of the vitamin.
- Measurement of urinary metabolites of a substance, the metabolism of which requires the vitamin after administration of a test load of the substance.

Reduced serum concentrations of a vitamin do not always indicate a deficiency that interrupts cellular function. Conversely, values within the reference interval do not always reflect adequate function. Interpretation of

TABLE 31-1. VITAMIN AND DEFICIENCY STATES

VITAMIN NAME	CLINICAL DEFICIENCY
Fat-Soluble Vitamins	
Vitamin A_1	Night blindness, growth retardation, abnormal taste response, dermatitis, recurrent infections
Vitamin E	Mild hemolytic anemia (newborn), red blood cell fragility, ataxia
Vitamin D	Rickets (young), osteomalacia (adult)
Vitamin K	Hemorrhage (ranging from easy bruising to massive bruising), especially post-traumatic bleeding
Water-Soluble Vitamins	
Vitamin B_1	Infants: dyspnea, cyanosis, diarrhea, vomiting Adults: beriberi (fatigue, peripheral neuritis), Wernicke-Korsakoff syndrome (apathy, ataxia, visual problems)
Vitamin B_2	Angular stomatitis (mouth lesions), dermatitis, photophobia, neurologic changes
Vitamin B_6	Infants: irritability, seizures, anemia, vomiting, weakness Adults: facial seborrhea
Niacin/niacinamide	Pellagra (dermatitis, mucous membrane inflammation, weight loss, disorientation)
Folic acid	Megaloblastic anemia
Vitamin B_{12}	Megaloblastic anemia, neurologic abnormalities
Vitamin C	First, vague aches and pains; if long-term, scurvy (hemorrhages into skin, alimentary and urinary tract, anemia, wound healing delayed)

laboratory values must be done with knowledge of the biochemistry and physiology of vitamins.[7–9]

Fat-Soluble Vitamins

Vitamin A

Retinol and retinoic acid are derived directly from dietary sources, primarily as retinyl esters, or from metabolism of dietary carotenoids (provitamin A), primarily β-carotene. Major dietary sources of these compounds include animal products and pigmented fruits and vegetables (carotenoids). Vitamin A is stored in the liver and transported in the circulation complexed to retinol-binding protein (RBP) and transthyretin. Vitamin A and related retinoic acids are a group of compounds essential for vision, cellular differentiation, growth, reproduction, and immune system function. A clearly defined physiologic role for retinol is in vision. Retinol is oxidized in the rods of the eye to retinal, which, when complexed with opsin, forms rhodopsin, allowing dim-light vision. This vitamin and vitamin D act through specific nuclear receptors in the regulation of cell proliferation. Vitamin A deficiency leads to night blindness (nyctalopia) and, when prolonged, may cause total blindness. In vitamin A deficiency states, epithelial cells (cells in the outer skin layers and cells in the lining of the gastrointestinal, respiratory, and urogenital tracts) become dry and keratinized. Fruits and vegetables contain carotene, which is a precursor of retinol. Carotenes provide more than one half of the retinol requirement in the American diet. Vitamin A deficiency is most common among children living in nonindustrialized countries and is usually a result of insufficient dietary intake. Deficiency may also occur as a result of chronic fat malabsorption or impaired liver function or may be associated with severe stress and protein malnutrition. Premature infants are born with lower serum retinol and RBP levels, as well as lower hepatic stores of retinol; therefore, these newborns are treated with vitamin A as a preventive measure.[10]

When ingested in high doses, either chronically or acutely, vitamin A causes many toxic manifestations and may ultimately lead to liver damage due to *hypervitaminosis*. High doses of vitamin A may be obtained from excessive ingestion of vitamin supplements or large amounts of liver or fish oils, which are rich in vitamin A. Carotenoids, however, are not known to be toxic because of a reduced efficiency of carotene absorption at high doses and limited conversion to vitamin A. The *recommended dietary allowance (RDA)* of vitamin A is 1000 μg/day for adult males and 800 μg/day for adult females. Measurement of retinol is the most common means of assessing vitamin A status in the clinical setting. Retinol is most commonly measured by high-performance liquid chromatography (HPLC). Toxicity is usually assessed by measuring retinyl ester levels in serum rather than retinol, which is accomplished by HPLC.[11]

Vitamin E

Vitamin E is a powerful *antioxidant* and the primary defense against potentially harmful oxidations that cause disease and aging, protecting unsaturated lipids from peroxidation (cleavage of fatty acids at unsaturated sites by oxygen addition across the double bond and formation of free radicals). The role of vitamin E in protecting the erythrocyte membrane from oxidant stress is presently the major documented role of vitamin E in human physiology. It has been shown to strengthen cell membranes and augment such functions as drug metabolism, heme biosynthesis, and neuromuscular function. The generic name for vitamin E is *tocopherol*, which includes several biologically active isomers. Alpha-tocopherol is the predominant isomer in plasma and the most potent isomer by current biologic assays. About 40% of ingested tocopherol is absorbed, affected mainly by the amount and degree of unsaturated dietary fat, largely determining the physiologic requirement. Absorbed vitamin E is associated with circulating chylomicrons, very-low-density lipoprotein, and chylomicron remnants. Dietary sources of tocopherols include vegetable oil, fresh leafy vegetables, egg yolk, legumes, peanuts, and margarine. Diets suspect for vitamin E deficiency are those low in vegetable oils or fresh green vegetables or those low in unsaturated fats.

The major symptom of vitamin E deficiency is hemolytic anemia. Although the use is still controversial, premature newborns are commonly supplemented with vitamin E to stabilize red blood cells and prevent hemolytic anemia. There is evidence for preventive roles of vitamin E in retrolental fibroplasia; intraventricular hemorrhage; and mortality of small, premature infants. Premature infants receiving vitamin E in amounts that sustain serum levels above 30 mg/L have an increased incidence of sepsis and necrotizing enterocolitis.[10]

Patients with conditions that result in fat malabsorption, especially cystic fibrosis and abetalipoproteinemia, are also susceptible to vitamin E deficiency.[10] A relationship exists between vitamin E deficiency and progressive loss of neurologic function in infants and children with chronic cholestasis.[10] Absorption of dietary vitamin E is most efficient in the jejunum, where it combines with lipoproteins and is transported through the lymphatics. Vitamin E is stored in the liver and other tissues with high lipid content and excreted principally in the feces. Assessment of vitamin E status is, therefore, primarily indicated in newborns, patients with fat-malabsorption states, and patients receiving synthetic diets. Synergistic with two other essential nutrients, selenium and ascorbic acid, vitamin E is also necessary for the maintenance of normal vitamin A levels.[10] This vitamin deficiency commonly occurs in two groups: premature, very-low-birth-weight infants, and patients who do not absorb fat normally. Although megadoses of vitamin E do not produce toxic effects, high doses have no proven health benefit; the RDA is 10 mg/day for adult males and 8 mg/day for adult females.[12] The most widely distributed and most biologically active form of vitamin E is alpha-tocopherol, which is the form commonly measured in the laboratory using HPLC methods.

Vitamin D

Vitamin D refers to a group of related metabolites used for proper skeleton formation and mineral homeostasis. Exposure of the skin to sunlight (ultraviolet light) catalyzes the formation of cholecalciferol from 7-dehydrocholesterol. The other major form of vitamin D is ergocalciferol (vitamin D_2). Vitamin D occurs in foods as cholecalciferol or ergocalciferol. The most active metabolite of vitamin D is $1,25(OH)_2D_3$. It stimulates intestinal absorption of calcium and phosphate for bone growth and metabolism and, together with parathyroid hormone, stimulates bone to increase the mobilization of calcium and phosphate. $1,25(OH)_2D_3$ has an important proapoptotic effect, acting through a vitamin D hormonal system, that depends on binding of the active ligand to a vitamin D receptor. This led to important drug discovery developments in which calcium and phosphate release is minimized and proliferative and anti-inflammatory effects of D-analogues are modulated.

In northern climates, it is difficult to receive enough ultraviolet exposure to fully meet minimum requirements (2 hours/day). Major dietary sources of vitamin D include irradiated foods and commercially prepared milk. Small amounts occur in butter, egg yolks, liver, sardines, herring, tuna, and salmon. The RDA of vitamin D for adults is 5 μg/day. Absorbed in the small intestine, vitamin D requires bile salts for absorption. It is stored in

---

CASE STUDY 31-1

A 4-year-old boy is brought to an Alaskan children's clinic by the Social Services System of Alaska. The child was living in a foster home. Infrequently outdoors, his diet consisted of few green vegetables, dairy products, or meats. He began walking at 14 months; his legs showed some bowing. There is tetany or convulsions. He is small for his age: 27 pounds; 90.6-cm tall; third percentile. His laboratory test results are shown in Case Study Table 31-1.1.

Questions

1. This disorder is probably related to:
   a. Wilson's disease.
   b. maple syrup urine disease.
   c. galactosemia and galactosuria.
   d. some form of vitamin or mineral metabolism disorder, probably related to some vitamin D deficiency.

2. The causative agent in this disease is:
   a. inadequate intake of lipids and fatty acids.
   b. a viral disease related to rhinovirus.
   c. an abnormality related to vitamin D or inadequate intake or vitamin D resistance.
   d. inadequate intake of sugar.

3. The therapy that might help in this situation is:
   a. vitamin D, 10,000 IU/day.
   b. 5% glucose and water.
   c. normal Ringer's lactate solution.
   d. a diet with a high level of unsaturated fatty acids.

CASE STUDY TABLE 31-1.1. LABORATORY RESULTS

TEST	RESULT	REFERENCE RANGE
Hgb	14.1 g/dL	12.0–18.0 g/dL
Hct	46%	34.0–52.0%
WBC	8.4 × 10³/μL Normal differential	4.0–11.0 μL
Urinalysis		
Specific gravity	1.010	1.003–1.030
pH	6.8	5.0–9.0
Glucose	Negative	Negative
Protein	Negative	Negative
Microscopic	Negative	Negative
Amino acid screen	Negative	Negative
Serum		
Na	140 mEq/L	132–143 mEq/L
K	4.0 mEq/L	3.2–5.7 mEq/L
Cl	101 mEq/L	98–116 mEq/L
CO_2	14.3 mg/dL	13–29 mg/dL
Ca	7.0 mg/dL	8.9–10.3 mg/dL
Phosphate	1.1 mg/dL	3.4–5.9 mg/dL
Alkaline phosphatase	23 units	15–20 units
Total protein	6.6 g/dL	5.6–7.7 g/dL
Albumin	3.4 g/dL	3.1–4.8 g/dL

the liver and excreted in the bile. Severe deficiency in children causes a failure to calcify cartilage at the growth plate in metaphysial bone formation, leading to the development of *rickets*. In adults, the deficiency leads to undermineralization of bone matrix in remodeling, resulting in *osteomalacia*. Low levels of vitamin D are reported with the use of anticonvulsant drugs and in small bowel disease, chronic renal failure, hepatobiliary disease, pancreatic insufficiency, and hypoparathyroidism. Vitamin D can be toxic, especially in children. Elevated levels of vitamin D are present in hyperparathyroidism and hypophosphatemia and during pregnancy. Excess vitamin D produces hypercalcemia and hypercalciuria, which can lead to calcium deposits in soft tissue and irreversible renal and cardiac damage.[10]

It is important to measure the metabolic form of vitamin D ($1,25(OH)_2D_3$), parathyroid hormone, and calcium levels when diagnosing primary hyperparathyroidism and different types of rickets, when monitoring patients with chronic renal failure, and when assessing patients on $1,25(OH)_2D_3$ therapy. Two forms are most commonly measured in the clinical laboratory: $25(OH)D_3$ and $1,25(OH)_2D_3$. $25(OH)D_3$ is the major circulating form of vitamin D; its measurement is a good indicator of vitamin D nutritional status, as well as vitamin D intoxication. The reference range is 22–42 ng/mL for $25(OH)D_3$ and 30–53 pg/mL for $1,25(OH)_2D_3$. Quantitation of the metabolites of vitamin D should be performed using radioimmunoassay (RIA) or HPLC in conjunction with competitive protein binding.[13]

Vitamin K

Vitamin K (German, *koagulation*) is the group of substances essential for the formation of prothrombin and at least five other coagulation proteins, including factors VII, IX, and X and proteins C and S. The quinone-containing compounds are a generic description for menadione and derivatives exhibiting this activity. Vitamin K helps convert precursor forms of these coagulation proteins to functional forms; this transformation occurs in the liver. Dietary vitamin K is absorbed primarily in the terminal ileum and, possibly, the colon. Vitamin K is synthesized by intestinal bacteria; this synthesis provides 50% of the vitamin K requirement. Major dietary sources are cabbage, cauliflower, spinach and other leafy vegetables, pork, liver, soybeans, and vegetable oils. Uncomplicated dietary vitamin K deficiency is considered rare in healthy children and adults.

Vitamin K deficiency may be caused by antibiotic therapy, which results from decreased synthesis of the vitamin by intestinal bacteria. When vitamin K antagonists, such as warfarin sodium (Coumadin), are used for anticoagulant therapy, anticoagulant factors II, VII, IX, and X are synthesized but nonfunctional. An apparent vitamin K deficiency may lead to a hemorrhagic episode

or may result when anticoagulants, such as warfarin sodium, are used.[14,15]

Prothrombin time (velocity of clotting after addition of thromboplastin and calcium to citrated plasma) determination is an excellent index of prothrombin adequacy. Prothombin time is prolonged in vitamin K deficiency and in liver diseases characterized by decreased synthesis of prothrombin. Vitamin K deficiency also results in prolongation of the partial thromboplastin time, but the thrombin time is within the reference interval.

Toxicity from vitamin K is not commonly seen in adults. Large doses in infants may result in hyperbilirubinemia. The adult RDA of vitamin K is 80 μg/day for males and 65 μg/day for females.[16] For most laboratories, vitamin K is not assayed; however, prothrombin time is used as a functional indicator of vitamin K status.[12] The normal prothrombin time is 11–15 seconds, which varies with method. With a vitamin K deficiency, the prothrombin time is prolonged. Several herbal supplements (*eg*, garlic, gingko, and ginseng) may enhance the effects of coumadin or interact with platelets, increasing the risk of bleeding.

Water-Soluble Vitamins

Thiamine

Thiamine (vitamin B_1) acts as a coenzyme in decarboxylation reactions in major carbohydrate pathways and in branched-chain amino acid metabolism. It is rapidly absorbed from food in the small intestine and excreted in the urine. The clinical condition associated with chronic thiamine deficiency is *beriberi*. Although usually found in underdeveloped countries of the world, beriberi may be found in the United States among persons with chronic alcoholism. Decreased intake, impaired absorption, and increased requirements all appear to play a role in the development of thiamine deficiency in persons with alcoholism. The RDA of thiamine is 1.5 mg/day for adult males and 1.1 mg/day for adult females.[17] Thiamine functional activity is best measured by erythrocyte transketolase (ETK) activity, before and after the addition of thiamine pyrophosphate (TPP). Thiamine deficiency is present if the increase in activity after the addition of TPP is greater than 25%.

Riboflavin

Riboflavin (vitamin B_2) functions primarily as a component of two coenzymes, flavin mononucleotide and flavin adenine dinucleotide (FAD). These two coenzymes catalyze various oxidation-reduction reactions. Dietary riboflavin is absorbed in the small intestine. The body stores of a well-nourished person are adequate to prevent riboflavin deficiency for 5 months. Excess riboflavin is excreted in the urine and has no known toxicity. Foods high in riboflavin include milk, liver, eggs, meat, and leafy vegetables. Riboflavin deficiency occurs with other nutritional deficiencies, alcoholism, and chronic diarrhea and malabsorption. Certain drugs antagonize the action or metabolism of riboflavin, including phenothiazine, oral contraceptives, and tricyclic antidepressants.[18] The RDA of riboflavin is 1.7 mg/day for adult males and 1.3 mg/day for adult females.[18] Reduced glutathione reductase activity greater than 40% is an indication of deficiency.

Pyridoxine

Pyridoxine (vitamin B_6) is ubiquitous. Vitamin B_6 is three related compounds: pyridoxine, occurring mainly in plants; and pyridoxal and pyridoxamine, which are present in animal products. The major dietary sources of vitamin B_6 are meat, poultry, fish, potatoes, and vegetables; dairy products and grains contribute lesser amounts. Readily absorbed from the intestinal tract, vitamin B_6 is excreted in the urine in the form of metabolites.[19] Vitamin B_6 deficiency rarely occurs alone; it is more commonly seen in patients deficient in several B vitamins. Those particularly at risk for deficiency are patients with uremia, liver disease, absorption syndromes, malignancies, or chronic alcoholism. High intake of proteins increases the requirements for vitamin B_6. Deficiency is associated with hyperhomocystinemia. Vitamin B_6 has low toxicity because of its water-soluble nature; however, extremely high doses may cause peripheral neuropathy. The RDA of vitamin B_6 is 2.0 mg/day for adult males and 1.6 mg/day for adult females.[19]

Niacin

The requirement for niacin in humans is met, to some extent, by the conversion of dietary tryptophan to niacin. Niacin is the generic term for both nicotinic acid and nicotinamide. Niacin functions as a component of the two coenzymes (NAD) and (NADP), which are necessary for many metabolic processes, including tissue respiration, lipid metabolism, fatty acid metabolism, and glycolysis. Reduction of the coenzyme yields dihydronicotinamide (NADH or NADPH), which has a strong absorption at 340 nm, a feature widely used in assays of pyridine nucleotide-dependent enzymes.

Niacin is absorbed in the small intestine, and excess is excreted in the form of metabolites in the urine.[20] *Pellagra,* the clinical syndrome resulting from niacin deficiency, is associated with diarrhea, dementia, dermatitis, and death. Niacin deficiency may result from alcoholism. To decrease lipid levels, pharmacologic doses of nicotinic acid are given therapeutically. The toxicity of niacin is low. When large doses are ingested, however, as often occurs during lipid-lowering therapies, flushing of the skin and vasodilation may occur. The RDA of niacin is 19 mg/day for adult males and 15 mg/day for an adult females.[20] Blood or urinary niacin levels are of value in assessing niacin nutritional status.

Folate

Folate is the generic term for components nutritionally and chemically similar to folic acid. Folate functions metabolically as coenzymes involved in various one-carbon transfer reactions. Folate and vitamin B_{12} are closely related metabolically. The hematologic changes that result from deficiency of either vitamin are indistinguishable. Folate in the diet is absorbed in the jejunum, and the excess is excreted in the urine and feces. Large quantities of folate are also synthesized by bacteria in the colon. Structural relatives of pteroylglutamic acid (folic acid) are metabolically active compounds usually referred to as *folates*. Food folates are primarily found in green and leafy vegetables, fruits, organ meats, and yeast. Boiling food and using large quantities of water result in folate destruction. The average American diet may be inadequate in folate for adolescents and for pregnant or lactating women.[21]

The major clinical symptom of folate deficiency is megaloblastic anemia. Chemical indices of deficiency are, in order of occurrence, low serum folate, hypersegmentation of neutrophils, high urinary formiminoglutamic acid (FIGLU) (a histidine metabolite accumulating in the absence of folate), low erythrocyte folate, macroovalocytosis, megaloblastic marrow, and anemia. Serum folate levels, although an early index of deficiency, can frequently be low despite normal tissue stores. Because most folate storage occurs after the vitamin B_{12}-dependent step, erythrocyte folate can also be reduced in deficiency of either vitamin B_{12} or folate. Despite this overlap, erythrocyte folate concentration is accepted as the best laboratory index of folate deficiency.[22] Most physicians order both serum and erythrocyte folate levels because serum levels indicate circulating folate and erythrocyte levels better approximate stores. Homocysteine elevation in serum and urine occurs in folate deficiency.[22] Total homocysteine is generally measured, which is the sum of all homocysteine species, both free and protein-bound forms.[23]

Folate requirement is increased during pregnancy and especially during lactation. The increase during lactation results, in part, from the presence of high-affinity folate binders in milk. Dietary supplementation of folate in pregnant women reduces the incidence of fetal neural tube defects. Other instances of increased folate requirement include hemolytic anemia, iron deficiency, prematurity, and multiple myeloma. Patients receiving dialysis treatment rapidly lose folate. Clinical conditions[22,24] associated with folate deficiency include megaloblastic anemia, alcoholism, malabsorption syndrome, carcinoma, liver disease, chronic hemodialysis, and hemolytic and sideroblastic anemia. Certain anticonvulsants and other drugs that interfere with folate metabolism include sulfasalazine, isoniazid, and cycloserine. Folate deficiency of dietary origin commonly occurs in older persons. Phenytoin (Dilantin) therapy accelerates folate excretion and interferes with folate absorption and metabolism. Alcohol interferes with folate's enterohepatic circulation, and methotrexate, a chemotherapeutic agent, inhibits the enzyme dihydrofolate reductase. Low levels of serum folate can occur with use of oral contraceptives.

There are no known cases of folate toxicity; the RDA is 200 μg/day for adult males and 180 μg/day for adult females. Reference ranges are as follows:

Serum: 3–16 ng/mL
Erythrocyte: 130–630 ng/mL
Deficient stores: less than 140 ng/mL

Folate levels may be measured in serum using a microbiologic assay employing *Lactobacillus casei* or a competitive protein-binding assay for levels in serum and erythrocytes. When folate deficiency develops, serum levels fall first, followed by a decrease in erythrocyte folate levels and ultimate hematologic manifestation.[24] Measuring both serum and erythrocyte levels is helpful because serum levels indicate circulating folate and erythrocyte levels better approximate stores.[22,24]

Serum contains endogenous binding proteins that can bind folate and result in falsely low serum folate concentration measurements. Although measurement of red blood cell folate concentration has advantages over the serum assay for the diagnosis of megaloblastic anemia, analytic problems may result from the various forms of folate in erythrocytes. Folate in serum is almost exclusively present in the monoglutamate form; however, in red blood cells, it is in the polyglutamate form and as high-molecular-weight complexes.[24]

Vitamin B₁₂

Vitamin B_{12} (cobalamin) refers to a large group of cobalt-containing compounds. Intestinal absorption of vitamin B_{12} takes place in the ileum and is mediated by a unique binding protein called *intrinsic factor,* which is secreted by the stomach. Vitamin B_{12} participates as a coenzyme in enzymatic reactions necessary for hematopoiesis and fatty acid metabolism. Excess vitamin B_{12} is excreted in the urine. Vitamin B_{12} bears a corrin ring (containing pyrroles similar to porphyrin) linked to a central cobalt atom. Different corrinoid compounds, or cobalamins, are distinguished by the substituent linked to the cobalt. The active cofactor forms of vitamin B_{12} are methylcobalamin and deoxyadenosylcobalamin. The dietary sources for vitamin B_{12} are from animal products (*eg,* meat, eggs, and milk) and few plant products. Total vegetarian diets are, therefore, likely to have deficiencies of vitamin B_{12}. Animals derive vitamin B_{12} from intestinal microbial synthesis. The average daily diet contains 3–30 μg of vitamin B_{12}, of which 1–5 μg is absorbed. The frequency of dietary deficiency increases with age, occurring in more

than 0.5% of people older than age 60,[24] although the symptoms resulting from dietary deficiency are rare.

Most vitamin B_{12} absorption occurs through a complex with intrinsic factor, a protein secreted by gastric parietal cells. This intrinsic factor–B_{12} complex binds with specific ileal receptors. "Blocking" intrinsic factor antibodies prevent binding of vitamin B_{12} to intrinsic factor, and "binding" antibodies can combine with either free intrinsic factor or the intrinsic factor–B_{12} complex, preventing attachment of the complex to ileal receptors and intestinal uptake of the vitamin. Parietal cell antibodies have also been identified as a cause of pernicious anemia. After release from the intrinsic factor complex within the mucosal cell, vitamin B_{12} circulates in plasma bound to specific transport proteins and is deposited in liver, bone marrow, and other tissue. There is a significant enterohepatic circulation of vitamin B_{12}. Plasma contains both types of transport proteins, transcobalamins, and the three forms of vitamin B_{12} (hydroxycobalamin, methylcobalamin, and deoxyadenosylcobalamin).

In the Schilling test, the patient receives a small, oral dose of radiolabeled vitamin B_{12}. Parenteral B_{12} is given simultaneously to saturate binding sites. Serum and urine are collected at intervals, and labeled B_{12} is measured in the specimens. Patients who cannot absorb vitamin B_{12} (usually a deficiency of intrinsic factor, as in pernicious anemia) cannot absorb the labeled B_{12} and, therefore, have low levels in the blood and urine.

The term *pernicious anemia* is now most commonly applied to vitamin B_{12} deficiency resulting from lack of intrinsic factor. Antibodies to intrinsic factor and parietal cells are common in patients with pernicious anemia, their healthy relatives, and patients with other autoimmune disorders. Deficiency of B_{12} can occasionally occur in strict vegetarians as a result of dietary deficiency. A loss of B_{12} also occurs in individuals infected with fish tapeworm or as a result of malabsorption diseases, such as sprue or celiac disease. Low vitamin B_{12} levels occur with folate deficiency, and B_{12} deficiency can be masked by large doses of folate. Toxicity of vitamin B_{12} has not been reported. The RDA of vitamin B_{12} for adults is 2 μg/day. Assay methods for B_{12} are either microbiologic assay using *Lactobacillus leichmanii* competitive protein-binding radioimmunoassay or an enzyme immunoassay.

Deficiency of vitamin B_{12} causes two major disorders—megaloblastic anemia (pernicious anemia) and a neurologic disorder called *combined systems disorder.*[24] The neurologic manifestations are variable and may be subtle. For this reason, vitamin B_{12} deficiency should be considered a cause of any unexplained macrocytic anemia or neurologic disorder, especially in an older person. Serum vitamin B_{12} may be used in the initial assessment.[24] Methylmalonic acid levels may be more definitive because the lower reference limit is unclear. Patients with pernicious anemia usually have atrophic gastritis and

CASE STUDY 31-2

A 65-year-old woman was admitted to the hospital in mild congestive heart failure. She had been seen in the family practice clinic with complaints of numbness, tingling in the calves and feet, and weight loss. The physical examination revealed a slightly confused, depressed, pale woman. Her blood pressure was 110/70 mm Hg. Faint scleral icterus was present. There was 1+ pitting and ankle edema. The neurologic examination revealed loss of vibratory sensation in both legs with exaggerated ankle and knee reflexes. Initial laboratory results are shown in Case Study Table 31-2.1.

Questions

1. What is a biologically active form of cobalamin in plasma?
   a. Cyanocobalamin
   b. Hydrocobalamin
   c. Deoxyadenosylcobalamin
   d. Aquocobalamin
   e. Transcobalamin

2. Where is intrinsic factor made in the body?
   a. Stomach
   b. Esophagus
   c. Small intestine
   d. Large intestine

3. What is the binding protein for vitamin B_{12}?
   a. Retinol-binding protein
   b. Extrinsic factor
   c. Corticotropin
   d. Transcobalamin II

4. List food substances that contain vitamin B_{12}.

5. List food substances that contain folate.

CASE STUDY TABLE 31-2.1. LABORATORY RESULTS

TEST	RESULT	REFERENCE RANGE
Hemoglobin	9.3 g/dL	12–16 g/dL
Hematocrit	28%	38–47%
MCH	35 pg	27–31 pg
MCV	108 fL	80–96 fL
MCHC	32.4 g/dL	32–36 g/dL
Na	141 mEq/L	136–145 mEq/L
K	4.2 mEq/L	3.5–5.3 mEq/L
Cl	102 mEq/L	96–106 mEq/L
CO_2	26 mg/dL	22–33 mg/dL
Ca	9.7 mg/dL	8.4–10.3 mg/dL
Glucose	100 mg/dL	70–110 mg/dL
BUN	14 mg/dL	10–20 mg/dL
Creatine	1.0 mg/dL	0.4–1.4 mg/dL
Serum B_{12}	130 pg/mL	180–900 pg/mL
Serum folate	6 ng/mL	5–12 ng/mL
RBC folate	105 ng/mL	200–700 ng/mL

have an increased incidence of gastric carcinoma. The reference range for vitamin B_{12} is 110–800 pg/mL.[24,25] The most common methods for determination of vitamin B_{12} are the competitive protein-binding radioimmunoassays, which are based on the principle that vitamin B_{12} released from endogenous binding proteins can be measured by its competition with colabeled B_{12} for a limited amount of specific binding protein. The binding proteins typically used are animal intrinsic factors. Special measures must be taken to eliminate interference caused by other, nonspecific protein binders of vitamin B_{12}. Several nonradioisotopic assays for vitamin B_{12} have been developed for routine laboratory use.

Biotin

Biotin is a coenzyme for several enzymes that transport carboxyl units in tissue and plays an integral role in gluconeogenesis, lipogenesis, and fatty acid synthesis. Dietary biotin is absorbed in the small intestine, but it is also synthesized in the gut by bacteria. Numerous foods contain biotin, although no food is especially rich (up to 20 μg/100 g). Dietary intake, low in the neonatal period, increases as newborns switch from colostrum to mature breast milk. Biotin deficiency can be produced by ingestion of large amounts of avidin, found in raw egg whites that bind to biotin. Biotin deficiency has been noted in patients receiving long-term parenteral nutrition and in infants with genetic defects of carboxylase and biotinidase enzymes. The RDA of biotin has not been established; however, a provisional range of 30–100 μg/day is recommended.[26] Levels of biotin are rarely measured in the clinical setting.[26]

Pantothenic Acid

A growth factor occurring in all types of animal and plant tissue was first designated *vitamin B₃* and later named *pantothenic acid* (Greek, *from everywhere*). Dietary sources include liver and other organ meats, milk, eggs, peanuts, legumes, mushrooms, salmon, and whole grains. Approximately 50% of pantothenate in food is available for absorption. Pantothenate is metabolically converted to 4′-phosphopantetheine, which becomes covalently bound to either serum acyl carrier protein or coenzyme A. Coenzyme A is a highly important acyl-group transfer coenzyme involved in many reactions of many reaction types. Whole blood pantothenate of less than 1000 mg/L and urinary excretion of less than 10 mg/day are regarded as indicative of deficiency.

Ascorbic Acid

The most commonly discussed vitamin, ascorbic acid (vitamin C) is a strong reducing compound that has to be acquired by dietary ingestion. Major dietary sources include fruits (especially citrus) and vegetables (*eg*, tomatoes, green peppers, cabbage, leafy greens, and potatoes). Ascorbic acid is important in formation and stabilization of collagen by hydroxylation of proline and lysine for cross-linking and conversion of tyrosine to catecholamines (by dopamine β-hydrolase). It increases the absorption of certain minerals, such as iron, and is absorbed in the upper small intestine and distributed throughout the water-soluble compartments of the body.[27] The deficiency state, known as *scurvy*, is characterized by hemorrhagic disorders, including swollen, bleeding gums, as well as impaired wound healing and anemia.[27,28]

Although urine is the primary route of excretion, measurement of urinary ascorbate is not recommended for status assessment. Drugs known to increase urinary excretion of ascorbate include aspirin, aminopyrine, barbiturates, hydantoin, and paraldehyde. Ascorbic acid requirements are more increased with acute stress injury and chronic inflammatory states, but are also increased with pregnancy and oral contraceptive use. Excessive intake may interfere with vitamin B₁₂ metabolism and drug actions (*eg*, aminosalicylic acid, tricyclic antidepressants, and anticoagulants).[27,28]

The most widely used assay for ascorbic acid is the 2,4-dinitrophenylhydrazine method. In this procedure, ascorbic acid is first oxidized to dehydroascorbic acid and 2,3-diketogulonic acid with the formation of a colored product that absorbs at 520 nm. This method measures the total vitamin C content of the sample because ascorbic acid, dehydroascorbic acid, and diketogulonic acid are also measured, and it is subject to interference from amino acids and thiosulfates. HPLC has been developed to give increased sensitivity and specificity. The reference range for ascorbic acid is 0.4–0.6 mg/dL.[28]

Carnitine

Carnitine, which includes L-carnitine and its fatty acid esters (acylcarnitine), is described as a conditionally essential nutrient.[29] Meat, poultry, fish, and dairy products are the major dietary sources. Foods of plant origin generally contain little carnitine, except for peanut butter and asparagus.[29] Normal diets provide more than half the human requirement, but strict vegetarian diets provide only 10% of the total carnitine needed by humans.[29] Synthesis occurs in liver, brain, and kidney. L-Carnitine facilitates entry of long-chain fatty acids into mitochondria for oxidation and energy production.[29] The major signs of carnitine deficiency are muscle weakness and fatigue. Total carnitine is measured after hydrolysis of ester forms to free carnitine. Human deficiency can be either hereditary or acquired—by inadequate intake, increased requirement (pregnancy and breast-feeding), or increased urinary loss (valproic acid therapy). Infants and patients following a course of long-term parenteral nutrition and those on hemodialysis are most vulnerable to deficiency.[29]

Recommended Dietary Allowance

For use in the United States, the recommended dietary allowance (RDA) is the level of intake of essential nutrients sufficient to meet the nutritional needs of practically all healthy individuals in the general population, based on available scientific knowledge.[6] The RDA is not considered adequate for premature infants; to cover the special therapeutic needs of people who have infections, metabolic disorders, or chronic diseases; or people who use certain pharmaceutical preparations, such as oral contraceptives.[6]

The RDA should not be interpreted as nutrient requirements for individuals; however, they may be used in assessing individual dietary intakes. Because they are intended to meet the nutritional needs of practically everybody, it must be understood that the RDA may be in excess of the needs for some people. Therefore, although an individual's diet does not meet the recommended allowances, it must not be assumed that the person is malnourished or has a deficient diet unless there is evidence of clinical or biochemical abnormalities.

Vitamin Metabolism

Although all people are somewhat equal with respect to nutrient requirements, there are numerous factors affecting vitamin and nutritional requirements, including genetic differences, acquired factors (*eg*, pregnancy, disease, hypermetabolic states), and others (*eg*, surgery, drugs, alcohol).

TABLE 31-2. ACTIONS OF DRUGS AND ORAL CONTRACEPTIVES ON VITAMINS

Drug or Nutrient

Pyridoxine—antagonized by isoniazid, steroids, penicillamine

Riboflavin—antagonized by phenothiazines, some antibiotics

Folate—antagonized by phenytoin, alcohol, methotrexate, trimethoprim

Ascorbate—antagonized by (increased excretion) aspirin, barbiturates, hydantoins

Ascorbate excess—interferes with actions of aminosalicylic acid, tricyclic antidepressants, anticoagulants; may cause "rebound scurvy" on withdrawal

Oral Contraceptive Agents Cause

Increased serum vitamin A, RBP

Decreased requirement for vitamins K and C

Decreased vitamin B_6 status indices

Decreased riboflavin use

Increased niacin pathway of tryptophan

Decreased induction of thiamin deficiency

Decreased serum folate (cycle-day dependent)

Decreased induction of cervical folate deficiency

The primary cause of latent malnutrition is inadequate food intake. Secondary causes must also be considered, including problems related to nutrient needs, such as poor absorption, inefficient utilization, impaired transportation, increased requirement, and excessive excretion of nutrients.

Drugs and oral contraceptives also impact vitamin metabolism. Table 31-2 summarizes the actions of oral contraceptives and drugs on vitamin metabolism.

Special Diets

The quality of protein in plant foods, notably cereal grains, is generally lower than that of animal proteins. If mixing of plant proteins is done judiciously, combinations of lower-quality protein foods can give mixtures of about the same nutritional value as high-quality animal protein foods.[7,8] Vitamin B_{12} intake is usually low in most vegetarian diets.

ESSENTIAL FATTY ACIDS

Fatty acids (FA) are classified according to two characteristics:

- Chain length (ie, short, medium, or long chain).
- Number of double bonds (ie, saturated, monounsaturated, or polyunsaturated).

The essential fatty acids discussed here are the polyunsaturated fatty acids and their derivatives. Polyunsaturated FA belong to the omega-6 (ω6) and to the omega-3 (ω3) families.[30,31] Omega-3 FA are anti-inflammatory and have proved beneficial in special enteral formulas to modulate the systemic inflammatory response syndrome (SIRS). Omega-6 FA are proinflammatory. These act through eicosanoid pathways; ω3 FA affects platelet adhesiveness.[32,33] Omega-3 FA form prostaglandins and leukotrienes (in particular, PG_3 and LT_5) known to reduce inflammation and reduce immunosuppression, while ω6 fatty acids create PG_2 and LT_4, which induce inflammation and immunosuppression. Polyunsaturated FA may be attacked by free radicals and oxidized into lipid peroxides. The role of FA in the progression of atherosclerosis and nonalcoholic steatosis is currently under investigation, with a potential link to type 2 diabetes through TNF-α. The complement of ω3/ω6 throughout the body is reflected in membrane fluidity.[33]

Measurement of essential fatty acids is done using gas chromatography-mass spectrometry (GC-MS). Because of enormous improvements in technology, a normal triene:tetrene ratio has been brought from 0.4 to 0.02.

Essential fatty acid composition of plasma and red cells is shown in Table 31-3. A low triene:tetraene ratio measures a relative ω3 FA deficiency. An absolute FA deficiency occurs in Crohn's disease, but a relative insufficiency occurs with imbalanced intake of carbohydrate and polyunsaturated fatty acid (PUFA), ω3 in particular.

TABLE 31-3. MEAN REFERENCE VALUES FOR PERCENTAGES OF KEY FATTY ACIDS IN PLASMA AND RBCs[a]

FATTY ACID	PLASMA	RBCs
16:1ω7	<2.1	<0.4
18:2ω6	30–40	8–12
18:3ω3	0.3–1.5	0.5
DFA_6	8–14	7–25
DFA_3	>3	>5
20:3ω9/20:4ω6	<0.02	<0.01
SFA	<30	<35–40
MUFA	<28	<14–20
ω6	40–55	30–35
ω3	2–4	5–8
PUFA	45–55	45–55

(Reprinted with permission from Siguel E. Deficiencies and abnormalities of essential fats in gastrointestinal and coronary artery disease. J Clin Ligand Assay 2000;23[12]:104–111.)
[a]Reference values not well established; depends on methods used and reference population. Values are approximate to illustrate differences between plasma and RBCs.

CASE STUDY 31-3

A 27-year-old man was diagnosed with a carcinoid tumor in the lower portion of the small intestine. The tumor was debulked, with removal of a portion of the lower section of the small intestine. His recovery course was somewhat complicated by weight loss. Seven months after surgery, he underwent a laparotomy, which showed that the carcinoid tumor had not been entirely removed; more of the small bowel was removed because of the obstructing adhesions. He recovered from the second surgery, and tube feeding was discontinued. He came back to the clinic 18 months after the initial surgery slightly pale and stating that he was having trouble maintaining weight. His laboratory evaluation showed slight hypochromic, macrocytic anemia, normal renal function, and normal liver function. A stool specimen was negative for ova, parasites, and enteric pathogens. He was readmitted for intravenous fluid and electrolyte replacement.

Questions

1. What biochemical evidence exists for fat malabsorption?

2. What nutritional parameters would be affected by fat malabsorption?

3. Identify the fat-soluble vitamins.

4. What condition results from vitamin B_{12} deficiency?

CASE STUDY TABLE 31-3.1. LABORATORY RESULTS

TEST	RESULT	REFERENCE RANGE
Albumin	3.4 g/dL	3.5–5 g/dL
Prealbumin	15 mg/dL	18–40 mg/dL
Sodium	139 mmol/L	136–145 mmol/L
Potassium	3.7 mmol/L	3.5–5 mmol/L
Chloride	101 mmol/L	99–109 mmol/L
Bicarbonate	23 mmol/L	22–28 mmol/L
Calcium	8.6 mg/dL	8.5–10.5 mg/dL
Magnesium	1.7 mg/dL	1.5–2.5 mg/dL
Phosphate	3 mg/dL	2.8–4 mg/dL
Prothrombin time	17 seconds	
Ferritin	22 ng/mL	20–250 ng/mL
Vitamin A	207 μg/L	300–800 mg/L
Vitamin D	6 ng/mL	30–53 ng/mL
Vitamin E	2 mg/L	5–18 mg/L
Vitamin C	0.4 mg/dL	0.4–0.6 mg/dL
Vitamin B_{12}	100 pg/mL	110–800 pg/mL
Fecal fat (72 hours)	30 g/day	<6 g/day

Omega-3 FA insufficiency is associated with increased platelet adhesiveness and a hypercoagulable state[33]; these patients are at particular risk for stroke and coronary artery disease. Omega-3 FA is supplemented by fish (eg, tuna, salmon, cod) and fish oil, flaxseed and flaxseed oil, nuts, and tofu.

THE MALNUTRITION RISK

Malnutrition is a state of involuntary inadequate intake or use of calories, proteins or essential fats, or micronutrients (vitamins and trace elements), which results in a risk of impaired physiologic function associated with increased morbidity and mortality.[34–40] Patients who are chronically calorie malnourished suffer from a loss of both adipose and muscle tissue as a result of increased lipolytic and gluconeogenic activity, respectively.[41] These patients, however, do not demonstrate protein deficiency as reflected by normal levels of serum transport proteins. This malnourished state is referred to as *marasmus*. Acute

protein-calorie malnutrition is also strongly associated with severe muscle loss (proteolysis)[42] from an obligatory cytokine-driven response referred to as *nutritionally dependent adaptive dichotomy (NDAD)*,[42,43] with significant nitrogen loss from the proteolysis.[44,45] Patients who are obese and catabolic and who would not be considered malnourished are at high risk for malnutrition-associated complications—particularly, impaired wound healing. This state is also marasmic. *Kwashiorkor,* a state associated with chronic malnutrition and liver disease or with physiologic stress, results in impaired protein synthesis and lower serum transport proteins.

Those at Risk for Malnutrition

Malnutrition affects more than 1.3 billion people worldwide, ranging from 10 million to 20 million individuals in the United States. The prevalence of significant malnutrition in the United States among nursing home patients, older people, and medically and surgically hospitalized patients is no longer challenged. Those at risk for malnutrition are listed in Table 31-4.

It has been repeatedly documented for 30 years that 30–50% of hospitalized patients may be malnourished.[35,37,38] This occurs in the hospital setting when oral nutritional intake is inadequate or impossible because of treatment procedures or complications that follow surgery. Chronic malnutrition may occur before hospitalization as a result of a chronic disease process or a medical condition that leads to poor food choices, protein depletion, or low protein intake. Chronic diseases leading to chronic malnutrition include malignancy; gastrointestinal disease, including malabsorption syndrome; infectious diseases, such as acquired immunodeficiency syndrome (AIDS) and tuberculosis; alcoholism; and end-stage renal or liver disease. The hospitalized patient may also have recent decreased food intake secondary to disease, chemotherapy, or depression or reduced intake due to nausea. The hypermetabolic state associated with major trauma, burns, surgery, multiple organ failure, acute renal failure, septicemia, and systemic inflammatory response syndrome is the most important cause of acute malnutrition from increased energy expenditure.[46]

A patient severely ill with hypermetabolism (kwashiorkor-like) and multiorgan failure is metabolically different from the starved hypometabolic patient (marasmus-like), although a clear distinction in clinical presentation is not frequently seen. The long-term malnourished hypometabolic patient with primary loss of body fat uses ketogenic fatty acid, not carbohydrates, as a primary fuel. These individuals tend to be thin, with a wasted appearance, and have little adipose tissue reserves. In the hypometabolic starved patient, aggressive feeding, especially with carbohydrates, may not be desirable. In these patients, with the body's ability to adapt to chronic starvation by reducing the *basal metabolic rate (BMR)*, cardiac output, temperature, and physical activity, overzealous provision of energy substrate may induce a refeeding syndrome.[43] In the refeeding syndrome, life-threatening fluid and electrolyte shifts occur after the initiation of aggressive nutritional support therapies. Refeeding syndrome can induce hypophosphatemia and hypokalemia as these electrolytes move with glucose out of the circulation into the tissue. The hypermetabolic patient, however, needs energy and protein, requiring aggressive nutritional support to minimize *catabolism* and protein losses and support the immune response.[47] When malnutrition is not detected and treated in patients during their hospital stay, there is increased morbidity and mortality.[36] This is especially the case with patients who are severely injured and have prior liver disease and chronic inanition; these patients have impaired wound healing and increased rates of infection,[36] with extended lengths of hospital stay and higher mortality rates. Of those patients identified as malnourished, too few receive timely nutritional support. The early identification of malnourished patients and the establishment of nutritional intervention have become a quality of care issue.[48]

Systemic Inflammatory Response and the Nutritionally Dependent Adaptive Dichotomy[42,43]

Injury of any cause mediated by cytokines, mainly interleukins 1 and 6 (IL-1, IL-6) and tumor necrosis factor-α (TNF-α), triggers a cascade effect evolving in 3 successive steps[42]: (1) the hemodynamic or ebb phase, dominated by fever, anorexia, tachycardia, and circulatory changes in the first 12 hours; (2) the flow phase, occurring over several days and associated with catabolic processes with massive urinary nitrogen loss; and (4) the anabolic phase, ensuing as the starting point of repair activities and coinciding with a decreased loss and retention of nitrogen.[44]

Stress Hypermetabolism

The increased metabolism associated with stress injury is termed *hypermetabolic state*.[2–4,42,43]

The catabolic state associated with trauma and sepsis is a cytokine-driven metabolic event that must be distinguished from the loss that occurs with starvation. It is driven by interleukin-1 (IL-1), interleukin-6 (IL-6), and tumor necrosis factor-α (TNF-α). The release of these mediators is proportionate to the amount of injury. The release of cytokines is linked to upregulation of hor-

TABLE 31-4. GROUPS AT RISK FOR MALNUTRITION

Depressed or mentally ill people who fail to eat
Older people, especially those in nursing homes
People of low socioeconomic status
Population with loss of fluids and nutrients from long-term diarrhea, draining fistula, or wounds
Persons who have experienced stroke
Patients in the postoperative state and those with ileus with long periods without oral intake
Patients with hypermetabolic conditions: head trauma, multiple trauma, major burns, organic failure, and sepsis
Patients with cancer of the gastrointestinal tract or cachexia
Patients with unintentional weight loss exceeding 10% in 6 months
Patients with chronic disease; long-term dialysis
Patients with pancreatitis

monal and humoral events. The hormonal events include the release of glucagon and catecholamines, thyroid hormone, growth hormone, and cortisol and their effects—hyperglycemia, metabolic rate, release of free fatty acids and associated ketosis, insulin-like growth factor-1 (IGF-1), and negative nitrogen balance from gluconeogenesis. The increased metabolic rate, proportional to the severity of the condition, results in massive proteolysis, with conversion of lean body protein to amino acids for gluconeogenic precursors. This is associated with hyperglycemia, insulin resistance, mobilization of triglycerides, and ketosis. Marasmus is the gradual loss of adipose tissue (fat) alone associated with starvation; the acute loss of muscle tissue in stress injury is marasmic. Kwashiorkor, identified by visceral protein losses, is also present in stress injury. This phase lasts for 3–10 days, but may be extended. The anabolic flow phase emerges as metabolism shifts to synthetic activities and reparative processes.

The earliest hormonal event within 24 hours is the action of catecholamines and glucagon on the conversion of hepatic glycogen to glucose, raising the plasma glucose level. Thyroid hormone (T_4) has an effect on target organs through free thyroxine (FT_4). The catabolic effect of growth hormone on lipid metabolism is reciprocal to and dissociated from an anabolic effect through IGF-1. An adrenal cortisol secretory response opposes the action of insulin and promotes a diabetogenic response. Hypercortisolemia results in muscle proteolysis. Amino acids, especially branched-chain amino acids from skeletal muscle, provide gluconeogenic precursors through alanine. These hormones, released by the stress response, drive the metabolic pathways necessary for the use of carbohydrate and fatty acid fuels and are necessary to support the repair of damaged tissue. The humoral events include the changes in and interactions between serum proteins in the inflammatory response. The systemic effects of fever, tachycardia, increased energy expenditure, and muscle weakness and wasting are associated with elevations of acute-phase reactants (APRs) (*eg*, C-reactive protein, TNF-α, and α₁-acid glycoprotein) and hormonal changes.

Nutritionally Dependent Adaptive Dichotomy
The stress response immediately suppresses synthetic activity by the liver, which has a sole synthetic function with NADP dominated pathways. Serum cholesterol decreases as does production of essential transport proteins, such as albumin, transferrin, cortisol-binding globulin (CBG), thyroxine-binding globulin (TBG), transthyretin or thyroxine-binding prealbumin (TTR), insulin growth factor-1 (IGF-1). Although transport proteins decline abruptly by as much as 40%, APR synthesis is unaffected. The essentially controlling and adaptive role they exert through binding to and effects on active ligands. Ingen-

bleek refers to the relationship between the binding proteins and their respect ligands, under the influence of cytokines, as nutritionally-dependent adaptive dichotomy (NDAD).[42] NDAD is illustrated in Table 31-5. It should also be considered that this adaptive relationship in stress injury is affected by protein malnutrition prior to the injurious state. Why? Because the basal level of binding proteins is set low and the adaptive response is blunted.

The metabolic effect of stress injury in the catabolic phase increases the flow of fuel substrates for energy using processes by its effect on the liver. The decrease in CBG, TBG, TTR and RBP increases the hypermetabolic effect. The free hormone hypothesis states that hormonal effect on target tissue is a result of the free hormone. The adrenal gland is releasing increased cortisol, which has an amplified effect with its binding to a lower plasma concentration of CBG. The liver is the repository for extrathyroidal T_4. The extrathyroidal T_4 is released with a decreased circulating TBG and TTR,[42] resulting in an increased thyroidal activity measured by increased free T_4 (FT_4). This is referred to as the sick euthyroid syndrome. The TSH is not affected or slightly decreased, but not in the hyperthyroid range. Vitamin A is stored in the liver, and it is transported in the circulation in a complex with TTR and RBP. Vitamin A and RBP are dependent on the level of TTR.

Energy intake at birth is approximately 120 kcal/kg per day for both males and females. During the first 2 years of life, there is a gradual drop to 90–100 kcal/kg per day. From 2 to 14 years of age, energy requirements decrease gradually to approximately 40 kcal/kg per day, with males requiring 5 kcal/kg per day more than females.

Downregulation of Healthy Tissue
These metabolic events, proportionate to the amount of the injury, are characterized by the cytokine-induced release of glucagon, catecholamines, and cortisol, which re-

TABLE 31-5. RECIPROCAL ALTERATIONS OF THE PLASMA CONCENTRATIONS OF THE VISCERAL PROTEINS AND THEIR TRANSPORTED LIGANDS IN THE NDAD[a]

BINDING PROTEIN		HORMONAL CHANGE	
Albumin	▽		
TBG	▽	Free T_4	△
CBG	▽	Free Cortisol	△
Transthyretin	▽	Free T_4	△
RBP	▽	Free Retinol	△
IGF-1-BP3	▽	Free IGF-1	△

[a]This adaptive pattern is blunted in the case of preexisting malnutrition.

sult in plasma hyperglycemia, increased catabolic rate, release of fatty acids and ketones, and negative nitrogen balance. The systemic effects of fever, tachycardia, increased energy expenditure, muscle weakness and wasting are associated with the elevations of APRs. TNF-α and hypercortisolemia drive loss of muscle mass, accounting for muscle weakness and wasting associated with severe stress. The counter-regulatory hormones override the action of insulin, reinforced by tissue insulin resistance. Thyroid function is concomitantly altered as decreased conversion of T_4 to T_3 and the production of T_3 declines to minimal levels compatible with euthyroidism. Insulin resistance working in concert with low T_3 syndrome, create the milieu for muscle loss with increased energy expenditure associated with this systemic response.

Upregulation of Inflamed Territories

The liver is central to these adaptive changes, a salient feature involving IL-6 mediated reprioritization of syntheses. Although APR production is strongly enhanced by

---

CASE STUDY 31-4

A 66-year-old postmenopausal woman complained of severe weakness and dyspnea during the past 6 months on exertion. She noted that her appetite had decreased, with resultant weight loss. Her past medical history revealed ulcers. On admission to the hospital, she had normal blood pressure and pulse. Skin, conjunctiva, and mucous membranes were pale. Lungs were clear at auscultation. A grade 3/6 systolic murmur was present, heard best at the lower left sternal border and radiating to the carotids and axilla. Stool guaiac examination was 2+. Nail beds were pale, with no pedal edema. Laboratory data on admission are shown in Case Study Table 31-4.1.

Questions

1. This patient's anemia is probably best explained by:
   a. dietary habits.
   b. chronic blood loss.
   c. chronic intravascular hemolysis.
   d. chronic inflammatory disease.

2. Clinical manifestations of her anemia may include all of the following EXCEPT:
   a. glossitis.
   b. pica.
   c. spoon nail (koilonychia)
   d. peripheral neuropathy.

3. The bone marrow iron stores are:
   a. reduced.
   b. normal.
   c. absent.
   d. increased but present only in reticuloendothelial cells.

4. If the correct treatment for this anemia is with oral ferrous sulfate, the treatment should:
   a. be stopped as soon as the hematocrit returns to normal.
   b. be continued indefinitely, even if the cause of the deficiency has been corrected.
   c. be continued for 3–6 months after the hematocrit returns to normal to replace body iron stores.
   d. be continued only until there is a brisk response in the reticulocyte index and hematocrit.

CASE STUDY TABLE 31-4.1. LABORATORY RESULTS

TEST	RESULT	REFERENCE RANGE
CBC		
Hct	15%	36–48%
Hb	3.8 g/dL	12–16 g/dL
RBC	2.79×10^6/mL	3.6–5.0×10^6/mL
MCV	53.8 FL	82–98 FL
MCHC	25.3 g/dL	31–37 g/dL
WBC	8.2×10^3/mL	4.0–11.0×10^3/mL
Neutrophil	80%	40–80%
Lymph	20%	15–40%
Retic Ct	5.5%	0.5–1.5%
Reticulocyte index	0.8%	>3
Chemistry		
BUN	15 mg/dL	7–18 mg/dL
Glucose	150 mg/dL	Fasting, 70–100 mg/dL
		Nonfasting, 70–150 mg/dL
Electrolytes	Normal	
Bilirubin	1.0 mg/dL	0.2–1 mg/dL
Direct	0.4 mg/dL	0–0.2 mg/dL
T_3 and T_4	Normal	
Serum Fe	15 µg%	30–150 µg/dL
TIBC	439 µg%	241–421 µg%

the provision of amino acids derived from muscle breakdown, most visceral proteins (albumin, transferrin, TTR, RBP, TBG, CBG, and insulin-like growth factor-1–binding proteins [mainly, IGF-1-BP3]) are suppressed. The decline in concentration of these carrier-proteins, with dissociation of the protein-ligand complex, increases the availability of free ligands to the target site so that all thyroxine-, retinol-, and cortisol-dependent processes are amplified during a transient hypermetabolic flow phase. In addition, TBG and CBG are degraded at the site of inflammation, allowing release of their ligand. Other mediators involved in immune response and tissue repair and cell lines contributing to tissue rebuilding are stimulated in this reactive state,[46] and the cleavage of BP3 releases significantly augmented fractions of IGF-1 in free form. Anabolic processes are, therefore, strongly promoted in inflamed tissue. The energy requirements of diseased tissue are fulfilled by anaerobic glycolysis (RQ ~ 1). The site of injury is supported by the breakdown of whole body protein to support the immune response.

NUTRITIONAL ASSESSMENT

Nutritional assessment, the evaluation of a patient's metabolic and nutritional needs, is performed by clinical, laboratory, and other means. Clinical evaluation is the basis for subjective global assessment (SGA), which uses past nutritional intake, disease process, the extent of catabolic disease, functional status.[49] However, SGA is skill dependent and hasn't been proved to be reliable for wide use in identifying the hospitalized malnourished patient.

Because it was shown that a preoperative weight loss of more than 20% was associated with 33% mortality, whereas a 4% mortality rate occurred in those with less than a 20% weight loss, the estimation of weight loss is a key indicator in the nutritional assessment of surgical patients.[50] Recent weight change is a commonly used index of malnutrition. More than 10% loss over any time period has been taken as evidence of malnutrition, and a useful correlation has been proposed between the extent of weight loss and the time over which it develops,[51] as illustrated in Table 31-6. A weight loss 10 days prior to surgery of more than 4.5 kg is highly predictive of surgical mortality.[52]

TABLE 31-6. WEIGHT CHANGE EVALUATION[a]

TIME	SIGNIFICANT WEIGHT LOSS (%)	SEVERE WEIGHT LOSS (%)
1 week	1–2	>2
1 month	5	>5
3 months	7.5	>7.5
6 months	10	>10

[a]Values used are percent weight change (%W): %W = (Usual weight = Actual Weight)/(Usual weight) × 100.

Malnutrition Risk Prevention Program

Hospital malnutrition can be systematically identified, and its identification can be connected to implementation of a structured, timely plan for nutrition care; such implementation yields definite cost benefits. Brugler[53] and Mears[54] have demonstrated workable hospital systems for nutrition screening that might be considered as models for other hospitals. The final outcome for an integrated project is a cost-effective system by the hospital and adaptability to other hospitals.

These systems demonstrate that:

1. early screening and assessment of patients at risk for developing nutrition-related complications can effectively identify patients who are protein-energy malnourished (PEM).
2. identifying these patients, combined with early intervention, reduces nutrition-related complications and length of stay (LOS) by at least one day.
3. notification has a positive effect on effecting timely provision of nutritional support.
4. the costs of allocating the needed resources are, at worse, small compared with the costs of failure to implement such a system.
5. a system can be established that will enhance communication between MDs and other health care providers.

Creatinine/Height Index

Creatine, present almost entirely within muscle (as creatine phosphate), is converted to creatinine at a relatively constant rate, and the amount of urinary creatinine excreted may be indicative of total muscle mass.[55] This inaccurate measure of lean body mass has been replaced for study designs by measurement of urinary excretion of 3-methylhistidine, an amino acid specific for skeletal muscle proteolysis.

Immunologic Testing

Immunologic testing is an insensitive method to identify the effects of malnutrition in disease states. An absolute lymphocyte count below 300/mm^3 reflects life-threatening immune deficiency[52] and is associated with a negative response to an injected antigen. In surgical patients studied, those who were anergic and showed no skin response to injected antigens preoperatively had a 29% incidence of sepsis and a 29.9% mortality rate, compared with 7.5% and 4.6%, respectively, for those classified as immunologically normal.[56–60]

Body Composition

The composition of an adequately nourished adult man (75-kg) is illustrated in Figure 31-1 in both biochemical and cellular terms.[61]

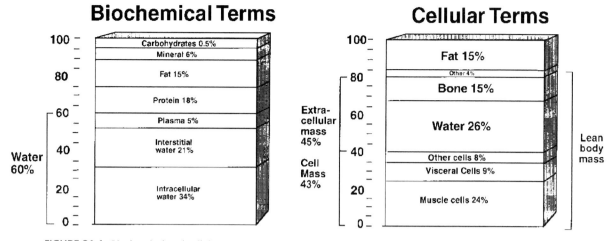

FIGURE 31-1. Biochemical and cellular terms used to describe body mass and the percentage contribution to total mass in a well-nourished 75-kg man.

Body mass described in cellular terms is divided into two mass components: lean body mass (tissue devoid of all fat) and body fat. Lean body mass comprises the metabolically active tissue, known as *body cell mass*, and the metabolically inactive *extracellular mass*. The body cell mass accounts for all oxygen consumption and carbon dioxide production.[61] The primary function of the extracellular mass is intracellular transport and structural support. Malnourished hospitalized patients have a body cell mass 40.5% less than healthy nonhospitalized patients of the same age-group. Obesity, greatly expanded body fat, may be associated with decreased lean body mass. Lean body mass, which declines with age, is greater in men than women and is significantly decreased in obese patients with sarcopenia.

Functional Tests

Muscle function is susceptible to the effects of withdrawing nutrients and refeeding. One method of evaluating muscle function is handgrip dynamometry.[62] In this approach, grip strength had a sensitivity of 90% in predicting postoperative complications. Handgrip dynamometry uses the electrical stimulation technique of the ulnar nerve of the wrist. The rate of relaxation of the electrically stimulated abductor pollicis longus muscle mea-

sures nutrient status in both chronic states and anorexia and during nutrient withdrawal and refeeding in the postoperative period.

Protein Markers in Nutritional Assessment

The primary objective of nutritional assessment is to identify the patient who is malnourished and then, through nutritional therapy, to preserve or replenish the protein component of the body. Laboratory nutritional assessment is best accomplished by monitoring selected serum proteins. The ideal proteins have a short biologic half-life and reflect changes in protein status by measuring concentration changes in the serum. The concentration of protein markers of malnutrition are affected by protein malnutrition associated with end-stage liver and renal disease and severe infection and, most significantly, by stress injury. Because the effect of the inflammatory response is closely associated with the decline of essential transport proteins, a separation of the inflammatory state from protein malnutrition can be problematic, except by using an APR, such as C-reactive protein. The prognostic inflammatory nutritional index (PINI), using the ratio of the CRP-orosomucoid (α_1-acid glycoprotein) product to the albumin–transthyretin product, is intended to resolve this issue.[63] Table 31-7 offers detailed information about these protein markers.

TABLE 31-7. CHARACTERISTICS OF PLASMA PROTEINS OF NUTRITIONAL INTEREST

PROTEIN	MOLECULAR WEIGHT (kD)	HALF-LIFE	REFERENCE RANGE
Albumin	65,000	20 days	33–48 g/L
Fibronectin	250,000	15 hours	220–400 mg/L
Prealbumin (transthyretin)	54,980	48 hours	160–350 mg/L
Retinol-binding protein	21,000	12 hours	30–60 mg/L
Insulin growth factor-1	7,650	2 hours	0.10–0.40 mg/L
Transferrin	76,000	9 days	1.6–3.6 g/L

Albumin

Albumin has long been used in the assessment of hospitalized patients. The albumin concentration in the body is influenced by albumin synthesis, degradation, and distribution. Low levels of serum albumin may reflect low hepatic production or loss from transfer of albumin between the extravascular and the vascular compartment. The long biologic half-life of albumin (20 days) allows changes in the serum concentration only after long periods of malnutrition. Low albumin levels have been identified as a predictor of mortality in patients in long-term-care facilities. Hospitalized patients with low serum albumin levels experience a fourfold increase in morbidity and a 6-fold increase in mortality.[64,65]

Serum albumin is not a good indicator of short-term protein and energy deprivation; however, albumin levels are good indicators of chronic deficiency. Traditionally, albumin has been used to help determine two important nutritional states. First, it helps identify chronic protein deficiency under conditions of adequate non–protein-calorie intake, which leads to marked hypoalbuminemia. This may result from the net loss of albumin from both the intravascular and extravascular pools, causing kwashiorkor. Second, albumin concentrations may help define marasmus. Because this is caused by caloric insufficiency without protein insufficiency, the serum albumin level remains normal but there is considerable loss of body weight.

Studies have classified various levels of malnutrition by using albumin levels. Serum albumin levels of ≥35 g/L are considered normal. Albumin levels of 28–30 to 35 g/L indicate mild malnutrition, levels of 23–25 to 28–30 g/L indicate moderate malnutrition, and levels less than 23–25 g/L indicate severely depleted levels of albumin. Serum albumin is an accurate marker of the catabolic stress of infection. A level of ≤32 g/L indicates that if a patient is in the hospital for up to 10 days, there is a 75% chance of developing decubitus ulcers. Serum albumin levels of less than 25 g/L can be used as an accurate measure of predicting survival prognosis in 90% of critically ill patients.

Transferrin

Transferrin is a glycoprotein with a biologic half-life of 9 days (shorter than albumin). It is synthesized in the liver and binds and transports ferric iron. Transferrin synthesis is regulated by iron stores. When hepatocyte iron is absent or low, transferrin levels rise in proportion to the deficiency. It is an early indicator of iron deficiency, and the elevated transferrin is the last analyte to return to normal when iron deficiency is corrected.

The half-life of transferrin is one half that of albumin, and the body pool is smaller than that of albumin; therefore, transferrin is more likely to indicate protein deple-

tion before serum albumin concentration changes. The usefulness of transferrin in diagnosis of subclinical, marginal, or moderate malnutrition is questionable, however, because a wide range of values have been reported in various studies. Transferrin levels can be lowered by factors other than protein or energy deficiency, such as nephrotic syndrome, liver disorders, anemia, and neoplastic disease.

In hospital and nursing home settings, transferrin levels have been used as indices of morbidity and mortality.[66] Information shows, however, that serum transferrin concentrations are not sufficiently sensitive to detect a change in nutritional status that occurs after 2 weeks of total parenteral nutrition.[67] In addition to being responsive to serum iron concentrations, transferrin is uniquely sensitive to some antibiotics and fungicides.

Transthyretin

Transthyretin is sometimes called *prealbumin* because it migrates ahead of albumin in the customary electrophoresis of serum or plasma proteins. In normal situations, each transthyretin subunit contains one binding site for RBP. Transthyretin and RBP are considered the major transport proteins for thyroxine and vitamin A, respectively.

Because of its short half-life and small body pool, transthyretin is a better indicator of visceral protein status and positive nitrogen balance than albumin and transferrin.[67] Transthyretin is a superior indicator for monitoring short-term effects of nutritional therapy. The features of an ideal protein marker of malnutrition risk are shown in Table 31-8. The concentration of transthyretin and RBP complex, greatly decreased in protein-energy malnutrition,[68] returns toward normal values after nutritional replenishment. Transthyretin has a low pool concentration in the serum, a half-life of 2 days, and a rapid response to low energy intake, even when protein intake is inadequate for as few as 4 days.[69] Serum transthyretin concentrations are decreased postoperatively by 50–90 mg/L in the first week, with the ability to double in 1 week or at least increase 40–50 mg/L in response to adequate nutritional support. If the transthyretin response increases less than 20 mg/L in 1 week as an outcome measure, this indicates either inadequate nutritional support or inadequate response.[67,70]

TABLE 31-8. FEATURES OF AN IDEAL MARKER

Identifies clinically significant depletion
Reflects severity of deficits
Indicates current status and change in status
Sensitive to decline
Sensitive to improvement
Minimal interference

When transthyretin decreases to levels of less than 80 mg/L, severe protein-calorie malnutrition develops; however, nutritional support can cause a daily increase in transthyretin of up to 10 mg/L.[67] These concentrations do not appear to be significantly influenced by fluctuations in the hydration state. Although end-stage liver disease appears to affect all protein levels in the body, liver disease does not affect transthyretin as early or to the same extent as it affects other serum protein markers, particularly RBP. Although transthyretin levels may be elevated in patients with renal disease, if a trend in the direction of change is noted, the changes are likely to reflect alteration in nutritional status and nitrogen balance. Steroids can cause a slight elevation in transthyretin, but the nutritional trend can still be followed because transthyretin responds to both overfeeding and underfeeding.

Transthyretin is also used as an indicator of the adequacy of a nutritional feeding plan[67] because changes in plasma protein are correlated with nitrogen balance. Transthyretin concentrations increase in patients with positive nitrogen balance and decrease in patients with negative nitrogen balance. When the transthyretin level is at ≥180 mg/L, this correlates with a positive nitrogen balance and indicates a return to adequate nutritional status. It has been shown in both the pediatric and neonate population to be a highly accurate and relatively inexpensive marker for nutritional status[71,72] and has been found to be the most sensitive and helpful indicator when looking at the nutritional status of very ill patients.[73]

In summary, transthyretin effectively demonstrates an anabolic response to feeding and is a good marker for visceral protein synthesis in patients receiving metabolic or nutritional support.[73–75]

Retinol-Binding Protein

RBP has been used in monitoring short-term changes in nutritional status.[76–78] Its usefulness as a metabolic marker is based on its biologic half-life of 12 hours and its small body pool size. As a single polypeptide chain, RBP interacts strongly with plasma transthyretin and circulates in the plasma as a 1:1 mol/L transthyretin–RBP complex.[79] A potential problem exists in using RBP as a nutritional marker, however. Although RBP has a shorter half-life than transthyretin (12 hours, compared with 2 days), it is excreted in urine, and its concentration increases more significantly than transthyretin in patients with renal failure. In contrast to RBP, transthyretin concentration is only moderately elevated in advanced chronic renal insufficiency.

Insulin Growth Factor-1

Insulin growth factor-1 (IGF-1) (formerly termed somatomedin C) is important for stimulation of growth. The molecular size and structure of IGF-1 is similar to proinsulin.[80] IGF-1 serum concentrations are regulated by growth hormone and nutritional intake. Growth hormone stimulates the liver to produce IGF-1, which circulates bound to IGF-BP3. IGF-BP3 modulates the biologic effect of IGF-1 in the stress response, causing both decreases and increases in biologic activity. IGF-1 has been used as a nutritional marker in adults and children.[81–83]

Fibronectin

Fibronectin is an opsonic glycoprotein with a half-life in humans of about 15 hours. This protein has repeating blocks of a homogeneous sequence of amino acids and is an α_2-glycoprotein that serves important roles in cell-to-cell adherence and tissue differentiation, wound healing, microvascular integrity, and opsonization of particulate matter. It is considered the major protein regulating phagocytosis. Synthesis sites include endothelial cells, peritoneal macrophages, fibroblasts, and the liver. Fibronectin concentrations may decrease after physiologic damage caused by severe shock, burns, or infection. Levels return to normal on recovery. Fibronectin is of interest because it is not exclusively synthesized in the liver,[84] and it is an indicator of sepsis in burn patients. Fibronectin levels have been shown to decrease during infection or severe stress, partly due to its opsonic property. The infection or trauma, however, does not significantly decrease fibronectin concentration.[85] Fibronectin only increases in severe infection, in which it remains flat and does not increase as soon as IGF-1. It is not routinely used as a nutritional marker.

Nitrogen Balance

Another nutritional evaluation tool, *nitrogen balance,* is the difference between nitrogen intake and nitrogen excretion. It is one of the most widely used indicators of protein change. In the healthy population, anabolic and catabolic rates are in equilibrium, and the nitrogen balance approaches zero. During stress, trauma, or burns, the nutritional intake decreases, and nitrogen loss may exceed intake, leading to a negative nitrogen balance. During recovery from illness, the nitrogen balance should become positive with nutritional support. In humans, 90–95% of the daily nitrogen loss is accounted for by elimination through the kidneys. About 90% of this loss is in the form of urea. Therefore, the determination of 24-hour urinary urea nitrogen is a method for estimating the amount of nitrogen excretion. The nitrogen balance is calculated as follows[86]:

$$\text{Nitrogen balance} = \frac{\text{24-hour protein intake (g)}}{6.25}$$

$$-\frac{\text{24-hour UUN} + 4}{\text{Total volume (L)}} \quad \text{(Eq. 31–1)}$$

Protein intake includes grams of protein that are provided by intravenous amino acids or by *enteral feeding.*

Protein intake is converted into grams of nitrogen by dividing by 6.25. The factor of 4 in the equation represents an estimation of nonurinary nitrogen loss (*eg*, from skin, feces, hair, and nails).[86] Nitrogen balance, as calculated by this equation, is not valid in patients with severe stress or sepsis, as can be seen in critical care areas or in patients with renal disease. Determining the validity of this equation in other clinical conditions involving normally high nitrogen losses may be difficult or even incorrect.

C-Reactive Protein

C-reactive protein is an acute-phase protein that increases dramatically under conditions of sepsis, inflammation, and infection. C-reactive protein can increase dramatically up to 1,000 times after tissue injury, which is more than two or three orders of magnitude greater than any other acute-phase reactant. C-reactive protein rises in concentration 4–6 hours before other acute-phase reactants begin to rise.[87,88]

The flow phase of marked catabolism presents clinically with tachycardia, fever, increased respiratory rate, and increased cardiac output. During this time, synthesis rates of C-reactive protein and other acute-phase proteins increase and albumin and prealbumin decrease[89] (Fig. 31-2). Even with this increase in acute-phase proteins, a significant negative nitrogen balance usually occurs secondary to the greater protein catabolism.[90] Whether this catabolic state produces a clinically defined malnutrition or a separate entity is unknown, but it certainly produces weight loss with decreased albumin and prealbumin levels.

Interleukins

Nutrition research has focused on the interleukins, a complex group of proteins and glycoproteins that can exert pleiotropic effects on several different target cells. Most interleukins are produced by macrophages and T lymphocytes, in response to antigenic or mitogenic stimulation, and affect primary T-lymphocyte function. Most nutritional investigations have been performed on interleukin-1 (IL-1), IL-6, and TNF-α.

Total Parenteral Nutrition

Total parenteral nutrition (TPN) is a widely used means of intense nutritional support for patients who are malnourished, or in danger of becoming malnourished, because they are unable to consume required nutrients or to take nutrients enterally. Parenteral nutrition therapy involves administering appropriate amounts of carbohydrate, amino acid, and lipid solutions, as well as electrolytes, vitamins, minerals, and trace elements to meet the caloric, protein, and nutrient requirements while maintaining water and electrolyte balance.[91] Parenteral nutritional preparations are usually administered through a subclavian catheter. Enterally, a nasogastric tube delivers nutrients directly into the stomach or duodenum, or patients having gastrointestinal surgery may have a feeding gastro-

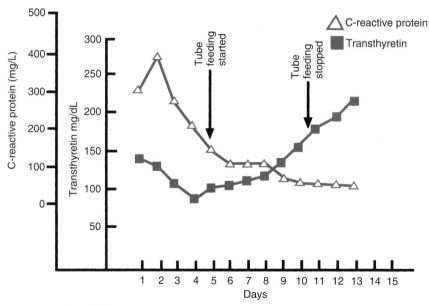

FIGURE 31-2. Sequential levels of C-reactive protein and transthyretin were obtained on a 26-year-old man who was involved in an automobile accident. This pattern shows an initial elevation of C-reactive protein, which is increasing because of the inflammatory response due to the automobile accident. As it begins to decrease, transthyretin, an inverse acute-phase reactant, decreases. At day 5, acute-phase response is over, and transthyretin becomes a nutritional marker. At this time, tube feeding is started because the patient shows both biochemical and physical signs of malnutrition. Tube feeding is stopped when the transthyretin reaches a level of 180 mg/L. This illustrates the use of transthyretin in an acute-phase response situation.

stomy or jejunostomy catheter put in place during the surgical procedure. Because TPN administration bypasses normal absorption and circulation routes, careful laboratory monitoring of these patients is critical. The goal is to provide optimal nutritional status by whatever routes nutrients are administered. An unintended weight loss of more than 10–12% leads to suspicion of either disease or malnutrition. The patient's height, age, and activity level are also considered.[92]

It is important to monitor the TPN patient to avoid possible complications. Such laboratory monitoring provides necessary information needed to properly administer TPN therapy.

Urine Testing

In small premature infants, glycosuria during the early phase of TPN is a signal that glucose infusion is too rapid. If glucose appears in the urine of small infants after glucose tolerance has been established, however, the clinician should question the presence of respiratory disease, sepsis, or cardiovascular changes.

Tests to Monitor Electrolyte Disturbances

Sodium regulation is a problem in children during TPN. Daily sodium requirements may vary depending on renal maturity and the ability of the child's body to regulate sodium. Factors that increase the amount of sodium necessary to maintain normal serum sodium concentrations in both children and adults are glycosuria, diuretic use, diarrhea or other excessive gastrointestinal losses, and increased postoperative fluid losses.

Hyperkalemia is a common problem in children when blood is obtained by heel stick. The squeezing of the heel may cause red cell hemolysis, resulting in falsely high serum potassium levels. Although adequate nutrition may be supplied to promote *anabolism,* hypokalemia may develop as the extracellular supply is used for cell synthesis.

The primary function of chloride is osmotic regulation. Hyperchloremia metabolic acidosis is a problem when crystal amino acid solutions are used, but such acidosis can be prevented or treated by altering the amount of chloride salt in the parenteral nutrition solution. Supplying some of the sodium and potassium requirements as acetate or phosphate salts can reduce the required amount of chloride. The reformulation of synthetic amino acid solutions by commercial manufacturers has helped to avoid this serious complication. If hyperchloremia metabolic acidosis does occur, treatment with sodium and potassium acetate solutions is used because acetate is metabolized rapidly to bicarbonate. Acetate salts are compatible with all other common parenteral nutrition components and are ideal to use when acidosis is present. Sodium bicarbonate cannot be used in parenteral nutrition solutions containing calcium because calcium carbonate readily precipitates. The use of acetate

not only increases serum bicarbonate but also decreases the amount of chloride delivered to the patient.

Mineral Tests to Monitor

One of the most important aspects of TPN monitoring is determining deficiencies and excesses of calcium, phosphorus, and magnesium. When regulated inadequately, these minerals not only affect bone mass but also can precipitate life-threatening situations. Calcium and phosphorus are related closely in the important role of bone mineralization. Calcium is present in serum in two forms—protein-bound, or nondiffusible, and ionized diffusible calcium. Ionized calcium is the physiologically active form and constitutes only 25% of total serum calcium. Regardless of total serum calcium, a decrease in ionized calcium may result in tetany. Decreased ionized calcium often is caused by an increase in blood pH (alkalosis). It is important to monitor ionized serum calcium and blood pH, especially in a patient on TPN who is receiving calcium supplementation along with ingredients in the TPN solution that may alter blood pH. Although calcium imbalance is frequent in newborns undergoing TPN, it is much less common in adolescents and adults. Hypercalciuria with nephrolithiasis has been reported, however, as a complication in patients on long-term TPN.

A reciprocal relationship exists between calcium and phosphorus. Intracellular phosphate is necessary to promote protein synthesis and other cellular functions. Calcium and phosphorus must be monitored carefully to maintain the correct balance between these two minerals. Severe hypophosphatemia has been reported in patients undergoing prolonged TPN.[93,94] Magnesium, as a TPN solution additive, is closely related to calcium and phosphorus. A reciprocal relationship exists between magnesium and calcium and, in certain situations, between magnesium and phosphorus. Low levels of magnesium can cause tetany, whereas high levels can increase cardiac atrioventricular conduction time. Certain electrolyte and mineral abnormalities associated with parenteral nutrition are shown in Table 31-9.

Trace Elements to Monitor

The diets of most patients on TPN must be supplemented to maintain optimal levels of several trace elements; these elements also must be monitored to prevent deficiency or toxicity. Copper and zinc are the most common trace elements added to TPN solutions. Pallor, decreased pigmentation, vein enlargement, and rashes resembling seborrheic dermatitis are the major clinical signs of copper deficiency, which at times go unnoticed. Some other abnormalities include recurrent leukopenia (white blood cell count, less than 5×10^9/L) and neutropenia (neutrophils, less than 1.5×10^9/L).

The diagnosis of copper deficiency is confirmed when both serum copper and ceruloplasmin (the copper-

TABLE 31-9. ELECTROLYTE AND MINERAL ABNORMALITIES ASSOCIATED WITH TPN

ABNORMALITY	MANIFESTATIONS	USUAL CAUSES
Hypernatremia	Edema, hypertension, thirst, intracranial hemorrhage	Inappropriate sodium intake
Hyponatremia	Weakness, hypotension, oliguria, tachycardiaintake	Inadequate sodium intake relative to water
Hyperkalemia	Weakness, paresthesia, cardiac arrhythmias	Acidosis, renal failure, excessive potassium intake
Hypokalemia	Weakness, alkalosis, cardiac abnormalities	Insufficient potassium intake associated with protein anabolism
Hyperchloremia	Metabolic acidosis	Excessive chloride intake, amino acid solutions with high chloride content
Hypocalcemia	Tetany, seizures, rickets, bone demineralization	Inadequate calcium, phosphorus, and/or vitamin D intake
Hypophosphatemia	Weakness, bone pain, bone demineralization	Insufficient phosphorus intake
Hypomagnesemia	Seizure, neuritis	Inadequate intake of magnesium

binding glycoprotein) are low. It is difficult to make this diagnosis in premature infants, however, because their serum copper levels remain depressed until about 9 weeks of age. Low copper levels have also been reported in malabsorption syndrome, protein-wasting intestinal diseases, nephrotic syndrome, severe trauma, and burns.

Patients on TPN may develop acute zinc deficiency.[95,96] They initially suffer from a massive urinary loss of zinc during phases of catabolism. When weight gain begins, the zinc-deficient patient may experience diarrhea, perioral dermatitis, and alopecia. Premature newborns are particularly predisposed to zinc deficiency because zinc normally is acquired at the rate of about 500 mg/day during the final month of gestation. To compensate for this deficiency, zinc supplements for the premature newborn should be 50% higher than for the full-term newborn. This concentration is then gradually decreased until it is the same as for a full-term infant.

Serum zinc and copper levels should be monitored weekly or, at least, bimonthly. Zinc should be monitored even more frequently in patients with ongoing gastrointestinal losses, even if they are receiving zinc supplements in their parenteral solutions.[97]

Chromium deficiency has been described in patients on long-term parenteral nutrition.[98] Initial signs and symptoms include weight loss, increased carbohydrate intolerance, and neuropathy. The diagnosis is supported by low levels of serum chromium and by the clinical response to chromium administration. Evidence indicates that plasma chromium levels are reduced, not only in deficiency but also in acute illnesses.[99] They are elevated by increased insulin and glucose loads.

Selenium deficiency has been described in long-term TPN.[100] It has been associated with both cardiomyopathy and malabsorption. Cardiomyopathy can be severe, and

death has been reported. More work is needed, however, to establish its significance in TPN.

Use of Panel Testing

To regulate the metabolic state of critically ill patients on TPN, it is necessary to monitor their nutritional therapy consistently. The constant demand for monitoring these patients produces an ideal situation for laboratory panels. By requesting these panels, a group of tests can be performed in the most cost-efficient manner. This allows the laboratory the option of test batching and automated analysis, which results in less specimen processing, more efficient chemical analysis, and, therefore, cost containment. Panels only should consist of repeatedly ordered routine tests.

SUMMARY

The current emphasis on nutrition and health has resulted in the increasing importance of vitamin and nutritional assessment in the clinical laboratory. Vitamins, low-molecular-weight compounds with a wide range of functions in biologic tissue, must be partially or completely obtained from food sources and, in some instances, bacterial synthesis. Nutritional assessment is the evaluation of a patient's metabolic and nutritional needs. It is best performed by clinical and laboratory measurements of nutritional status. Nutritional assessment has become increasingly important in medical care, especially in the treatment of critically ill and chronically emaciated patients. It is uncommon to identify patients at risk of developing nutritionally related complications in the course of an illness; however, this does not have to be the case. Standards are available for identifying patients at high risk and monitoring the effectiveness of feeding to replace nutritional losses.

REVIEW QUESTIONS

1. Match the vitamin with its appropriate category:
   a. Fat soluble; b. Water soluble
   Vitamin A ____
   Vitamin E ____
   Folate ____
   Biotin ____
   Vitamin K ____

2. Which of the following describes the correct source, function, and deficient state of the vitamin listed?
   a. Vitamin E—plant tissue, antioxidant, osteomalacia
   b. Thiamine (B_1)—whole grains, carbohydrate metabolism, beriberi
   c. Niacin—meat, oxidation-reduction reactions, scurvy
   d. Folic acid—dairy products, myelin formation

3. Which vitamin would be affected if a patient was diagnosed with a disorder involving fat absorption?
   a. Vitamin B_{12}
   b. Ascorbic acid
   c. Thiamine
   d. Vitamin K

4. Which vitamin is a powerful antioxidant, found primarily in vegetable oils, that protects the erythrocyte membrane from oxidative stress?
   a. Vitamin K
   b. Vitamin C
   c. Vitamin E
   d. Folic acid

5. A 70-year-old man presented to his physician with a broken arm. Laboratory work indicated an elevated prothrombin time, with all other laboratory results being normal. The man was taking an antibiotic for an earlier respiratory infection. Which, if any, of the following vitamins might be involved?
   a. Vitamin K
   b. Vitamin D
   c. Biotin
   d. None of the above

6. The most commonly used method for determination of vitamin B_{12} is:
   a. chemiluminescence assay.
   b. magnetic-separation immunoassay.
   c. competitive protein-binding radioimmunoassay.
   d. HPLC.

7. The term describing chronically calorie-malnourished patients who lose adipose and muscle tissue but do not demonstrate a protein deficiency is:
   a. kwashiorkor.
   b. marasmus.
   c. debilitated.
   d. none of the above.

8. The percentage of hospitalized patients who may be malnourished is:
   a. 5–8%.
   b. 10–15%.
   c. 20–25%.
   d. 30–50%.

9. Which nutritional marker has been found to be the most sensitive and helpful indicator of nutritional status in very ill patients?
   a. Transthyretin
   b. Transferrin
   c. Albumin
   d. Insulin growth factor-1

10. Laboratory monitoring of the patient on TPN therapy is important to avoid possible complications. Which trace element should be monitored on a weekly basis?
    a. Copper
    b. Selenium
    c. Molybdenum
    d. Chromium

REFERENCES

1. World Health Organization: Energy and protein requirements. A joint FAO/WHO/UNU expert consultation technical report. Series 724. Geneva, Switzerland: WHO, 1985.
2. Kinney JM. Metabolic responses to injury. In: Winters RW, Greene HL, eds. Nutritional Support of the Seriously Ill Patient. New York: Academic Press, 1983:5–12
3. Wilmore DW, Black PR, Muhlbacher F. Injured man: trauma and sepsis. In: Winters RW, Greene HL, eds. Nutritional Support of the Seriously Ill Patient. New York: Academic Press, 1983:33–52.
4. Kinney JM. Energy metabolism: heat, fuel and life. In: Kinney JM, Jeejeebhoy KN, Hill GL, Owen OE, eds. Nutrition and Metabolism in Patient Care. Philadelphia: WB Saunders, 1988:3–34.
5. Briggs MH, ed. Vitamins in Human Biology and Medicine. Boca Raton, FL: CRC Press, 1981.
6. Food and Nutrition Board. Recommended Dietary Allowances, 10th ed. Washington, D.C.: National Academy of Science, 1989.
7. Calabrese EJ. The vitamins. In: Nutrition and Environmental Health, Vol. 1. New York: John Wiley & Sons, 1980.

8. Ensminger AH, Ensminger ME, Konlande JE, et al. Foods and Nutrition Encyclopedia, 2nd ed. Boca Raton, FL: CRC Press, 1994:2257–2260.

9. Garry PJ. Vitamin A. In: Labbe RF, ed. Clinics in Laboratory Medicine, Vol 1. Laboratory Assessment of Nutritional Status. Philadelphia: WB Saunders, 1981.

10. Book LS. Fat soluble vitamins and essential fatty acids in total parenteral nutrition. In: Lebenthal E, ed. Total Parenteral Nutrition: Indications, Utilization, Complications. New York: Raven Press, 1986:59–81.

11. Underwood BA. Methods for assessment of vitamin A status. J Nutr 1990;120(Suppl 11):1459–1463.

12. Bieri JG, Evarts RP, Thorp S. Factors affecting the exchange of tocopherol between red cells and plasma. Am J Clin Nutr 1977; 30:686.

13. Holick MF. The use and interpretation of assays for vitamin D and its metabolites. J Nutr 1990;120(Suppl 11):1464–1469.

14. Suttie JW. Role of vitamin K in the synthesis of clotting factors. In: Draper HH, ed. Advances in Nutritional Research, Vol 1. New York: Plenum, 1977.

15. Hazell K, Baloch KH. Vitamin K deficiency in the elderly. Gerontol Clin 1970;12:10–17.

16. Sitren H. Vitamin K. In: Baumgartner TG, ed. Clinical Guide to Parenteral Micronutrition. New York: Fujizawa USA, 1991:411–430.

17. Sitren HS, Bailey LB, Cerda JJ, Anderson CR. Thiamin (vitamin B₁). In: Baumgartner TG, ed. Clinical Guide to Parenteral Micronutrition. New York: Fujizawa USA, 1991:431–449.

18. Sitren HS, Bailey LB, Cerda JJ, Anderson CR. Riboflavin (vitamin B₂). In: Baumgartner TG, ed. Clinical Guide to Parenteral Micronutrition. New York: Fujizawa USA, 1991:451–468.

19. Bailey LB. Pyridoxine (vitamin B₆). In: Baumgartner TG, ed. Clinical Guide to Parenteral Micronutrition. New York: Fujizawa USA 1991:521–539.

20. Sitren HS, Bailey LB, Cerda JJ, Anderson CR. Niacin (vitamin B₃). In: Baumgartner TG, ed. Clinical Guide to Parenteral Micronutrition. New York: Fujizawa USA, 1991:469–486.

21. Bailey LB. Folic Acid. In: Baumgartner TG, ed. Clinical Guide to Parenteral Micronutrition. New York: Fujizawa USA, 1991:573–590.

22. Bailey LB. Folate status assessment. J Nutr 1990;120(Suppl 11): 1508–1511.

23. Ueland PM, Refsum H, Stabler SP, et al: Total homocysteine in plasma or serum: methods and clinical applications. Clin Chem 1993;39:1764–1779.

24. Steinkamp RC. Vitamin B₁₂ and folic acid: clinical and pathophysiological considerations. In: Brewster MA, Naito IIK, eds. Nutritional Elements and Clinical Biochemistry. New York: Plenum, 1980.

25. Bailey LB. Cobalamine (vitamin B₁₂). In: Baumgartner TG, ed. Clinical Guide to Parenteral Micronutrition. New York: Fujizawa USA, 1991:541–572.

26. Roth KS. Biotin in clinical medicine: a review. Am J Clin Nutr 1981;34:1967.

27. England S, Seifter S. The biochemical functions of ascorbic acid. Annu Rev Nutr 1986;6:265–304.

28. Jacob RA. Assessment of human vitamin C status. J Nutr 1990;120(Suppl 11):1480–1485.

29. Tanphaichitr V, Leelahagul P. Carnitine metabolism and human carnitine deficiency. Nutrition 1993;9:246–254.

30. Simopolis AP. Evolutionary aspects of diet: essential fatty acids. In: Mostofsky D, Yehuda S, Salem Jr N, eds. Fatty Acids: Physiological and Behavioral Functions. Totowa, NJ: Humana Press, 2001;3–22.

31. Huang MC, Brenna JT. On the relative efficacy of α-linolenic acid and preformed docosahexaenoic acid as substrates for tissue docohexaenoate during perinatal development. In: Mostofsky D, Yehuda S, Salem Jr N, eds. Fatty Acids: Physiological and Behavioral Functions. Totowa, NJ: Humana Press, 2001;99–113.

32. Lindgren JA, Edenius C, Samuelsson B. Eicosanoid metabolism and function–nutritional modulation. In: Kinney J, Borum P, eds. Perspectives in Clinical Nutrition. Baltimore: Urban & Schwartzenberg, 1989:379–391.

33. Spielmann D. Metabolism of unsaturated fatty acids: role of n-3 and n-6 fatty acids in clinical nutrition. In: Kinney J, Borum P, eds. Perspectives in Clinical Nutrition. Baltimore: Urban & Schwartzenberg, 1989:351–378.

34. Meguid MM, Mughal MM, Meguid V, et al. Risk-benefit analysis of malnutrition and preoperative nutrition support: a review. Nutr Int 1987;3:25.

35. Bistrian BR, Blackburn GL, Vitale J, et al. Protein status in general medical patients. JAMA 1976;235:1567.

36. Reilly JJ Jr, Hull SF, et al. Economic impact of malnutrition: a model system for hospitalized patients. J Parenter Enteral Nutr 1988;12:371.

37. Weinsier RL, Hunker EM, Krumdieck GL, et al. A prospective evaluation of general medical patients during the course of hospitalization. Am J Clin Nutr 1979;32:419.

38. Bistrian BR, Blackburn GL, Hollwell H, et al. Protein status of general surgical patients. JAMA 1974;230:858.

39. Reinhardt GF, Myskofski JW, Wilkins DB, et al. Incidence and mortality of hypoalbuminemic patients in hospitalized veterans. J Parenter Enteral Nutr 1980;4:357.

40. Cannon PR, Wissler RW, Woolridge RL, et al. The relationship of protein deficiency to surgical infection. Ann Surg 1944;120:514.

41. Cahill GF, Jr. Starvation: some biological aspects. In: Kinney JM, Jeejeebhoy KN, Hill GL, Owen OE, eds. Nutrition and Metabolism in Patient Care. Philadelphia: WB Saunders, 1988:193–204.

42. Ingenbleek Y, Bernstein L. The stressful condition as a nutritionally dependent adaptive dichotomy. Nutrition 1999;15(4): 305–320.

43. Ingenbleek Y, Bernstein LH. The nutritionally-dependent adaptive dichotomy (NDAD) and stress hypermetabolism. In: Bernstein LH, Ingenbleek Y, eds. Nutrition-Disease Interactions, Part I. J Clin Ligand Assay 1999;22(3):259–267.

44. Kinney JM. Metabolic responses to injury. In: Winters RW, Greene HL, eds. Nutritional Support of the Seriously-Ill Patient. New York: Academic Press, 1983:5–12.

45. Kinney JM, Elwyn DH. Protein metabolism and injury. Annu Rev Nutr 1983;3:433–466.

46. Molawer LL, Fong Y, Marano MA, Lowry SF. Role of interleukins and tumor necrosis factor in regulating skeletal protein mass during inflammation. In: Kinney JM, Borum PR. Perspectives in Clinical Nutrition. Baltimore: Urban & Schwartzenberg, 1989:307–321.

47. Jeejeebhoy KN. Nutritional support in the malnourished patient. Nutritional Support of the Seriously Ill Patient. New York: Academic Press, 1983:207–222.

48. Bernstein LH, Shaw-Stiffel TA, Schorow M, et al. Financial implications of malnutrition. In: Labbe R, ed. Clinics in Laboratory Medicine. Philadelphia: WB Saunders, 1993:1.

49. Detsky AS, Baker JP, Mendelson RA, et al. Evaluation of accuracy of nutritional assessment techniques applied to hospitalized patients: methodology and comparisons. J Parenter Enteral Nutr 1984;8:153.

50. Studley HO. Percentage of weight loss: a basic indicator of surgical risk in patients with chronic peptic ulcer. JAMA 1936;106: 458.

51. Morgan DB, Hill GL, Burkinshaw L. The assessment of weight loss from a single measurement of body weight: the problems and limitations. Am J Clin Nutr 1980;33:210.

52. Blackburn GL, Bistrian BR, Maini BS, et al. Nutritional and metabolic assessment of the hospitalized patient. J Parenter Enteral Nutr 1977;1:11.

53. Brugler L, DiPrinzio MJ, Bernstein LH. The five year evolution of a malnutrition treatment program in a community hospital. Joint Comm J Qual Improvement 1999;25(4):191–206.

54. Mears E. Linking serum prealbumin measurements to managing a malnutrition clinical pathway. J Clin Ligand Assay 1999;22(3): 296–303.

55. Forbes GB, Bruining GJ. Urinary creatinine excretion and lean body mass. Am J Clin Nutr 1976;20:1359.

56. Christou NV, Meakins JL. Neutrophil function in anergic surgical patients: neutrophil adherence and chemotaxis. Ann Surg 1979; 190:557.

57. Moore FD, Oleson KH, McMurphy JD, et al. The body cell mass and its supporting environment: body composition in health and disease. Philadelphia: WB Saunders, 1963.

58. Klidjian AM, Foster KJ, Kammerling RM, et al. Anthropometric and dynamometric variables to serious postoperative complications. Br Med J 1980;281:899.

59. Ingenbleek Y, Carpentier YA. Prognostic inflammatory and nutritional index scoring critically ill patients. Int J Vitam Nutr Res 1985;55:91.

60. Seltzer MH, Bastidas JA, Cooper DM, et al. Instant nutritional assessment. J Parenter Enteral Nutr 1979;3:157.

61. Forse RA, Shizgal HM. Serum albumin and nutritional status. J Parenter Enteral Nutr 1980;4:450.

62. Grant JP, Custer PB, Thurlow J. Current techniques of nutritional assessment. Surg Clin North Am 1981;61:437.

63. Royle GT, Kettlewell MGW. Liver function tests in surgical infection and malnutrition. Ann Surg 1980;192:459.

64. Apelgren KN, Rombeau JL, Twomey PL, et al. Comparison of nutritional indices and outcome in critically ill patients. Crit Care Med 1982;10:305.

65. Ingenbleek Y, Van Den Schrieck H-G, De Nayer P, et al. Albumin, transferrin and thyroxine-binding prealbumin/retinol-binding protein (TBPA-RBP) complex in assessment of malnutrition. Clin Chem Acta 1975;63:61.

66. Georgieff MK, Amarnath UM, Murphy EL, et al. Serum transferrin levels in the longitudinal assessment of protein-energy status in preterm infants. J Pediatr Gastroenterol Nutr 1989;8:234.

67. Ingenbleek Y, De Visscher M, De Nayer P. Measurement of prealbumin as an index of protein-calorie malnutrition. Lancet 1972; 2:106.

68. Smith FR, Goodman DS, Zaklama MS, et al. Serum vitamin A, retinol-binding protein, and prealbumin concentrations in protein calorie malnutrition. I. Functional defect in hepatic retinol release. Am J Clin Nutr 1973;26:973.

69. Bernstein LH, Leukhardt-Fairfield CJ, Pleban W, et al. Usefulness of data on albumin and prealbumin concentrations in determining effectiveness of nutritional support. Clin Chem 1989;35:271.

70. Large S, Neal G, Glover J, et al. The early changes in retinol-binding protein and prealbumin concentrations in plasma of protein-energy malnourished children after treatment with retinol and an improved diet. Br J Nutr 1980;43:393.

71. Georgieff MK, Sasanow SR, Pereira GR. Serum transthyretin levels and protein intake as predictors of weight gain velocity in premature infants. J Pediatr Gastroenterol Nutr 1987;6:775.

72. Giacoia GP, Watson S, West K. Rapid turnover transport proteins, plasma albumin, and growth in low birth weight infants. J Parenter Enteral Nutr 1984;8:367.

73. Moskowitz SR, Pereira G, Spitzer A, et al. Prealbumin as a biochemical marker of nutritional adequacy in premature infants. J Pediatr 1983;102:749.

74. Church JM, Hill GL. Assessing the efficacy of intravenous nutrition in general surgical patients: dynamic nutritional assessment with plasma proteins. J Parenter Enteral Nutr 1987;11:135.

75. Tuten MB, Wogt S, Dasse F, et al. Utilization of prealbumin as a nutritional parameter. J Parenter Enteral Nutr 1985;9:709.

76. Cavarocchi NC, Au FC, Dalal FR, et al. Rapid turnover proteins as nutritional indicators. World J Surg 1986;10:468.

77. Carlson DE, Cioffi WG Jr, Mason AD Jr, et al. Evaluation of serum visceral protein levels as indicators of nitrogen balance in thermally injured patients. J Parenter Enteral Nutr 1991; 15:440.

78. Ingenbleek Y, Van Den Schrieck HG, De Nayer P, et al. The role of retinol-binding protein in protein-calorie malnutrition. Metabolism 1975;24:633.

79. Smith FR, Suskind R, Thanangkul O, et al. Plasma vitamin A, retinol-binding protein and prealbumin concentrations in protein-calorie malnutrition. III. Response to varying dietary treatments. Am J Clin Nutr 1975;28:732.

80. Baxter RC. The somatomedins: Insulin-like growth factors. Adv Clin Chem 1986;25:49.

81. Isley WL, Lyman B, Pemberton B. Somatomedin-C as a nutritional marker in traumatized patients. Crit Care Med 1990; 18:795.

82. Clemmons DR, Underwood LE, Dickerson RN, et al. Use of plasma somatomedin-C/insulin-like growth factor I measurements to monitor the response to nutritional repletion in malnourished patients. Am J Clin Nutr 1985;41:191.

83. Unterman TG, Vazquez RM, Slas AJ, et al. Nutrition and somatomedin. XIII. Usefulness of somatomedin-C in nutritional assessment. Am J Med 1985;78:228.

84. Mosher DF. Physiology of fibronectin. Annu Rev Med 1984; 35:561.

85. Saba TM, Blumenstock FA, Shah DM, et al. Reversal of opsonic deficiency in surgical, trauma, and burn patients by infusion of purified human plasma fibronectin. Am J Med 1986;80:229.

86. Spiekerman AM. Laboratory tests for monitoring total parenteral nutrition (TPN). Clin Chem 1987;27:1.

87. Deodhar SD. C-Reactive protein: the best laboratory indicator available for monitoring disease activity. Cleve Clin J Med 1989;56:126.

88. Hokama Y, Nakamura RM. C-Reactive protein: current status and future perspectives. J Clin Lab Anal 1987;1:15.

89. Wilmore DW, Black PR, Muhlbacher F. Injured man: trauma and sepsis. In: Winters RW, Greene M, eds. Nutritional support of the seriously ill patient. New York: Academic Press, 1983:33–52.

90. Cerra FB. Hypermetabolism, organ failure, and metabolic support. Surgery 1987;101:1.

91. Dudrick SJ. A clinical review of nutritional support of the patient. J Parenter Enteral Nutr 1979;3:444.

92. Howard L, Meguid MM. Nutritional assessment in total parenteral nutrition. Clin Lab Med 1981;1:611.

93. Takala J, Neuvonen P, Klossner J. Hypophosphatemia in hypercatabolic patients. Acta Anaesthesiol Scand 1985;29:65.

94. Tovey SJ, Benton KGF, Lee HA. Hypophosphatemia and phosphorus requirements during intravenous nutrition. Postgrad Med 1977;53:289.

95. Gordon EF, Gordon RC, Passal DB. Zinc metabolism: basic clinical and behavioral aspects. J Pediatr 1981;99:341.

96. Jeejeebhoy KN. Zinc and chromium in parenteral nutrition. Bull N Y Acad Med 1984;60:118.

97. Lockitch G, Godophin W, Pendray MR, et al. Serum zinc, copper, retinol-binding protein, prealbumin and ceruloplasmin concentrations in infants receiving intravenous zinc and copper supplement. J Pediatr 1983;102:304.

98. Freund H, Atamian S, Fischer JE. Chromium deficiency during total parenteral nutrition. JAMA 1979;241:496.

99. Jeejeebhoy KN, Chu RC, Marliss EB, et al. Chromium deficiency, glucose intolerance, and neuropathy reversed by chromium supplementation in a patient receiving long-term total parenteral nutrition. Am J Clin Nutr 1977;30:531.

100. Sjils ME, Levander OA, Alcock NW. Selenium levels in long-term TPN patients. Am J Clin Nutr 1982;35:838.

Clinical Chemistry and the Geriatric Patient

Larry H. Bernstein

OBJECTIVES

Upon completion of this chapter, the clinical laboratorian should be able to:
• Define aging, apoptosis, atherosclerosis, free radical, geriatrics, gerontology, homeostasis, menopause, and osteoporosis.
• Discuss the impact of geriatric patients on the clinical laboratory.
• Describe the current theories of aging.
• Appraise the physiologic changes that occur with the aging process.

• Identify the age-related changes in clinical chemistry analytes.
• Explain the problems associated with establishing reference intervals for the elderly.
• Describe the effects of medication on clinical chemistry results in the elderly.
• Discuss the effects of exercise and nutrition on chemistry results in the elderly.
• Correlate age-related physiologic changes and laboratory results with pathologic conditions.

KEY TERMS

Aging
Apoptosis
Atherosclerosis

Free radical
Geriatrics

Gerontology
Homeostasis

Menopause
Osteoporosis

Aging is a complex process that is not well understood. There is no universally accepted definition of aging. One definition of *aging* is, "a progressive, unfavorable loss of adaptation, leading to increased vulnerability, decreased viability, and decreased life expectancy."[1] The problem with this definition is that the aging process is variable with respect to age and loss of function. Indeed, there may be early loss or marginal and delayed loss at a late age. In addition, mental function may be maintained independent of physical functioning loss rate. How is this "progressive, unfavorable loss of adaptation" reflected in clinical laboratory results, specifically clinical chemistry results? This chapter focuses on the clinical chemistry laboratory and the biochemical and physiologic processes of aging.

THE IMPACT OF GERIATRIC PATIENTS ON THE CLINICAL LABORATORY

In addition to the definition of aging, the reader should be familiar with the terms *gerontology* and *geriatrics*. *Gerontology* is the study of the aging process. *Geriatrics* is the branch of general medicine dealing with physiologic, psychological, economic, and sociologic problems of the elderly. Although there is no specific physiologic basis, such as puberty or menopause, for the distinction in our society, the terms *elderly people, seniors,* and *geriatric patients* are generally considered to include anyone older than age 65. However, because we are confronted with significant variation in age-associated loss, there is also

young-old and young and old geriatric, ranging from 60 to 75 years, or even a well-functioning age 85. For the purpose of this chapter, information primarily relates to individuals 65 years of age and older, except where indicated.

Because of improved medical care, better nutrition, and an emphasis on exercise, an ever-growing number of people are living to age 65 and older. Therefore, the overall percentage of elderly people in the United States population continues to increase. Among the elderly, the oldest-old (ie, those age 85 and older) is the fastest growing age-group. According to a U.S. Census Bureau report, the number of people 65 years of age and older increased by a factor of 11 between 1900 and 1994, from 3.1 million to 33.2 million. In 1994, 1 of 8 Americans was elderly, but the projection for the year 2030 is that 1 of 5 Americans will be elderly.[2] Figure 32-1 shows the increase in the percentage of the U.S. population aged 65 years and older from 1900 to 2040.

The increase in the percentage of elderly people presents a major challenge to the nation's health care and social systems, as well as to the clinical laboratory. The establishment of Medicare benefits at age 65 years was based on an estimate that 1% of the population would be age 65 when the benefits were needed, having no effect on the economy. That view has changed.

Clinical laboratorians must familiarize themselves with problems unique to or especially common in the geriatric population. They must become aware of special considerations regarding the collection of blood samples,

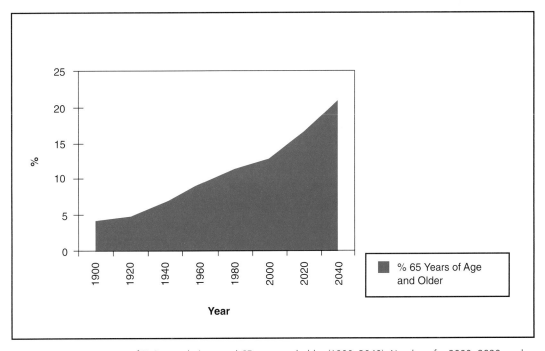

FIGURE 32-1. Percentage of U.S. population aged 65 years and older (1900–2040). Numbers for 2000, 2020, and 2040 are projections. (Source: U.S. Bureau of the Census. Current Population Reports, Special Studies, P23-190, 65+ in the United States. Washington, D.C.: U.S. Government Printing Office, 1996.)

development of reference intervals, effect of medications on chemistry results, and diagnosis of diseases in the elderly. Most important, however, they must thoroughly understand the effects of aging on laboratory values.

THEORIES OF AGING

Theories of aging have described both intrinsic (genetic) and extrinsic (environmental) factors that are associated with change in structure and cell damage, a combination of which can be attributed to the aging process. Table 32-1 includes: (1) random genetic damage, (2) glycation, (3) developmental processes involving the immune and neuroendocrine systems, (4) genetic programming, and (5) free radical damage.[3,4]

The theory involving damaged DNA is not random, involving damage or alteration of genetic materials by mutagens, such as background radiation (ultraviolet), and causing chromosome or DNA damage.[3] This damage is cumulative, but the failure associated with aging is a diminished capacity for repair of damaged DNA.[3,5] The "error catastrophe" theory, requires posttranslational modification of proteins that lead to genetic abnormalities and ultimate death of the cell.[3] The loss of a nonessential amino acid in a protein, as with isoforms of CK-MM, is a nonfunctional change. The glycation theory contends that the nonenzymatic interaction of glucose with numerous proteins forms glycated end products and cross-linked protein molecules. These modified proteins may eventually accumulate and interfere with both cell structure and function. This process may then result in various problems characteristic of the elderly, (eg, stiffening or loss of flexibility).[3,6]

The developmental theories of aging involve the immune and neuroendocrine systems, neither of which provides a plausible explanation for aging. Immune system capability declines with age.[3] Thymic atrophy occurs early in the aging process. Reduction of the T-cell population with an associated loss of B cells leads to a decreased response to new antigens. However, the exposure to neoantigens is highest at an early age. In addition, misfolding abnormalities, which occur in various forms of amyloidosis, are not merely associated with chronic infection and autoimmune disorders. Familial amyloid polyneuropathy associated with polymerization of the transthyretin molecule (55 mutants) is an example of this disorder limited to communities in Portugal, Brazil, Japan, and Sweden. This and the endocrine model are not sufficient to explain various infectious diseases and disorders (eg, autoimmune disorders, lymphocytic leukemia, and cancer) in the elderly.[3,6,7] The aging theory involving the neuroendocrine system focuses on the hypothalamic–pituitary system and its target glands. The most notable changes involving decline in endocrine function occur in postmenopausal women and include a loss of estrogen and bone calcium. In men, plasma testosterone levels decrease with age.[1]

The genetically programmed theory of aging suggests that genes play a role in the aging process and that everyone is "programmed" by their genes to live a certain number of years.[3] Support for this theory is based on general observations of life span in families and various aging syndromes, such as progeria, Werner's syndrome, and Down's syndrome.[3] There is more compelling work in basic science that has opened a large scope of study of cell signaling and cell death. Genes carry instructions not only for growth and development but also for cell destruction, causing decline of the body and ultimate death. Preprogrammed cell death is called *apoptosis*, from the Greek term *for dropping out*. Apoptosis was first described in 1972 as a process in cellular development and aging distinct from necrosis.[8] While necrotic cells swell, apoptotic cells typically shrink and detach from surrounding parenchymal cells. Concurrently, cell volume decreases and chromatin condenses at the edge of the nucleus. Apoptotic cells die by design, whereas necrotic cells die by accident and lethal injury.[8] The investigation of apoptosis was driven by its observation in the nematode *Caenorhabditis elegans*, followed by the identification of death gene homologs in other organisms.[9] Aberrant regulation of apoptosis contributes to well-known pathologies, such as autoimmune diseases, cancer, and viral infections.[10] During apoptosis, the cell is killed by a class of proteases called *caspases*. Certain caspases (ie, caspase 8 and 10) are involved in the initiation of apoptosis, others (caspase 3, 6, and 7) execute the death order by destroying essential proteins in the cell. The apoptotic process can be summarized as follows:

Activation of initiating caspases by specific signals.
Activation of executing caspases by the initiating caspases, which can cleave inactive caspases at specific sites.

TABLE 32-1. SOME CURRENT THEORIES OF AGING

Random genetic damage
Mutagen or background radiation damage
Errors in chromosomal translation or transcription
Glycation of proteins
Developmental
Immune system decline
Neuroendocrine
Genetically programmed
Preprogrammed cell death (apoptosis)
Free radical (eg, OH·, $O_2 \cdot^-$) damage

Adapted from Knight JA. Laboratory Medicine and the Aging Process. Chicago: American Society of Clinical Pathologists, 1996.

Degradation of essential cellular proteins by the protease activity of executing caspases.

Mitochondria have a central role in the mechanism of apoptosis.

Changes also occur from the action of reactive oxygen species generated and scavenged incompletely throughout the cell cycle that affect between cell interactions via alterations in the intercellular matrix, the intercellular exchange of trophic factors, the release of inflammatory cytokine mediators, and other effects. The basis of the free radical theory is that oxygen-free radicals cause progressive, random damage to cellular components. A *free radical* is an atom or molecule with one or more unpaired electrons; therefore, free radicals have an odd number of electrons, resulting in an open bond, or a half bond, making them highly reactive. A free radical may be represented by a superscript dot which signifies the unpaired electron, for example, $H_2O = HO\cdot + H\cdot$. The hydroxyl ion ($HO\cdot$) is a highly reactive free radical and perhaps one of the most damaging to cells. Free radicals are also electrophilic and attack sites of increased electron density (*eg*, DNA, RNA, proteins, membranes). Eventually, free radical damage to cellular components causes death of the cell.[3,5,11]

Superoxide ($O_2\cdot^-$) is another free radical generated in the body by several reactions, including oxidative phosphorylation and cytoplasmic reactions. Fortunately, the body has a way of handling most of these free radicals. For example, superoxide dismutase, an enzyme present in all body cells, converts superoxide to hydrogen peroxide. Other enzymes (*eg*, glutathione peroxidase and catalase) then inactivate the hydrogen peroxide. Hydroxyl radicals are neutralized by nonenzymatic compounds, such as vitamins C and E and the provitamin A and β-carotene (the antioxidants).[3,6,11] Recently, there has been much support for and research into this particular theory of aging.[11]

Although many theories of aging have been proposed, no one mechanism has been fully borne out by research.

TABLE 32-2. DISEASES AND DISORDERS COMMONLY ASSOCIATED WITH AGING[3,11]

Atherosclerosis (*eg*, myocardial infarct, renal disease, stroke)

Cancer

Diabetes mellitus

Hyperparathyroidism

Hyperthyroidism

Hypothyroidism

Monoclonal gammopathies (*eg*, multiple myeloma)

Osteoporosis

In fact, in studies of multiple species, the only intervention known to delay aging is caloric restriction. In rodents, for example, caloric restriction increased average life expectancy and maximum life span and delayed the onset of some typical age-associated diseases, as well as the deterioration of physiologic processes (*eg*, immune system responsiveness and glucose metabolism).[4] The reasons for these effects appear to be related solely to caloric restriction and *not* to the reduction of any one dietary factor, such as fat intake, or dietary supplement, such as vitamins or antioxidants. Unfortunately, the impact of caloric restriction on aging in humans is still not known.[4]

BIOCHEMICAL AND PHYSIOLOGIC CHANGES OF AGING

The theories of aging have points of intersection and are not mutually exclusive. There are many biochemical and physiologic changes associated with aging. In general, aging is associated with a decreasing efficiency in adaptation to stress. Aging systems continue to function adequately as long as they are not subjected to excessive physiologic stress. The ability of the body to successfully cope with stress decreases with advancing age and varies among individuals. The extent and rate at which the ability to adapt declines depends on many factors, including heredity, lifestyle, and nutrition; therefore, it becomes difficult to generalize about the complex process of aging. There is an aging associated decrease in total body water, muscle mass, increased bone density with remodeling (and decreased mass with osteoporosis); an increase in lipids (*eg*, cholesterol, high-density lipoprotein [HDL] cholesterol, and triglycerides); and a gradual decline in respiratory, cardiovascular, kidney, liver, gastrointestinal, immune, neurologic, and endocrine system functions.[1,4,6,12,13]

Aging is also typically associated with the development of several diseases and disorders.[4,14] Table 32-2 shows some common diseases and disorders associated with the aging process. The leading causes of death in people 65 years of age and older are shown in Table 32-3.

The specific biochemical and physiologic changes of the aging process, as they relate to clinical chemistry tests, are discussed in the following sections. Table 32-4 summarizes changes in chemistry analytes associated with the aging process. Changes in analytes are those generally cited in the literature.[4,13] Whenever possible, laboratorians should examine the possibility of establishing age-adjusted reference intervals based on analyte values determined for healthy, older adults.

Endocrine Function Changes

It has long been known that endocrine-related abnormalities are common in the elderly and tend to increase in frequency during the aging process. Not only are there

TABLE 32-3. THE TOP TEN LEADING CAUSES OF DEATH (AGE 65 AND OLDER)

1. Disease of the heart
2. Malignant neoplasm
3. Cerebrovascular disease
4. Chronic obstructive pulmonary disease and related conditions
5. Pneumonia and influenza
6. Diabetes mellitus
7. Accidents and adverse effects
8. Nephritis, nephrotic syndrome, and nephrosis
9. Alzheimer's disease
10. Septicemia

From Birth and Deaths: United States, 1996. Mon Vital Stat Rep 1997;46(1 Suppl 2):1–40.

TABLE 32-4. CHANGES IN SELECTED CLINICAL CHEMISTRY ANALYTES WITH AGE[1,3,4,6,18–20,25,28]

INCREASE	DECREASE	UNCHANGED
GGT	Albumin	Chloride
Alkaline phosphatase, women	Aldosterone	Cortisol
α_1-Antitrypsin	Bilirubin	Free T_4
Amylase	Creatinine clearance	Haptoglobin
AST	DHEA	Insulin, fasting
BUN	Growth hormone	PCO_2, or slight increase
Creatine kinase, slight	PO_2	pH, or slight decrease
γ-Globulin, slight	T_3	Sodium
Glucose, fasting	Total protein	T_4, or slight decrease
HDL	Transferrin	Thyroid-binding globulin (TBG)
Inorganic phosphate		
Lactate dehydrogenase (LD)		
PCO_2		
Potassium, slight		
Total cholesterol		
Triglycerides		
TSH, slight		
Uric acid		

Note: Changes in analytes are those generally cited in the literature. Some variability in the results of studies on aging and laboratory results may exist (ie, one author may report no significant change for an analyte; another may report a slight decrease or increase for the same analyte).

obvious changes in the production of hormones by the sex organs, there are also changes in thyroid, pituitary, and adrenal function. The most notable changes relate to the gonadal and thyroid hormones.

A variety of significant and complex hormonal changes relating to gonadal function occur in both men and women, including a decrease in the gonadal production of estrogen in women (menopause) and testosterone in men (andropause); the adrenal production of dehydroepiandrosterone (DHEA) and DHEA sulfate (DHEAS) (adrenopause); and a decrease in the activity of growth hormone (GH)/insulin-like growth factor (IGF) axis (somatopause).[15,16] As a result, hormone replacement regimens are being developed as a strategy to delay or prevent some of the consequences of aging. Between 60 and 80 years of age, the ratio of testosterone to estradiol falls from 12:1 to 2:1.[1,4] The decrease in testosterone is linked primarily to diminished testicular function.[1,17] In women, endocrine system changes are primarily related to menopause, when there is a cessation of ovarian estrogen production. *Menopause* is the permanent cessation of menstruation caused by a decline in ovarian follicular activity; it generally occurs between 35 and 58 years of age. The process of apoptosis, nontraumatic and noninflammatory cell death, balances cell proliferation and maintains *homeostasis*. Aging disrupts the orderly neuroendocrine feedback regulation of the secretion of GH, luteinizing hormone (LH), follicle-stimulating hormone (FSH), and adrenocorticotropin hormone (ACTH).[17] Specific gene products either promote (Bax) or oppose (Bcl-2) regulated cell death via mitochondrial effects. Dysregulation of apoptosis has been implicated in the development of diseases that are more prevalent in older individuals, such as cancer and neurodegenerative disorders (Alzheimer's and Parkinson's disease). The major consequences of estrogen deficiency are osteoporosis and coronary heart disease (CHD).[18,19]

Osteoporosis is a problem in both older men and women, but particularly in women after menopause (at about 50 years of age). It is estimated that about 30% of elderly women and 20% of elderly men have osteoporosis.[18,19] Osteoporosis involves a gradual loss of bone mass; the skeleton becomes weak and less dense as a result of increased bone resorption unbalanced by bone remodeling. The osteoblast cell maintains bone homeostasis. Bone resorption and bone formation are carried out in orderly sequence throughout life by osteoclasts and osteoblasts. The osteoclasts remove bone matrix at a rate of 150 μm/day; refill is carried out by osteoblasts at a rate of 1 μm/day. The refill of bone increases the strength of the bone by the structure of the osteon. Partly driven by muscle tension, refill is affected by estrogen. The uncompensated loss of skeletal mass may lead to microfractures and pain. Common clinical chemistry values in osteoporosis are generally normal, including serum calcium, phosphorus, magnesium, alkaline phosphatase, and the parathyroid and thyroid hormones,[18,19] because bone loss is not associated with massive, rapid removal of mineral, as for hyperparathyroidism (parathyroid hypercalcemia) or Paget's disease (uncontrolled bone turnover). After a diagnosis of osteoporosis has been made, laboratory tests to assess bone metabolism (turnover) are helpful in following its progress in response to therapy. Major risk factors include diet, inactive lifestyle, genetic predisposition, smoking, endocrine disturbances, and medications.[20] The greatest problem secondary to osteoporosis is hip fracture, which is disabling and associated with nonhealing in the older population. Osteoporosis, therefore, is a significant problem among the elderly, resulting in increased morbidity and health care costs. A significant association also exists between hypovitaminosis D and secondary hyperparathyroidism (elevated alkaline phosphatase and osteoporotic changes) in the elderly.[21,22] This would presumably be related to both dietary intake, lack of exposure to sunlight, and to reduced conversion of 25-hydroxy vitamin D_3 to the 1,25 form by the kidney.

The thyroid gland is central to the regulation of metabolic processes (*ie*, regulation of metabolic rate). Although there is little evidence of changes in thyroid function in the elderly, the incidence of both hypothyroidism and hyperthyroidism increases.[1,3,4] It has been reported that the prevalence of hypothyroidism in the elderly is between 0.5% and 4.4%, whereas the prevalence of hyperthyroidism is between 0.5% and 3%.[23] Hypothyroidism, although more common in the elderly, is often more difficult to diagnose.[24] Typically, the signs and symptoms of hypothyroidism may be easily misinterpreted as just "old age."[3] In subclinical hypothyroidism, for example, patients have few or no clinical symptoms, but have a normal thyroxine (T_4) level with an elevated thyroid-stimulating hormone (TSH) level.[24] Whether these patients should be treated with thyroid hormone or followed with periodic thyroid tests is controversial. Interpretation of thyroid function in hospitalized and very ill patients is also difficult because of the effect of non–thyroid-related illness on common thyroid function

tests.[24] Illness can depress the serum concentrations of both triiodothyronine (T_3) and T_4, whereas TSH remains normal or is even decreased. Alterations in protein binding, thyroid hormone metabolism, and suppression of the pituitary release of TSH may account for these findings in non–thyroid-related illness. Generally, these patients are considered to be euthyroid (*ie*, have normal thyroid function) and no hormone supplementation is prescribed.[23] Many early studies attributed changes in thyroid function to the natural aging process. More recent studies, however, indicate that abnormal thyroid function is probably secondary to some underlying or associated disorder and not just old age.[3] Because thyroid disorders may present subtly and are often difficult to diagnose, laboratory evaluation becomes important. In healthy elderly people, there is essentially no change in T_4, free T_4, thyroid-binding globulin, and reverse T_3 levels.[6,23,24] However, some studies have shown a significant decrease in T_3 levels after 50 years of age, with a slight increase in TSH levels, perhaps as a normal response to the low T_3 level. It is still unclear whether these changes are age related or the result of underlying disease.[6,23]

There are few morphologic changes of the pancreas in the elderly, other than some degree of atrophy and an increased incidence of tumors.[25] Although other aspects of endocrine function, such as the hypothalamus–anterior pituitary system and adrenal glands, exhibit no change in cortisol production, both aldosterone and DHEA decline with age.[26,27] The prevalence of hypertension also increases with age, with about 60% of people older than 60 years having the condition.[27] Causes include increased peripheral resistance due to atherosclerosis, chronic renal and endocrine disorders, and multiple medications. In general, there is also a decline in the efficiency of homeostatic regulation.[4,27]

Diabetes Mellitus and Insulin Resistance

Glucose tolerance declines with age, with elderly people having a slightly higher fasting serum glucose level than younger adults. Fasting glucose increases about 1–2

CASE STUDY 32-1

A 65-year-old woman hospitalized for pneumonia and uncontrolled diabetes had the thyroid test results shown in Case Study Table 32-1.1.

Questions

1. Based on the patient's status and the laboratory test results, how might the thyroid data be explained?

2. Should any additional testing be done?

CASE STUDY TABLE 32-1.1. LABORATORY RESULTS

TEST	RESULT	REFERENCE RANGE
Serum TSH	1.5 μU/mL	0.5–5 μU/mL
Total T_4	3.8 μg/dL	4.5–12 μg/dL
Total T_3	55 ng/dL	60–220 ng/dL

mg/dL (0.11 mmol/L) per decade throughout life.[6,28] The renal threshold (the point at which glucose spills in the urine) also increases with age; there is also an altered insulin response to glucose.[1,3] Diabetes mellitus is a common problem in the elderly, with a prevalence of about 18.4% in persons 65 years of age and older. The above observations about expected values for healthy elderly can be misleading. The definition of diabetes and prediabetes has been revised to glucose values above 126 mg/dL and to 100–126 mg/dL, respectively. There has been an alarming increase in obesity with increased type 2 diabetes and associated increase in hypertension and cardiovascular risk. This syndrome is characterized by varying degrees of glucose intolerance, abnormal cholesterol and/or triglyceride levels, high blood pressure, and upper body obesity, all independent risk factors for cardiac disease. The PROCAM (Prospective Cardiovascular Munster) study, which examined the relationship between various cardiac risk factors and the incidence of heart attack in 2754 men aged 40–65 years over a 4-year period, showed that the presence of diabetes or high blood pressure alone increased heart attack risk by 2.5 times. When diabetes and high blood pressure were both present, risk increased 8 times. An abnormal lipid profile increased the risk 16 times; when abnormal lipid levels were present with high blood pressure and/or diabetes, the risk was 20 times higher. These abnormalities constitute the insulin resistance syndrome. The insulin resistance syndrome was first described in 1988, when it was suggested that the defect was related to insulin.[29] This syndrome is estimated to affect 70–80 million Americans.[30] Because resistance usually develops long before these diseases appear, identifying and treating insulin-resistant patients has potentially great preventive value. The condition is common among persons with obesity (defined as a body mass index [BMI] of 30 kg per m[2] or more). The pattern of obesity is also extremely important. There is a strong relationship between abdominal obesity and degree of insulin resistance, independent of total body weight.[31] The degree of abdominal obesity can be estimated by use of waist circumference or the waist–hip ratio. The waist is usually measured at its narrowest point and the hips at the fullest point around the buttocks. A waist–hip ratio of greater than 1.0 in men or 0.8 in women is strongly correlated with abdominal obesity and insulin resistance and confers an increased risk of associated diseases. Advanced glycation end products (AGEs) are assumed to play a key role in diabetic nephropathy (DN) and other diabetic complications. These exert marked effects on endothelial cells, monocytes, macrophages, and bind to AGE receptors (RAGEs). AGEs are formed by the binding of aldoses on free NH_2 groups on proteins. The binding of AGEs to RAGEs activates endothelial cells, monocytes, and macrophages, which when activated, produce cytokines and express adhesion molecules and tissue factors. These have a role in increased oxidative stress and the microvascular lesions in diabetes.[32] There is also a complex relationship between fat mass, tumor necrosis factor-α (TNF-α) and insulin resistance; however, the mechanism(s) by which TNF-α induces insulin resistance is not understood. TNF-α-induced genes include transcription factors implicated in preadipocyte gene expression or nuclear factor-κ B activation, cytokines and cytokine-induced proteins, growth factors, enzymes, and signaling molecules.[33] Based on this, type 2 diabetes is more suspect as a chronic inflammatory disease than as a disease of pancreatic endocrine dysfunction.

Renal Function Changes

All aspects of renal function are affected by the aging process; it is age of onset, specific changes, and consequences that vary in elderly people.[34] Renal function begins to decline after the age of 30 years and, by age 60, is further reduced to one half.[34] This decline is attributed to the gradual loss of nephrons, decreased enzymatic and

---

CASE STUDY 32-2

An otherwise healthy 70-year-old man entered the hospital for abdominal surgery. Preoperative chemistry test results are shown in Case Study Table 32-2.1.

Questions

1. What is the BUN/creatinine ratio for this patient?

2. What do these data suggest?

3. Which test results support this conclusion?

4. How common is this condition in the elderly?

CASE STUDY TABLE 32-2.1. LABORATORY RESULTS

TEST	RESULT	REFERENCE RANGE
Albumin	53 g/L	35–50 g/L
BUN	40 mg/dL	8–26 mg/dL
Creatinine	1.6 mg/dL	0.9–1.5 mg/dL
Serum osmolality	330 mOsm/kg	275–295 mOsm/kg
Sodium	150 mmol/L	135–145 mmol/L

metabolic activity of tubular cells, and increased incidence of pathologic processes (eg, atherosclerosis).[34]

Renal function may be assessed at any age by a number of clinical tests, including urine volume, analysis of constituents and concentration, blood urea nitrogen (BUN), uric acid, and several clearance tests.[34] Creatinine clearance, glomerular filtration rate (GFR), and renal plasma flow all decrease with age.[6,34] The analytes, BUN, uric acid, and inorganic phosphate that reflect GFR are found to increase.[6]

In general, elderly people have a decreased capacity to conserve water through the kidneys and a significantly lower sensation of thirst.[35] This, of course, can lead to dehydration, a common and underappreciated problem in the elderly. Not only is dehydration a common finding in the elderly, it also can be serious, leading to increased mortality rates.[3] Clinical laboratory tests indicative of dehydration include hypernatremia, increased BUN/creatinine ratio, increased serum osmolality, and increased urine specific gravity.[3]

In addition to the previously mentioned renal changes of aging, there is an increased incidence of renal disease and a reduced ability to handle the excretion of drugs. Problems affecting renal function are related to damage from infections or drugs (medications), hypertension, or disorders such as diabetes mellitus, tuberculosis, and nephritis.[34]

Hepatic Function Changes

In general, atrophy and decreased liver weight, as well as a decline in liver function, are common in the elderly.[3,36] Although the liver performs many functions (Chapter 22, *Liver Function*), three important functions—synthetic, excretory and secretory, and detoxification and drug metabolism—are addressed in this section in relation to the aging process.

The synthetic function of the liver can be monitored by means of concentrations of plasma proteins. Tietz and colleagues reported a slight decrease of total protein in "fit" aging people.[28] Albumin and transferrin show a decline as well. This observation has to be taken with some reservation. The homogeneity of the fit aging population sample must be taken with reservation. The decline in albumin and transferrin are probably attributable to a significant degree of malnutrition and liver disease in the population studied. The existence of malnutrition, alcoholic liver disease, depression, and poor nutrient intake in the ambulatory elderly population can not be discounted. In the nursing home population, protein energy malnutrition rates are as high as 40–50%. If the malnutrition rate were 10% and the ambulatory aged people had an albumin of 2.8 g/dL, the serum albumin concentration for a sample of 10,000 people at a level of 3.5 g/dL would decrease to 3.4 g/dL. In addition, type 2 diabetes can be associated with nonalcoholic steatosis and steato-

hepatitis, which would lead to decreased albumin and transferrin and increased alkaline phosphatase. γ-Globulin and α$_1$-antitrypsin, however, increase slightly with age, whereas haptoglobin remains essentially the same as in young adults.[28] Likewise, immunoglobulins are decreased in a part of the population.

Certain enzymes also change. Alkaline phosphatase (ALP) and lactate dehydrogenase (LD), for example, increase in both men and women, but it is unlikely that these are age-related changes. Urea synthesis, a process that occurs in the hepatocytes, and bilirubin metabolism both decline with age.[3,36] The liver's detoxification or drug metabolism function is important when considering the increased numbers of medications that are usually prescribed to elderly patients. Although people 65 years of age and older compose about 12% of the U.S. population, they receive about one third of all prescribed medications.[3] In addition to possible drug interactions, drug toxicity is a potential problem. As mentioned previously, there is some atrophy of the liver as well as reduced hepatic blood flow with the aging process. This, in turn, may lead to the accumulation of some drugs (eg, lidocaine and morphine) and the possibility of toxicity.[3] Medications and the elderly are discussed in more detail later.

Pulmonary Function and Electrolyte Changes

Several known anatomic and physiologic changes occur in cardiopulmonary function during the aging process. Pulmonary function actually begins to decline after the age of 25 as a result of changes in the lung, thoracic cage, respiratory muscles, and respiratory centers in the central nervous system.[37] Of course, pulmonary function is, perhaps, more affected by personal habits, such as smoking, and by environmental pollution.[37]

The more frequently described changes relating to pulmonary function in the elderly include the PO$_2$ and PCO$_2$ values. These changes reflect the decreased vital (lung) capacity found in most elderly people.[37] Arterial PO$_2$, for example, decreases during the aging process, whereas PCO$_2$ is reported to increase slightly or remain the same.[4,37] The blood pH value is reported to remain fairly constant or to decrease only slightly.[6,37]

The electrolytes sodium, potassium, and chloride all show little change in healthy elderly people from values seen in younger adults.[27] Sodium remains fairly constant from young adulthood to older age. Chloride values are also fairly constant but have been found to be slightly higher in people older than 90 years. Potassium, however, increases slightly from age 60 to 90.[27]

Respiratory-related diseases are prevalent in elderly people and account for 25% of all deaths in those older than 85.[37] Respiratory diseases of the elderly include chronic bronchitis, emphysema, neoplasia, and lung infections, particularly tuberculosis and pneumonia.[37]

Cardiovascular and Lipid Changes

Cardiovascular disease continues to be an important cause of death in old age in both men and women. Atherosclerosis, a type of arteriosclerosis, is the major cause of death from cardiovascular disease in the United States.[3] *Atherosclerosis,* a progressive disease process that begins early in life, involves vascular alterations characterized by fatty accumulations in the vascular walls.[3] Atherosclerosis develops slowly over the years. Results of atherosclerosis include hypertension, hemorrhage, thrombosis, stroke, and coronary heart disease (CHD). CHD, also called *ischemic heart disease,* continues to be a major cause of disability and death in the United States, its prevalence increasing with advancing age.[38] Risk factors for CHD include age, gender, genetic predisposition, obesity, hypertension, poor fitness, diabetes mellitus, cigarette smoking, and hyperlipidemia.[3]

Lipids shown to play a major role in the atherosclerotic process and risk for CHD are HDL and low-density lipoprotein (LDL) cholesterol, total cholesterol, and triglycerides. In a study by Tietz and colleagues of fit elderly, total cholesterol, HDL cholesterol and triglycerides were found to increase as a part of the aging process.[28] HDL cholesterol, or "good" cholesterol, however, is considered as an important *inverse* risk factor for CHD, with values less than about 35 mg/dL indicating a high risk and values more than 35 mg/dL indicating a low risk.[3]

Enzyme Changes

Changes in enzyme levels during the aging process have been studied extensively; they are varied and complex. Enzyme concentration and synthesis are under genetic control and are affected by hormones, substrates, and other factors. Enzymes do not appear to follow any particular age-related pattern; they may increase, decrease, or remain the same during the aging process. However, the ability to initiate adaptive changes in the activity of enzymes has been found to be impaired with increasing age.[3]

Enzymes reported to change in healthy, elderly people include aspartate aminotransferase (AST), alanine aminotransferase (ALT), ALP, γ-glutamyltransferase (GGT), creatine kinase (CK), lactate dehydrogenase, and amylase.[28] AST, GGT, LD, and amylase show increases in both men and women. ALT levels show only a marginal increase in men, whereas values in women show no change. ALP, however, shows a significant increase in women, whereas men show no increase until age 90. CK values in men increase slightly between 60 and 69 years of age; however, between 70 and 90 years of age, the values decrease. In women, CK values also increase slightly from 60 to 70 years of age but decrease in those older than age 70. Lipase increases only slightly, if at all, in those aged 60–90, but definitely increases in those older than age 90.[28]

CLINICAL CHEMISTRY RESULTS AND AGING

In addition to a knowledge of basic biochemical and physiologic changes of aging, clinical laboratorians must understand other factors that may affect clinical chemistry results in the elderly. For example: Does the aging process affect laboratory test results sufficiently to warrant separate reference intervals for the elderly? What preanalytic variables (*eg,* diet, posture, medications) relating to the elderly affect clinical chemistry results? How does the aging process affect interpretation of drug levels in the elderly? What are the effects of exercise and nutrition on the elderly and chemistry results? Table 32-5 shows some factors laboratorians should consider when interpreting laboratory values for the elderly.

Establishing Reference Intervals for the Elderly

Interpretation of test results and reference intervals for the elderly can be confusing and complex. In addition, there appears to be some confusion on the topic of reference intervals for the elderly among experts in the field of clinical chemistry and aging.

TABLE 32-5. FACTORS TO CONSIDER IN THE INTERPRETATION OF CLINICAL LABORATORY RESULTS FOR THE ELDERLY[3,22,33]

Exercise
Duration
Type
Medications
Polypharmacy
Mobility
Immobility
Posture
Nutritional status
Personal habits
Alcohol use
Smoking
Presence of multiple chronic or subclinical disorders
Reference interval validity
Specimen collection variables
Site
Trauma
Volume

As previously discussed, many reference intervals for analytes vary from the reference intervals of younger adults. Certain analytes, such as the levels of male and female hormones, are the undisputed result of aging organs. With other analytes, however, the case may not be so clear.[3] Some variance in analyte levels may be a result of various secondary conditions (eg, subclinical diseases, drugs, inactivity, nutrition) and not the aging process alone; for example, the relationship between non–insulin-dependent diabetes mellitus and a rise in serum glucose levels.

Frequently, abnormal test results in the elderly are interpreted as "normal" for the individual's age and not a sign of a disorder or disease.[11] Research is now showing, however, that in many instances, abnormal laboratory results in so-called healthy individuals, may, in fact, be associated with unrecognized subclinical disorders or with other secondary conditions.[3,11] The fact that reference intervals are not easily determined, even for younger healthy adult populations, adds to the problem. Frequently, reference intervals are poorly defined and not always determined by a uniform process.[39] The establishment of reference intervals involves a well-defined protocol, including careful selection of reference individuals, control of preanalytic factors, a comprehensive list of analytic interferences, careful and consistent collection of specimens for a given analyte, analysis of specimens under well-defined conditions, and identification of data errors.[39] It is apparent that determination of reference intervals for the elderly can be problematic because a large percentage of elderly have some subclinical or obvious pathologic abnormality. The National Committee for Clinical Laboratory Standards (NCCLS) published an important guideline (C28-A), regarding the determination of valid reference intervals for quantitative clinical laboratory tests[40]; however, the guideline is inadequate for validating or determining reference intervals because of inadequate power, sample bias, and failure to control for confounding conditions in the sample population.

Although the aging process does affect certain selected analytes, the relationship between aging and changes in other analytes is less understood. Generally, clinicians and laboratorians agree that separate reference intervals for the elderly are needed to prevent false abnormal results. Knight recommends that until we have a better understanding of the relationships among true aging, age-associated disorders, and various laboratory results, clinicians and laboratorians should maintain the normal reference intervals established for healthy, younger adults.[3] It is also useful to compare a person's current values with values obtained throughout their adult life. In any case, clinicians and clinical laboratory scientists should keep in mind all factors affecting the interpretation of laboratory test results for the elderly.

Preanalytic Variables, the Elderly, and Chemistry Results

Many preanalytic variables may affect the interpretation of chemistry results; however, preanalytic variables may have a much greater effect on the elderly. Preanalytic variables relating to the patient include diet, gender, posture (eg, sitting or lying), personal habits (eg, smoking and alcohol consumption), body composition, physical activity, and prescribed medications.[41] Any of these may affect the concentration of various analytes; for example, body composition changes with age. In healthy people, body fat increases and lean muscle mass decreases with age. In view of the increase in type 2 diabetes, body fat, and inherent health risks, a reference to "healthy" people may be unwarranted. Body mass and height also decrease after about age 60.[41] These changes, in turn, may affect the levels of various analytes (eg, creatinine).

Other preanalytic variables affecting laboratory results for the elderly involve the collection of specimens for analysis.[42] Several physical and physiologic changes of aging can affect the collection and quality of a specimen and make phlebotomy a challenge to the phlebotomist. Because elderly patients may have diseases such as arthritis, malnutrition, or dehydration, in addition to the aging process itself, there may be a decrease in muscle tone and skin elasticity (ie, flabby skin). Veins may be difficult to find or inappropriate to use, making phlebotomy difficult and causing hemolysis and an increased likelihood of elevated plasma hemoglobin and lactate dehydrogenase level.[42] The veins of elderly patients may also provide poor blood flow, resulting in a less-than-adequate sample for some laboratory tests.[42]

Therapeutic Drug Monitoring in the Elderly

Elderly people, 12% of the U.S. population, use 30% of prescription medications and often are on multiple medications.[43] Unfortunately, overdosing and adverse drug reactions (from multiple medications) are problematic in the elderly. With the normal aging process, there are many changes in how the body handles drugs.[43] Absorption, distribution, metabolism, and excretion of a drug are all affected by the aging process. (See Chapter 28, *Therapeutic Drug Monitoring*, for more information on the pharmacokinetics of drugs.) For example, gastric emptying time may be prolonged in the elderly, causing a delay in drug absorption.[44,45] Absorption by intramuscular injections may also be impaired because of decreased blood flow.[44] Metabolism or biotransformation of drugs, which is handled primarily by the liver, may be impaired as a result of an age-related decrease in hepatic mass and blood flow.[44]

The most significant pharmacokinetic change in the elderly is related to the elimination of drugs through the kidneys. Renal mass and blood flow both decrease with advancing age.[44] Serum albumin may also be decreased because of protein energy malnutrition, which affects drugs that are transported bound to albumin. Glomerular filtration rate (as measured by creatinine clearance) also declines linearly with age.[4,44] For drugs principally excreted in the urine, caution should be exercised in treatment to prevent any overdosing or toxic effects.[44]

Drug dosing is adjusted for creatinine clearance using the Cockroft-Gault formula[43]:

$$Cl_{cr} = \frac{(140 - age)(wt\ in\ kg)}{(72)(serum\ creatinine)} \qquad \text{(Eq. 32–1)}$$

Multiply by 0.85 for women. Ideal weight, rather than usual weight, corrects for weight in obese individuals. Because serum creatinine below 0.9 gives a spuriously high clearance creatinine, creatinine must be rounded.

Psychosocial factors common among the elderly, such as depression, dementia, poverty, and loneliness, are also factors contributing to medication problems. Elderly patients, for example, may be less compliant (eg, because of poverty) or incapable of following medication instructions, adding to the problem.[44] Because the effects of drugs are more likely to be exaggerated in the elderly, laboratorians should be knowledgeable of the principles of therapeutic drug monitoring and the affects of aging on therapeutic drug monitoring. To provide the best quality care to the elderly, frequent drug monitoring and the development of therapeutic ranges for the elderly may be necessary.[45]

The Effects of Exercise and Nutrition on the Elderly and Chemistry Results

Many studies indicate that exercise is an excellent way for the elderly to maintain health and increase longevity. Rowe, in a study of more than 40,000 postmenopausal women during a 7-year period, reported that those who exercised regularly were 20% less likely to die than those who were sedentary.[35] Shephard concludes that exercise may benefit the sedentary elderly population (75–80 years of age) by improving overall health, increasing social contacts, and improving cerebral function.[46] Obesity, as a result of metabolic changes, reduced activity, and age-related alterations in muscle, is a common problem in elderly people that is also helped by exercise.[47,48] Other studies indicated that: (1) the more frequent the exercise, the greater the benefit, (2) moderate exercise (eg, walking) is nearly as beneficial as vigorous exercise, and (3) exercise can negate the adverse effects of other risk factors, such as high blood pressure and hyperglycemia.[27] The health benefits from exercise include reduced cardiovascular risk, weight control, increased functional capacity, improved nutrient intake, and better sleep.[3,47,48]

As increasing numbers of elderly people are encouraged to participate in exercise programs, laboratorians will need a better understanding of how exercise affects the test results of these individuals; for example, exercise affects lipids by lowering triglycerides and increasing HDL cholesterol, insulin is lowered, and growth hormone increased.[47]

Consideration should also be given to type of exercise, timing of specimen collection, and prescribed medications. Glucose and insulin, for example, do not respond in the same manner to different types of exercise. Both essentially remain stable during isometric exercise with large muscle groups, whereas insulin decreases during dynamic exercise of moderate to high intensity.[47] Timing of specimen collection is important because glucagon secretion is stimulated after intense exercise in patients with type 2 diabetes, which results in a transient elevation of glucose levels for about 1 hour after exercise.[47]

Nutritional problems are common in elderly patients. There is a growing body of information on the nutritional needs of the elderly population. Elderly people are at increased risk for poor nutritional status (eg, protein-calorie malnutrition) compared with younger adults, as a result of both physiologic and psychological factors, including age-related changes in taste and smell; malabsorption caused by medications or changes in stomach acidity; and mobility, disability, depression, and poverty.[46,49,50] The incidence of malnutrition among elderly residents in long-term-health care facilities is reported to range from 50% to 85%; in acute care hospitals, the percentage may range from 17% to 65%.[51]

The relationships among nutrition, general health, aging, and disease are important and need to be investigated further. A protein-calorie deficit can lead to decreased resistance to infection and lymphopenia. Excessive calories result in obesity and the probability of type 2 diabetes. Deficiencies in vitamins A, C, and E (the antioxidants) may lead to atherosclerosis and an increased risk for cancer.[8] Low-fiber diets may lead to diverticulitis and colon cancer.[3]

Through nutritional assessment, it may be possible to prevent and identify nutritional deficiencies in elderly people, preventing many chronic diseases of aging and promoting better health.[38,52,53] In the clinical laboratory, nutritional assessment includes the measurement of various proteins (eg, albumin, prealbumin, transferrin, and retinol-binding protein) and vitamin levels. A detailed discussion of nutritional assessment and vitamins can be found in Chapter 31, *Vitamins, Essential Fats, and Macronutrients.*

SUMMARY

The proportion of elderly persons is increasing in the U.S. population, presenting a major challenge for the health care system.[38] With this increase, it will become increasingly important for clinical laboratorians to be knowledgeable of the aging process and its effects on clinical chemistry results.[3] The aging process has been described as a loss of adaptation with a decrease in viability and life expectancy. Knowledge of the aging process and chronic diseases associated with aging is the basis for understanding changes in laboratory values. Although theories of aging have been described, none is adequate.

Aging is associated with several physiologic changes—decreasing efficiency in maintenance of homeostasis; reduction in muscle mass; and decline in respiratory, cardiovascular, kidney, liver, immune, neurologic, and endocrine system functions. Carbohydrate, protein, lipid, and calcium metabolism all change with age. The specific changes in selected chemistry analytes are shown in Table 32-4. In addition to a knowledge of the basic biochemical and physiologic changes of aging, clinical laboratorians must understand other factors that may affect clinical chemistry test results, including establishment and interpretation of reference intervals, certain preanalytic variables, prescribed medications, and the effects of exercise and nutrition.

The clinical laboratorian should remember, however, that aging is not fixed by an individual's biology or by a specific time frame. There is extensive individuality among people in regard to the rate at which aging occurs. Environmental and social factors are also important and play a role in the aging process. With an increasing proportion of elderly in the population, it will become even more important to research the physiology *and* psychosocial aspects of aging.

REVIEW QUESTIONS

1. Which of the following serum analytes essentially remains unchanged in healthy, elderly adults?
   a. Triglycerides
   b. Glucose
   c. Chloride
   d. Bilirubin

2. Which of the following is a common and underappreciated condition in the elderly?
   a. Hyponatremia
   b. Dehydration
   c. Amyloidosis
   d. Multiple myeloma

3. Which of the following is NOT one of the top ten causes of death in people older than age 65?
   a. Alzheimer's disease
   b. Pneumonia
   c. Diabetes mellitus
   d. Diverticulitis

4. When interpreting laboratory test results from the elderly, the clinical laboratorian must consider all of the following EXCEPT:
   a. multiple medications (polypharmacy).
   b. poor nutrition or malnutrition.
   c. subclinical disorders.
   d. intelligence quotient (IQ).

5. Which of the following theories of aging involves the accumulation of waste products that prevent the cell from carrying out its normal functions?
   a. Genetic programming theory
   b. Glycation of protein theory
   c. Random genetic damage theory
   d. Free radical theory

REFERENCES

1. Liew CC. Biochemical aspects of aging. In: Gornall AG, ed. Applied Biochemistry of Clinical Disorders, 2nd ed. Philadelphia: Lippincott-Raven, 1986:558–565.
2. U.S. Bureau of the Census. Current Population Reports, Special Studies, P23-190, 65+ in the United States. Washington, D.C.: U.S. Government Printing Office, 1996.
3. Knight JA. Laboratory Medicine and the Aging Process. Chicago, IL: American Society of Clinical Pathologists, 1996.
4. Resnick NM. Part 1: Introduction to Clinical Medicine. Chapter 9. Geriatric Medicine. Harrison's on-line available at: www.harrisonsonline.com. New York: McGraw-Hill, 1998.
5. Strehler BL. A critique of theories of biological aging. In: Dietz AA, ed. Aging: Its Chemistry. Washington, D.C.: American Association of Clinical Chemistry, 1980:25–45.
6. Gorman LS. Aging: laboratory testing and theories. Clin Lab Sci 1995;8:24–30.
7. Cearlock DM, Laude-Flaws M. Stress, immune function and the older adult. Med Lab Observer 1997;29(10):36–46.
8. Kerr JFR, Wyllie AH, Currie AR. Apoptosis: a basic biological phenomenon with wide-ranging implications in tissue kinetics. Brit J Cancer 1972;26:239–257.
9. Sulston JE, Horvitz HR. Post-embryonic cell lineages of the nematode, *Caenorhabditis elegans*. Develop Biol 1977;56:110–156.
10. Carson DA, Ribeiro JM. Apoptosis and disease. Lancet 1993; 341(885):1251–1254.
11. Miller SM. Antioxidants and aging. Med Lab Observer 1997; 29:42–51.
12. Etnyre-Zacher P, Isabel JM. The impact of an aging population on the clinical laboratory. MLO Med Lab Observer 1997;29(4): 48–54.

13. Young, DS. Effects of Preanalytical Variables on Clinical Laboratory Tests. Washington, D.C.: AACC Press, 1993.

14. Knight JA. Laboratory issues regarding geriatric patients. Lab Med 1997;28(7):458–461.

15. Merry BJ, Holehan AM. Aging of the male reproductive system. In: Timiras PS, ed. Physiological Basis of Aging and Geriatrics, 2nd ed. Boca Raton, FL: CRC Press, 1994:171–178.

16. Merry BJ, Holehan AM. Aging of the female reproductive system: the menopause. In: Timiras PS, ed. Physiological Basis of Aging and Geriatrics, 2nd ed. Boca Raton, FL: CRC Press, 1994:147–170.

17. Pincus S, Mulligan T, Iranmanesh A, et al. Older males secrete luteinizing hormone and testosterone more irregularly, and jointly more asynchronously, than younger males. Proc Natl Acad Sci USA 1996;93:14100–14105.

18. Kane RL, Ouslander JG, Abrass IB. Essentials of Clinical Geriatrics, 3rd ed. New York: McGraw-Hill, 1994.

19. Meier DE. Osteoporosis and other disorders of skeletal aging. In: Cassel CK, et al, eds. Geriatric Medicine, 3rd ed. New York: Springer-Verlag, 1997:411–432.

20. Davies MD, Bliziotes M. Osteoporosis: risk factors, diagnosis and therapy. Lab Med 1998;29:418–421.

21. Komar L, Nieves J, Cosman F, et al. Calcium homeostasis of an elderly population upon admission to a nursing home. J Am Geriatr Soc 1993;41:1057–1064.

22. Perry HM III, Miller DK, Morley JE, et al. A preliminary report of vitamin D and calcium metabolism in older African Americans. J Am Geriatr Soc 1993;41:612–616.

23. Timiras PS. Aging of the thyroid gland and basal metabolism. In: Timiras PS, ed. Physiological Basis of Aging and Geriatrics, 2nd ed. Boca Raton, FL: CRC Press, 1994:179–189.

24. Simons RJ, Demers LM. Thyroid disorders in the elderly. In: Faulkner WR, Meites S, eds. Geriatric Clinical Chemistry: Reference Values. Washington, D.C.: AACC Press, 1994:103–116.

25. Timiras PS. The endocrine, pancreas and carbohydrate metabolism. In: Timiras PS, eds. Physiological Basis of Aging and Geriatrics, 2nd ed. Boca Raton, FL: CRC Press, 1994:191–197.

26. Timiras PS. Aging of the adrenals and pituitary. In: Timiras PS, ed. Physiological Basis of Aging and Geriatrics, 2nd ed. Boca Raton, FL: CRC Press, 1994:133–146.

27. Timiras PS. Cardiovascular alterations with age: atherosclerosis, coronary heart disease, hypertension. In: Timiras PS, ed. Physiological Basis of Aging and Geriatrics, 2nd ed. Boca Raton, FL: CRC Press, 1994:199–214.

28. Tietz NW, Shuey DF, Wekstein DR. Laboratory values in fit aging individuals: sexagenarians through centenarians. In: Faulkner WR, Meites S, eds. Geriatric Clinical Chemistry: Reference Values. Washington, D.C.: AACC Press, 1994:145–184.

29. Reaven GM. Role of insulin resistance in human disease. Banting lecture 1988. Diabetes 1988;37:1595–607.

30. American Diabetes Association. Consensus Development Conference on Insulin Resistance. November 5–6, 1997. Diabetes Care 1998;21:310–314.

31. Karter AJ, Mayer-Davis EJ, Selby JV, et al. Insulin sensitivity and abdominal obesity in African-American, Hispanic, and non-Hispanic white men and women. The Insulin Resistance and Atherosclerosis Study. Diabetes 1996;45:1547–1555.

32. Wautier JL, Guillausseau PJ. Advanced glycation end products, their receptors and diabetic angiopathy (review). Diabetes Metab (Paris) 2001;27:535–542.

33. Ruan H, Hacohen N, Golub TR, et al. Tumor necrosis factor-alpha suppresses adipocyte-specific genes and activates expression of preadipocyte genes in 3T3-L1 adipocytes: nuclear factor-kappa B activation by TNF-alpha is obligatory. Diabetes 2002;51:1319–1336.

34. Timiras ML. The kidney, the lower urinary tract, the prostate, and body fluids. In: Timiras PS, ed. Physiological Basis of Aging and Geriatrics, 2nd ed. Boca Raton, FL: CRC Press, 1994:235–246.

35. Rowe JW, Kahn RL. Successful Aging. New York: Pantheon Books, 1998.

36. Timiras PS. Aging of the gastrointestinal tract and liver. In: Timiras PS, ed. Physiological Basis of Aging and Geriatrics, 2nd ed. Boca Raton, FL: CRC Press, 1994:247–257.

37. Timiras PS. Aging of respiration, erythrocytes, and the hematopoietic system. In: Timiras PS, ed. Physiological Basis of Aging and Geriatrics, 2nd ed. Boca Raton, FL: CRC Press, 1994:225–233.

38. Institute for Health and Aging Report. University of California, San Francisco. Chronic Care in America: A 21st Century Challenge. Princeton, NJ: Robert Wood Johnson Foundation, 1996. (Best-Assembly@worldnet.att.net)

39. Sasse EA. The determination of reference intervals. In: Faulkner WR, Meites S, eds. Geriatric Clinical Chemistry: Reference Values. Washington, D.C.: AACC Press 1994:6–17.

40. NCCLS Approved Guideline. How to define and determine reference intervals in the clinical laboratory. Villanova, PA: National Committee for Clinical Laboratory Standards, 1995.

41. Young DS. Pre-analytical variability in the elderly. In: Faulkner WR, Meites S, eds. Geriatric Clinical Chemistry: Reference Values. Washington, D.C.: AACC Press, 1994:19–39.

42. Klosinski DD. Collecting specimens from the elderly patient. Lab Med 1997;28(8):518–522.

43. Bloom HG, Shlom EA. Drug Prescribing for the Elderly. New York: Raven Press, 1993.

44. Beizer JL, Timiras ML. Pharmacology and drug management in the elderly. In: Timiras PS, ed. Physiological Basis of Aging and Geriatrics, 2nd ed. Boca Raton, FL: CRC Press, 1994:279–284.

45. Warner A. Therapeutic drug monitoring in the elderly. In: Faulkner WR, Meites S, eds. Geriatric Clinical Chemistry: Reference Values. Washington, D.C.: AACC Press, 1994:134–144.

46. Shephard RJ. The scientific basis of exercise prescribing for the very old. J Am Geriatr Soc 1990;38:62–70.

47. Cearlock DM, Nuzzo NA. Evaluating the benefits and hazards of exercise in the older adult. Med Lab Observer 1997;29(6):40–49.

48. Holloszy JO. Health benefits of exercise in middle-aged and older people. In: Kotsonis FN, Mackey MA, eds. Nutrition in the '90s: Current Controversies and Analysis. New York: Marcel Dekker, 1994:81–97.

49. Blair SN. Physical activity, fitness, and health. In: Kotsonis FN, Mackey MA, eds. Nutrition in the '90s: Current Controversies and Analysis. New York: Marcel Dekker, 1994:61–79.

50. Ham RJ. The signs and symptoms of poor nutritional status. In: Ham JR, ed. Primary Care: Nutrition in Old Age. Philadelphia: WB Saunders, 1994:33–54.

51. Garry PJ. Nutrition and aging. In: Faulkner WR, Meites S, eds. Geriatric Clinical Chemistry: Reference Values. Washington, D.C.: AACC Press, 1994:48–72.

52. Miller SM. Nutrition, the elderly, and the laboratory. Med Lab Observer 1997;29(3):23–30.

53. Gallagher-Allred CR, Emley S. Specific dietary interventions: diabetes, osteoporosis, renal disease. In: Ham JR, ed. Primary Care: Nutrition in Old Age. Philadelphia: WB Saunders, 1994:175–89.

Pediatric Clinical Chemistry

Michael J. Bennett

OBJECTIVES

Upon completion of this chapter, the clinical laboratorian should be able to:
- Define the adaptive changes that occur in the newborn.
- Describe the developmental changes that occur throughout childhood.
- Discuss the problems associated with collecting blood from small children.
- Understand the role of point-of-care testing in pediatric settings.

- Summarize the changes that occur in children with regard to electrolyte and water balance, endocrine function, liver function, and bone metabolism.
- Explain how drug treatment and pharmacokinetics differ between children and adults.
- Discuss the procedures used to diagnose inherited metabolic diseases.
- Describe the development and disorders of the immune system.

Drug metabolism
Endocrine system
Genetic disease

Growth
Immunity
Physiologic development

Point-of-care testing
Sexual maturation

Tandem mass
 spectrometry

DEVELOPMENTAL CHANGES FROM NEONATE TO ADULT

Pediatric laboratory medicine provides us with many unique opportunities to study how the homeostatic and physiologic mechanisms that control normal human development evolve. With these opportunities to study development, comes a completely new set of challenges, many based on failure of some component of the normal development process and resulting disease. With this scenario in mind, it becomes clear that the environment for the specialist pediatric laboratorian is different from the environment encountered in adult practice, in which *physiologic development* is not a major issue. The diseases encountered in pediatric practice, therefore, differ considerably from those in adult situations. Moreover, the nature of body size and, hence, available blood volume creates additional problems for the analyst with regard to choice of instrumentation and testing menu.

The greatest pediatric challenge relates to the birth of an infant. There is a requirement at this time for rapid adaptation from intrauterine life, in which homeostasis is maintained by maternal and placental means, to the self-maintenance needed to adapt to extrauterine life. Issues related to this adaptation are further complicated by prematurity or intrauterine growth retardation (IGR), when many organ systems have not reached sufficient maturity to enable the newborn to adapt to the necessary changes at the time of delivery.[1]

Respiration and Circulation

At birth, the normal infant rapidly adapts by initiating active respiration. The stimuli for this process include clamping of the umbilicus, cutting off maternal delivery of oxygen, and the baby's first breath. Initiation of breathing requires the normal expression of surfactant in the lungs. Surfactant is necessary for the normal expansion and contraction of alveoli and allows gaseous exchange to take place.

Initiation of respiration and expansion of lung volume causes increased pulmonary blood flow and reduced blood pressure. This, in turn, results in closure of the ductus arteriosus and a shift in blood flow through the heart that allows newly oxygenated blood from the lungs to be directed through the left side of the heart to the body. Blood flow now goes from the right side of the

heart to the lungs for oxygenation. Closure of the ductus arteriosus is essential for this process to take place.

Growth

A normal baby delivered at term weighs about 3.2 kg. A baby weighing less than 2.5 kg at term is regarded as small for gestational age (SGA), which is usually a result of IGR. Babies of low birth weight born before term are regarded as premature. In the first days of life, weight loss is a result of insensible water loss through the skin. This is generally offset by weight gain of 6 g/kg per day as feeding is initiated. An infant's body weight will double in 4–6 months. Premature babies tend to grow at a slower rate and often still weigh less than a term baby at the equivalent of term.

Organ Development

Most organs are not fully developed at birth. Glomerular filtration rate of the kidney and renal tubular function mature during the first year of life at which point laboratory markers of renal function approximate adult values. Liver function can take 2–3 months to fully mature. Motor function and visual acuity develop during the first year of life. This development is accompanied by changes in the electroencephalogram until the normal "adult" picture is seen. There are dramatic changes in hematopoiesis as the switch from fetal hemoglobin to adult hemoglobin takes place. This coincides with significant hyperbilirubinemia as fetal hemoglobin is broken down coincident with immature hepatic pathways of bilirubin metabolism. Bone growth in the rapid growth phases in the first few years of life and at puberty results in cyclical changes in bone growth markers. *Sexual maturation* results in significant endocrine changes, particularly of the hypothalamic–pituitary–gonadal hormone pathway, which eventually lead to the constitutive development of adult secondary sexual characteristics and eventually to the adult.

Problems of Prematurity and Immaturity[1]

Intrauterine development is programmed for a normal 38- to 40-week gestation. Many organs are not fully ready to deal with extrauterine life before this time. This organ immaturity results in many of the clinical problems that we see associated with prematurity, which include respiratory distress (lung immaturity), electrolyte and water imbalance (kidney immaturity), and excessive jaundice (liver immaturity). Infants born before their due date constitute a major burden on the laboratory. They not only have abnormal biochemical parameters that require frequent blood drawing, they also have small blood volumes from which to draw on.

PHLEBOTOMY AND CHOICE OF INSTRUMENTATION FOR PEDIATRIC SAMPLES

Phlebotomy

Blood collection from infants and young children is complicated by the patient's size and frequently by the ability of the patient to communicate with the phlebotomist. The small blood volume of small patients dictates both the number of tests that can safely be performed on the patient and the number of times that blood can safely be drawn for repeat analysis.[2] Table 33-1 shows the percentage of total body blood that is drawn from an individual with a 10-mL blood draw. This volume is standard in adult laboratory medicine but the table clearly shows that this amount of blood represents about 5% of total blood volume in a premature neonate. Clearly, frequent blood draws of this nature will quickly lead to anemia and the need for blood transfusion. Table 33-2 shows the guidelines for blood volume collection developed at Children's Medical Center of Dallas. It is necessary on occasion to advise the physician that a particular set of orders may result in excessive blood depletion and transfusion requirement.

Infants and children have smaller veins than adults; to ensure that small veins do not collapse, narrow-gauge needles are generally used for venipuncture. Smaller needles increase the risk of hemolysis and hyperkalemia.

Frequently, good access to veins is impossible in a pediatric patient with intravenous and central lines in place. Capillary samples are often collected when suitable veins are not available. Capillary samples, either by heel or by thumb stick, should be collected by phlebotomists with pediatric expertise. The heel should be warmed and well perfused to "arterialize" the capillaries. This can be achieved by gently rubbing the area or by immersion in warm water. The lancet puncture should be in an area of the heel away from bone. Stabbing into bone may result in osteomyelitis. Excessive squeezing or milking of the lancet site can result in both hemolysis and factitious hyperkalemia from tissue fluid leakage.

Preanalytic Concerns

There is a growing trend toward complete front-end automation in clinical chemistry laboratories. The clear advantage with automation of sample handling is that traditional bottlenecks at sites of data entry and centrifugation are removed and turnaround times reduced. Several issues have retarded the introduction of automation in pediatrics. A typical pediatric chemistry laboratory receives samples in tubes of many different sizes, varying from standard adult tubes to small "peditubes." At this time, no automated systems have been developed that can handle this range of tubes.

A second important issue relates to evaporation of sample from open tubes. Most automated sample handling systems require open-topped tubes for processing. With large sample volumes, the effect of evaporation is minimal. With small volumes that have relatively large surface areas to total volume, evaporation can be significant and may effect results by as much as 10%.

TABLE 33-1. IMPLICATIONS OF A 10-mL BLOOD DRAW IN AN INFANT POPULATION

AGE	WEIGHT (kg)	TOTAL BLOOD VOLUME (%)
26 weeks gestation	0.9	9.0
32 weeks gestation	1.6	5.5
34 weeks gestation	2.1	4.0
Term	3.4	2.5
3 months	5.7	2.0
6 months	7.6	1.6
12 months	10.1	1.4
24 months	12.6	1.0

TABLE 33-2. RECOMMENDED BLOOD DRAW VOLUMES FOR PEDIATRIC PATIENTS[a]

WEIGHT (lb)	VOLUME PER EVENT (mL)	VOLUME PER HOSPITALIZATION (mL)
<2	1.0	8
2–4	1.5	12
4–6	2.0	17
6–8	2.5	23
8–10	3.5	30
10–15	5.0	40
15–20	10	60
20–25	10	70
25–30	10	80
30–35	10	100
35–40	10	130
40–45	20	140

[a]Children's Medical Center of Dallas, Dallas, TX.

Choice of Analyzer

Careful inspection and choice of analytic systems remains crucial for handling pediatric samples. Until recently, only a few analyzers were capable of performing multiple analytic procedures on small sample volumes (5–50 μL). Today, most analyzers can perform this function. Choice of analyzer becomes dependent on issues such as:

1. How much dead volume is there in the system? The smaller the dead volume, the greater number of tests that can be run.
2. Does clot or bubble detection allow for salvage of sample? All analyzers can detect a clot, but not all will allow retrieval of sample.
3. Is the system truly random access? This allows selectivity of menu for a given sample.

Typically, sample throughput time is less of an issue, as pediatric facilities tend to run fewer samples than busy adult services.

POINT-OF-CARE ANALYSIS IN PEDIATRICS[3]

Point-of-care testing (POCT), or near-patient testing, plays an important and expanding role in pediatric practice. Testing devices that are portable and easy to use, require small specimen volume, do not require sample preparation, and provide rapid results at the bedside are providing the momentum for increased POCT. To provide cost effective and appropriate quality assurance for POCT, several factors need to be addressed.

1. Does the analyte really require immediate turnaround for optimal patient management? Analyzers are becoming available that measure increasing numbers of different analytes at the patient's bedside. Typically, the cost of POCT measurement is higher than the traditional laboratory measurement. The idea of instant results is so seductive that nonlaboratorian users often discount economic factors. In the author's institution, the clinical laboratory has played a leading role in determining which POCT assays will be available and in which clinical settings they have real value (Table 33-3)
2. Who chooses the POCT device? As the field of POCT expands, the number of devices on the market is also increasing. The clinical laboratory should be the setting in which POCT devices for institutional use should be first evaluated. The laboratory should make choices for instrumentation. Important features of a good POCT device should include the following:
   - The ability to lock out untrained users. Only individuals accredited to use the device should be allowed access via a personal code.

TABLE 33-3. IMPORTANT PEDIATRIC POINT-OF-CARE TESTS AND TESTING SITES

Tests
Blood gas
Electrolyte
Glucose
Activated clotting time
Hemoglobin
Glycated hemoglobin
Pregnancy
Urinalysis
Prothrombin time
Rapid streptococcus
Testing Sites
Coronary care unit/Intensive care unit
Trauma unit/Emergency department
Diabetes clinic
Transport
Surgery
Extracorporeal membrane oxygenation sites

   - The device should not be allowed to proceed to patient sample analysis without running and validating appropriate quality assurance procedures.
   - The data should be downloadable to the hospital laboratory information system (LIS) for evaluation by the hospital quality assurance officer. Downloading the data also allows for billing and data entry into patient charts, features readily lost when analyzers are used that cannot be linked to the LIS.

The data generated by POCT devices have limitations. Typical analytic performance is not as good as the main laboratory analyzer. POCT data is less precise and not suited to monitoring therapy in instances where small changes are important. The linear range for most POCT devices is not as broad as the main chemistry analyzer, and users need to be aware of these limitations. A prime example in the author's institution is the use of POCT glucose analyzers. The instrument used for acute diabetic management loses linearity above 400 mg/dL, particularly in patients who are hemoconcentrated. We recommend that any POCT glucose level above 400 mg/dL be immediately checked in the main laboratory. Hypoglycemia is also particularly common in pediatrics and characteristically difficult to accurately quantitate using POCT devices. Low glucose levels should also be checked using a more sensitive main laboratory analyzer.

REGULATION OF BLOOD GASES AND pH IN NEONATES AND INFANTS

Primary maintenance of blood gas and pH homeostasis following birth requires that the lungs and kidneys are sufficiently mature to regulate acid and base metabolism. At about 24 weeks of gestation, the lung expresses two distinct types of cells: type 1 and type 2 pneumocytes. Type 2 pneumocytes are responsible for the secretion of surfactant, which contains the phospholipids lecithin and sphingomyelin. Surfactant is required for the lungs to expand and the transfer of blood gases following delivery. Oxygen crosses into the circulation and carbon dioxide is removed and expired. Immaturity of the surfactant system as a result of prematurity or IGR results in respiratory distress syndrome (RDS). In RDS, there is failure to excrete carbon dioxide and, as a result, CO_2 levels rise, causing respiratory acidosis; oxygen levels are low and result in additional oxygen requirements for the baby.

The relative amounts of lecithin and sphingomyelin are critical for normal surfactant function. The measurement of amniotic fluid lecithin/sphingomyelin (L/S ratio) has been used for many years to predict fetal lung maturity. A ratio of less than 1.5 is considered indicative of surfactant deficiency.

The fetal fibronectin (fFibronectin) test is a promising new test designed to determine the likelihood of premature delivery and risk for fetal maturity.[4] fFibronectin is a protein secreted uniquely by the fetus; toward term, it is found in maternal cervical fluid. A POCT device is available which has been designed for use in the obstetrician's office. It has a high predictive value for impending early delivery of the baby and can be used to alert the pediatrician to the potential for RDS.

The trauma and relative anoxia during delivery can also induce acidosis in the newborn. This is typically a metabolic acidosis associated with increased lactic acid production. Serum bicarbonate levels are reduced in this situation compared with the respiratory acidosis in RDS. Persistent metabolic acidosis in the newborn that is difficult to correct with bicarbonate replacement is an indication for further intensive evaluation for possible inborn error of metabolism or other etiologies that require differentiation (Table 33-4).

Alkalosis is an unusual finding in pediatric medicine. One important cause of alkalosis is hyperammonemia, which may be secondary to a number of etiologies, including liver disease and inborn errors of metabolism (Table 33-4).

Blood Gas and Acid-Base Measurement

Oxygen status can readily be measured using noninvasive transcutaneous monitoring. Good correlation has been demonstrated between the arterial pressure of oxy-

TABLE 33-4. CAUSES OF ACIDOSIS AND ALKALOSIS IN NEONATES AND INFANTS

RESPIRATORY ACIDOSIS	HYPOVENTILATION/CO$_2$ RETENTION
Metabolic acidosis	Renal tubular bicarbonate wasting
	Anoxia
	Poor tissue perfusion
	Metabolic disease
Respiratory alkalosis	Hyperventilation
	High blood ammonia/metabolic disease
Metabolic alkalosis	Pyloric stenosis/loss of gastric acid
	Excessive bicarbonate administration
	Low blood potassium

gen and transcutaneous measurement. Transcutaneous CO_2 monitors are also in widespread use. The measurement of acid-base status requires blood sampling. Most blood gas/acid-base analyzers can be adapted to take the small capillary samples routinely collected in pediatric settings. It is important for the person drawing the capillary blood to do so anaerobically, which requires thorough warming of the capillary site and collection of a freely flowing blood sample from a lancet stick. The sample needs to be sealed to ensure minimal gas exchange. Analysis should be performed immediately to not compromise the sample integrity. The author's laboratory maintains a goal of a 10-minute turnaround time from the sample receipt.

Most blood gas analyzers measure PO_2, PCO_2, and pH by ion-specific electrodes and calculate bicarbonate concentration by the Henderson-Hasselbalch equation. The Henderson-Hasselbalch equation is less valid when pH is far outside the normal physiologic range (extreme acidosis or alkalosis). On these occasions, it may become important to measure the bicarbonate concentration using a direct measurement.

Many blood gas analyzers have been upgraded in recent years to measure additional analytes, including blood sodium, potassium, and chloride, using ion-specific electrodes and lactate and urea. The major advantage of this type of analyzer in pediatrics is that whole blood can be used. The volumes are typically smaller than those required for the main chemistry analyzer, and the lack of need for centrifugation shortens the turnaround time. One disadvantage of using whole blood is that the analyst cannot detect if a sample is hemolyzed.

TABLE 33-5. DEVELOPMENT OF GLOMERULAR FILTRATION IN THE NEWBORN

AGE	GLOMERULAR FILTRATION RATE (mL/minute per 1.73 m² MEAN)	RANGE
1 day	24	3–38
2–8 days	38	17–60
10–22 days	50	32–68
37–95 days	58	30–86
1–2 years	115	95–135[a]

[a]Adult values.

REGULATION OF ELECTROLYTES AND WATER: RENAL FUNCTION

From the 35th week of gestation, the fetal kidneys develop rapidly in preparation for extrauterine life.[1] The kidneys, critical organs for the maintenance of electrolyte and water homeostasis, control the rate of salt and water loss and retention. At term, neither the glomeruli nor the renal tubules function at the normal rate. The glomerular filtration rate is about 25% of the rate seen in older children and does not reach full potential until age 2 years (Table 33-5). Tubular function also develops at a similar rate. The maximal concentrating power of the kidney is only about 78% of that of the adult kidney at this time, although the tubular response to antidiuretic hormone appears to be normal. This gradual process of renal development in the newborn results in diminished filtration and impaired reabsorption of salt and water; therefore, in the newborn period and early infancy, large shifts in serum electrolyte levels can be observed. These problems are exacerbated in the preterm infant with renal function that is even less mature.

The kidneys also primarily maintain water loss and retention. However, in the newborn period, insensible water loss through the skin is also an important cause of water and electrolyte imbalance. Water loss and consequent hemoconcentration frequently result from the use of radiant heaters that are used to maintain body temperature. Increased water loss also occurs via respiration in children with RDS. Up to one third of insensible water loss may occur through this route. The total body water content of a newborn is about 80%; 55% is intracellular fluid and 45% is extracellular fluid. The extracellular water is 20% plasma water and 80% interstitial. During the first month of extrauterine life, the total body water content decreases to about 60%, mostly a result of loss of the interstitial component.[1]

Disorders Effecting Electrolytes and Water Balance

The causes of hypernatremia (sodium, >145 mEq/L) and hyponatremia (sodium, <130 mEq/L) are listed in Table 33-6. Both disturbances can have dire outcomes, with a high risk of seizures. This is a result of the shift of water out of or into brain cells, with concurrent shrinkage or expansion of these cells. Hypernatremia results from hypotonic fluid loss, and hyponatremia results from hypertonic fluid loss. Hyponatremia may also be a result of excessive body water content and needs to be distinguished from hypertonic loss. Clinical evaluation and measurement of other components, including hematocrit, serum albumin, creatinine, and blood urea nitrogen, can be used to differentiate these etiologies. All of these compounds will be elevated with hemoconcentration. Clinically, it is usually possible to distinguish dehydration from excessive hydration.

Treatment of electrolyte and water loss is directed at replacing the loss to regain normal physiologic levels. Care must be taken to avoid too rapid a replacement, particularly with hypertonic dehydration. If water replacement is done too quickly, a rapid expansion of neuronal cell volume can occur, which results in seizures.

The causes of hyperkalemia and hypokalemia are listed in Table 33-7. The symptoms of hyperkalemia (serum potassium, >6.5 mEq/L) include muscle weakness and cardiac conduction defects that may lead to heart failure. In pediatrics, it is particularly important to recognize factitious hyperkalemia as a result of hemolysis and bad capillary blood collection, without hemolysis but with high potassium tissue leakage.

Because the situation regarding electrolyte and water homeostasis can change rapidly in small infants, it is important to monitor therapeutic intervention on a frequent basis.[1,2] The availability of POCT devices that use small volumes of whole blood helps with management of

TABLE 33-6. CAUSES OF HYPERNATREMIA AND HYPONATREMIA

Hypernatremia

Excessive loss of water through overhead heater

Gastrointestinal fluid loss

Fluid deprivation

Renal loss of water/nephrogenic diabetes insipidus

Administration of hypertonic fluids containing sodium

Hyponatremia

Inappropriate ADH secretion due to trauma or infection

Administration of hypotonic fluids

Renal tubular acidosis

Salt-losing congenital adrenal hyperplasia (21-hydroxylase deficiency)

Cystic fibrosis

Diuretics

Renal failure

TABLE 33-7. CAUSES OF HYPERKALEMIA AND HYPOKALEMIA

Hyperkalemia

Fluid deprivation/dehydration causing tissue leakage

Intravascular hemorrhage causing release from red cells

Trauma/tissue damage

Acute renal failure

Salt-losing adrenal hyperplasia (see *hyponatremia*)

Exchange transfusion using stored blood

Hypokalemia

Inappropriate ADH secretion

Diuretics, particularly frusemide

Alkalosis

Pyloric stenosis

Renal tubular acidosis secondary to bicarbonate loss

these imbalances, with the only caution being that it is impossible to detect hemolysis and factitious hyperkalemia on a whole blood sample.

DEVELOPMENT OF LIVER FUNCTION

Physiologic Jaundice

The liver is an essential organ for many metabolic processes. The processing of many normal metabolic pathways and the metabolism of exogenous compounds, in particular pharmacologic agents, proceed slower in neonates. The most striking effect of an immature liver, even in a normal term baby, is the failure to adequately metabolize bilirubin. Bilirubin is an intermediate of the breakdown of the heme molecules, which accumulate as fetal hemoglobin is rapidly destroyed and replaced by adult hemoglobin. Normally, the liver conjugates bilirubin to glucuronic acid using the enzyme bilirubin UDP-glucuronoyltransferase. Conjugated bilirubin can be readily excreted in the bile or through the kidneys. At birth, this enzyme is too immature to complete the process and increased levels of unconjugated bilirubin and "physiologic" jaundice result. At this time, a normal baby may have a serum bilirubin level of up to 15 mg/dL, most of which is unconjugated. This level, which would be alarming in adult practice, should fall back to baseline by about 10 days of age. Because excessive jaundice can lead to kernicterus and result in severe brain damage, the measurement of blood conjugated and unconjugated bilirubin has an important role in pediatrics. An alternative means of reducing high-unconjugated circulating bilirubin levels is phototherapy with ultraviolet light, which causes bilirubin to be converted to a potentially less toxic and more readily excreted metabolite. Severe

cases may require an exchange transfusion. Complete absence of the bilirubin-conjugating enzyme results in severe persistent jaundice and Crigler-Najjar disease, a rare *genetic disease*. It is important to differentiate Crigler-Najjar from physiologic immaturity because treatment options vary considerably.

Energy Metabolism

The liver plays an essential role in energy metabolism for the whole body (Table 33-8). Carbohydrates derived from the diet as disaccharides or polysaccharides form the bulk of our energy sources. They are broken down into simpler monosaccharides, which reach the liver via the portal blood system. The primary sugars in newborns and infants come from the breakdown of disaccharide lactose in milk. Lactose is broken down to glucose and galactose. When it reaches the hepatocytes, galactose is converted to glucose by a series of enzymic reactions that have unique pediatric significance. Genetic deficiency of any of the reactions results in failure to convert galactose to glucose and essentially reduce the energy content of milk by 50%. The most common cause of failure to convert galactose to glucose results in galactosemia or deficiency of galactose-1-phosphate uridyltransferase, a serious genetic disease of the newborn. In this disease, galactose-1-phosphate accumulates inside liver cells and causes hepatocellular damage and rapid liver failure. Other organs are also involved with this disease, including the renal tubules and the eyes. Galactose-1-phosphate accumulation causes acute renal tubular failure and tubular loss of glucose, phosphate, and amino acids. The loss of glucose in cooperation with the liver damage results in severe hypoglycemia. Accumulation of galactose in the eye results in cataract forma-

TABLE 33-8. IMPORTANT BIOCHEMICAL PATHWAYS IN THE LIVER

Catabolic

Transamination

Amino acid oxidation to make ketones and acetyl-CoA

Fatty acid oxidation to make ketones

Urea cycle to remove ammonia

Bilirubin metabolism (hemoglobin breakdown)

Drug and exogenous xenobiotic compounds metabolized

Anabolic

Albumin synthesis

Clotting factor synthesis

Lipoprotein synthesis, very-low-density lipoprotein

Gluconeogenesis (synthesis of glucose)

Bile acid synthesis

CASE STUDY 33-1

A 30-week premature infant developed progressive hyperbilirubinemia that did not respond immediately to phototherapy. Because there was a risk of developing kernicterus, the baby received two exchange transfusions. Following the second transfusion, it was noted that the baby was jittery and had a seizure.

Questions

1. What is the most likely biochemical cause of the seizure?

2. What is the mechanism for this abnormality?

3. What other metabolic abnormality might result in a neonatal seizure?

tion. A simple test that directs us to the diagnosis of galactosemia is the urine reducing substance test. This detects the presence of non–glucose-reducing sugars (galactose) in urine when a child is symptomatic. The clinical significance of establishing a diagnosis is clear; galactosemia is often fatal if undiscovered but completely treatable by dietary lactose restriction when diagnosis is made.

Another critical pathway of carbohydrate energy metabolism in the newborn involves the pathway of gluconeogenesis. At birth, a term baby has sufficient liver glycogen stores to provide glucose as an energy source and maintain euglycemia. If the delivery is particularly stressful, these reserves of energy may become depleted prematurely. At this time, the normal physiologic role of gluconeogenesis, which essentially converts the amino acid alanine into glucose, becomes critical in maintaining glucose homeostasis. This pathway is not always mature at birth and suboptimal operation results in what is termed *physiologic hypoglycemia*. Newborns can survive blood glucose levels below 30 mg/dL, although adults would fall into rapid hypoglycemic coma and risk sudden death at these levels. Physiologic hypoglycemia usually corrects quickly as the enzyme systems mature or by simple intravenous glucose infusion. Persistent and severe hypoglycemia should alert the physician toward a possible inborn error of metabolism, such as galactosemia, gluconeogenesis, or disorders of fatty acid oxidative metabolism.

Diabetes

Blood glucose homeostasis and hepatic metabolism of glucose is maintained by the concerted actions of several hormones.[5] Following a meal, the level of glucose in the circulation rises, which triggers increased synthesis and release of insulin by the pancreatic β-cells of the islets of Langerhans. Increased levels of insulin in the circulation cause glucose to be taken up by certain cells, such as hepatocytes and muscle cells, and be converted into glycogen as a future source of energy. As a result of the insulin action, blood glucose levels begin to fall to the preprandial level. Glucagon, a hormone secreted by the α-cells of the islets of Langerhans, has an opposing effect to that of insulin. It is generally believed that the insulin/glucagon ratio, rather than absolute amounts of either, is the primary endocrine modulator of circulating glucose levels. Other hormones, including cortisol, epinephrine, and insulin-like growth factor, can also affect glucose levels. These hormones are secreted in response to stress and can affect glucose measurement when samples are collected under stressful situations.

Diabetes mellitus, a condition in which the endocrine control of glucose metabolism is abnormal, is usually related to failure of the insulin regulatory pathway. Type 1 diabetes (insulin-dependent) is the most common in pediatrics. This may be caused by failure of the pancreas to secrete insulin or by the presence of circulating insulin antibodies that reduce the ability for endocrine action. A patient typically presents with diabetic ketoacidosis, with profound hyperglycemia and metabolic acidosis that results from the liver increasing fatty acid metabolism and producing excess ketone bodies.

Type 2 diabetes (non–insulin-dependent) has a much lower incidence in the pediatric population and is normally associated with increased resistance to normally secreted insulin in obese individuals. Sadly, type 2 diabetes is being recognized more frequently in children as the number of obese children increases in the population. It may soon become more prominent in our children than type 1.

It is important to recognize diabetes as a cause of hyperglycemia in children and to distinguish it from other medical causes of high blood sugar, including acute pancreatic disease or hypersecretion of counter-regulatory hormones such as growth hormone, cortisol, or catecholamines. Chronic hyperglycemia can be readily distinguished from acute causes by simply measuring the blood concentration of glycated hemoglobin or hemoglobin $A1_c$, a well-established marker for long-term hyperglycemia. This assay also has great value in monitoring diabetic compliance in patients on treatment.

Nitrogen Metabolism

The liver plays a central role in nitrogen metabolism. It is involved with the metabolic interconversions of amino acids and the synthesis of nonessential amino acids. The liver synthesizes many body proteins, including most proteins found in the circulation, such as albumin, transferrin, and the complement clotting factors. The liver does not synthesize immunoglobulins. The liver is also responsible for complete metabolism of the breakdown products of nitrogen turnover, such as ammonia and urea through the urea cycle and creatinine and uric acid from energy stores and nucleic acids, respectively. Blood ammonia levels are higher in the newborn period than in later life, presumably due to immaturity of urea cycle enzymes and the portal circulation. A blood ammonia level of 100 μmol/L in a newborn would be regarded as less significant than the same level in a 1 year old. Persistently elevated ammonia levels should alert the investigator to possible liver damage and secondary failure of the urea cycle. High ammonia levels suggest a possible primary defect in the urea cycle, and patients should be evaluated for such a defect.

Nitrogenous End Products as Markers of Renal Function

In contrast to the high neonatal ammonia levels, creatinine and uric acid levels are lower in newborns. Both metabolites rise eventually to normal adult ranges. Creatinine concentrations in blood increase with muscle mass and are independent of diet. It is filtered at the glomerulus and not extensively reabsorbed by the renal tubules. Its measurement as a clearance ratio in blood and in a 24-hour urine sample has been used as a marker for glomerular filtration for many years. Serum cystatin C, a new and possibly more sensitive marker, has recently appeared on the market as a potential replacement for creatinine.[6] This marker awaits further evaluation in pediatric populations, but could potentially replace the creatinine clearance assay and remove the need for difficult 24-hour urine collections from children. Incomplete collections form the basis of most errors in this assay.

Liver Function Tests

As discussed above, the liver is responsible for performing a large number of synthetic and catabolic processes, and normal liver function is central to maintaining body homeostasis. Several laboratory tests have emerged that are generally classified as liver function tests.

The measurement of serum albumin and total and conjugated bilirubin are true tests of liver function because they measure the synthetic and metabolic pathways for these compounds. In protein–calorie malnutrition, the reduced of availability of amino acids for synthesis of new proteins results in diminished functional synthetic rate and low levels of newly synthesized proteins, such as albumin. Very low levels of albumin indicate a long exposure to protein restriction, and its measurement in blood is often used as a guide to nutritional status and chronic liver disease of other etiologies. Impaired hepatocellular function also results in reduced ability to conjugate bilirubin, with subsequent increase in the unconjugated form, which is normally barely detectable.

Other tests, such as measurement of liver enzymes, more truly reflect tests of liver cell integrity and are not strictly functional assays. Large elevations in serum AST and ALT indicate hepatocellular damage and subsequent leakage of cellular contents into the serum, and elevated ALP suggests hepatic biliary damage but gives little functional information.

CALCIUM AND BONE METABOLISM IN PEDIATRICS

Normal bone *growth*, which parallels body growth, requires integration of calcium, phosphate, and magnesium metabolism with endocrine regulation from vitamin D, parathyroid hormone (PTH), and calcitonin.[5] The active metabolite of vitamin D is 1,25-dihydroxy vitamin D. Hydroxylation of vitamin D from the diet takes place in the liver and in the kidneys and requires normal functioning of these organs. Absorption of vitamin D from the gastrointestinal tract, conversion to its active form in the kidney, and incorporation of calcium and phosphate into growing bone requires normally active PTH. Secretion of PTH is, in turn, modulated by serum calcium and magnesium levels. Low levels of both divalent cations inhibit PTH secretion. Calcitonin has an antagonistic effect on PTH action.

The rapid bone growth that occurs during infancy, and later during puberty, requires optimal coordination of mineral absorption, transport, and endocrine-controlled incorporation of the minerals into growing bone. Approximately 98% of total body calcium content is present in bone and less than 1% is measurable in the blood. Serum calcium is present as the unbound ionized fraction (about 50% of total in blood), with the rest bound to protein (40%) or chelated to anions in the circulation, such as phosphate and citrate. Serum ionized and bound calcium levels are highly regulated and maintained within strict homeostatic limits. Abnormalities in any of the regulatory components have profound clinical effects on children.

Hypocalcemia and Hypercalcemia

Hypocalcemia is defined as total serum calcium below 7.0 mg/dL or ionized calcium below 3.0 mg/dL. In the newborn and particularly the immature newborn, these levels may be commonly encountered with few symptoms. However, hypocalcemia can result in irritability, twitching, and seizures. Serum calcium is usually measured in infants with seizures of unknown etiology. Prolonged hypocalcemia can result in reduced bone growth and rickets. The causes of hypocalcemia are listed in Table 33-9. Hypomagnesemia frequently occurs with hypocalcemia. Because low levels of serum magnesium

TABLE 33-9. CAUSES OF HYPOCALCEMIA

Prematurity
Metabolic acidosis
Vitamin D deficiency
Liver disease (failure to activate vitamin D)
Renal disease (failure to activate vitamin D)
Hypoparathyroidism
Low calcium intake
High phosphorus intake
Diuretic use
Hypomagnesemia
Exchange transfusion (anticoagulants in transfused blood)

TABLE 33-10. CAUSES OF HYPERCALCEMIA[a]

Hyperparathyroidism
Acute renal failure
Excessive intake of vitamin D
Idiopathic hypercalcemia of infancy

[a]Less common than hypocalcemia in infants.

also inhibit PTH secretion, it is important to consider the possibility of concurrent hypomagnesemia in a child with hypocalcemic seizures and to correct any abnormalities that may be identified in the magnesium status as calcium is also corrected.

Hypercalcemia is defined as total serum calcium of greater than 11.0 mg/dL. This is an unusual finding in pediatrics (Table 33-10) but has potentially severe clinical implications. Patients with hypercalcemia have poor muscle tone, constipation, failure to thrive, and may develop kidney stones leading to renal failure.

ENDOCRINE FUNCTION IN PEDIATRICS

The field of endocrinology provides numerous examples of the "differences" that occur in clinical chemistry between children and adults.[2] The process of maturation into a sexually fertile adult, for example, requires a complex, endocrine-mediated, developmental process switching on during childhood. As addressed in the previous section, the bone growth that accompanies systemic growth also requires a complex process, which is under endocrine control.

Hormone Secretion

The endocrine system relates to a group of hormones that are typically produced and secreted by one cell type into the circulation, where their effect is exerted in other target cells. Certain of these hormones are polypeptides, others are amino acid derivatives or steroids.

Four major *endocrine systems* have been described, all of which play critical roles in normal human development. These systems all involve the hypothalamus as a major higher brain control center, the pituitary gland as a major secretor of hormones, and then various end organs, which have responsive elements for the pituitary hormone and affect many metabolic and developmental functions. These end organs include the thyroid gland, adrenal cortex, liver, and gonads. Each system involves regulated secretion of a trophic hormone by the hypothalamus, which, in turn, controls endocrine secretion by the pituitary and, occasionally, secondary hormonal secretion by the end organ, which then produces the appropriate endocrine effect. There is feedback on the hypothalamus by the final product of the pathway (long-loop feedback) and also by the endocrine product of the pituitary (short-loop feedback). The feedback regulates hypothalamic control of the pathway. Clearly, there are many areas that can go wrong in each of these pathways, all of which result in disease. Certain disease conditions are uniquely pediatric and they will be discussed further.

Hypothalamic–Pituitary–Thyroid System[5]

The hypothalamus secretes thyrotropin-releasing hormone (TRH), a 3-amino acid peptide. TRH causes specialized cells in the anterior pituitary to secrete thyroid-stimulating hormone (TSH), a polypeptide made up of two chains (α and β). TSH is released into the circulation and targets its end organ, the thyroid gland. Unique TSH-receptors on the thyroid gland, when occupied by a TSH molecule, cause the thyroid gland to synthesize and release thyroid hormones into the circulation. The synthesis of thyroid hormone involves several complex steps in which iodine is trapped within the thyroid tissue and used to convert the amino acid tyrosine into triiodothyronine (T_3) and tetraiodothyronine (T_4). Thyroid hormones are greater than 99% bound to specific transporter proteins in the blood called *thyroid-binding globulins*. Free thyroid hormone, in particular free T_3, is active and reacts with many peripheral tissues to cause increased metabolism and simulates normal growth and development. T_4, T_3 (long loop), and TSH (short loop) levels feed back on the hypothalamus to regulate TRH production.

Two major areas of dysfunction in this endocrine pathway need consideration in pediatrics: primary hypothyroidism and secondary hypothyroidism. Primary hypothyroidism results from any defect that causes failure of the thyroid gland to synthesize and secrete thyroid hormone. This results in a common disease known as *congenital hypothyroidism*, which is present in one of 4000 births. Untreated patients with this disease have severe mental retardation with unusual facial appearances. Treatment by thyroid replacement therapy is usually successful when diagnosis is established. The best diagnostic test is to measure serum TSH levels, which are high as a result of failure of the long feedback loop. Thyroid hormone levels in untreated patients are very low.

Secondary hypothyroidism is a result of the pituitary gland failing to secrete TSH, which results in lack of thyroid gland stimulation and subsequent production of thyroid hormone. The differential diagnosis is established by measuring low circulating TSH levels. Because the pituitary is involved with all major endocrine systems, it is important to study the other pathways below to determine if the hypothyroidism is the result of an isolated TSH defect or to panhypopituitarism involving all other pathways. Panhypopituitarism is a clinically complex situation, which may include hypoglycemia, salt loss, poor somatic and bone growth, failure to thrive, and failure to develop secondary sexual characteristics.

Hypothalamic–Pituitary–Adrenal Cortex System[5]

This system is essential for regulating mineral and carbohydrate metabolism. The hypothalamus secretes corticotrophin-releasing hormone (CRH), a 41-amino acid polypeptide, which reacts with the anterior pituitary, resulting in the release of corticotrophin or adrenocorticotropic hormone (ACTH). ACTH is released into the circulation and reaches its end organ, the adrenal cortex, which is then stimulated to secrete the steroid hormones, cortisol and aldosterone. This pathway is also stimulated by stress at the higher cerebral center. ACTH acts as a short-loop feedback control; the steroid hormones secreted by the adrenal cortex are long-loop regulators. Aldosterone functions in the kidneys and regulates salt and water balance. Cortisol acts in many peripheral tissues and has many reactions, including regulation of carbohydrate, protein, and lipid metabolism. It also functions by providing resistance to infection and inflammation, a poorly understood mechanism that accounts for the therapeutic use of steroids in these clinical situations. As with all endocrine systems, diseases occur that result from hyperfunction or hypofunction of that pathway. Diseases may be primary, resulting from end organ dysfunction, or secondary, resulting from pituitary or hypothalamic disease. Pediatric diseases associated with primary disorders of the adrenal cortex are shown in Table 33-11. Many disorders listed are rare, genetic diseases; however, one particular disease, the steroid 21-hydroxylase deficiency, is sufficiently common (about 1 of 5000 births) to merit whole population screening by state screening laboratories. This disorder results in failure to adequately synthesize both aldosterone and cortisol. Aldosterone deficiency results in salt-losing crises, and patients in the newborn period can be profoundly hyponatremic and hyperkalemic. Failure to synthesize cortisol results in stress-induced hypoglycemia. Furthermore, intermediates of steroid metabolism, which build up as a result of the metabolic block, cause androgenization. Girls born with this disorder frequently have ambiguous genitalia and may be first classed as boys. Boys may not have such pronounced abnormalities at birth, but may still develop electrolyte crises. This disorder is usually detected by measuring 17-hydroxyprogesterone levels in neonatal blood samples.

Growth Factors

The hypothalamus secretes two regulatory hormones that effect growth. Growth hormone-releasing hormone is a 40-amino acid polypeptide that stimulates release of growth hormone (GH) from the anterior pituitary. Growth hormone-inhibiting factor, also known as *somatostatin,* inhibits GH secretion. Additional factors from higher cerebral centers, including catecholamines, serotonin, and endorphins, have a positive effect on GH secretion. Inhibition of GH secretion also occurs when infants are socially deprived. The mechanism for this reversible inhibition is not known but neglect and potential child abuse are major differentials in infants with retarded growth.

GH is a 191-amino acid polypeptide, with the liver as its primary site of action. GH receptors on the liver that are occupied by a GH molecule cause the liver to secrete a group of related polypeptide hormones, called *insulin-like growth factors (IGF),* and their binding proteins, called *IGF-binding proteins.* IGF-1 and IGF-BP3 are the most significant products of GH activity on the liver. IGF-1 has a molecular structure similar to insulin; however, it is a much more potent stimulator of linear growth and increased metabolism in infants.

This growth pathway probably represents the most important endocrine pathway responsible for normal growth; deficiencies of any component of the pathway are known to result in poor growth, resulting in short statured adults.

Because it is difficult to measure GH in serum as a result of diurnal variation and various stress-related effec-

TABLE 33-11. CONGENITAL DISEASES OF THE ADRENAL CORTEX

	METABOLIC PROFILE
21-Hydroxylase[a]	↑ 17-hydroxyprogesterone, ↓ cortisol
3β-Hydroxy dehydrogenase	↑ dehydroepiandrosterone (DHEA)
11β-Hydroxylase	↑ 11-deoxycortisol, ↓ cortisol
17α-Hydroxylase	↑ 17-ketosteroids, ↓ testosterone
18-Hydroxylase	↓ aldosterone, ↑ renin

[a]Common disorder screened for in all newborns.

A 5-year-old boy is taken to his pediatrician because of growth delay. He was below the third percentile in height and weight. There was no history of trauma and no other pertinent family history or clinical findings.

Questions

1. What conditions may be associated with growth delay?

2. What condition should be primarily considered in this patient?

3. What tests should be performed to confirm the diagnosis?

4. Is the patient likely to respond to therapy?

tors (*eg*, catecholamines), a single, low level of GH may not be sufficient to confirm GH deficiency. It is important to determine true organic deficiency, caused by hypothalamic or pituitary disease, from emotional deficiency because only organic deficiency responds to expensive GH replacement therapy, while nonorganic GH deficiency will respond to emotional lifestyle changes. Trauma to the head may also cause failure of GH secretion by the pituitary through direct anoxic damage to GH secreting cells. This type of growth failure will respond to GH therapy. Several stimulation tests have been devised to test the capacity of the pituitary to secrete GH, including inducement of hypoglycemia with insulin or direct stimulation with glucagon. These tests require that up to five blood samples be collected in the 2 hours poststimulation and the peak level of GH secretion determined. If this is less than 10 ng/mL, the patient has organic GH deficiency and is likely to respond to GH therapy.

Recently, tests for IGF-1 and IGF-BP3 have become available that show great promise in the identification of GH deficiency because these compounds are not released by the liver in GH deficiency states and their basal levels do not seem to have the large variation that occurs for GH. In addition, defects of both IGF and IGF-BP synthesis and secretion have been recognized as a cause of growth failure in certain infants. Individuals with these defects are unlikely to respond to GH replacement.

Endocrine Control of Sexual Maturation

The hypothalamus secretes a 10-amino acid peptide called *gonadotropin-releasing hormone (GnRH)*. This hormone causes the release of two larger polypeptide hor-

mones, called *follicle-stimulating hormone (FSH)* and *luteinizing hormone (LH)*, in both males and females. FSH and LH are structurally similar to TSH and also to human chorionic gonadotropin (hCG), which is not discussed further in this chapter.

Baseline levels of FSH and LH are low in infants as a result of GnRH suppression and require sensitive immunoassays based on chemiluminescence for accurate detection.

FSH and LH have different effects in males and females, both before and during puberty. In males, the hormonal activity is directed to the testis, which causes the release of androgens, primarily testosterone and androstenedione. In females, the primary site of action is the ovary, which results in the excretion of a different family of steroid hormones—estrogens; primarily, estradiol. Prior to puberty, the circulating levels of androgens and estrogens are low, although the pediatric clinical laboratory is often requested to measure these hormones when a child appears to be going into premature puberty. Testosterone is particularly difficult to measure in prepubertal children as most commercial assays detect an interfering compound, which results in false elevation of the hormone level.

At puberty, the GnRH suppression is removed and there is a gradual increase in FSH and LH secretion, with concomitant increase in androgens in males and estrogens and progesterone in females. This results in the development of secondary sexual characteristics and onset of menarche in females. This period is also associated with a major surge in linear and bone growth until adult proportions are achieved.

Disorders of this endocrine pathway are associated with either premature or precocious puberty or delayed onset of puberty. The measurement of FSH, LH, testosterone, and estradiol is useful in evaluating disordered puberty. Often, disorders of other endocrine systems effect puberty. Congenital adrenal hyperplasia, the disorder described under adrenal cortex diseases, results in excess secretion of androgen-like steroids that can effect puberty. Disorders of the hypothalamus and pituitary can effect secretion of FSH and LH and cause delayed puberty.

DEVELOPMENT OF THE IMMUNE SYSTEM

In pediatric clinical facilities, the vast majority of hospital visits and admissions are related to complications arising from infectious diseases. At the same time, although the parents or caregivers may be exposed to the same infectious etiologies, they do not become so ill as to require medical attention. This is because the child does not have the same degree of *immunity* to disease at birth or during infancy.[1]

Basic Concepts of Immunity

The immune system is divided into two functional divisions; the innate immune system and the adaptive immune system. The innate immune system is the first line of defense, particularly in the newborn and infant not exposed to infection. The adaptive immune system generates a specific reaction following exposure to an infectious agent and provides greater immunity with subsequent exposure to that agent. Initially, however, the first response to exposure may be suboptimal and result in illness related to that exposure.

Components of the Immune System[5]

Skin

The skin is normally an effective barrier to most microorganisms, although in premature babies this barrier is less well developed and can easily become a source of infection. Most infectious agents enter the body by the nasopharynx, gastrointestinal tract, lungs, and genitourinary tract. Surgical incisions and intravenous or central lines are also potential sites of entry. Normally, various physical and biochemical defenses protect the nonsurgical sites of entry. Lysozyme, an enzyme widely distributed in different secretions, for example, is capable of partially digesting a chemical bond in the membrane of many bacterial cell walls.

Phagocytes

Phagocytes are present in many cell types. When a foreign organism penetrates an epithelial surface, it encounters phagocytic cells, which are derived from bone marrow and recruited into tissue in response to the organism. These cells engulf and digest particles. Phagocytic cells include polymorphonuclear cells, which are short-lived in the circulation, and monocytes that, when exposed to a foreign particle, develop into macrophages that subsequently recognize the organism when the individual is reexposed.

B Cells

B cells are lymphocytes that are characterized by the presence of surface immunoglobulins. These cells can differentiate into plasma cells that are able to respond to foreign antigens in the circulation by producing neutralizing antibodies. Activation, proliferation, and differentiation of B cells are assisted by cytokine secretion from T-cell lymphocytes, which do not produce antibodies. On binding antigen, antibodies can activate a cascade involving complement, which ultimately produces lysis and cellular death of foreign organisms.

Natural Killer Cells

Natural killer (NK) cells are leukocytes capable of recognizing cell-surface changes on host cells infected by virus particles. The NK cells bind to these target cells and can kill them and the virus. The NK cells respond to interferons, which are cytokine molecules produced by the host cells when infected by virus. Interferons are also part of the innate immune system capable of providing resistance to infection in host cells not virally infected.

Acute-Phase Proteins

Acute-phase proteins are defense proteins produced by the liver in response to infection, particularly bacterial infection. Certain proteins can increase in the serum by twofold to 100-fold. The most significant acute-phase protein is called *C-reactive protein (CRP)* because of its ability to bind to the C-protein of *pneumococci*. CRP bound to bacteria promotes the binding of complement that, in turn, aids phagocytosis. Serum CRP levels are routinely measured to determine degree of infection in pediatric patients. The required sensitivity of the CRP assay for this clinical purpose is less than that used for the high-sensitivity CRP assay used clinically as an independent risk factor for cardiac disease. In the pediatric application of this assay, rapid turnaround of results is most important. The complement system consists of at least 20 proteins, most of which are acute-phase proteins. They interact sequentially with each other, with antigen–antibody complexes, and with cell membranes in a coordinate manner to ultimately destroy bacteria and viruses. Clinically, the complement proteins that are measured most often are C3 and C4. Low levels of either of these proteins indicate poor ability to destroy foreign particles.

Antibody Production

Immunoglobulins are classified into five major groups, based on structure and function: IgG, IgM, IgA, IgD, and IgE. Secreted by plasma cells derived from B-lymphocytes, their properties are listed in Table 33-12. IgG is the major immunoglobulin subclass providing antibody response in adults and represents 70–75% of total immunoglobulin content. IgG is further broken down into four additional subclasses: IgG_{1-4}. Each immunoglobulin is built from similar structural units, based on two heavy polypeptide chains (A, G, M, D, and E) and two light chains (kappa and lambda). The ability to recognize large numbers of foreign antigens is a result of the infinite ability of the genes for the so-called variable region of the immunoglobulin molecule to rearrange. This area recognizes foreign antigens, and a gene rearrangement and production of a unique antibody covers each new antigen exposed to the body. Because of the large number of different immunoglobulin species, electrophoretic separation of these serum proteins on an isoelectric-focusing gel during serum protein electrophoresis (SPEP) analysis is diffuse, unlike albumin or transferrin separation, which generates distinct bands.

TABLE 33-12. PROPERTIES OF IMMUNOGLOBULIN (IG) CLASSES

	IgG[a]	IgA	IgM	IgD	IgE
Mass (kD)	160	160	970	184	188
% of total Ig	70–75	10–15	5–10	<1	Trace
Crosses placenta	Yes	No	No	No	No
In breast milk	Yes	Yes	No	Unknown	Unknown
Activates complement	Yes	Yes	Yes	No	No
In secretions	No	Yes	No	No	No
Binds to mast cells	No	No	No	No	Yes

[a]Present as four subclasses (IgG$_{1-4}$).

Neonatal and Infant Antibody Production

The human fetus is able to synthesize a small amount of IgM and, to a lesser degree, IgA. IgG has a lower molecular weight than IgM and is readily able to cross the placenta. IgG is also transferred from mother to baby in breast milk. Transplacental and breast milk-derived IgG offer the baby a passive immunologic protection until endogenous IgG production takes place. The half-life of IgG is about 30 days and, with prolonged breast-feeding, the infant can derive additional protection. The process of antibody production in infants takes several years to complete when based on total serum levels of the immunoglobulin subclasses, which take up to 4 years to be attained. Premature babies have an even greater immunoglobulin deficit because of diminished transplacental delivery of antibodies.

Immunity Disorders[7]

Given the complexity of the immune system, there are many stages at which acquired or genetically inherited defects can result in inappropriate infectious disease in the pediatric population. Transient hypogammaglobulinemia of infancy may occur in prematurity or, in certain infants, may be a result of delayed onset of immunoglobulin production of unknown etiology. These infants eventually develop a normal immune system, but will be prone to repeated bouts of severe infection. At the opposite end of the spectrum, complete absence of γ-globulins occurs in boys in an X-linked disorder known as *agammaglobulinemia,* or Bruton's disease. This disorder presents early in life with recurrent febrile infections. Patients do not have B-cells and have low levels of all endogenous immunoglobulin subclasses. The disease process probably begins the moment that any maternally derived immunoglobulins have been lost. The most common infections are of the upper and lower respiratory tracts, causing otitis, pneumonia, sinusitis, meningitis, sepsis, and osteomyelitis. Without early γ-globulin therapy, these children die from respiratory complications. Other immune pathways are normal in these children.

Severe Combined Immune Deficiency (SCID)

One of the most graphic examples of unique pediatric disease comes from infants who lack both humoral and cellular pathways for killing bacteria and viruses. These children are at risk of severe infection each time they are exposed to an infectious agent. The vivid image is of the "boy in the bubble," existing in a completely sterile environment to avoid contact with any bacteria or virus particles. SCID may be inherited as an X-linked disorder only seen in boys, or it may be autosomal recessive and girls may also inherit the disease. There are several causes of SCID, including genetic diseases of purine metabolism and disorders of lymphocyte development and maturation, in which both T cells and B cells, if present, are nonfunctional. The most common purine disorder, adenosine deaminase deficiency, is responsible for 15% of SCID cases. It is diagnosed by measuring elevated levels of adenosine in body fluids. Establishing this diagnosis is important because enzyme replacement therapy using recombinant enzyme has been successfully used to treat the disorder.

GENETIC DISEASES

Analytic methods for the identification of genetic disease play an important part in the pediatric clinical chemistry laboratory.[1,8] Most genetic diseases are unique to the pediatric population and require specialized knowledge and training. Most diseases that present with clinical signs in the pediatric population are inherited in an autosomal recessive mode, which means that the patient has two disease-causing mutations in the gene for that disorder, one inherited maternally and one inherited paternally. Several examples of diseases with this inheritance pattern have already been introduced in this chapter, including galactosemia and congenital adrenal hyperplasia as a result of steroid 21-hydroxylase deficiency. Certain other diseases are recessive but are inherited on the X chromosome. Typically, boys inherit a mutated X-chromosome from their mothers; because they do not inherit a paternal X chromosome, they show signs of disease with only one mutation. For both inheritance patterns, the parent with one normal gene will be, for the most part, asymptomatic. Dominantly inherited diseases, which can be inherited as a single mutation through either parental line, tend not to present in childhood and do not impact fertility. Examples include familial hypercholesterolemia, Huntington disease, and factor V Leiden thrombophilia, all of which are diseases of the adult population. Recently, a new mode of genetic inheritance was identified. All of the diseases described above are diseases of DNA that replicates in the cell nucleus. Mitochondria, the organelles responsible for generating cellular energy and other important metabolic pathways, contain a small molecule of DNA (mtDNA) that encodes proteins involved in energy generation. mtDNA has a high rate of spontaneous mutation and results in a large number of energy wasting diseases. Mitochondria is only inherited from the mother, so that mutations that are not spontaneous can only come from the maternal lineage.

Cystic Fibrosis

Cystic fibrosis (CF) is one of the most commonly inherited genetic diseases encountered by pediatric clinical chemistry laboratories. One of 2400 live births have this debilitating disease, which results from recessively inherited mutations in the cystic fibrosis transmembrane regulator (CFTR) gene. Patients may present in the newborn period with severe pancreatic insufficiency caused by accumulated thick mucous secretions in the pancreatic ducts, which inhibit the secretion of pancreatic digestive enzymes. These babies have steatorrhea and fail to thrive. Patients with CF do not always develop pancreatic symptoms; however, in most patients, the thick mucous that accumulates in the lungs causes respiratory disease and makes them particularly susceptible to rare infectious diseases, such as *pseudomonas*. Although palliative therapies have improved over the last few generations because of the availability of better antibiotics, CF is still regarded as untreatable.

The gold standard diagnostic test for CF has been available for many years. It involves measurement of chloride content in sweat collected after pilocarpine iontophoresis. This type of testing is time consuming and requires specialist experience from the operator. The genetic basis for CF has been established. Although there are some mutations that are frequently encountered in the population, such as the ΔF508, there are hundreds of other mutations. Recently, the American College of Medical Genetics and the American College of Obstetrics and Gynecology recommended heterozygote screening in selected couples.[9] This recommendation poses an analytic challenge because of the large number of mutations, and it will probably require the development of a clinically acceptable microchip technology before they can be fully implemented (see Chapter 26, *Gastrointestinal Function*).

Newborn Screening for Whole Populations

Certain inherited diseases are sufficiently common in the population to be considered candidates for whole population screening. Phenylketonuria was the first genetic metabolic disorder to be screened in every baby born in the western world. Other diseases that are readily treatable were added to the list in following years, including steroid 21-hydroxylase deficiency, sickle cell disease, and congenital hypothyroidism and, in some states, galactosemia. These genetic diseases respond well to simple therapy, often dietary. In most states, this process takes place in the state-screening laboratory, a facility that has the ability to easily follow up abnormal test results. The nature of the testing procedure requires a sensitive screening test that has few false-negative results. There should then be confirmation using a test that is more specific to rule out false-positive results. A new technology, *tandem mass spectrometry*, allows 25–30 different biochemical genetic diseases to be screened on a single sample at the same time (Table 33-13). This technique allows whole groups of similar compounds to be analyzed on small sample volumes without complex sample preparation. The analytic time is about 2 minutes per sample, which means that it is possible to readily perform analysis for an entire state. The birthrate in the United States is approximately 3.5–4 million births per year. Tandem mass spectrometry has been shown to be capable of this workload. At the time of writing, nine states have already endorsed this process and other states are in advanced stages of evaluation.

Diagnosis of Metabolic Disease in the Clinical Setting

At the present time, the clinical laboratory is needed to confirm the diagnosis in most of the diseases listed in Table 33-13 and also for the rest of the 500 single gene defects that result in biochemical genetic disease not detectable by tandem mass spectrometry. These inborn errors of metabolism can be broken down generally into two main types.

Large Molecule Diseases

Large molecule diseases have an accumulating intermediate of metabolism comprised of large complex molecules; examples are listed in Table 33-14. Many of these diseases involve intracellular accumulation of the abnormal chemical with relatively small excretion in body fluids. In glycogen storage diseases, the glycogen accumulates in liver and muscle but cannot be seen in blood or urine samples. The histopathologist, using microscopic

TABLE 33-13. METABOLIC DISEASES DETECTABLE BY EXPANDED NEWBORN SCREENING

Amino Acids

Phenylketonuria (PKU)

Maple syrup urine disease (MSUD)

Tyrosinemia, types 1 and 2

Homocystinuria

Hypermethioninemia

Urea Cycle

Argininemia

Citrullinemia

Argininosuccinic aciduria (ASA)

Organic Acids

Propionic acidemia (PA)

Methylmalonic acidemia (MMA)

Isovaleric acidemia (IVA)

Glutaric acidemia, types 1 and 2 (GA1, GA2)

β-Ketothiolase deficiency

3-Hydroxy-3-methylglutaryl-CoA lyase deficiency (HMG-CoA lyase)

3-Methylcrotonyl-CoA carboxylase deficiency (MCC)

Malonyl-CoA decarboxylase deficiency

2-Methyl-3-hydroxybutyryl-CoA dehydrogenase

Fatty Acids

Medium-chain acyl-CoA dehydrogenase deficiency (MCAD)

Short-chain acyl-CoA dehydrogenase deficiency (SCAD)

Very-long-chain acyl-CoA dehydrogenase deficiency (VLCAD)

Carnitine palmitoyltransferase, types 1A and 2 (CPT1A, CPT2)

Carnitine acylcarnitine translocase deficiency (CAT)

Long-chain 3-hydroxyacyl-CoA dehydrogenase deficiency (LCHAD)

Mitochondrial trifunctional protein deficiency (MTP)

examination of tissue, often makes these diagnoses. A few, mostly urine, tests are available for gathering clues to large molecule diseases, including glycosaminoglycan analysis using high voltage electrophoresis to identify unusual metabolites associated with the mucopolysaccharide storage diseases. These tests are relatively insensitive and confirmation of the diagnosis requires measurement of deficient enzyme activity on a body tissue. Fortunately, many enzymes that result in large molecule storage diseases can be found in white blood cells, enabling confirmation to be made on a blood sample. Enzymic confirmation can be difficult to establish in small babies because large blood samples are frequently required for diagnostic testing.

Small Molecule Diseases

Small molecule diseases result from defects in metabolic pathways of intermediary metabolism. Usually, the abnormal compounds that are present in these diseases are low-molecular-weight compounds that are readily excreted in body fluids; the types of pathways involved are listed in Table 33-15. Initially, the clinical chemistry laboratory had few diagnostic tools capable of identifying the large number of metabolic intermediates that may accumulate in these diseases, and a number of simple, colorimetric urine tests, such as the dinitrophenylhydrazine (DNPH) test for ketoacids, were developed to establish diagnosis. These methods lack both sensitivity and specificity and have no role to play in the modern clinical chemistry laboratory. They have been superseded by assays with greater sensitivity and specificity, often based on mass spectrometry.

Small molecule diseases have a variable clinical presentation and could present to almost any medical subspecialty with any organ system involved. (Table 33-16 lists certain diseases and which specialist may be consulted). Biochemical testing for these diseases is usually described in two phases. First, it is important to recognize the degree of tissue compromization at presentation. This requires routine chemistry evaluation for

TABLE 33-14. EXAMPLES OF LARGE MOLECULE STORAGE DISORDERS

Mucopolysaccharide (MPS) or Glycosaminoglycan Storage Diseases

Hurler disease (MPS, type I)

Hunter disease (type II)

Morquio disease (type IV)

Complex Lipid Storage

Gaucher disease

Tay-Sachs disease

Niemann-Pick disease (types A, B, C)

Glycogen Storage Diseases

Von Gierke (type 1)

Pompe (type 2)

McArdle (type 5)

Peptide Storage

Neuronal Ceroid Lipofuscinoses, Types 1–8 (Batten Disease)

TABLE 33-15. PATHWAYS INVOLVED WITH SMALL MOLECULE METABOLIC DISEASE

Amino acids
Fatty acids
Organic acids
Urea cycle
Oxidative phosphorylation
Vitamin metabolism
Steroid biosynthesis and breakdown
Cholesterol synthesis
Purine and pyrimidine metabolism
Neurotransmitter metabolism
Plasmalogen synthesis
Glutathione metabolism
Oxalate metabolism

CASE STUDY 33-3

An infant presented to the pediatrician with failure to thrive and steatorrhea (foul smelling, fatty stool). An older sibling with the same clinical presentation has a confirmed genetic disease.

Questions

1. What is the likely diagnosis?

2. How is the disease inherited?

3. What is the long-term prognosis for the patients?

4. What is the gold standard diagnostic test?

blood gas status, if acidotic; anion gap measurement; liver function testing; analysis of muscle markers, such as CK; lactic acid; and ammonia measurement. All of these analyses should be available stat and used to monitor management. The second phase of analysis should be to look for metabolic markers that pinpoint the site of a defect. These tests involve a form of separation technology, such as ion-exchange chromatography for amino acids. The preferred material for amino acid analysis is serum because the renal tubules have efficient transport systems for reabsorbing filtered amino acids. It is possible to miss an amino acid abnormality if urine is analyzed. Urine amino acid analysis is only of value if a tubular defect such as cystinuria is suspected. The most useful test for detecting abnormal metabolic intermediates is organic acid analysis. This test is performed on urine and should only be performed using the technique of gas chromatography mass spectrome-

try. It is a method that is capable of identifying metabolic markers for up to 200 genetic diseases. Tandem mass spectrometry is another technique seeing rapid growth in the metabolic disease diagnosis field. This technique is being applied to newborn screening and is also playing an increasing role in analysis of multiple different metabolites. Currently, this technology is mainly found in research and cutting-edge clinical chemistry laboratories, but it will find a place in all chemistry laboratories in the near future.

DRUG METABOLISM AND PHARMACOKINETICS[1,10]

There are several important differences in the way that infants and children handle pharmacologic agents when compared with adults. This area of pediatric laboratory medicine provides many good examples of why children

TABLE 33-16. DRUGS WITH WELL-DEFINED THERAPEUTIC INDICES

DRUG	THERAPEUTIC RANGE	TOXICITY
Phenytoin	10–20 mg/L	>40 causes seizures; ataxia
Phenobarbital	10–40 mg/L	>40 causes drowsiness; >60 coma
Carbamazepine	4–10 mg/L	>10 causes drowsiness
Theophylline[a]	5–15 mg/L	>20 can cause cardiac arrhythmia
Caffeine[a]	5–15 mg/L	Less toxic than theophylline
Methotrexate	Depends on therapy	High levels cause myelosuppression
Gentamycin	5–10 mg/L (peak)[b]	>12 ototoxic; renal toxicity

[a]Theophylline is metabolized to caffeine in neonates but not in adults. Used to treat apnea.
[b]Peak level should be drawn 30 minutes after last dose for aminoglycoside drugs. Children are particularly prone to hearing loss at toxic levels.

should not be regarded as "small adults." It is not clinically appropriate to prorate the amount of drug prescribed to a child based on relative body weight when compared with an adult dose.

Drug metabolism depends upon the following factors: absorption, circulation and distribution, and metabolism and clearance. Often, the medium in which a drug is provided to a child differs from that in which an adult may take the same drug. Syrups, for instance, provide a more rapid release of a drug and greater availability for gastrointestinal absorption than tablets, which have the drug trapped in a solid matrix that requires digestion. Children are more likely to be given medication in a palatable form, such as syrup, and to require lower doses. The pH of gastric secretions differs in infants. At birth, the gastric pH is nearly neutral, not reaching the adult level of acidity for several years. This pH difference can affect the absorption of certain drugs, including some frequently prescribed penicillins. The distribution of drugs often differs between adults and children. Lipid-soluble drugs are taken up into lipid reserves and only slowly released into the circulation. Because infants have relatively little adipose tissue, these drugs are not stored as efficiently. The overall effect is that lipid-soluble drugs reach a higher level more quickly than in individuals with sizable fat stores; however, the drug is also cleared more rapidly. It becomes appropriate for drugs to be provided in smaller, more frequent doses to optimize the effect. Hepatic metabolism of many drugs is immature in young infants. This may delay the metabolic conversion to an active drug or increase the time in which an active drug is circulating. Good hepatic function is important for clearing those drugs metabolized by the liver, as good renal function is important for clearing drugs that have water-soluble end products.

Therapeutic Drug Monitoring

The principles of therapeutic drug monitoring remain the same in adult and pediatric clinical chemistry. It is important to measure the blood levels of various drugs if that information can provide important guidance to the physician with regard to optimal dosing. This is most important if a drug has a well-defined therapeutic index. This means that the drug is known to be ineffective if the blood level is below a certain value, that there is a well-defined therapeutic range over which the drug is effective, and that there is a higher level at which the drug becomes toxic. It is important to monitor levels of drugs with these characteristics. Table 33-16 lists drugs for which the importance of therapeutic monitoring is established.

Toxicologic Issues in Pediatric Clinical Chemistry

Issues related to the provision of a toxicologic service can be divided into two distinct groups in pediatrics. The first group involves infants and young children who unknowingly consume pharmacologic and other chemical agents. This usually involves the child finding access to medication belonging to another individual in the household and consuming the medication as if it were candy. It is relatively easy for the investigator to ascertain the nature of the medication by identifying what is available in the household. Toxicologic investigation can usually be restricted to a few specific tests.

A rare, but potentially dangerous condition, is that of Munchausen disease by proxy. In this condition, mental illness in a caregiver causes them to give unnecessary and illness-causing drugs to an otherwise well child. This can go unrecognized and result in multiple hospitalizations and even death of the child. Clinical suspicion of this form of child abuse should involve performing a comprehensive drug screen to identify causative agents. Because of the intermittent nature of clinical presentation of Munchausen syndrome by proxy, it can often be confused with metabolic disease. Metabolic studies, in addition to comprehensive toxicologic studies may be necessary.

Because the likelihood of self-ingestion of street drugs of abuse is present in older children, pediatric clinical chemistry laboratories should make assays available for street drugs similar to those in adult practice.

SUMMARY

Pediatrics is a branch of medicine that deals with the diagnosis and treatment of disease in children. This involves investigation of small individuals, from birth to teenagers. The most significant difference between this population and the adult population is related to physiologic development of children. Immature organ systems can have profound effects on biochemical parameters.

Children present to the hospital with different disease profiles. There are many more presentations with infectious disease as a result of undeveloped immunity. Metabolic genetic diseases are almost unique to pediatrics, and the pediatric clinical chemist is required to understand the analytic processes involved with diagnosis.

The small size of many patients in a pediatric center necessitates a different approach to chemistry test menus and choice of instrumentation.

REVIEW QUESTIONS

1. Which of the following occurs in an infant immediately after birth?
   a. Normal hepatic function and bilirubin metabolism
   b. Closure of the ductus arteriosus and adult respiration
   c. Adult rates of glomerular filtration by the kidneys
   d. Normal water homeostasis

2. How much blood should be drawn at any one time from a 7-pound baby?
   a. No more than 10 mL
   b. No more than 20 mL
   c. No more than 1.0 mL
   d. No more than 2.5 mL

3. When choosing a chemistry analyzer for a pediatric laboratory, it is necessary to:
   a. have rapid turnaround.
   b. be able to analyze from small volumes.
   c. have an extensive menu.
   d. have front-end automation.

4. High blood ammonia levels result in:
   a. metabolic acidosis.
   b. metabolic alkalosis.
   c. respiratory alkalosis.
   d. respiratory acidosis.

5. Point-of-care testing is helpful when:
   a. results are needed quickly.
   b. only small sample sizes are available.
   c. the device can be linked to the hospital LIS.
   d. quality control samples are not needed.

6. Which of the following immunoglobulins are provided to a new baby by the mother?
   a. IgG
   b. IgD
   c. IgM
   d. IgA

7. The pituitary secretes which of the following hormones?
   a. Growth hormone
   b. Testosterone
   c. Insulin-like growth factor
   d. Thyroid-stimulating hormone

8. Tandem mass spectrometry can be used to detect:
   a. cystic fibrosis.
   b. combined immune deficiency.
   c. 25–30 metabolic diseases.
   d. panhypopituitarism.

9. Aminoglycoside drug levels, such as gentamycin, should be measured:
   a. 30 minutes after a dose.
   b. 3 hours after a dose.
   c. at steady state.
   d. at any time.

REFERENCES

1. Green A, Morgan I, Gray J. Neonatology and Laboratory Medicine. London: ACB Venture Publications, 2003.
2. Soldin SJ, Rifai N, Hicks JMB, eds. Biochemical Basis of Pediatric Disease. Washington, D.C.: American Association for Clinical Chemistry, 1992.
3. Gill FN, Bennett MJ. The pediatrics unit. In: Price CP, Hicks JM, eds. Point of Care Testing. Washington, D.C.: American Association for Clinical Chemistry, 1999.
4. Goldenberg RL, Mercer BM, Iams JD. The preterm prediction study: patterns of cervicovaginal fetal fibronectin as predictors of spontaneous preterm delivery. Am J Obstet Gynecol 1997;177: 8–12.
5. Burtis CA, Ashwood ER, eds. Tietz Fundamentals of Clinical Chemistry, 5th ed. Philadelphia: WB Saunders, 2001.
6. Newman DJ. Cystatin C. Ann Clin Biochem 2002;39:89–104.
7. Scriver CR, Beaudet AL, Valle D, Sly WS, eds. The Metabolic and Molecular Bases of Inherited Disease, 8th ed. New York: McGraw-Hill, 2001.
8. Hommes FA, ed. Techniques in Diagnostic Human Biochemical Genetics. New York: Wiley-Liss, 1991.
9. Baskin LB, Wians FH, Elder F. Preconception and prenatal screening for cystic fibrosis. MLO Med Lab Observer 2002;34(10):8–12.
10. Hallworth M, Capps N. Therapeutic Drug Monitoring and Clinical Biochemistry. London: ACB Venture Publications, 1993.

Appendices

For additional information, refer to the latest edition of one of the following excellent references:
Bold AM, Wilding P. Clinical Chemistry Companion. Oxford, UK: Blackwell Scientific Publications.
Weast RC. CRC Handbook of Clinical Chemistry. Boca Raton, FL: CRC Press.
Werner M. CRC Handbook of Clinical Chemistry. Boca Raton, FL: CRC Press.

APPENDIX A. BASIC SI UNITS

MEASUREMENT	NAME	SYMBOL
Length	Meter	m
Mass	Kilogram	kg
Quantity of substance	Mole	mol
Time	Second	s
Electric current	Ampere	A
Thermodynamic temperature	Kelvin	K
Luminous intensity	Candela	cd

Note: SI (Système Internationale d'Unités) units are those having a definition recognized by international agreement. Note that some SI units have capitalized symbols. This is to avoid confusion with SI prefixes using the same letter symbol.

APPENDIX B. PREFIXES TO BE USED WITH SI UNITS

FACTOR	PREFIX	SYMBOL
10^{-18}	atto	a
10^{-15}	femto	f
10^{-12}	pico	p
10^{-9}	nano	n
10^{-6}	micro	μ
10^{-3}	milli	m
10^{-2}	centi	c
10^{-1}	deci	d
10^{1}	deka	da
10^{2}	hecto	h
10^{3}	kilo	k
10^{6}	mega	M
10^{9}	giga	G
10^{15}	peta	P
10^{18}	exa	E

Note: Prefixes are used to indicate a subunit or multiple of a basic SI unit.

APPENDIX C. BASIC CLINICAL LABORATORY CONVERSIONS

LENGTH, VOLUME, WEIGHT CONVERSIONS

TO CONVERT	INTO	MULTIPLY BY
Inches	Centimeters	2.54
Centimeters	Inches	.39
Yards	Meters	.91
Meters	Yards	1.09
Gallons (U.S.)	Liters	3.78
Liters	Gallons (U.S.)	.26
Fluid ounces (U.S.)	Milliliters	29.6
Milliliters	Fluid ounces (U.S.)	.034
Ounces	Grams	28.4
Grams	Ounces	.035
Pounds	Kilograms	.45
Kilograms	Pounds	2.2

TEMPERATURE CONVERSIONS

TO CONVERT	INTO	USE
Centigrade (°C)	Kelvin (°K)	$°K = °C + 273$
Centigrade (°C)	Fahrenheit (°F)	$°F = (°C \times 1.8) + 32$
Fahrenheit (°F)	Centigrade (°C)	$°C = (°F - 32) \times 0.556$

CONCENTRATION CONVERSIONS

TO CONVERT	INTO	USE
% w/v	Molarity (M)	$M = \dfrac{\% \text{ w/v} \times 10}{\text{GMW}}$
% w/v	Normality (N)	$N = \dfrac{\% \text{ w/v} \times 10}{\text{eq wt}}$
mg/dL	mEq/L	$\text{mEq/L} = \dfrac{\text{mg/dL} \times 10}{\text{eq wt}}$
Molarity	Normality	$N = M \times \text{valence}$

APPENDIX D. CONVERSION OF TRADITIONAL UNITS TO SI UNITS FOR COMMON CHEMISTRY ANALYTES[a]

	CONVENTIONAL/CURRENT	SI UNIT	CONVERSION FACTOR
Albumin	g/100 mL	g/L	10
Aspartate aminotransferase (AST)	U/L (mU/mL)	μkat/L	0.0167
Ammonia	μg/dL	μmol/L	0.587
Bicarbonate (HCO_3)	mEq/L	mmol/L	1.0
Bilirubin	mg/dL	μmol/L	17.1
BUN	mg/dL	mmol/L	0.357
Calcium	mg/dL	mmol/L	0.25
Chloride	mEq/L	mmol/L	1.0
Cholesterol	mg/dL	mmol/L	0.026
Cortisol	μg/dL	μmol/L	0.0276
Creatinine	mg/dL	μmol/L	88.4
Creatinine clearance	mL/min	mL/s	0.0167
Folic acid	ng/mL	nmol/L	2.27
Glucose	mg/dL	mmol/L	0.0555
Hemoglobin	g/dL	g/L	10
Iron	mg/dL	μmol/L	0.179
Lithium	mEq/L	μmol/L	1.0
Magnesium	mEq/L	mmol/L	0.5
Osmolality	mOsm/kg	mmol/kg	1.0
Phosphorus	mg/dL	mmol/L	0.323
Potassium	mEq/L	mmol/L	1.0
Sodium	mEq/L	mmol/L	1.0
Thyroxine (T_4)	μg/dL	nmol/L	12.9
Total protein	g/dL	g/L	10
Triglyceride	mg/dL	mmol/L	0.0113
Uric acid	mg/dL	mmol/L	0.0595
Vitamin B_{12}	ng/mL	pmol/L	0.0738
PCO_2	mm/Hg	kPa	0.133
PO_2	mm/Hg	kPa	0.133

[a]To obtain SI unit, multiply current unit by conversion factor. To obtain the conventional or current unit, divide the SI unit by the conversion factor.

APPENDIX E. CONCENTRATIONS OF COMMONLY USED ACIDS AND BASES WITH RELATED FORMULAS

CHEMICAL SUBSTANCE	CHEMICAL FORMULA	FORMULA WEIGHT/GMW	EQUIVALENT WEIGHT	AVERAGE SPECIFIC GRAVITY CONC REAGENT[a]	AVERAGE % PURITY CONC REAGENT[a]	NORMALITY CONC REAGENT (APPROXIMATE)
Ammonium hydroxide	NH_4OH	35.05	35.05	0.90	28.0	15
Acetic acid (glacial)	CH_5COOH	60.05	60.05	1.06	99.5	18
Formic acid	$HCOOH$	46.03	46.03	1.20	88.0	23
Hydrochloric acid	HCL	36.46	36.46	1.19	37.0	12
Nitric acid	HNO_3	63.02	63.02	1.42	70.0	16
Perchloric acid	$HCLO_4$	100.46	100.46	1.67	71.0	12
Phosphoric acid	H_3PO_4	98.00	32.67	1.69	85.0	44
Sulfuric acid	H_2SO_4	98.08	49.04	1.84	96.0	36

Conc = concentration.

[a]Varies according to lot and/or manufacturer. Related formulas:

Molarity (M) = g/L/GMW

Equivalent weight (eq wt) = GMW/valence

Normality (N) = g/L/ef wt

Specific gravity (sp gr): sp gr $\times$ % purity (in decimal form) = g of solute/mL

APPENDIX F. EXAMPLES OF INCOMPATIBLE CHEMICALS

CHEMICAL	IS INCOMPATIBLE WITH
Acetic acid	Chromic acid, nitric acid, hydroxyl compounds, ethylene glycol, perchloric acid, peroxides, permanganates
Acetylene	Chlorine, bromine, copper, fluorine, silver, mercury
Acetone	Concentrated nitric and sulfuric acid mixtures
Alkali and alkaline earth metals (such as powdered aluminum or magnesium, calcium, lithium, sodium, potassium)	Water, carbon tetrachloride or other chlorinated hydrocarbons, carbon dioxide, halogens
Ammonia (anhydrous)	Mercury (in manometers, for example), chlorine, calcium hypochlorite, iodine, bromine, hydrofluoric acid (anhydrous)
Ammonium nitrate	Acids, powdered metals, flammable liquids, chlorates, nitrites, sulfur, finely divided organic or combustible materials
Aniline	Nitric acid, hydrogen peroxide
Arsenical materials	Any reducing agent
Azides	Acids
Bromine	See Chlorine
Calcium oxide	Water
Carbon (activated)	Calcium hypochlorite, all oxidizing agents
Carbon tetrachloride	Sodium
Chlorates	Ammonium salts, acids, powdered metals, sulfur, finely divided organic or combustible materials
Chromic acid and chromium trioxide	Acetic acid, naphthalene, camphor, glycerol, alcohol, flammable liquids in general
Chlorine	Ammonia, acetylene, butadiene, butane, methane, propane (or other petroleum gases), hydrogen, sodium carbide, benzene, finely divided metals, turpentine
Chlorine dioxide	Ammonia, methane, phosphine, hydrogen sulfide
Copper	Acetylene, hydrogen peroxide
Cumene hydroperoxide	Acids (organic or inorganic)
Cyanides	Acids
Flammable liquids	Ammonium nitrate, chromic acid, hydrogen peroxide, nitric acid, sodium peroxide, halogens
Fluorine	Everything
Hydrocarbons (such as butane, propane, benzene)	Fluorine, chlorine, bromine, chromic acid, sodium peroxide
Hydrocyanic acid	Nitric acid, alkali
Hydrofluoric acid (anhydrous)	Ammonia (aqueous or anhydrous)
Hydrogen peroxide	Copper, chromium, iron, most metals or their salts, alcohols, acetone, organic materials, aniline, nitromethane, combustible materials

APPENDIX F. EXAMPLES OF INCOMPATIBLE CHEMICALS (continued)

CHEMICAL	IS INCOMPATIBLE WITH
Hydrogen sulfide	Fuming nitric acid, oxidizing gases
Hypochlorites	Acids, activated carbon
Iodine	Acetylene, ammonia (aqueous or anhydrous), hydrogen
Mercury	Acetylene, fulminic acid, ammonia
Nitrates	Sulfuric acid
Nitric acid (concentrated)	Acetic acid, aniline, chromic acid, hydrocyanic acid, hydrogen sulfide, flammable liquids, flammable gases, copper, brass, any heavy metals
Nitrites	Acids
Nitroparaffins	Inorganic bases, amines
Oxalic acid	Silver, mercury
Oxygen	Oils, grease, hydrogen, flammable liquids, solids, or gases
Perchloric acid	Acetic anhydride, bismuth and its alloys, alcohol, paper, wood, grease, oils
Peroxides, organic	Acids (organic or mineral), avoid friction, store cold
Phosphorus (white)	Air, oxygen, alkalis, reducing agents
Potassium	Carbon tetrachloride, carbon dioxide, water
Potassium chlorate	Sulfuric and other acids
Potassium perchlorate (see also chlorates)	Sulfuric and other acids
Potassium permanganate	Glycerol, ethylene glycol, benzaldehyde, sulfuric acid
Selenides	Reducing agents
Silver	Acetylene, oxalic acid, tartaric acid, ammonium compounds, fulminic acid
Sodium	Carbon tetrachloride, carbon dioxide, water
Sodium nitrite	Ammonium nitrate and other ammonium salts
Sodium peroxide	Ethyl or methyl alcohol, glacial acetic acid, acetic anhydride, benzaldehyde, carbon disulfide, glycerin, ethylene glycol, ethyl acetate, methyl acetate, furfural
Sulfides	Acids
Sulfuric acid	Potassium chlorate, potassium perchlorate, potassium permanganate (similar compounds of light metals, such as sodium, lithium)
Tellurides	Reducing agents

Reprinted with permission from National Research Council, Committee on Hazardous Substances in the Laboratory. Prudent Practices for Handling Hazardous Chemicals in Laboratories. Washington, D.C.: National Academy Press, 1981. For additional information, see Pipitone DA. Safe Storage of Laboratory Chemicals, 2nd ed. New York: John Wiley & Sons, 1991.

APPENDIX G. NOMOGRAM FOR THE DETERMINATION OF BODY SURFACE AREA

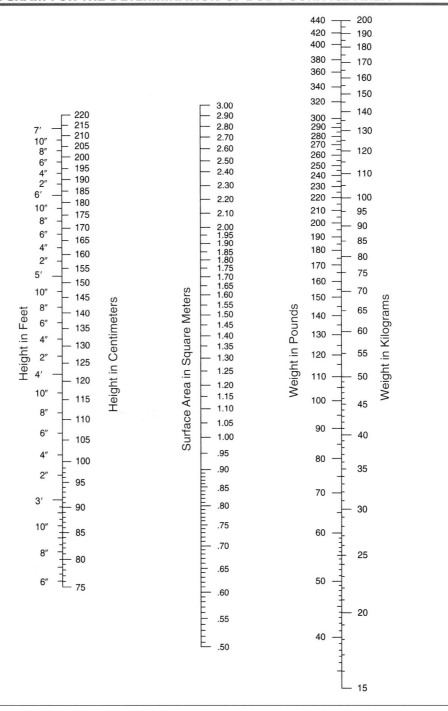

Reprinted by permission from N Engl J Med 1921;185:337.

APPENDIX H. RELATIVE CENTRIFUGAL FORCE NOMOGRAM

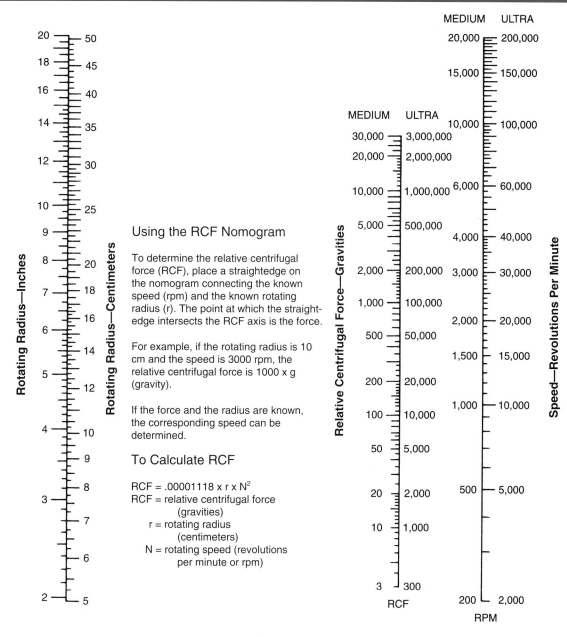

Using the RCF Nomogram

To determine the relative centrifugal force (RCF), place a straightedge on the nomogram connecting the known speed (rpm) and the known rotating radius (r). The point at which the straightedge intersects the RCF axis is the force.

For example, if the rotating radius is 10 cm and the speed is 3000 rpm, the relative centrifugal force is 1000 x g (gravity).

If the force and the radius are known, the corresponding speed can be determined.

To Calculate RCF

$RCF = .00001118 \times r \times N^2$
RCF = relative centrifugal force (gravities)
  r = rotating radius (centimeters)
  N = rotating speed (revolutions per minute or rpm)

Rotating Tip Radius

The distance measured from the rotor axis to the tip of the liquid inside the tubes at the greatest horizontal distance from the rotor axis is the rotating tip radius.

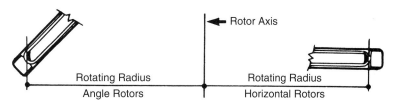

Reprinted by permission from International Equipment Co., Damon Corporation.

APPENDIX I. CENTRIFUGATION—SPEED AND TIME ADJUSTMENT

Use the following formula to calculate the new speed necessary to achieve the relative centrifugal force specified in the original procedure, given a different rotor with a different radius.

$$RPM = 1000 \sqrt{\frac{RCF}{1.12\ r}}$$

where RPM = revolutions per minute (speed)
RCF = relative centrifugal force
r = rotating tip radius in millimeters (check manufacturer's rotor specifications)

Use this formula to calculate the new centrifugation time necessary when a different rotor is used.

$$t_N = \frac{t_0 \times RCF_0}{RCF_N}$$

where t_N = centrifugation time necessary with different rotor
t_0 = time (minutes) specified in original procedure
RCF_N = relative centrifugal force of different rotor
RCF_0 = relative centrifugal force specified in original procedure

APPENDIX J. PERCENT TRANSMITTANCE–ABSORBANCE CONVERSION TABLE

%T	ABSORBANCE[a]				%T	ABSORBANCE[a]			
	.00	.25	.50	.75		.00	.25	.50	.75
1	2.000	1.903	1.824	1.757	52	.284	.282	.280	.278
2	1.690	1.648	1.602	1.561	53	.276	.274	.272	.270
3	1.523	1.488	1.456	1.426	54	.268	.266	.264	.262
4	1.398	1.372	1.347	1.323	55	.260	.258	.256	.254
5	1.301	1.280	1.260	1.240	56	.252	.250	.248	.246
6	1.222	1.204	1.187	1.171	57	.244	.242	.240	.238
7	1.155	1.140	1.126	1.112	58	.237	.235	.233	.231
8	1.097	1.083	1.071	1.059	59	.229	.227	.226	.224
9	1.046	1.034	1.022	1.011	60	.222	.220	.218	.216
10	1.000	.989	.979	.969	61	.215	.213	.211	.209
11	.959	.949	.939	.930	62	.208	.206	.204	.202
12	.921	.912	.903	.894	63	.201	.199	.197	.196
13	.886	.878	.870	.862	64	.194	.192	.191	.189
14	.854	.846	.838	.831	65	.187	.186	.184	.182
15	.824	.817	.810	.803	66	.181	.179	.177	.176
16	.796	.789	.782	.776	67	.174	.172	.171	.169
17	.770	.763	.757	.751	68	.168	.166	.164	.163
18	.745	.739	.733	.727	69	.161	.160	.158	.157
19	.721	.716	.710	.704	70	.155	.153	.152	.150
20	.699	.694	.688	.683	71	.149	.147	.146	.144
21	.678	.673	.668	.663	72	.143	.141	.140	.138
22	.658	.653	.648	.643	73	.137	.135	.134	.132
23	.638	.634	.629	.624	74	.131	.129	.128	.126
24	.620	.615	.611	.606	75	.125	.124	.122	.121
25	.602	.598	.594	.589	76	.119	.118	.116	.115
26	.585	.581	.577	.573	77	.114	.112	.111	.100
27	.569	.565	.561	.557	78	.108	.107	.105	.104
28	.553	.549	.545	.542	79	.102	.101	.100	.098
29	.538	.534	.530	.527	80	.097	.096	.094	.093

APPENDIX J. PERCENT TRANSMITTANCE–ABSORBANCE CONVERSION TABLE (continued)

| %T | ABSORBANCE[a] | | | | %T | ABSORBANCE[a] | | | |
	.00	.25	.50	.75		.00	.25	.50	.75
30	.523	.520	.516	.512	81	.092	.090	.089	.088
31	.509	.505	.502	.498	82	.086	.085	.084	.082
32	.495	.491	.488	.485	83	.081	.080	.078	.077
33	.482	.478	.475	.472	84	.076	.074	.073	.072
34	.469	.465	.462	.459	85	.071	.069	.068	.067
35	.456	.453	.450	.447	86	.066	.064	.063	.062
36	.444	.441	.438	.435	87	.061	.059	.058	.057
37	.432	.429	.426	.423	88	.056	.054	.053	.052
38	.420	.417	.414	.412	89	.051	.049	.048	.047
39	.409	.406	.403	.401	90	.046	.045	.043	.042
40	.398	.395	.392	.390	91	.041	.040	.039	.037
41	.387	.385	.382	.380	92	.036	.035	.034	.033
42	.377	.374	.372	.369	93	.032	.030	.029	.028
43	.367	.364	.362	.359	94	.027	.026	.025	.024
44	.357	.354	.352	.349	95	.022	.021	.020	.019
45	.347	.344	.342	.340	96	.018	.017	.016	.014
46	.337	.335	.332	.330	97	.013	.012	.011	.010
47	.328	.325	.323	.321	98	.009	.008	.007	.006
48	.319	.317	.314	.312	99	.004	.003	.002	.001
49	.310	.308	.305	.303	100	.0000	.0000	.0000	.0000
50	.301	.299	.297	.295					
51	.292	.290	.288	.286					

[a]Absorbance = 2 – log % T.

APPENDIX K. SELECTED ATOMIC WEIGHTS

ELEMENT	SYMBOL	ATOMIC NUMBER	ATOMIC WEIGHT*	VALENCE
Aluminum	Al	13	26.98	3
Antimony	Sb	51	121.75	3,5
Argon	Ar	18	39.95	0
Arsenic	As	33	74.92	3,5
Barium	Ba	56	137.34	2
Beryllium	Be	4	9.01	2
Bismuth	Bi	83	208.98	3,5
Boron	B	5	10.81	3
Bromine	Br	35	79.90	1,3,5,7
Cadmium	Cd	48	112.40	2
Calcium	Ca	20	40.08	2
Carbon	C	6	12.01	2,4
Cerium	Ce	58	140.12	3,4
Cesium	Cs	55	132.91	1
Chlorine	Cl	17	35.45	1,3,5,7
Chromium	Cr	24	51.99	2,3,6
Cobalt	Co	27	58.93	2,3
Copper	Cu	29	63.55	1,2
Fluorine	F	9	18.99	1
Gold	Au	79	196.97	1,3
Helium	He	2	4.00	0
Hydrogen	H	1	1.01	1
Iodine	I	53	126.90	1,3,5,7
Iron	Fe	26	55.85	2,3
Lead	Pb	82	207.19	2,4
Lithium	Li	3	6.94	1
Magnesium	Mg	12	24.31	2
Manganese	Mn	25	54.94	2,3,4,6,7
Mercury	Hg	80	200.59	1,2
Molybdenum	Mo	42	95.94	3,4,6
Nickel	Ni	28	58.71	2,3
Nitrogen	N	7	14.01	3,5
Oxygen	O	8	16.00	2
Phosphorus	P	15	30.97	3,5
Platinum	Pt	78	195.09	2,4
Potassium	K	19	39.10	1
Rubidium	Rb	37	85.47	1
Selenium	Se	34	78.96	2,4,6
Silicon	Si	14	28.09	4
Silver	Ag	47	107.87	1
Sodium	Na	11	22.99	1
Strontium	Sr	38	87.62	2

APPENDIX K. SELECTED ATOMIC WEIGHTS (continued)

ELEMENT	SYMBOL	ATOMIC NUMBER	ATOMIC WEIGHT[a]	VALENCE
Sulfur	S	16	32.06	2,4,6
Tellurium	Te	52	127.60	2,4,6
Tin	Sn	50	118.69	2,4
Tungsten	W	74	183.85	6
Uranium	U	92	238.03	4,6
Xenon	Xe	54	131.30	0
Zinc	Zn	30	65.37	2
Zirconium	Zr	40	91.22	4

[a]Atomic weights are based on C^{12} and have been rounded to two decimal places.

APPENDIX L. CHARACTERISTICS OF TYPES OF GLASS

CATEGORY	TYPE OF MATERIAL	COMMON OR BRAND NAMES	ROUTINE USES	LIMITATIONS
High thermal resistance	Borosilicate with low alkaline content	Pyrex Kimax	All purpose, all types of beakers, flasks, etc. Can tolerate heating and sterilization for lengthy periods of time to 510°C	Should not be cooled too quickly after heating. May cloud after use with a strong alkali. Subject to scratching
	Aluminosilicate	Corex	Centrifuge tubes and thermometers. Extremely strong and hard. Temperature stability to 672°C; short-term use to 850°C	Resists scratching. Subject to some acid or alkali attack at temperature of 100°C
		Vycor	Ashing and ignition techniques. Can withstand very high temperature (900–1200°C), as well as drastic changes in temperature. Most are alkali resistant in this category.	
High silica	96% silica		Cuvets and thermometers. Can be used at high temperatures (900–1200°C) and withstand a sharp change in temperature. Can be considered optically pure (cuvets, thermometers)	
High resistance to alkali	Aluminosilicate		Can be used with strong alkali and suffer minimal attack (0.09 mg/cm² vs. 1.4 mg/cm² for borosilicate or 0.35 mg/cm² for regular aluminosilicate)	Must be heated and cooled with care. Highest temperature for safe use is 578°C

APPENDIX M. CHARACTERISTICS OF TYPES OF PLASTIC

PLASTIC	TEMPERATURE LIMIT (°C)	TRANSPARENCY	AUTOCLAVABLE	FLEXIBILITY	USAGE EXAMPLES
Polystyrene (PS)	70	Clear	No	Rigid	Disposables
Polyethylene Conventional (CPE)	80	Translucent	No	Excellent	All-purpose Reagent bottles Test-tube rack Carboys Droppers
Linear (LPE)	120	Opaque	With caution	Rigid	Specimen transport containers Reagent bottles
Polypropylene (PP)	135	Translucent	Yes	Rigid	Screw-cap closures Bottles
Tygon	95	Translucent	Yes	Excellent	Tubing
Teflon FEP	205	Clear Translucent	Yes	Excellent	Stopcocks Wash bottles Beakers
Polycarbonate (PC)	135	Very clear	Yes	Rigid	All-purpose Large reagent containers Carboys Test-tube rack
Polyvinyl chloride[a] (PVC)	70	Clear	No	Rigid	Bottles/tubing

[a]PVC tubing can be heated to 120°C, can be autoclaved, and is very flexible.

APPENDIX N. CHEMICAL RESISTANCE OF TYPES OF PLASTIC

PLASTIC	CHEMICAL RESISTANCE[a]
Polystyrene	Useful with water and aqueous salt solutions. It is not recommended for use with acids, aldehydes, ketones, ethers, hydrocarbons, or essential oils. Alcohols and bases can be used, but storage beyond 24 h is discouraged.
Polyethylene	Both classifications of polyethylene (*i.e.*, conventional and linear) have similar chemical resistances. They have excellent chemical resistance to most substances, with the exception of aldehydes, amines, ethers, hydrocarbons, and essential oils. For conventional polyethylene, the exceptions should also include lubricating oil and silicones. The usage of any of the above-named chemical groups should be limited to 24 h at room at room temperature.
Polypropylene	Has the same chemical resistance as linear polyethylene.
Teflon	This resin possesses excellent chemical resistance to almost all chemicals used in the clinical laboratory.
Polycarbonate	Very susceptible to damage by most chemicals. It is resistant to water, aqueous salts, food, and inorganic acids for a long period of time.

[a]It should be noted that this information is based on room temperature (22°C) and normal atmospheric pressure. Resistance to chemicals decreases as the temperature of the resin nears its maximum. Chemical resistance will also vary as the concentration of the chemical increases.

APPENDIX O. CLEANING LABWARE

GLASSWARE "PROBLEM"	CLEANING TECHNIQUE
General usage (procedure 1 is recommended for routine washing needs)	1. *Dirty* glassware should be immediately placed in a soapy or dilute bleach solution and allowed to soak. Wash using any detergent designed for labware. Rinse with tap water 3 times, followed by 1 rinse with distilled water. Dry in an oven at temperature less than 140°C.
	2. *Acid dichromate.* Dissolve 50 g technical-grade sodium dichromate in 50 mL of distilled water. Add this mixture to 500 mL of technical-grade concentrated sulfuric acid. This solution is useful until a green color develops. Store in a covered glass jar. Soak glassware overnight and then rinse with dilute ammonia. Rewash glassware according to procedure 1.
	3. *Nitric acid* (20%). Soak for 12–24 hours. Wash according to procedure 1.
Blood clots	4. *Sodium hydroxide* (10%). Soak for 12–24 hours; then follow routine procedure. Dry micropipets using an acetone rinse.
New pipets (S1 alkaline)	5. *Rinse* with 5% hydrochloric acid or 5% nitric acid. Wash following routine procedure.
Metal ion determinations	6. *Acid soak* (20% nitric acid), for 12–24 hours. Rinse with distilled water 3–4 times. Water should be fresh for each rinsing step. Dry.
Grease	7. *Soak* in any organic solvent.
	8. *Dissolve* 100 g potassium hydroxide in 100 mL of distilled water. Allow to cool. Add 900 mL commercial-grade 10% ethanol. Not to be used for delicate glassware.
	9. *Contrad 70* (manufactured by Decon Labs).
Permanganate stains	10. *50% Hydrochloric acid.* Rinse with tap water. Wash.
	11. *Dissolve* 1% ferrous sulfate in 25% sulfuric acid.

APPENDIX P. SUMMARY TABLE OF PHARMACOKINETIC PARAMETERS

	THERAPEUTIC RANGE PER mL PLASMA	TOXIC CONC. PER mL PLASMA	TIME TO PEAK CONC. (HOURS)	HALF-LIFE (HOURS)	% PROTEIN BOUND	VOLUME OF DISTRIBUTION (L/kg)	% ORAL BIOAVAILABILITY	% EXCRETED IN URINE UNCHANGED
Cardioactive drugs								
Amiodarone	1.0–3 μg		2–6	15–100 days	95–98	70–150	22–88	0
Digitoxin	15–30 ng	>35		2.4–16.4 days	90	0.6	95	30–50
Digoxin	0.8–2 ng	>2.4	1–5	36–51	20–40	5–10	Tablets, 60–75 Elixir, 80 Capsules, 95 IM, 80	60–80
Disopyramide	2–5 μg	>7	0.5–3.0	5–6	10–80	0.8–2	80	
Lidocaine	1.5–5 μg 0.5–1.5 free	>5	15–30[a]	1–2	70	1.3	25–50[b]	5–10
Procainamide	4–10 μg	>12	1–2	2.5–4.7	15	1.7–2.2	70–95	50
NAPA	15–25 μg			4.3–15				
Total	5–30 μg							
Propranolol	50–100 ng	Variable	1–2	2–6	90–95	4–6	20–40[b]	1–4
Quinidine	2–6 μg	>6	1–2 4–8[c]	6–8	70–90	2–3	70–80[b]	10–30
Antiepileptic drugs								
Carbamazepine	6–12 μg	>15	6–12	18–54[d] 10–25[e]	72–75	0.8–1.4	75–85	2
Ethosuximide	40–100 μg	>150	1–4	40–60	<10	0.6–0.9	100	10–20
Phenobarbital	15–40 μg	>40	6–18	50–120	49–58	0.6	80–100	10–30
Phenytoin	10–20 μg	>20	4–8	7–42	87–93	0.5–0.8	85–95	5
Primidone	5–12 μg	>15	2–4	3.3–19	0–20	0.6–1	80–90	45–50
Valproic Acid	50–100 μg	>100	1–2	8–20	85–95	0.1–0.5	85–100	3
Bronchodilator								
Theophylline	10–20 μg	>20	2–3	6–12	55–65	0.3–0.7	95–100	9–11
Antibiotics								
Aminoglycosides			0.5–IM[a]					
Amikacin	5–12 μg							
Peak	50–100 μg	>32						
Trough	10–20 μg	>5						
Gentamicin								
Peak	20–25 μg	>12						
Trough	1–4 μg	>2						
Kanamycin								
Peak	5–10 μg	>30						
Trough	0.5–1.5 μg	>10						
Netilmicin								
Peak	5–12 μg	>12						
Trough	0.5–1.5 μg	>2						

APPENDIX P. SUMMARY TABLE OF PHARMACOKINETIC PARAMETERS (continued)

	THERAPEUTIC RANGE PER mL PLASMA	TOXIC CONC. PER mL PLASMA	TIME TO PEAK CONC. (HOURS)	HALF-LIFE (HOURS)	% PROTEIN BOUND	VOLUME OF DISTRIBUTION (L/kg)	% ORAL BIOAVAILABILITY	% EXCRETED IN URINE UNCHANGED
Antibiotics (continued)								
Streptomycin								
Peak	20–25 μg	>30						
Trough	1–3 μg	>10						
Tobramycin								
Peak	5–12 μg	>12						
Trough	0.5–1.5 μg	>2						
Vancomycin								
Peak	30–40 μg	>80		3–9	50	0.5–0.8	<2	80–90
Trough	5–10 μg	>20						
Chloramphenicol	10–20 μg	>25	2	1.5–3	50	0.5–1	90	10
Psychoactive drugs								
Amitriptyline	125–250 ng	>500	1–5	17–40	82–96	6.4–36	56–70	
Nortriptyline	50–150 ng	>500	3–12	16–88	87–95	14–38	46–70	2–5
Imipramine	150–250 ng	>500[f]	1.5–3	6–34	63–96	9–23	29–77	1–4
Desipramine	150–300 ng	>500	3–6	11–46	73–92	15–60	31–51	1–4
Doxepin	110–250 ng		1–4	8–36	68–82	9–52	13–45	
Protriptyline	70–260 ng		6–12	54–198	90–94	15–31	75–90	
Lithium	0.8–1.4 μEq	>2	1–3	8–35[g]	0	0.5–1.0	85–95	100
Immunosuppressants								
Cyclosporine (HPLC)	100–300 ng	>400	1–8	4–60	98	3.5–4.5	4–90	<6
Antineoplastics								
Methotrexate	After 24 hours > 10^{-5} M		1–2	Variable	50–70	0.75–0.8	30	90
	After 48 hours > 10^{-6} M							
	After 72 hours > 10^{-7} M							

[a]Varies dependent on dosage regimen, immediately after IV infusion.
[b]Much of the drug metabolized on first pass through the liver.
[c]Slow-release preparation.
[d]After single dose.
[e]After multiple doses.
[f]Imipramine + desipramine.
[g]Variable with renal function.

APPENDIX Q. SELECTED INFORMATION ON COMMONLY ABUSED DRUGS

DRUG	STREET NAME (TRADE NAME)	ROUTE OF INGESTION	DURATION OF EFFECT (HOURS)	HALF-LIFE (HOURS)	EXCRETED UNCHANGED IN URINE	PRINCIPAL URINARY METABOLITES	SYMPTOMATOLOGY
Stimulants							
Cocaine	Coke, crack, snow flake	Nasal, oral, IV, smoked	1–2	2–5	<10%	Benzoylecgonine; ecgonine; ecgonine methyl ester	Anesthesia, euphoria, confusion, depression, convulsions, cardiotoxicity
Amphetamine	Bennies, dexies, uppers	Oral, IV	2–4	4–24	~30%	Benzoic acid; p-hydroxyamphetamine; p-hydroxynorephedrine; phenylacetone	Insomnia, anorexia, euphoria, tolerance and dependence, paranoid psychosis
Methamphetamine	Meth, speed, crystal	Oral, IV	2–4	9–24	10–20%	4-Hydroxymethamphetamine; amphetamine; 4-thyroxy-amphetamine; norephedrine	Euphoria, agitation, psychosis, depression, exhaustion
Narcotics							
Heroin	Horse, smack, white lady, scag	IV, nasal, smoked	3–6	1–1.5	<1%	6-Acetylmorphine; morphine; morphine glucuronide	Euphoria, drowsiness, respiratory depression, convulsions, coma
Codeine	C; Co-Dine; Lean and dean; School Boy; Syrup	Oral, IV, IM	3–6	2–4	5–20%	Morphine; norcodeine; conjugates	Sedation, convulsions, respiratory failure
Morphine	Junk, white stuff, morpho, M	IV, IM, oral, smoked	3–6	2–4	<10%	Morphine-3-glucuronide; morphine-6-glucuronide; morphine sulfate; nor-morphine; codeine	Analgesia, euphoria, nausea, respiratory coma
Methadone	Methadose	Oral, IV, IM	12–24	15–60	5–50%	2-Ethylidene-1, 5-dimethyl-3,3-diphenylpyrroline; 2-ethyl-5methyl-3,3-diphenyl-pyrroline methadol; normethadol; conjugates	Analgesia, sedation, respiratory depression, coma
Meperidine	(Demerol)	IV, oral	3–6	2–5	5%	Normeperidine; meperidinic acid; normeperidinic acid	Analgesia, stupor, respiratory depression, hypotension, coma
Propoxyphene	Yellow footballs (Darvon)	Oral	1–6	8–24	<1%	Norpropoxyphene; dinor-propoxyphene	Analgesia, stupor, respiratory depression, coma
Hallucinogens							
Phencyclidine (PCP)	PCP, angel dust, hog, killer weed	IV, oral, nasal, smoked	2–4; psychoses may last weeks	7–16	30–50%	4-Phenyl-4-piperidinocyclohexanol; 1-(1-phenylcyclohexyl)-4-hydroxy-piperidine; glucuronide conjugates	Dissociative anesthesia, depression, psychosis, stupor, coma, seizures

Drug	Slang names	Route	Peak	Duration	%	Metabolites	Effects
LSD	Acid, LSD-25, white lightning, microdots	Oral	8–12	3–4	1%	N-Desmethyllysergide; 13-hydroxylysergide	Hallucinations, flashbacks, psychosis, vomiting, paralysis, respiratory depression
Marijuana, hashish	Pot, THC, mary jane, grass, hash	Oral, smoked, IV	2–4	14–38	<1%	11-Nor-9-carboxy-Δ^9-THC; 11-hydroxytetrahydrocannabinol	Altered perception, memory loss, disorientation, psychosis
Benzodiazepines							
Chlordiazepoxide	(Librium)	Oral, IM	4–8	6–27	<1%	Norchlordiazepoxide; demoxepam; nordiazepam; oxazepam; glucuronide conjugates	Drowsiness, muscle relaxation, coma
Diazepam	(Valium)	Oral, IV, IM	4–8	20–50	<1%	Nordiazepam; oxazepam; 3-hydroxydiazepam; glucuronide conjugates	Drowsiness, dizziness, muscle relaxation
Sedatives/Depressants							
Pentobarbital	Yellow, nembies, yellow jackets	Oral, IV, IM	3–6	15–48	1%	3-Hydroxypentobarbital; N-hydroxpentobarbital; 3-carboxypentobarbital	Sedation, respiratory collapse
Amobarbital	Rainbows, blues, bluebirds	Oral, IV, IM	3–24	12–60	<1%	3-Hydroxyamobarbital; N-glucosyl amobarbital	Exhilaration, sedation, disorientation, respiratory depression, coma
Secobarbital	Reds, seccies, red devils, M & M's	Oral, IV, IM	3–6	15–40	5%	3-Hydroxysecobarbital secodiol; 5-(1-methylbutyl) barbituric acid	Sedation, lethargy, coma, respiratory collapse
Ethanol		Oral	2–6	2–14	2–10%	Acetaldehyde; acetic acid glucuronide	Slurred speech, loss of equilibrium, drowsiness, coma, respiratory collapse
Methaqualone	Ludes, soapers	Oral	4–8	20–60	<1%	3',4'-, and 6-Hydroxymethatesqualone; respective glucuronide	Sedation, dizziness, paresthesias, convulsions, respiratory and circulatory depression
Chloral hydrate	Joy juice	Oral, rectal	5–8	<1	<1%	Trichloroethanol; trichloroacetic acid; conjugates	Sedation, GI distress, hypotension, respiratory depression

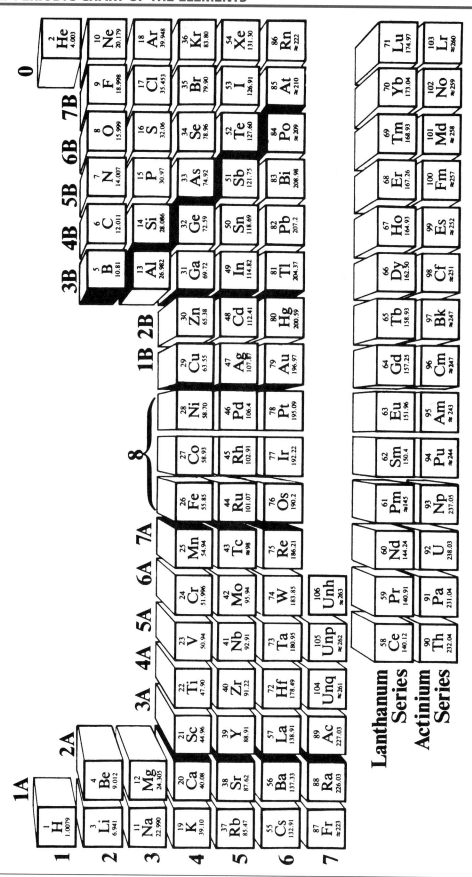

Source: Monroe M, Abrams K. Experimental Chemistry: A Laboratory Course. Belmont, CA: Star Publishing Company, 1991. Reprinted with permission.

Glossary

A

Accuracy: without error; closeness to the true value.

Acid: a substance that can yield a hydrogen ion or hydronium ion when dissolved in water.

Acidemia: a pH of blood less than the reference range.

Acidosis: a pH below the reference range.

Acromegaly: chronic disease of middle-aged individuals typified by elongation and enlargement of the extremities and certain head bones.

ACTH: see Adrenocorticotropic hormone.

Activation energy: energy required to raise all molecules in 1 mole of a compound at a certain temperature to the transition state at the peak of the energy barrier.

Activator: a substance that converts an inactive substance to an active one; induces activity.

Active transport: a mechanism that requires energy in order to move ions across cellular membranes.

Activity coefficient (AC): relating to the study of vitamins, an expression indicating the enhancement of enzyme activity upon saturation with a vitamin. The greater the AC, the more likely the patient is to be deficient in the vitamin.

Acute coronary syndromes: a progression of pathologic conditions involved in ischemic heart disease, including erosion and rupture of coronary artery plaques, activation of platelets, and thrombi. This progression is termed the acute coronary syndromes and ranges from unstable angina to extensive tissue necrosis in acute myocardial infarction.

Acute renal failure: a sudden, sharp decline in renal operation as a result of an acute toxic or hypoxic insult to the kidneys. This has been defined as occurring when the glomerular filtration rate (GFR) is reduced to <10 mL/minute.

Adaptive immune system: one of two functional parts of the immune system; it produces a specific reaction to each infectious agent, then normally eradicates that agent and remembers that particular infectious agent, preventing it from causing disease later. For example, measles and diphtheria produce a lifelong immunity following an infection.

Addison's disease: disease stemming from a deficiency in the secretion of adrenocortical hormones.

ADH: see Antidiuretic hormone.

Adrenal glands: paired organs located with one at the upper pole of each kidney. Each gland consists of an outer cortex and an inner medulla, which have different embryological origins, different mechanisms of control, and different products.

Adrenocorticotropic hormone (ACTH): a peptide hormone secreted by the anterior pituitary. It stimulates the cortex of the adrenal glands to produce adrenal cortical hormones.

Affinity: attraction or force causing two substances to unite.

Aging: maturing; a progressive loss of adaptation leading to decreased viability and life expectancy and increased vulnerability.

Airborne pathogen: any infectious agent transmissible by air, *eg,* tuberculosis.

Albumin: the main protein in plasma.

Aldosterone: the principal mineralocorticoid (electrolyte-regulating hormone) produced by the zona glomerulosa of the adrenal cortex.

Alkalemia: a blood pH greater than the reference range ($\sim$7.35–7.45).

Alkalosis: a pH above the reference range.

Allantoin: produced by the oxidation of uric acid by the enzyme uricase. It is the end product of purine metabolism.

Allograft: transplant tissue from the same species (*eg,* kidney).

Amenorrhea: cessation of menstruation.

Amine: any one of a group of nitrogen-containing organic compounds. The amine hormones include epinephrine, norepinephrine, thyroxine, and triiodothyronine.

Amino acid: small biomolecules with a tetrahedral carbon covalently bound to an amino group, a carboxyl group, a variable (R) group, and a hydrogen atom.

Aminoacidopathies: inherited disorders of amino acid metabolism.

Ammonia: NH_3; formed *in vivo* from breakdown of amino acids.

Amniocentesis: puncture of the amniotic sac to obtain fluid for analysis.

Amniotic fluid: a fluid in which the fetus is suspended; it provides a cushioning medium for the fetus and serves as a matrix for influx and efflux of constituents.

Amphoteric: having two or more ionizable sites that can result in either a net positive or a net negative charge depending on the pH of the environment.

Amplicon: amplified target DNA sequences.

Analgesic: a drug that relieves pain.

Analyte: a biologic solute or constituent (*eg,* calcium, glucose, sodium).

Analytical error: error due to the instrument's, procedure's, or laboratory scientist's handling of a specimen during testing.

Analytical variations: nonidentical measurements that have diverse causes, including instrument, reagent, and operator variations.

Androgen: any substance (hormone) stimulating the development of male characteristics (*eg,* testosterone).

Anneal: the action of pairing complementary sequences to form a double-stranded molecule, usually DNA or RNA molecules.

Angina pectoris: pain and a feeling of constriction around the heart; may radiate down the arm and into the jaw and is caused by deficiency of oxygen to heart muscle.

Angiotensin: a polypeptide produced when renin is released from the kidney; a vasopressor substance.

Anhydrous: without water.

Anion: a negatively charged ion; anions move toward the anode (positive pole) because of its positive charge.

Anion gap: the difference between unmeasured anions and unmeasured cations.

Antecubital fossa: area of forearm at the bend of the elbow; most commonly used for venipuncture.

Anterior pituitary: adenohypophysis. The pituitary is located in a small cavity in the sphenoid bone of the skull called the sella turcica. The tropic hormones of the anterior pituitary are mediated by negative feedback, which involves interaction of the effector hormones with the hypothalamus, as well as with cells of the anterior pituitary.

Anthropometric methods: used to assess the general nutritional status of a patient. Includes skin fold test and arm circumference and height and weight measurements.

Antibody: glycoproteins (immunoglobulins) secreted by plasma cells, which in turn are under the control of many lymphocytes and their cytokines. Antibodies are produced in response to antigens.

Anticoagulant: inhibits the blood's clotting action; yields specimens containing intact clotting factors.

Antidiuretic hormone (ADH): vasopressin; produced by the hypothalamus.

Antigen: agents that are recognized as foreign by the immune system. The immune system produces antibodies in response.

Antigenic determinant: a part of an antigens structure that is recognized as foreign by the immune system. This structural domain is also referred to as an epitope.

Antioxidant: substance (*eg,* vitamin) that inhibits or prevents oxidation.

Antiplatelet therapy: therapy to destroy platelets.

Apoenzyme: protein portion of an enzyme.

Apoptosis: programmed death of cells; disintegration of body cells into membrane-bound particles that can then be phagocytized by other cells.

Arrhythmia: irregular heartbeat or action.

Arterial blood: blood from arteries.

Arterial septal defect: heart abnormality that causes left-to-right shunting of blood between the atria.

Arteriosclerosis: includes a number of pathological conditions in which there is a thickening or hardening of the walls of the arteries.

Ascites: excess fluid in the peritoneal cavity; the fluid is called ascitic fluid.

Atherosclerosis: a disease in which there is an accumulation of lipid material in the veins and arteries.

Autocrine system: cell secretions that act to influence only their own development.

Atomic absorption: analytical technique that measures concentration of analyte by detecting absorption of electromagnetic radiation by atoms rather than by molecules. Instrument is atomic absorption spectrophotometer.

Autoimmune disorder: disease or disorder in which the body produces antibodies (immunological response) against itself.

Automation: mechanization of the steps in a procedure. Manufacturers of clinical chemistry analyzers design their instruments to mimic the manual techniques in an analytical procedure.

Atrial septal defects (ASD): abnormality causing left-to-right shunting of blood between the atria.

Avidity: strength of bond of antigen-antibody complex; attraction.

Azotemia: elevated level of urea in blood.

B

Bar code: a set of vertical bars of varying width used to encode information. Used most frequently in the clinical laboratory for patient and specimen information.

Basal state: early morning before the patient has eaten or become physically active. This is a good time to draw blood specimens because the body is at rest and food has not been ingested during the night.

Base: a substance that can yield hydroxyl ions (OH^-).

Base excess (BE): the theoretical amount of titratable acid or base required to return the plasma pH to 7.40 at a PCO_2 of 40 mm Hg at 37°C.

Beer's law: mathematically establishes the relationship between concentration and absorbance in photometric determinations; expressed as: A = *abc*.

Beriberi: chronic deficiency of the vitamin thiamin produces the disease beriberi.

Bicarbonate: the HCO_3^- anion.

Bile: a fluid produced by the liver and composed of bile acids or salts, bile pigments (primarily bilirubin esters), cholesterol, and other substances extracted from the blood. Total bile production averages about 3 L/day, although only 1 L is excreted.

Bilirubin: the principal pigment in bile; derived from the breakdown of hemoglobin when aged red blood cells are phagocytized by the reticuloendothelial system, primarily in the spleen, liver, and bone marrow.

Biohazard: anything harmful or potentially harmful to man, other organisms, or the environment. Examples include blood or blood products and contaminated laboratory waste.

β-Blocking drug: drug that reduces heart rate and/or the force of contractions, reducing the oxygen demand of the heart by blocking the β receptors in the sinus mode and the myocardium (*eg,* propranolol).

Bloodborne pathogen: any infectious agent or pathogen transmissible by means of blood or blood products.

Bone mineral densitometry (DXA): x-ray procedure that measures bone mineral density, measure grams of calcium per square centimeter of cross sectional area of bone (g/cm^2).

Bone turnover: coupled process that takes place throughout life in bone with bone formation and bone resorption.

Buffer: a substance that minimizes any change in hydrogen ion concentration; a weak acid or base and its conjugate salt.

BUN/creatinine ratio: ratio of plasma or serum urea nitrogen (mg/dL) to plasma or serum creatinine (mg/dL).

Buret: a wide, long, graduated pipet with a stopcock at one end.

C

CAH: see Congenital adrenal hyperplasia.

Calcitonin: hormone produced by the thyroid gland; important in bone and calcium metabolism.

Calibration: standardization or the determination of the accuracy of an instrument.

Cancer: the uncontrolled growth of cells from normal tissue. Cancer cells can grow and spread, killing the host.

Capillary blood: blood from minute blood vessels.

Carbohydrate: polyhydroxy aldehydes or polyhydroxy ketones, or multimeric units of such compounds. The general formula of a carbohydrate is $(CH_2O)_n$.

Carbonic acid: H_2CO_3.

Carcinogen: cancer causing agent.

Carcinoid syndrome: syndrome produced by metastatic carcinoid tumors that secrete excessive amounts of serotonin.

Cardiac catheterization: invasive technique where a catheter is placed into a peripheral vessel and advanced into the heart.

Cardiac glycosides: drugs used to increase the contractility of the heart and slow the conduction impulses (*eg*, digoxin).

Cardiac markers: diagnostic test or analyte used to assess cardiac function.

Cardiac radiology: use of x-rays to assess heart size and position, etc.

Cardiomyopathy: disease of the myocardium.

Cardiovascular nuclear imaging: technique using radionuclides to assess cardiovascular performance and perfusion of the myocardium and viability of the cardiac muscle.

Cation: a positively charged ion; cations migrate in the direction of the cathode because of their positive charge.

CCK: see Cholecystokinin.

Centrifugal analysis: analytical technique that uses the force generated by centrifugation to transfer and then contain liquids in separate cuvets for measurement at the perimeter of a spinning rotor.

Centrifugation: a process whereby centrifugal force is used to separate solid matter from a liquid suspension.

Cerebrospinal fluid (CSF): a selective ultrafiltrate of the plasma that surrounds the brain and spinal cord.

Ceruloplasmin: an α_2-glycoprotein to which copper is attached; more than 90–95% of the circulating copper in the plasma is bound to ceruloplasmin.

Chain-of-custody: records each step and each person who handled a sample (for toxicological analysis) from time of collection to time of analysis.

Channel: on an automated analyzer, a path or passage for reagents, specimens or electrical impulses. Automated analyzers may be single or multiple channel analyzers.

Character: the number to the left of the decimal point in a logarithmic expression.

Chelator: causing the joining of an ion (*eg*, metal) and a ring structured chemical.

Chemical hygiene: procedures and work practices for regulating exposure of laboratory personnel to hazardous chemicals.

Chemical toxin: a substance that is a poison.

Chemiluminescence: light produced as a result of a chemical reaction. Most important chemiluminescence reactions are oxidation reactions of luminol, acridinium esters, and dioxetanes and are characterized by a rapid increase in intensity of emitted light followed by a gradual decay.

Cholecystokinin: CCK, formerly called pancreozymin; a hormone produced by the pancreas. CCK, in the presence of fats and/or amino acids in the duodenum, is produced by the cells of the intestinal mucosa and responsible for release of enzymes from the acinar cells by the pancreas into the pancreatic juice.

Cholesterol: an unsaturated steroid alcohol of high molecular weight, consisting of a perhydrocyclopentanthroline ring and a side chain of eight carbon atoms. In its esterified form, it contains one fatty acid molecule.

Chronic renal failure: a clinical syndrome that occurs when there is a gradual decline in renal operation over time.

Chylomicrons: large triglyceride rich particles.

Cirrhosis: derived from the Greek word that means ``yellow.'' However, in current usage, cirrhosis refers to the irreversible scarring process by which normal liver architecture is transformed into abnormal nodular architecture.

CK isoforms: produced as a part of the normal clearance mechanism for CK isoenzymes and are present in all sera.

Clearance: volume of plasma filtered by glomeruli per unit time.

Clinical Laboratory Improvement Amendments (CLIA): regulations signed into federal law in 1988; mandate standards in clinical laboratory operations and testing.

Closed collection system: a type of collection system in which blood is taken directly from a patient's vein into a stoppered tube; the sample is completely contained, thereby reducing the risk of outside contaminants to the sample and reducing the hazard of the collector's exposure to the blood; also known as the evacuated-tube system.

Closed tube sampling: an instrument's ability to remove the patient's sample for analysis from the primary collection tube by piercing through the stopper.

Coarctation of aorta: narrowing of the aorta at the insertion of the ductus arteriosus.

Coenzyme: an enzyme activator (*eg*, coenzyme a).

Cofactor: a nonprotein molecule that may be necessary for enzyme activity.

Colligative property: the properties of osmotic pressure, freezing point, boiling point, and vapor pressure.

Common variable agammaglobulinemia: also known as acquired agammaglobulinemia. This disorder represents a group of disorders characterized by hypogammaglobulinemia.

Compensation: the body's attempt to return the pH toward normal whenever an imbalance occurs.

Competitive immunoassay: see Competitive protein binding.

Competitive protein binding: also competitive immunoassay. Labeled and unlabeled antigen compete for limited antibody sites. Labeled antigen bound to antibody will be inversely proportional to the concentration of antigen.

Conductivity: relates to the ease in which electricity passes through a solution.

Congenital adrenal hyperplasia (CAH): results from the lack of an enzyme necessary for the production of cortisol.

Congenital agammaglobulinemia: X-linked agammaglobulinemia, also called Bruton disease. This disorder presents with early onset of recurrent pyogenic infections. These patients have no circulating B cells, low concentrations of all circulating immunoglobulin classes, and absence of plasma cells in all lymphoid tissue. T cells are not involved.

Congestive heart disease: (also congestive heart failure) results from an inability of the heart to pump blood effectively.

Conjugated bilirubin: bilirubin diglucuronide; it is water-soluble and is secreted from the hepatic cell into the bile canaliculi and then passes along with the rest of the bile into larger bile ducts and eventually into the intestines.

Conjugated protein: composed of a protein (amino acids) and a nonprotein moiety.

Conn's syndrome: aldosterone-secreting adrenal adenoma.

Continuous flow: an approach to automated analysis in which liquids (reagents, diluents, and samples) are pumped through a system of continuous tubing. Samples are introduced in a sequential manner, following each other through the same network. A series of air bubbles at regular intervals serve as separating and cleaning media.

Control: a substance or material of determined value, used to monitor the accuracy and precision of a test. Controls are run with the patient's specimens.

Control rule: criterion for judging whether an analytical process is out of control; error detection criteria.

Corpus albicans: fibrous tissue that replaces a degenerating corpus luteum.

Corpus luteum: small body that develops within a ruptured ovarian follicle; secretes progesterone.

Corrosive chemical: chemicals injurious to the skin or eyes by direct contact or to the tissues of the respiratory and gastrointestinal tracts if inhaled or ingested. Examples include acids (acetic, sulfuric, nitric, and hydrochloric) and bases (ammonium hydroxide, potassium hydroxide, and sodium hydroxide).

Cortical bone: type of bone that is very strong in the axial and cross-sectional dimensions, very well suited to the needs of the long bones.

Corticotropin-releasing hormone (CRH): A hormone released from the hypothalamus that acts on the anterior pituitary to increase ACTH secretion.

Cortisol: a steroid hormone produced by the adrenal glands.

Countercurrent multiplier system: process occurring in the loop of Henle whereby a high osmolality is maintained within the kidney and a hypoosmolal urine is produced.

Coupled enzymatic method: use of several sequential enzymatic reactions that produce a product which can be detected spectrophotometrically and whose concentration will be related to the analyte in question.

Creatine: compound found in muscle synthesized from several amino acids. It combines with high-energy phosphate to form creatine phosphate, which functions as an energy compound in muscle.

Creatinine: compound formed when creatine or creatine phosphate spontaneously loses water or phosphoric acid. It is excreted into the plasma at a relatively constant rate in a given individual and excreted in the urine.

Creatinine clearance: rate of removal of creatinine from plasma. Calculated as urine creatinine concentration times 24-hour urine volume divided by serum creatinine concentration or UV/P, expressed in mL/minute. Usually corrected to normal body surface area.

CRH: see Corticotropin-releasing hormone.

Cross-reactivity: capability of an antibody to react with an antigen that is structurally similar to the homologous antigen.

Cryogenic material: material brought to low temperatures, such as liquefied gases.

CSF: see Cerebrospinal fluid.

Cushing's syndrome: syndrome resulting from excessive production of glucocorticoids by adrenal cortex.

Cyclosporine: a cyclic polypeptide of fungal origin. It consists of 11 amino acids and has a molecular weight of 1203. It inhibits the immune response selectively by inhibiting the interleukin-2-dependent proliferation of activated T cells that destroy the allograft. The immune response is frozen and unresponsive.

Cytochrome: a pigment that plays a role in respiration, such as hemoglobin or myoglobin.

Cytokines: extracellular factors produced by a variety of cells including monocytes, lymphocytes and other nonlymphoid cells. They are important in controlling local and systemic inflammatory responses.

D

Dehydroepiandrosterone (DHEA): an androgen primarily derived from the adrenal gland.

Deionized water: water purified by ion exchange.

Deliquescent substances: compounds that absorb enough water from the atmosphere to cause dissolution.

Delta absorbance: difference in absorbance, known as delta absorbance or ΔA.

Delta check: an algorithm in which the most recent result of a patient is compared with the previously determined value.

Denaturation: alteration of a substance (eg, proteins) to alter physical and chemical properties.

Density: weight of a substance compared with a standard; expressed in terms of mass per unit volume.

Descriptive statistics: statistics or values (eg, mean, median, mode) used to summarize the important features of a group of data.

Desiccant: causing dryness; materials that can remove moisture from the air as well as from other materials.

Desiccator: a closed chamber for drying substances.

DHEA: see Dehydroepiandrosterone.

Diabetes mellitus: a diverse group of hyperglycemic disorders with different etiologies and clinical pictures.

Dialysis: a method for separating macromolecules from a solvent.

Diffusion: the movement of the molecules of a substance from a location of higher concentration to one of lesser concentration; as in gel diffusion precipitation.

Dilution: a dilution represents the ratio of concentrated or stock material to the total final volume of a solution and consists of the volume or weight of the concentrate plus the volume of the diluent (the concentration units remaining the same).

Direct effector: hormone that acts directly on peripheral tissues.

Direct immunofluorescence: detection of antigens with fluorescent labeled antibody.

Disaccharide: separate carbohydrates, or monosaccharides joined together.

Discrete analysis: an approach to automated analysis in which each sample and accompanying reagents is in a separate container. Discrete analyzers have the capability of running multiple tests one sample at a time or multiple samples one test at a time.

Dispersion: the spread of data; most simply estimated by the range, the difference between the largest and smallest observations. The most commonly used statistic for describing the dispersion of groups of single observations is the standard deviation, which is usually represented by the symbol s.

Distal tubule: portion of renal tubule extending from ascending limb of loop of Henle to the collecting duct.

Distilled water: water solely purified by distillation results

Diuretics: agents that increase the secretion of urine.

DNA index (DI): ploidy status of malignancies; the amount of measured DNA in cancer cells relative to that in normal cells.

DNA probe: a known fragment of DNA molecule used to join with or locate an unknown or comparable DNA strand. Human papilloma virus DNA has been detected using DNA probes.

Done nomogram: a chart that approximates drug toxicity, given the time of ingestion and blood drug level.

Dopamine: the only neuroendocrine signal that inhibits prolactin.

Dose-response relationship: comparison of the dose of a substance (ie, drug or chemical) with its potential pathologic effects. Dose-response relationship implies that there will be an increase in toxic response with an increased dose.

Drug absorption: uptake of a drug in the gastrointestinal tract into the body.

Drug disposition: the way in which the body handles a foreign compound, the drug. The mechanisms used by the body to handle a drug can be explained in terms of four general processes: absorption, distribution, metabolism, and excretion.

Drug distribution: the circulation and diffusion of a drug into the interstitial and intracellular spaces.

Drug elimination: clearance of a drug from the body by a variety of mechanisms.

Drugs of abuse: drugs used illegally or inappropriately; many drugs have the potential for abuse.

Dry chemistry slide: a multilayered film technology (dry chemicals) used by the Vitros series of automated analyzers. All reagents necessary for a particular test are contained on the "slide."

Dual-energy x-ray absorptiometry (DEXA): x-ray procedure that measures bone mineral density by measuring grams of calcium per square centimeter of cross-sectional area of bone (g/cm²).

Duplex: a hybrid formed from complementary strands of nucleic acid from unrelated sources bound together.

Dyslipidemias: diseases associated with abnormal lipid concentrations.

E

ECG: see Electrocardiography.

Echocardiography: noninvasive diagnostic technique that uses high-frequency sound waves to show the heart structure on a CRT screen.

Ectopic: in an abnormal position or location.

Ectopic hormone production: hormones produced by cells in sites other than the gland from which they are usually derived.

EDTA: ethylenediaminetetraacetic acid; anticoagulant used in lavender and royal blue stopper blood collection tubes. Commonly used for whole blood hematology studies.

Effusion: abnormal accumulations of pleural or pericardial fluid.

Electrocardiography (ECG): test used to evaluate the electrical stimulation of the heart.

Electrochemistry: the use of galvanic and electrolytic cells (electrochemical cells) for chemical analysis. Examples include potentiometry, amperometry, coulometry, and polarography.

Electrodes: electronic sensing devices to measure PO_2, PCO_2, and pH.

Electrolyte: ions capable of carrying an electric charge.

Electrophoresis: migration of charged solutes or particles in an electrical field.

Embden-Myerhof pathway: series of steps involving the anaerobic metabolism of glucose, glycogen or starch to lactic acid; principal means of producing energy in man.

Encephalopathy: disorder or dysfunction of brain.

Endocrine gland: a ductless gland that produces a secretion (hormone) into the blood or lymph to be carried by the circulation to other parts of the body.

Endogenous: triglycerides synthesized in liver and other tissues.

Enzyme: specific biologically synthesized proteins that catalyze biochemical reactions without altering the equilibrium point of the reaction or being consumed or undergoing changes in composition.

Enzyme-substrate complex: a physical binding of a substrate to the active site of an enzyme.

Epinephrine: an amine hormone. The adrenal medulla primarily produces epinephrine.

Epitope: component of an antigen that functions as an antigenic determinant, allowing the attachment of certain antibodies.

Equivalent weight: equal to the molecular weight of a substance divided by its valence.

Erectile dysfunction: inability to have or maintain an erection.

Erythropoietin: a hormone that stimulates red blood cell production.

Essential element: an element that is absolutely necessary for life. Deficiency or absence of the element will cause a severe alteration of function and/or eventually lead to death.

Essential hypertension: hypertension with no known cause.

Estimated glomerular filtration rate (EGFR): equation used to predict the Glomerular Filtration Rate and is based on serum creatinine, age, body size, gender and race, without the need of a urine creatinine.

Estriol: an estrogenic hormone; estriol is not produced in significant quantities in the mother and is solely a reflection of fetoplacental function. Thus estriol measurement provides valuable information about fetal well-being.

Estrogen: any of the group of substances (hormones) that induces estrogenic activity; specifically the estrogenic hormones, estradiol and estrone produced by the ovary.

Estrone: an estrogenic hormone found in the urine of pregnant women.

Evacuated tube: sample collection tube with a vacuum.

Exocrine gland: any gland that excretes externally through a duct. Secretions of exocrine glands do not directly enter the circulation.

Exogenous: triglycerides obtained from dietary sources.

Extracellular fluid: water (fluid) outside the cell; can be subdivided into the intravascular extracellular fluid (plasma) and the interstitial cell fluid (ISCF) that surrounds the cells in the tissues.

Extrauterine: outside the uterus or womb.

Exudate: accumulation of fluid in a cavity; also the production of pus or serum. In comparison with a transudate, an exudate contains more cells and protein. Exudates demand immediate attention.

F

F-test: statistical test used to compare the features of two or more groups of data.

Fasting specimens: a blood specimen taken after the patient has not eaten for at least 12 hours.

Fatty acids: major constituents of triglycerides and phospholipids. There are short-chain (4–6 carbon atoms), medium-chain (8–12 carbon atoms), and long-chain fatty acids (>12 carbon atoms).

Feedback loops: a control system of a physiologic function that allows for feedback and correction based on conditions or circulating levels of a hormone or substance.

Ferritin: a spherical protein shell composed of 24 subunits with a molecular mass of 500 kDa. The protein can bind up to 4,000 iron molecules, making it a large potential source of iron.

Filtrate: liquid that passes through filter paper is called the filtrate.

Filtration: separation of solids from liquids.

FIO$_2$: the fraction of inspired oxygen; can be as much as 100% when oxygen is being supplied.

Fire tetrahedron: a three-dimensional pyramid representing the element of fire; previously the fire triangle.

First-order kinetics: point in enzyme reaction in which the rate of the reaction is dependent on enzyme concentration only.

Fisher projection: diagrammatic model that can be used to represent carbohydrates. The Fisher projection of a carbohydrate has the aldehyde or ketone at the top of the drawing. The carbons are numbered starting at the aldehyde or ketone end, and the compound can be represented either as a straight chain or in a cyclic, hemiacetal form.

Flag: on automated analyzers, a computerized printed warning of an error or instrument problem.

Flame photometry: analytical technique that measures the wavelength and intensity of light emitted from a burning solution (patient specimen).

Fluorescence resonance energy transfer (FRET): the nonradioactive transfer of energy from a donor molecule to an acceptor molecule.

Flow cytometry: the use of immunofluorescent labels to identify specific antigens on live cells in suspension. Stained cell suspensions are transported under pressure past a laser beam, and emitted fluorescence (at 90° relative to the beam) is measured and computer analyzed with this technique. Using multiple labels, cells can be identified and sorted either electronically or physically. The technique has been used to analyze a subpopulation of lymphocyte cells in various clinical diagnoses.

Fluorescence polarization immunoassay (FPIA): a technique in which a fluorescein-labeled antigen rotates rapidly in solution and, when excited, does not emit polarized light. After binding to antibody the label rotates much slower and emits polarized light. When polarized light is used as a source of excitation, emitted fluorescence is measured in two planes. The difference in fluorescence polarization (calculated) before and after the addition of labeled analyte is inversely proportional to the concentration of unknown analyte. This methodology is most useful for small antigens (drugs, hormones, etc.).

Fluorometry: analytical technique used to measure fluorescence (light emitted as a result of energy absorbed).

Follicular cells: (or cuboidal) one of two types of cells of the thyroid; they are secretory cells and produce thyroxine (T$_4$) and triiodothyronine (T$_3$).

Follicular phase: the first half of the menstrual cycle, when estrogen effect is unopposed by progesterone, also called the proliferative phase.

Follicle-stimulating hormone (FSH): a protein hormone secreted by the anterior pituitary.

Forensic: pertaining to the law or legal matters (eg, toxicology and the law).

Forensic medicine: medical knowledge or results that apply to questions of law affecting life or property. A specimen result might be used as evidence in a court of law to prove cause of death, an accused individual's innocence or guilt, or possibly alcohol or drug abuse.

FPIA: see fluorescence polarization immunoassay.

Fractional oxyhemoglobin (FO$_2$Hb): is the ratio of the concentration of oxyhemoglobin to the concentration of total hemoglobin (ctHb).

Free radical: a highly reactive molecule containing an open bond or half a bond; free radicals are harmful to the body (eg, OH·).

Free thyroxine index (FT$_4$I): an indirect measure of free hormone concentration and is based on the equilibrium relationship of bound T$_4$ and FT$_4$. The FT$_4$I is calculated by the following formula: $FT_4I = T_4 \times T_3U$ ratio.

Friedewald calculation: calculation used to estimate LDL cholesterol in routine clinical practice.

Fructosamine: any glycated serum protein.

FSH: see Follicle-stimulating hormone.

G

Gas chromatography: analytical technique used to separate mixtures of compounds that are volatile or can be made volatile. Gas chromatography may be gas-solid chromatography (GSC), with a solid stationary phase, or gas-liquid chromatography (GLC), with a nonvolatile liquid stationary phase.

Gastrin: a gastrointestinal hormone. It is a peptide secreted by the G cells of the antrum (lower third) of the stomach. It is released in response to contact of food.

Geriatrics: branch of general medicine dealing with remedial and preventable clinical problems in the elderly, as well as the social consequences of such illness.

Gerontology: study of the aging process in the human body.

GFR: see Glomerular filtration rate.

GH: see Growth hormone.

Globulins: heterogeneous group of proteins that can be separated by electrophoresis into α_1, α_2, and γ fractions.

Glomerular filtrate: plasma filtrate containing water and small molecules but lacking cells and large molecules such as most proteins.

Glomerular filtration rate (GFR): rate at which plasma is filtered by glomerulus, expressed in mL/minute.

Glomerulonephritis: inflammation of the glomeruli of the kidney. May be acute, subacute, or chronic.

Glomerulus: small blood vessels in the nephron that project into the capsular end of the proximal tubule and serve as a filtering mechanism.

Glucagon: a protein hormone that is involved in the regulation of carbohydrate, fat, and protein metabolism. It is synthesized by the α cells of the pancreatic islet and is composed of 29 amino acids.

Glucocorticoid: a general classification of hormones synthesized in the zona fasciculata of the adrenal cortex. Cortisol is the principal glucocorticoid hormone.

Gluconeogenesis: the conversion of amino acids by the liver and other specialized tissues, such as the kidney, to substrates that can be converted to glucose. Gluconeogenesis also encompasses the conversion of glycerol, lactate, and pyruvate to glucose.

Glycogen: a polysaccharide similar to starch; form in which carbohydrates are stored.

Glycogenolysis: process by which glycogen is converted back to glucose 6-phosphate for entry into the glycolytic pathway.

Glycolysis: hydrolysis of glucose by an enzyme into pyruvate or lactate; the process is anaerobic.

Glycolytic inhibitor: a substance that prevents the hydrolysis of sugar. Sodium fluoride is a glycolytic inhibitor.

Gout: arthritis associated with increased levels of uric acid in the blood, which then become deposited in the joints or tissues causing painful swelling. It is more common in men than in women.

Graft: tissue that is transplanted.

Grave's disease: diffuse toxic goiter. Graves' disease occurs six times more commonly in women than in men. It occurs frequently at puberty, during pregnancy, at menopause, or following severe stress.

Growth hormone (GH): a peptide composed of 191 amino acids. In contrast to most of the other protein hormones, GH does not act through cAMP. Binding of GH to its membrane receptor leads to glucose uptake, amino acid transport, and lipolysis. Secreted by the anterior pituitary.

Gynecomastia: abnormally large mammary gland development in the male.

H

Half-life: time needed for 50% of a radionuclide to decay and become more stable.

Hapten: a substance that can bind with an antibody but cannot initiate an immune response unless bound to a carrier.

Hashimoto's disease: chronic autoimmune thyroiditis; it is the most common cause of primary hypothyroidism.

Haworth projection: represents glucose in a cyclic form that is more representative of the actual structure. When glucose is drawn in a Haworth projection, the a form of D-glucopyranose is represented by the hydroxy group of carbon-1 oriented downwards or below the plane of the paper.

Hazard communication: based on the fact that all employees must be informed of any health risks involving the use of chemicals; from the Hazardous Communication Standard of 1987 (Right to Know Law).

Hazardous material: a material that may potentially cause personal injury or damage if handled.

Hazardous waste: any potentially dangerous waste material.

HbA$_{1c}$: see Hemoglobin A$_{1c}$.

hCG: see Human chorionic gonadotropin.

HDL: see High-density lipoproteins.

Hemodialysis: a technique or procedure that provides the function of the kidneys when one or both are damaged. The patient's blood is circulated through membranes to remove wastes.

Hemofiltration: an ultrafiltration procedure or technique (similar to hemodialysis) used to remove an excess accumulation of normal metabolic products from the blood.

Hemoglobin A$_{1c}$ (HbA$_{1c}$): largest subfraction of normal HbA in both diabetic and nondiabetic subjects. It is formed by the reaction of the β chain of HbA with glucose. It reflects the concentration of glucose present in the body over a prolonged time period related to the 60-day half-life of erythrocytes.

Hemoglobin-oxygen (binding) capacity: the maximum amount of oxygen that can be carried by hemoglobin in a given quantity of blood.

Hemoglobin–oxygen dissociation curve: a graphic representation ("S"-shaped) of oxygen content as percent oxygen saturation against PO$_2$; based on the principle that oxygen dissociates from adult hemoglobin in a characteristic fashion.

Hemoglobinopathy: a disorder associated with the presence of an abnormal hemoglobin.

Hemolysis: damage to erythrocyte membranes, causing release of cellular constituents (eg, hemoglobin) into the blood plasma or serum.

Henderson-Hasselbalch equation: equation that mathematically describes the dissociation characteristics of weak acids and bases and the effect on pH; pH = pK$_a$ (6.1) + log of the ratio of bicarbonate to carbon dioxide (HCO$_3$/H$_2$CO$_3$)

HEPA filter: high-efficiency particulate air filter; a respirator.

Heparin: an anticoagulant used in blood collection.

Hepatitis: "inflammation of the liver;" may be caused by a virus, bacteria, parasites, radiation, drugs, chemicals, or toxins. Among the viruses causing hepatitis are hepatitis types A, B, C, D (or delta), and E, cytomegalovirus, Epstein-Barr virus, and probably several others.

Hepatoma: primary malignant tumors of the liver; also known as hepatocellular carcinoma or hepatocarcinoma.

Heterogeneous assay: a technique (*eg*, radioimmunoassay) where it is necessary to physically separate labeled antigen or hapten bound to antibody from a labeled antigen or hapten that remains free in solution.

High-density lipoproteins (HDL): a "clean-up crew" that gathers up extra cholesterol for transport back to the liver.

Hirsutism: excessive and abnormal hair growth

Histogram: graphical representation of data where the number or frequency of each result is placed on the y axis and the value of the result is plotted on the x axis.

Holoenzyme: enzyme consisting of a protein portion and a non–amino acid portion or prosthetic group.

Homeostasis: state of equilibrium in the body maintained by dynamic processes.

Homogeneous assay: a technique (*eg*, EMIT) that does not require the physical separation of the bound and free labeled antigen.

Hormone: a chemical substance that is produced and secreted into the blood by an organ or tissue and has a specific effect on a target tissue.

HPL: see Human placental lactogen.

HPTA: see Hypothalamic–pituitary–thyroid axis.

Human chorionic gonadotropin (hCG): a protein hormone produced by the placenta and consisting of α and β subunits.

Human placental lactogen (HPL): a protein hormone that is structurally, immunologically, and functionally very similar to growth hormone and prolactin. Like hCG, it is produced by the placenta and can be measured in maternal urine and serum as well as amniotic fluid.

Hybridization: the production of hybrids.

Hydrate: compound and its associated water.

Hydrolase: an enzyme that catalyzes hydrolysis of ether, ester, acid–anhydride, glycosyl, C–C, C–halide, or P–N bonds.

Hygroscopic: substances that take up water on exposure to atmospheric conditions.

Hyperaldosteronism: excessive production of aldosterone by the adrenal gland. It may be primary (due to an adrenal lesion) or secondary to abnormalities in the renin-angiotensin system.

Hyperandrogenemia: excessive production of androgens in women.

Hypercalcemia: elevated levels of calcium in the blood.

Hyperchloremia: elevated levels of chloride in the blood.

Hypercoagulability: increased ability (*ie*, of blood) to coagulate.

Hypercortisolism: increased levels of cortisol.

Hyperglucagonemia: excessive production of glucagon. Hyperglucagonemia due to tumors must be differentiated from other causes of increased glucagon, which include diabetes, pancreatitis, and trauma.

Hyperglycemic: increased level of blood sugar.

Hyperinsulinemia: excessive and/or inappropriate release of insulin.

Hyperkalemia: elevated levels of potassium in the blood.

Hypermagnesemia: elevated levels of magnesium in the blood.

Hypernatremia: elevated levels of sodium in the blood.

Hyperoxemia: increased oxygen in the blood.

Hyperparathyroidism: condition resulting from the increased activity of the parathyroid glands.

Hyperphosphatemia: elevated levels of phosphorus in the blood.

Hyperprolactinemia: excess secretion of prolactin due to hypothalamic-pituitary dysfunction. Generally due to a pituitary neoplasm.

Hyperproteinemia: total protein level in the blood that is higher than the reference interval.

Hypertension: abnormally elevated blood pressure

Hyperthyroidism: excessive secretion of the thyroid glands.

Hyperuricemia: plasma levels of uric acid greater than 7.0 mg/dL in males and 6.0 mg/dL in females.

Hypervitaminosis: a condition that results from excessive intake of a vitamin(s).

Hypoaldosteronism: decreased level of aldosterone.

Hypocalcemia: decreased levels of calcium.

Hypochloremia: decreased levels of chloride in the blood.

Hypocortisolism: low or decreased levels of cortisol.

Hypogonadism: aberrant internal secretion of the gonads.

Hypoglycemic: decreased level of blood sugar.

Hypoglycorrhachia: decreased CSF glucose levels.

Hypoinsulinemia: decreased level of insulin.

Hypokalemia: decreased levels of potassium.

Hypomagnesemia: decreased levels of magnesium in the blood.

Hyponatremia: decreased levels of sodium in the blood.

Hypoparathyroidism: most often due to destruction of the adrenal glands and, as such, is associated with glucocorticoid deficiency.

Hypophosphatemia: decreased levels of phosphorus in the blood.

Hypoproteinemia: total protein level in the blood that is below the reference interval.

Hypothalamic-pituitary-thyroid axis (HPTA): the neuroendocrine system that regulates the production and secretion of thyroid hormones.

Hypothalamus: the portion of the brain located in the walls and floor of the third ventricle. It is directly above the pituitary gland and is connected to the posterior pituitary by the pituitary stalk.

Hypothyroidism: decreased thyroid secretion.

Hypouricemia: plasma levels of uric acid less than 2.0 mg/dL.

Hypovitaminosis: a condition that results from a lack or deficiency of vitamins in the diet.

Hypovolemia: decreased blood volume.

Hypoxemia: insufficient or decreased oxygenation of the blood.

Hypoxia: physiologic condition caused by a deficiency of the amount of oxygen reaching the tissues.

I

ICF: see intracellular fluid.

Icterus: yellow pigmentation in the skin or sclera (including tissues, membranes, and secretions); also known as jaundice. A result of excess bilirubin concentration in the blood.

Icterus index: a test that involves diluting serum with saline until it visually matches the color of a 0.01% potassium dichromate solution. The number of times the serum must be diluted is called the icterus index.

Immune system: a complex series of events in the body that protect the individual from external, harmful agents. Individual survival depends on a properly functioning system.

Immunity: resistance to infection by a pathologic agent.

Immunoassay: a technique that measures the rate of immune complex formation. Immunoassays can be labeled or nonlabeled.

Immunoblot: a technique for analysis and identification of antigens; western blot.

Immunocytochemistry: use of antibodies to detect antigens in cells.

Immunoelectrophoresis: a technique combining electrophoresis of proteins and immunodiffusion.

Immunofixation: or immunofixation electrophoresis (IFE); a technique in which an immune precipitate is trapped (fixed) on the an electrophoretic support medium. This method has superseded immunoelectrophoresis because of ease and speed.

Immunohistochemistry: use of antibodies to detect antigens in tissue.

Immunophenotyping: use of flow cytometer to detect intracellular and cell surface antigens.

In situ hybridization: a technique performed on cells, tissue, or chromosomes that are fixed on a microscope slide. After the dna is heat denatured, a labeled probe is added and will hybridize the target sequence after the slide is cooled. Colorimetric or fluorescent products are generally used.

Indirect immunofluorescence: technique in which serum antibody reacts with antigen fixed on a slide and the antibody in turn reacts with conjugated antihuman globulins. If the patient serum contains antibody of interest this will be observed under a fluorescent microscope.

Infancy: infant; period in life where child is unable to walk or feed itself.

Infectious endocarditis: inflammation of the inner lining of the heart chambers and valves; caused by a number of microorganisms.

Inferential statistics: values or statistics used to compare the features of two or more groups of data.

Infertility: inability or diminished ability to produce offspring.

Inhibin: a testicular hormone that inhibits luteinizing hormone.

Innate immune system: one of two functional divisions of the immune system; it is the first line of defense.

Insulin: a peptide hormone that is synthesized in the B cells of the islets of Langerhans in the pancreas.

International unit: IU, the amount of enzyme that will catalyze the reaction of 1 μmole of substrate per minute under specified conditions of temperature, pH, substrates, and activators.

Intracellular fluid (ICF): fluid inside the cells.

Intrinsic factor: a substance normally present in gastric juice that allows absorption of vitamin B_{12}.

Inulin: an exogenous plant polysaccharide derived from artichokes and dahlias. It is completely filtered by the glomeruli and neither secreted nor reabsorbed by the tubules. It is the most accurate of all GFR assays.

Ion selective electrodes: the half-cell or electrode (indicator) that responds to a specific ion in a solution.

Ionic strength: concentration or activity of ions in a solution or buffer.

Islets of Langerhans: clusters of cells (α, β, and δ) in the pancreas; insulin is a peptide hormone that is synthesized by the β cells of the pancreatic islets.

Isoelectric point (pI): the pH at which the molecule has no net change.

Isoenzyme: different forms of an enzyme that may originate from genetic or nongenetic causes and may be differentiated from each other based on certain physical properties, such as electrophoretic mobility, solubility, or resistance to inactivation.

K

Ketone: a compound containing a carbonyl group (C=O) attached to two carbon atoms.

Kinetic assay: a type of test or procedure in which there is a reaction proceeding at a particular rate.

Kinetic method of measurement: quantitation by determining the rate at which a reaction occurs or a product is formed.

K_m: see Michaelis-Menten constant.

Kupffer cells: phagocytic macrophages capable of ingesting bacteria or other foreign material from the blood that flows through the sinusoids.

Kwashiorkor: acute protein calories malnutrition.

L

Laboratory standard: a rule or criterion related to the laboratory.

Lactescence: resembling milk; milky appearance.

Lactose tolerance test: an assay to determine the lactase content in the intestinal mucosa. The enzyme lactase is essential to the absorption of lactose from the intestinal tract.

Lancet: a surgical device used to puncture the skin for blood collection.

Lateral: to the side.

Lactate dehydrogenase flipped pattern: situation in which serum levels of LD-1 increase to a point where they are present in greater concentration than LD-2.

LDL: see Low-density lipoproteins.

Lecithins/sphingomyelins ratio (L/S ratio): a classic test that assesses the ratio of lecithins to sphingomyelins to determine fetal lung maturity.

Leuteinizing hormone (LH): a glycoprotein hormone secreted by the anterior pituitary.

Leydig cells: cells of the testicles that produce testosterone.

LH: see Leuteinizing hormone.

Ligase chain reaction: probe amplification technique that uses two pairs of labeled probes that are complementary for two short target DNA sequences in close proximity.

Lipoprotein: protein bound with lipid components, ie, cholesterol, phospholipid, and triglyceride. May be classified as very low density (VLDL), low density (LDL), and high density (HDL).

Lipoprotein a [Lp(a)]: LDL-like lipoprotein particles.

Liquid chromatography: separation technique in which the mobile phase is a liquid.

Lobule: forms the structural unit of the liver, which measures 1–2 mm in diameter, It is composed of cords of liver cells (hepatocytes) radiating from a central vein.

Loop of Henle: descending and ascending loops of the renal tubule.

Low-density lipoproteins (LDL): "empty tankers" rich in cholesterol that remain after the triglycerides have been deposited.

Lp(a): see Lipoprotein A.

L/S ratio: see Lecithins/Sphingomyelins ratio.

Luteal phase: phase in menstrual cycle; progesterone is synthesized by the corpus luteum during this phase. Also secretory phase

M

Malnutrition: a state of decreased intake of calories or micronutrients (vitamins and trace elements) resulting in a risk of impaired physiologic function; associated with increased morbidity and mortality.

Mantissa: that portion of the logarithm to the right of the decimal point, derived from the number itself.

Marasmus: a condition caused by caloric insufficiency without protein insufficiency so that, the serum albumin level remains normal; there is considerable loss of body weight.

Material safety data sheets (MSDS): a major source of safety information for employees who may use hazardous materials in their occupations.

Mechanical hazard: any potential danger from equipment such as centrifuges, autoclaves, and homogenizers.

Medial: in the middle.

Medical waste: material that is infectious or physically dangerous; includes discarded blood, tissues, fluids, body parts, sharps, etc.

Megavitamin: intake of a vitamin or vitamins in extreme excess of daily requirements.

MEN: see Multiple endocrine neoplasia.

Menopause: the permanent cessation of menstrual activity.

Metabolic (nonrespiratory) acidosis and alkalosis: a disorder due to a change in the bicarbonate level (a renal or metabolic function).

Metabolite: any product of metabolism as in the derivative of a drug.

Metalloenzyme: trace element associated with an enzyme as an essential component or cofactor.

Metalloprotein: trace element associated with an protein as an essential component or cofactor.

Metanephrine: a metabolic product of epinephrine and norepinephrine.

Michaelis-Menten constant (K_m): Constant for a specific enzyme and substrate under defined reaction conditions and is an expression of the relationship between the velocity of an enzymatic reaction and substrate concentration.

Microalbuminuria: small quantities of albumin in the urine; microalbumin concentrations are between 20 and 300 mg/day.

Microchemistry: clinical chemistry analyses involving only several microliters of sample.

β_2-Microglobulin: a small, nonglycosylated peptide; used as an indicator of GFR.

Mineralocorticoid: a group of substances produced by the adrenal cortex. Aldosterone is the principal mineralocorticoid (electrolyte-regulating hormone) produced by the zona glomerulosa.

Modular analyzers: flexible laboratory instruments that can be expanded and modified by adding or removing components in order to meet the laboratory's changing testing requirements.

Molality: represents the amount of solute per kilogram of solvent.

Molarity: number of moles per liter of solution.

Monoclonal: arising from one line of cells.

Monosaccharide: a simple carbohydrate; it cannot be decomposed by hydrolysis. Examples include glucose, galactose, and fructose.

MSDS: see Material safety data sheets.

Multiple endocrine neoplasia (MEN): the occurrence of several tumors or hyperplasias involving diverse endocrine organs.

Myocardial infarction: also heart attack; occurs when blood flow to an area of the cardiac muscle is suddenly blocked, leading to ischemia and death of myocardial tissue.

Myocarditis: inflammation of the myocardium.

Myoglobin: myoglobin is a heme protein found only in skeletal and cardiac muscle in humans. It can reversibly bind oxygen in a manner similar to the hemoglobin molecule, but myoglobin is unable to release oxygen, except under very low oxygen tension.

Myosin heavy/light chains: myocardial proteins.

Myxedema: condition resulting from hypofunction of the thyroid. The term is used to describe the peculiar nonpitting swelling of the skin.

N

Nanofiltration: filtration technique for removing particulate matter, microorganisms and any pyrogens or endotoxins.

Narcotic: any group of substances (drug) that produces the opioid group of substances; encompass not only heroin, morphine, and codeine, but also several synthetic compounds such as meperidine, methadone, propoxyphene, pentazocine, and others. All have some potential for addiction.

NCCLS: National Committee for Clinical Laboratory Standards; an agency that establishes laboratory standards.

Neonate: a newborn up to six weeks of age.

Neoplasm: a new and abnormal growth of cells or tissue; also tumor.

Nephelometry: analytical technique that measures the amount of light scattered by particles (immune complexes) in a solution. Measurements are made at 5°–90° incident to the beam.

Nephrotic syndrome: glomerular injury; an abnormally increased permeability of the glomerular basement membrane. Can be a result of many different etiologies.

Neuroblastoma: malignant tumors of the adrenal medulla that occur in children. They produce catecholamines and may occasionally be associated with hypertension.

Neurohypophysis: posterior portion of the pituitary gland.

NFPA: National Fire Protection Association.

Nitrogen balance: equilibrium between protein anabolism and catabolism.

Noncompetitive immunoassay: use of labeled reagent antibody to detect an antigen; also immunometric immunoassay.

Nonprotein nitrogen (NPN): nitrogen-containing compounds remaining in a blood sample after the removal of protein constituents.

Norepinephrine: a hormone (and catecholamine) produced by the adrenal medulla. As hormones, both norepinephrine and epinephrine serve to mobilize energy stores and prepare the body for muscular activity (increase heart rate and blood pressure, increase blood sugar, etc.). They are secreted in increased amounts with stress (pain, fear, etc.).

Normality: number of gram equivalent weights per liter of solution.

Normetanephrine: a metabolite of epinephrine.

Northern blot: technique for detection of RNA molecules or species with defined sequences.

NPN: see Nonproetin nitrogen.

Nucleic acid probes: use of nucleic acids to investigate cellular changes; nucleic acids store all genetic information and direct the synthesis of specific proteins.

Nutritional assessment: evaluation of a patient's metabolic and dietary (nutritional) needs.

Nyctalopia: poor vision in dim light due to vitamin A deficiency. This condition is also known as night blindness.

O

Oncofetal antigen: a protein produced in large amounts during fetal life and released into the fetal circulation. After birth, the production of oncofetal antigens is repressed, and only minute quantities are present in the circulation of adults.

Oncogenes: viral DNA segments that can transform normal cells into malignant cells.

One point calibration (or calculation): a term that refers to the calculation of the comparison of a known standard/calibrator concentration and its corresponding absorbance to the absorbance of an unknown value.

Opsonization: action of opsonins to facilitate phagocytosis.

OSHA: Occupational Safety and Health Act; enacted by Congress in 1970. The goal of this federal regulation was to provide all employees (clinical laboratory personnel included) with a safe work environment.

Osmolal gap: difference between the measured osmolality and the calculated osmolality. The osmolal gap indirectly indicates the presence of osmotically active substances other than sodium, urea, or glucose, such as ethanol, methanol, ethylene glycol, lactate, or β-hydroxybutyrate.

Osmolality: physical property of a solution, based on the concentration of solutes (expressed as millimoles) per kilogram of solvent.

Osmolarity: concentration of osmotically active particles in solution reported in milliosmoles per liter; not routinely used.

Osmometer: laboratory instrument used to measure osmolality, or concentration of solute per kilogram of solvent.

Osmotic pressure: pressure that allows solvent flow between a semipermeable membrane to establish an equilibrium between compartments of different osmolality.

Osteoblast: cells that build bone when triggered by the appropriate hormonal signals.

Osteoclast: cells that causes reabsorption of bone when triggered by the appropriate hormonal signals.

Osteomalacia: condition resulting from a deficiency of vitamin D. Deficiency of vitamin D causes bones to be soft and brittle. It is the adult form of rickets.

Osteoporosis: a disease involving the gradual loss of bone mass resulting in a less dense and weak skeleton.

Otorrhea: discharge from the ear; also leakage of CSF from the ear.

Ovulation: the periodic discharge of an ovum from the ovary.

Oxidized: loss of electrons; combined with oxygen.

Oxidizing agent: substance that accepts electrons.

Oxidoreductase: an enzyme that catalyzes an oxidation—reduction reaction between two substrates.

Oxygen content: sum of the oxygen bound to hemoglobin as O_2Hb and the amount dissolved in the blood.

Oxygen saturation: (SO_2) represents the ratio of oxygen that is bound to the carrier protein—hemoglobin—compared with the total amount that the hemoglobin could bind.

Oxytocin: a hormone produced in the hypothalamus. It stimulates contraction of the gravid uterus at term and also results in contraction of myoepithelial cells in the breast, causing ejection of milk.

P

P_{50}: represents the partial pressure of oxygen at which the hemoglobin oxygen saturation (SO_2) is 50%. The P_{50} is a measure of the O_2Hb binding characteristics and identifies the position of the oxygen—hemoglobin dissociation curve at half saturation.

Pancreatitis: inflammation of the pancreas ultimately caused by autodigestion of the pancreas as a result of reflux of bile or duodenal contents into the pancreatic duct.

Panhypopituitarism: a condition resulting from pituitary hormone deficiencies; it usually involves more than one and eventually all the anterior pituitary hormones. These hormones are lost in a characteristic order, with growth hormone and gonadotropins disappearing first, followed by TSH, ACTH, and prolactin.

Paracentesis: aspiration of fluid through the skin; as in removal or aspiration of pericardial, pleural, and peritoneal fluids.

Paracrine: secretion of a hormone from other than a endocrine gland.

Parathyroid glands: four glands adjacent to the thyroid gland. Two of these glands are found in the upper portion and two are found near the lower portion of the thyroid gland. The parathyroid glands produce parathyroid hormone, which controls calcium and phosphate metabolism.

Parathyroid hormone (PTH): hormone synthesized as a prohormone containing 115 amino acids. The active form of the hormone contains 84 amino acids and is secreted by the chief cells of the parathyroid glands.

Parenteral nutrition: intense nutritional support for patients who are malnourished, or in danger of becoming malnourished, because they are unable to consume required nutrients or to take nutrients entirely. Parenteral nutrition therapy involves administering appropriate amounts of carbohydrate, amino acid, and lipid solutions as well as electrolytes, vitamins, minerals, and trace elements to meet the caloric, protein, and nutrient requirements while maintaining water and electrolyte balance.

Partial pressure: the pressure exerted by an individual gas in the atmosphere; equal to blood pressure at a particular altitude times the appropriate percentage for each gas.

PCO_2: partial pressure of carbon dioxide.

PCR: see Polymerase chain reaction.

Peak drug level: the time after administration until a drug reaches peak concentration in the body. A rule of thumb suggests that, for peak drug levels, the specimen should be collected 1 hour after the dose is administered.

Pediatric: regarding the treatment of children.

Pellagra: a condition resulting from a deficiency of niacin. Initial signs of pellagra include anorexia, headaches, weakness, irritability, indigestion, and sleeplessness. This progresses to the classic four Ds of advanced pellagra: dermatitis, diarrhea, dementia, and death.

Pepsin: a group of relatively weak proteolytic enzymes, with pH optima from about 1.6–3.6, that catalyze all native proteins except mucus.

Peptide bond: linkage combining the carboxyl group of one amino acid to the amino group of another amino acid.

Peptides: compounds formed by the cleavage of peptones, which contain two or more amino acids. The peptide hormones include insulin, glucagon, parathyroid hormone, growth hormone, and prolactin.

Percent solution: the amount of solute per 100 total units of solution.

Pericardial fluid: fluid surrounding and protecting the heart. The frequency of pericardial sampling and laboratory analysis is rare.

Pericarditis: inflammation of the pericardium.

Perifollicular cells: one of two types of cells forming the thyroid gland. Also C cells; they are situated in clusters along the interfollicular or interstitial spaces. The C cells produce the polypeptide calcitonin, which is involved in calcium regulation.

Peritoneal fluid: a clear to straw-colored fluid secreted by the cells of the peritoneum (abdominal cavity). It serves to moisten the surfaces of the viscera.

PG: see Prostaglandins.

pH: represents the negative or inverse log of the hydrogen ion concentration; $-\log [H^+]$.

Phalanx: any of the bones of the fingers or toes.

Pharmacokinetics: characterization, mathematically of the disposition of a drug over time in order to better understand and interpret blood levels and to effectively adjust dosage amount and interval for best therapeutic results with minimal toxic effects.

Phenylketonuria (PKU): phenylpyruvic acid in the urine; a recessive hereditary disease.

Pheochromocytoma: tumors of the adrenal medulla or sympathetic ganglia that produce and release large quantities of catecholamines.

Phlebotomist: an individual who obtains or draws blood samples.

Phlebotomy: procedure for withdrawing blood from the body.

Phospholipids: formed by the conjugation of two fatty acids and a phosphorylated glycerol. Phospholipids are amphipathic, which means they contain polar hydrophilic (water-loving) head groups and nonpolar hydrophobic (water-hating) fatty acid side chains.

Pipet: utensils made of glass or plastic that are used to transfer liquids; they may be reusable or disposable.

pK: the negative log of the ionization constant.

PKU: see Phenylketonuria.

Placenta: a structure in the uterus through which the fetus derives nourishment. The placenta synthesizes and secretes a variety of protein hormones, as well as the steroids estrogen and progesterone. Evaluation of maternal serum and urine concentration of these hormones may be of value not only in diagnosing pregnancy but also in monitoring placental development and fetal well-being.

Plasma: liquid portion of blood that contains clotting factors.

Plasma renal flow: renal secretory capability.

Pleural fluid: essentially interstitial fluid of the systemic circulation; it is contained in a membrane that surrounds the lungs.

PO₂: the partial pressure of oxygen.

Point-of-care testing (POCT): analytical testing of patient specimens performed outside the physical laboratory and at the site of patient care.

Poison: any substance that causes a harmful effect upon exposure.

Polyclonal: arising from different cell lines.

Polydipsia: excess H_2O intake due to chronic thirst.

Polymerase chain reaction (PCR): an in vitro process used to replicate unlimited specific short regions of DNA

Polysaccharide: complex carbohydrates; polysaccharides are the most abundant organic molecules in nature.

Porphyria: disorders that result from disturbances in heme synthesis.

Porphyrin: chemical intermediates in the synthesis of hemoglobin, myoglobin, and other respiratory pigments called cytochromes.

Porphyrinogens: the reduced form of porphyrins.

Porphyrinuria: increased amount of porphyrins in the urine.

Postrenal: obstruction in the flow of urine from kidney to bladder and its excretion.

Posterior pituitary: a portion of the pituitary; also the neurohypophysis.

Posthepatic: extrahepatic disturbance in the excretion of bilirubin. Posthepatic jaundice results from the impaired excretion of bilirubin caused by mechanical obstruction of the flow of bile into the intestines. This may be due to gallstones or a tumor.

Postzone: in immunoprecipitation reactions, antigen concentration is in excess and cross-linking is decreased.

Prerenal: prior to plasma reaching the kidney.

Preanalytical error: mistakes introduced during the collection and transport of samples prior to analysis.

Precision: the closeness of repeated results; quantitatively expressed as standard deviation or coefficient of variation.

Precocious puberty: onset of puberty (normal sexual development) earlier than the expected time (generally 10–14 years old).

Predictive value theory: referring to diagnostic sensitivity, specificity and predictive value. The predictive value of a test can be expressed as a function of sensitivity, specificity, and disease prevalence.

Prehepatic: before the liver. Prehepatic jaundice results when an excessive amount of bilirubin is presented to the liver for metabolism, such as in hemolytic anemia. This type of jaundice is characterized by unconjugated hyperbilirubinemia.

Primary standard: a highly purified chemical that can be measured directly to produce a substance of exact known concentration.

Probe: on an automated analyzer, a mechanized device that automatically dips into a sample cup and aspirates a portion of the liquid.

Proficiency testing: confirmation of the quality of laboratory testing by means of "unknown" samples.

Progesterone: a steroid hormone produced by the corpus luteum and placenta. Progesterone serves to prepare the uterus for pregnancy and the lobules of the breast for lactation.

Prohormone: a precursor to the active hormone.

Proinsulin: precursor to insulin; it is packaged into secretory granules, where it is broken down into equimolar amounts of insulin and an inactive C-peptide.

Prolactin: a protein hormone whose amino acid composition is similar to that of GH. It is produced by the pituitary gland. In humans, it appears to function solely in the initiation and maintenance of lactation.

Prostaglandins (PG): a group of biologically active unsaturated fatty acids; metabolites of arachidonic acid.

Protein-free filtrate: clear filtrate of whole blood or plasma prepared by adding acid or other ions to remove proteins.

Proteinuria: protein in the urine.

Proto-oncogenes: normal cellular genes that play essential roles in cell differentiation and proliferation and potentially can become oncogenic are known as proto-oncogenes. Transformation of proto-oncogenes into oncogenes can occur by single-point mutations, translocation, and amplification.

Proximal tubule: portion of renal tubule beginning at Bowman's capsule and extending to loop of Henle.

Prozone: in immunoprecipitation reactions, antibody concentration is in excess and cross-linking is decreased.

PTH: see Parathyroid hormone.

Pyrrole: a heterocyclic structure or compound that is the basis for substances such as hemoglobin.

Q

Quality assurance: system or process that encompasses (in the laboratory) preanalytical, analytical, and postanalytical factors. Quality control is part of a quality-assurance system.

Quality control: system for recognizing and minimizing (analytical) errors. The purpose of the quality-control system is to monitor analytical processes, detect analytical errors during analysis, and prevent the reporting of incorrect patient values. Quality control is one component of the quality-assurance system.

Quality improvement: activities and systems designed to evaluate and improve patient care.

Quaternary structure: the arrangement of two or more polypeptide chains to form a functional protein molecule.

R

Radial immunodiffusion (RID): immune precipitation technique used to quantitate a protein (the antigen).

Radioactive material: any material capable of emitting radiant energy (rays or particles).

Random access: the capability of an automated analyzer to process samples independently of other samples on the analyzer. Random access analyzers may be programmed to run individual tests or a panel of tests without operator intervention.

Random error: a type of analytical error; random error affects precision and is the basis for disagreement between repeated measurements. Increases in random error may be caused by factors such as technique and temperature fluctuations.

Random urine specimen: a urine specimen in which collection time and volume are not important. The first morning void

is often requested because it is the most concentrated; generally used for routine urinalysis (pH, glucose, protein, specific gravity, and osmolality).

RDA: see Recommended dietary allowance.

Reabsorption: process of absorbing again.

Reactive chemical: substances that, under certain conditions, can spontaneously explode or ignite or that evolve heat and/or flammable or explosive gases.

Receptor: site of hormone action on a cell; receptors provide for target-organ specificity, since not all cells have receptors for all hormones.

Recommended dietary allowance (RDA): The amount of a vitamin that should be ingested by a healthy individual to meet routine metabolic needs and allow for biologic variation, maintain normal serum concentrations, prevent depletion of body stores, and thus preserve normal function and health.

Redox potential: a measure of a solution's ability to accept or donate electrons.

Reduced: substance that has gained electrons.

Reference interval: the usual values for a healthy population; also normal range.

Reference method: an analytical method used for comparison. It is a method with negligible inaccuracy in comparison with its imprecision.

Renal threshold: plasma concentration above which a substance appears in the urine.

Renal tubular secretion: process that transports substances from plasma into tubular filtrate for excretion into urine.

Renin: enzyme produced by the kidney that acts on angiotensin to form angiotensin I.

Respiratory acidosis and alkalosis: a disorder due to ventilatory dysfunction (a change in the PCO_2, the respiratory component).

Respiratory distress syndrome: a condition that may occur upon the changeover to air as an oxygen source at birth if the proper quantity and type of phospholipid (surfactant) is not present. Also referred to as *hyaline membrane disease* because of the hyaline membrane found in affected lungs.

Restriction fragment length polymorphisms (RFLP): a technique to evaluate differences in genomic DNA sequences.

Retinoids: derivatives of vitamin A

Reverse transcriptase-polymerase chain reaction: conversion of RNA to DNA by reverse transcriptase; the complementary DNA (cDNA) can then be analyzed by PCR.

Rhabdomyolysis: destruction of skeletal muscle cells

Rheumatic heart disease: affects all layers of the heart. Inflammation of the inner surface of the heart (endocarditis), especially the valves of the left heart, leads to ulceration and growth of vegetations on the heart lining and eventually to irreversible valve damage

Rhinorrhea: discharge from the nose; also leakage of CSF into the nose.

RID: see Radial immunodiffusion.

Rickets: the classic vitamin D deficiency disease of children. It may be nutritional or metabolic in origin.

Robotics: front end automation to "handle" a specimen through the processing steps and load the specimen onto the analyzer.

Rotor: a round device on some automated analyzers that holds sample cups and is capable of spinning.

S

Secondary hypertension: hypertension with an identified source.

Secondary standard: a substance of lower purity whose concentration is determined by comparison with a primary standard.

Secretagogue: an agent that stimulates or causes secretion.

Secretin: secretin is synthesized by cells in the small intestine in response to the acidic contents of the stomach reaching the duodenum. It can control gastrin activity in the stomach and cause the production of alkaline bicarbonate rich pancreatic juice thereby protecting the lining of the intestine from damage.

Secretion: process whereby glandular organ cells produce substances from blood.

Self-sustained sequence replication: target amplification method that detects target RNA and involves continuous isothermic cycles of reverse transcription.

Sella turcica: a small cavity in the sphenoid bone of the skull; the pituitary is located in this cavity.

Serial dilution: multiple progressive dilutions ranging from more concentrated solutions to less concentrated solutions.

Serotonin (5-OH tryptamine): an amine derived from hydroxylation and decarboxylation of tryptophan. It is synthesized by enterochromaffin cells, which are located primarily in the gastrointestinal tract and, to a lesser degree, in the bronchial mucosa, biliary tract, and gonads.

Serous fluid: liquid of the body similar to blood serum; in part secreted by serous membranes.

Sertoli cell: cell of seminiferous tubules that nourish spermatids.

Serum: liquid portion of the blood without clotting factors.

Sheehan's syndrome: hypopituitarism arising from an infarct (necrosis) of the pituitary.

Shift: a sudden change in data and the mean.

SI: see Systéme internationale d'unités.

SIADH: syndrome of inappropriate ADH; it results when ADH is released despite low serum osmolality in association with a normal or increased blood volume.

Significant figures: the minimum number of digits needed to express a particular value in scientific notation without loss of accuracy.

Simple protein: composed only of amino acids.

Sinusoids: spaces between the cords of liver cells; they are lined by endothelial cells and Kupffer cells.

Skin puncture: an open collection system. Blood is brought to the surface of the skin by applying pressure to the site. The sample is dripped into a capillary blood collector (instead of vacuum pressure pulling the sample into the tube). Specimen contains both venous and arterial blood.

Solid phase: in radioimmunoassay (RIA), solid particles or tubes onto which antibody is adsorbed.

Solute: a substance that is dissolved in a liquid or solvent.

Solution: a liquid containing a dissolved substance; the combination of solute and solvent.

Solvent: liquid in which the solute is dissolved.

Southern blot: a technique for detecting specific DNA sequences using a mixture of DNA molecules.

Specific gravity: term used to express density.

Specificity: in regard to quality control, the ability of an analytical method to quantitate one analyte in the presence of others in a mixture such as serum.

Spectrophotometry: analytical technique to measure the light absorbed by a solution. A spectrophotometer is used to measure the light transmitted by a solution in order to determine the concentration of the light-absorbing substance in the solution.

SRM: see Standard reference materials.

Staging: determination of the period in the course of a disease. The major clinical value of tumor markers is in tumor staging, monitoring therapeutic responses, predicting patient outcomes, and detecting cancer recurrence.

Standard: a substance or solution in which the concentration is determined. Standards are used in the calibration of an instrument or method.

Standard precautions: guidelines that consider blood and other body fluids from all patients as infective; include hand washing, gloves, eye protection, etc.

Standard reference materials (SRM): established by authority; used for comparison of measurement.

Steatorrhea: failure to digest and/or absorb fats.

Steroids: classification of hormones; they are all synthesized from cholesterol, using the same initial biochemical pathways. The end result depends on the enzymatic machinery that is predominant in a particular organ.

Subacute thyroiditis: one of the simplest classification schemes of thyroiditis. Conditions are often associated with a thyrotoxic phase when thyroid hormone is leaking into the circulation, a hypothyroid phase when the thyroid gland is repairing itself and a euthyroid phase once the gland is repaired. These phases can last weeks to months

Synovial fluid: fluid formed by ultrafiltration of plasma across the synovial membrane of a joint. The membrane also secretes into the dialysate a mucoprotein rich in hyaluronic acid, which causes the synovial fluid to be viscous.

Systematic error: a type of analytical error that arises from factors that contribute a constant difference, either positive or negative, and directly affects the estimate of the mean. Increases in systematic error can be caused by poorly made standards or reagents, failing instrumentation, poorly written procedures, etc.

Système internationale d'unités (SI): internationally adopted system of measurement. Established in 1960 and is the only system used in many countries. The units of the system are referred to as SI units.

T

TBA: see Thyroxine-binding albumin.

TBG: see Thyroxine-binding globulin.

TBPA: see Thyroxine-binding prealbumin.

TD_{50}: dose of a drug that would be predicted to produce a toxic response in 50% of the population.

TDM: see Therapeutic drug monitoring.

T-test: used to determine whether there is a statistically significant difference between the means of two groups of data.

T_3 uptake: assay used to measure the number of available binding sites of the thyroxine-binding proteins, most notably TBG. It should not be confused with the T_3 assay.

Tandem mass spectrometry: analytical technique that allows whole groups of similar compounds to be analyzed on very small sample volumes without complex sample preparation.

Teratogen: anything that may cause abnormal development of an embryo.

Testosterone: a steroid hormone synthesized from cholesterol. It causes growth and development of the male reproductive system, prostate, and external genitalia.

Tetany: irregular muscle spasms.

Tetralogy of Fallot: a congenital condition of the heart that includes septal defects, stenosis of the pulmonary artery, dextroposition of the aorta, and hypertrophy of the right ventricle.

Thalassemia: disorder involving a defect in rate and quantity of production of hemoglobin.

THBR: see Thyroid hormone-binding ratio.

Therapeutic drug monitoring (TDM): the determination of serum drug levels in order to produce a desirable effect.

Therapeutic range: concentration range of a drug that is beneficial to the patient without being toxic.

Thermistor: electronic thermometer.

Thoracentesis: removal of fluid from the pleural space by needle and syringe after visualization by radiology.

Thrombolytic agents: substances that break up a thrombus (blood clot) (*eg*, streptokinase).

Thyroglobulin: an iodine containing protein secreted by the thyroid gland.

Thyroid: a gland consisting of two lobes located in the lower part of the neck. The lobes are connected by a narrow band called an isthmus and are typically asymmetrical, with the right lobe being larger than the left.

Thyroid hormone-binding ratio (THBR): test used to measure available binding sites of the thyroxine-binding proteins; also T_3-uptake test.

Thyroiditis: inflammation of the thyroid gland.

Thyroperoxidase (TPO) antibodies: thyroid antibodies; formerly known as Thyroid Antimicrosomal antibodies.

Thyrotoxicosis: a group of syndromes caused by high levels of free thyroid hormones in the circulation. Thyrotoxicosis means only that the patient is suffering the metabolic consequences of excessive quantities of thyroid hormones.

Thyrotropin (TSH): thyrotropin, or thyroid-stimulating hormone (TSH), is a glycoprotein consisting of two subunits, α and β, linked noncovalently. It is released by the anterior pituitary.

Thyrotropin receptor (TSHR) antibodies: thyroid antibodies associated with hyperthyroid or hypothyroid states.

Thyrotropin-releasing hormone (TRH): a tripeptide released by the hypothalamus. It travels along the hypothalamic stalk to the β cells of the anterior pituitary, where it stimulates the synthesis and release of thyrotropin or thyroid-stimulating hormone (TSH).

Thyroxine-binding albumin (TBA): a protein that binds thyroxine.

Thyroxine-binding globulin (TBG): a protein that binds thyroid hormones. The TBG assay is used to confirm results of FT_3 or FT_4 or abnormalities in the relationship of the TT_4 and T_3U test; or as a postoperative marker of thyroid cancer.

Thyroxine-binding prealbumin (TBPA): transport protein of thyroxine; also transthyretin (TTR).

Thyroxine (T_4): hormone produced by the thyroid gland.

TIBC: see Total iron-binding capacity.

Timed urine specimen: specimens collected at specific intervals, such as before and after meals, or specimens to be collected over specific periods of time. For example, discrete samples collected over a period of time are used for tolerance tests (*eg*, glucose).

Titer: the highest dilution of serum that shows a positive reaction in the presence of antigen (*eg*, precipitation of antigen–antibody complex).

Total iron-binding capacity (TIBC): an estimate of serum transferrin levels; obtained by measuring the total iron binding capability of a patient's serum. Since transferrin represents most of the iron-binding capacity of serum, TIBC is generally a good estimate of serum transferrin levels.

Total laboratory automation: automated devices and robots integrated with existing analyzers to perform all phases of laboratory testing.

Total parenteral nutrition (TPN): a widely used means of intense nutritional support for patients who are malnourished, or in danger of becoming malnourished, because they are unable to consume required nutrients.

Toxicology: the study of poisons, their actions, their detection, and the treatment of the conditions produced by them.

Trace element: an element that occurs in biological systems at concentrations of mg/kg amounts or less (parts per million). Typically the daily requirement of such an element is a few milligrams per day.

Tracer: radioactive isotope used to tag or mark a molecule; also called label.

Transferase: an enzyme that catalyzes the transfer of a group other than hydrogen from one substrate to another.

Transferrin saturation: percent of transferrin molecules that have iron bound. A ratio of serum iron (actual iron in the serum) and serum transferrin or TIBC (potential quantity of iron that can be bound). Also Percent Saturation.

Transudate: fluid that passes through a membrane; in comparison to an exudate it has fewer cells and is of lower specific gravity. Transudates are secondary to remote (nonpleural) pathology and indicate that treatment should begin elsewhere.

Trend: a gradual change in data and the mean.

TRH: see Thyrotropin-releasing hormone.

Triglyceride: consists of one molecule of glycerol with three fatty acid molecules attached (usually three different fatty acids including both saturated and unsaturated molecules).

Triiodothyronine (T_3): a hormone produced by the thyroid gland.

Triose: a monosaccharide having three carbons.

Troponin I: globular protein; specific marker for cardiac disease.

Troponin T: asymmetrical globular protein; cardiac marker that allows for both early and late diagnosis of AMI.

Trough drug level: the lowest concentration of drug obtained in the blood. Trough levels should be drawn immediately before the next dose.

TSH: see Thyrotropin.

Tubular reabsorption: process in which movement of a substance (eg, calcium) is from the tubular lumen to the peritubular capillary plasma.

Tubular secretion: movement of substances from peritubular capillary plasma to tubular lumen; also secretion of some products of cellular metabolism into the filtrate in the tubular lumen.

Tubules: tubes or canals that make up a part of the kidney; as in convoluted tubules.

Tumor-associated antigen: an antigen associated with a tumor; it is derived from the same or closely related tissue. Oncofetal proteins are an example of tumor-associated antigens. They are present in both embryonic/fetal tissue and cancer cells.

Tumor marker: biological substances synthesized and released by cancer cells or substances produced by the host in response to cancerous tissue. Tumor markers can be present in the circulation, body cavity fluids, cell membranes, or the cytoplasm/nucleus of the cell.

Tumor-specific antigen: a tumor antigen; thought to be a direct product of oncogenesis induced by viral oncogenes, radiation, chemical carcinogens, or unknown risk factors.

Turbidimetry: an analytical technique that measures the decreased amount of light transmitted through a solution as a result of light scatter by particles. Measurements are made at 180° to the incident beam (unscattered light).

U

Ultrafiltration: filtration technique for removing particulate matter, microorganisms and any pyrogens or endotoxins

Ultratrace element: present in tissues at concentrations of mg/kg amounts or less (parts per billion) and has extremely low daily requirements (usually less than 1 mg).

Urea: compound synthesized in the liver from ammonia and carbon dioxide and excreted in the urine.

Uremia or uremic syndrome: very high levels of urea in blood accompanied by renal failure.

Uric acid: end product of the breakdown of purines from nucleic acids in humans.

Urinalysis: a group of screening tests generally performed as part of a patient's admission workup or physical examination. It includes assessment of physical characteristics, chemical analyses, and a microscopic examination of the sediment from a (random) urine specimen.

Urobilinogen: colorless product or derivative of bilirubin formed by the action of bacteria.

V

Valence: mass of material that can combine with or replace 1 mole of hydrogen ions.

Vanillylmandelic acid (VMA): epinephrine and norepinephrine are metabolized by the enzymes monoamine oxidase and catechol-O-methyltransferase to form metanephrines and vanillylmandelic acid.

Vasodilator drugs: drugs that dilate the peripheral arteries and veins, decreasing the amount of effort that the heart expends to pump blood.

Vasopressin: a hormone secreted by the hypothalamus. Involved in blood pressure regulation.

Venipuncture: puncture of a vein. For example, to obtain blood for analysis.

Venous blood: blood obtained from a vein.

Ventricular septal defect: defect in the septum between the left and right ventricles of the heart.

Very-low-density lipoproteins (VLDL): a group of lipoproteins that carry triglycerides assembled in the liver out to cells for energy needs or storage as fat.

Virilization: development of masculine sex characteristics in the female.

Vitamer: related compounds that interconvert to or substitute for the functional form of the vitamin.

Vitamin: organic molecules required by the body in amounts ranging from micrograms to milligrams per day for maintenance of structural integrity and normal metabolism. They perform a variety of functions in the body.

VLDL: see very-low-density lipoproteins.

VMA: see vanillylmandelic acid.

W

Waived tests: the simplest complexity listing in CLIA. It involves primarily test systems approved by the Food and Drug Administration for home use. The requirements are that there is no reasonable risk of harm to the patient if the test is performed incorrectly. The likelihood of erroneous results is negligible; the test method be simple and uncomplicated; and it is available for home use.

Western blot: transfer technique used for analyzing protein antigens. Antigens are separated by electrophoresis and transferred to a new medium by absorption or covalent bonding and then detected by a wide range of antibody probes. The probe could be labeled with a radioactive tag, an enzyme that can produce a visual product or a fluorescent or chemiluminescent label. Detection would be accomplished with specialized instrumentation, spectrophotometer, fluorometer and luminometer, respectively. Used to detect the presence of human immunodeficiency virus (HIV).

Whole blood: complete blood, containing the liquid portion (plasma) and the cellular elements.

X

D-Xylose absorption test: an analytical technique that assesses the ability to absorb D-xylose; it is of value in differentiating malabsorption of intestinal etiology from that of exocrine pancreatic insufficiency.

Z

Zero-order kinetics: point in enzyme reaction when product is formed and the resultant free enzyme immediately combines with excess free substrate; the reaction rate is dependent on enzyme concentration only.

Zollinger-Ellison syndrome: a gastrin-secreting neoplasm, usually located in the pancreatic islets, associated with exceptionally high plasma gastrin concentrations. The fasting plasma gastrin levels typically exceed 1,000 pg/mL and can reach 400,000 pg/mL, compared with the normal range of 50–150 pg/mL.

Zona fasciculata: the adrenal cortex.

Zona glomerulosa: outer portion of the adrenal cortex.

Zona reticularis: inner layer of the cortex of the adrenal gland.

Zymogens: inactivated forms of enzymes; must be converted into active forms for biological function.

Index

Page numbers in *italics* denote figures; those followed by a *t* denote tables.

A

ABCA1 transporter, 289–290
Absolute specificity, 239
Absorbance (A)
  in automated analysis measurement, 136–137
  and Beer's law, 25, 92
  delta, 26
  of hemoglobin, *354*
  and percent transmittance, 682*t*–683*t*
Absorption
  of copper, 369
  of drugs, 571–572
  of energy, 91, *92*
  in fluorometry, 98
  intestinal, 549, 550–551
  of iron, 366
  of lipids, 288
  ultraviolet, 205
  of D-xylose, 545, 550–551
  of zinc, 370
Absorptivity, molar (ϵ), 26, 92–93
Abused drugs, 598–601, 690*t*–691*t*
  amphetamines, 599–600
  anabolic steroids, 600
  cannabinoids, 600
  cocaine, 600–601
  opiates, 601
  phencyclidine, 601
  prevalence of, 599*t*
  sedative hypnotics, 601
ACA (Automated Clinical Analyzer) Star
  automated column chromatography in, 135
  calibration of, 139
  delay stations in, 136
  history of, 125
  mixing in, 134–135
  photometer in, 137
  reagents in, 132–133, *134*
  specimen measurement and delivery in, 132
Accidents, 45–46
Accreditation, 35
Accuracy
  estimation of, 65–66
  in lipid analysis, 298, 304–305
  of wavelength, 96
Acetaminophen, 481, 597–598
Acetylcholinesterase (AChE), 555, 596
Acetylsalicylic acid, 597
Acid elution stain, 392
α_1-Acid glycoprotein (orosomucoid), 190*t*, 195
Acid phosphatase (ACP), 253–255
  assay for, 254
  diagnostic significance of, 254
  reference range for, 255
  sources of error, 255
  tissue sources of, 254
Acid-base balance
  assessment of, 346, 348–349
  blood gas measurement, 353–358
  buffer systems in, 344–345
  disorders of, 348–349

kidneys in, 345, 346, *347*, 348, 523
lungs in, 345
maintenance of H^+, 344
oxygen and gas exchange in, 349–353
in pediatric patients, 659
quality assurance in assessments, 358–361
Acidemia, 185, 348
Acidosis
  defined, 344
  ketoacidosis, 271
  lactic, 336
  metabolic (nonrespiratory), 324, 348, 349, 358
  in pediatric patients, 659
  renal tubular, 530
  respiratory, 348, 349
Acids (*See also* Acid-base balance)
  concentrations of, 677*t*
  defined, 344
  excretion of, 523
  pH of, 9, 344
ACP (*See* Acid phosphatase)
Acridinium esters, 152
Acromegaly, 404–405, 526
ACTH (*See* Adrenocorticotropic hormone)
Activated clotting time (ACT), 175–176
Activation energy, 238, *239*
Activators, 237, 241
Active sites of enzymes, 237
Active transport, 315
Activity units, 243
Actual percent oxyhemoglobin (O_2Hb), 353–354
Acute coronary syndrome, 501–503 (*See also* Coronary heart disease)
Acute intermittent porphyria (AIP), 379, 380
Acute renal failure (*See* Renal failure)
Acute-phase proteins/reactants
  α-antitrypsin, 190*t*, 194–195
  C-reactive protein, 190*t*, 198, 636, 667
  fibrinogen, 190*t*, 198, 509, 513*t*
  in immunity, 667
  in protein electrophoresis, 210
Adaptive immune system, 667
Adenocarcinoma, *429*
Adenohypophysis (anterior pituitary), 400
Adenomas
  adrenal, 417–418
  aldo-producing, 417
  toxic, 453
Adenosine triphosphate (ATP), 265–266
Adenylate kinase (AK), 247
ADH (*See* Antidiuretic hormone)
Adhesion molecules, 607
Administration routes of drugs, 571
ADP (ALA dehydratase deficiency porphyria), 379–380
Adrenal function, 413–429
  adrenal cortex in, 414–424
  adrenal insufficiency, 418–419
  adrenal medulla in, 424–426, 428–429
  androgen excess, 423–424
  catecholamines in, 424–426, 428, *429*
  causes of sympathetic hyperactivity, 426
  congenital adrenal hyperplasia, 415–418, 666
  cortex steroidogenesis, 414–415
  Cushing's syndrome, 419–422

  embryology and anatomy in, 413–414
  hypercortisolism, 419–423
  incidentaloma, 427, *429*
  in pediatric patients, 665
  pheochromocytoma, 424, 426, 428
  primary aldosteronism, 417–418, *429*
Adrenal imaging, 417–418
Adrenal insufficiency, 418–419
Adrenal vein sampling, 418
β-Adrenergic blocking drugs, 512, 513*t*
Adrenocorticotropic hormone (ACTH)
  and cortisol, 418, 421–422, 665
  and diurnal rhythms, 402
  in glucose regulation, 267
  in steroid hormone biosynthesis, 414–415
  and vasopressin, 402
Adsorption chromatography, 108
Adsorption in immunoassays, 155
Advanced glycation end products (AGEs), 648
Advia analyzers, 125, 128*t*, 138
Aerobic pathway, 265, *266*
Aeroset analyzers, 125, 128*t*
Affinity
  of antibodies, 146–147
  of hemoglobin and oxygen, 353
Affinity chromatography, 277
Affinity constant (K_a), 147
AFP (*See* α_1-Fetoprotein)
A/G (albumin-globulin) ratio, 205
Agammaglobulinemia, 668
Agarose gel
  in electrophoresis, 106, 208, 300
  in immune precipitation, 147–150
Age
  and atherosclerosis, 501
  gestational, 557
  and reference intervals, 57, 58
  and testosterone levels, 440
Aging, 643–652
  biochemical and physiologic changes in, 645–650
    analytes, 646*t*
    cardiovascular function, 650
    diabetes and insulin resistance, 647–648
    electrolytes, 649
    endocrine function, 645–647
    enzymes, 650
    hepatic function, 649
    lipids, 650
    pulmonary function, 649
    renal function, 648–649
  defined, 643
  diseases and disorders associated with, 645*t*
  and laboratory results, 650–652
    exercise and nutrition in, 652
    preanalytic variables in, 651
    reference intervals, 650–651
    therapeutic drug monitoring, 651–652
  and leading causes of death, 646*t*
  theories of, 644–645
AIP (acute intermittent porphyria), 379, 380
Airborne pathogens, 39
Air-displacement pipets, 13
ALA (*See* Aminolevulinic acid)

CLINICAL CHEMISTRY TESTS

TEST	ABBREVIATION	TUBE, SAMPLE CONSIDERATION	CLINICAL CORRELATION
Acid phosphatase	Acid p'tase	SST; centrifuge, separate and freeze serum; transport frozen	Prostate cancer
Alanine transferase	ALT (SGPT)	SST; centrifuge for complete separation and refrigerate	Evaluate hepatic disease
Alcohol	ETOH for forensic studies	Gray; use nonalcohol germicidal solution to cleanse skin; chain-of-custody required if for legal purposes	Intoxication
Aldosterone		Plain red top; centrifuge, separate, and refrigerate serum; draw "upright" sample at least $1/2$ hour after patient sits up	Aldosterone overproduction
Alkaline phosphatase	ALP or Alk phos	SST; centrifuge for complete separation; fasting 8–12 hours is required	Liver function
Aluminum	Al	Royal blue tube; EDTA; submit original, unopened tube; avoid all sources of external contamination. If no additive royal blue is used, serum must be transferred to a plastic tube within 45 minutes of collection.	Trace metal contamination; dialysis complication
Ammonia	NH_4	Green-top tube placed immediately on ice slurry; centrifuge within 15 minutes without removing stopper; separate plasma and freeze in plastic vial using dry ice	Evaluate liver function. High levels in the blood lead to hepatic encephalopathy.
Amylase		SST; centrifuge and refrigerate serum; avoid hemolysis and lipemia	Acute pancreatitis
Aspartate transferase	AST	SST; centrifuge for complete separation and refrigerate	Acute and chronic liver disease
B_{12} and folate		SST; centrifuge, separate and refrigerate; avoid hemolysis. If testing is delayed, freeze specimen in plastic vial.	Macrocytic anemia
Bilirubin, total and direct	Bili	Wrap in foil to protect from light; refrigerate	Increased with types of jaundice (ie, obstructive, hepatic, hemolytic), hepatitis, or cirrhosis
Blood urea nitrogen	BUN	SST; centrifuge for complete separation and refrigerate	Kidney function
Calcitonin		Plain red; centrifuge, separate, and freeze immediately in plastic vial; overnight fasting preferred	Evaluate suspected medullary carcinoma of the thyroid characterized by hypersecretion of calcitonin
Carbon monoxide (carboxyhemoglobin)	CO level	Fill lavender tube completely; submit at room temperature	Carboxyhemoglobin intoxication
Cancer antigen	CA 125	Refrigerate; freeze if testing is delayed	Tumor marker primarily for ovarian carcinoma
Calcium, ionized		Allow blood to clot for 20 minutes; centrifuge with cap on; do not pour over; refrigerate	Bone cancer; nephritis; multiple myeloma
Carcinoembryonic antigen	CEA	Refrigerate serum	Monitor patients with diagnosed malignancies; malignant or benign liver disease; indicator of tumors

TEST	ABBREVIATION	TUBE, SAMPLE CONSIDERATION	CLINICAL CORRELATION
Carotene		Refrigerate serum; wrap in aluminum foil to protect from light; overnight fasting preferred	Carotenemia
Cholesterol	Chol	Refrigerate serum	Evaluates risk of coronary heart disease (CHD)
Chromium	Cr level	Royal blue, no additive; metal-free, separate and refrigerate immediately	Associated with diabetes and aspartame toxicity
Copper	Cu level	Royal blue, no additive; separate and refrigerate immediately	Wilson's disease or nephritic syndrome
Cortisol, timed		Refrigerate serum; clearly note time drawn	Cushing's syndrome
Creatine kinase	CK	Refrigerate serum	Muscular dystrophy; muscle trauma
Creatine kinase MB	CK-MB	Refrigerate serum	Organ differentiation; rule out myocardial infarction
Creatinine		Refrigerate serum	Kidney function
Cyclosporin		Whole blood or serum refrigerated (NOTE: use same specimen type each time analyte is measured)	Immunosuppressive drug for organ transplants
Cryoglobulin		Draw and process at room temperature; should be fasting	Associated with immunologic diseases (eg, multiple myeloma, rheumatoid arthritis)
Electrolytes	Na^+, K^+, Cl, CO_2,	Spun barrier tube; centrifuge within 30 minutes after drawing; avoid hemolysis and lipemia	Fluid balance; cardiotoxicity; heart failure; edema
α-Fetoprotein	AFP	SST; avoid hemolysis; do not freeze; can be performed on amniotic fluid	Fetal abnormalities, adult hepatic carcinomas
Ferritin		Refrigerate serum	Hemachromatosis; iron deficiency
Gastrin		Overnight fasting required; separate serum from cells within 1 hour after collection; freeze serum	Stomach disorders
Glucose	FBS (fasting blood sugar); RBS (random blood sugar)	Separate from cells within 1 hour or use gray-top tube	Diabetes; hypoglycemia
Glycosylated hemoglobin	HbA_{1c}	Lavender tube	Monitor diabetes mellitus
Glucose-6-phosphate dehydrogenase	G-6-PD	Lavender tube; do not freeze	Drug-induced anemia
γ-Glutamyl transpeptidase	GGTP	Refrigerate serum	Diagnosis of liver problems; specific for hepatobiliary problems
HLA typing A and B		Yellow-top (ACD) tubes; do not freeze or refrigerate; ethnic origin must be included	Disease association; bone marrow; platelet capability; liver or heart transplant
Human chorionic gonadotropin	hCG	Refrigerate serum	Pregnancy; testicular cancer
Immunoglobulins	IgA IgG IgM	Refrigerate serum	Measurement of proteins capable of becoming antibodies; chronic liver disease; myeloma

TEST	ABBREVIATION	TUBE, SAMPLE CONSIDERATION	CLINICAL CORRELATION
Iron + iron-binding capacity	TIBC and Fe	Refrigerate serum; separate from cells within 1 hour of collection; fasting morning specimen preferred	Diagnosis of anemia
Lactic acid (blood lactate)		Draw whole blood from a stasis-free vein into a gray-top tube; centrifuge and separate plasma within 15 minutes of collection	Measurement of anaerobic glycolysis as a result of strenuous exercise; increased lactic acid can occur in liver disease
Lactic dehydrogenase	LD	Serum; avoid hemolysis; do not freeze or refrigerate	Cardiac injury; other muscle damage
Lead	Pb	Royal blue EDTA or tan-top lead-free tube; other evacuated tubes or transfer tubes may produce falsely elevated results due to contamination	Lead toxicity that can lead to neurologic dysfunction and possible permanent brain damage
Lipase		Refrigerate serum	Distinguish between abdominal pain and pain resulting from acute pancreatitis
Lipoproteins		Refrigerate serum	
High-density	HDL	Minimum 12-hour fast	Evaluates lipid disorders and coronary artery disease risk
Low-density	LDL	Minimum 12-hour fast	Evaluates lipid disorders and coronary artery disease risk
Magnesium	Mg	Separate from cells within 45 minutes; maintain specimen at room temperature	Mineral metabolism; kidney function
Phosphorus	P	Separate from cells within 45 minutes; maintain specimen at room temperature	Thyroid function; bone disorders; kidney disease
Prostatic-specific antigen; total and free	PSA	Separate and freeze immediately in a plastic vial.; transport frozen	Screen for prostate cancer; monitor disease progression and response to prostate cancer treatment
Serum protein electrophoresis	SPEP or PEP	Refrigerate serum	Abnormal protein detection
Sweat electrolytes (iontophoresis)		Fluid collected is sweat	Cystic fibrosis
Thyroid profile (comprehensive)	FTI, T_3, T_4, TSH	SST or red stopper tube that must be separated to plastic transfer tube	Hyperthyroid or hypothyroid conditions
Triglycerides		Refrigerate serum; strict 12–14 hour fasting (water only) required	Evaluate coronary heart disease risk
Uric acid	UA	SST or red stopper tube that must be separated within 45 minutes; maintain specimen at room temperature	Gout
Zinc	Zn	Royal blue, no additive or EDTA; if serum, should be separated within 45 minutes and transferred to plastic transport tube	Liver dysfunction